PERLOFF'S
Clinical Recognition of Congenital Heart Disease

PERLOFF'S
Clinical Recognition of Congenital Heart Disease

Sixth Edition

Joseph K. Perloff, MD

Emeritus
Streisand American Heart Association
Professor of Medicine and Pediatrics
Ahmanson/UCLA Adult Congenital Heart Disease Center
University of California–Los Angeles School of Medicine
Los Angeles, California

Ariane J. Marelli, MD, FRCP(C), MPH

Associate Professor of Medicine
Director, McGill Adult Unit for Congenital Heart Disease
McGill University
Montreal, Quebec
Canada

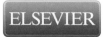

1600 John F. Kennedy Blvd.
Ste 1800
Philadelphia, PA 19103-2899

CLINICAL RECOGNITION OF CONGENITAL HEART DISEASE   ISBN: 978-1-4377-1618-4

Library of Congress Cataloging-in-Publication Data
Perloff, Joseph K., 1924-
    Clinical recognition of congenital heart disease / Joseph K. Perloff, Ariane J. Marelli. – 6th ed.
        p. ; cm.
    ISBN 978-1-4377-1618-4 (hardcover : alk. paper)
    I. Marelli, Ariane. J. II. Title.
    [DNLM: 1. Heart Defects, Congenital–diagnosis. WG 220]
    616.1′2043–dc23

                                                                    2011032130

Executive Content Strategist: Dolores Meloni
Content Development Specialist: Julie Mirra
Publishing Services Manager: Anne Altepeter
Project Manager: Cindy Thoms
Design Direction: Ellen Zanolle

Printed in China

Last digit is the print number: 9 8 7 6 5 4 3 2 1

In memory of my parents,
Rose and Richard,
and with high hopes for
Alexandra, Benjamin, and Nicholas
Joseph K. Perloff

To students past and future,
whose privilege it has been and will be
to learn from Joseph K. Perloff
Ariane J. Marelli

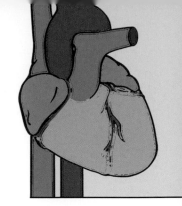

Preface

The objective set forth in the first five editions of *Clinical Recognition of Congenital Heart Disease* remains the same: to stimulate clinicians to use the basic diagnostic tools at their disposal, the history, physical examination, electrocardiogram, and chest x-ray. When the second edition was published, two-dimensional echocardiography was in its infancy, but it is now virtually routine. Cardiac catheterization and angiography were major steps forward, followed by transthoracic and transesophageal echocardiography. Magnetic resonance imaging and computed tomography provide exquisite anatomic detail and refined physiologic information.

In light of these advances, and with more in the offing, emphasis on basic diagnostic tools is more relevant than ever. Intelligent selection from the increasing array of currently available procedures requires far more sophisticated judgment than when the choices were limited. The basic tools provide the basis for this judgment. The bedside diagnosis of congenital heart disease is a clinical syllogism, an exciting discipline in logical thinking, and a gratifying source of self-education.

Joseph K. Perloff
Los Angeles, California

Ariane J. Marelli
Montreal, Quebec, Canada

Acknowledgments

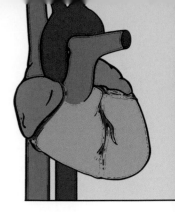

The Ahmanson Foundation generously supported the preparation of this edition. Natasha Andjelkovic, our editor at Elsevier, was exemplary. A collaboration of pediatric cardiology colleagues at UCLA and McGill fostered an atmosphere of interchange that made congenital heart disease a continuum from the fetus to the extended ages that survival now permits.

The scholarly integrity and academic achievements of Marjorie Gabrielle Perloff, PhD, Professor Emerita, Stanford University, determined my standards.

Joseph K. Perloff
Los Angeles, California

It is a privilege to have stood on the shoulders of giants at UCLA, including Joseph Perloff, John Child, Pamela Miner, Hillel Laks, and Roberta Williams. The legacy of knowledge, compassion, and vision drives me to this day. I am grateful to have the opportunity to participate in the life of this singular book.

I thank Dr. Luc Jutras, for his creativity as exemplified by the magnetic resonance imaging of the Holmes heart included in this edition. The numerous fellows we have the pleasure of working with stimulate our imaginations. Among these, Dr. Boris Lowe of New Zealand and Dr. Noriko Kitamura of Japan participated in the preparation of the images included in this edition.

The intellectual curiosity, substance, and stability that my husband, Julian Falutz, and our children, Jacob and Rebecca, have given to each of our endeavors enable me in my efforts daily. For this, I can never be thankful enough.

Ariane J. Marelli
Montreal, Quebec, Canada

Contents

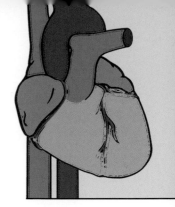

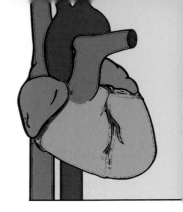

Video Contents

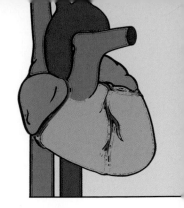

Chapter 1

Introduction: Formulation of the Problem

"The heart is the youngest, most diverse, most fluid, most changeable, most versatile part of creation."

Goethe[1]

Congenital heart disease (*con*, together; *genitus*, born) is often viewed as a group of gross structural abnormalities that are present at birth. Although not incorrect, this definition requires elaboration and qualification.

Prenatal diagnoses have been possible for more than 25 years.[2] At about embryonic day 20 in the human fetus, progenitor cells within the mesoderm become committed to a cardiogenic destination.[3] Most malformations compatible with 6 months of intrauterine life permit live offspring at term. A given malformation may exist in relative harmony with the fetal circulation, only to be modified considerably, at least physiologically, by dramatic circulatory changes at birth.[4] Weeks, months, or years may then elapse before an anomaly reveals itself as *characteristic* or *typical*. A functionally normal aortic valve that is congenitally bicuspid at birth may take decades to fibrose, calcify, and present as overt aortic stenosis. Conversely, a malformation may *disappear*, as is the case with spontaneous closure of a ventricular septal defect.

Congenital malformations of the heart and circulation are not fixed anatomic defects that appear at birth but instead are anomalies in flux that originate in the early embryo, evolve during gestation, survive the dramatic circulatory alterations at birth, and change considerably during the course of extrauterine life. Congenital heart disease was once the exclusive and legitimate domain of pediatrics, but survival patterns have changed appreciably.[5,6] In the United States today, there are more adults with congenital heart disease than there are infants and children; these new generations of patients are best cared for by specially trained cardiologists.[7] Clinical presentations, especially in adults,[8,9] can be exceptionally complex.[10–12]

Furthermore, certain defects that are actually or potentially of functional significance are not gross structurally, such as congenital complete heart block, either isolated (see Chapter 4) or with congenitally corrected transposition of the great arteries (see Chapter 6) or left isomerism (see Chapter 3); Wolff-Parkinson-White preexcitation, either isolated or complicated (see Chapter 13); absence of a sinus node, as with a superior vena caval sinus venosus atrial septal defect (see Chapter 15) or left isomerism (see Chapter 3); ventricular tachycardia with the long QT syndromes[13]; or arrhythmogenic right ventricular

dysplasia. Still other abnormalities, such as Marfan syndrome, which is the result of mutations in the gene that encodes fibrillin-1, are actually or potentially of functional significance but are not necessarily manifest at birth as gross structural malformations and, as a matter of convention, are usually not classified as congenital.[14] And a handful of odd defects tend to escape inclusion, such as congenital kinking of the internal carotid artery.[15]

Because of the intimate interplay between congenital malformations of the heart and the fetal substrate, we now turn to the fetal circulation per se and the remarkable circulatory changes that occur at birth.[4,16] In utero patterns of blood flow have been defined in fetal lambs after insertion of catheters into limb vessels,[4] and in utero left and right ventricular outputs and flow distributions through the foramen ovale, ductus arteriosus, and pulmonary bed have been measured in human fetuses with high-resolution color Doppler ultrasound scan.[16,17] The right and left ventricles do not function in series in the fetus as they do in the extrauterine circulation. Gas exchange occurs in the placenta, not in the lungs. About two thirds of the right ventricular output is diverted away from the lungs through a widely patent ductus arteriosus into the descending thoracic aorta, from which a large portion enters the umbilical circulation for oxygenation in the placenta. Pulmonary blood flow is low but meets nutritional requirements for growth of the lungs. Inferior vena cava blood, which is a composite from the umbilical vein, the left and right hepatic veins, the ductus venosus, and the distal inferior vena cava, streams in the direction of the foramen ovale into the left atrium and then into the left ventricle, assisted by the eustachian valve. About 60% of the umbilical venous return that is oxygenated in the placenta bypasses the liver through the ductus venosus and enters the inferior vena cava and right atrium. Blood from the superior vena cava is deflected within the right atrium toward the tricuspid valve, across which it reaches the right ventricle. About 70% of the relatively oxygen-rich blood ejected from the left ventricle is distributed to the coronary circulation (and thus the myocardium), to the head and neck (and thus the brain), and to the forelimbs. Almost 90% of the relatively oxygen-poor blood ejected by the right ventricle passes through the ductus arteriosus into the descending aorta to be oxygenated in the placenta. Accordingly, the fetal circulation is designed so that blood with higher oxygen saturation preferentially reaches the myocardium and brain and less saturated blood preferentially reaches the placenta.

The profound circulatory changes at birth occur almost simultaneously. The umbilical/placental circulation is eliminated, the lungs expand, rhythmic ventilation commences, oxygen tension rises as alveolar fluid is eliminated and ambient air is breathed, pulmonary vascular resistance falls, and pulmonary blood flow increases eight to 10 fold. Venous return to the left atrium increases, left atrial pressure rises, the valve of the foramen ovale closes, and the ductus arteriosus functionally closes (constricts) within hours after birth, effectively separating the pulmonary and systemic circulations.[4]

A number of important delayed events complete the transition from the fetal to the maturing circulation after birth. During the course of gestation, pulmonary vascular resistance falls progressively as new resistance arterioles develop. Regulation of the perinatal pulmonary circulation reflects a complex interplay between vasoconstrictor and vasodilator factors, but the net effect is a dramatic increase in pulmonary blood flow initiated by expansion of the lungs and rhythmic ventilation that reflects a shift from active pulmonary vasoconstriction in the fetus to active vasodilation in the neonate.[4] Failure of this shift to occur results in persistent fetal circulation of the newborn. Thick-walled fetal pulmonary arterioles are designed to meet the full force of systemic right ventricular pressure the instant the lungs expand. As respiration commences, a marked increase in alveolar and systemic arterial oxygen tension occurs, to which pulmonary arterioles are exquisitely sensitive, setting the stage for dilation and involution. Large pulmonary arteries also play a role, although much lesser, in determination of the total drop in pressure across the lungs.

Maturational changes have an impact on the neonatal disparity in size between the main and branch pulmonary arteries and on the angulation at the origins of the right and left pulmonary arterial branches (see Chapter 11). Both of these factors are responsible for a physiologic drop in pressure distal to the pulmonary trunk. Another important change relates to the fetal right ventricle, which slowly loses its relative mass. With the stimulus of afterload eliminated, a gradual reduction is seen in right ventricular wall thickness relative to the ventricular septum and left ventricle. The neonatal right ventricle does not undergo regression but instead does not increase its mass as rapidly as the left ventricle. Normal physiologic adaptations at birth are remarkable in their own right. Therefore, that congenital malformations of the heart or circulation will, to varying degrees, interact with and be modified by extrauterine life is not surprising.

"One of the most wondrous features of animate nature must surely be the perfect harmony existing between structure and function."[17] No organ system exemplifies this harmony as well as the heart and circulation. In the presence of congenital heart disease, both the morphology and the physiology of the heart and circulation change with the passage of time from the fetus to the neonate to the infant, to the child, to the adolescent, and to the adult. Some of these changes result in neonatal death, and others express themselves gradually over weeks, months, years, or even decades. The clinical manifestations of congenital heart disease are dealt with herein in terms of anatomic and physiologic mechanisms. The

method of assessment used in the process of *clinical recognition* is a syllogism of applied logic. When conclusions are drawn from accurate observations, correct diagnoses emerge with gratifying frequency, even when the malformations are complex. Logic is encouraged; memorization is minimized. In each chapter, the gross morphology is first established to shed light on the physiologic derangements. The question is then asked: What clinical manifestations might result from these anatomic and physiologic derangements? The stage is now set for *clinical recognition*—the thesis of this book—which depends on a synthesis of information from the history, the physical examination, the electrocardiogram, and the chest x-ray. Contemporary imaging techniques serve as important supplements.

The *history*, which is an interview, is designed to secure background information. The physical examination includes physical appearance, arterial pulse, jugular venous pulse, precordial percussion, movement and palpation, and auscultation.[18] The stethoscope is the oldest cardiovascular diagnostic instrument in continuous clinical use. The *electrocardiogram*, developed in 1903 by Willem Einthoven, when read closely and interpreted in clinical context, provides gratifying diagnostic insights, even in complex congenital heart disease.[19] Meticulous attention should be devoted to the P wave, the P duration, the PR interval, the QRS, the QT interval, and the T wave. The electrocardiographic waves are thought to have been so-named by Rene Descartes, an 18th century French philosopher and scientist[20] who was surely known to Einthoven. The x-ray was developed in 1895 by Wilhelm Konrad Roentgen. Chest x-rays must be read closely and interpreted in clinical context. Posteroanterior and lateral views should be read according to a planned sequence: namely, penetration, rotation, degree of inhalation, age and sex, right/left orientation, thoracic and abdominal situs, positions and malpositions above and below the diaphragm, the bones, extrapulmonary soft tissue densities, vascular and parenchymal intrapulmonary soft tissue densities, the great arteries and great veins, the atria, and the ventricles. Much can be said for learning interpretation by reading chest x-rays with a trained chest radiologist. As with the electrocardiogram, so too with the chest x-ray—the amount of information that can be extracted is gratifying, even in complex congenital heart disease.

It is axiomatic that emphasis should be placed on the relationship of the parts to the whole, a relationship that results in a harmonious picture devoid of contradictions rather than a collection of loosely related observations. Maximum information should be extracted from each source while information from one source is related to that of another. Each step should advance our thinking and narrow the diagnostic possibilities. By the end of the clinical assessment, *untenable* considerations should have been discarded, *possibilities* retained for further consideration, and probabilities brought into sharper focus. The process reflects Herophilus' adage that the best physician is one who distinguishes between the possible and the impossible.

A diagnostic impression, once entertained, unnecessarily influences the objectivity with which subsequent impressions are appraised. If the same sequence of clinical evaluation is always used, the latter steps cannot be objectively assessed. Varying the sequence with which information is assembled is therefore useful. Begin, for example, with the chest x-ray or electrocardiogram. With infants, the practical approach often is to take advantage of temporary periods of calm and start with the physical examination, which may shortly be difficult to perform. It is not the sequence that matters, but the depth and synthesis of analysis. Irrespective of how the order of information is arranged, two questions must always be asked: How does one step relate to the next? How do the parts relate to the whole?

Diagnostic thinking benefits from the use of *anticipation* and *supposition*. After conclusions are drawn from the history, it is useful to pause and ask: If these assumptions are correct, what can I anticipate from the physical examination? Or what specific points can I *anticipate* in the electrocardiogram or x-ray to support or refute my initial impressions? Anticipation heightens interest as the clinical assessment progresses. Confirmation comes as a source of satisfaction, and error stands out in bold relief. Nor should we be afraid of mistakes. *Truth emerges sooner from error than from confusion.*

Decades ago, Paul Wood proposed that we answer five clinical questions (Box 1-1). When approached according to this proposal, the clinical recognition of congenital heart disease becomes a stimulating challenge, a satisfying discipline in logical thinking, and a constant source of self education. The intensity of enquiry and the analytic standards used at the bedside should be the same as those in diagnostic laboratories.

The Preface to the first edition stated, "I hope to stimulate clinicians to use the basic tools readily at their disposal—the history, the physical examination, the electrocardiogram, and the chest x-ray." The Preface to the third edition stated, "Two-dimensional echocardiography was in its infancy when the second edition appeared, but now is a routine laboratory procedure." Cardiac catheterization and angiography were followed by transthoracic and transesophageal echocardiography, and magnetic resonance imaging, magnetic resonance angiography, and computed tomography now provide exquisite anatomic detail and refined physiologic information.[21-24]

Given these advanced imaging techniques, and with more in the offing, has emphasis on the history, physical examination, electrocardiogram, chest x-ray, and echocardiogram become irrelevant? *Intelligent selection of investigative procedures from an ever increasing array requires far more sophisticated decision making than was necessary when choices were limited to the electrocardiogram and chest x-ray. The basic clinical assessment provides the information necessary for most of these decisions. With increasing emphasis on the cost of medical care, a resurgence of interest in the inexpensive and safe clinical examination is likely.*[25]

SOME ADDITIONAL POINTS

The term *natural history* is not used. Julien Hoffman's definition is relevant: "The natural history of any disease is a description of what happens to people with the disease who do not receive treatment for it."[26] Natural history is therefore not synonymous with unoperated, and unnatural history is not synonymous with postoperative. Nonsurgical therapeutic interventions can hardly be considered natural. A second point: differential diagnoses are not used. Instead, each chapter ends with a summary that permits clinical recognition of the congenital anomaly covered in the chapter. These summaries bring together clinical highlights and serve as reminders for the reader's convenience.

Finally, a comment on *terminology* is needed. The First International Summit on Nomenclature for Congenital Heart Disease was held in 2001 in Toronto and ended with virtually unanimous support for the development of a unified system for describing congenial cardiac malformations.[27] The terms used herein to describe congenital malformations of the heart and circulation include older Latinized forms and more recent Anglicized forms.[28-30] The vocabulary of congenital heart disease is replete with abbreviations understood only by the initiated. Accordingly, when abbreviations are used, they are first defined for the reader's convenience, but full terms are subsequently used. New terms are not used when old terms suffice. Acronyms are avoided.

I have tried to ensure that the material in this book is accessible to a broad audience. The terminology was assiduously addressed and based on decades of personal experience. My objective remains to excite interest and to be understood.

BOX 1-1 **FIVE BASIC QUESTIONS**

1. Is the patient's condition acyanotic or cyanotic?
2. Is pulmonary arterial blood flow increased?
3. Does the malformation originate in the left or the right side of the heart?
4. Which is the dominant ventricle?
5. Is pulmonary hypertension present?

REFERENCES

1. Williams JR. *The life of Goethe*. Oxford: Blackwell Publishers; 1998.
2. Allan L. Prenatal diagnosis of structural cardiac defects. *Am J Med Genet C Semin Med Genet*. 2007;145C:73–76.
3. Olson EN, Srivastava D. Molecular pathways controlling heart development. *Science*. 1996;272:671–676.
4. Moller JH, Hoffman JIE, eds. *Pediatric cardiovascular medicine*. New York: Churchill Livingstone; 2000.
5. Marelli AJ, Mackie AS, Ionescu-Ittu R, Rahme E, Pilote L. Congenital heart disease in the general population: changing prevalence and age distribution. *Circulation*. 2007;115:163–172.
6. Khairy P, Ionescu-Ittu R, Mackie AS, Abrahamowicz M, Pilote L, Marelli AJ. Changing mortality in congenital heart disease. *J Am Coll Cardiol*. 2010;56:1149–1157.
7. Child JS, Freed MD, Mavroudis C, Moodie DS, Tucker AL. Task force 9: training in the care of adult patients with congenital heart disease. *J Am Coll Cardiol*. 2008;51:389–393.
8. Sommer RJ, Hijazi ZM, Rhodes Jr JF. Pathophysiology of congenital heart disease in the adult: part I: shunt lesions. *Circulation*. 2008; 117:1090–1099.
9. Rhodes JF, Hijazi ZM, Sommer RJ. Pathophysiology of congenital heart disease in the adult, part II. Simple obstructive lesions. *Circulation*. 2008;117:1228–1237.

10. Sommer RJ, Hijazi ZM, Rhodes JF. Pathophysiology of congenital heart disease in the adult: part III: complex congenital heart disease. *Circulation.* 2008;117:1340–1350.

11. Ellis CR, Graham Jr TP, Byrd 3rd BF. Clinical presentations of unoperated and operated adults with congenital heart disease. *Curr Cardiol Rep.* 2005;7:291–298.

12. Perloff JK, Child JS, Aboulhosn J, eds. *Congenital heart disease in adults.* 3rd ed. Philadelphia: Saunders/Elsevier; 2009.

13. Chiang CE, Roden DM. The long QT syndromes: genetic basis and clinical implications. *J Am Coll Cardiol.* 2000;36:1–12.

14. Milewicz DM. Molecular genetics of Marfan syndrome and Ehlers-Danlos type IV. *Curr Opin Cardiol.* 1998;13:198–204.

15. Le Bret E, Pineau E, Folliguet T, et al. Congenital kinking of the internal carotid artery in twin brothers. *Circulation.* 2000;102: E173–E174.

16. Mielke G, Benda N. Cardiac output and central distribution of blood flow in the human fetus. *Circulation.* 2001;103: 1662–1668.

17. Alcazar JL, Rovira J, Ruiz-Perez ML, Lopez-Garcia G. Transvaginal color Doppler assessment of fetal circulation in normal early pregnancy. *Fetal Diagn Ther.* 1997;12:178–184.

18. Perloff JK. *Physical examination of the heart and circulation.* 4th ed. Shelton, Connecticut: People's Medical Publishing House; 2009.

19. Khairy P, Marelli AJ. Clinical use of electrocardiography in adults with congenital heart disease. *Circulation.* 2007;116: 2734–2746.

20. Hurst JW. Naming of the waves in the ECG, with a brief account of their genesis. *Circulation.* 1998;98:1937–1942.

21. Hlavacek AM, Baker GH, Shirali GS. Innovation in three-dimensional echocardiography and cardiac computed tomographic angiography. *Cardiol Young.* 2009;19(suppl 2):35–42.

22. Crean A. Cardiovascular MR and CT in congenital heart disease. *Heart.* 2007;93:1637–1647.

23. Valente AM, Powell AJ. Clinical applications of cardiovascular magnetic resonance in congenital heart disease. *Cardiol Clin.* 2007;25:97–110.

24. Marx GR, Su X. Three-dimensional echocardiography in congenital heart disease. *Cardiol Clin.* 2007;25:357–365.

25. Braunwald E. Foreword. In: Perloff JK, ed. *Physical examination of the heart and circulation.* 4th ed. Shelton, Connecticut: People's Medical Publishing House; 2009.

26. Hoffman JIE. Reflections on the past, present and future of pediatric cardiology. *Cardiol Young.* 1994;4:208–223.

27. Beland MJ, Franklin RCG, Jacobs JP, et al. Update from the International Working Group for Mapping and Coding of Nomenclatures for Paediatric and Congenital Heart Disease. *Cardiol Young.* 2004; 14:225–229.

28. Botto LD, Lin AE, Riehle-Colarusso T, Malik S, Correa A. National Birth Defects Prevention S. Seeking causes: classifying and evaluating congenital heart defects in etiologic studies. *Birth Defects Research.* 2007;79:714–727.

29. Carr C. Congenital nomenclature: a cause of confusion during literature search. *Ann Thorac Surg.* 2007;84:716.

30. Jacobs JP, Anderson RH, Weinberg PM, et al. The nomenclature, definition and classification of cardiac structures in the setting of heterotaxy. *Cardiol Young.* 2007;17(suppl 2):1–28.

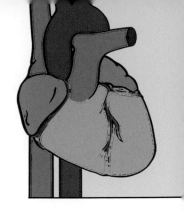

Chapter 2

Normal or Innocent Murmurs

Murmurs that occur in the absence of either morphologic or physiologic abnormalities of the heart or circulation have been called *normal, innocent, functional, physiologic,* or *benign. Normal* is perhaps the best term because it is unambiguous. Normal murmurs are common, are virtually ubiquitous in children, and can with few exceptions be recognized with a physical examination alone. The index of suspicion is the murmur itself. Auscultation is otherwise normal, and the history, physical appearance, arterial pulse, jugular venous pulse, precordial palpation, the electrocardiogram, x-ray, and echocardiogram are all normal.

Seven types of normal *systolic* murmurs and three types of normal *continuous* murmurs are known (Box 2-1).[1] Normal *systolic* murmurs include the vibratory murmur, the main pulmonary artery murmur, the branch pulmonary artery murmur of the neonate, the supraclavicular systolic murmur, the systolic mammary souffle, the aortic systolic murmur of older adults, and the cardiorespiratory systolic murmur. All normal systolic murmurs are *midsystolic*, except the mammary souffle, and are *not loudest at the right base.*[2] Normal *continuous* murmurs include the venous hum, the continuous mammary souffle, and the continuous cephalic (cranial) murmur (see Box 2-1).

Normal murmurs are never solely diastolic, with one exception—the transient left basal holodiastolic or middiastolic ductus arteriosus murmur, sometimes heard during the first 3 or 4 days of life.[3] A valve-like structure at the pulmonary arterial end of the ductus (see Chapter 20) is responsible for selective diastolic flow.[3,4]

NORMAL SYSTOLIC MURMURS

Vibratory Systolic Murmur

The normal vibratory midsystolic murmur was described by George F. Still in 1909 (Figures 2-1 and 2-2).[5] Still wrote, "It is heard usually just below the level of the nipple, and about halfway between the left margin of the sternum and the vertical nipple line. . . . It's characteristic feature is a twanging sound very like that made by twanging a piece of tense string. . . . Whatever may be it's origin, I think it is clearly functional, that is to say, not due to any organic disease either congenital or acquired."

Still's murmur is seldom heard in infants[6] but is prevalent after age 3 years, with diminishing frequency toward adolescence.[7,8–10] The murmur ranges from grade 1 to 3/6 and is loudest between the apex and lower left sternal edge

in the supine position.[9,11–14] During exercise, excitement, or fever, the murmur intensifies (see Figure 2-1).[9] The quality is distinctive:[9,15] vibratory or buzzing with a uniform, medium, pure frequency (70 to 130 cycles per second)[16] that requires the stethoscopic bell for best assessment.[11] The closest acoustic analogy is Still's twanging of a taut rubber band or string (see previous quotation).[17] The murmur begins shortly after the first heart sound and is typically confined to the first half of systole with a relatively long gap between the end of the murmur and the second heart sound (see Figures 2-1 and 2-2).

The mechanism of Still's murmur remains to be established, but theories take into account the distinctive frequency composition and configuration, location on the chest wall, and incidence according to age. The pure medium frequency implies that a cardiac structure is set into periodic vibration during ventricular systole. *Origin in the right side of the heart* has been assigned to the pulmonary valve itself when "trigonoidation" of the leaflets results in periodic vibrations of the base of the cusps.[10] A catheter across the pulmonary valve can tense the cusps and generate a transient pure-frequency midsystolic murmur (Figure 2-3A). The relatively low right ventricular ejection pressure and velocity are thought to cause the attachments of the pulmonary cusps to vibrate at a low to medium frequency. A murmur produced by a vibrating semilunar valve at its arterial attachment tends to be transmitted into the cavity of the concordant ventricle,[2,18,19] which could account for the thoracic location of Still's murmur between the apex and lower left sternal edge (i.e., topographically over the right ventricle). In children with Still's murmur, Doppler echocardiocardiography has been used to identify systolic vibrations in *the aortic valve* and higher maximal acceleration of flow in the left ventricular outflow tract.[14,20] However, a murmur that originates in a vibrating aortic valve is transmitted into the *left* ventricular cavity and heard best over the *left* ventricular impulse. Midsystolic murmurs in adults have been ascribed to high intraventricular velocities generated by vigorous left ventricular contraction associated with an increase in left ventricular mass.[21] Origin of Still's murmur has also been assigned to the *left ventricular cavity*, a location that is in accord with delayed response to the Valsalva's maneuver.[22] Left ventricular bands or false tendons (Figure 2-3B) are thought to vibrate periodically during ventricular systole and transmit their vibrations to the chest wall.[23–25] A high percentage of patients with Still's murmur reportedly have left ventricular bands, especially

BOX 2-1 **NORMAL MURMURS**

A. Systolic
1. The vibratory systolic murmur of Still
2. The pulmonary artery systolic murmur
3. The branch pulmonary artery systolic murmur
4. The supraclavicular systolic murmur
5. The systolic mammary souffle
6. The aortic sclerotic systolic murmur
7. The cardiorespiratory systolic murmur

B. Continuous
1. The venous hum
2. The continuous mammary souffle
3. The cephalic continuous murmur

in the outflow tract.[23-26] However, the prevalence rate of Still's murmur declines from childhood to adolescence,[9,10] whereas the prevalence rate of left ventricular bands is the same in children, adolescents, and adults.[23,24,27] The incidence rate of Still's murmur is thought to exceed the incidence rate of left ventricular bands,[14] although incidence rate depends largely on the avidity with which bands are sought with echocardiography.

Pulmonary Artery Systolic Murmur

The normal systolic murmur in the main pulmonary artery is most prevalent in children, adolescents, and young adults.[9,11,28] The murmur is midsystolic with maximal intensity in the second left intercostal space next to the sternum (Figure 2-4) and ranges from bare audibility to grade 3/6 in response to exercise, fever, or excitement. The frequency composition is medium pitched and impure, best heard in the supine position with the stethoscopic diaphragm or moderate pressure of the bell during full held exhalation.[9,11,29] The murmur represents normal ejection vibrations that reach the threshold of audibility from within the main pulmonary artery during right ventricular systole. The chest wall location is appropriate for origin in the pulmonary trunk, and intracardiac phonocardiograms record midsystolic murmurs within the pulmonary trunk in healthy young subjects.[29]

These murmurs are commonly heard during pregnancy and in subjects with anemia or hyperthyroidism. Loss of thoracic kyphosis increases proximity of the pulmonary trunk to the chest wall and increases the incidence rate of pulmonary systolic murmurs in the second left interspace.[30]

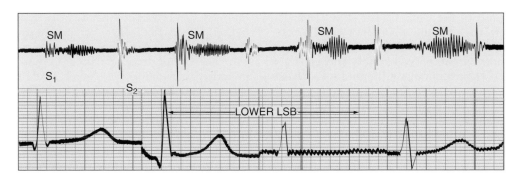

FIGURE 2-1 Vibratory midsystolic murmurs (SM) from four healthy children. The murmurs are pure frequency, relatively brief, and maximal along the lower left sternal border (LSB). The last of the four murmurs was from a 5-year-old febrile girl. After defervescence, the murmur decreased in loudness and duration.

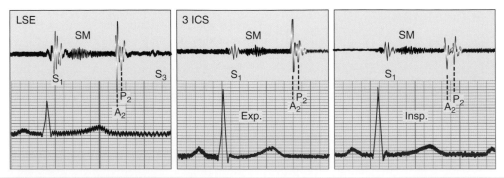

FIGURE 2-2 A vibratory midsystolic murmur (SM) from a healthy 7-year-old boy. The murmur is maximal along the lower left sternal edge (LSE) and is accompanied by a physiologic third heart sound (S_3) and normal respiratory splitting of the second heart sound (A_2/P_2 = aortic and pulmonary components; 3 ICS = third intercostal space).

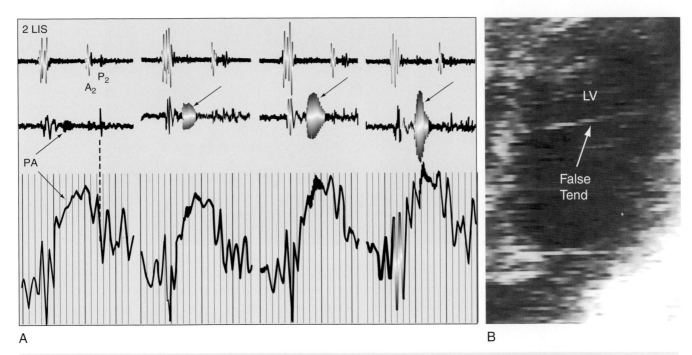

A

B

FIGURE 2-3 A, Phonocardiocardiogram recorded from within the pulmonary trunk (PT). **B,** Echocardiogram (apical view) from a 12-year-old boy with a left ventricular (LV) false tendon that was an incidental finding. The boy did *not* have Still's murmur distal to a normal pulmonary valve. The catheter transiently tensed the pulmonary cusps, setting them into pure-frequency periodic vibration *(arrow).*

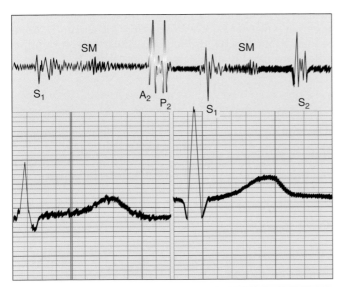

FIGURE 2-4 Pulmonary artery systolic murmurs (SM) recorded from the second left intercostal space of two healthy children aged 8 and 11 years. The murmurs are brief, midsystolic, and mixed frequency.

Branch Pulmonary Artery Systolic Murmur

Branch pulmonary artery systolic murmurs are occasionally heard in healthy neonates, especially premature neonates.[28,31–33] These murmurs are typically grade 1 to 2/6 and are medium pitched and impure but most importantly, are distributed to the left and right anterior chest, axillae, and back. The similarity of frequency composition to breath sounds, the rapid respiratory rate of infants, and the widespread thoracic locations of pulmonary artery systolic murmurs cause these murmurs to be overlooked. Audibility is improved if respiration is temporarily arrested with pinching the nostrils while the infant sucks a pacifier. Auscultation is best carried out with examination of the infant in both supine and prone positions and with use of the stethoscopic diaphragm applied to the right and left anterior chest, back, and axillae. The murmurs are typically confined to neonates, are usually absent at the first well-baby examination, and seldom persist beyond 3 to 6 months of age.[13,28,34] The transient branch pulmonary artery systolic murmur in healthy neonates is indistinguishable from the peripheral murmur of fixed stenosis of the pulmonary artery and its branches (see Chapter 10). The analogy sheds light on the mechanism of production.[28,32,33] The pulmonary trunk in the fetus is a relatively dilated domed structure because it receives the output of the high-pressure right ventricle. Proximal right and left pulmonary arteries arise from the pulmonary trunk as comparatively small lateral branches that receive a paucity of intrauterine blood flow. When the lungs expand at birth, the difference in size between the pulmonary trunk and its right and left branches transiently persists, especially in premature infants (Figure 2-5).[34] In addition to the disparity in size, the branches arise at relatively sharp angles from the inferior and posterior walls of the pulmonary trunk. These anatomic arrangements account for both the turbulence and the physiologic drop in systolic pressure from pulmonary trunk to proximal branches and for the branch pulmonary artery systolic murmur.[28,33]

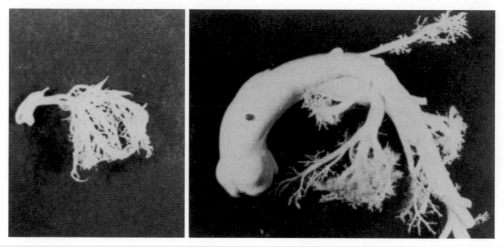

FIGURE 2-5 Casts from the pulmonary arteries of two lambs at ages 12 hours and 4 months. There is a decrease in the ratio of the size of the pulmonary trunk to its branches and a loss of acute angulation of the branches. *(From Danilowicz DA, Rudolf AM, Hoffman JIE, Heymann M. Circulation 1972;45:410, with permission; and the American Heart Association, Inc, with permission.)*

Supraclavicular Systolic Murmur

Normal supraclavicular systolic arterial murmurs are typically heard in children and young adults, are always *maximal above the clavicles*, tend to be louder on the right, are generally bilateral, and are prominent in the suprasternal notch (Figure 2-6).[2,35] The weight of evidence assigns supraclavicular systolic murmurs to the aortic origins of major brachiocephalic arteries, especially the subclavians.[36] Intensity can reach grade 4/6, may generate a thrill, and may be sufficient for radiation below the clavicles but with distinct attenuation (see Figure 2-6). The configuration of the supraclavicular systolic murmur is crescendo-decrescendo, the onset is abrupt, the duration is brief, and the timing is maximal in the first half or two thirds of systole (see Figure 2-6). The frequency composition is uneven, but the murmur is seldom noisy even when loud. Partial compression of the subclavian artery intensifies the murmur, whereas compression sufficient to obliterate the ipsilateral radial pulse has the opposite effect. Auscultation is most effectively carried out when the patient is sitting upright and looking straight ahead with shoulders relaxed and forearms and hands on the lap (Figure 2-7A).[2,37] The stethoscopic bell is applied above the medial aspect of the right clavicle. The shoulders are then hyperextended, with elbows brought sharply behind the back until shoulder girdle muscles are taut (Figure 2-7B). When this maneuver is done smoothly but rapidly, the supraclavicular murmur diminishes considerably or disappears altogether.[37]

Systolic Mammary Souffle

The souffle either is confined to systole or is louder in systole even when continuous (see subsequent discussion). As the name implies, the murmur is heard over the breasts late in pregnancy but especially postpartum

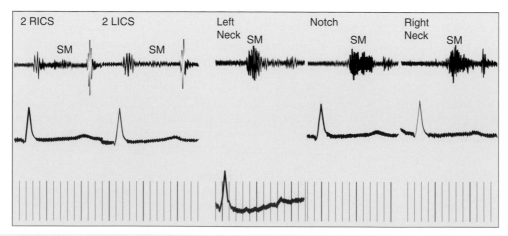

FIGURE 2-6 A supraclavicular systolic murmur (SM) in a healthy 8-year-old girl. Maximal intensity is above the clavicles (left neck, right neck). Onset is abrupt, duration is brief, and timing is maximal in the first half of systole. The murmur is well recorded in the suprasternal notch. There is radiation to the second right and left intercostal spaces (2 RICS, 2 LICS) but with considerable attenuation.

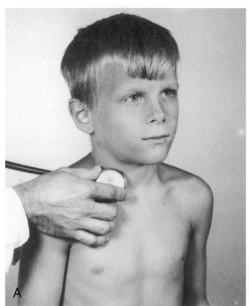
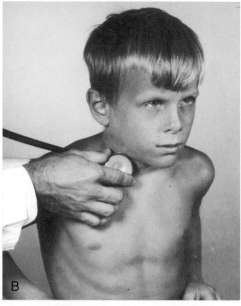

FIGURE 2-7 Shoulder maneuvers for assessment of normal supraclavicular systolic murmurs. **A,** Auscultation is initially performed while the patient sits with shoulders relaxed and arms in front of the chest. **B,** When the elbows are brought well behind the back, hyperextending the shoulders, the supraclavicular murmur diminishes or disappears.

in lactating women (Figure 2-8). The systolic component was recognized by van den Bergh in 1908.[38] The murmur begins distinctly after the first heart sound because sufficient time must elapse from left ventricular ejection to arrival at the artery of origin. The length of the murmur ranges from short (midsystolic), to long (up to the second heart sound), to beyond the second heart sound into diastole (continuous; see subsequent discussion).

Aortic Systolic Murmur in Older Adults

The most common form of normal midsystolic murmur in older adults is caused by fibrous or fibrocalcific thickening of the bases of inherently normal aortic cusps as they insert into the sinuses of Valsalva (Figure 2-9).[39,40] As long as the fibrous or fibrocalcific thickening is confined to the *base* of the leaflets, the cusps move well, so no functional deficit is seen. These structural alterations of inherently normal trileaflet aortic valves affect 20% to 25% of adults over age 65 years.[2,39–44] The fibrous, ridge-like thickenings that are initially confined to the base of the aortic cusps may subsequently extend to the free edges as fibrocalcific changes without commissural fusion. Because the initial morphologic changes do not impair cusp mobility and therefore do not cause obstruction, the accompanying murmur has been called the *aortic sclerotic* systolic murmur of older age. Intraarterial phonocardiography has identified midsystolic murmurs above the aortic valve before audibility on the chest wall occurs in clinically healthy adults over age 40 years.[44] The fully developed aortic sclerotic murmur has *two mechanisms* and represents a *combination of two murmurs*. The murmur in the second right intercostal space is midsystolic, impure, and grade 2 or 3/6 and originates within the aortic root (mixed-frequency ejection vibrations of

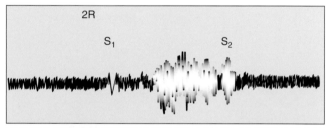
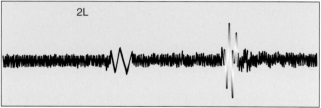
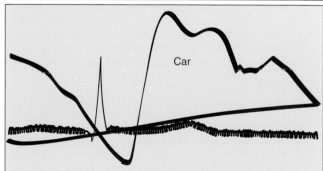

FIGURE 2-8 Systolic mammary souffle in the second right intercostal space (2R) of a healthy 24-year-old lactating woman. The murmur begins at a distinct interval after the first heart sound (S_1), is crescendo-decrescendo, and fades toward the second heart sound (S_2). (2L = second left intercostal space; Car = carotid.)

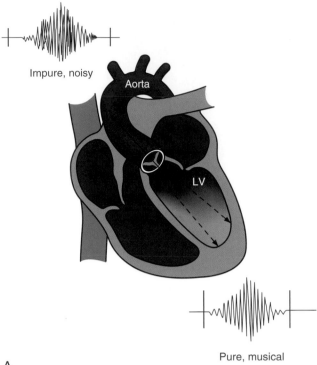

Impure, noisy

Aorta

LV

Pure, musical

A

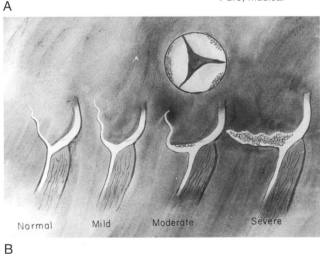

Normal   Mild   Moderate   Severe

B

FIGURE 2-9 A, Illustration of *Gallavardin dissociation* of the two murmurs associated with fibrocalcific aortic stenosis of an inherently normal trileaflet aortic valve.[68] The impure midsystolic murmur at the right base originates within the aortic root because of turbulence caused by the high-velocity jet. The pure musical midsystolic murmur at the apex originates from periodic high-frequency vibrations of the fibrocalcific aortic leaflets and radiates into the left ventricle cavity (LV). **B,** Schematic illustrations that begin with the normal attachment of an aortic cusp to its sinus of Valsalva *(left).* The initial alteration is a ridge-like fibrous thickening at the base of the aortic cusp as it inserts into its sinus. Calcium is subsequently deposited on the aortic surface of the leaflet (moderate) and ultimately extends to the free edge of the leaflet (severe), converting an inherently normal trileaflet valve into calcific aortic stenosis.

nonlaminar flow). The murmur heard over the left ventricular impulse is midsystolic, high-frequency musical, pure, and grade 2 to 3/6 and originates from periodic vibrations of the stiffened bases of aortic cusps at the sinus of Valsalva attachments (see Figure 2-9).[2,18,19,39] These periodic vibrations have been recorded from aortic valve leaflets with M mode echocardiography.[2] Intracardiac phonocardiography is used to detect the musical high-frequency murmur *within* the left ventricular cavity and the harsh impure right basal murmur *within* the aortic root (Gallavardin dissociation; see Figure 2-9).[2] What begins as an aortic sclerotic murmur can culminate in severe calcific aortic stenosis. In adults with increased anteroposterior chest dimensions, the *precordial* murmur of calcific aortic stenosis can be deceptively soft and is best heard in the *suprasternal notch.*

There is reason to believe that the essential morphologic substrate for the development of aortic sclerosis on an inherently normal trileaflet aortic valve is *cuspal inequality*—a congenital variation of normal—as originally proposed by Roberts.[45] The ideal aortic valve is equipped with cusps of identical size so that closing forces are equally distributed on the aortic surfaces of the three leaflets. Congenital variations in aortic leaflet size—cuspal inequality—is the rule rather than the exception and results in unequal distribution of tension during valve closure, the long-term effects of which are thought to culminate in the morphologic changes of aortic sclerosis/stenosis.[46] At its inception, the process is *functionally benign,* although there is an association between aortic valve sclerosis and cardiovascular mortality and morbidity.[41,47] Echocardiography can be used to detect focal areas of increased echogenicity and thickening at aortic cusp attachments to the sinuses of Valsalva without restriction of leaflet motion.[41] The *auscultatory* diagnosis of aortic sclerosis (see previous discussion) requires nothing more than proper use of a stethoscope.

Functionally Normal Bicuspid Aortic Valve

More than 400 years ago, Leonardo da Vinci sketched and described the bicuspid aortic valve.[48] He wrote, "Diagrams to illustrate . . . the triangular shape of the aortic aperture. In figure 2-2 the customary three cusps are illustrated. In figure 2-3, only two cusps fill the orifice."[48] *Functionally normal* refers to a bicuspid aortic valve that has the trivial gradient and the trivial regurgitation inherent in a mechanism equipped with two rather than three leaflets. A bicuspid aortic valve at birth is either functionally normal or intrinsically stenotic; it can become "thick and unyielding" or conversely can become incompetent so that "blood which has entered the aorta is allowed to regurgitate into the ventricle,"[49] as Thomas Peacock observed in 1858. It was William Osler in 1866 who called attention to the susceptibility of bicuspid aortic valves to infective endocarditis.[50]

Because of potential hazards, it is important to distinguish the murmur of a functionally normal congenitally bicuspid aortic valve from normal systolic murmurs that prevail in the same age group. Normal systolic murmurs in the *young*, with the exception of a systolic mammary souffle, are not heard *maximally* at the right base. A midsystolic murmur that is most prominent in the second right intercostal space in children or young adults arouses suspicion of a functionally normal bicuspid aortic, especially in males (relative male prevalence rate, 70% to 75%).[45] Auscultation should then seek the confirmatory evidence of an aortic ejection sound that is most prominent at the apex where it is readily mistaken for the second component of a split first heart sound.[2,51] The first component of a normally split first heart sound is louder at the apex, and the second component is louder at the lower left sternal border.[2] Additional evidence of a functionally normal bicuspid aortic valve is the soft high-frequency early diastolic murmur of bicuspid aortic regurgitation that adds materially to the diagnosis. The murmur is heard best when firm pressure of the stethoscopic diaphragm is applied at the mid left sternal edge during held exhalation as the patient sits and leans forward. Isometric exercise (clenched fists), squatting, and Valsalva's maneuver are used to improve audibility.[2,52]

The combination of a midsystolic murmur at the right base, an aortic ejection sound at the apex, and a soft high-frequency early diastolic murmur at the left sternal border in a young male is used to establish the diagnosis of bicuspid aortic valve. When the ejection sound is equivocal and the aortic regurgitation murmur is absent, clinical suspicion rests on the right basal midsystolic murmur alone. The echocardiogram then plays a pivotal role. The normal trileaflet aortic valve in the short axis resembles the letter Y during diastole (Figure 2-10A) and resembles an inverted triangle during systole.[53] A congenitally bicuspid aortic valve appears as a single linear band in diastole (Figure 2-10B) and appears as a *fish mouth* in systole. Color flow imaging is used to detect mild inaudible aortic regurgitation.

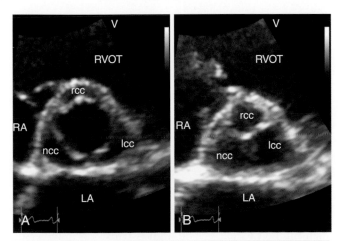

FIGURE 2-10 Echocardiogram (short axis) of a normal trileaflet aortic valve in diastole (**A**) and a functionally normal congenitally bicuspid aortic valve (**B**). (LA = Left atrium; lcc = left coronary sinus; ncc = noncoronary sinus; RA = right atrium; rcc = right coronary sinus; RVOT = right ventricular outflow tract) (Video 2-1).

Cardiorespiratory Murmur

In 1915, Richard Cabot wrote, "Such murmurs may be heard under the left clavicle or below the angle of the left scapula, as well as near the apex of the heart—less often in other parts of the chest. . . . Cardiorespiratory murmurs may be either systolic or diastolic, but in the vast majority of cases are systolic. The area over which they are audible is usually a very limited one. They are generally affected by a position and by respiration, and are heard most distinctly if not exclusively during inspiration, especially at the end of that act."[54]

Cardiorespiratory murmurs were known to Laënnec, but James Hope's description is the most colorful. Hope described his examination of two university students: "Both wore very tight waistcoats, preventing the expansion of the lower ribs. During this state of breathing, a bellows murmur . . . existed in both. In both, the murmur ceased entirely when, unbuttoning their waistcoats and waistbands of their trousers, they breathed with the lungs naturally inflated. By altering the circumstances, the murmur could be created or removed at pleasure. I presume therefore that it proceeded from a cause exterior to the heart."[55]

The mechanism responsible for the cardiorespiratory murmur is unclear, but its benign nature as well as its location, timing, and relation to respiration remain as Cabot originally described.[54]

NORMAL CONTINUOUS MURMURS

Venous Hum

The venous hum was described by Potain[56] in 1867 and is the most common type of normal continuous murmur. It is universal in children and occurs in healthy young adults,[57,58] even in the absence of thyrotoxicosis, anemia, or pregnancy.[2] Maximal intensity is in the supraclavicular fossa just lateral to the sternocleidomastoid muscle. The hum may radiate widely and is often bilateral but is usually more prominent on the right (Figure 2-11). A loud venous hum, especially in children, may radiate below the clavicles and be mistaken for a patent ductus arteriosus. Abolition of the hum with digital compression prevents this error (Figures 2-11 and 2-12). Intensity varies from faint to grade 6/6, and occasionally, patients are subjectively and unpleasantly aware of a loud hum that is sensed as audible pulsatile tinnitus.[59–61]

A venous hum is best elicited with the patient sitting upright. The stethoscope is held in the right hand of the examiner and the bell is applied to the medial aspect of the supraclavicular fossa (Figure 2-12A) while the examiner's left hand grasps the patient's chin from behind and pulls it tautly to the left and upward (see Figure 2-12A).[2] Occasionally, the hum develops or increases when the chin is simply tilted upward, and a prominent hum is sometimes audible without neck maneuvers and irrespective of position. In a child who is either sitting or supine, a venous hum may appear when the patient's

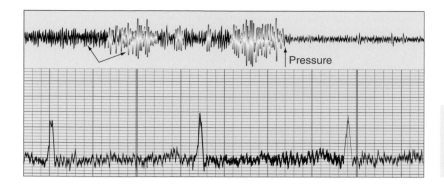

FIGURE 2-11 Continuous venous hum in a healthy 24-year-old woman. The *diastolic* component of the hum is louder *(paired arrows)*. Digital pressure on the right internal jugular vein *(vertical arrow)* abolished the murmur.

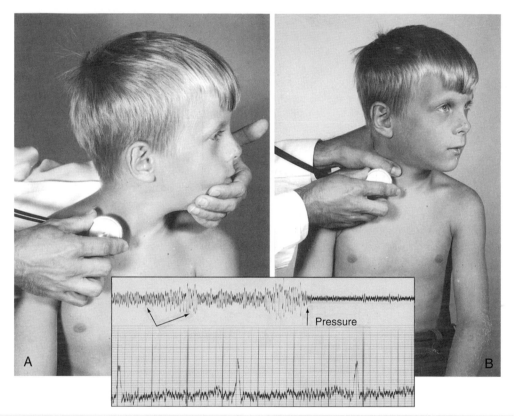

FIGURE 2-12 Maneuvers for eliciting or abolishing a venous hum. **A,** The bell of the stethoscope is applied to the medial aspect of the right supraclavicular fossa. The left hand grasps the patient's chin from behind and pulls it tautly to the left and upward. **B,** Digital compression of the right internal jugular vein obliterates the hum. The head has returned to a more neutral position.

head is voluntarily turned to the left or tilted upward. The hum may appear when the child looks up at the examiner and may disappear when the child looks down at the stethoscope. The hum is reduced or abolished with digital compression of the ipsilateral internal jugular vein (Figure 2-12B), with removal of the stretch on the neck as the head is returned to a neutral position, with the Valsalva's maneuver, and with recumbency. The simplest procedure for abolishing the hum is compression of the deep jugular vein with the thumb of the free hand (see Figure 2-12B). Compression causes instantaneous obliteration of the hum (see Figure 2-11),

which suddenly and transiently intensifies as pressure is released.[2,58]

The term *hum* does not necessarily characterize the quality of these cervical venous murmurs, which can be rough and noisy and are occasionally accompanied by a high-pitched whine.[58] The hum is truly continuous (see Figure 2-11) although typically louder in diastole, as is the case with venous continuous murmurs in general (Figure 2-13). The mechanism responsible for the venous hum is unclear. Laminar flow in the internal jugular vein may be disturbed by deformation at the level of the transverse process of the atlas during head rotation.[62]

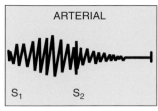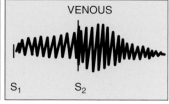

FIGURE 2-13 Schematic illustration of *arterial* and *venous* continuous murmurs. The arterial murmur is louder in systole, and the venous murmur is louder in diastole.

Continuous Mammary Souffle

A second but far less common benign continuous murmur occurs during late pregnancy and early postpartum in healthy lactating women. A consensus supports the view that the mammary souffle is arterial in origin,[63-65] an opinion originally held by both van den Bergh[38] and Jones.[66] Origin in superficial veins of the breast has less credibility.[67] The delay in onset, accentuation in systole, relatively high frequency, and persistence during Valsalva's maneuver are in accord with arterial origin.

The *continuous* mammary souffle was included in Jones' 1951 book *Heart Disease in Pregnancy*.[66] *Soufflare* is Latin, meaning *to blow*. Maximal intensity of the souffle can be anywhere over either breast, but the souffle tends to be louder in the second or third right or left intercostal space, and occasionally the souffle is bilateral.[65] A distinct gap between the first heart sound and the onset of the murmur represents the interval between ejection of blood from the left ventricle and arrival of blood at the artery that gives rise to the souffle.[63-65] The murmur is typically louder in systole, as is usually the case with continuous murmurs of arterial origin, with the diastolic portion often fading completely before the subsequent first heart sound (Figures 2-13 and 2-14). The pitch may be relatively high, but the murmur is not musical.[65] Audibility is best with the patient supine, and the murmur may vanish in the upright position.[65] Light pressure with the stethoscope tends to augment the murmur and bring out its continuous features.[64] Firm pressure with the stethoscope or digital pressure adjacent to the site of auscultation can abolish the murmur completely.[10,64,65]

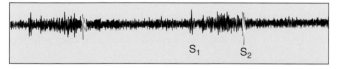

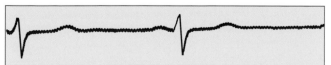

FIGURE 2-14 Continuous mammary souffle recorded at the upper left chest in a healthy 26-year-old lactating woman. The murmur is continuous but is louder in systole and does *not* peak around the second heart sound (S₂). (S₁ = first heart sound.)

Intensity may vary from beat to beat, from hour to hour, and from day to day.[65] Valsalva's maneuver does not affect the intensity.[64]

The location of a continuous mammary souffle may arouse suspicion of patent ductus arteriosus or of an arteriovenous fistula. However, the typical ductus murmur peaks *at* the second heart sound, whereas the mammary souffle peaks much earlier (see Figure 2-14); and obliteration with local compression excludes patent ductus. An arteriovenous fistula may generate a continuous murmur that is maximal in systole and attenuates with pressure, but the cycle-to-cycle or day-to-day variation of the mammary souffle and its invariable disappearance after termination of lactation resolve the issue.

Cephalic (Cranial) Continuous Murmur

Low-intensity cephalic murmurs, which are usually continuous and less often systolic, are occasionally detected over the cranium of normal children under 4 years of age, especially in association with a febrile illness.[13] These murmurs tend to be most prominent over the anterior fontanel, the temporal regions, or the orbits and are best heard with the diaphragm of the stethoscope. Because auscultation is not routinely applied to the head, cephalic murmurs are overlooked. Their mechanism is unknown.

REFERENCES

1. Pelech AN. The physiology of cardiac auscultation. *Pediatr Clin North Am.* 2004;51:1515–1535.
2. Perloff JK, ed. *Physical examination of the heart and circulation.* 4th ed. Shelton, Connecticut: People's Medical Publishing House; 2009.
3. Papadopoulos GS, Folger Jr GM. Transient solitary diastolic murmurs in the newborn. *Clin Pediatr (Phila).* 1983;22:548–550.
4. Keith TR, Sagarminaga J. Spontaneously disappearing murmur of patent ductus arteriosus. A case report. *Circulation.* 1961;24:1235–1238.
5. Still GF. *Common disorders and diseases of childhood.* London: Frowde, Hodder & Stoughton; 1909.
6. Braudo M, Rowe RD. Auscultation of the heart: early neonatal period. *Am J Dis Child.* 1961;101:575–586.
7. Advani N, Menahem S, Wilkinson JL. The diagnosis of innocent murmurs in childhood. *Cardiol Young.* 2000;10:340–342.
8. De Monchy C, Van Der Hoeven GM, Beneken JE. Studies on innocent praecordial vibratory murmurs in children. 3. Follow-up study of children with an innocent praecordial vibratory murmur. *Br Heart J.* 1973;35:685–690.
9. Fogel DH. The innocent systolic murmur in children: a clinical study of its incidence and characteristics. *Am Heart J.* 1960;59:844–855.
10. Humphries JO, McKusick VA. The differentiation of organic and "innocent" systolic murmurs. *Prog Cardiovasc Dis.* 1962;5:152–171.
11. Castle RF, Craige E. Auscultation of the heart in infants and children. *Pediatrics.* 1960;26:511–561.
12. Lessof M, Brigden W. Systolic murmurs in healthy children and in children with rheumatic fever. *Lancet.* 1957;273:673–674.
13. Rosenthal A. How to distinguish between innocent and pathologic murmurs in childhood. *Pediatr Clin North Am.* 1984;31:1229–1240.
14. Van Oort A, Hopman J, De Boo T, Van Der Werf T, Rohmer J, Daniels O. The vibratory innocent heart murmur in schoolchildren: a case-control Doppler echocardiographic study. *Pediatr Cardiol.* 1994;15:275–281.
15. Goldblatt E. Diseases of the heart and blood-vessels. Innocent systolic murmurs in childhood. *Br Med J.* 1966;2:95–98.
16. Harris TN, Lisker L, Needleman HL, Saltzman HA. Spectrographic comparison of ranges of vibration frequency among some innocent

cardiac murmurs in childhood and some murmurs of valvular insufficiency. *Pediatrics*. 1957;19:57–67.

17. Guntheroth WG. Innocent murmurs: a suspect diagnosis in non-pregnant adults. *Am J Cardiol*. 2009;104:735–737.

18. Perloff JK. Clinical recognition of aortic stenosis: the physical signs and differential diagnosis of the various forms of obstruction to left ventricular outflow. *Prog Cardiovasc Dis*. 1968;10:323–352.

19. Roberts WC, Perloff JK, Costantino T. Severe valvular aortic stenosis in patients over 65 years of age. A clinicopathologic study. *Am J Cardiol*. 1971;27:497–506.

20. Klewer SE, Donnerstein RL, Goldberg SJ. Still's-like innocent murmur can be produced by increasing aortic velocity to a threshold value. *Am J Cardiol*. 1991;68:810–812.

21. Spooner PH, Perry MP, Brandenburg RO, Pennock GD. Increased intraventricular velocities: an unrecognized cause of systolic murmur in adults. *J Am Coll Cardiol*. 1998;32:1589–1595.

22. Barlow JB, Bosman CK. The origin of the innocent vibratory systolic murmur. *S Afr J Med Sci*. 1965;30:96.

23. Darazs B, Hesdorffer CS, Butterworth AM, Ziady F. The possible etiology of the vibratory systolic murmur. *Clin Cardiol*. 1987;10:341–346.

24. Malouf J, Gharzuddine W, Kutayli F. A reappraisal of the prevalence and clinical importance of left ventricular false tendons in children and adults. *Br Heart J*. 1986;55:587–591.

25. Perry LW, Ruckman RN, Shapiro SR, Kuehl KS, Galioto Jr FM, Scott 3rd LP. Left ventricular false tendons in children: prevalence as detected by 2-dimensional echocardiography and clinical significance. *Am J Cardiol*. 1983;52:1264–1266.

26. Gerlis LM, Wright HM, Wilson N, Erzengin F, Dickinson DF. Left ventricular bands. A normal anatomical feature. *Br Heart J*. 1984;52:641–647.

27. Gardiner HM, Joffe HS. Genesis of Still's murmurs: a controlled Doppler echocardiographic study. *Br Heart J*. 1991;66:217–220.

28. Rodriguez RJ, Riggs TW. Physiologic peripheral pulmonic stenosis in infancy. *Am J Cardiol*. 1990;66:1478–1481.

29. Lewis DH, Ertugrul A, Deitz GW, Wallace JD, Brown Jr JR, Moghadam AN. Intracardiac phonocardiography in the diagnosis of congenital heart disease. *Pediatrics*. 1959;23:837–853.

30. Deleon Jr AC, Perloff JK, Twigg H, Majd M. The straight back syndrome: clinical cardiovascular manifestations. *Circulation*. 1965;32:193–203.

31. Arlettaz R, Archer N, Wilkinson AR. Closure of the ductus arteriosus and development of pulmonary branch stenosis in babies of less than 32 weeks gestation. *Arch Dis Child Fetal Neonatal Ed*. 2001;85:F197–F200.

32. Barrillon A, Havy G, Scebat L, Baragan J, Gerbaux A. Congenital pressure gradients between main pulmonary artery and its primary branches. *Br Heart J*. 1974;36:669–675.

33. Danilowicz DA, Rudolph AM, Hoffman JI, Heymann M. Physiologic pressure differences between main and branch pulmonary arteries in infants. *Circulation*. 1972;45:410–419.

34. Arlettaz R, Archer N, Wilkinson AR. Natural history of innocent heart murmurs in newborn babies: controlled echocardiographic study. *Br Med J*. 1998;78:F166.

35. Stapleton JF, El-Hajj MM. Heart murmurs simulated by arterial bruits in the neck. *Am Heart J*. 1961;61:178–183.

36. Kawabori I, Stevenson JG, Dooley TK, Phillips DJ, Sylvester CM, Guntheroth WG. The significance of carotid bruits in children: transmitted murmur or vascular origin, studies by pulsed Doppler ultrasound. *Am Heart J*. 1979;98:160–167.

37. Nelson WP, Hall RJ. The innocent supraclavicular arterial bruit—utility of shoulder maneuvers in its recognition. *N Engl J Med*. 1968;278:778.

38. Van Den Bergh AaH. Een Schijnbaar Hartgeruisch. *Ned Tijdschr Geneeskd*. 1908;52:1104.

39. Bruns DL, Van Der Hauwaert LG. The aortic systolic murmur developing with increasing age. *Br Heart J*. 1958;20:370–378.

40. Pomerance A. Cardiac pathology and systolic murmurs in the elderly. *Br Heart J*. 1968;30:687–689.

41. Otto CM, Lind BK, Kitzman DW, Gersh BJ, Siscovick DS. Association of aortic-valve sclerosis with cardiovascular mortality and morbidity in the elderly. *N Engl J Med*. 1999;341:142–147.

42. Howard TH. Cardiac murmurs in old age: a clinico-pathological study. *J Am Geriatr Soc*. 1967;15:509.

43. Perez GL, Jacob M, Bhat PK, Rao DB, Luisada AA. Incidence of murmurs in the aging heart. *J Am Geriatr Soc*. 1976;24:29–31.

44. Stein PD, Sabbah HN. Aortic origin of innocent murmurs. *Am J Cardiol*. 1977;39:665–671.

45. Roberts WC. The congenitally bicuspid aortic valve. A study of 85 autopsy cases. *Am J Cardiol*. 1970;26:72–83.

46. Vollebergh FE, Becker AE. Minor congenital variations of cusp size in tricuspid aortic valves. Possible link with isolated aortic stenosis. *Br Heart J*. 1977;39:1006–1011.

47. Nightingale AK, Horowitz JD. Aortic sclerosis: not an innocent murmur but a marker of increased cardiovascular risk. *Heart*. 2005;91:1389–1393.

48. O'Malley CD, Saunders JB. *Leonardo on the human body*. New York: Dover Publications; 1983.

49. Peacock TB. *On malformations of the human heart*. London: John Churchill; 1858.

50. Osler W. The bicuspid condition of the aortic valve. *Trans Assoc Am Physicians*. 1886;2:185.

51. Leech G, Mills P, Leatham A. The diagnosis of a non-stenotic bicuspid aortic valve. *Br Heart J*. 1978;40:941–950.

52. Nishimura RA, Tajik AJ. The Valsalva maneuver-3 centuries later. *Mayo Clin Proc*. 2004;79:577–578.

53. Child JS. Transthoracic and transesophageal echocardiographic imaging: anatomic and hemodynamic assessment. In: Perloff JK, Child JS, eds. *Congenital heart disease in adults*. Phildelphia: W.B. Saunders Company; 1998.

54. Cabot RC. *Physical diagnosis*. New York: William Wood and Company; 1915.

55. Hope J. *A treatise on the diseases of the heart and great vessels*. London: William Kidd; 1839.

56. Potain SC. Des mouvements et des bruits qui se passent dans les veines jugulaires. *Bull Mem Soc Med Hop Paris*. 1867;4:3.

57. Hardison JE. Cervical venous hum. A clue to the diagnosis of intracranial arteriovenous malformations. *N Engl J Med*. 1968;278:587–590.

58. Jones Jr FL. Frequency, characteristics and importance of the cervical venous hum in adults. *N Engl J Med*. 1962;267:658–660.

59. Cary FH. Symptomatic venous hum. Report of a case. *N Engl J Med*. 1961;264:869–870.

60. Chandler JR. Diagnosis and cure of venous hum tinnitus. *Laryngoscope*. 1983;93:892–895.

61. Rothstein J, Hilger PA, Boies Jr LR. Venous hum as a cause of reversible factitious sensorineural hearing loss. *Ann Otol Rhinol Laryngol*. 1985;94:267–268.

62. Cutforth R, Wiseman J, Sutherland RD. The genesis of the cervical venous hum. *Am Heart J*. 1970;80:488–492.

63. Grant RP. A precordial systolic murmur of extracardiac origin during pregnancy. *Am Heart J*. 1965;52:944.

64. Scott JT, Murphy EA. Mammary souffle of pregnancy: report of two cases simulating patent ductus arteriosus. *Circulation*. 1958;18:1038–1043.

65. Tabatznik B, Randall TW, Hersch C. The mammary souffle of pregnancy and lactation. *Circulation*. 1960;22:1069–1073.

66. Jones AM. *Heart disease in pregnancy*. London: Harvey & Blythe; 1951.

67. Hurst JW, Staton J, Hubbard D. Precordial murmurs during pregnancy and lactation. *N Engl J Med*. 1958;259:515–517.

68. Gallavardin L, Ravault P. Le souffle de retrecissement aortique peut changer de timbre et devenir musical dans sa propagation apexienne. *Lyon Med*. 1925;135:523.

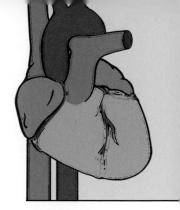

Chapter 3

Cardiac Malpositions

"The heart may be congenitally misplaced in various ways, occupying either an unusual position within the thorax, or being situated external to that cavity."

Thomas B. Peacock, 1858

Dextrocardia in situ inversus was known to the anatomist-surgeon Marco Aurelio Severino in 1643 and was one of the first recognized congenital malformations of the heart.[1] Nearly a century and a half elapsed before Matthew Baillie's[2] account of "complete transposition in the human subject, of the thoracic and abdominal viscera, to the opposite side from what is natural."

Cardiac malpositions, which have a prevalence rate of 0.10 per 1000 live births,[3] refer to hearts that are located abnormally *within* the thoracic cavity or that are located *outside* the thoracic cavity—*ectopia cordis*.[4] In 1901, Paltauf[5] published remarkable illustrations that distinguished the various types of dextrocardia; and in 1928, the first useful classification of cardiac malpositions was proposed.[6] Subsequent observations by Lichtman[7] and by de la Cruz[8] shed light on the embryologic bases of the malpositions; the landmark observations of van Praagh[9] confirmed the validity of those assumptions. Campbell's[10–12] diagrams in the 1950s and 1960s, and Elliott's[13] radiologic classification in 1966, set the stage for the *clinical recognition* of cardiac malpositions.

The genetics of cardiac midline and lateral defects occur along three geometric axes: anteroposterior, dorsal-ventral, and left-right.[14] Genes expressed in dorsal midline cells coordinate the development of the three embryonic axes, driving the cardiac tube to loop in the appropriate direction relative to body axes. The left-right axis is established at approximately the 18th day after fertilization.[14] Both bilateral left-sidedness and bilateral right-sidedness have been reported in members of the same family, which implies that the two conditions are different manifestations of a primary defect in lateralization.[15]

The first section of this chapter deals with the *three basic cardiac malpositions* in the presence of *bilateral asymmetry*. The second section of the chapter deals with cardiac malpositions in the presence of *bilateral symmetry*. Certain organs or structures are in fact bilateral but asymmetrical, such as the bronchi and lungs. Certain essentially unilateral organs, such as the liver, are transverse. Parts of certain structures, such as the atrial appendages, are symmetrical, and the remainders of the atria are morphologically different.

The literature on cardiac malpositions is replete with an arcane vocabulary that often confounds rather than clarifies. Terms have been fully abbreviated, minimally abbreviated, or unabbreviated. In this chapter, unabbreviated terms are used because they are accessible to the widest audience.[16]

DEFINITIONS AND TERMINOLOGY*

Cardiac position: Refers to the intrathoracic location of the heart as left-sided (levocardia), right-sided (dextrocardia), or midline (mesocardia).

Cardiac malposition: An abnormal intrathoracic location of the heart or a location that is abnormal (inappropriate) relative to the position (situs) of the abdominal viscera.

Situs: Site or position.

Solitus: Usual or normal.

Situs solitus: Normal position (Figure 3-1).

Inversus: Reverse or opposite.

Situs inversus: Opposite or reverse of normal (Figure 3-2).

Ambiguus: Uncertain, indeterminant.

Situs ambiguus: Uncertain, indeterminant, or ambiguous position.

Cardiac displacement: A *secondary* shift in intrathoracic cardiac position in response to eventration of a hemidiaphragm (Figure 3-3B), agenesis of a lung (Figure 3-3A,C), or congenital complete absence of the pericardium (see Chapter 5).

Ectopia cordis: (Gr) *ektopos* = displaced. *Extrathoracic* location of the heart (Figure 3-4).

Chamber designations: Right and left refer to morphology rather than position, as right or left atrium and right or left ventricle.

Great arterial designations: Ascending aorta and pulmonary trunk are defined in terms of their ventricular alignments or their spatial relations to each other.

Heterotaxy: (Gr) *heteros* = other, different; *taxis* = arrangement.

Isomerism: (Gr) *isos* = equal; *meros* = part. Refers to the morphologic similarity of bilateral structures that are normally dissimilar, such as right and left atrial appendages, right and left bronchi, and right and left lungs.

*References 16–18

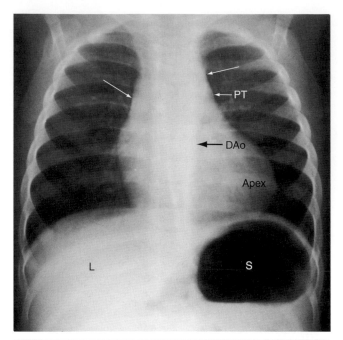

FIGURE 3-1 Normal heart and viscera in *situs solitus*. The stomach bubble (S) is on the *left*, the liver (L) is on the *right*, and the heart is left-sided with its base to apex axis pointing to the left. Despite a large stomach bubble (S), the left hemidiaphragm is lower than the right hemidiaphragm because the cardiac apex is on the left. The ascending aorta, the aortic knuckle *(unmarked white arrows)*, and the pulmonary trunk (PT) are in normal positions. The descending aorta (DAo) is concordant on the left.

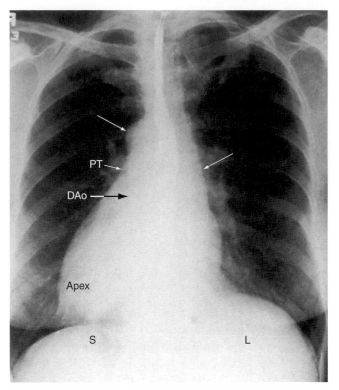

FIGURE 3-2 Chest x-ray from a 65-year-old woman with complete *situs inversus*. The stomach bubble (S) is on the *right*, the liver (L) is on the *left*, the heart (Apex) is on the *right* (dextrocardia), and the hemidiaphragm is lower on the side of the cardiac apex *(right)*. The ascending aorta, the aortic knuckle *(unmarked white arrows)*, and the pulmonary trunk (PT) are in their mirror image positions. The descending aorta (DAo) is concordant on the *right*.

Right isomerism: Refers to bilateral structures in which both have morphologic *right* characteristics, such as morphologic right atrial appendages, morphologic right bronchi, and bilateral trilobed lungs.

Left isomerism: Refers to bilateral structures in which both have morphologic *left* characteristics, such as morphologic left atrial appendages, morphologic left bronchi, and bilateral bilobed lungs.

Asplenia: Congenital absence of the spleen. Splenic tissue is either entirely absent or is rudimentary and nonfunctional.

Polysplenia: *Many spleens*, each of which is appreciably smaller than one normal-sized spleen. Multiple spleens of *polysplenia* differ from *accessory spleens* (splenules) that accompany one normal-sized spleen.

Ventricular loop: The right or left bend (loop) that forms in the straight heart tube of the embryo.

d-Loop: The normal *rightward* (dextro = d) bend in the embryonic heart tube. The d-loop designation as applied to the developed heart indicates that the sinus or inflow portion of the morphologic right ventricle lies to the right of the morphologic left ventricle.

l-Loop: A *leftward* (levo = l) bend in the embryonic heart tube. The l-loop designation as applied to the developed heart indicates that the sinus or

inflow portion of the morphologic right ventricle lies to the left of the morphologic left ventricle.

Concordant: (L) *concordare* = to agree (i.e., agreeing or appropriate).

Concordant loop: Refers to a ventricular loop that agrees with (is appropriate for) the visceroatrial situs (i.e., d-loop in situs solitus, l-loop in situs inversus).

Atrioventricular concordance: Refers to appropriate (concordant) connection of a morphologic *right* atrium to morphologic *right* ventricle via a morphologic *tricuspid* valve and appropriate (concordant) connection of a morphologic *left* atrium to a morphologic *left* ventricle via a morphologic *mitral* valve. Each atrioventricular valve is normally *concordant* with the morphologic ventricle to which it is attached.

Infundibulum (conus): The ventriculo/great arterial segment that is normally subpulmonary.

Ventriculoarterial concordance: Refers to appropriate (concordant) connection of a morphologic *right* ventricle to a *pulmonary trunk* and appropriate (concordant) connection of a morphologic *left* ventricle to an aorta.

Discordant: Not agreeing, inappropriate.

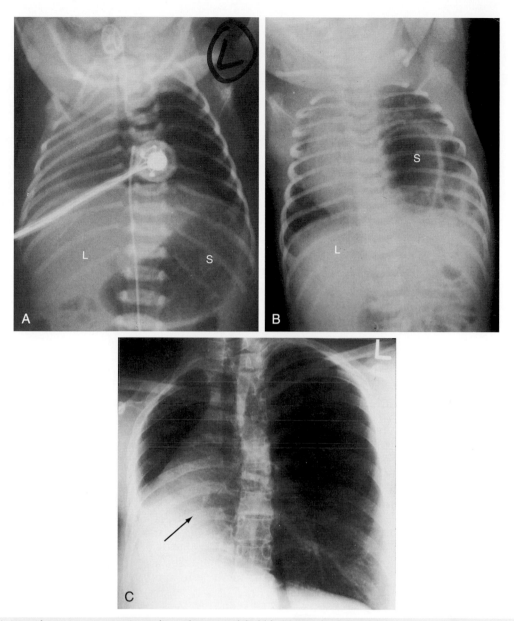

FIGURE 3-3 A, X-ray from a neonate in *situs solitus*. The stomach bubble (S) is on the *left* and the liver (L) is on the *right,* but the heart is in the right thoracic cavity because of displacement caused by congenital agenesis of the right lung. The proximity of the posterior ribs reflects the reduced size of the right hemithorax. **B,** X-ray from a neonate in *situs solitus*. The heart is displaced into the right hemithorax because of congenital eventration of the left hemidiaphragm through which the stomach (S) has entered the left thoracic cavity. The liver (L) is in its normal position on the *right*. **C,** Chest x-ray from a 29-year-old woman in *situs solitus*. The heart is displaced into the right thoracic cavity because of congenital agenesis of the right lung. The right posterior ribs are in close proximity, and the right hemidiaphragm is elevated because the right hemithorax is reduced in size (arrow).

Transposition of the great arteries: Each great artery is connected to a morphologically discordant ventricle (ventriculoarterial *discordance*). The *aorta* arises from a morphologic *right* ventricle, and the *pulmonary trunk* arises from a morphologic *left* ventricle.

Malposition of the great arteries: Refers to abnormal *spatial* relationships of the aorta and the pulmonary trunk to each other. Malpositions can be in either the lateral or the anteroposterior plane.

The great arteries are *malposed* but not *transposed* because ventriculo/great arterial concordance is maintained.

Inversion: Refers to *right/left* reversal with no change in anteroposterior or superoinferior relationships.

Atrioventricular discordance with ventriculoarterial discordance: *Atrioventricular* discordance applies when a morphologic *right* atrium connects to a morphologic *left* ventricle via a morphologic *mitral* valve and when a morphologic *left* atrium connects to a morphologic *right* ventricle via a morphologic *tricuspid* valve. *Ventriculoarterial* discordance applies when a morphologic *right* ventricle gives rise to the *aorta* and a morphologic *left* ventricle gives rise to the *pulmonary trunk. Congenitally corrected*

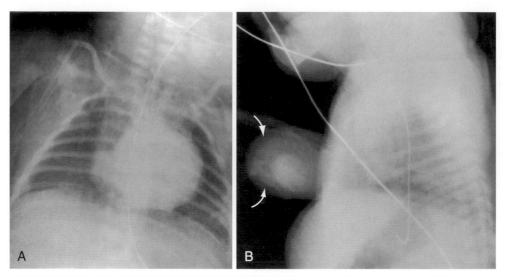

FIGURE 3-4 X-rays from a 2-day-old male with *ectopia cordis*. **A,** The external position of the heart cannot be inferred from the frontal projection, but is obvious (arrows) in the lateral projection **(B).**

transposition applies when a *double* discordance (atrioventricular and ventriculoarterial) results in *physiologic correction*, so right atrial blood reaches the pulmonary artery through a morphologic left ventricle and left atrial blood reaches the aorta through a morphologic right ventricle.

A systematic approach: Refers to sequential attention to the atria, the atrioventricular valves, the atrioventricular connections, the ventricles, the ventriculoarterial connections, the great arteries, and the positions or malpositions of the heart and abdominal viscera.[16–18]

Let us first focus on *normal* cardiac and *normal* abdominal visceral positions *(situs solitus)*, and then on the three major cardiac *malpositions* in the presence of right/left *asymmetry*.

Situs Solitus

Because *atrial situs* and *abdominal situs* are usually concordant, *atrial situs solitus* can be inferred at the bedside with percussion of a left-sided stomach, a right-sided liver, and a left-sided heart. The chest x-ray confirms the positions of the stomach, liver, and heart (see Figure 3-1) and discloses bronchial morphology, which is a reliable predictor of atrial situs.[19] A morphologic *right* bronchus is relatively short and straight, whereas a morphologic *left* bronchus is relatively long and curved (Figure 3-5). A morphologic *right* bronchus is concordant with a *trilobed* morphologic *right* lung, and a morphologic *left* bronchus is concordant with a *bilobed* morphologic *left* lung. The chest x-ray establishes the direction of the base to apex axis, which points to the left because

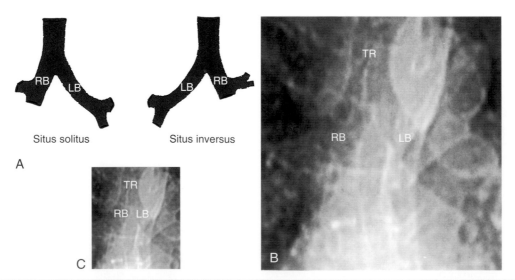

FIGURE 3-5 A, In *situs solitus*, the morphologic right bronchus (RB) is short, wide, and relatively straight and is right-sided. The morphologic left bronchus (LB) is long, thin, and curved and is left-sided. In *situs inversus* (mirror image), the morphologic right bronchus is left-sided and the morphologic left bronchus is right-sided. **B** and **C,** Tomographic scans show the morphologic right bronchus (RB) and morphologic left bronchus (LB) in *situs solitus*. (TR = trachea.)

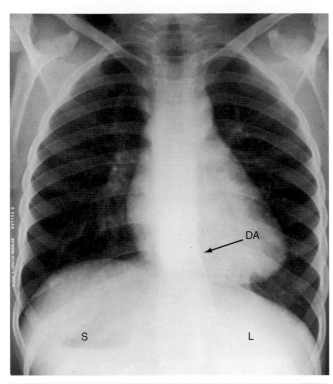

FIGURE 3-6 X-ray from an 8-year-old girl with *thoracoabdominal discordance* represented by abdominal *situs inversus* but thoracic *situs solitus* with a left-sided heart. The stomach (S) lies in the right upper quadrant, and the liver (L) lies in the left upper quadrant. (DA = descending aorta).

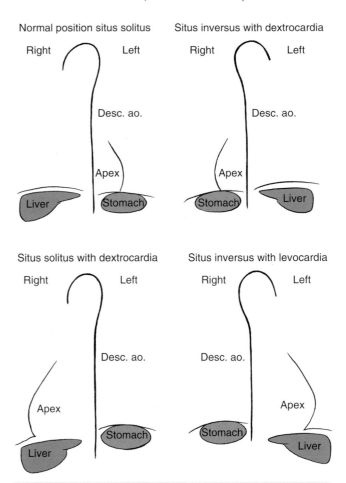

FIGURE 3-7 Schematic illustrations of the four basic cardiac positions (normal and three malpositions) and the relationships of descending aorta, cardiac apex, stomach, and liver. The drawings are shown as projected from the frontal view of a chest x-ray. In *situs solitus*, the descending aorta, cardiac apex, and stomach are all on the *left*. In *situs inversus* with *dextrocardia*, the descending aorta, cardiac apex, and stomach are all on the *right*. In *situs solitus* with *dextrocardia*, the descending aorta and stomach are on the *left* (normal), but the cardiac apex is on the *right*. In *situs inversus* with *levocardia*, the descending aorta and stomach are on the *right* (situs inversus), but the cardiac apex is on the *left*.

the straight heart tube of the embryo initially bends to the right (d-loop) and then pivots to the left until the ventricular portion comes to occupy its normal left thoracic position (see Figure 3-1).[9,20] The relative levels of the two hemidiaphragms are determined by the location of the cardiac apex, not by the location of the liver, so the left hemidiaphragm is normally lower than the right hemidiaphragm.[21] Thoracoabdominal *discordance* is represented by *thoracic situs solitus*, a *left* thoracic heart, and *abdominal situs inversus* (Figure 3-6)[22,23] or by *thoracic situs inversus*, a *right* thoracic heart (dextrocardia), and *abdominal situs solitus*.

The next step in the systematic analysis concerns the *great arteries*. The chest x-ray provides information on the spatial relationships of aorta and pulmonary trunk and on ventriculoarterial alignments. In *situs solitus* with atrioventricular and ventriculo/great arterial concordance, the ascending aorta forms a convex shadow at the right basal aspect of the cardiac silhouette, the aortic arch forms a left basal knuckle below which lies the slightly convex main pulmonary artery segment, and the descending thoracic aorta runs parallel to the left border of the vertebral column (see Figure 3-1).

MALPOSITIONS

Three major cardiac malpositions occur in the presence of right/left asymmetry (Figures 3-7 and 3-8): (1) visceroatrial *situs inversus* with dextrocardia; (2) visceroatrial

situs solitus with dextrocardia; and (3) visceroatrial *situs inversus* with levocardia. *Mesocardia*, a midline heart, is sometimes regarded as a fourth malposition. A midline heart in *situs solitus* with a d-bulboventricular loop is a variation of normal, but a midline heart with visceroatrial *situs inversus* and an l-bulboventricular loop occurs with major congenital malformations.[18]

Situs Inversus with Dextrocardia

The incidence rate in the general population is estimated at 1/8000 to 1/25,000.[24] The heart and the thoracic and abdominal viscera are mirror images of normal (see Figure 3-2).[25] The bronchi are inverted (see Figure 3-5A), with the morphologic *right bronchus* concordant with the morphologic *right atrium* and the *trilobed lung* and with the morphologic *left bronchus* concordant

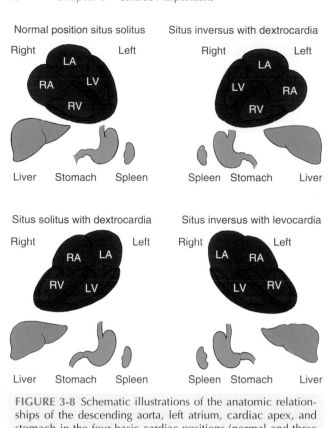

Normal position situs solitus

Situs inversus with dextrocardia

Situs solitus with dextrocardia

Situs inversus with levocardia

FIGURE 3-8 Schematic illustrations of the anatomic relationships of the descending aorta, left atrium, cardiac apex, and stomach in the four basic cardiac positions (normal and three malpositions). In *situs solitus*, the descending aorta, left atrium, cardiac apex, and stomach are all on the *left*. In *situs inversus* with *dextrocardia*, the descending aorta, left atrium, cardiac apex, and stomach are all on the *right*. In *situs solitus* with *dextrocardia*, the descending aorta, left atrium, and stomach are on the *left* (normal), but the cardiac apex is on the *right*. In *situs inversus with levocardia*, the descending aorta, left atrium, and stomach are on the *right* (situs inversus), but the cardiac apex is on the *left*. (RA = right atrium; LA = left atrium; RV = right ventricle; LV = left ventricle; spleen as shown.)

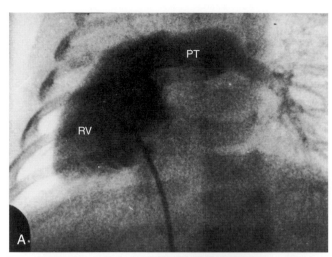

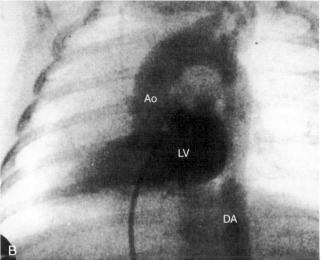

FIGURE 3-9 **A,** Right ventriculogram (anteroposterior) in a 2-month-old female in *situs solitus* with dextrocardia and no associated congenital heart disease. The morphologic right ventricle (RV) occupies the apex on the right and gives rise to the pulmonary trunk (PT). The hemidiaphragm is lower on the side of the apex. **B,** The morphologic left ventricle (LV) is in a medial position and gives rise to a normally positioned ascending aorta (Ao) and a left-sided descending aorta (DA).

with the morphologic *left atrium* and the *bilobed lung* (see Figure 3-5). The heart is right-sided, and the right hemidiaphragm is lower than the left hemidiaphragm (see Figure 3-2). The descending aorta is on the right; the ascending aorta, aortic knuckle, and pulmonary trunk are in their mirror image positions; and the anatomic right ventricle lies to the left of the anatomic left ventricle (l-bulboventricular loop), which is normal for *situs inversus* just as a d-bulboventricular loop is normal for *situs solitus*.

Situs Solitus with Dextrocardia

The lungs and abdominal viscera are *situs solitus*, but the heart is right thoracic (dextrocardia) (Figures 3-7 through 3-10).[25] The ascending aorta and aortic knuckle occupy their normal positions and the descending aorta runs its normal course along the left vertebral border (see Figure 3-9), but the major cardiac shadow lies to the *right* of midline (dextrocardia), the base to apex axis points to the *right*, and the *right* hemidiaphragm is lower than the left hemidiaphragm (see Figure 3-9). In the type

of *situs solitus* with dextrocardia shown in Figure 3-9, the anatomic right ventricle lies to the right of the anatomic left ventricle (d-loop) because the straight heart tube of the embryo initially bends in a rightward direction (d-loop) but then fails to pivot into the left chest. Varying degrees of incomplete pivoting determine the degree to which the ventricular portion of the heart lies to the right of midline (see Figure 3-10).

Situs Inversus with Levocardia

The defining characteristics of this malposition are *situs inversus* of thoracic and abdominal viscera in the presence of a left thoracic heart (levocardia; Figures 3-7 and 3-11). The left hemidiaphragm is lower than the right hemidiaphragm because the apex is on the left (see Figure 3-11). Inversion of the bronchi (see Figure 3-5A)

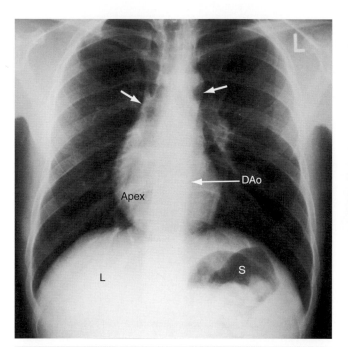

FIGURE 3-10 Chest x-ray from a 20-year-old man in *situs solitus* with dextrocardia and no associated congenital heart disease. The stomach (S) is on the *left,* and the liver (L) is on the *right.* The base to apex axis points to the *right* and the cardiac shadow is chiefly to the right of midline, but the hemidiaphragms are at the same level. The ascending aorta and aortic knuckle *(unmarked white arrows)* are in their normal positions, and the descending thoracic aorta (DAo) is normally positioned along the left border of the vertebral column.

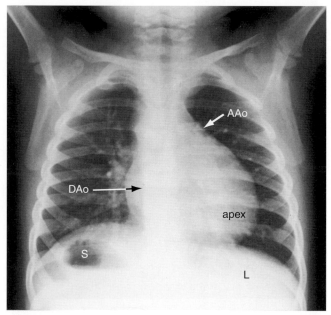

FIGURE 3-11 X-ray from a 2-year-old girl in *situs inversus* with levocardia. The stomach (S) is on the *right* and the liver (L) is on the *left,* but the heart (apex) is to the left of midline. The left hemidiaphragm is lower than the right hemidiaphragm because the cardiac apex is on the left. The descending thoracic aorta (DAo) is on the *right* (concordant for *situs inversus*), but the position of the ascending aorta (AAo) indicates a discordant d-bulboventricular loop.

coincides with inversion of the atria and lungs. The stomach is on the right, and the liver is on the left (abdominal *situs inversus;* see Figure 3-11). The major cardiac mass lies in the left chest for one of two morphogenetic reasons. First, an embryonic l-loop, which is *concordant* for *situs inversus,* fails to pivot into the right side of the chest. Second, an embryonic d-loop, which is *discordant* for *situs inversus,* fails to pivot into the left side of the chest. When a d-loop in *situs inversus* is associated with congenitally corrected transposition of the great arteries (ventricular inversion), the ascending aorta forms a smooth shadow at the left basal aspect of the heart (see Figure 3-11).

Midline Heart (Mesocardia)

The example shown in Figure 3-12 is a midline cardiac position in the presence of thoracic and abdominal *situs solitus.* The cardiac silhouette extends equally to the right and left of midline (Figure 3-12A). A d-bulboventricular loop stops in the midline as it pivots to the left (Figure 3-12B).[18,26] Much less commonly, mesocardia is associated with *situs inversus* and an l-loop that stops in the midline as it incompletely pivots to the *right*.[18,26]

In brief, two varieties of *right-thoracic hearts* exist (see Figures 3-7 and 3-8): namely, *situs inversus* with dextrocardia and *situs solitus* with dextrocardia. And two varieties of *left-thoracic hearts* exist: namely, *situs solitus* with levocardia (normal) and *situs inversus* with

levocardia. A midline heart (mesocardia) is exceptional but occurs either in *situs solitus* or rarely in *situs inversus.* Once the cardiac malposition has been defined, clinical assessment turns to the presence and type of associated congenital heart disease.

Situs inversus with *dextrocardia* (complete *situs inversus,* mirror image dextrocardia; see Figure 3-2) usually occurs without coexisting congenital heart disease. Isolated atrial inversion is rare.[27] *Situs solitus* with *dextrocardia* is only occasionally associated with a structurally normal heart (see Figures 3-9 and 3-10); left-to-right shunts at atrial level or ventricular level usually coexist. When *situs solitus* with *dextrocardia* occurs with a bulboventricular loop that initially bends to the *left* and then pivots to the *right* (where an l-loop *belongs*),[18] ventricular inversion, ventricular septal defect, and obstruction to venous ventricular outflow usually coexist.[13,18,28]

Situs inversus with *levocardia* is consistently associated with coexisting congenital heart disease (see Figure 3-11),[18] whether the left thoracic heart results from a discordant d-loop that pivots into the left hemithorax or from a concordant l-loop that fails to pivot into the right hemithorax. A discordant d-loop in *situs inversus* results in ventricular inversion, as does a discordant l-loop in *situs solitus.*[18] Coexisting congenital heart disease is invariable and complex but occurs without prevailing patterns.[13,18]

A *midline cardiac position* (mesocardia) occurs in *situs solitus* (see Figure 3-12) or in *situs inversus.*[18,26] If the bulboventricular loop is discordant, ventricular inversion coexists.

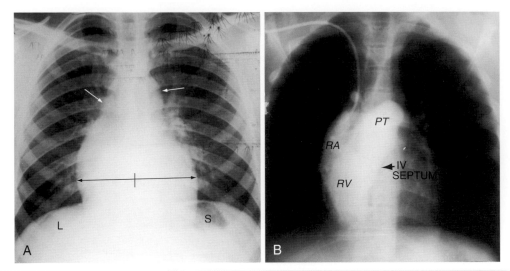

FIGURE 3-12 A, X-ray from a 16-year-old boy in *situs solitus* with a midline heart (mesocardia) and no associated congenital heart disease. The stomach (S) is on the *left,* and the liver (L) is on the *right.* Identical extension of the heart to the right and left of center *(equal black arrows)* is seen. The ascending aorta and aortic knuckle *(white arrows)* are in their normal positions. The cardiac silhouette is hump-shaped because the right atrium (RA) and right ventricle (RV) are superimposed (see angiogram; **B**). The right hemidiaphragm is lower than the left hemidiaphragm because the base to apex axis points to the right. **B,** The position of the right ventricle (RV) and the interventricular septal plane (IV SEPTUM) indicate that mesocardia resulted from a d-bulboventricular loop in which leftward pivoting stopped at the midline. (RA = right atrium; PT = pulmonary trunk.)

History

Situs inversus with *dextrocardia* and a structurally normal heart is usually discovered by chance in a chest x-ray, which is often considered normal because the film is inadvertently reversed when first read. A tendency for left handedness in complete *situs inversus* is reported,[1] but Matthew Baillie[2] wrote: "The person seems to have used his right hand in preference to his left . . . which was readily discovered by the greater bulk and hardness of that hand as well as the greater fleshiness of the arm." Baillie's conclusion has been confirmed.[29]

Investigations of the human brain, which is asymmetric in both structure and function, are important.[29] The developmental factors that determine *functional* asymmetry of the brain independently recognize laterality (asymmetry) in visceral situs.[29] Developmental factors that determine *anatomic* asymmetry of the brain are distinct from those that determine visceral asymmetry and lateralization of language.[29]

Situs inversus with dextrocardia is the malposition most likely to occur with an otherwise structurally normal heart and with normal longevity. Symptoms caused by coexisting acquired cardiac or noncardiac disease may lead to the discovery of hitherto unsuspected *situs inversus.* The pain of ischemic heart disease is located in the *right* anterior chest with radiation to the *right* shoulder and *right* arm. The pain of appendicitis is referred to the *left* lower quadrant,[30] and the pain of biliary colic presents in the *left* upper quadrant (Figure 3-13).

In 1933, Kartagener[31] called attention to the association of sinusitis, bronchiectasis, and *situs inversus,* a combination subsequently called Kartagener's syndrome or triad.[32] In the first English-language publication of the syndrome (1937), as many as one fifth of patients with *situs inversus* had bronchiectasis, underscoring that the association was not fortuitous.[33] In 1986, a blinded controlled study of cilia ultrastructure in Kartagener's syndrome found a widespread inherited ciliary disorder[34] that included the upper and lower respiratory tracts (bronchitis, bronchiectasis, sinusitis)[32] and the testis (immobile sperm, male infertility).[35,36] *Situs inversus* is common in infertile men, an observation that contributed to the identification of a generalized disorder of ciliary motility.[36] Respiratory symptoms are a significant part of the history and may lead to the discovery of *situs inversus.* Familial *situs inversus* has been reported,[37] and Kartagener's syndrome is sometimes familial.[34] One family of six siblings included two cases of Kartagener's syndrome and two cases of isolated bronchiectasis.

Situs solitus with *dextrocardia* occasionally occurs without coexisting congenital heart disease and escapes recognition. A routine chest x-ray may provide the first evidence (see Figure 3-10). As a rule, accompanying congenital cardiac malformations bring the patient to medical attention. *Situs inversus* with *levocardia* (see Figure 3-11) invariably occurs with coexisting congenital heart disease that leads to the discovery of the cardiac malposition.

Physical Appearance, Arterial Pulse, and Jugular Venous Pulse

These features are determined by coexisting congenital heart disease rather than the cardiac malposition. The left testicle in the healthy upright male is lower than the right testicle, whereas the opposite is the case in *situs inversus.* Poland's syndrome, which is characterized by the absence of a pectoralis major muscle (usually right-sided),

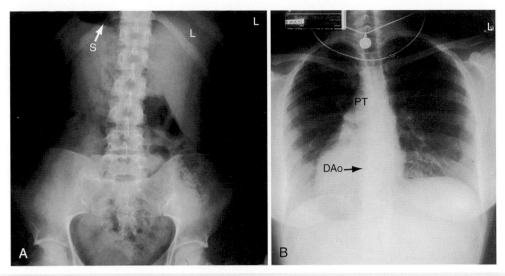

FIGURE 3-13 X-rays from a 28-year-old woman who presented with acute *left* upper quadrant colic. **A,** The abdominal x-ray disclosed the stomach bubble (S) on the *right* and the liver (L) on the *left,* establishing the diagnosis of abdominal *situs inversus,* which was appropriate for biliary colic referred to the *left* upper quadrant. **B,** The chest x-ray disclosed thoracic *situs inversus* with dextrocardia and abdominal situs inversus with the stomach (S) on the *right* and the liver (L) on the *left.* The pulmonary trunk (PT) is in its mirror image position, and the descending aorta (DAo) is along the right side of the vertebral column.

ipsilateral syndactyly, brachydactyly, and hypoplasia of a hand, (see Chapter 15, Figure 15-16) has been reported with *situs solitus* and dextrocardia[38]; and Goldenhar's syndrome (oculoauricular vertebral dysplasia, hemifacial microsomia) has been reported with complete *situs inversus.*[39]

Percussion and Palpation

A *right* anterior chest bulge with asymmetry arouses suspicion of dextrocardia. Percussion and palpation are useful in the clinical recognition of cardiac malpositions because these physical signs are influenced by the malposition *per se* and establish the right or left thoracic location of the heart and the abdominal location of hepatic dullness and gastric tympany. If the stomach is not sufficiently air-filled to generate a tympanitic percussion note, a carbonated beverage or deliberate aerophagia (an infant can suck an empty bottle) solves the problem. Percussion begins over the sternum and then is used to compare left and right parasternal sites. The side of major cardiac dullness is more accurately established with percussion with the patient turned moderately to the left and then moderately to the right. The heart tends to fall to the side toward which the base to apex axis points. *Situs inversus* with *dextrocardia* is characterized by gastric tympany on the right, hepatic dullness on the left, and cardiac dullness on the right (see Figures 3-2 and 3-7). *Situs solitus* with *dextrocardia* is characterized by normal locations of gastric tympany and hepatic dullness and by cardiac dullness on the right (see Figures 3-7 and 3-10). *Situs inversus* with *levocardia* is the converse of *situs solitus* with dextrocardia (see Figures 3-7 and 3-11).

Palpation is undertaken with the patient supine and then in both left and right lateral decubitus positions. The normal *situs solitus* heart (see Figure 3-1) is represented by a morphologic left ventricle that occupies the apex and a morphologic right ventricle that underlies the lower left sternal border.[40] *Situs inversus* with *dextrocardia* (see Figure 3-2) is represented by a morphologic left ventricle that occupies the apex in the *right* hemithorax and a morphologic right ventricle that underlies the lower *right* sternal border. *Situs solitus* with *dextrocardia* is represented by a right thoracic apical low-pressure morphologic *right* ventricle that retracts and a high-pressure systemic morphologic *left* ventricle that generates outward systolic movement adjacent to the lower right sternal border (see Figures 3-9 and 3-10). *Situs inversus* with *levocardia* and l-bulboventricular loop is represented by a left thoracic apical low-pressure morphologic right ventricle that retracts and a high-pressure systemic morphologic left ventricle that generates outward systolic movement adjacent to the lower left sternal border (see Figures 3-11).

Auscultation

The relative prominence of auscultatory events should be compared in the left and right anterior hemithorax, more specifically along the left and right sternal borders and at the apices (Figure 3-14). The stethoscope should alternate from one side to the other for comparison of analogous right and left thoracic sites. With dextrocardia, the first and second heart sounds are louder in the right anterior chest (see Figure 3-14); splitting of the second sound in the second *right* intercostal space is a feature of dextrocardia just as splitting of the second heart sound in the second *left* interspace is a feature of a left thoracic heart. In *situs solitus* with dextrocardia and a d-bulboventricular loop (see Figures 3-9 and 3-10), the position of the pulmonary valve results in splitting of the second sound in the second *right* interspace and the anterior position of

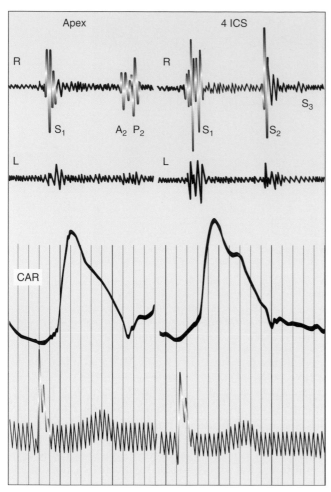

FIGURE 3-14 Phonocardiograms from a 7-year-old boy in *situs solitus* with dextrocardia and an ostium secundum atrial septal defect. Heart sounds are louder on the right (R). The pulmonary component of the second sound (P₂) was recorded at the right cardiac apex because the apex was occupied by the right ventricle. (L = left; 4 ICS = fourth intercostal space; CAR = carotid pulse.)

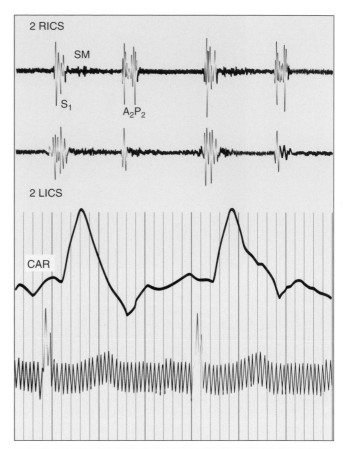

FIGURE 3-15 Phonocardiograms from the 7-year-old boy referred to in Figure 3-14. A short soft pulmonary midsystolic murmur was recorded in the second right interspace (2 RICS) together with persistent splitting of the second heart sound. (A₂ = aortic component; P₂ = pulmonary component; CAR = carotid pulse; 2 LICS = second left intercostal space.)

the aorta results in amplification of the aortic component (Figure 3-15). In *situs inversus* with levocardia, splitting of the second sound is more prominent in the second *left* interspace.

The location and radiation of murmurs are governed by the type of cardiac malposition. In *situs inversus* with dextrocardia, murmur sites are the mirror images of normal. In *situs solitus* with dextrocardia, a pulmonary stenotic murmur is louder to the *right* of the sternum (Figure 3-16) and radiates upward and to the *left* because of the direction taken by the pulmonary trunk (see Figure 3-9A).

Electrocardiogram

As early as 1889, well before the advent of electrocardiography, it was postulated that ventricular potentials in *complete situs inversus* should be diametrically opposite the ventricular potentials of the normal heart.[41] In *situs inversus* with dextrocardia, a mirror image sinus node lies at the junction of a *left* superior vena cava and the mirror image *left-sided* morphologic right atrium. The right and left bundle branches supply their corresponding mirror image right and left ventricles.[42] Certainty that the limb leads are properly attached is essential before proceeding with interpretation of the 12-lead electrocardiogram.[43] Interpretation in mirror image dextrocardia is easier when the arm leads are *intentionally* reversed and when *right* precordial leads are *intentionally* recorded from locations that are the exact opposites of standard left precordial lead positions (Figure 3-17).[11] In *situs solitus* with *dextrocardia*, the limb leads are best left unchanged, and the precordial leads are recorded from the right anterior chest (Figure 3-18). This recommendation is appropriate because atrial situs is normal (sinus node is at the junction of the right superior vena cava and morphologic right atrium on the right)[42] and because the base to apex axis points to the right whether the bundle branches supply their corresponding ventricles as d-loop or l-loop.[42] In *situs inversus* with *levocardia*, standard limb lead and precordial lead positions suffice (Figure 3-19).

Analysis of the electrocardiogram commences with the P wave direction, which is determined by atrial situs unless the atrial pacemaker is ectopic.[44-46] In *situs solitus*

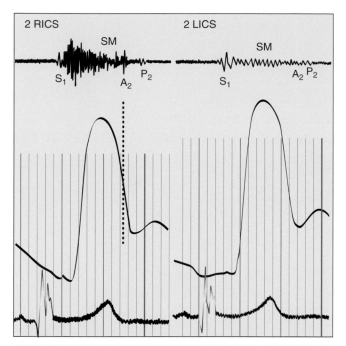

FIGURE 3-16 Phonocardiograms, carotid pulse, and electrocardiogram from a 15-year-old boy in *situs solitus* with dextrocardia. Pulmonary stenosis was found with a right-to-left shunt through a ventricular septal defect. The pulmonary stenotic murmur (SM) was appreciably louder in the second right intercostal space (2 RICS) compared with the second left intercostal space (2 LICS). A soft, delayed pulmonary component of the second (P₂) was more apparent on the right.

with either levocardia or dextrocardia, atrial depolarization proceeds from a normally positioned right sinus node, so upright P waves appear in leads 1 and aVL and an inverted P wave appears in lead aVR (Figure 3-20).[11,12,45,47] Conversely, in *situs inversus* with either dextrocardia or levocardia, atrial depolarization proceeds from a *left* sinus node, so *inverted* P waves appear in leads 1 and aVL and an *upright* P wave appears in lead aVR (see Figures 3-17 and 3-19).[12] In the presence of a right sinus

node, the direction of the P wave can be altered by a left atrial ectopic focus.[12,47–49] Valsalva's maneuver, ocular pressure, or exercise may transiently shift the ectopic focus to the right sinus node.[49] Left atrial ectopic rhythm is manifested by a negative P wave in lead 1 and isoelectric or negative P waves in left precordial leads (see Figure 3-18). A less common but more distinctive configuration is the *dome and dart* P wave in lead V_1 (Figure 3-21).[49] A negative P wave in lead 1 or lead V_1 does not distinguish *situs solitus* with a left atrial ectopic rhythm from *situs inversus*, but a dome and dart P wave in lead V_1 or V_2 confirms a left atrial ectopic focus irrespective of atrial situs.[48–50]

In *situs inversus* with *dextrocardia*, ventricular activation and repolarization are the reverse of normal as predicted in 1889 (see Figure 3-17).[41] In lead 1, the major QRS deflection is negative and the T wave is inverted; lead aVR resembles lead aVL, and vice versa; and right precordial leads resemble leads from corresponding left precordial sites (see Figure 3-17). Septal Q waves appear in *right* lateral precordial leads rather than in left lateral precordial leads because septal depolarization proceeds from right to left (see Figure 3-17). The electrocardiogram can be "corrected" when limb leads are reversed and chest leads are recorded from right precordial sites (see previous discussion).

In *situs solitus* with *dextrocardia* and a d-loop, the left ventricle is relatively anterior and the right ventricle lies to the right (see Figure 3-10); left ventricular electrical activity is directed anteriorly, and right ventricular activity is directed to the right. Depolarization in the frontal plane is counterclockwise, so Q waves appear in leads 1 and aVL (see Figures 3-18 and 3-20). Precordial leads display relatively prominent R waves in leads V_1 and V_2 (anterior left ventricular forces) and display prominent RS complexes in most of the remaining right precordial leads (see Figure 3-18). Normal left-to-right septal depolarization (d-loop) results in Q waves in standard *left* precordial locations (see Figures 3-18 and 3-20). The converse is the case for an l-loop with which Q waves are *absent* in *left* precordial leads and are present in *right* precordial leads, indicating right-to-left septal depolarization (Figure 3-22).

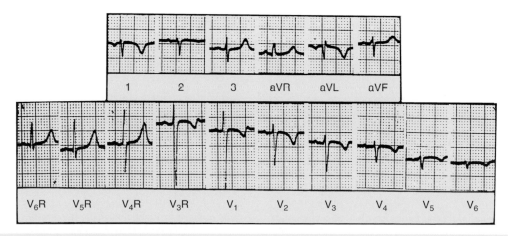

FIGURE 3-17 Electrocardiogram from an 11-year-old girl in *situs inversus* with dextrocardia and no coexisting congenital heart disease. The P wave and T wave are inverted in lead 1, and the major QRS deflections are negative. Lead aVR and lead aVL are mirror images of normal. Precordial leads V_2 through V_6R resemble normal *left* precordial leads (mirror image).

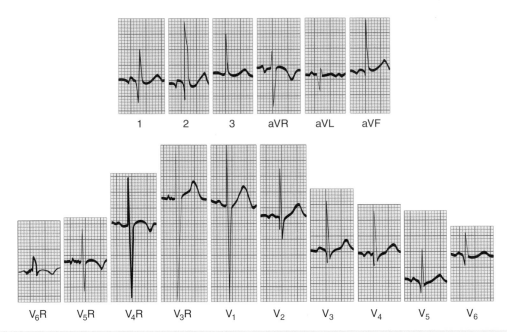

FIGURE 3-18 Electrocardiogram from the 7-year-old boy in *situs solitus* with dextrocardia referred to in Figure 3-14. The direction of the P wave is abnormal because of a left atrial ectopic focus. The frontal QRS axis is vertical. The deep Q wave in lead 1 is a sign of right ventricular hypertrophy. Septal depolarization proceeds from left to right as in normally positioned hearts. *Septal Q waves* in left precordial leads indicate that ventricular inversion does not coexist. The dominant R wave in V$_6$R is evidence of right ventricular hypertrophy because the right-sided right ventricle occupies the apex.

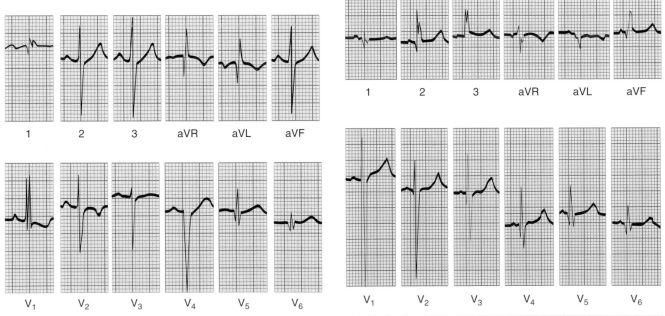

FIGURE 3-19 Electrocardiogram from an 11-year-old boy in *situs inversus* with levocardia, severe pulmonary stenosis, ventricular septal defect, ventricular inversion, and a Blalock-Taussig shunt. Negative P waves in leads 1 and aVL indicate atrial situs inversus. Q waves in left precordial leads identify left-to-right septal depolarization of ventricular inversion.

FIGURE 3-20 Electrocardiogram from a 15-year-old boy in *situs solitus* with dextrocardia, pulmonary stenosis, and a ventricular septal defect. The upright P wave in lead 1 indicates normal atrial situs. Right ventricular hypertrophy is responsible for a vertical QRS axis with a prominent Q wave and a small r wave in lead 1. Septal depolarization proceeds from left to right as in the normal heart, so septal Q waves appear in left precordial leads.

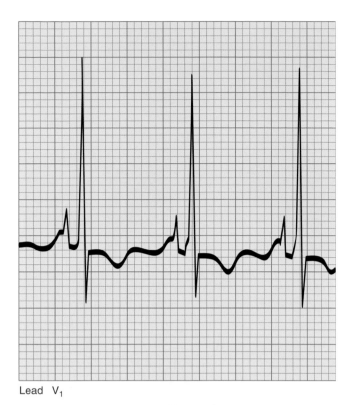

Lead V₁

FIGURE 3-21 Lead V₁ from a 5-year-old boy in *situs solitus* with dextrocardia. The dome and dart P wave is characteristic of a left atrial ectopic rhythm.

X-Ray

The x-ray permits confident recognition of cardiac malpositions.[13,18,19,51] The first necessity is to identify the orienting letters L and R or analogous symbols that designate left and right. From the radiologic point of view, this is all that is required to diagnose *situs inversus* with dextrocardia (see Figure 3-2). The aorta is in its inverted position with the arch deviating the trachea toward the *left*, the descending thoracic aorta runs as a fine line along the right vertebral border, and the major cardiac shadow to the right of midline (Figures 3-2 and 3-23A). *Situs inversus* is missed if the film is inadvertently read in a reversed position because it then appears *correct* except for the L and R designations that are on the wrong side (Figure 3-23B). Complete *situs inversus* implies atrial situs inversus (visceroatrial concordance; see Figures 3-8 and 3-23), which is established by identifying the inverted morphologic right and left bronchi (see Figure 3-5).[19]

Situs solitus with *dextrocardia* (Figures 3-9, 3-10, and 3-24) is represented by normal positions of the stomach, liver, descending thoracic aorta, and right and left bronchi; by the major cardiac shadow to the right of midline; and by the right hemidiaphragm positioned lower than the left hemidiaphragm because the cardiac apex is on the right.[21,52] The position of the ascending aorta permits identification of a d-bulboventricular loop (Figure 3-24A).

Situs inversus with *levocardia* is represented by inverted positions of the stomach, liver, descending aorta, and bronchi; the major cardiac shadow is to the *left* of midline; and the *left* hemidiaphragm is lower than the right hemidiaphragm because the cardiac apex is on the *left* (Figures 3-11, 3-25, and 3-26). When the bulboventricular loop is discordant for *situs inversus* (d-loop), the ascending aorta forms a smooth contour at the left basal aspect of the heart (see Figure 3-25).

A *midline cardiac position*, mesocardia, is uncommon and is usually represented by *situs solitus* with a d-bulboventricular loop that stops at midline as it pivots

Left ventricular hypertrophy is manifested by tall R waves in leads V₁ and V₂, and *right* ventricular hypertrophy is manifested by tall R waves in leads V₅R and V₆R and deep Q waves in lead 1 (see Figures 3-18 and 3-20). In *situs inversus* with *levocardia* and l-loop, septal depolarization is right to left, so precordial Q waves are present at right thoracic sites and are absent on the left.

FIGURE 3-22 Electrocardiogram from a 26-year-old woman in *situs solitus* with dextrocardia, ventricular inversion, pulmonary stenosis, and a ventricular septal defect. The upright P wave in lead 1 indicates normal atrial situs. Q waves in *right* precordial leads and *absent* Q waves in *left* precordial leads indicate the reversed septal depolarization of ventricular inversion.

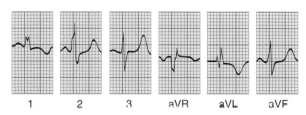

1   2   3   aVR   aVL   aVF

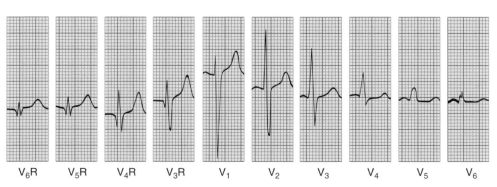

V₆R   V₅R   V₄R   V₃R   V₁   V₂   V₃   V₄   V₅   V₆

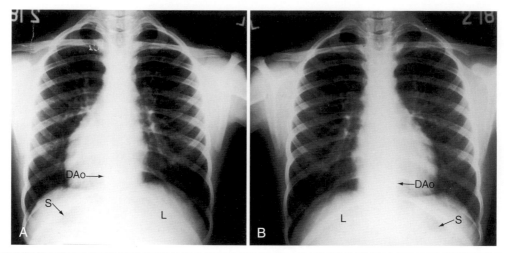

FIGURE 3-23 X-rays from an 11-year-old girl in *situs inversus* with dextrocardia and no associated congenital heart disease (see Figure 3-17). **A,** The L in the upper right corner of the film indicates that the x-ray is viewed properly. The stomach (S) and liver (L) are inverted. **B,** When the x-ray is reversed, it normalizes except for the L designation. (DAo = descending aorta.)

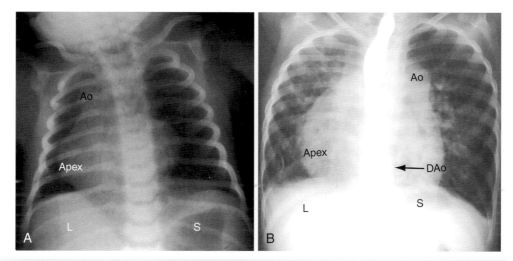

FIGURE 3-24 A, X-ray from a 3-week-old female in *situs solitus* with dextrocardia, d–bulboventricular loop, and a ventricular septal defect with pulmonary atresia. The liver (L) and stomach (S) are in normal positions, but the heart (Apex) is on the *right*, so the right hemidiaphragm is lower than the left hemidiaphragm. The ascending aorta (Ao) is concordant with a d-bulboventricular loop and is relatively prominent because of pulmonary atresia. **B,** X-ray from a 4-year-old acyanotic boy in *situs solitus* with dextrocardia, an l-bulboventricular loop, and ventricular and atrial septal defects. The liver, stomach, and descending aorta (DAo) are in normal positions, but the base to apex axis points to the right and the ascending aorta (Ao) forms a prominent leftward shadow appropriate for an l-loop.

from right to left (see Figure 3-12). A hump-shaped contour of the right cardiac border is to the result of superimposition of right ventricular and right atrial shadows (see Figure 3-12B).

Echocardiogram

Echocardiography with color flow imaging lends itself to systematic segmental analysis of visceroatrial situs, atrioventricular connections, ventricular locations, and the spatial relationships and ventricular alignments of the great arteries.[53,54] Atrial morphology and atrial situs are established with identification of the right atrial appendage with its broad junction and the left atrial appendage with its narrow junction. However, atrial morphology and situs are easier to infer from the abdominal echocardiogram. The normal *situs solitus with left thoracic heart* is represented by an aorta on the *left* side of the spinal column and an inferior cava on the *right* side of the spinal column (Figure 3-27). The morphologic right atrium resides on the same side as the inferior vena cava (atrial situs solitus). The inferior vena cava and aorta are distinguished from each other with color flow imaging because the aorta pulsates. The liver is on the right and the stomach on the left—normal positions (see Figure 3-27). Hepatic venous connections to the

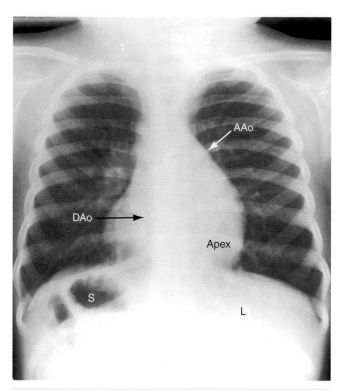

FIGURE 3-25 X-ray from a 4-year-old boy in *situs inversus* with a left thoracic heart and discordant d-bulboventricular loop. The stomach (S), liver (I), and descending aorta (DAo) are in inverted positions, but the major cardiac shadow is to the left of midline. The smooth leftward silhouette of the *ascending* aorta (AAo) indicates a d-bulboventricular loop in *situs inversus* (ventricular inversion).

inferior vena cava can be identified as can the course of the inferior vena cava to the right-sided morphologic right atrium.

Situs inversus with *dextrocardia* is the reverse (mirror image) of the normal arrangements.[53,54] The short-axis view recognizes the left atrial appendage with its narrow junction to the right of the aorta and recognizes the right atrial appendage with its broad junction to the left of the aorta. The abdominal echocardiogram identifies the aorta to the right of the spinal column and identifies the inferior vena cava to the left of the spinal column (Figure 3-28A and Video 3-1). Color flow imaging refines identification of the aorta and inferior vena cava (Figures 3-28B and 3-28C). The echocardiogram is then used to determine hepatic venous connections to the inferior vena cava and determine the course of the left-sided inferior vena cava to the left-sided morphologic right atrium.[54] *Situs solitus* with *dextrocardia* has echocardiographic features of normal atrial situs. *Situs inversus* with *levocardia* has the echocardiographic features of atrial situs inversus. Once atrial situs is established, echocardiography focuses on the atrioventricular junction, ventricular morphology, ventricular location, and ventricular/great arterial connections.

Summary

The three basic cardiac malpositions in the presence of right/left asymmetry are *situs inversus* with *dextrocardia*, *situs solitus* with *dextrocardia*, and *situs inversus* with *levocardia*. *Situs inversus* with *dextrocardia* is characterized by a right thoracic heart, a right-sided stomach, a left-sided liver, a left-sided morphologic right bronchus and trilobed lung, a right-sided morphologic left bronchus and bilobed lung, and inverted positions of the atria. *Situs inversus* with *dextrocardia* (mirror image) is likely to be

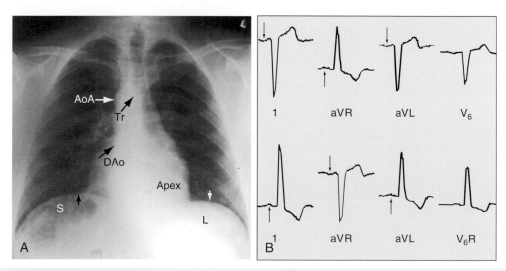

FIGURE 3-26 **A,** X-ray from a 35-year-old man in *situs inversus* with a left thoracic heart and ventricular inversion. The stomach (S) is on the right, the liver (L) is on the *left,* a right aortic arch (AoA) indents the right side of the trachea (Tr), and the aorta descends on the *right* (DAo = descending aorta), appropriate positions for *situs inversus*. The hemidiaphragm is lower on the side of the cardiac apex *(left)*. **B,** Limb leads and precordial lead V₆. The P wave is inverted in leads 1 and aVL and upright in lead aVR, appropriate for atrial *situs inversus*. Reversed limb leads together with precordial lead V₆R. The P wave is now upright in leads 1 and aVL and inverted in lead aVR. The Q wave in lead V₆ and the absent Q wave in lead V₆R indicate the reversed septal depolarization of ventricular inversion.

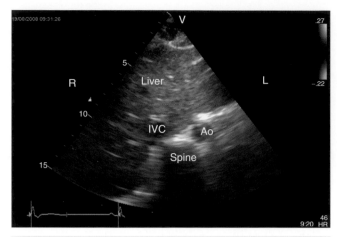

FIGURE 3-27 Abdominal echocardiogram from a healthy 5-year-old boy in *situs solitus*. The liver and inferior vena cava (IVC) are on the *right*, and descending aorta (Ao) are on the *left*. L = left; R= right; Spine = spinal column.

discovered incidentally on a routine chest x-ray, especially when the heart is structurally normal, as is usually the case. On physical examination, gastric tympany and cardiac dullness are on the right, hepatic dullness is on the left, and heart sounds are louder on the right side of the chest. The x-ray confirms the stomach bubble on the right, the liver on the left, and the cardiac silhouette to the right of midline. The electrocardiogram shows an inverted P wave, negative QRS complex and inverted T wave in lead 1, reversal of the QRS pattern in lead aVR and lead aVL, and reversal of corresponding right and left precordial leads. Echocardiography visualizes the inferior vena cava and the liver to the left of the spine and the stomach and descending aorta to the right of the spine.

Situs solitus with *dextrocardia* is characterized by a right thoracic heart with normal locations of the stomach, liver, bronchi, lungs and atria. The malposition usually comes to light because of coexisting congenital heart disease. Gastric tympany is on the left and hepatic dullness is on the right (normal), but cardiac dullness is on the *right* and heart sounds are louder in the right anterior chest (dextrocardia). The x-ray confirms normal positions of the stomach and liver, with the cardiac silhouette to the right of midline and the right hemidiaphragm lower than the left hemidiaphragm. The electrocardiogram shows an upright P wave in lead 1 with normal P wave patterns in leads aVR and aVL (atrial situs solitus), but the major precordial QRS voltage lies in the right hemithorax. Echocardiography visualizes normal positions of the liver and inferior vena cava to the right of the spine and normal positions of the stomach and aorta to the left of the spine.

Situs inversus with *levocardia* is characterized by reversed locations of the stomach, liver, bronchi, lungs and atria, with the heart to the left of midline. The malposition comes to attention because of invariably coexisting congenital heart disease. Gastric tympany is on the right, hepatic and cardiac dullness are on the left, and heart sounds are louder in the left hemithorax. The

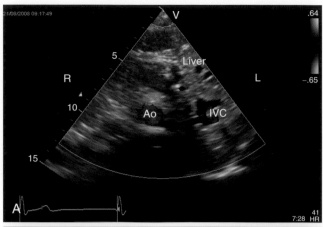

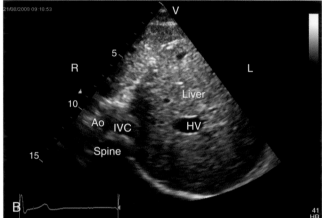

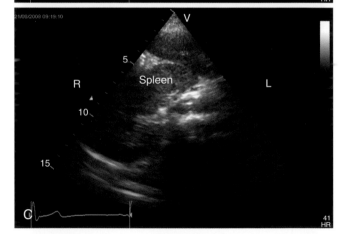

FIGURE 3-28 **A,** Abdominal echocardiogram from a 4-year-old boy *situs inversus*. The descending aorta (Ao) is on the *right*, and the liver and inferior vena cava (IVC) are on the *left* (Video 3-1). **B** and **C,** Abdominal echocardiogram from a 12-year-old boy with *situs inversus* and dextrocardia. The liver (HV = hepatic vein) is on the *left*, and the spleen is on the *right*. The Ao lies on the right side of the spine, and the IVC lies on the left of the spine.

x-ray confirms the heart to the left of midline, the stomach on the right, the liver on the left, and the left hemidiaphragm lower than the right hemidiaphragm. The electrocardiogram shows inverted P waves in lead 1 and lead aVL and an upright P wave in lead aVR (atrial situs inversus). The major precordial QRS voltage resides to the left of midline. Echocardiography identifies the liver and inferior vena cava to the left of the spine and the stomach and descending aorta to the right of the spine (inverted).

VISCERAL HETEROTAXY

Visceral heterotaxy[18,55,56] occurs in 0.8% of cases of congenital heart disease.[3] Isolated congenital asplenia in otherwise healthy individuals is rare. Right and left bronchi are normally asymmetric (Figures 3-29A and 3-30A); the right lung is trilobed, the left lung is bilobed, and the right and left atrial appendages are morphologically distinctive. The spleen is the only organ that is normally left-sided from its inception because it develops in the left side of the dorsal mesogastrium.[57] Unpaired structures such as the liver, spleen, and stomach are normally confined to either the right or left upper quadrant of the abdomen.

The two bronchi can be morphologically right or morphologically left (Figures 3-29 and 3-30B), the two lungs can be bilaterally trilobed or bilaterally bilobed (Figure 3-29B), and the two atrial appendages can exhibit right or left morphologic features. A relationship exists, albeit imperfect, between *right isomerism* and *asplenia* and *left isomerism* and *polysplenia*.[58] In right isomerism (asplenia) and left isomerism (polysplenia), the liver is typically transverse (bilaterally symmetric; Figures 3-31 and 3-32) and the superior vena cavae are typically bilateral (Figure 3-33). There is strong but not invariable concordance between a morphologic *right* bronchus (see Figures 3-30A), a morphologic *right* atrial appendage, and a trilobed morphologic *right* lung (see Figure 3-29B).[58] There is similar strong but not invariable concordance between a morphologic *left* bronchus (see Figure 3-30A), a morphologic *left* atrial appendage, and a bilobed morphologic *left* lung.[58] Accordingly, and with few exceptions,[58] *bilaterally symmetric* morphologic *right* bronchi (see Figures 3-29 and 3-30B) are coupled with bilateral morphologic right atrial appendages and with bilateral trilobed right lungs (see Figure 3-29B), and *bilaterally symmetric* morphologic *left* bronchi (see Figures 3-29A and 30A) are coupled with bilateral morphologic left atrial appendages and with bilateral

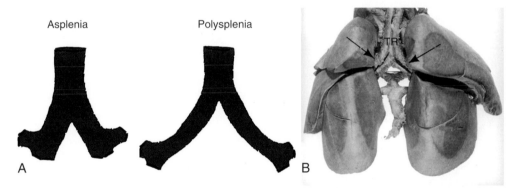

FIGURE 3-29 A, Schematic illustrations of bilateral morphologic *right* bronchi that are features of right isomerism, and bilateral morphologic *left* bronchi that are features of left isomerism. **B,** Gross specimen from an asplenic male neonate with bilateral morphologic right bronchi *(arrows)* and right isomerism. (TR = trachea.)

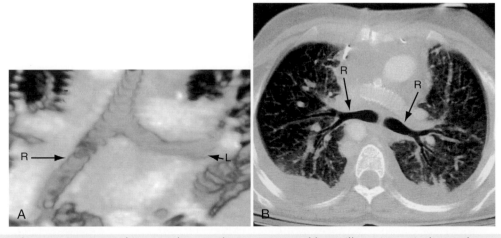

FIGURE 3-30 A, Thoracic computerized tomographic scan from an 18-year-old man illustrating typical normal asymmetric morphologic right (R) and left (L) bronchi. **B,** Magnetic resonance image illustrating symmetric morphologic right bronchi (R and R) in a 4-year-old girl with right isomerism.

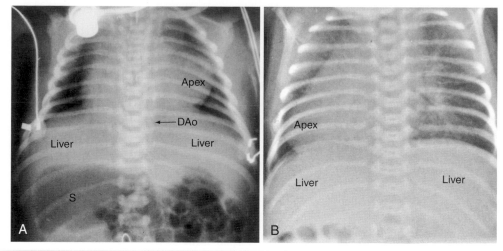

FIGURE 3-31 **A,** X-ray from an asplenic male neonate with right isomerism. The liver is transverse, the stomach (S) is on the right, and the heart is midline, but the base to apex axis points to the left. **B,** X-ray from an asplenic male neonate with right isomerism. The liver is transverse, the base to apex axis points to the right, and heart is to the right of midline. The ground-glass appearance of the lungs was caused by total anomalous pulmonary venous connection with obstruction.

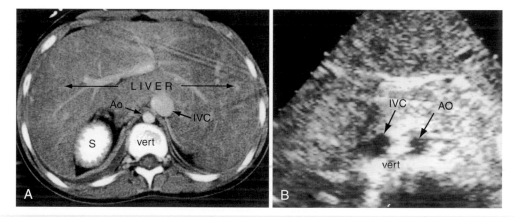

FIGURE 3-32 **A,** Abdominal magnetic resonance image from a 5-year-old boy with left isomerism. The liver is transverse. The aorta (Ao) lies directly anterior to the vertebral column (vert), the inferior vena cava (IVC) is leftward, and the stomach (S) is on the right. **B,** Abdominal echocardiogram from an asplenic female neonate with right isomerism. The inferior vena cava (IVC) and aorta (Ao) are both anterior to the vertebral column (vert).

bilobed left lungs. In about 15% of cases, splenic tissue does not coincide with the type of isomerism; and in about 5% of necropsy cases, a normal-sized spleen is located in the *right* upper quadrant. Rarely, bronchial morphology is not concordant with atrial morphology.[58,59]

Asplenia can be diagnosed with ultrasound or computed tomographic scan and has been diagnosed with fetal ultrasound scan.[60] A simple and readily accessible method for identification of asplenia is the presence of Howell-Jolly bodies in peripheral blood smears (Figure 3-34),[61] although Howell-Jolly bodies are occasionally found in healthy infants during the first week of life.[46,62] *Pitted* red cells are also evidence of asplenia, but visualization of the pits requires examination of wet preparations with a special optical system. A *wandering spleen* is highly mobile and may be located anywhere in the abdomen or pelvis. Oversight has been mistaken for absent spleen.[59,63] What is important in a *clinical*

setting is not the presence, absence, or multiplicity of the spleen, but the relatively consistent relationships that exist between the type of isomerism and the type of congenital heart disease.[59] It is this relationship that forms the basis of the following sections.

Visceral Heterotaxy with Right Isomerism

Right isomerism as characterized in Box 3-1 is accompanied by the congenital cardiovascular malformations listed in Box 3-2. The heart is likely to reside to the left of midline.[64,65] The liver is transverse (Figures 3-31 and 3-35). The superior vena cavae are bilateral,[66] hence the tendency for bilateral sinus nodes.[42,67] Exceptionally, one vena cava is partially or completely atretic.[00] Bilateral morphologic right bronchi (see Figures 3-29 and 3-30)

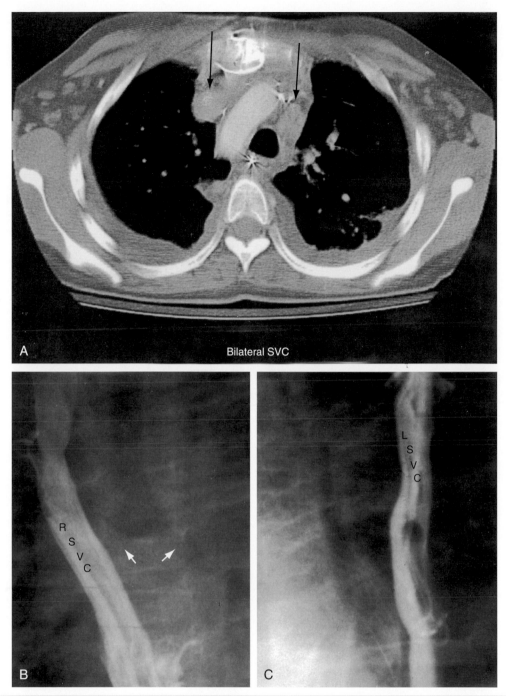

FIGURE 3-33 A, Magnetic resonance image from a 4-month-old female with left isomerism and bilateral superior vena cavae *(vertical arrows).* **B,** Angiographic visualization of the right superior vena cava (RSVC) and, **C,** of the left superior vena cava (LSVC). *Paired arrows* in **B** point to bilaterally symmetric morphologic left bronchi.

are closely coupled with bilateral morphologic right atrial appendages and bilateral trilobed lungs (see Figure 3-29B).[59,68] Ventricular/great arterial connections are usually discordant.[64] Total anomalous pulmonary venous connection is a common arrangement.[57,59,62,66,67] The ductus arteriosus may be bilateral.[69] Intracardiac malformations approximate a bilocular heart (see Figure 3-35), namely, common atrium, common atrioventricular valve, functionally single ventricle (hypoplastic right or left

ventricle) or anatomically single ventricle, and severe pulmonary stenosis or atresia.[59,62,64,67]

Extracardiac malformations have focused chiefly on the spleen, the largest lymphoid organ in the body. Because of the spleen's manifold immunologic functions, *asplenia* is accompanied by recurrent, serious, and even life-threatening infections.[70] Gastrointestinal abnormalities are the rule. Biliary atresia[71] and midline defects such as tracheoesophageal fistula are prevalent,[58] but the most

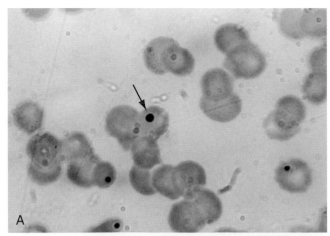

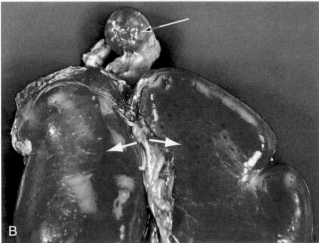

FIGURE 3-34 **A,** Peripheral blood smear in right isomerism with asplenia showing Howell-Jolly bodies *(arrow).* **B,** A normally formed sectioned spleen *(paired arrows)* with a splenule *(single arrow).*

BOX 3-1 **RIGHT ISOMERISM**

Bilateral superior vena cavae
Bilateral sinoatrial nodes
Paired atrioventricular nodes
Bilateral morphologic right atria (appendages)
Bilateral morphologic right bronchi
Bilateral morphologic right lungs
Dextrocardia or levocardia
Asplenia
Transverse liver
Right-sided or left-sided stomach

common gastrointestinal disorder is intestinal malrotation that predisposes to volvulus.[58,64] Midline defects also include central nervous system (meningomyelocele, cerebellar agenesis, encephalocele), craniofacial (cleft lip and palate), genitourinary (horseshoe kidney), and musculoskeletal (kyphoscoliosis, pectus deformity) defects.[58,64]

BOX 3-2 **RIGHT ISOMERISM**

Congenital Cardiac Malformations
Common atrium
Common atrioventricular valve
Morphologic or functional single ventricle
Pulmonary stenosis or atresia
Total anomalous pulmonary venous connection
Absent coronary sinus

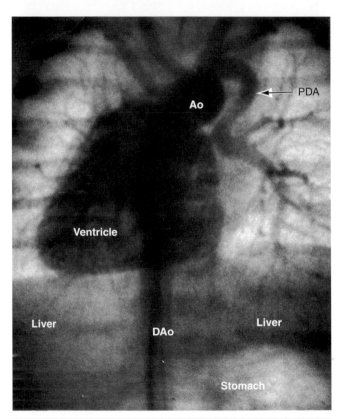

FIGURE 3-35 Angiocardiogram from an asplenic male neonate with right isomerism. The liver is transverse, and the stomach and descending aorta (DAo) are on the same side. The heart was right-sided with single ventricle and pulmonary atresia. (Ao = dilated aorta.)

History

The gender distribution of visceral heterotaxy with right isomerism is approximately equal[65] or with male predominance.[57,58,62] Asplenia has been reported in siblings and in families.[62,72] Cyanosis is often evident in the first 24 hours.[64] Survival is determined chiefly by coexisting congenital heart disease (see Box 3-2), but extracardiac anomalies (see previous discussion) weigh heavily in determination of morbidity and mortality. Most deaths are within the first few months of life, with only sporadic survivals after the first year[57,62,73] and a single remarkable survival to age 21 years.[74] Because asplenia increases the risk of bacterial infection and septicemia,[70] the clinical presentation may be characterized by high fever, vomiting, hypotension, coma, and death shortly after the onset of symptoms.

Physical Appearance

Infants with visceral heterotaxy and right isomerism are usually born at term, are normally formed, and have normal birth weights.[62] Neonatal cyanosis is invariable (see previous discussion) and conspicuous.

Palpation and Percussion

Palpation of a transverse liver edge crossing the upper abdomen (see Figure 3-35) is presumptive evidence of visceral heterotaxy. Percussion is likely to reveal a left rather than a right thoracic heart.[57,64,65] The location of the stomach is variable (see subsequent discussion).

Electrocardiogram

The sinus node is normally at the junction of a morphologic right atrium and a right superior vena cava. In right isomerism, paired sinus nodes are seen because each of the bilateral morphologic right atria is equipped with a junction to each of the bilateral superior vena cavae.[67,73,75,76] The P wave axis is usually normal, however, which indicates that the *right* sinus node is the dominant atrial pacemaker.[75] AP wave axis that is directed inferior and to the *right* implies that atrial depolarization is from the *left* sinus node. The conduction system is also equipped with two atrioventricular nodes that are connected by a sling of conducting tissue.[77] Supraventricular tachycardia has been attributed to reentry between the paired atrioventricular nodes.[76] Atrioventricular block is rare in contrast to left isomerism.[65,73]

X-Ray

The x-ray is especially valuable when the upper abdomen is included (see Figure 3-31). A transverse liver (see Figure 3-32A) implies visceral heterotaxy but not its type. In right isomerism, the position of the stomach is variable (right, left, or occasionally central; see Figures 3-31 and 3-34),[57] and the heart can be either to the right or left of midline (see Figure 3-31). Once visceral heterotaxy is suspected because of a transverse liver, bilateral symmetry (isomerism) is confirmed by bilaterally symmetric bronchi (see Figure 3-5A).[19,65] The next step is determination of whether the symmetric bronchi are morphologic right or morphologic left. Overpenetrated films or tomographic scans serve to make this distinction (see Figures 3-5B,C and 3-30).

Echocardiogram

Echocardiography can be used to identify morphologic right and morphologic left atrial appendages with their respective broad and narrow junctions. Abdominal imaging of the liver, aorta, inferior vena cava, and hepatic veins provides a reliable basis for the diagnosis of visceral heterotaxy.[53,54,65,78] The liver is transverse, and the inferior vena cava and aorta are anterior to or on the same side of the spinal column (Figures 3-32 and 3-36). Hepatic veins drain into the inferior vena cava, which joins the right-sided atrium. Imaging of the upper quadrants fails in identification of a spleen. Visceral heterotaxy has been diagnosed with fetal echocardiography.[79] The largely predictable coexisting cardiac malformations are as in Box 3-2.

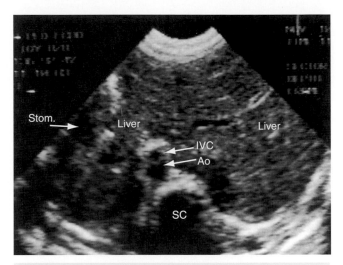

FIGURE 3-36 Echocardiogram from an asplenic male neonate with right isomerism. The liver is transverse, the stomach is on the right (Stom), and the aorta (Ao) and inferior vena cava (IVC) are on the same side of the spinal column (SC).

Summary

Visceral heterotaxy with right isomerism usually comes to light because of complex cyanotic congenital heart disease or because of the septicemia associated with asplenia. Howell-Jolly bodies on peripheral blood smears after the first week of life are evidence of asplenia. Palpation of a transabdominal liver edge in a cyanotic neonate or infant implies visceral heterotaxy but not its type. Sinoatrial nodes are bilateral, but the right sinus node is usually dominant so the P wave axis is normal. The x-ray confirms the transverse liver and may disclose bilaterally symmetric morphologic right bronchi. Abdominal echocardiography visualizes a transverse liver but no spleen. The aorta and inferior vena cava are anterior to or on the same side of the spinal column, and the inferior vena cava joins the right-sided atrium after receiving the hepatic veins.

Visceral Heterotaxy with Left Isomerism

Left isomerism as characterized in Box 3-3 is associated with the cardiovascular anomalies represented in Box 3-4. *Polysplenia* is a common but not invariable feature of left isomerism.[59,65,80,81] Matthew Baillie[2] wrote, "There were three spleens, nearly of the size of

BOX 3-3 **LEFT ISOMERISM**
Bilateral superior vena cavae
Bilateral morphologic left atria (appendages)
Absent or atretic sinoatrial node
Bilateral morphologic left bronchi
Bilateral morphologic left lungs
Transverse liver
Polysplenia
Stomach usually right-sided

a pullet's egg, found adhering to the larger spleen by short adhesions, besides two other still smaller spleens which were involved in the epiploon at the great end of the stomach." Baillie's *larger spleen* was accompanied by additional spleens of different size and was an example of a normally formed spleen with *accessory spleens*. Accessory spleens or splenules are present in about 10% of the general population and are usually located in the vicinity of a normally formed spleen (see Figure 3-34B) but may reside elsewhere in the abdomen.[82] Two well-formed spleens may be accompanied by one or more splenules.[57] Because splenic tissue develops in the dorsal mesogastrium, accessory spleens tend to be located along the greater curvature of the stomach.[57] Normal single spleens are occasionally bilobed, trilobed, or multilobed.[73,81] *Polysplenia* is characterized by a cluster of multiple splenules that collectively approximates the mass of one normal spleen.[73,81]

Left isomerism—bilateral left-sidedness—is characterized by bilateral morphologic left bronchi, bilateral morphologic left atria,[83] and bilateral morphologic bilobed left lungs. The superior vena cavae are bilateral (see Figure 3-33) and attach to morphologic left atria.[68,84] Paired morphologic left atria seemingly preclude the existence of an atrial septum, but attention has been called to a divided left-sided atrium, an intact atrial septum, and a sinus venosus atrial septal defect.[85] The answer may lie in the nature of atrial isomerism in which the appendages are morphologically the same, but bilateral similarity (isomerism) may not include the rest of the atria.[58]

However, it is *interruption of the inferior vena cava* with *azygous continuation* that is distinctive and diagnostically important.[57,59,62,81,86] The suprarenal segment of the inferior cava is absent, and the infrarenal segment continues as the azygos or hemiazygous vein (Figure 3-37).[59] Rarely, isolated inferior caval interruption with azygos continuation occurs without visceral heterotaxy, without isomerism, with normal hearts, and with a normal single spleen (Figure 3-38).

Anomalous pulmonary venous connection in left isomerism is partial, ventriculo/great arterial alignments are concordant, and the pulmonary valve is occasionally stenotic but rarely atretic. The atrioventricular orifices are guarded by two valves or a common valve with an atrioventricular septal defect or a separate inlet ventricular septal defect.[57,67,73,81] Two normally formed noninverted ventricles are present, as is a moderate increase in incidence of left ventricular outflow obstruction.[87]

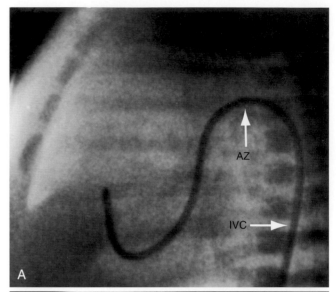

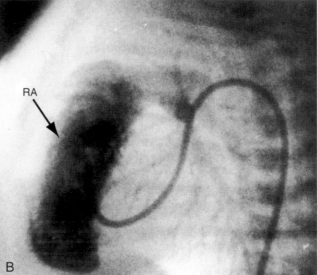

FIGURE 3-37 Angiocardiograms (anteroposterior projection) from a 5-month-old polysplenic female with left isomerism, inferior vena caval interruption with azygos continuation, and a right thoracic heart. **A,** The course of the catheter is through the interrupted inferior vena cava (IVC) into the azygos vein (AZ) and into the right atrium where the tip lies. **B,** Contrast material visualized in the right atrium (RA).

The most prevalent *extracardiac anomalies* in left isomerism are gastrointestinal and, apart from the ubiquitous transverse liver, include intestinal malrotation,[58,85] biliary atresia,[58,71,85] esophageal atresia, and congenital short pancreas.[88] Nongastrointestinal extracardiac anomalies are analogous to those with right isomerism, namely, musculoskeletal, neurologic, and craniofacial.[58,85]

History

Visceral heterotaxy with *left isomerism* tends to occur in females,[83] and *right isomerism* tends to occur in males.[83] The clinical course (morbidity and mortality) of left isomerism is determined by coexisting cardiovascular

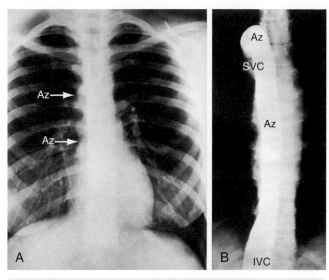

FIGURE 3-38 A, X-ray from a healthy 28-year-old woman with isolated inferior vena caval interruption and azygos continuation to a right superior vena cava. The spleen was present and single. The azygos vein (Az) ascends along the right vertebral border, forming a knuckle as it courses anterior to join the right superior cava. **B,** Inferior vena cavagram (IVC) showing the course of azygos continuation to the right superior vena cava (SVC).

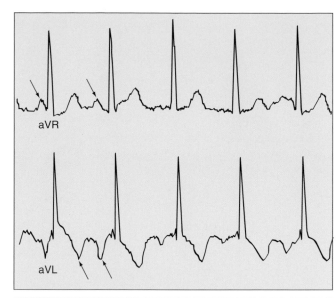

FIGURE 3-39 Leads aVR and aVL from a 16-month-old male with left isomerism, bilateral superior vena cavae, and absent sinus node. The upright P wave in lead aVR (arrows) and the inverted P wave in lead aVL (arrows) reflect an ectopic atrial focus.

malformations (see Box 3-4) and by extracardiac anomalies but not by the septicemia of asplenia (see previous discussion). An investigation of fetal bradycardia from complete heart block serves to identify intrauterine left isomerism.[89,90] Most patients present as neonates with congestive heart failure or cyanosis,[73,81,85] but an important minority present with symptoms related to an extracardiac malformation, especially biliary atresia.[85] Approximately 20% die as neonates, and 50% survive adolescence.[85] Adult survival is uncommon but not unknown.[62,81,91,92] Reports exist of familial polysplenia and familial asplenia,[27,62,93] and attention has been called to sibling pairs[94] in which one had polysplenia and the other had asplenia.[95]

Physical Appearance

Infants are normally formed and usually acyanotic. Abnormal physical appearance is likely to reflect the extracardiac anomalies, such as biliary atresia (jaundice), myelomeningocele, or cleft lip/palate.[85]

Percussion and Palpation

Palpation of a *transverse liver* in an *acyanotic* infant is presumptive evidence of *left* isomerism.

Electrocardiogram

The normal sinus node is a *right*-sided structure that arises at the junction of a right superior vena cava and a morphologic right atrium (see previous discussion). In left isomerism, a sinus node is absent or hypoplastic because vena caval connection is to a morphologic *left*

atrium. The atrial pacemaker is therefore ectopic (Figure 3-39), located in the atrial wall or near the ostium of a coronary sinus,[67,75,86,96] so the P wave axis is abnormal.[57,62,73,75,97] The ectopic pacemaker may shift from one site to another[85,96] or may fire slowly (ectopic atrial bradycardia).[85] Atrial fibrillation or atrial flutter occasionally develops.[85,98] Complete atrioventricular block occurs in approximately one in five cases of left isomerism and can be present in the fetus and neonate (see previous discussion)[77] with a significant impact on morbidity and mortality.[57,62,97] Conduction is interrupted at the level of the penetrating bundle, producing nodoventricular discontinuity and a narrow QRS complex.[77]

X-Ray

A transverse liver is an important radiologic sign of visceral heterotaxy (see previous discussion; Figure 3-40), and when accompanied by symmetric morphologic left bronchi (see Figure 3-29A), the diagnosis of heterotaxy with left isomerism is secure.[57,62,81] The heart is usually left-sided,[62,81] and the stomach tends to be on the side opposite the descending aorta (see Figure 3-40). A distinctive radiologic feature of left isomerism is *inferior vena caval interruption with azygous continuation* that is best seen in the frontal projection (see Figure 3-38).[62,85] Absence of an inferior vena caval shadow in the lateral projection is not a reliable sign of interruption because azygos continuation may create the impression of a normal uninterrupted inferior cava.[86,99] The lung fields usually show increased pulmonary blood flow because left-to-right shunts occur without obstruction to right ventricular outflow. A transverse liver is a feature of conjoined twins without heterotaxy (Figure 3-41).

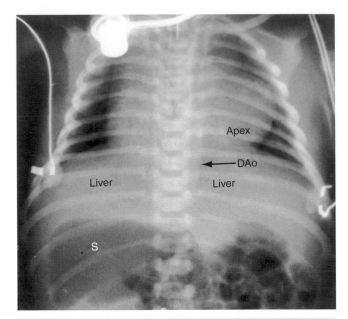

FIGURE 3-40 X-ray from a polysplenic female neonate with left isomerism. The liver is transverse, the apex is on the left, the stomach (S) is on the right, and the descending aorta (DAo) is on the left. This opposite-sided arrangement tends to occur in left isomerism.

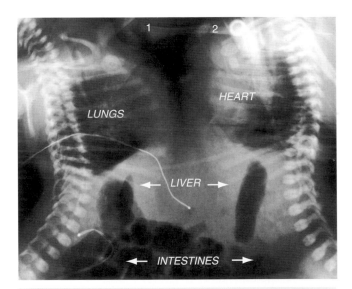

FIGURE 3-41 X-ray of conjoined twins with a single shared liver and shared intestines. Twin 1 had adequate lungs but an inadequate cardiac mass. Twin 2 had hypoplastic lungs but an adequate cardiac mass with a ventricular septal defect and pulmonary atresia.

Echocardiogram

The echocardiogram confirms a transverse liver (Figure 3-42).[53,54] The aorta and inferior vena cava lie anterior to or on the same side of the spinal column (Figures 3-42 and 3-43). When inferior vena caval interruption with azygous continuation is seen, the hepatic veins connect directly to the atria and do not join the inferior cava (Figure 3-43B). Echocardiographic diagnosis can be made in the fetus.[79]

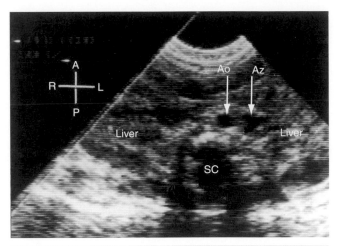

FIGURE 3-42 Abdominal echocardiogram from a polysplenic female infant with left isomerism. The liver is transverse. The aorta (Ao) and azygos vein (Az) are on the same side of the spinal column (SC). The inferior vena cava was interrupted with azygous continuation. (A = anterior; L = left; P = posterior; R = right.)

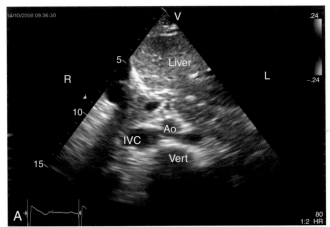

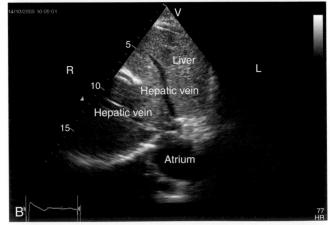

FIGURE 3-43 Abdominal echocardiogram from a polysplenic neonate with isomerism. **A,** The liver is transverse. The aorta (Ao) and the inferior vena cava (IVC) are on the same side of the vertebral column (Vert). **B,** Hepatic veins connect directly to an atrium because of inferior caval interruption with azygos continuation.

Summary

Visceral heterotaxy with left isomerism presents in an acyanotic infant with congestive heart failure because a left-to-right shunt exists without obstruction to right ventricular outflow. Physical examination discloses a transverse liver and a left-sided heart. The x-ray confirms the transverse liver and reveals bilaterally symmetric morphologic left bronchi. A distinctive radiologic feature is inferior vena caval interruption with azygous continuation. The electrocardiogram discloses the abnormal P wave axis of an ectopic atrial pacemaker because the sinus node is absent. A diagnostically useful electrocardiographic combination is an abnormal P wave axis, complete atrioventricular block, and narrow QRS complexes. Abdominal echocardiography is used to confirm the transverse liver and identify an inferior vena cava and aorta anterior to or on the same side of the spinal column. When the inferior cava is interrupted, hepatic veins do not join the caval vein but instead connect to the atria.

REFERENCES

1. Brown JW. *Congenital heart disease.* London: Staples Press; 1950.
2. Baillie M. Of a remarkable transposition of the viscera. *Philos Trans R Soc Lond B Biol Sci.* 1785–1790;16:483.
3. Fyler DC, Buckley LP, Hellenbrand WE. Report of the New England Regional Infant Cardiac Program. *Pediatrics.* 1980;65:375–461.
4. Khoury MJ, Cordero JF, Rasmussen S. Ectopia cordis, midline defects and chromosome abnormalities: an epidemiologic perspective. *Am J Med Genet.* 1988;30:811–817.
5. Paltauf R. Dextrocardie und Dextroversio Cardis. *Wien Klin Wochenschr.* 1901;14:1032.
6. Mandelstam ME, Reinberg SA. Die Dextrokardie. *Ergeb Med Kinderheilkd.* 1928;34:154.
7. Lichtman SS. Isolated congenital dextrocardia: report of two cases with unusual electrocardiographic findings; anatomic, clinical, roentgenologic and electrocardiographic studies of the cases reported in the literature. *Arch Intern Med.* 1931;48:866–903.
8. De La Cruz MV, Da Rocha JP. An ontogenetic theory for the explanation of congenital malformations involving the truncus and conus. *Am Heart J.* 1956;51:782–805.
9. Van Praagh R, Van Praagh S, Vlad P, Keith JD. Anatomic types of congenital dextrocardia: diagnostic and embryologic implications. *Am J Cardiol.* 1964;13:510–531.
10. Campbell M, Deuchar DC. Dextrocardia and isolated laevocardia. I. Isolated laevocardia. *Br Heart J.* 1965;27:69–82.
11. Campbell M, Deuchar DC. Dextrocardia and isolated laevocardia. II. Situs inversus and isolated dextrocardia. *Br Heart J.* 1966;28:472–487.
12. Campbell M, Reynolds G. The significance of the direction of the P wave in dextrocardia and isolated laevocardia. *Br Heart J.* 1952;14:481–488.
13. Elliott LP, Jue KL, Amplatz K. A roentgen classification of cardiac malpositions. *Invest Radiol.* 1966;1:17–28.
14. Yost HJ. The genetics of midline and cardiac laterality defects. *Curr Opin Cardiol.* 1998;13:185–189.
15. Casey B, Devoto M, Jones KL, Ballabio A. Mapping a gene for familial situs abnormalities to human chromosome Xq24-q27.1. *Nat Genet.* 1993;5:403–407.
16. Van Praagh R. Terminology of congenital heart disease. Glossary and commentary. *Circulation.* 1977;56:139–143.
17. Anderson RH, Macartney FJ, Shinebourne EA, Tynan M. Terminology. In: *Paediatric Cardiology.* Edinburgh: Churchill Livingstone; 1987:65.
18. Van Praagh R, Weinberg PM, Smith SD. Malpositions of the heart. In: Moss AJ, Adams FH, Emmanouilides GC, Riemenschneider TA, eds. *Heart disease in infants, children and adolescents.* 4th ed. Baltimore: Williams & Wilkins; 1989.
19. Van Mierop LH, Eisen S, Schiebler GL. The radiographic appearance of the tracheobronchial tree as an indicator of visceral situs. *Am J Cardiol.* 1970;26:432–435.
20. Stalsberg H. Development and ultrastructure of the embryonic heart. II. Mechanism of dextral looping of the embryonic heart. *Am J Cardiol.* 1970;25:265–271.
21. Reddy V, Sharma S, Cobanoglu A. What dictates the position of the diaphragm—the heart or the liver? A review of sixty-five cases. *J Thorac Cardiovasc Surg.* 1994;108:687–691.
22. Hastreiter AR, Rodriguez-Coronel A. Discordant situs of thoracic and abdominal viscera. *Am J Cardiol.* 1968;22:111–118.
23. Sacks LV, Rifkin IR. Mirror image arrangement of the abdominal organs with a left-sided morphologically normal heart. *Br Heart J.* 1987;58:534–536.
24. Douard R, Feldman A, Bargy F, Loric S, Delmas V. Anomalies of lateralization in man: a case of total situs inversus. *Surg Radiol Anat.* 2000;22:293–297.
25. Garg N, Agarwal BL, Modi N, Radhakrishnan S, Sinha N. Dextrocardia: an analysis of cardiac structures in 125 patients. *Int J Cardiol.* 2003;88:143–155; discussion 155–156.
26. Lev M, Liberthson RR, Golden JG, Eckner FA, Arcilla RA. The pathologic anatomy of mesocardia. *Am J Cardiol.* 1971;28:428–435.
27. Santoro G, Masiello P, Farina R, Baldi C, Di Leo L, Di Benedetto G. Isolated atrial inversion in situs inversus: a rare anatomic arrangement. *Ann Thorac Surg.* 1995;59:1019–1021.
28. Schiebler GL, Edwards JE, Burchell HB, Dushane JW, Ongley PA, Wood EH. Congenital corrected transposition of the great vessels: a study of 33 cases. *Pediatrics.* 1961;27(suppl 5):849–888.
29. Kennedy DN, O'craven KM, Ticho BS, Goldstein AM, Makris N, Henson JW. Structural and functional brain asymmetries in human situs inversus totalis. *Neurology.* 1999;53:1260–1265.
30. Nagaratnam N, Kotagama LS. Dextrocardia, situs inversus totalis and appendicular abscess. *Postgrad Med J.* 1957;33:287–288.
31. Kartagener M. Zur Pathogenese der Bronchiektasien; Bronchiektasien bei Situs Viscerum Inversus. *Beitr Klin Tuberk.* 1933;83:489.
32. Katz M, Benzier E, Nangeroni L, Sussman B. Kartagener's syndrome (situs inversus, bronchiectasis and chronic sinusitis). *N Engl J Med.* 1953;248:730–731.
33. Adams R, Churchill E. Situs inversus, sinusitis, bronchiectasis. *J Thorac Surg.* 1937;7:206.
34. Narayan D, Krishnan SN, Upender M, et al. Unusual inheritance of primary ciliary dyskinesia (Kartagener's syndrome). *J Med Genet.* 1994;31:493–496.
35. Abu-Musa A, Hannoun A, Khabbaz A, Devroey P. Failure of fertilization after intracytoplasmic sperm injection in a patient with Kartagener's syndrome and totally immotile spermatozoa: case report. *Hum Reprod.* 1999;14:2517–2518.
36. Gershoni-Baruch R, Gottfried E, Pery M, Sahin A, Etzioni A. Immotile cilia syndrome including polysplenia, situs inversus, and extrahepatic biliary atresia. *Am J Med Genet.* 1989;33:390–393.
37. Campbell M. The mode of inheritance in isolated laevocardia and dextrocardia and situs inversus. *Br Heart J.* 1963;25:803–813.
38. Fraser FC, Teebi AS, Walsh S, Pinsky L. Poland sequence with dextrocardia: which comes first? *Am J Med Genet.* 1997;73:194–196.
39. Gorgu M, Aslan G, Erdooan B, Karaca C, Akoz T. Goldenhar syndrome with situs inversus totalis. *Int J Oral Maxillofac Surg.* 1998;27:404.
40. Perloff JK. *Physical examination of the heart and circulation.* 4th ed. Shelton, Connecticut: People's Medical Publishing House; 2009.
41. Waller AD. On the electromotive charges connected with the beat of the mammalian heart and of the human heart in particular. *Philos Trans R Soc Lond B Biol Sci.* 1889;180:169–194.
42. Bharati S, Lev M. The course of the conduction system in dextrocardia. *Circulation.* 1978;57:163–171.
43. Edenbrandt L, Rittner R. Recognition of lead reversals in pediatric electrocardiograms. *Am J Cardiol.* 1998;82:1290–1292, A1210.
44. Blieden LC, Moller JH. Analysis of the P wave in congenital cardiac malformations associated with splenic anomalies. *Am Heart J.* 1973;85:439–444.
45. Momma K, Linde LM. Cardiac rhythms in dextrocardia. *Am J Cardiol.* 1970;25:420–427.
46. Rao PS. Dextrocardia: systematic approach to differential diagnosis. *Am Heart J.* 1981;102:389–403.
47. Mirowski M, Neill CA, Bahnson HT, Taussig HB. Negative P waves in lead I in dextroversion: differential diagnosis from mirror-image

dextrocardia, with a report of a successful closure of a ventricular septal defect in a patient with dextroversion associated with agenesis of the right lung. *Circulation.* 1962;26:413–420.

48. Frankl WS, Soloff LA. Left atrial rhythm. Analysis by intra-atrial electrocardiogram and the vectorcardiogram. *Am J Cardiol.* 1968; 22:645–656.

49. Mirowski M, Neill CA, Taussig HB. Left atrial ectopic rhythm in mirror-image dextrocardia and in normally placed malformed hearts: Report of twelve cases with" dome and dart" P waves. *Circulation.* 1963;27:864.

50. Harris BC, Shaver JA, Gray 3rd S, Kroetz FW, Leonard JJ. Left atrial rhythm. Experimental production in man. *Circulation.* 1968;37:1000–1014.

51. Maldjian PD, Saric M. Approach to dextrocardia in adults: review. *AJR Am J Roentgenol.* 2007;188:S39–S49; quiz S35–38.

52. Martinez E, Divekar A. Which diaphragm is lower and why? *Pediatr Cardiol.* 2007;28:243.

53. Huhta JC, Hagler DJ, Seward JB, Tajik AJ, Julsrud PR, Ritter DG. Two-dimensional echocardiographic assessment of dextrocardia: a segmental approach. *Am J Cardiol.* 1982;50:1351–1360.

54. Huhta JC, Smallhorn JF, Macartney FJ. Two dimensional echocardiographic diagnosis of situs. *Br Heart J.* 1982;48:97–108.

55. Jacobs JP, Anderson RH, Weinberg PM, et al. The nomenclature, definition and classification of cardiac structures in the setting of heterotaxy. *Cardiol Young.* 2007;17(suppl 2):1–28.

56. Van Praagh R, Van Praagh S. Atrial isomerism in the heterotaxy syndromes with asplenia, or polysplenia, or normally formed spleen: an erroneous concept. *Am J Cardiol.* 1990;66:1504–1506.

57. Van Mierop LHS, Gessner IH, Schiebler GL. Asplenia and polysplenia syndromes. *Birth Defects.* 1972;8:36.

58. Ticho BS, Goldstein AM, Van Praagh R. Extracardiac anomalies in the heterotaxy syndromes with focus on anomalies of midline-associated structures. *Am J Cardiol.* 2000;85:729–734.

59. Anderson C, Devine WA, Anderson RH, Debich DE, Zuberbuhler JR. Abnormalities of the spleen in relation to congenital malformations of the heart: a survey of necropsy findings in children. *Br Heart J.* 1990;63:122–128.

60. Chitayat D, Lao A, Wilson RD, Fagerstrom C, Hayden M. Prenatal diagnosis of asplenia/polysplenia syndrome. *Am J Obstet Gynecol.* 1988;158:1085–1087.

61. Corazza GR, Ginaldi L, Zoli G, et al. Howell-Jolly body counting as a measure of splenic function. A reassessment. *Clin Lab Haematol.* 1990;12:269–275.

62. Rose V, Izukawa T, Moes CA. Syndromes of asplenia and polysplenia. A review of cardiac and non-cardiac malformations in 60 cases withspecial reference to diagnosis and prognosis. *Br Heart J.* 1975; 37:840–852.

63. Abell I. Wandering spleen with torsion of the pedicle. *Ann Surg.* 1933;98:722–735.

64. Hashmi A, Abu-Sulaiman R, Mccrindle BW, Smallhorn JF, Williams WG, Freedom RM. Management and outcomes of right atrial isomerism: a 26-year experience. *J Am Coll Cardiol.* 1998; 31:1120–1126.

65. Sapire DW, Ho SY, Anderson RH, Rigby ML. Diagnosis and significance of atrial isomerism. *Am J Cardiol.* 1986;58:342–346.

66. Rubino M, Van Praagh S, Kadoba K, Pessotto R, Van Praagh R. Systemic and pulmonary venous connections in visceral heterotaxy with asplenia. Diagnostic and surgical considerations based on seventy-two autopsied cases. *J Thorac Cardiovasc Surg.* 1995; 110:641–650.

67. Macartney FJ, Zuberbuhler JR, Anderson RH. Morphological considerations pertaining to recognition of atrial isomerism. Consequences for sequential chamber localisation. *Br Heart J.* 1980;44: 657–667.

68. Uemura H, Ho SY, Devine WA, Anderson RH. Analysis of visceral heterotaxy according to splenic status, appendage morphology, or both. *Am J Cardiol.* 1995;76:846–849.

69. Formigari R, Vairo U, De Zorzi A, Santoro G, Marino B. Prevalence of bilateral patent ductus arteriosus in patients with pulmonic valve atresia and asplenia syndrome. *Am J Cardiol.* 1992;70:1219–1220.

70. Wang JK, Hsieh KH. Immunologic study of the asplenia syndrome. *Pediatr Infect Dis J.* 1991;10:819–822.

71. Herman TE. Special imaging casebook. Left-isomerism (polysplenia) with congenital atrioventricular block and biliary atresia. *J Perinatol.* 1999;19:155–157.

72. Eronen M, Kajantie E, Boldt T, Pitkanen O, Aittomaki K. Right atrial isomerism in four siblings. *Pediatr Cardiol.* 2004;25:141–144.

73. Stanger P, Rudolph AM, Edwards JE. Cardiac malpositions. An overview based on study of sixty-five necropsy specimens. *Circulation.* 1977;56:159–172.

74. Wolfe MW, Vacek JL, Kinard RE, Bailey CG. Prolonged and functional survival with the asplenia syndrome. *Am J Med.* 1986;81: 1089–1091.

75. Wren C, Macartney FJ, Deanfield JE. Cardiac rhythm in atrial isomerism. *Am J Cardiol.* 1987;59:1156–1158.

76. Wu MH, Wang JK, Lin JL, et al. Supraventricular tachycardia in patients with right atrial isomerism. *J Am Coll Cardiol.* 1998;32: 773–779.

77. Ho SY, Fagg N, Anderson RH, Cook A, Allan L. Disposition of the atrioventricular conduction tissues in the heart with isomerism of the atrial appendages: its relation to congenital complete heart block. *J Am Coll Cardiol.* 1992;20:904–910.

78. Arisawa J, Morimoto S, Ikezoe J, et al. Cross sectional echocardiographic anatomy of common atrioventricular valve in atrial isomerism. *Br Heart J.* 1989;62:291–297.

79. Atkinson DE, Drant S. Diagnosis of heterotaxy syndrome by fetal echocardiography. *Am J Cardiol.* 1998;82:1147–1149, A1110.

80. Merklin RJ. Cardiac lesions associated with visceral inversion. A study of 185 cases. *J Int Coll Surg.* 1964;41:597–606.

81. Peoples WM, Moller JH, Edwards JE. Polysplenia: a review of 146 cases. *Pediatr Cardiol.* 1983;4:129–137.

82. Dodds WJ, Taylor AJ, Erickson SJ, Stewart ET, Lawson TL. Radiologic imaging of splenic anomalies. *AJR Am J Roentgenol.* 1990;155: 805–810.

83. Pepes S, Zidere V, Allan LD. Prenatal diagnosis of left atrial isomerism. *Heart.* 2009;95:1974–1977.

84. Roguin N, Aydinalp A. Isomeric arrangement of the left atrial appendages and visceral heterotaxy. *Cardiol Young.* 2000;10:668.

85. Gilljam T, Mccrindle BW, Smallhorn JF, Williams WG, Freedom RM. Outcomes of left atrial isomerism over a 28-year period at a single institution. *J Am Coll Cardiol.* 2000;36:908–916.

86. Roguin N, Hammerman H, Korman S, Riss E. Angiography of azygos continuation of inferior vena cava in situs ambiguus with left isomerism (polysplenia syndrome). *Pediatr Radiol.* 1984;14: 109–112.

87. Van Praagh S, Geva T, Friedberg DZ, et al. Aortic outflow obstruction in visceral heterotaxy: a study based on twenty postmortem cases. *Am Heart J.* 1997;133:558–569.

88. Sener RN, Alper H. Polysplenia syndrome: a case associated with transhepatic portal vein, short pancreas, and left inferior vena cava with hemiazygous continuation. *Abdom Imaging.* 1994;19:64–66.

89. Phoon CK, Villegas MD, Ursell PC, Silverman NH. Left atrial isomerism detected in fetal life. *Am J Cardiol.* 1996;77: 1083–1088.

90. Schmidt KG, Ulmer HE, Silverman NH, Kleinman CS, Copel JA. Perinatal outcome of fetal complete atrioventricular block: a multicenter experience. *J Am Coll Cardiol.* 1991;17:1360–1366.

91. Gayer G, Apter S, Jonas T, et al. Polysplenia syndrome detected in adulthood: report of eight cases and review of the literature. *Abdom Imaging.* 1999;24:178–184.

92. Hojo Y, Kuroda T, Yamasawa M, et al. Polysplenia accompanied by major cardiovascular anomalies with prolonged survival. *Internal Medicine.* 1994;33:357–359.

93. De La Monte SM, Hutchins GM. Sisters with polysplenia. *Am J Med Genet.* 1985;21:171–176.

94. Thacker D, Gruber PJ, Weinberg PM, Cohen MS. Heterotaxy syndrome with mirror image anomalies in identical twins. *Congenit Heart Dis.* 2009;4:50–53.

95. Toriello HV, Kokx N, Higgins JV, Hofman R, Waterman DF. Sibs with the polyasplenia developmental field defect. *Am J Med Genet Suppl.* 1986;2:31–36.

96. Momma K, Takao A, Shibata T. Characteristics and natural history of abnormal atrial rhythms in left isomerism. *Am J Cardiol.* 1990; 65:231–236.

97. Garcia OL, Metha AV, Pickoff AS, et al. Left isomerism and complete atrioventricular block: a report of six cases. *Am J Cardiol.* 1981;48:1103–1107.

98. Wang TD, Tseng CD, Lee YT. Left isomerism in a middle-aged woman with early-onset atrial fibrillation. *Int J Cardiol.* 1997;58: 269–272.

99. Bartram U, Fischer G, Kramer HH. Congenitally interrupted inferior vena cava without other features of the heterotaxy syndrome: report of five cases and characterization of a rare entity. *Pediatr Dev Pathol.* 2008;11:266–273.

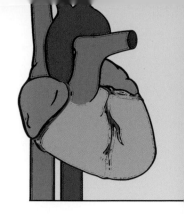

Chapter 4

Isolated Congenital Complete Heart Block

Congenital complete atrioventricular block was recognized in 1901 when Morquio[1] described familial recurrence with Stokes-Adams attacks and death in childhood. In 1908, van den Heuvel[2] published the electrocardiogram of a patient with complete heart block and syncopal episodes that dated from infancy. Thirteen years later, White and Eustis[3] described slow *fetal* heart rate; at birth, the electrocardiogram disclosed complete heart block.[3] Davis and Stecher[4] distinguished congenital from acquired complete heart block; shortly thereafter, Yater[5–7] established criteria for the clinical diagnosis of the congenital form. Currently, complete atrioventricular block is regarded as congenital when it is diagnosed in utero, at birth, or within the neonatal period.[8]

Complete heart block is characterized by a random relationship between atrial and ventricular activation. Atrial impulses are not conducted to the ventricles, which are depolarized in response to a subsidiary pacemaker.[9] The electrocardiogram is a simple but secure means of identifying complete heart block (Figures 4-1 and 4-2). *Atrioventricular dissociation* is a disorder of both conduction *and* impulse formation[9] and is not considered in this chapter.

Fetal echocardiography permits intrauterine diagnosis, and *isolated* complete heart block can be distinguished from cases with coexisting congenital heart disease, most commonly ventricular inversion (see Chapter 6) and left isomerism (see Chapter 3). The incidence rate of congenital high-degree heart block, either complete or with more than 50% of blocked atrial impulses, has been estimated at 1 in 2500 to 1 in 20,000 live births.[9–12] Block can be within the atrioventricular (AV) node or within the His bundle (or infra-Hisian), and the discontinuity in conduction can be anatomic or functional.[13,14] Narrow QRS complexes indicate that the subsidiary pacemaker is above the bifurcation of the His bundle,[9] but morphologic abnormalities have been identified at multiple levels.[7,13,15,16] The connection between atrial muscle and atrioventricular node is deficient or absent.[13,16] The node can be congenitally absent or defective[13,14,16,17] and separated from the His bundle,[18] which supports the view that the AV node and bundle of His originate as separate structures that normally are destined to join during early fetal development.[15] Disruption can be within the His bundle,[13,19] at the origins of the bundle branches, or in the right or left bundle branch.[16] Anatomic defects occasionally exist in the AV node itself or at the junction of AV node and atrial muscle.[15] The fetal sinoatrial and

atrioventricular nodes can calcify.[20] Nevertheless, spontaneous changes from complete to incomplete heart block[21,22] or even to sinus rhythm[23,24] indicate that interruption of the conduction pathways is not necessarily anatomic, complete, or permanent (Figure 4-3).

Myocardial contractile force is augmented by the slow heart rate, the long diastolic filling period, and the increased end-diastolic volume and fiber length,[9,25] so stroke volume increases and basal cardiac output is maintained.[26,27] An increase in cardiac output with exercise is chiefly rate dependent.[26] Submaximal isotonic exercise generally provokes an appropriate increase in ventricular rate and cardiac output, but higher workloads are accompanied by blunted hemodynamic and rate responses.[26] An increase in stroke volume and, to a lesser degree, an increase in arteriovenous oxygen difference partially compensate for the blunted rate response.[25] Despite compensatory mechanisms, oxygen consumption during submaximal exercise is significantly lower than in healthy age-matched and sex-matched control subjects.[25] A subset of patients with congenital complete heart block has development of dilated cardiomyopathy for which no definite cause has been found.[28]

An association between maternal lupus erythematosus and congenital complete heart block was reported in 1966 and confirmed a decade later.[9,29–32] Congenital heart block is a passively transferred autoimmune disease that affects the offspring of mothers with Ro/SSA autoantibodies.[33] Sinus node disease may occur in children with prenatal exposure to anti-Ro or anti-La antibodies.[34] Complete heart block in utero or at birth is strongly associated with the neonatal lupus syndrome and with maternal antibodies to 48-kD SSB/La, 52-kD SSA/Ro, and 60-kD SSA/Ro ribonucleoproteins.[35] Congenital heart block is an important model of passive autoimmunity, with cardiac injury believed to be in response to active transport of maternal immunoglobulin G (IgG) autoantibodies into the fetal circulation.[35] Anti-SSA/Ro associated with third-degree heart block is irreversible.[36] Dilation of the ascending aorta is present in a large proportion of pediatric patients with isolated congenital complete heart block.[37]

HISTORY

Congenital complete heart block necessarily begins in utero[10,38] and must be distinguished from the bradycardia of fetal distress,[39,40] a distinction that is more certain

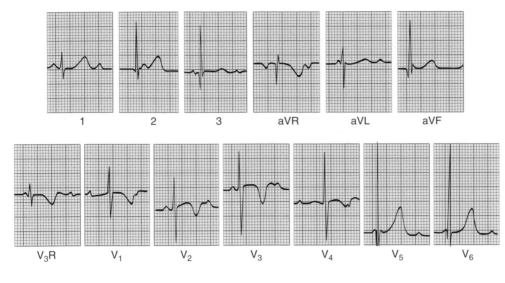

FIGURE 4-1 Electrocardiogram from a 7-year-old boy with isolated complete heart block. P waves are independent of QRS complexes. The QRS complex is normal in configuration and duration, and its axis is normal. Deep Q waves and tall R waves are found in leads V_5 and V_6. The R wave in lead V_1 is relatively tall, with an R/S ratio of 1:1. T waves are deeply inverted in right precordial leads and are tall and peaked in left precordial leads. See Figure 4-5 for rhythm strip.

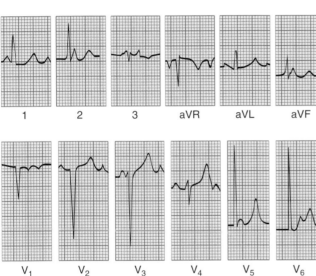

FIGURE 4-2 Electrocardiogram of a 25-year-old man with congenital complete heart block. P waves are independent of QRS complexes. The QRS complex is narrow, and its axis is normal. Tall R waves and relatively tall, peaked T waves are found in leads V_5 and V_6.

Fetal echocardiography is used to establish the diagnosis and determine whether the heart block is isolated or associated with congenital heart disease, which is usually left isomerism or ventricular inversion (see previous discussion). Only 14% of fetuses with coexisting congenital heart disease survive as neonates.[10] Conversely, 85% of fetuses with *isolated* intrauterine complete heart block live beyond the neonatal period.[10,26,38] This survival rate is similar to that of isolated congenital complete heart block diagnosed after birth, in which approximately 90% of infants and children are alive at long-term follow-up.[10] The fetal cardiac rhythm may change from sinus to second-degree atrioventricular block to complete heart block within hours or weeks after birth, which suggests that immunologic damage occurs early, develops slowly, or appears late.[10]

A tendency for female preponderance in congenital complete heart block has been found,[41] and approximately 76% of mothers of affected children are white.[35] *Familial* heart block has been well established.[9,22,39,42–45] In Morquio's[1] original description, atrioventricular block recurred in five of eight siblings (see previous mention). Osler[46] reported Stokes-Adams attacks in a patient who had relatives with slow pulses. Familial congenital heart block can become overt years after birth[43,47] and can be characterized by right or left bundle branch block.[48] Almost all degrees and forms of heart block have occurred in different members of the same family. Four generations of a single family had right bundle branch block, left anterior fascicular block, bifascicular block,

when the slow heart rate is detected before the onset of labor.[40] However, congenital complete heart block usually comes to attention because an inappropriately slow heart rate is detected in an otherwise healthy neonate or infant (see subsequent section, Arterial Pulse).

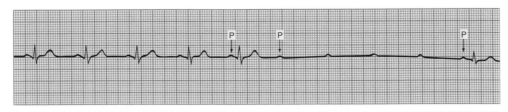

FIGURE 4-3 Rhythm strip from a 28-year-old man with intermittent congenital complete heart block. Sinus rhythm with normal PR intervals and normal QRS complexes is followed by sudden absence of AV conduction (see second P wave). The next sinus beat conducts with a slightly prolonged PR interval (see 3rd P wave). *(Courtesy Dr. R. J. Burger, Fairbanks, Alaska.)*

and complete heart block.[49] Mothers with systemic lupus erythematosus and one child with neonatal heart block are at greater risk of having subsequent offspring with heart block.[45] Children of mothers with lupus not only can have congenital heart block but subsequently can have development of the overt connective tissue disease.[50] Maternal lupus may not become manifest for years after birth of an infant with congenital complete heart block.[51] Long-term outlook for the mothers is more reassuring, however.[52,53]

The key determinants of clinical stability in isolated congenital complete heart block are the ventricular rate, the hemodynamic adjustments at rest and with exercise (previously discussed), and the presence of inherently normal myocardium.[9,54] Nevertheless, patients can have development of dilated cardiomyopathy attributed to bradycardia, and a strong relationship exists between SSA/Ro and SSB/La antibodies and cardiomyopathy.[28,52] Although subnormal exercise performance has been reported in children and adolescents with congenital complete atrioventricular block,[23,55,56] exercise tolerance is generally normal or nearly so, and endurance performance is occasionally normal.[25,57] One patient was an ardent ice hockey player, and other patients have included Air Force pilots,[58,59] a cricket player,[55] a 56-year-old woman who for 20 years walked 2 miles to her daily job on a farm,[24] a 38-year-old man who had won boxing matches in his youth,[24] and a 48-year-old man who experienced a normal response to a Royal Canadian Air Force decompression chamber at age 23 years and subsequently flew jet aircraft.[54] High levels of physical activity are not desirable but are at least possible despite the exercise limitations described previously. Pregnancy is generally uneventful in otherwise healthy women with congenital heart block,[60,61] but Stokes-Adams attacks occasionally occur during gestation or the puerperium.[61]

A substantial majority of young patients with isolated congenital complete heart block are asymptomatic, but the mortality rate even in infancy and childhood is estimated at 8%,[62] and longevity in adolescents and adults is less than normal.[23,41,62] The heart may not respond adequately to increased circulatory demands, especially in the vulnerable neonatal period.[9,41,54,62] Infants with slow ventricular rates may succumb to congestive heart failure before physiologic adaptation is achieved.[62] Metabolic acidosis slows the heart rate,[63] and the stress of febrile illnesses in infancy are poorly tolerated. Congenital complete heart block may come to light in toddlers because of night terrors or irritability.[9] Stokes-Adams episodes are uncommon in the young but pose tangible hazards, with symptoms that range from mild dizziness to syncope and convulsions.[24,55] Neurologic sequelae follow cardiac arrest. A Stokes-Adams episode with sudden death can occur in previously asymptomatic patients (Figure 4-4). Fatal Stokes-Adams seizures occasionally occur in childhood, but death rarely accompanies the initial episode.[23,41] One patient experienced recurrent Stokes-Adams episodes between 2 and 4 years of age, but the attacks gradually diminished and finally vanished, leaving him able to participate in cricket, football, and swimming.[23,55] Syncope and sudden death are usually caused by bradycardia, but ventricular tachycardia and

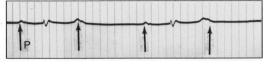
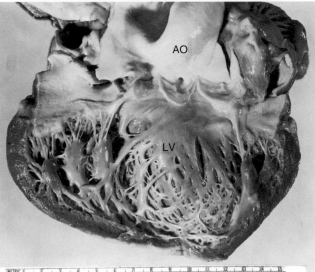

FIGURE 4-4 Electrocardiogram and gross specimen from an 18-year-old laboratory technician with isolated congenital complete heart block who experienced a fatal Stokes-Adams episode. The rhythm strip shows broad, independent P waves and a narrow QRS. The left ventricle (LV) is dilated but otherwise normal. (AO = aorta.)

fibrillation also play a role.[25] Frequent ventricular ectopic beats have been recorded during nocturnal monitoring, and young patients sometimes experience unifocal, multifocal, or repetitive ventricular ectopic beats during treadmill exercise.[57] Serious symptoms and complications are more likely in patients with daytime heart rates below 50 beats per minute, wide QRS complexes, a blunted rate response to graded exercise, a disproportionate increase in left ventricular internal dimensions, or subnormal left ventricular function.[64]

PHYSICAL APPEARANCE

Growth, development, and general appearance are normal. Cyanosis can accompany congestive heart failure in infants who are bradycardic.

ARTERIAL PULSE

A pulse rate *inappropriately* slow for age often leads to the diagnosis of congenital complete heart block. At birth, the heart rate in affected patients is seldom more than 90 beats per minute, and in infants, the rate is seldom more than 65 to 70 beats per minute.[9] After infancy, the basal rate generally exceeds 50 beats per minute (Figure 4-5) and not uncommonly reaches 60, 70, or even 80 beats per minute.[23] The pulse rate in congenital complete heart block is slow but is relatively rapid compared with *acquired* complete heart block.[23,24] In healthy

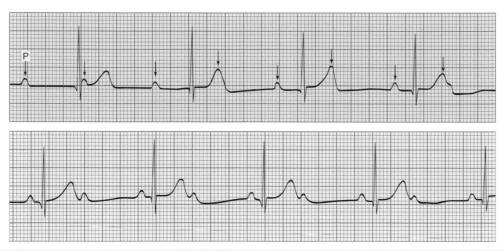

FIGURE 4-5 Long strip of lead 2 of the electrocardiogram shown in Figure 4-1. Independent P waves are identified with *arrows*. The PP intervals are shorter when separated by a QRS complex (positive chronotropic effect). The ventricular rate is 48 to 50 beats per minute. The QRS complexes are narrow.

young adults, rates of 40 to 60 beats per minute may be mistaken for sinus bradycardia.[23] A Royal Canadian Air Force veteran described by Mathewson and Harvie[58] was a case in point. His slow heart rate was initially attributed to the sinus bradycardia of physical conditioning. Strenuous exercise was tolerated without difficulty. Complete heart block thought to be congenital was subsequently recognized.

Three features other than rate deserve comment: namely, upstroke, pulse pressure, and *atrial waves*. The upstroke is brisk, and the pulse pressure is relatively wide.[55] Rapid ejection of a large stroke volume from a functionally normal left ventricle increases the rate of rise and increases the systolic pressure, while prolonged diastole permits a pressure decline to relatively low levels. Small waves synchronous with atrial contraction appear on the diastolic portion of the arterial pressure pulse[65] and can sometimes be detected with meticulous palpation. These waves are believed to result from external impact of the left atrium on the aorta and are analogous to waves that have been recorded on the pulmonary arterial pressure pulse. Sinus arrhythmia is conspicuous by its absence and weighs in favor of sinus bradycardia.

JUGULAR VENOUS PULSE

The jugular venous pulse alone is a reliable indication of complete heart block. Independent A waves occur at a rate more rapid than the arterial pulse and intermittently increase in amplitude (see subsequent discussion). Small regular A waves during diastole occur more rapidly than the arterial pulse rate, which indicates that atrial and ventricular contractions are independent. When the right atrium contracts against a tricuspid valve that has been fortuitously closed during a ventricular systole, the A wave abruptly amplifies—a *cannon wave* (Figure 4-6).[66] Precise timing of cannon waves localizes their maximal amplitude at isovolumetric ventricular systole.[67] The first heart sound that accompanies a cannon

wave is comparatively soft because atrial systole *follows* rather than precedes ventricular contraction (see subsequent discussion).

PRECORDIAL MOVEMENT AND PALPATION

The left ventricular impulse is prominent because a large stroke volume is ejected rapidly from a volume-overloaded but functionally normal chamber. A right ventricular impulse is absent despite equivalent volume overload. Variations in intensity of the first heart sound can be detected with the fingertips with palpation of the left ventricular impulse, and mid-diastolic distention is sensed when atrial contraction coincides with the rapid filling phase.

AUSCULTATION

Auscultation is a means of suspecting *fetal* complete heart block.[40] Intrauterine diagnosis was made in a twin when two fetal heart rates were detected, one at 52 beats per minute and the other at 150 beats per minute.[40]

The following auscultatory signs are useful in the diagnosis of congenital complete heart block: (1) variable intensity of the first heart sound; (2) a midsystolic murmur; (3) normal respiratory splitting of the second heart sound; (4) a third heart sound; (5) a fourth heart sound; (6) a summation sound; (7) an atrial murmur; (8) a mid-diastolic murmur; and (9) vascular sounds over the carotid, subclavian, and femoral arteries. Variation in intensity of the first heart sound is an auscultatory hallmark of complete heart block (Figures 4-7 through 4-10).[66,68] When the variation occurs with a slow heart rate and a regular rhythm, the diagnosis of complete heart block can be entertained with considerable confidence.

The PR relationship is an important determinant of the intensity of the first heart sound, an observation

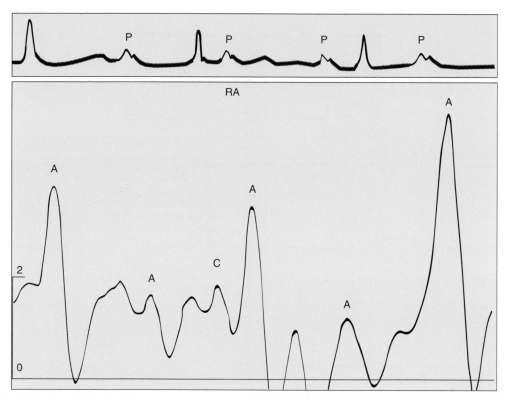

FIGURE 4-6 Electrocardiogram (lead 2 rhythm strip) and right atrial pressure pulse from a 13-year-old boy with isolated congenital complete heart block. The A waves intermittently increase (cannon waves) when a P wave falls between QRS complex and T wave. The increase occurs because the right atrium contracts against a closed tricuspid valve. The A waves are small when a P wave falls between T wave and QRS complex (i.e., when the tricuspid valve is open). (RA = right atrium.)

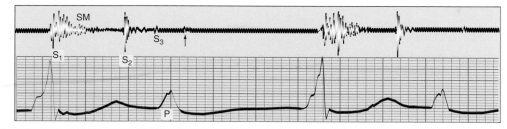

FIGURE 4-7 Phonocardiogram (apex) and electrocardiogram (lead 2) from the 25-year-old man referred to in Figure 4-2. The first heart sound (S_1) is loud and constant because each QRS complex is immediately preceded by a P wave, to which it is fused. The independent P waves are tall and notched. A grade 2/6 systolic murmur (SM), a third heart sound (S_3), and a short, soft diastolic murmur *(arrow)* follow the independent P waves.

made by Wolferth and Margolies in 1930.[69] In complete heart block, the PR relationship changes from beat to beat because the atria and ventricles contract independently, so the first sound varies in intensity from cycle to cycle, ranging from booming *(bruit de canon)* to virtual inaudibility (see Figures 4-7, 4-9, and 4-10). The first heart sound is loud when the PR interval is short (120 msec or less), soft when the PR interval is long (200 to 300 msec), and louder again when PR prolongation exceeds 500 msec.[66,68] When the PR interval exceeds 500 msec, reopening of the mitral valve is followed by secondary closure at the onset of ventricular systole, resulting in reappearance of the first heart sound.[68]

A grade 2/6 to 3/6 midsystolic murmur is related principally if not exclusively to rapid ejection of a large stroke volume from the *right* ventricle (see Figures 4-7, 4-8, and 4-9). Maximal intensity is at the mid to upper left sternal border. The murmur is relatively short, occupying the first half to two thirds of systole and always ending well before the second heart sound.[66]

Normal respiratory splitting of the second heart sound is a useful sign of congenital as opposed to acquired complete heart block.[66] Physiologic splitting implies a normal sequence of ventricular activation that is in accord with a narrow QRS complex and a subsidiary pacemaker above the bifurcation of the His bundle (see subsequent section, Electrocardiogram).

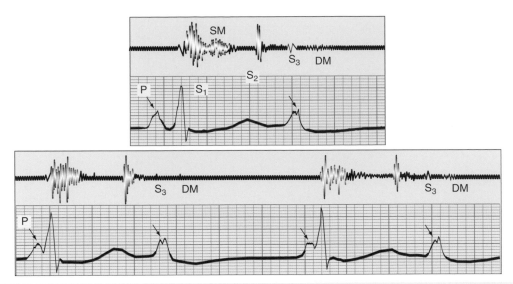

FIGURE 4-8 Phonocardiogram (cardiac apex) and electrocardiogram (lead 2) from the 25-year-old man whose 12-lead tracing is shown in Figure 4-2. The first heart sound (S_1) is loud (short interval between P wave and QRS complex). A grade 2/6 to 3/6 systolic murmur (SM) ends well before the second heart sound (S_2). The murmur was maximal at the mid left sternal border. A third heart sound (S_3) and a short diastolic murmur (DM) follow the subsequent P wave, which is notched.

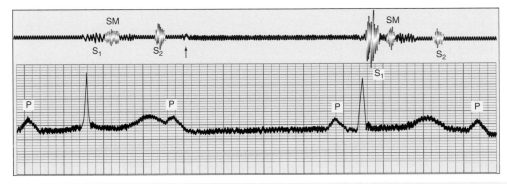

FIGURE 4-9 Phonocardiogram (apex) and electrocardiogram (lead 2) from a 12-year-old girl with isolated congenital complete heart block. The first heart sound (S_1) varies from soft (long PR interval) to loud (short PR interval). A short grade 2/6 midsystolic murmur (SM) is seen. A soft fourth heart sound *(arrow)* follows the second P wave.

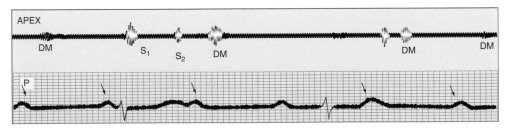

FIGURE 4-10 Phonocardiogram and electrocardiogram from a 15-year-old boy with isolated congenital complete heart block. *Arrows* point to independent P waves. The first heart sound (S_1) varies from loud to soft. The short diastolic murmurs (DM) are especially prominent when atrial contraction (P wave) coincides with the rapid filling phase (shortly after the T wave).

Third heart sounds are indistinguishable from normal third heart sounds in the young (see Figures 4-7 and 4-8). However, fourth heart sounds—aptly called *gallop du bloc* by Gallavardin[70]—are of special interest because they are *not* heard in healthy young people. Timing in diastole is variable because the atria and ventricles beat independently. The fourth sounds have the brevity of a sound per se (see Figure 4-9) or the prolongation of a short murmur (see Figure 4-8). When atrial contraction coincides with rapid ventricular filling, third and fourth heart sounds either summate or generate a short mid-diastolic murmur (see Figure 4-10). Summation sounds and mid-diastolic murmurs are detected more often than isolated fourth heart sounds or atrial murmurs. *Systolic vascular sounds* attributed to high-velocity ejection are occasionally heard over the carotid, subclavian, and femoral arteries.

ELECTROCARDIOGRAM

The definitive diagnosis of complete heart block depends on nothing more than an electrocardiogram. Fetal electrocardiography is an extension of this simple accurate diagnostic tool.[40]

The P wave of atrial activity and the QRS of ventricular activity occur independently, with no arithmetical relationship between the two (see Figure 4-5). In acquired complete heart block, periods of synchronization—*accrochage*—sometimes occur.[16,71] This phenomenon is seldom witnessed in congenital complete heart block (see Figure 4-7). Although atrial depolarization does not activate the ventricles, examples of a change from *partial* to *complete* heart block,[21] as well as from *complete* to *partial* heart block, are occasionally encountered (see Figure 4-3).[23,24] A neonate with congenital complete heart block experienced intermittent 1/1 atrioventricular conduction through a Wolff-Parkinson-White accessory pathway.[53]

The atrial rate tends to decrease with age but remains rapid compared with the ventricular rate, which is relatively constant after infancy until well into adulthood.[23,24] During exercise, a stepwise increase is seen in *atrial* rate with slow return to normal, whereas the *ventricular* rate increases irregularly with a more rapid return to baseline levels. The flat exercise response of the subsidiary junctional pacemaker[56] was mentioned previously. Rarely, atrial flutter coexists with congenital complete heart block.[72]

The PP intervals vary in both congenital and acquired complete heart block. PP intervals that are separated by a QRS complex tend to be shorter (positive chronotropic effect) and less commonly longer (negative chronotropic effect) than PP intervals that are not separated by a QRS (Figure 4-11).

Sinus P waves are tall and broad, reflecting volume overload of the atria (see Figures 4-4, 4-7, and 4-8). A normal QRS duration indicates a normal sequence of ventricular activation because the pacemaker is located *above* the bifurcation of the His bundle (see Figures 4-1 and 4-2).[24] In *acquired* complete heart block, the QRS duration is prolonged because the idioventricular pacemaker is located *below* the His bundle and its major branches. In *congenital* complete heart block, the QRS occasionally resembles right or left bundle branch block because the block is infra-Hisian. The lower the pacemaker is in the conduction system, the greater the vulnerability to Stokes-Adams syncope. When QRS prolongation coincides with a slow heart rate, Stokes-Adams attacks are more likely.

In *familial* complete heart block with *adult onset*, the QRS duration is prolonged and the outlook is unfavorable.[44] Ambulatory electrocardiograms of isolated congenital complete heart block have recorded multiple arrhythmias: junctional exit block, exercise-related ventricular ectopic beats, blunted ventricular rate responses, and marked nocturnal bradycardia.[56,57,73]

Voltage criteria for left ventricular hypertrophy are sometimes present, together with prominent left precordial Q waves of volume overload (see Figures 4-1 and 4-2). Right ventricular hypertrophy or biventricular hypertrophy is occasional.

The T wave configuration is likely to be normal, but deep T wave inversions or coving sometimes occur in right or midprecordial leads, and T waves may be peaked in left chest leads (see Figures 4-1 and 4-2). QT interval prolongation increases the risk of torsades de pointes.[74]

His bundle electrograms in congenital complete heart block are used to identify the location of the conduction defect and the site of the subsidiary pacemaker (see previous discussion).[62,75–78] The block is typically proximal to the site at which His bundle potentials are recorded.[77–79] A normal HV interval and a normal QRS complex indicate that the conduction system is normal distal to the site of block.[78] His electrograms do not permit identification of where in the AV junction the escape rhythm originates because block proximal to the His potential can be within the AV node, between the AV node and atrial muscle, or in the AV node–His bundle junction.[13,77,78]

Escape rhythms in congenital complete heart block are likely to originate in the bundle of His because

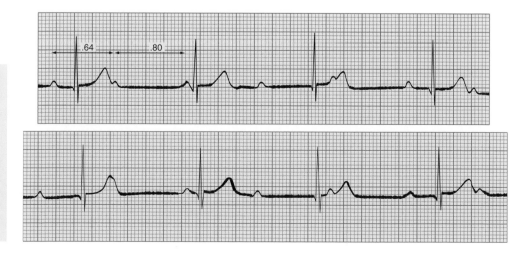

FIGURE 4-11 Rhythm strips of lead 2 of the electrocardiogram shown in Figure 4-1. The P waves are independent, and the ventricular rate is 47 beats per minute. The first PP interval is separated by a QRS complex and is relatively short (0.64 second; positive chronotropic effect). The second PP interval is *not* separated by a QRS complex and is relatively long (0.80 second).

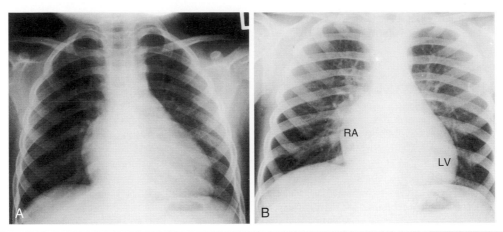

FIGURE 4-12 X-rays from the child whose electrocardiogram is shown in Figure 4-1. **A,** At age 4 years, the heart size was a moderately increased (LV = left ventricle; RA = right atrium). **B,** At age 7 years, a further increase in heart size coincided with a decrease in heart rate to 50 beats per minute.

automaticity is a property of His/Purkinje cells but not of AV nodal cells. Origin is probably in the *proximal* His bundle in light of observations on complete heart block from *intra-His* discontinuity.[76,78] Electrophysiologic studies have recorded split His potentials proximal and distal to the site of block,[76] so the escape pacemaker can be in the distal His bundle at the site of the second His potential. The distal pacemaker is associated with a slower ventricular rate and little or no acceleration in response to atropine.

X-RAY

The radiologic appearances of the heart, great arteries, and lungs tend to be normal in congenital complete heart block.[24] Ventricular chamber size usually remains constant through adulthood.[23] A mild to moderate increase in heart size reflects prolonged diastolic filling periods and increased ventricular volume because of the slow heart rate (Figures 4-4 and 4-12).[80]

ECHOCARDIOGRAM

Echocardiography with Doppler interrogation and color flow imaging are used to establish that the congenital complete heart block is isolated,[64] and fetal echocardiography is used to establish the diagnosis of isolated intrauterine complete heart block. Complete heart block can be diagnosed in utero with pulsed Doppler and color flow recordings of left ventricular inflow and outflow signals.[10,38,81,82]

SUMMARY

Isolated congenital complete heart block is a model of passive autoimmunity with the conduction defect caused by injury from active transplacental transport of maternal IgG antibodies into the fetal circulation. The conduction

defect is usually discovered incidentally in otherwise healthy children, or an obstetrician may detect a slow fetal heart rate. The diagnosis of complete heart block is straightforward based on nothing more than a standard scalar electrocardiogram. If liberal use were made of the electrocardiogram in infants and children with inappropriately slow heart rates, few cases would be missed. Fetal electrocardiography and echocardiography are used to establish the intrauterine diagnosis. Stokes-Adams attacks are uncommon but can occur even in the young. The arterial pulse rate is inappropriately slow for age, the upstroke is brisk, the pulse pressure is wide, and the rhythm is regular. The jugular venous pulse exhibits intermittent cannon waves and independent asynchronous A waves that are more rapid than the carotid pulse, which indicates that atrial and ventricular activity are independent. The electrocardiogram records independent P waves, and the QRS complexes are of normal duration because the block is above the bifurcation of the His bundle.

REFERENCES

1. Morquio L. Sur une maladie infantile et familiale caractérisée par des modifications permanentes du pouls, des attaques syncopales et epileptiforme et la mort subite. *Archives médicales d'enfants.* 1901;4:467.
2. Van den Heuvel G. De zeikte van Stokes-Adams eneen geval van aangeborenen hartblock. *Groningen Proefschrift Rijks Universitait.* 1908;12:142.
3. White P, Eustis R. Congenital heart block. *Am J Dis Child.* 1921; 22:299.
4. Davis H, Stecher R. Congenital heart block. *Am J Dis Child.* 1928; 36:115.
5. Yater W. Congenital heart block; review of the literature; report of case with incomplete heterotaxy; electrocardiogram in dextrocardia. *Am J Dis Child.* 1929;38:112.
6. Yater W, Leamon W, Cornall V. Congenital heart block; report of third case of complete heart block studied by serial section through conduction system. *J Am Med Assoc.* 1934;102:1660.
7. Yater W, Lyon J, Mcnabb P. Congenital heart block; review and report of second case of complete heart block studied by serial sections through conduction system. *J Am Med Assoc.* 1933;100:1831.
8. Brucato A, Jonzon A, Friedman B, et al. Proposal for a new definition of congenital complete atrioventricular block. *Lupus.* 2003;12: 427–435.

9. Ross BA. Congenital complete atrioventricular block. *Pediatr Clin North Am.* 1990;37:69–78.
10. Schmidt KG, Ulmer HE, Silverman NH, Kleinman CS, Copel JA. Perinatal outcome of fetal complete atrioventricular block: a multicenter experience. *J Am Coll Cardiol.* 1991;17:1360–1366.
11. Anderson RH, Wenick AC, Losekoot TG, Becker AE. Congenitally complete heart block. Developmental aspects. *Circulation.* 1977;56:90–101.
12. Suarez-Penaranda JM, Munoz JI, Rodriguez-Calvo MS, Ortiz-Rey JA, Concheiro L. The pathology of the heart conduction system in congenital heart block. *J Clin Forensic Med.* 2006;13:341–343.
13. Bharati S, Lev M. Pathology of atrioventricular block. *Cardiol Clin.* 1984;2:741–751.
14. Lev M. The normal anatomy of the conduction system in man and its pathology in atrioventricular block. *Ann N Y Acad Sci.* 1964;111:817–829.
15. James TN. Cardiac conduction system: fetal and postnatal development. *Am J Cardiol.* 1970;25:213–226.
16. Lev M, Silverman J, Fitzmaurice FM, Paul MH, Cassels DE, Miller RA. Lack of connection between the atria and the more peripheral conduction system in congenital atrioventricular block. *Am J Cardiol.* 1971;27:481–490.
17. Lev M, Benjamin JE, White PD. A histopathologic study of the conduction system in a case of complete heart block of 42 years' duration. *Am Heart J.* 1958;55:198–214.
18. Lev M. The anatomic basis for disturbances in conduction and cardiac arrhythmias. *Prog Cardiovasc Dis.* 1960;2:360–369.
19. Lev M, Cuadros H, Paul MH. Interruption of the atrioventricular bundle with congenital atrioventricular block. *Circulation.* 1971;43:703–710.
20. Angelini A, Moreolo GS, Ruffatti A, Milanesi O, Thiene G. Images in cardiovascular medicine. Calcification of the atrioventricular node in a fetus affected by congenital complete heart block. *Circulation.* 2002;105:1254–1255.
21. Dunn HG. Congenital partial heart block. *Proc R Soc Med.* 1952;45:456–458.
22. Khorsandian RS, Moghadam AN, Mueller OF. Familial congenital A-V dissociation. *Am J Cardiol.* 1964;14:118–124.
23. Campbell M, Emanuel R. Six cases of congenital complete heart block followed for 34–40 years. *Br Heart J.* 1967;29:577–587.
24. Campbell M, Thorne MG. Congenital heart block. *Br Heart J.* 1956;18:90–101.
25. Reybrouck T, Vanden Eynde B, Dumoulin M, Van Der Hauwaert LG. Cardiorespiratory response to exercise in congenital complete atrioventricular block. *Am J Cardiol.* 1989;64:896–899.
26. Manno BV, Hakki AH, Eshaghpour E, Iskandrian AS. Left ventricular function at rest and during exercise in congenital complete heart block: a radionuclide angiographic evaluation. *Am J Cardiol.* 1983;52:92–94.
27. Thilenius OG, Chiemmongkoltip P, Cassels DE, Arcilla RA. Hemodynamics studies in children with congenital atrioventricular block. *Am J Cardiol.* 1972;30:13–18.
28. Udink Ten Cate FE, Breur JM, Cohen MI, et al. Dilated cardiomyopathy in isolated congenital complete atrioventricular block: early and long-term risk in children. *J Am Coll Cardiol.* 2001;37:1129–1134.
29. Chameides L, Truex RC, Vetter V, Rashkind WJ, Galioto Jr FM, Noonan JA. Association of maternal systemic lupus erythematosus with congenital complete heart block. *N Engl J Med.* 1977;297:1204–1207.
30. Litsey SE, Noonan JA, O'Connor WN, Cottrill CM, Mitchell B. Maternal connective tissue disease and congenital heart block. Demonstration of immunoglobulin in cardiac tissue. *N Engl J Med.* 1985;312:98–100.
31. Mccue CM, Mantakas ME, Tingelstad JB, Ruddy S. Congenital heart block in newborns of mothers with connective tissue disease. *Circulation.* 1977;56:82–90.
32. Nolan RJ, Shulman ST, Victorica BE. Congenital complete heart block associated with maternal mixed connective tissue disease. *J Pediatr.* 1979;95:420–422.
33. Ottosson L, Salomonsson S, Hennig J, et al. Structurally derived mutations define congenital heart block-related epitopes within the 200-239 amino acid stretch of the Ro52 protein. *Scand J Immunol.* 2005;61:109–118.
34. Menon A, Silverman ED, Gow RM, Hamilton RM. Chronotropic competence of the sinus node in congenital complete heart block. *Am J Cardiol.* 1998;82:1119–1121, A1119.
35. Buyon JP, Hiebert R, Copel J, et al. Autoimmune-associated congenital heart block: demographics, mortality, morbidity and recurrence rates obtained from a national neonatal lupus registry. *J Am Coll Cardiol.* 1998;31:1658–1666.
36. Friedman DM, Kim MY, Copel JA, et al. Utility of cardiac monitoring in fetuses at risk for congenital heart block: the PR Interval and Dexamethasone Evaluation (PRIDE) prospective study. *Circulation.* 2008;117:485–493.
37. Radbill AE, Brown DW, Lacro RV, et al. Ascending aortic dilation in patients with congenital complete heart block. *Heart Rhythm.* 2008;5:1704–1708.
38. Gembruch U, Hansmann M, Redel DA, Bald R, Knopfle G. Fetal complete heart block: antenatal diagnosis, significance and management. *Eur J Obstet Gynecol Reprod Biol.* 1989;31:9–22.
39. Connor AC, McFadden JF, Houston BJ, Finn JL. Familial congenital complete heart block; case report and review of the literature. *Am J Obstet Gynecol.* 1959;78:75–79.
40. Dunn HP. Antenatal diagnosis of congenital heart block. *J Obstet Gynaecol Br Empire.* 1960;67:1006–1007.
41. Reid JM, Coleman EN, Doig W. Complete congenital heart block. Report of 35 cases. *Br Heart J.* 1982;48:236–239.
42. Gazes PC, Culler RM, Taber E, Kelly TE. Congenital familial cardiac conduction defects. *Circulation.* 1965;32:32–34.
43. Morgans CM, Gray KE, Robb GH. A survey of familial heart block. *Br Heart J.* 1974;36:693–696.
44. Sarachek NS, Leonard JL. Familial heart block and sinus bradycardia. Classification and natural history. *Am J Cardiol.* 1972;29:451–458.
45. Scheib JS, Waxman J. Congenital heart block in successive pregnancies: a case report and evaluation of risk with therapeutic consideration. *Obstet Gynecol.* 1989;73:481–484.
46. Osler W. On the so-called Stokes-Adams disease. *Lancet.* 1903;2:516.
47. James TN, Spencer MS, Kloepfer JC. De Subitaneis Mortibus. XXI. Adult onset syncope. with comments on the nature of congenital heart block and the morphogenesis of the human atrioventricular septal junction. *Circulation.* 1976;54:1001–1009.
48. Esscher E, Hardell LI, Michaelsson M. Familial, isolated, complete right bundle-branch block. *Br Heart J.* 1975;37:745–747.
49. Stephan E. Hereditary bundle branch system defect: survey of a family with four affected generations. *Am Heart J.* 1978;95:89–95.
50. Lanham JG, Walport MJ, Hughes GR. Congenital heart block and familial connective tissue disease. *J Rheumatol.* 1983;10:823–825.
51. Kasinath BS, Katz AI. Delayed maternal lupus after delivery of offspring with congenital heart block. *Arch Intern Med.* 1982;142:2317.
52. Eronen M. Long-term outcome of children with complete heart block diagnosed after the newborn period. *Pediatr Cardiol.* 2001;22:133–137.
53. Mcleod KA, Rankin AC, Houston AB. 1:1 atrioventricular conduction in congenital complete heart block. *Heart.* 1998;80:525–526.
54. Corne RA, Mathewson FA. Congenital complete atrioventricular heart block. A 25 year follow-up study. *Am J Cardiol.* 1972;29:412–415.
55. Campbell M. Congenital complete heart block. *Br Heart J.* 1943;5:15–18.
56. Dewey RC, Capeless MA, Levy AM. Use of ambulatory electrocardiographic monitoring to identify high-risk patients with congenital complete heart block. *N Engl J Med.* 1987;316:835–839.
57. Winkler RB, Freed MD, Nadas AS. Exercise-induced ventricular ectopy in children and young adults with complete heart block. *Am Heart J.* 1980;99:87–92.
58. Mathewson FA, Harvie FH. Complete heart block in an experienced pilot. *Br Heart J.* 1957;19:253–258.
59. Turner LB. Asymptomatic congenital complete heart block in an Army Air Force pilot. *Am Heart J.* 1947;34:426–431.
60. Groves AM, Allan LD, Rosenthal E. Outcome of isolated congenital complete heart block diagnosed in utero. *Heart.* 1996;75:190–194.

61. Perloff J. Pregnancy and congenital heart disease. In: Perloff J, Child J, Aboulhosn J, eds. *Congenital heart disease in adults.* 3rd ed. Philadelphia: WB Saunders; 2009.

62. Michaelsson M, Engle MA. Congenital complete heart block: an international study of the natural history. *Cardiovasc Clin.* 1972; 4:85–101.

63. Spach MS, Scarpelli EM. Circulatory dynamics and the effects of respiration during ventricular asystole in dogs with complete heart block. *Circ Res.* 1962;10:197–207.

64. Sholler GF, Walsh EP. Congenital complete heart block in patients without anatomic cardiac defects. *Am Heart J.* 1989;118:1193–1198.

65. Howarth S. Atrial waves on arterial pressure records in normal rhythm, heart block, and auricular flutter. *Br Heart J.* 1954; 16:171–176.

66. Perloff J. *Physical examination of the heart and circulation.* 4th ed. Philadelphia: WB Saunders; 2009.

67. Lagerlof H, Werko L. Studies on circulation in man: auricular pressure pulse. *Cardiologia.* 1948;13:240.

68. Burggraf GW, Craige E. The first heart sound in complete heart block. Phono-echocardiographic correlations. *Circulation.* 1974;50: 17–24.

69. Wolferth CC, Margolies A. The influence of auricular contraction on the first heart sound and the radial pulse. *Arch Intern Med.* 1930;46:1048–1071.

70. Gallavardin L. Contractions auriculaires perceptibles à l'oreille dans le bloc total. *Arch Mal Coeur Vaiss.* 1914;7:171.

71. Marriott HJ. Atrioventricular synchronization and accrochage. *Circulation.* 1956;14:38–43.

72. Schuster B, Imm CW. Congenital atrial flutter with complete heart block. *Am J Cardiol.* 1963;12:575–578.

73. Nagashima M, Nakashima T, Asai T, et al. Study on congenital complete heart block in children by 24-hour ambulatory electrocardiographic monitoring. *Jpn Heart J.* 1987;28:323–332.

74. Kernohan RJ, Froggatt P. Atrioventricular dissociation with prolonged QT interval and syncopal attacks in a 10-year-old boy. *Br Heart J.* 1974;36:516–519.

75. Abella JB, Teixeira OH, Misra KP, Hastreiter AR. Changes of atrioventricular conduction with age in infants and children. *Am J Cardiol.* 1972;30:876–883.

76. Bharati S, Lev M, Wu D, Denes P, Dhingra R, Rosen KM. Pathophysiologic correlations in two cases of split His bundle potentials. *Circulation.* 1974;49:615–623.

77. Kelly DT, Brodsky SJ, Mirowsri M, Krovetz J, Rowe RD. Bundle of His recordings in congenital complete heart block. *Circulation.* 1972;45:277–281.

78. Rosen KM, Mehta A, Rahimtoola SH, Miller RA. Sites of congenital and surgical heart block as defined by His bundle electrocardiography. *Circulation.* 1971;44:833–841.

79. Smithen CS, Sowton E. His bundle electrograms. *Br Heart J.* 1971; 33:633–638.

80. Moss AJ. Congenital complete atrioventricular block. Clinical features, hemodynamic findings, and physical working capacity. *Lancet.* 1961;81:542–547.

81. Arbeille P, Paillet C, Chantepie B. In utero ultrasonic diagnosis of atrioventricular block. *J Cardiovasc Ultrasonogr.* 1984;3:313.

82. Kleinman CS, Hobbins JC, Jaffe CC, Lynch DC, Talner NS. Echocardiographic studies of the human fetus: prenatal diagnosis of congenital heart disease and cardiac dysrhythmias. *Pediatrics.* 1980;65:1059–1067.

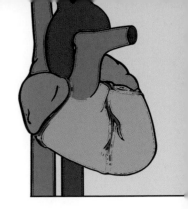

Chapter 5

Congenital Abnormalities of the Pericardium

The *pericardium* (*peri*, around; *cardium*, heart) consists of two layers with nerves, lymphatics and a blood supply. The layer attached to the surface of the heart is the *visceral* pericardium. The layer that is not attached to the surface of the heart is the *parietal* pericardium; it is separated from the visceral pericardium by 20 to 30 mL of a serous ultrafiltrate of plasma. It is with the *parietal* pericardium that this chapter is concerned.

Congenital absence of the pericardium was recognized by M. Realdus Columbus[1] in 1559 and by Matthew Baille[2] in 1793, but the anomaly was not clinically diagnosed in a chest x-ray until 1959.[3] The pericardial abnormality varies from a localized defect to complete absence.[4–6] The sternum, abdominal wall, pericardium, and part of the diaphragm arise from somatic mesoderm. Morphogenesis of congenital defects of the left pericardium has been attributed to premature atrophy of the left duct of Cuvier that results in deficient blood supply to the left pleuropericardial membrane.[7,8]

The necropsy incidence rate of congenital absence of the pericardium has been estimated at 1/14,000.[9] About two thirds of cases are represented by partial absence of the *left* pericardium (Figure 5-1).[9–11] Congenital absence of the right pericardium is rare (Figure 5-2).[6,12] Approximately one third of congenital pericardial defects occur in conjunction with other congenital malformations, both cardiac (Figure 5-3) and noncardiac.[4,13,14] A case in point is the *Cantrell's syndrome* described in 1958[13] (also called the Cantrell-Heller-Ravitch syndrome) that consists of two major defects, *ectopia cordis* and *epigastric omphalocele*, and three lesser defects, *cleft of the distal sternum* and defects of the anterior diaphragm and diaphragmatic pericardium.[13,15,16]

The parietal pericardium exerts contact stress that contributes to ventricular diastolic pressure and limits acute dilation.[17] The stress is greater on the relatively thin right ventricle and right atrium whose dimensions and pressures depend chiefly on pericardial constraint.[17] Accordingly, congenital complete absence of the parietal pericardium is accompanied by alterations in systemic venous return[18] and an increase in right ventricular size.[17] Alternans of the right ventricular diastolic pressure has been reported during cardiac catheterization in a patient with congenital complete absence of the pericardium.[19]

HISTORY

Partial or complete absence of the pericardium usually comes to light because of an abnormality on the routine chest x-ray of an asymptomatic patient or in a chest x-ray taken as part of the cardiovascular evaluation of a symptomatic patient with coexisting cardiac defects.[4] The most common symptom is chest pain that appears suddenly in a previously asymptomatic adult and that varies from mild and occasional to frequent, prolonged, and debilitating.[4] The pain is stabbing; left-sided; brief, if not fleeting; unrelated to exertion but aggravated by position, especially the left lateral decubitus; awakens the patient from sleep; and is relieved with an upright position.[6,20] The pain associated with *partial* absence of the left pericardium (see Figure 5-1) is attributed to herniation of the left atrial appendage through the pericardial defect. The pain associated with complete absence of the pericardium (see Figure 5-2) is believed to originate from torsion of the thoracic inlet.[20] In light of evidence of transient compression of coronary arteries, myocardial ischemia is also a consideration.[21,22]

Additional symptoms include dyspnea, palpitations, dizziness, syncope, and most ominously, sudden death.

Familial congenital partial absence of the left pericardium has been reported.[7] The male:female prevalence ratio is reportedly 3:1. Longevity is not affected by congenital partial absence of the pericardium[20] but has not been established with congenital complete absence. However, one patient reportedly survived to the eighth decade.[23]

PHYSICAL APPEARANCE

Congenital partial absence of the left pericardium has been reported with abnormal facies and growth hormone deficiency[24] and with VATER defects (*V*, vertebral defects; *A*, anal atresia; *T*, tracheo; *E*, esophageal fistula; *R*, radial atresia and renal dysplasia).[25]

ARTERIAL PULSE AND JUGULAR VENOUS PULSE

The *arterial pulse* is normal with congenital complete absence of the pericardium despite alternans of diastolic pressure.[19] The *jugular venous pulse* is normal with

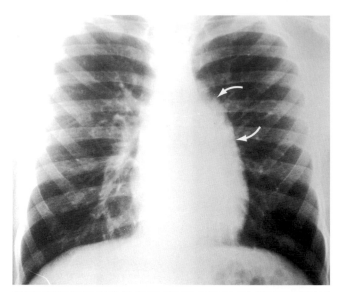

FIGURE 5-1 X-ray from a 12-year-old girl with congenital partial absence of the pericardium. Note the typical localized convexity of a protruding left atrial appendage *(arrows)*. The x-ray is otherwise normal.

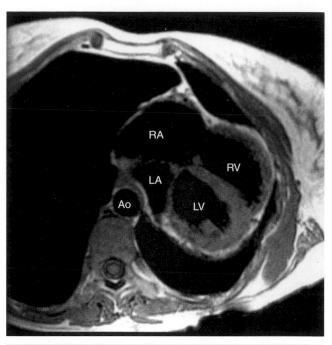

FIGURE 5-2 Magnetic resonance image with axial view from a 38-year-old woman with congenital complete absence of the pericardium and hypoplasia of the left lower lobe and the left pulmonary artery (see Figure 5-3). The strikingly mobile heart is displaced far into the left thoracic cavity. (LA/RA = left and right atrium; LV/RV = left and right ventricle; Ao = aorta.)

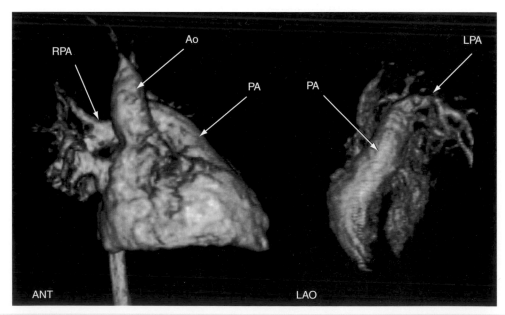

FIGURE 5-3 Three-dimensional reconstruction of gadolinium-enhanced magnetic resonance angiography of the heart and great arteries from the 38-year-old woman with congenital complete absence of the pericardium with hypoplasia of the left lower lobe and left pulmonary artery (see Figure 5-2 for magnetic resonance image). The left anterior oblique view (LAO) discloses a hypoplastic left pulmonary artery (LPA). The anterior view (ANT) discloses a well-formed main pulmonary artery (PA) and a well-formed right pulmonary artery (RPA). (Ao = ascending aorta.)

congenital *partial* absence of the pericardium and is normal with congenital *complete* absence, despite the decrease in contact stress exerted on the right atrium and right ventricle.

PRECORDIAL MOVEMENT AND PALPATION

With congenital partial absence of the left pericardium, the position and movements of the heart are normal. With complete absence, a striking mobility of the heart shifts dramatically to the left (see Figure 5-2), a position that can be detected with percussion. Displacement is accompanied by major rotation (see Figure 5-2),[6] so identification of a left or right ventricular impulse is not feasible.

AUSCULTATION

Congenital complete absence of the pericardium is accompanied by torsion of the thoracic inlet and great arteries that may generate basal midsystolic murmurs, especially in the left lateral decubitus position.

ELECTROCARDIOGRAM

With congenital *partial* absence of the left pericardium, the electrocardiogram results are normal because the heart is not displaced and is inherently normal apart from the pericardial defect. With congenital *complete* absence of the pericardium, standard precordial lead placements show delayed transition that reflects the leftward position of the heart.[4] Axis deviation, generally right, probably results from rotation.[4] Incomplete right bundle branch block is frequently mentioned.[4] Individual reports are found of complete heart block[26] and sinus node dysfunction.[27]

X-RAY

The posteroanterior chest x-ray is a major key to the diagnosis and was the basis for the earliest clinical recognition of congenital absence of the pericardium.[3] Congenital *partial* absence of the left pericardium is accompanied by herniation of the left atrial appendage, represented in the x-ray by a convexity immediately below the pulmonary trunk or, if herniation is larger, by extension of the convexity to the second *and* third left interspaces (see Figure 5-1). The heart is not displaced, and the cardiac silhouette is otherwise normal. The x-ray of an *intrapericardial* congenital aneurysm of the left atrial appendage (Figure 5-4)[28] is similar if not indistinguishable from the x-ray of partial absence of the left pericardium (see Figure 5-1). A *congenital pericardial cyst* typically presents as a smooth homogeneous radiodensity in the right cardiophrenic angle, touching the anterior chest wall and the anterior portion of the right hemidiaphragm (Figure 5-5).[29] The distinction between congenital partial absence of the pericardium is less clear when the cyst presents along the *left* cardiac border above the *left* hemidiaphragm.[29]

Congenital *complete* absence of the pericardium is characterized by dramatic mobility of the heart that results in striking leftward and posterior displacement (see Figure 5-5)[4] that is even more striking if hypoplasia of the left pulmonary artery and left lung coexist (Figures 5-2 and 5-6). A cardiac shadow to the right of the vertebral column is absent. A tongue of lung tissue is typically interposed between the pulmonary trunk and aorta (see Figure 5-6).[4] The definitive clinical diagnosis is based on computed tomographic scan and magnetic resonance imaging (see Figure 5-2).[8,30,31]

ECHOCARDIOGRAM

The echocardiogram may strongly suggest the diagnosis of congenital absence of the pericardium and can be used to identify coexisting cardiac defects, but magnetic

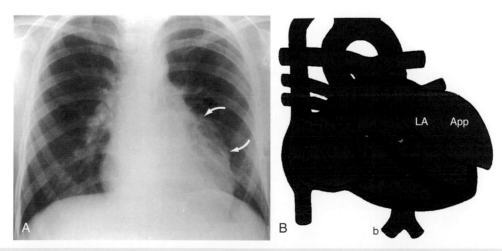

FIGURE 5-4 A, X-ray from a 10-year-old girl shows a relatively long left paracardiac convexity (arrows) caused by a congenital *intrapericardial* aneurysm of the left atrial appendage. **B,** Schematic illustration of the congenital intrapericardial aneurysm of the left atrial appendage (LAA App).

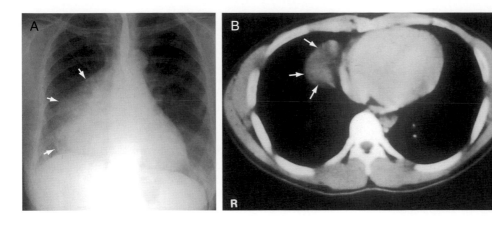

FIGURE 5-5 A, X-ray from a 23-year-old woman with an unusually large congenital pericardial cyst *(arrows)* that occupies the entire right cardiac border. **B,** Magnetic resonance image from an 18-year-old man with a typical congenital pericardial cyst *(arrows)* that originated at the right cardiophrenic angle.

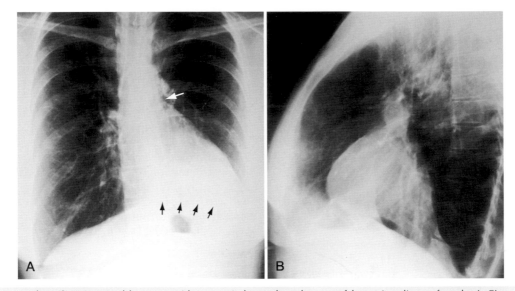

FIGURE 5-6 X-rays from the 38-year-old woman with congenital complete absence of the pericardium referred to in Figures 5-2 and 5-3. **A,** The frontal projection shows the marked leftward position of the mobile heart with no cardiac shadow to the right of the vertebral column. The leftward shift was exaggerated by hypoplasia of the left lung indicated by the elevated left hemidiaphragm *(black arrows).* The *white arrow* identifies a tongue of lung tissue interposed between the pulmonary trunk and aorta. **B,** The lateral projection shows the striking posterior position of the mobile heart.

resonance imaging and computerized tomographic scan are definitive.[32] Distinctive features of the echocardiogram in congenital *complete* absence of the pericardium are the unorthodox windows required for imaging, leftward and posterior displacement and rotation of the heart, hypermobility with an abnormal swinging movement, paradoxical motion of the ventricular septum, and enlargement of the right ventricle and right atrium.[4,33] Lack of normal pericardial constraint has a greater effect on the relatively thin-walled right ventricle, which accounts for right ventricular dilation, for a selective increase in systemic venous return, and for paradoxical motion of the ventricular septum.[4,18,33] Congenital *partial* absence of the pericardium is not an echocardiographic diagnosis. A fetal echocardiogram was used to detect an intrapericardial aneurysm.[34]

SUMMARY

Congenital absence of the pericardium can be partial or complete. Congenital partial absence is typically left-sided. The x-ray discloses a convex shadow in the topographic location of the left atrial appendage. The diagnosis is entertained when this abnormality is identified in a routine chest x-ray in an asymptomatic patient or in a patient who comes to attention because of chest pain. Right-sided partial absence of the pericardium is rare. Also rare is congenital *complete* absence, which typically presents in adulthood. The heart is strikingly mobile and markedly displaced to the left and posterior. Stabbing left-sided chest pain is provoked or aggravated by position, especially the left lateral decubitus. Additional symptoms include dyspnea, palpitations, dizziness, syncope, and most ominously, sudden death. Thoracic magnetic resonance imaging and computerized tomographic scan are used to make a definitive diagnosis.

REFERENCES

1. Columbus MR. De re anatomica. In: Beurlaque N, ed. Venice: 1559:265–269.
2. Baille M. On the want of a pericardium in the human body. *Transactions of the Society for Improved Medical and Chirurgical Knowledge*. 1793;1:91.
3. Ellis K, Leeds NE, Himmelstein A. Congenital deficiencies in partial pericardium: review with two new cases including successful diagnosis by plain roentgenography. *AJR Am J Roentgenol*. 1959; 82:125–137.
4. Gatzoulis MA, Munk MD, Merchant N, Van Arsdell GS, Mccrindle BW, Webb GD. Isolated congenital absence of the pericardium: clinical presentation, diagnosis, and management. *Ann Thorac Surg*. 2000;69:1209–1215.
5. Nasser WK, Helmen C, Tavel ME, Feigenbaum H, Fisch C. Congenital absence of the left pericardium. Clinical, electrocardiographic, radiographic, hemodynamic, and angiographic findings in six cases. *Circulation*. 1970;41:469–478.
6. Ratib O, Perloff JK, Williams WG. Congenital complete absence of the pericardium. *Circulation*. 2001;103:3154–3155.
7. Taysi K, Hartmann AF, Shackelford GD, Sundaram V. Congenital absence of left pericardium in a family. *Am J Med Genet*. 1985; 21:77–85.
8. Faridah Y, Julsrud PR. Congenital absence of pericardium revisited. *Int J Cardiovasc Imaging*. 2002;18:67–73.
9. Southworth H, Stevenson CS. Congenital defects of the pericardium. *Arch Intern Med*. 1938;61:223.
10. Mehta SM, Myers JL. Congenital Heart Surgery Nomenclature and Database Project: diseases of the pericardium. *Ann Thorac Surg*. 2000;69:S191–S196.
11. Van Son JA, Danielson GK, Schaff HV, Mullany CJ, Julsrud PR, Breen JF. Congenital partial and complete absence of the pericardium. *Mayo Clin Proc*. 1993;68:743–747.
12. Karakurt C, Oguz D, Karademir S, Sungur M, Ocal B. Congenital partial pericardial defect and herniated right atrial appendage: a rare anomaly. *Echocardiography*. 2006;23:784–786.
13. Cantrell JR, Haller JA, Ravitch MM. A syndrome of congenital defects involving the abdominal wall, sternum, diaphragm, pericardium, and heart. *Surg Gynecol Obstet*. 1958;107:602–614.
14. Rais-Bahrami K, Granholm T, Short BL, Eichelberger MR. Absence of pericardium in an infant with congenital diaphragmatic hernia. *Am J Perinatol*. 1995;12:172–173.
15. Vazquez-Jimenez JF, Muehler EG, Daebritz S, et al. Cantrell's syndrome: a challenge to the surgeon. *Ann Thorac Surg*. 1998; 65:1178–1185.
16. Meeker TM. Pentalogy of Cantrell: reviewing the syndrome with a case report and nursing implications. *J Perinat Neonatal Nurs*. 2009;23:186–194.
17. Tyberg JV, Smith ER. Ventricular diastole and the role of the pericardium. *Herz*. 1990;15:354–361.
18. Fukuda N, Oki T, Iuchi A, et al. Pulmonary and systemic venous flow patterns assessed by transesophageal Doppler echocardiography in congenital absence of the pericardium. *Am J Cardiol*. 1995;75:1286–1288.
19. Shah RP. Diastolic pressure alternans: a new sign in congenital absence of the pericardium. *Singapore Med J*. 2001;42:78–79.
20. Beppu S, Naito H, Matsuhisa M, Miyatake K, Nimura Y. The effects of lying position on ventricular volume in congenital absence of the pericardium. *Am Heart J*. 1990;120:1159–1166.
21. Bennett KR. Congenital foramen of the left pericardium. *Ann Thorac Surg*. 2000;70:993–998.
22. Rees AP, Risher W, Mcfadden PM, Ramee SR, White CJ. Partial congenital defect of the left pericardium: angiographic diagnosis and treatment by thoracoscopic pericardiectomy: case report. *Cathet Cardiovasc Diagn*. 1993;28:231–234.
23. Hammoudeh AJ, Kelly ME, Mekhjian H. Congenital total absence of the pericardium: case report of a 72-year-old man and review of the literature. *J Thorac Cardiovasc Surg*. 1995;109:805–807.
24. Boscherini B, Galasso C, Bitti ML. Abnormal face, congenital absence of the left pericardium, mental retardation, and growth hormone deficiency. *Am J Med Genet*. 1994;49:111–113.
25. Lu C, Ridker PM. Echocardiographic diagnosis of congenital absence of the pericardium in a patient with VATER association defects. *Clin Cardiol*. 1994;17:503–504.
26. Varriale P, Rossi P, Grace WJ. Congenital absence of the left pericardium and complete heart block. Report of a case. *Dis Chest*. 1967;52:405–410.
27. Hano O, Baba T, Hayano M, Yano K. Congenital defect of the left pericardium with sick sinus syndrome. *Am Heart J*. 1996;132: 1293–1295.
28. Tanabe T, Ishizaka M, Ohta S, Sugie S. Intrapericardial aneurysm of the left atrial appendage. *Thorax*. 1980;35:151–153.
29. Feigin DS, Fenoglio JJ, Mcallister HA, Madewell JE. Pericardial cysts. A radiologic-pathologic correlation and review. *Radiology*. 1977;125:15–20.
30. Bogaert J, Francone M. Cardiovascular magnetic resonance in pericardial diseases. *J Cardiovasc Magn Reson*. 2009;11:14.
31. Kim JS, Kim HH, Yoon Y. Imaging of pericardial diseases. *Clin Radiol*. 2007;62:626–631.
32. Centola M, Longo M, De Marco F, Cremonesi G, Marconi M, Danzi GB. Does echocardiography play a role in the clinical diagnosis of congenital absence of pericardium? A case presentation and a systematic review. *J Cardiovasc Med*. 2009;10:687–692.
33. Connolly HM, Click RL, Schattenberg TT, Seward JB, Tajik AJ. Congenital absence of the pericardium: echocardiography as a diagnostic tool. *J Am Soc Echocardiogr*. 1995;8:87–92.
34. Fountain-Dommer RR, Wiles HB, Shuler CO, Bradley SM, Shirali GS. Recognition of left atrial aneurysm by fetal echocardiography. *Circulation*. 2000;102:2282–2283.

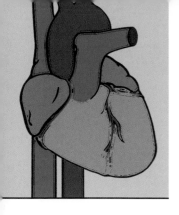

Chapter 6

Congenitally Corrected Transposition of the Great Arteries

More than a century elapsed before Karl von Rokitansky[1] applied the term *corrected* to a hitherto undescribed form of transposition of the great arteries: "The left atrioventricular valve and the left-sided ventricle resembled the usual right atrioventricular valve and right ventricle. The aorta is positioned somewhat left and anterior.... The right-sided ventricle ... is finely trabeculated, as usually seen in the left-sided ventricle. The venous atrioventricular ostium has a bivalve. From the right-sided ventricle arises a somewhat right and posteriorly positioned pulmonary artery.... The atria are normal, a right caval atrium and a left pulmonary venous atrium."

At the end of the 18th century, Mathew Baille[2] described a singular malformation characterized by discordant origins of the arterial trunks from the ventricular mass. In 1957, Anderson and coworkers described the clinical manifestations of Rokitansky's singular malformation; and 4 years later, Schiebler and coworkers[3] changed the term *corrected* to *congenitally corrected* to clarify that the correction was a gift of God and not a gift of the surgeon. The reader is referred to three seminal publications.[4-6]

Transposition of the great arteries is characterized by chambers that are joined *concordantly* at the atrioventricular junction but *discordantly* at the ventriculo-great arterial junction (see Chapter 27).[7,8] The pulmonary artery arises from a morphologic left ventricle, and the aorta arises from a morphologic right ventricle. The circulations are in parallel rather than in series. *Congenitally corrected transposition* is characterized by chambers that are joined discordantly at the atrioventricular junction and ventricles that are joined discordantly at the ventriculo-great arterial junction; atrioventricular alignments and ventriculoarterial alignments are both discordant (Figures 6-1 and 6-2).[3,4,9] The *double discordance*—atrioventricular and ventriculoarterial—*physiologically corrects* the discordance intrinsic to each (see Figure 6-1). Blood from a morphologic right atrium reaches the pulmonary artery by traversing a morphologic mitral valve and a morphologic left ventricle, and blood from a morphologic left atrium reaches the aorta by traversing a morphologic tricuspid valve and a morphologic right ventricle (Figures 6-1 and 6-3).[3,4,9] The terms *atrioventricular discordance, l-transposition, ventricular inversion*, and *congenitally corrected transposition* are used interchangeably. Atrioventricular discordance requires the presence of two morphologically distinct atria and two morphologically distinct ventricles. Hearts in which two morphologically distinct atria are aligned with one

ventricle (univentricular atrioventricular connection) are the subject of Chapter 26.

The terms used in this chapter were defined in Chapter 3 but are repeated here for the reader's convenience.

Transposition: Discordant origin of the arterial trunks from the ventricular mass. The aorta arises discordantly from a morphologic right ventricle, and the pulmonary trunk arises discordantly from a morphologic left ventricle. The pulmonary circulation and the systemic circulations are in parallel.

Congenitally corrected transposition: A morphologic right atrium is discordantly aligned with a morphologic left ventricle from which the pulmonary artery arises, and a morphologic left atrium is discordantly aligned with a morphologic right ventricle from which the aorta arises (see Figures 6-1 and 6-3). Systemic venous blood from the right atrium finds its way into the pulmonary artery, and pulmonary venous blood from the left atrium finds its way into the aorta, so the circulation is physiologically corrected. The pulmonary circulation and the systemic circulations are in series.

Ventricular inversion refers to atrioventricular discordance with ventriculoarterial concordance. A morphologic right atrium is aligned with a morphologic left ventricle that gives rise to the aorta, and a morphologic left atrium is aligned with a morphologic right ventricle that gives rise to the pulmonary trunk.[10,11]

l-Transposition: An l-loop in *situs solitus*. The sinus or inflow portion of the morphologic right ventricle is to the left of the morphologic left ventricle.

Inversion: Reversal of position but not mirror image. *Ventricular* inversion refers to a morphologic left ventricle in the right side of the heart and a morphologic right ventricle in the left side of the heart. Morphologic tricuspid and mitral valves are concordant with morphologic right and left ventricles, so inversion of the ventricles implies inversion of the atrioventricular valves. *Isolated infundibuloarterial inversion* is a rare anomaly in which the infundibulum and great arteries are inverted but the atria and ventricles are not inverted.[12] The inverted pulmonary trunk and its subpulmonary infundibulun originate from the morphologic left ventricle, and the inverted aorta originates from a morphologic right ventricle, so the physiology of the circulation is analogous to complete transposition of the great arteries (see Chapter 27).

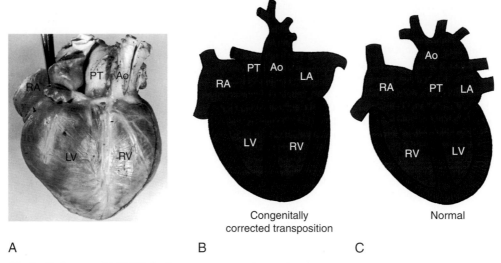

Congenitally
corrected transposition

Normal

A   B   C

FIGURE 6-1 A, Gross specimen of congenitally corrected transposition of the great arteries illustrates ventriculoarterial discordance. The pulmonary trunk originates from the morphologic left ventricle (LV) and the aorta (Ao) originates from the morphologic right ventricle (RV). **B** and **C,** Illustrations of congenitally corrected transposition of the great arteries for comparison with the normal heart. Congenitally corrected transposition is characterized by *atrioventricular discordance* and *ventriculoarterial discordance*. Blood from a morphologic *right* atrium (RA) traverses a morphologic *mitral* valve into a morphologic *left* ventricle (LV) and then enters a *pulmonary trunk* (PT) that is rightward and posterior. Blood from a morphologic *left* atrium (LA) traverses a morphologic *tricuspid* valve into a morphologic *right* ventricle (RV) and then enters an *aorta* (Ao) that is leftward and anterior. The double discordance means that right atrial blood finds its way into the pulmonary artery and left atrial blood finds its way into the aorta. *Anatomic* transposition of the great arteries is *physiologically* corrected. The great arteries run parallel to each other and do not cross as in the normal heart. Coexisting anomalies include a malformed left atrioventricular valve, a ventricular septal defect, and pulmonary stenosis. **B,** The normal heart is characterized by atrioventricular concordance, ventriculoarterial concordance, and a pulmonary artery that crosses anterior to the aorta.

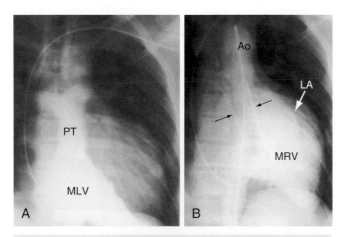

FIGURE 6-2 Angiocardiograms (anteroposterior) from a 34-year-old man with congenitally corrected transposition of the great arteries and a moderately incompetent left atrioventricular valve. **A,** Contrast material opacifies a morphologic left ventricle (MLV) from which a rightward and posterior pulmonary trunk arises (PT). **B,** Contrast material outlines a hump-shaped crescent morphologic right ventricle (MRV) from which a leftward and anterior ascending aorta (Ao) arises. Catheters in the pulmonary trunk and ascending aorta run parallel to each other and do not cross. The left atrium (LA) opacifies because of left atrioventricular valve regurgitation.

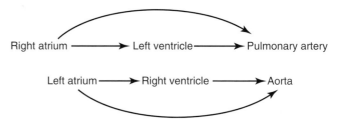

FIGURE 6-3 Simplified schematic illustration of the circulation in congenitally corrected transposition of the great arteries.

Chamber designations: *Right atrium* and *left atrium* and *right ventricle* and *left ventricle* refer to *anatomic* (morphologic) characteristics, not to position.

The great arteries: The ascending aorta and pulmonary trunk are defined by their ventricle of origin *and* by their lateral and anteroposterior spatial relationships.

d-Loop: Refers to the normal rightward (dextro = d) bend or loop in the developing straight heart tube of the embryo; indicates that the sinus or inflow portion of the morphologic right ventricle lies to the *right* of the morphologic left ventricle.

l-Loop: Refers to a leftward (levo = l) bend or loop in the straight heart tube of the embryo; indicates that the sinus or inflow portion of the morphologic right ventricle lies to the *left* of the morphologic left ventricle.

Concordant: Harmonious, appropriate.

Discordant: Disharmonious, inappropriate.

Discordant loop: An l-loop in *situs solitus* and a d-loop in *situs inversus*.

Atrioventricular discordance: Alignment of a morphologic right atrium with a morphologic left ventricle and alignment of a morphologic left atrium with a morphologic right ventricle.

Ventriculoarterial discordance: Origin of the pulmonary trunk from a morphologic left ventricle and origin of the aorta from a morphologic right ventricle.

Criss-cross hearts: Described by Lev and Rowlatt in 1961[13] and so-named by Anderson, Shinebourne, and Gerlis in 1974.[14] In normal hearts, the atrioventricular connections (inflow tracts) are parallel to each other when viewed from the front. In criss-cross hearts, the atrioventricular connections are not parallel but are angulated as much as 90 degrees.[14] Criss-cross hearts result from abnormal rotation of the ventricular mass around its long axis, resulting in relationships that could not be inferred from the inflow tracts. Several types of criss cross hearts exist. Those with discordant atrioventricular alignments and concordant ventriculoarterial alignments are called *isolated ventricular inversion* (see previous discussion). The physiology of the circulation is analogous to complete transposition of the great arteries.[10] Criss-cross hearts with ventricles that are in a *superoinferior* or *upstairs-downstairs* relationship reflect rotation of the ventricular mass along its *horizontal*. Criss-cross hearts and superoinferior ventricles may coexist (Figure 6-31) or occur separately. Morphologic patterns in criss-cross hearts include deficiency of the subpulmonary infundibulum, subpulmonary stenosis, a subaortic

infundibulum, a nonrestrictive ventricular septal defect, and visceroatrial *situs solitus*.[15]

Segmental approach: Analysis according to the heart's three major developmental segments: 1, visceroatrial situs; 2, ventricular loop; and 3, conotruncus. The atrioventricular valves and the infundibulum are the two connecting cardiac segments.

Congenitally corrected transposition of the great arteries typically occurs in *situs solitus*. The estimated prevalence rate is 0.5% of clinically diagnosed congenital malformations of the heart or approximately 1 in 13,000 live births.[16,17] Virtually all patients have coexisting cardiac malformations—ventricular septal defect, pulmonary stenosis, abnormalities of the left atrioventricular (AV) valve, and conduction defects.

The coronary artery arrangement is an important morphologic aspect of congenitally corrected transposition.[7] The Leiden Convention proposed a means of relating the origins of the coronary arteries to the aortic sinuses from which they originate.[7,18] The coronary arteries almost always arise from both, or one or the other, aortic sinuses that are adjacent to the pulmonary trunk[7] and are *morphologically concordant with the ventricles* (i.e., the right coronary artery perfuses the morphologic right ventricle and the left coronary artery perfuses the morphologic left ventricle; Figure 6-4; see Chapter 32).[3,4,19–22] Epicardial distribution is a guide to ventricular inversion because the course of the anterior descending artery establishes the location of the ventricular septum. Coronary artery abnormalities are common,[22] especially a single coronary artery (see Chapter 32).[20]

In congenitally corrected transposition of the great arteries, the anterior and leftward ascending aorta and the posterior and rightward pulmonary trunk are parallel and do not cross as in the normal heart[3] (see Figures 6-1 and 6-2). The aorta is either convex to the left or ascends vertically but is not border forming on the right. A subaortic conus is responsible for the anterior and leftward position

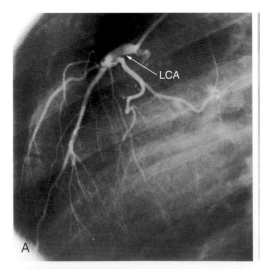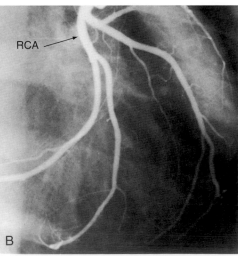

FIGURE 6-1 Coronary arteriograms from a 41-year-old man with congenitally corrected transposition of the great arteries. **A,** The left anterior oblique shows a morphologic *left* coronary artery (LCA) concordant with a morphologic *left* ventricle. **B,** The right anterior oblique shows a morphologic *right* coronary artery (RCA) concordant with a morphologic *right* ventricle.

of the ascending aorta and the posterior and medial position of the pulmonary trunk.[23] *Anatomically corrected malposition* refers to an anomaly in which the ascending aorta lies anterior and to the left of the pulmonary trunk in the presence of atrioventricular and ventriculoarterial concordance.[23,24]

The embryologic basis held responsible for atrioventricular discordance in congenitally corrected transposition resides in the *ventricular l-loop* of the embryonic heart tube. When the heart tube bends to the left in *situs solitus*, the morphologic right ventricle lies to the left of the morphologic left ventricle. The developing left atrium becomes aligned with the morphologic right ventricle, and the developing right atrium becomes aligned with the morphologic left ventricle. *Ventriculoarterial discordance* has a less well-defined embryologic basis, with one school of thought arguing that the developmental fault is in the infundibular segment of the embryonic heart tube and the other school arguing that the fault lies in the arterial segment of the embryonic heart tube.

The *physiologic consequences* of congenitally corrected transposition depend on the functional adequacy of a subaortic morphologic right ventricle and on coexisting congenital malformations.[4,16,25] The thick-walled subaortic right ventricle is concordant with a right coronary artery that is designed to perfuse a thin-walled low-resistance right ventricle. A normal subpulmonary right ventricle is designed to serve the low-resistance pulmonary circulation, and its geometry remains unchanged when it is inverted to the subaortic position. Regional strain, twist, and radial wall motion in a subaortic right ventricle differ considerably from a subaortic left ventricle.[26] An inverted subaortic right ventricle has a high prevalence of myocardial perfusion defects and abnormalities of regional wall motion.[27] A normal subpulmonary right ventricle has a relatively high end-diastolic volume, so normal stroke volumes are achieved with ejection fractions of 35% to 45%.[16,25] Importantly, the low ejection fraction does not increase when a morphologic right ventricle is inverted into the subaortic position, so the ejection fraction is considerably less than that of a normal subaortic left ventricle[16,25] and response to supine exercise is similar to the response of a *noninverted* right ventricle.[16,25] Ventricular septal defect, pulmonary stenosis, abnormalities of the left AV valve, and conduction defects have a considerable impact on the function of an inherently inadequate inverted right ventricle.[3,4]

A *ventricular septal defect* is present in 78% of necropsy cases (Figure 6-5), is usually nonrestrictive perimembranous, and typically extends into the inlet and trabecular septum.[4] The inlet septum is poorly aligned with the atrial septum, which results in a malalignment gap that is sometimes filled by tissue from the membranous septum. *Pulmonary stenosis or atresia* occurs in 50% of cases and represents obstruction to outflow of the morphologic *left* ventricle.[4] The stenosis is isolated in about 20% of cases and occurs with a ventricular septal defect in the remaining 80%. Fixed *subpulmonary stenosis*[4] takes several forms: (1) a fibrous subpulmonary diaphragm attached to the mitral valve, analogous to fixed subaortic stenosis in hearts with noninverted ventricles;

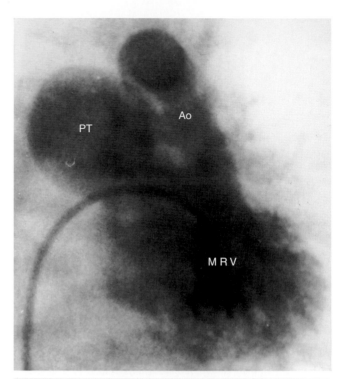

FIGURE 6-5 Angiocardiogram from a 4-year-old boy with congenitally corrected transposition of the great arteries and a nonrestrictive ventricular septal defect. The systemic ventricle has the shape and the coarse trabecular pattern of a morphologic right ventricle (MRV) and gives rise to an ascending aorta (Ao) that is convex to the left. An enlarged pulmonary trunk (PT) is visualized via the ventricular septal defect.

(2) aneurysms or fibrous tissue tags that originate from the relatively large membranous septum; and (3) accessory mitral leaflet tissue.[3] *Subaortic stenosis* (obstruction to outflow of the *morphologic right ventricle*) is caused by anterior deviation of the infundibulum septum or by hypertrophied infundibular muscle bundles.[1]

Abnormalities of the inverted *left atrioventricular valve* are present in more than 90% of cases.[4] The malformed valve usually functions normally in early life, but an age-related increase in regurgitation is seen. The abnormalities resemble those of Ebstein's anomaly of a right-sided tricuspid valve in hearts without ventricular inversion (Figure 6-6A),[3,4,28] but the anterior leaflet of the inverted Ebstein's valve is usually small and malformed[28] and the atrialized portion of the inverted right ventricle is poorly developed.[28] Left atrioventricular valve incompetence is not necessarily caused by an Ebstein's-like malformation, and the valve is occasionally stenotic rather than incompetent (see Chapter 13). Neonates with severe regurgitation of the inverted atrioventricular valve have an increased incidence of hypoplastic aortic arch, aortic atresia, and aortic coarctation.[29] Abnormalities of the *right-sided inverted mitral valve* have been reported in more than half of necropsy specimens and consist of multiple cusps, multiple or compound papillary muscles, anomalous chordal attachments, and a cleft valve or a common valve.[30]

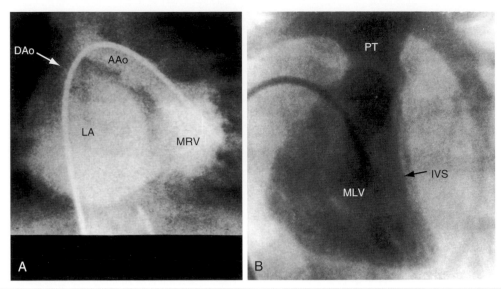

FIGURE 6-6 A, Angiocardiogram with contrast material injected into the small morphologic right ventricle (MRV) of a 7-month-old male with congenitally corrected transposition of the great arteries and severe incompetence of the left atrioventricular valve. Regurgitant flow opacifies a huge left atrium (LA). The ascending aorta (AAo) originates from the morphologic right ventricle, is convex to the left, and continues as a right-sided descending aorta (DAo). **B,** Angiocardiogram with contrast material injected into the morphologic left ventricle (MLV) of a 4-year-old boy with congenitally corrected transposition of the great arteries and no coexisting malformations. The plane of the interventricular septum (IVS) is vertical and close to the left sternal border. The morphologic left ventricle is finely trabeculated and gives rise to a rightward and posterior pulmonary trunk (PT) with right and left branches at the same level.

HISTORY

The male:female ratio is approximately 1.5:1.[3] The occurrence of congenitally corrected transposition and complete transposition among first-degree relatives in different families is believed to represent monogenic transmission and implies a pathogenetic link between the two malformations.[31,32] Symptoms and clinical course depend chiefly on the presence and degree of coexisting malformations (see previous discussion), but longevity principally hinges on the vulnerability of the subaortic morphologic right ventricle, even with no coexisting malformations.[33–35] Infant mortality is related to congestive heart failure. Survival is then relatively constant, with an attrition rate of approximately 1% to 2% year.[36] Young patients with isolated congenitally corrected transposition are often overlooked because symptoms are absent and clinical signs are subtle.[3] The diagnosis may come to light because of abnormalities in an x-ray (Figure 6-7) or an electrocardiogram (Figure 6-20) or because of symptomatic complete heart block (Figure 6-8).[3,37,38] High-degree heart block rarely occurs *in utero* but is occasionally present shortly after birth (see Figure 6-8),[39,40] or may announce itself later as a Stokes-Adams attack or sudden death.[39,41] The age-related risk of development of complete heart block is about 2% per year.[39] Left atrioventricular valve regurgitation is closely coupled to long-term survival.[36,38] The regurgitation is usually occult in infants, so late appearance prompts a mistaken diagnosis of acquired mitral regurgitation.

Survival to the sixth or seventh decade is infrequent,[3,17,21,33,42,43] but two patients reached their eighth decade.[36,44] In isolated congenitally corrected

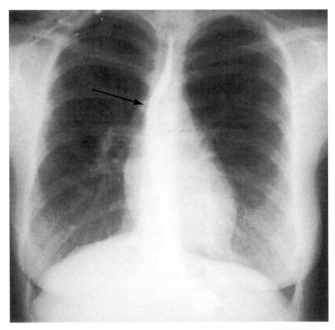

FIGURE 6-7 X-ray from a 23-year-old woman with congenitally corrected transposition of the great arteries and no coexisting malformations. The x-ray appears normal except for subtle evidence of an inverted ascending aorta that straightened the left superior cardiac border and a long indentation of the barium esophagram (*black arrow*).

transposition, failure of the subaortic right ventricle is uncommon but not rare and may occur during pregnancy in previously asymptomatic women.[45] Myocardial perfusion defects are prevalent.[27] Angina pectoris is attributed to a supply-demand imbalance between a

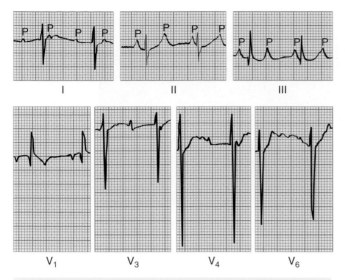

FIGURE 6-8 Electrocardiogram from a 20-month-old male with congenitally corrected transposition of the great arteries and complete heart block. P waves are independent of the narrow QRS complexes. Because of reversed septal depolarization, a prominent Q wave appears in lead V_1 but no Q wave appears in lead V_6.

thick-walled systemic right ventricle and its blood supply from a morphologic right coronary artery (see previous discussion).

The ventricular septal defect that accompanies congenitally corrected transposition is typically nonrestrictive with a clinical course analogous to a ventricular septal defect of analogous size in normally formed hearts (see Chapter 17).[3] Pulmonary stenosis exerts a protective effect by curtailing excessive pulmonary blood flow. An inverted subpulmonary left ventricle adapts to the systemic systolic pressure incurred by a nonrestrictive ventricular septal defect. Isolated *pulmonary stenosis* varies from mild to severe and has a clinical course analogous to equivalent pulmonary stenosis in hearts without ventricular inversion (see Chapter 11).

PHYSICAL APPEARANCE

Retarded growth and development are reserved for infants with a large ventricular septal defect and congestive heart failure. Cyanosis and clubbing appear when pulmonary stenosis or pulmonary vascular disease reverses the shunt.

ARTERIAL PULSE

Wave form is normal. Pulse rate reflects the bradycardia of 2/1 heart block or complete heart block (see section The Electrocardiogram).

JUGULAR VENOUS PULSE

PR interval prolongation is recognized by an increase in the interval between the jugular A wave and the carotid pulse, two-to-one heart block is recognized by A waves that occur with twice the frequency of the carotid pulse, and complete heart block is recognized by independent jugular A waves and random cannon A waves (see Chapter 4).[46]

Pulmonary stenosis is associated with A wave amplitudes that vary with the severity, as in isolated pulmonary stenosis in hearts without ventricular inversion (see Chapter 11). Pulmonary stenosis with a nonrestrictive ventricular septal defect is accompanied by a normal jugular venous pulse as in Fallot's tetralogy (see Chapter 18).

PRECORDIAL MOVEMENT AND PALPATION

Precordial movements are influenced by the spatial orientation of the ventricular septum and by the anterior and leftward position of the ascending aorta. The plane of the ventricular septum faces forward, and a vertical interventricular sulcus is closely aligned with the left sternal border (Figure 6-6B).[3,47] Accordingly, an inverted right ventricle occupies an anterior and leftward position, with its medial border adjacent to the left sternal edge and its lateral border at the apex (see Figure 6-2B), an arrangement that accounts for the large topographic area occupied by the right ventricular impulse, which is accentuated by left atrioventricular valve regurgitation and systolic expansion of the left atrium that causes anterior displacement of the heart (see Figure 6-6A). No retraction exists *medial* to the interventricular sulcus because the sulcus lies too close to the left sternal border (see Figure 6-6B). The inverted left ventricle occupies a posterior and rightward position behind the sternum[3] and cannot be palpated even in the presence of pulmonary hypertension or pulmonary stenosis (see Figures 6-2A and 6-6B). The ascending aorta is palpated when dilated and convex to the left (see Figure 6-5). The aortic component of the second heart sound is palpated because it is accentuated by the anterior position of the aortic root (Figures 6-5 and 6-9).

AUSCULTATION

A soft first heart sound reflects the PR interval prolongation of first-degree heart block, and variation in intensity is a sign of complete heart block (see Chapter 4).[46] An ejection sound at the left base (Figure 6-13B) originates in the anterior aorta, especially when the aortic root is dilated (see Figure 6-5). A short soft basal midsystolic murmur originates in the anterior aorta but may also originate in the posterior pulmonary trunk across the deeply wedged outflow tract of the morphologic left ventricle. The second heart sound is loud because the aortic valve is anterior (see section Palpation; see Figure 6-13B).[3,48] The loudness and location of the sound invite the mistaken diagnosis of pulmonary hypertension. The pulmonary component is attenuated by the posterior position of the pulmonary trunk, which makes splitting difficult to detect. When splitting is detected, it is heard in the second left interspace, despite the rightward position

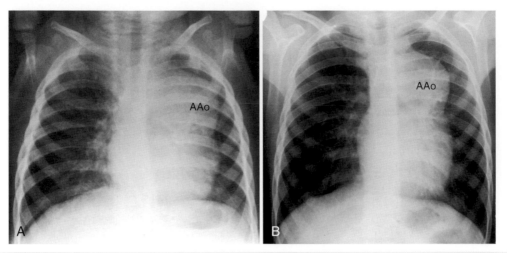

FIGURE 6-9 Virtually identical x-rays at ages 4 months **(A)** and 16 years **(B)** from a patient with congenitally corrected transposition of the great arteries, a nonrestrictive ventricular septal defect, pulmonary atresia, and reduced pulmonary blood flow. The ascending aorta (AAo) is dilated and strikingly convex to the left. No vascular shadow is seen at the right base. The heart size is normal.

of the posterior pulmonary valve.[49] A soft, high-frequency, early diastolic murmur at the mid left sternal border is more likely to be a Graham Steell murmur (Figure 6-10) than an early diastolic murmur of aortic regurgitation. The *ventricular septal defect* murmur is holosystolic (see Figure 6-10) or decrescendo (Figure 6-11), is

absent when the shunt is reversed, and is analogous in location, configuration, and quality to the murmur of ventricular septal defect in hearts without ventricular inversion (see Chapter 17). A mid-diastolic murmur is generated by increased flow across the left atrioventricular valve when the left-to-right shunt is large

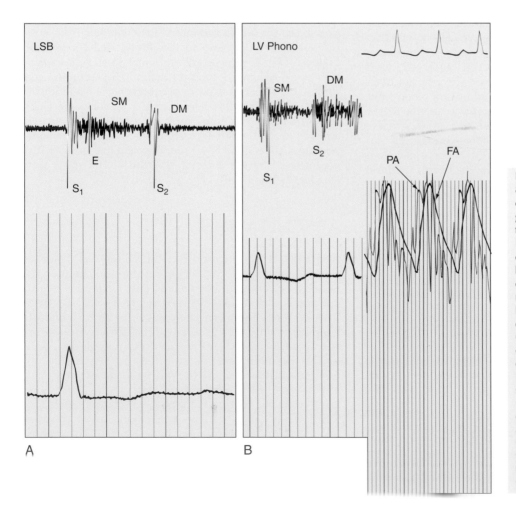

FIGURE 6-10 Tracings from an 8-year-old boy with congenitally corrected transposition of the great arteries, a nonrestrictive ventricular septal defect, and a large left-to-right shunt. **A,** Phonocardiogram from the lower left sternal border (LSB) shows a pulmonary ejection sound (E), a holosystolic murmur (SM), a loud single second heart sound (S$_2$), and an early diastolic Graham Steell murmur (DM). **B,** The intracardiac phonocardiogram (LV Phono) from the outflow tract of the subpulmonary left ventricle shows the ventricular septal defect murmur (SM) and the Graham Steell murmur (DM). Second panel shows equal pulmonary arterial (PA) and femoral arterial (FA) systolic pressures because the ventricular septal defect was nonrestrictive. (S$_1$ = first heart sound.)

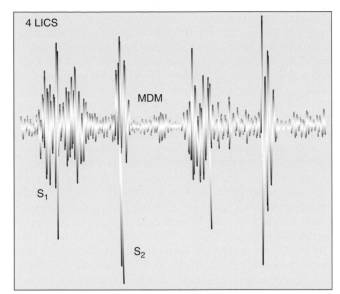

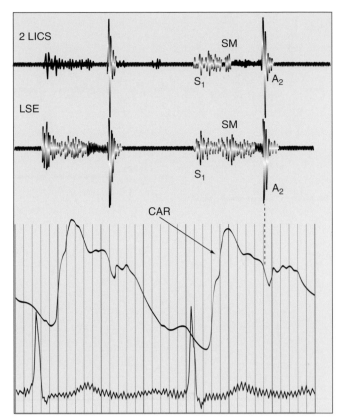

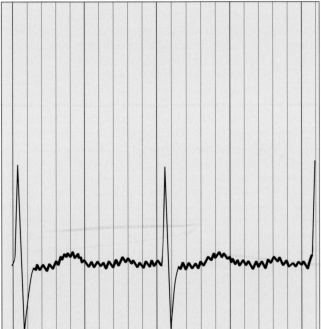

FIGURE 6-11 Phonocardiogram from the fourth left intercostal space (4 LICS) of a 4-month-old female with congenitally corrected transposition of the great arteries, a nonrestrictive ventricular septal defect, and a large left-to-right shunt. A decrescendo holosystolic murmur (SM) is followed by a loud single second heart sound (S_2) and a mid-diastolic flow murmur (MDM) across the left atrioventricular valve.

FIGURE 6-12 Tracings from a 15-year-old boy with congenitally corrected transposition of the great arteries and subpulmonary stenosis (gradient, 20 mm Hg). The pulmonary stenotic murmur (SM) is maximal at the mid left sternal edge (LSE) rather than in the second left intercostal space (2 LICS). Aortic valve closure (A_2) is loud and single because the aorta is anterior. (CAR = carotid pulse.)

(see Figure 6-11). A pulmonary ejection sound originates in a dilated hypertensive posterior pulmonary trunk (see Figures 6-5 and 6-10A). The intensity of an inherently loud aortic component of the second heart sound is augmented by pulmonary hypertension because the increased pulmonary component is synchronous with the prominent component from the anterior aortic valve (see Figures 6-10 and 6-11).

The murmur of *pulmonary stenosis* is maximal in the *third* left intercostal space because the stenosis is usually subpulmonary (Figure 6-12). It is relatively soft for a given degree of obstruction because of the attenuating effect of the anterior aorta. Radiation of the murmur is upward and to the *right* because the pulmonary trunk is oriented upward and to the right[3] (see Figure 6-2A). The loud second heart sound at the left base is aortic not pulmonary (see Figure 6-12).

Left atrioventricular valve regurgitation generates a systolic murmur analogous to mitral regurgitation in hearts without ventricular inversion (Figure 6-13).[13] Radiation tends to be toward the left sternal edge rather than into the axilla because the malformed tricuspid leaflets direct the jet medially within the left atrium. The first heart sound is not loud because in left-sided Ebstein's anomaly with congenitally corrected transposition, the malformed anterior tricuspid leaflet is small and poorly mobile.[28]

ELECTROCARDIOGRAM

In 1913, Monckeberg[50] described an anterior node that was responsible for atrioventricular conduction in congenitally corrected transposition of the great arteries. Walmsley[51] in 1931 and Yater, Lyon, and Mcnabb[52] in

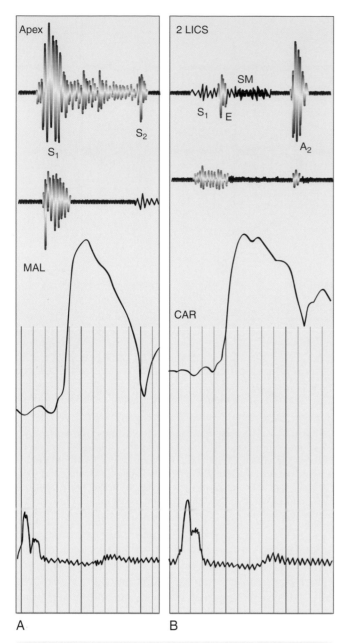

FIGURE 6-13 Tracings from a 34-year-old man with congenitally corrected transposition of the great arteries and moderate incompetence of the left atrioventricular valve. **A,** The apical decrescendo holosystolic murmur radiates poorly if at all to the axilla (MAL =midaxillary line). **B,** In the second left intercostal space, an aortic ejection sound (E) introduces a short systolic murmur (SM) and coincides with the onset of the carotid arterial pulse (CAR). Aortic valve closure (A_2) is loud and single because the aorta is anterior. (2 LICS = second left intercostal space.)

1933 established that the bundle branches were inverted. Elegant studies by Lev and Anderson[53] were major steps forward in advancing our knowledge of conduction tissues in hearts with ventricular inversion.

Because the atrial septum is malaligned with the inlet ventricular septum, the regular AV node does not make contact with infranodal right and left bundle branches. Instead, an anomalous anterior AV node with a bundle penetrates the atrioventricular fibrous annulus and descends onto the anterior aspect of the ventricular septum.[54] The penetrating atrioventricular bundle descends for a long distance down the septal surface before branching. The long penetrating atrioventricular bundle is well-formed in hearts of young children, but beginning in adolescence, the conduction fibers are replaced with fibrous tissue, which is responsible for atrioventricular block. Electrophysiologic studies have identified multiple levels of conduction defects that include the AV node, the penetrating bundle, and the bundle branches.[41] Complete heart block that is present at birth (see Figure 6-8)[54] results from discontinuity between the anterior AV node and the ventricular septum. A cordlike right bundle branch extends leftward to the morphologic right ventricle, and a left bundle branch descends down the septal surface of the morphologic left ventricle. The right bundle branch is *concordant* with the morphologic right ventricle, and the left bundle branch is *concordant* with the morphologic left ventricle. Ebstein's anomaly of left atrioventricular valve with left-sided accessory pathways provides the substrate for preexcitation between the morphologic left atrium and the morphologic right ventricle.[55] The arrhythmogenic atrialized morphologic right ventricle resides in the left side of the heart.

The *scalar electrocardiogram* exhibits three major features: 1, disturbances in conduction and rhythm; 2, QRS and T wave patterns that reflect ventricular inversion; and 3, modifications of the P wave, QRS, ST segment, and T wave caused by coexisting congenital heart disease. The P wave is normal in direction and configuration because the sinoatrial node is in its normal location, so the atria are normally activated. Broad notched left atrial P waves occur when the left atrium is volume overloaded by incompetence of the left atrioventricular valve or by a large left-to-right shunt through a ventricular septal defect (Figure 6-14). Tall peaked right atrial P waves occur with pulmonary hypertension (Figure 6-15) or pulmonary stenosis (Figure 6-16).

Atrioventricular conduction ranges from PR interval prolongation of first-degree heart block (see Figure 6-16) to complete heart block (Figures 6-8 and 6-17). More than 75% of patients with congenitally corrected transposition exhibit varying degrees of AV block when all ages are included, and the overall incidence rate of complete heart block is about 30%.[40,54,56] Normal conduction in the surface electrocardiogram coincides with normal conduction in intracardiac electrophysiologic studies and vice versa. The His electrogram does not necessarily localize the site of AV block because the long course of the nonbranching bundle precludes distinction between a distal AV nodal lesion and a proximal His bundle lesion.[54] Second-degree AV block is almost always 2/1. The degree of block varies from time to time in the same patient, and first-degree block can change to intermittent 2/1 block to complete heart block. Complete heart block is associated with a normal sequence of ventricular activation and a normal QRS duration (see Figures 6-8 and 6-17),[41] as is the case in isolated congenital complete heart block (see Chapter 4).

Accelerated conduction through bypass tracts occurs in congenitally corrected transposition with Ebstein's anomaly of the left AV valve. Delta waves in lead V_1

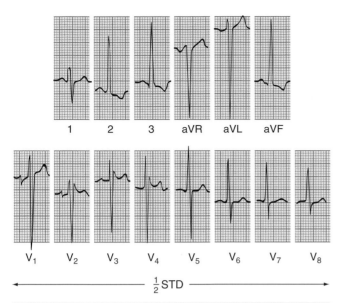

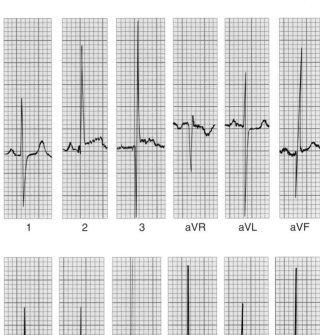

FIGURE 6-14 Electrocardiogram from an 8-year-old boy with congenitally corrected transposition of the great arteries, a nonrestrictive ventricular septal defect, and a large left-to-right shunt. Broad notched left atrial P waves appear in leads 1 and 2, and a prominent left atrial P terminal force appears in lead V_1. The QRS axis is rightward. Despite volume overload of the systemic ventricle, Q waves are absent in left precordial leads, including the lead V_8 position. T waves are upright in all precordial leads but are taller in *right* precordial leads. Large biphasic RS complexes of biventricular hypertrophy appear in leads V_{4-5}.

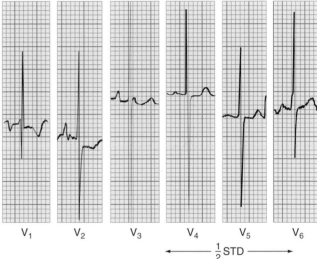

FIGURE 6-15 Electrocardiogram from a 4-month-old female with congenitally corrected transposition of the great arteries, a nonrestrictive ventricular septal defect, and a large left-to-right shunt. Peaked right atrial P waves appear in lead 2 and in lead V_{2-3}. The QRS axis is rightward. Q waves are prominent and are deeper in lead 3 than in lead aVF. Despite volume overload of the systemic ventricle, Q waves are absent in left precordial leads. Large biphasic RS complexes of biventricular hypertrophy appear in midprecordial leads.

indicate *left* bypass tracts,[54,55] and fusion beats indicate dual antegrade conduction via a bypass tract and an anterior AV node.[55] When discontinuity exists beyond the anterior AV node, antegrade conduction is occasionally achieved via an accessory pathway.[55] Supraventricular tachycardia, atrial fibrillation, and atrial flutter with left-sided Ebstein's anomaly do not necessarily coincide with the presence of Wolff-Parkinson-White accessory pathways.[54] Chronic atrial fibrillation occurs with chronic severe incompetence of the left atrioventricular valve.

QRS and T wave patterns are to be considered in light of the inverted right and left bundle branches and the coexisting cardiac malformations.[57] Activation of the ventricular septum in the normal heart proceeds from left to right, so Q waves appear in *left* precordial leads and an initial R wave appears in *right* precordial leads. In congenitally corrected transposition, the opposite is the case. Inversion of the right and left bundle branches results in reversed septal activation that proceeds from right to left. Q waves appear in right precordial leads (Figures 6-16 and 6-18 through 6-20) and are absent in left precordial leads (see Figures 6-14, 6-15, and 6-18 through 6-20). Absence of left precordial Q waves stands out in bold relief in the presence of volume overload of the systemic ventricle (see Figures 6-14 and 6-15). Presence or absence of left precordial Q waves can be confirmed with recording leads beyond the V_6 position (see Figure 6-14). Q waves in leads contiguous to lead V_1 can be detected in leads V_3R and V_4R. When supplementary lead placements are used, reversed septal activation is found in virtually all patients. An occasional

R wave in lead V_1 (see Figures 6-14 and 6-15) should not detract from the importance of consistent *absence* of Q waves in *left* precordial leads (see Figures 6-16 and 6-18 through 6-20). Septal activation in a superior direction is responsible for Q waves in leads 3 and aVF and for almost uniform absence of Q waves in leads 1 and aVL (see Figures 6-15 and 6-18 through 6-20).[3] Q waves are consistently deeper in lead 3 than in lead aVF and not uncommonly are very deep (see Figures 6-15 and 6-18 through 6-20).

Left axis deviation is diagnostically important (see Figures 6-18 through 6-20).[48,57] The mechanism responsible for the left superior axis is unsettled but cannot be the result of left anterior fascicular block because the left bundle branch is in the right side of the heart. In most cases, the atrioventricular conduction axis originates from an anomalous atrioventricular node rather

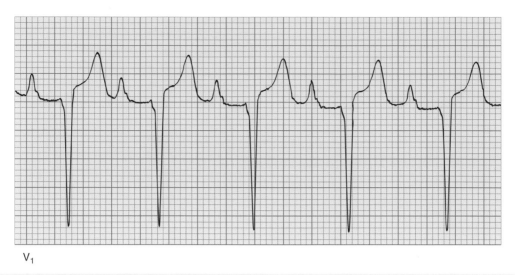

V_1

FIGURE 6-16 Lead V_1 from a 35-year-old woman with congenitally corrected transposition of the great arteries, a nonrestrictive ventricular septal defect, and subpulmonary stenosis. The P wave is tall and peaked (right atrial abnormality), the PR interval is 0.24 msec, and the QS wave indicates reversed septal depolarization.

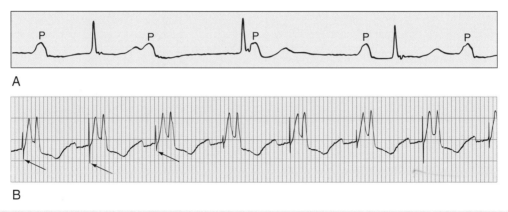

FIGURE 6-17 Monitor leads from a 41-year-old man with congenitally corrected transposition of the great arteries whose coronary arteriograms are shown in Figure 6-4. **A,** The rhythm strip identifies complete disassociation between P waves and QRS complexes that are of normal duration. **B,** Rhythm strip after insertion of a pacemaker into the subpulmonary left ventricle. *Arrows* identify the ventricular pacemaker spikes.

than the normal atrioventricular node located at the apex of the triangle of Koch.[58] Left axis deviation is most likely when systolic pressure in the subpulmonary left ventricle is not elevated (see Figures 6-18 through 6-20) and is least likely when systolic pressure is high (see Figures 6-14 and 6-15).[48,57] A left superior axis is occasionally associated with striking Q waves in leads 2, 3, and aVF and in Q waves in most if not all precordial leads (Figures 6-18, 6-20, and 6-21).

In more than 80% of cases, T waves are positive in all six precordial leads (see Figures 6-19, 6-20, and 6-21), a distinctive feature attributed to the side-by-side relationship of the inverted ventricles (see Figure 6-6). T waves are often taller in right precordial leads (see Figures 6-14, 6-17, 6-20, and 6-21).

Severe pulmonary stenosis with intact ventricular septum may produce a qR complex in lead V_1 and an rS complex in lead V_6.[57] Nonrestrictive ventricular septal defects with large left-to-right shunts are associated with large equidiphasic RS complexes in mid-precordial leads

and with increased R waves *without* Q waves in left precordial leads (see Figures 6-14 and 6-15).[57]

X-RAY

The normal heart in a posteroanterior chest x-ray is characterized by a distinctive triad of contours that consists of the ascending aorta on the right and the aortic knuckle and pulmonary trunk on the left. In congenitally corrected transposition, this triad is lost because the aorta does not ascend on the right and the pulmonary trunk is not border forming on the left (see Figure 6-2).[59] The most common relationship of the great arteries is side by side with the ascending aorta anterior and to the left of a medially and posteriorly positioned pulmonary trunk (see Figure 6-2). These relationships can usually be recognized even when subtle. The ascending aorta at the left base varies from absent (Figures 6-22 and 6-23) to straight (see Figure 6-7) to gently concave

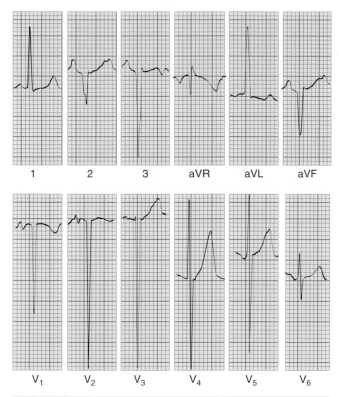

FIGURE 6-18 Electrocardiogram from a 2-year-old girl with congenitally corrected transposition of the great arteries, coarctation of the aorta, and systemic hypertension. Left axis deviation is seen. QS waves appear in leads V_{1-2}, but no Q waves are found in lead V_6 because septal depolarization is reversed. Deep S waves in right precordial leads, a tall R wave in lead aVL, and a deep S wave in lead 3 indicate hypertrophy of the after-loaded systemic subaortic right ventricle.

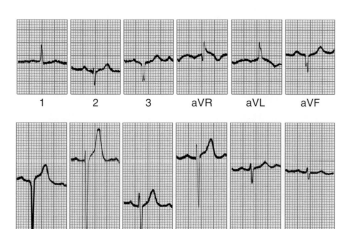

FIGURE 6-19 Electrocardiogram from a 15-year-old boy with congenitally corrected transposition of the great arteries and subpulmonary stenosis (gradient, 25 mm Hg). Left axis deviation is seen. A QS complex appears in lead V_1, but Q waves do not appear in left precordial leads because septal depolarization is reversed.

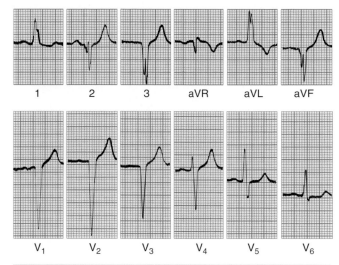

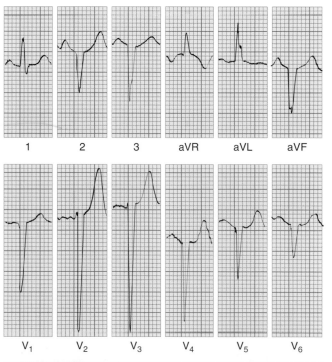

FIGURE 6-20 Electrocardiogram from a 34-year-old man with congenitally corrected transposition of the great arteries and mild incompetence of the left AV valve. Left axis deviation is seen. Prominent Q waves appear in leads 3 and aVF and in leads V_{1-3}, but no Q waves are found in left precordial leads because septal depolarization is reversed.

FIGURE 6-21 Electrocardiogram from a 23-year-old woman with congenitally corrected transposition of the great arteries and no coexisting malformations. Marked left axis deviation and marked posterior direction of ventricular depolarization result in QS waves in virtually all precordial leads.

(see Figure 6-22) to moderately convex (Figure 6-24) to strikingly convex (Figure 6-9).[9,59] Less commonly, the ascending aorta rises vertically and anterior to the posterior pulmonary trunk, so neither great artery is border forming (see Figure 6-23).

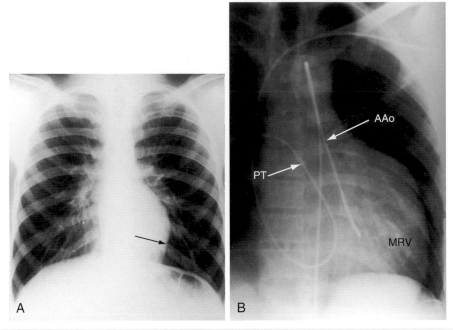

FIGURE 6-22 A, X-ray from a 15-year-old boy with congenitally corrected transposition of the great arteries and mild subpulmonary stenosis (gradient, 28 mm Hg). The left cardiac silhouette has a humped appearance and a *septal notch (arrow)*. The vascular pedicle is narrow because the ascending aorta is barely seen at the left base and is not seen at all at the right base. **B,** A retrograde femoral arterial catheter was advanced into a barely border-forming ascending aorta (AAo) and then into a hump-shaped subaortic morphologic right ventricle (MRV). A venous catheter was advanced into a subpulmonary morphologic left ventricle and then into the pulmonary trunk (PT). The ascending aorta and pulmonary trunk are parallel to each other and do not cross.

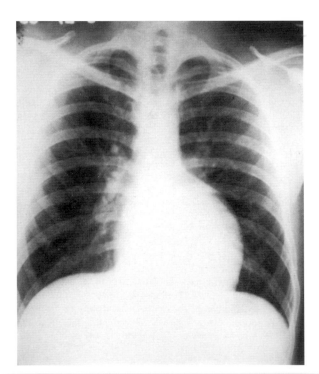

FIGURE 6-23 X-ray from a 34-year-old man with congenitally corrected transposition of the great arteries and mild incompetence of the left atrioventricular valve. The vascular pedicle is narrow because neither great artery is border forming. The left cardiac silhouette is hump-shaped.

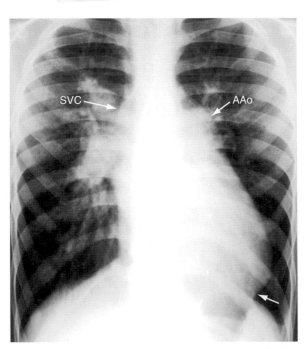

FIGURE 6-24 X-ray from an 8-year-old boy with congenitally corrected transposition of the great arteries, a nonrestrictive ventricular septal defect, and increased pulmonary blood flow. A *septal notch (unmarked arrow, lower right)* appears just above the left hemidiaphragm. The ascending aorta (AAo) is convex at the left base, and the dilated posterior pulmonary trunk causes rightward displacement of the superior vena cava (SVC).

The posterior and rightward pulmonary trunk tilts the right branch upward and the left branch downward, so that the two branches are at the same level (see Figure 6-6B).[48,59] A dilated posterior pulmonary trunk can displace the superior vena cava to the right, forming a right basal shadow (see Figure 6-24)[59] or may project as a right basal convexity that can be mistaken for the ascending aorta (Figure 6-25).[9] The leftward position of the aortic arch and proximal descending aorta produce a relatively bold indentation on the left side of the esophagus (see Figure 6-7).[59]

The silhouette of the morphologic right ventricle has two distinctive features: (1) a hump-shaped appearance caused by a prominent inverted infundibulum (see Figures 6-2B, 6-22, and 6-23);[59] and (2) a *septal notch*, which is a subtle indentation just above the left hemidiaphragm corresponding to the apical position of the interventricular groove (see Figures 6-22 and 6-24). The hump-shaped infundibular shadow occupies the site of the left atrial appendage (see Figures 6-2 and 6-23),[3] so left atrial enlargement is best identified in a lateral projection. A giant left atrium is presented as a huge ball suspended below a narrow vascular pedicle (Figure 6-26).

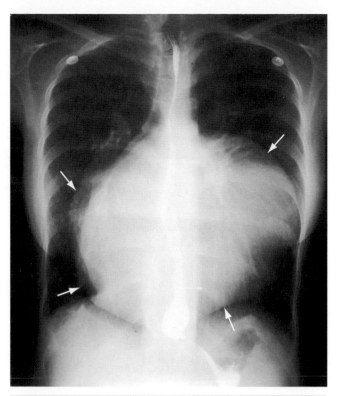

FIGURE 6-26 X-ray from a 17-year-old girl with congenitally corrected transposition of the great arteries and severe incompetence of the left atrioventricular valve. The cardiac silhouette resembles a huge suspended ball that consists almost entirely of a giant left atrium *(arrows).* Etiology of the giant left atrium may in part have been related to childhood rheumatic fever. The vascular pedicle is narrow because neither the ascending aorta nor the pulmonary trunk is border forming.

ECHOCARDIOGRAM

Echocardiography is used to identify atrioventricular and ventriculoarterial discordance, the morphologic right ventricle equipped with a tricuspid valve, the morphologic left ventricle equipped with a mitral valve, and the spatial relationships of the great arteries and their ventricles of origin, in addition to coexisting congenital heart disease. Echocardiographic criteria for determination of the morphology of a ventricular chamber and its atrioventricular valve include the level of attachment of each valve to the ventricular septum, valve leaflet configuration (bileaflet or trileaflet), papillary muscle arrangements, the presence of chordal attachments to the septum (tricuspid valve) or to the ventricular free wall (mitral valve), the type of ventricular trabeculations, the ventricular shape, and the presence or absence of fibrous continuity between mitral valve and a great artery.[60] A *morphologic left ventricle* is recognized by its ovoid or ellipsoid shape and its fine trabecular architecture (Figure 6-27), by an AV valve that inserts into the ventricular septum at a level more proximal than the septal insertion of the contralateral AV valve, by a bicommissural valve with a fish mouth appearance in diastole, by paired papillary muscles, by chordae tendineae that insert only into the ventricular free wall, and by continuity

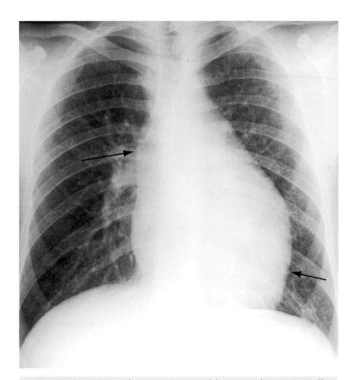

FIGURE 6-25 X-ray from a 22-year-old man with congenitally corrected transposition of the great arteries and pulmonary valve stenosis (gradient, 105 mm Hg). The convexity at the right hilus *(thin arrow)* is caused by rightward projection of the dilated posterior pulmonary trunk. An inverted ascending aorta straightens the left upper cardiac border. The cardiac silhouette is hump-shaped, and a subtle *septal notch* is found *(thick arrow).*

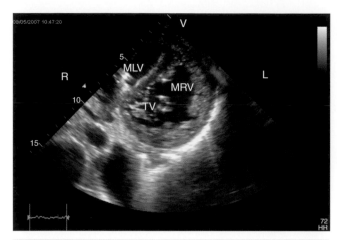

FIGURE 6-27 Echocardiogram (short axis) from a 4-year-old girl with congenitally corrected transposition of the great arteries. The morphologic right ventricle (MRV) is crescent-shaped and houses the tricuspid (TV). The morphologic left ventricle (MLV) is ovoid.

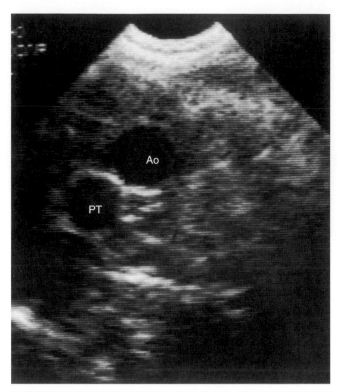

FIGURE 6-28 Echocardiogram (short axis) from a 4-year-old girl with congenitally corrected transposition of the great arteries. The figure shows cross sections of the anterior leftward aorta (Ao) and the posterior rightward pulmonary trunk (PT).

between an AV valve and a great artery. A *morphologic right ventricle* is recognized by its crescent shape and its coarse trabecular architecture, by a moderator band, by relatively distal insertion of the AV valve into the ventricular septum, by a tricommissural valve, by multiple irregular papillary muscles with chordal attachments to the ventricular septum, and by discontinuity between an AV valve and a great artery.

The crossed or spiral great arterial relationships of the *normal heart* (see Figure 6-1) are imaged in the short axis as a posterior circle, which is the aorta, and an anterior sausage, which is the right ventricular outflow tract and main pulmonary artery transected tangentially. The *transposed great arteries* of congenitally corrected transposition do not cross as in the normal heart (see Figure 6-1) and are imaged in the short axis as double circles that represent cross sections of the anterolateral aorta and poteromedial pulmonary trunk (Figure 6-28). Long-axis views image the aortic root and pulmonary trunk parallel to each other. The pulmonary trunk is identified by its bifurcation into right and left branches (Figure 6-29 and Videos 6-1 and 6-2), and the aorta is identified by its brachiocephalic branches.

A *ventricular septal defect* is typically nonrestrictive and perimembranous with extension into the inlet septum (Figure 6-29; see Chapter 17). When the defect is large, the relative levels of AV valve attachments to the ventricular septum are unreliable guides to ventricular inversion. Malformations of the left atrioventricular valve include Ebstein's anomaly (Figure 6-30 and Video 6-2) and multiple short chordae tendineae that attach to the septum and apex (see Chapter 13). Color flow imaging is used to determine the degree of left AV valve regurgitation.[61] Echocardiography with Doppler interrogation characterizes obstruction to outflow of the subpulmonary left ventricle.[4] Subpulmonary stenosis is caused by a fixed fibrous subpulmonary diaphragm, fibrous tags, a membranous septal aneurysm, or accessory mitral valve tissue.[4]

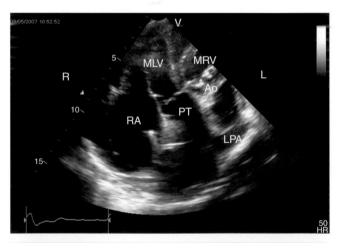

FIGURE 6-29 Echocardiogram (apical four-chamber) from a 5-year-old girl with congenitally corrected transposition of the great arteries. A morphologic right atrium (RA) is aligned with a morphologic left ventricle (MLV) that gave rise to the pulmonary trunk (PT) that is identified by its left pulmonary artery (LPA) (Videos 6-1 and 6-2). (MRV = morphologic right ventricle.)

Echocardiography defines the different types of crisscross hearts and superoinferior ventricles (Figures 6-31 and 6-32).[10] Atrioventricular discordance and ventriculoarterial discordance result in the physiology of congenitally corrected transposition.[10,15] Atrioventricular

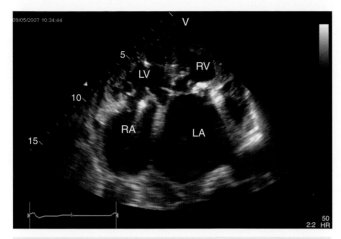

FIGURE 6-30 Echocardiogram (apical four-chamber) of a patient with congenitally corrected transposition of the great arteries (Video 6-3). (RA = Right atrium; RV = right ventricle; LA = left atrium; LV = morphologic LV.)

concordance with ventriculoarterial discordance and isolated ventricular inversion result in the physiology of complete transposition (see Figures 6-31 and 6-32).

SUMMARY

Congenitally corrected transposition of the great arteries without coexisting malformations is uncommon and initially can go unrecognized. The malformation may come to light in asymptomatic patients because of a loud second heart sound at the left base (anterior aortic valve); an electrocardiogram with PR interval prolongation, left axis deviation, reversed septal depolarization identified

by Q waves in right precordial leads but not in left precordial leads, or deep Q waves in lead 3 and lead aVF; or an x-ray with a narrow vascular pedicle, a straight left cardiac border, or a hump-shaped left cardiac silhouette. Echocardiography is used to establish ventricular inversion with atrioventricular and ventriculoarterial discordance. Congenitally corrected transposition may be

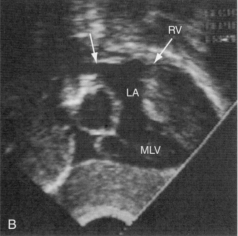

FIGURE 6-32 Echocardiogram from a 12-month-old female with a criss-cross heart. The right ventricle (RV) and left ventricle (LV) are superoinferior and harbor a nonrestrictive inlet ventricular septal defect (VSD arrow). The morphologic left atrium (LA) is concordant with a right-sided and inferior morphologic left ventricle (atrioventricular concordance). The morphologic left ventricle gives rise to the pulmonary trunk (PT), and the morphologic right ventricle gives rise to the aorta (Ao)(ventriculoarterial discordance).

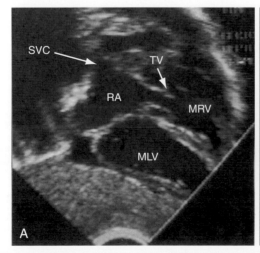

FIGURE 6-31 Echocardiograms (subcostal) in a criss-cross heart with superoinferior ventricles. **A,** The superior vena cava (SVC) joins a morphologic right atrium (RA) aligned with a concordant morphologic right ventricle (MRV) that is superior and to the left of a morphologic left ventricle (MLV). The tricuspid valve (TV) has a right-to-left orientation. **B,** Two pulmonary veins (PV; *arrows*) join the morphologic left atrium (LA), which is aligned with an inferior and rightward morphologic left ventricle (MLV). Atrioventricular *concordance* with ventriculoarterial *discordance* resulted in the physiology of complete transposition of the great arteries.

diagnosed during investigation of high-degree atrioventricular block or paroxysmal rapid heart action. Two to one heart block, especially when associated with intermittent complete heart block, is distinctive. Supraventricular tachycardia, atrial fibrillation, and atrial flutter occur with or without Ebstein's anomaly of the left atrioventricular valve. Accessory pathways are left-sided.

Ventricular septal defects are typically nonrestrictive and perimembranous and are analogous to comparable defects in hearts without ventricular inversion. Left precordial Q waves are absent despite volume overload of the systemic ventricle. The chest x-ray shows a convex shadow of the leftward ascending aorta, but the pulmonary artery segment is not border forming despite enlargement caused by increased pulmonary blood flow. The echocardiogram is used to identify atrioventricular and ventriculoarterial discordance and a large perimembranous ventricular septal.

Left atrioventricular valve regurgitation is the result of an Ebstein's-like malformation and is seldom present in infants. A holosystolic murmur may be incorrectly diagnosed as acquired mitral regurgitation, but error is avoided when the electrocardiogram exhibits PR interval prolongation, left axis deviation, and prominent Q waves in inferior leads and in right precordial leads, with absent left precordial Q waves despite volume overload of the systemic ventricle. The chest x-ray shows the ascending aorta at the left base varying in prominence from absent to straight to moderately convex to strikingly convex. Less commonly, the ascending aorta rises vertically and anterior to the posterior pulmonary trunk, so neither great artery is border forming. The posterior and rightward pulmonary trunk tilts its right branch upward and its left branch downward, so that the two branches are at the same level. A hump-shaped inverted infundibulum obscures enlargement of the left atrial appendage. The echocardiogram establishes the diagnosis of atrioventricular and ventriculoarterial discordance with left-sided Ebstein's anomaly.

Pulmonary stenosis regulates the left-to-right shunt through a ventricular septal defect. The pulmonary stenotic murmur is maximal at the mid left sternal border because the obstruction is subpulmonary, and the murmur radiates upward and to the right because of the rightward position and course of the pulmonary trunk. A loud second heart sound in the second left intercostal space is aortic because the aortic root is anterior. In the chest x-ray, the posterior pulmonary trunk is not border forming even if dilated. The echocardiogram identifies the type of pulmonary stenosis.

REFERENCES

1. Rokitansky KF. *Die Defekte der Scheidewande des Herzens*. Vienna: W. Braumuller; 1875.
2. Baille M. *The morbid anatomy of the most important parts of the human body.* 2nd ed. London: Johnson and Nicol; 1797.
3. Schiebler GL, Edwards JE, Burchell HB, Dushane JW, Ongley PA, Wood EH. Congenital corrected transposition of the great vessels: a study of 33 cases. *Pediatrics.* 1961;27(5)Suppl:849–888.
4. Allwork SP, Bentall HH, Becker AE, et al. Congenitally corrected transposition of the great arteries: morphologic study of 32 cases. *Am J Cardiol.* 1976;38:910–923.
5. Becker AE, Anderson RH. Conditions with discordant atrioventricular connections. In: Anderson RH, Shinebourne EA, eds. *Pediatric cardiology.* London: Churchill Livingstone; 1978.
6. Kurosawa H, Imai Y, Becker AE. Congenitally corrected transposition with normally positioned atria, straddling mitral valve, and isolated posterior atrioventricular node and bundle. *J Thorac Cardiovasc Surg.* 1990;99:312–313.
7. Anderson RH. Transposition—introduction. *Cardiol Young.* 2005; 15(Suppl 1):72–75.
8. Anderson RH, Weinberg PM. The clinical anatomy of transposition. *Cardiol Young.* 2005;15(Suppl 1):76–87.
9. Lester RG, Anderson RC, Amplatz K, Adams P. Roentgenologic diagnosis of congenital corrected transposition of great vessels. *Am J Roentgenol.* 1960;83:985–997.
10. Pasquini L, Sanders SP, Parness I, et al. Echocardiographic and anatomic findings in atrioventricular discordance with ventriculoarterial concordance. *Am J Cardiol.* 1988;62:1256–1262.
11. Quero-Jimenez M, Raposo-Sonnenfeld I. Isolated ventricular inversion with situs solitus. *Br Heart J.* 1975;37:293–304.
12. Foran RB, Belcourt C, Nanton MA, et al. Isolated infundibuloarterial inversion (S,D,I): a newly recognized form of congenital heart disease. *Am Heart J.* 1988;116:1337–1350.
13. Perloff JK, Roberts WC. The mitral apparatus. Functional anatomy of mitral regurgitation. *Circulation.* 1972;46:227–239.
14. Anderson RH, Shinebourne EA, Gerlis LM. Criss-cross atrioventricular relationships producing paradoxical atrioventricular concordance or discordance. Their significance to nomenclature of congenital heart disease. *Circulation.* 1974;50:176–180.
15. Hery E, Jimenez M, Didier D, et al. Echocardiographic and angiographic findings in superior-inferior cardiac ventricles. *Am J Cardiol.* 1989;63:1385–1389.
16. Benson LN, Burns R, Schwaiger M, et al. Radionuclide angiographic evaluation of ventricular function in isolated congenitally corrected transposition of the great arteries. *Am J Cardiol.* 1986;58:319–324.
17. Ikeda U, Furuse M, Suzuki O, Kimura K, Sekiguchi H, Shimada K. Long-term survival in aged patients with corrected transposition of the great arteries. *Chest.* 1992;101:1382–1385.
18. Gittenberger-De Groot AC, Sauer U, Quaegebeur J. Aortic intramural coronary artery in three hearts with transposition of the great arteries. *J Thorac Cardiovasc Surg.* 1986;91:566–571.
19. Mckay R, Anderson RH, Smith A. The coronary arteries in hearts with discordant atrioventricular connections. *J Thorac Cardiovasc Surg.* 1996;111:988–997.
20. Dabizzi RP, Barletta GA, Caprioli G, Baldrighi G, Baldrighi V. Coronary artery anatomy in corrected transposition of the great arteries. *J Am Coll Cardiol.* 1988;12:486–491.
21. Schwartz HA, Wagner PI. Corrected transposition of the great vessels in a 55-year-old woman; diagnosis by coronary angiography. *Chest.* 1974;66:190–192.
22. Ismat FA, Baldwin HS, Karl TR, Weinberg PM. Coronary anatomy in congenitally corrected transposition of the great arteries. *Int J Cardiol.* 2002;86:207–216.
23. Colli AM, De Leval M, Somerville J. Anatomically corrected malposition of the great arteries: diagnostic difficulties and surgical repair of associated lesions. *Am J Cardiol.* 1985;55:1367–1372.
24. Chen M-R. Anatomically corrected malposition of the great arteries. *Pediatr Cardiol.* 2008;29:467–468.
25. Graham Jr TP, Parrish MD, Boucek Jr RJ, et al. Assessment of ventricular size and function in congenitally corrected transposition of the great arteries. *Am J Cardiol.* 1983;51:244–251.
26. Fogel MA, Weinberg PM, Fellows KE, Hoffman EA. A study in ventricular-ventricular interaction. Single right ventricles compared with systemic right ventricles in a dual-chamber circulation. *Circulation.* 1995;92:219–230.
27. Hornung TS, Bernard EJ, Jaeggi ET, Howman-Giles RB, Celermajer DS, Hawker RE. Myocardial perfusion defects and associated systemic ventricular dysfunction in congenitally corrected transposition of the great arteries. *Heart.* 1998;80:322–326.
28. Anderson KR, Zuberbuhler JR, Anderson RH, Becker AE, Lie JT. Morphologic spectrum of Ebstein's anomaly of the heart: a review. *Mayo Clin Proc.* 1979;54:174–180.
29. Celermajer DS, Cullen S, Deanfield JE, Sullivan ID. Congenitally corrected transposition and Ebstein's anomaly of the systemic atrioventricular valve: association with aortic arch obstruction. *J Am Coll Cardiol.* 1991;18:1056–1058.

30. Gerlis LM, Wilson N, Dickinson DF. Abnormalities of the mitral valve in congenitally corrected transposition (discordant atrioventricular and ventriculoarterial connections). *Br Heart J*. 1986;55: 475–479.

31. Digilio MC, Casey B, Toscano A, et al. Complete transposition of the great arteries: patterns of congenital heart disease in familial precurrence. *Circulation*. 2001;104:2809–2814.

32. Piacentini G, Digilio MC, Capolino R, et al. Familial recurrence of heart defects in subjects with congenitally corrected transposition of the great arteries. *Am J Med Genet*. 2005;Part A. 137: 176–180.

33. Graham Jr TP, Bernard YD, Mellen BG, et al. Long-term outcome in congenitally corrected transposition of the great arteries: a multi-institutional study. *J Am Coll Cardiol*. 2000;36:255–261.

34. Skinner J, Hornung T, Rumball E. Transposition of the great arteries: from fetus to adult. *Heart*. 2008;94:1227–1235.

35. Warnes CA. Transposition of the great arteries. *Circulation*. 2006; 114:2699–2709.

36. Huhta JC, Danielson GK, Ritter DG, Ilstrup DM. Survival in atrioventricular discordance. *Pediatr Cardiol*. 1985;6:57–60.

37. Berman DA, Adicoff A. Corrected transposition of the great arteries causing complete heart block in an adult. Treatment with an artificial pacemaker. *Am J Cardiol*. 1969;24:125–129.

38. Beauchesne LM, Warnes CA, Connolly HM, Ammash NM, Tajik AJ, Danielson GK. Outcome of the unoperated adult who presents with congenitally corrected transposition of the great arteries. *J Am Coll Cardiol*. 2002;40:285–290.

39. Huhta JC, Maloney JD, Ritter DG, Ilstrup DM, Feldt RH. Complete atrioventricular block in patients with atrioventricular discordance. *Circulation*. 1983;67:1374–1377.

40. Walker WJ, Cooley DA, Mc ND, Moser RH. Corrected transposition of the great vessels, atrioventricular heart block, and ventricular septal defect: a clinical triad. *Circulation*. 1958;17:249–254.

41. Gillette PC, Busch U, Mullins CE, Mcnamara DG. Electrophysiologic studies in patients with ventricular inversion and "corrected transposition". *Circulation*. 1979;60:939–945.

42. Benchimol A, Sundararajan V. Congenital corrected transposition of the great vessels in a 58-year-old man. *Chest*. 1971;59:634–638.

43. Milici C, Bovelli D, Forlani D, et al. Images in cardiovascular medicine. An unusual case of congenitally corrected transposition of the great arteries in the elderly. *Circulation*. 2008;117:e485–e489.

44. Lieberson AD, Schumacher RR, Childress RH, Genovese PD. Corrected transposition of the great vessels in a 73-year-old man. *Circulation*. 1969;39:96–100.

45. Connolly HM, Grogan M, Warnes CA. Pregnancy among women with congenitally corrected transposition of great arteries. *J Am Coll Cardiol*. 1999;33:1692–1695.

46. Perloff JK. *Physical examination of the heart and circulation*. 4th ed. Shelton, Connecticut: People's Medical Publishing House; 2009.

47. Kraus Y, Yahini JH, Shem-Tov A, Neufeld HN. Precordial pulsations in corrected transposition of the great vessels. Diagnostic value of the electromechanical interval. *Am J Cardiol*. 1969;23: 684–689.

48. Cumming GR. Congenital corrected transposition of the great vessels without associated intracardiac anomalies. A clinical, hemodynamic and angiographic study. *Am J Cardiol*. 1962;10:605–614.

49. Gasul BM, Graettinger JS, Bucheleres G. Corrected transposition of the great vessels; demonstration of a new phonocardiographic sign of this malformation. *J Pediatr*. 1959;55:180–188.

50. Monckeberg JG. Zur Entwicklungsgeschichte des Atrioventrikularsystems. *Verh Dtsch Pathol Ges*. 1913;16:228.

51. Walmsley T. Transposition of the ventricles and the arterial stems. *J Anat*. 1931;65:528–540.

52. Yater WM, Lyon JA, Mcnabb P. Congenital heart block: review and report of the second case of complete heart block studied by serial sections through the conduction system. *JAMA*. 1933;100: 1831.

53. Anderson RH, Becker AE, Arnold R, Wilkinson JL. The conducting tissues in congenitally corrected transposition. *Circulation*. 1974; 50:911–923.

54. Daliento L, Corrado D, Buja G, John N, Nava A, Thiene G. Rhythm and conduction disturbances in isolated, congenitally corrected transposition of the great arteries. *Am J Cardiol*. 1986;58:314–318.

55. Bharati S, Rosen K, Steinfield L, Miller RA, Lev M. The anatomic substrate for preexcitation in corrected transposition. *Circulation*. 1980;62:831–842.

56. Marino B, Sanders SP, Parness IA, Colan SD. Obstruction of right ventricular inflow and outflow in corrected transposition of the great arteries (S,L,L): two-dimensional echocardiographic diagnosis. *J Am Coll Cardiol*. 1986;8:407–411.

57. Victorica BE, Miller BL, Gessner IH. Electrocardiogram and vectorcardiogram in ventricular inversion (corrected transposition). *Am Heart J*. 1973;86:733–744.

58. Anderson RH. The conduction tissues in congenitally corrected transposition. *Ann Thorac Surg*. 2004;77:1881–1882.

59. Carey LS, Ruttenberg HD. Roentgenographic features of congenital corrected transposition of the great vessels: a comparative study of 33 cases with a roentgenographic classification based on the associated malformations and hemodynamic states. *Am J Roentgenol Radium Ther Nucl Med*. 1964;92:623–651.

60. Meissner MD, Panidis IP, Eshaghpour E, Mintz GS, Ross J. Corrected transposition of the great arteries: evaluation by two-dimensional and Doppler echocardiography. *Am Heart J*. 1986; 111:599–601.

61. Lynch 3rd KP, Yan DC, Sharma S, Dhar PK, Fyfe DA. Serial echocardiographic assessment of left atrioventricular valve function in young children with ventricular inversion. *Am Heart J*. 1998; 136:94–98.

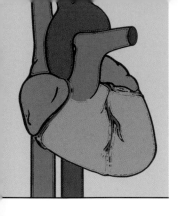

Chapter 7

Congenital Aortic Stenosis: Congenital Aortic Regurgitation

Clinical evaluation of congenital obstruction to left ventricular outflow seeks to establish the presence and degree of obstruction and the level and morphologic type.[1-6] Five varieties of congenitally abnormal aortic valves are based on the number and types of cusps and commissures (Box 7-1).[6] A *unicuspid* aortic valve is either acommissural[7] or unicommissural.[6] A *unicuspid acommissural* valve is characterized by a single leaflet with a central orifice that is usually stenotic but can be stenotic and regurgitant.[7] Traces of three rudimentary commissures do not divide the valve (Figure 7-1A, left upper).[6] This type of congenitally stenotic semilunar valve is found in the *pulmonary* location (see Chapter 11), but rarely in the aortic location.[6] A *unicommissural unicuspid* valve is characterized by a single commissural attachment to the aorta (Figures 7-1A, left middle, and 7-2A).[2,6] The single (unicuspid) leaflet originates from a single commissural attachment, proceeds across the aortic orifice without making contact with the aortic wall, bends on itself, and returns to reinsert at the same attachment site from which it originated.[2,6] Remnants of rudimentary raphes are occasionally present.[6] Viewed from above, the orifice resembles an exclamation point (see Figure 7-1A, left middle).[6] The typical unicommissural valve is intrinsically stenotic, but if the free edge is sufficiently redundant and the single commissure is not fused, obstruction is initially absent but subsequently appears when mobility is reduced by fibrosis and calcification.[2]

A *bicuspid aortic valve* is the most common congenital anomaly to which that structure is subject (see Figure 7-1A, left lower group)[1,2,6] and is the most common gross morphologic congenital abnormality of the heart or great arteries in adults.[8] Estimated frequency in the general population has been reported as 0.5% to 0.6%[9] and 0.9% to 1.36%,[10] with an overall prevalence rate in the United States of approximately four million.[4,11] The male:female ratio is 2:1. The bicuspid aortic valve is a genetic disorder, with a transmission pattern that suggests autosomal dominant inheritance.[10,12] A low prevalence rate of bicuspid aortic valve is found in African Americans.[13] Acquired calcification of a congenitally bicuspid aortic valve accounts for approximately half of surgical cases of isolated aortic stenosis in adults.[11,14] Hypercholesterolemia is an atherosclerotic risk factor for the development of calcification.[15]

The bicuspid aortic valve was first identified in the early 16th century by Leonardo da Vinci in his remarkable *Anatomical, Physiological, and Embryological Drawings,* released by Dover Publications in a facsimile edition.[16] *Normal aortic valves* are composed of a connective tissue framework of interstitial cells and a matrix covered by endothelial cells. During valvulogenesis, extracellular matrix proteins direct cell differentiation and cusp formation. Differentiation of mesenchymal cells into mature aortic valve cells correlates with the expression of the matrix protein fibrillin-1, which is deficient in bicuspid aortic valve tissue. Three morphologic types of a bicuspid aortic valve based on *cusp size* are characterized by two cusps of equal size, two cusps of unequal size, and a conjoined cusp twice the size of its nonconjoined mate.[11] Three morphologic types based on *commissural fusion* are characterized by fusion of the right and left coronary cusps (most common), fusion of the right and noncoronary cusps, and fusion of the left and noncoronary cusps (least common).[8] A false raphe can be well-formed, fenestrated, calcified, or absent.[11,17] If the free edges of the bicuspid leaflets are sufficiently long, if the cusps are thin and mobile, and if the commissures are not fused, the valve is functionally normal—unobstructed—which is the usual condition at birth (see Figure 7-1A, left lower).[4-6] Conversely, if the commissures are congenitally fused, or if the free edges of the cusps are not longer than the diameter of the aortic ring, the valve is inherently obstructed (see Figure 7-1A, left lower). Fusion of the right and left coronary cusps is strongly associated with coarctation of the aorta.[18] Fusion of the right and noncoronary cusps is associated with valve pathology.[18] Sclerosis of a bicuspid aortic valve begins as early as the second decade, and calcification as

---

BOX 7-1 CONGENITALLY ABNORMAL AORTIC VALVES

Number and Types of Cusps and Commissures

Unicuspid

A. Acommissural

B. Unicommissural

Bicuspid

Tricuspid

A. Miniature (small aortic ring)

B. Dysplastic

C. Cuspal inequality with or without equal commissures

Quadricuspid

Six-cuspid

early as the fourth decade.[19] The fibrocalcific process is more rapid in bicuspid aortic valves with cusps of unequal size because of maldistribution of tension during diastolic closure.[19] Rarely, a congenital bicuspid aortic valve is stenotic because of myxoid dysplasia.[20] Bicuspid aortic and bicuspid pulmonary valves coexist in the Syrian hamster,[21] but not in human subjects.

A functionally normal bicuspid aortic valve can continue to function normally throughout a long lifetime,[4] but more often than not, fibrocalcific thickening or acquired commissural fusion decreases mobility and renders the valve stenotic (see Figures 7-1A, left lower group,

and 7-2C).[1,4,11] Thomas Peacock[22] recognized this tendency in his *On Malformations of the Human Heart* (1858). Abnormal mechanical stress is an important factor in promotion of fibrosis and calcification of a bicuspid bicommissural aortic valve (see Figure 7-2C).[23] An important consequence of a functionally normal bicuspid aortic valve is progressive regurgitation, which may be accelerated by infective endocarditis to which a bicuspid valve is highly susceptible (see subsequent discussion). Rarely, a severely incompetent bicuspid aortic valve becomes stenotic with virtual loss of regurgitation.[24]

Dilation of the ascending aorta is consistently associated with a congenitally bicuspid aortic valve (Figures 7-1C, 7-3, and 7-4),[25–27] but the term *poststenotic dilation* is a misnomer because the ascending aorta is dilated whether the bicuspid valve is stenotic, incompetent, or functionally normal.[28] Dilation is the result of an inherent medial abnormality that expresses itself as an ascending aortic aneurysm with chronic aortic regurgitation (see Figure 7-4) or dramatically as a dissecting aneurysm (Figure 7-5).[28–32] A decrease in ascending aortic elasticity is independent of dilation.[33,34]

Trileaflet aortic valves are congenitally abnormal when three cusps and three commissures are miniaturized within a small aortic ring[35] or when an aortic valve is the site of myxoid dysplasia.[20] In a hydraulically ideal aortic valve with three equal cusps, diastolic force is equally distributed among the three cusps and their sinus attachments. Cuspal *inequality* is a common variation of normal in trileaflet aortic valves but results in unequal distribution of diastolic force (see Figure 7-1B).[5,36] The fibrocalcific process of aging proceeds more rapidly in the cusp or cusps that bear the greatest hemodynamic stress.[11,36]

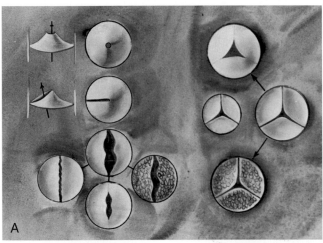

A

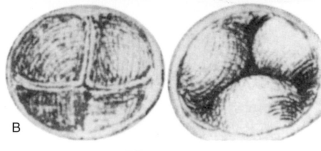

B

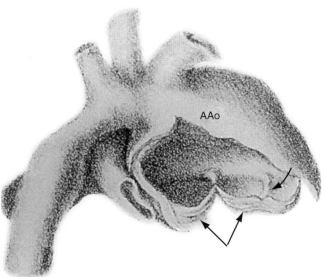

AAo

C

FIGURE 7-1 A, Illustrations of the various types of aortic valve stenosis. Figure on the left illustrates three types of congenitally abnormal aortic valves. The upper drawing shows a *unicuspid acommissural* valve. The middle drawing shows a *unicuspid unicommissural* valve with an eccentric orifice. The lower group of four drawings shows a functionally *normal bicuspid aortic valve* (upper center), a *fibrocalcific stenotic bicuspid aortic valve* (center right), a *bicuspid aortic that is inherently stenotic* because the free edges are not longer than the annular diameter (center left), and a *bicuspid aortic valve that is inherently stenotic* because of failure of commissural separation (lower center). Illustrations on the right show a *normal trileaflet aortic valve* with equal cusps and equal commissures (center right). A *congenitally hypoplastic trifleaflet aortic valve* (center left) is paired beside the normal trileaflet aortic valve (center left). Acquired aortic valve stenosis from fibrosis and calcification without commissural fusion (right lower) or from rheumatic fusion of commissures (upper) is shown. A *dysplastic trileaflet* valve is not shown. **B,** Congenital aortic cuspal inequality as represented by Leonardo da Vinci circa 1513.[16] His legend read: "Figures of the cusps (aorti) of the gateway which the left ventricle possesses when it closes itself." On the left is a trileaflet aortic valve as seen from above. On the right is a closed trileaflet aortic valve as seen from below. **C,** Dilation of the ascending aorta (AAo) above a congenitally bicuspid aortic valve (*paired arrows*) with a false raphe (*curved arrow*). (From Maude Abbott. Atlas of congenital cardiac disease. *Montreal: Osler Library, McGill University; 1936. Reproduced with permission.*)

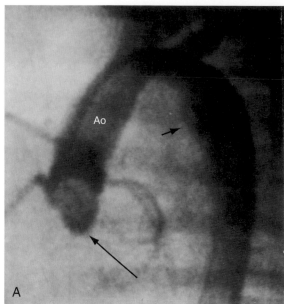

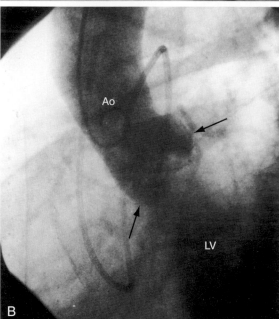

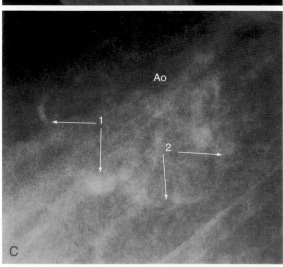

Accordingly, cuspal inequality in a normal trileaflet aortic valve enhances the aging process, converting a functionally normal trileaflet valve into fibrocalcific aortic stenosis.[5,36] Similarly, the tendency for a *bicuspid* aortic valve to become fibrocalcific (see Figure 7-2C) is related in part to the mechanical stress inherent in bicuspid cuspal inequality (see Figure 7-2B).[23] The *quadricuspid* aortic valve, first reported in 1862, can function normally or cause incompetence (Figures 7-35 and 7-42)[37] but is rarely stenotic.[6] *Six-cuspid* semilunar valves sporadically occur with truncus arteriosus (see Chapter 28).[6]

Fixed *subaortic* stenosis is the second most common variety of congenital obstruction to left ventricular outflow[6,38] and accounts for 15% to 20% of all types of congenital aortic stenosis.[39] It occurs in isolation (Figure 7-6) or with other congenital cardiac defects.[40,41] Nonfixed muscular subaortic stenosis can coexist with severe aortic valve stenosis and can account for as much as half the pressure gradient.[40–42]

This chapter deals with two principal varieties of fixed subaortic stenosis in hearts that are otherwise devoid of congenital heart disease. The first variety is characterized by a thin fibrous crescent-shaped membrane located immediately beneath the aortic valve (see Figure 7-6A).[6,40] The membrane is occasionally relatively thick and forms a fibrous or fibromuscular collar that extends across an otherwise normal left ventricular outflow tract[43] and inserts onto the anterior mitral leaflet. This form of fixed subaortic stenosis occurs in human hearts and in dogs, pigs, and cows.[44] The aortic root is not dilated.[28] Aortic regurgitation is associated with malformed leaflets that are damaged by the proximity of the subvalvular membrane or fibromuscular collar and by the impact of the eccentric systolic jet (see Figure 7-6B).[6] *Tubular subaortic stenosis* is a less common variety of fixed obstruction to left ventricular outflow and is represented by a fibromuscular channel that occupies several centimeters within the outflow tract (Figure 7-7).[40,41,45] A layer of fibrous tissue extends onto the ventricular surface of the anterior mitral leaflet. The aortic cusps show fibrous thickening as with discrete subaortic stenosis. The aortic root is not dilated (see Figure 7-7).[28,45]

Fixed subaortic stenosis as just defined is not present during intrauterine cardiac morphogenesis, is therefore not *con genitus*, and accordingly is uncommon if not rare in neonates and infants.[41] The disorder becomes manifest after the first year of life and then changes in both severity and morphology. In contrast to rapid progression in infants and children, fixed subaortic stenosis in adults

FIGURE 7-2 **A,** Lateral aortogram from a 5-day-old male with severe unicuspid unicommissural aortic stenosis *(long arrow).* The mobile valve is in its systolic (open) position doming upward. The aortic root (Ao) is not dilated. *Short arrow* points to a bulge at the aortic end of a closed ductus arteriosus. **B,** Lateral aortogram from a 78-year-old man with severe bicuspid aortic stenosis and moderate aortic regurgitation. *Arrows* point to two unequal cusps. **C,** Lateral chest x-ray from a 74-year-old man with calcific deposits in the two cusps (1 and 2) of a stenotic bicuspid aortic valve. (LV = left ventricle; Ao = aorta.)

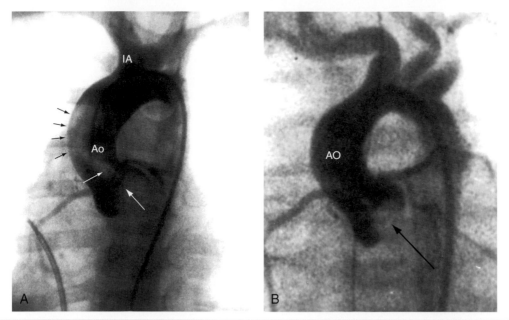

FIGURE 7-3 A, Aortogram from a 7-year-old boy with congenital bicuspid aortic stenosis *(thick white arrow).* An eccentric jet *(thin white arrow)* issues from the stenotic orifice. The jet adheres to the lateral aortic wall *(small black arrows,* Coanda effect). The aortic root (AO) is dilated. **B,** Left ventriculogram from a 9-year-old boy illustrating systolic doming of a mobile bicuspid aortic valve *(arrow).* (IA = innominate artery.)

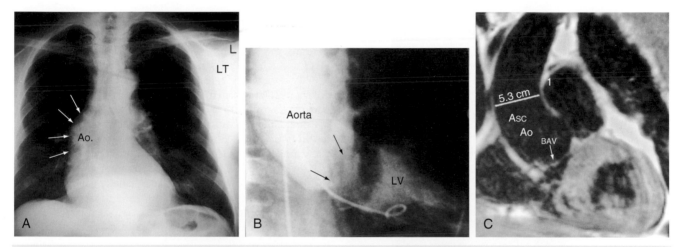

FIGURE 7-4 A, X-ray from a 66-year-old man with a bicuspid aortic valve, aneurysmal dilation of the ascending aorta (Ao), and moderate aortic regurgitation. **B,** Contrast material injected into the ascending aorta identifies the aneurysmal dilation, the bicuspid aortic valve *(black arrows),* and regurgitation into the left ventricle (LV). **C,** Magnetic resonance image from a 33-year-old man with a 5.3-cm ascending aorta (Asc Ao) above a bicuspid aortic valve (BAV).

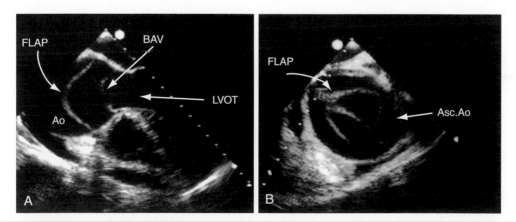

FIGURE 7-5 Transesophageal echocardiogram from a 37-year-old man with a bicuspid aortic valve (BAV) and a dissecting aneurysm of the ascending aorta (Ao). **A,** The flap of the dissection moved freely within the dilated ascending aorta. **B,** The flap is seen again within the ascending aorta. (LVOT = left ventricular outflow tract.)

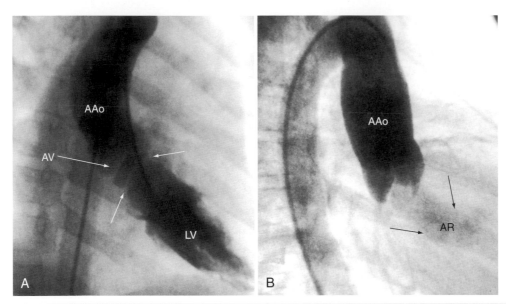

FIGURE 7-6 Angiocardiograms from a 3-year-old boy with fixed subaortic stenosis, a gradient of 40 mm Hg, and mild aortic regurgitation. **A,** Left ventriculogram (LV) shows the subaortic stenosis *(unmarked oblique arrows)* in close proximity to the aortic valve (AV). The ascending aorta (AAo) is mildly dilated. **B,** Contrast material injected into the ascending aorta discloses mild aortic regurgitation (AR).

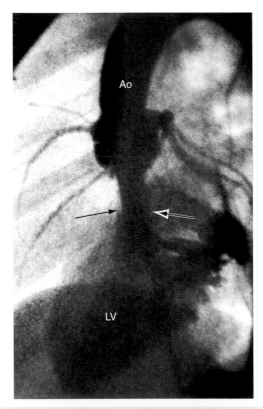

FIGURE 7-7 Left ventricular angiogram (LV) from a 9-year-old boy with tubular subaortic stenosis *(paired arrows)*. Five years previously, the patient underwent resection of a moderately obstructive discrete subaortic membrane. The ascending aorta (Ao) is not dilated.

progresses slowly.[40,41,45,46] Aortic regurgitation is common but is usually mild and nonprogressive (see Figure 7-6B).

Supravalvular aortic stenosis is the least common variety of congenital obstruction to left ventricular outflow.

The most frequent type is a localized segmental hourglass deformity immediately above the aortic sinuses with medial thickening and fibrous intimal proliferation (Figure 7-8A).[6] The size of the aorta distal to the obstruction is normal or reduced. The sinuses of Valsalva are enlarged.[47] Localized supravalvular aortic stenosis is occasionally caused by a fibrous membrane with a central opening.[6] An uncommon variety is represented by tubular hypoplasia of the ascending aorta beginning above the sinuses of Valsalva and associated with narrowing of the orifices of the brachiocephalic arteries (Figure 7-8B).[6,48] The *aortic leaflets* are usually thickened and adherent to the supravalvular stenosing ridge,[6,47] are occasionally dysplastic, and may fuse to a coronary ostium.[6] The aortic valve abnormalities usually cause no more than mild regurgitation.[6]

Three additional features of supravalvular aortic stenosis include: (1) the anatomy of the extramural *coronary arteries;* (2) the condition of the *aortic leaflets* and *aortic sinuses;* and (3) the association with Williams syndrome. Obstruction of a coronary ostium can be caused by adherence of a distorted aortic leaflet to the supravalvular stenotic ridge, by aortic medial proliferation, and by the supravalvular ridge itself, which can impede diastolic flow into an ostium.[49] Because the coronary ostia are proximal to the supravalvular obstruction, the coronary arteries are exposed to elevated left ventricular systolic pressure[6] and become thick-walled and dilated (see Figure 7-8). Coronary artery aneurysms have been described.[50] and hypertension is a risk factor for premature atherosclerosis.[6]

In 1961, Williams, Barratt-Boyes, and Lowe[51] described the association of supravalvular aortic stenosis with distinctive elfin facies and mental retardation. In 1962, Beuren, Apitz, and Harmjanz[52] expanded the syndrome to include pulmonary artery stenosis. Williams syndrome or Williams-Beuren syndrome now includes elfin facies, mental retardation, small stature, infantile

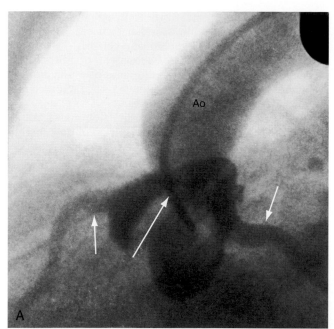

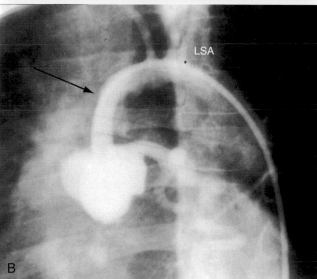

FIGURE 7-8 A, Lateral aortogram from a 15-year-old boy with supravalvular aortic stenosis. The *thin oblique arrow* points to the localized zone of obstruction just above the sinuses of Valsalva. The proximal coronary arteries are dilated *(paired thick arrows).* The size of the aortic root (Ao) is normal. **B,** Aortogram from a 15-year-old boy with tubular hypoplasia *(arrow)* of the ascending and transverse aorta, beginning above the sinuses and extending beyond the left subclavian artery (LSA). The origins of the brachiocephalic arteries are hypoplastic. The left coronary artery and its branches are enlarged.

hypercalcemia, supravalvular aortic stenosis, pulmonary artery stenosis, and important vascular abnormalities, especially in adults.[53,54] Renal abnormalities occur in nearly half of afflicted patients and are represented by renal artery stenosis, segmental scarring, cystic dysplasia, nephrocalcinosis, marked asymmetry in kidney size, solitary kidney, and pelvic kidney.[53,55] Systemic hypertension is not necessarily related to the renovascular abnormalities[56] but instead is related to stiffness of

arterial walls.[57] A generalized arteriopathy is characterized by medial thickening and luminal narrowing of systemic and pulmonary arteries.[58] Long segment narrowing of the aorta may occur with or without localized coarctation.[56] Involvement of cerebral arteries is responsible for strokes. Tortuous retinal arteries similar to those that accompany coarctation of the aorta (see Chapter 8, Figure 8-8) were described in the original report of Williams, Barratt-Boyes, and Lowe,[51] and in 1985, the observation was confirmed.[56]

The *physiologic consequences* of *congenital aortic valve stenosis* are reflected in the response of the left ventricle to increased afterload. An adaptive increase in left ventricular mass in the *immature heart* is chiefly the result of *hyperplasia* (replication) of cardiomyocytes. In contrast, the increase in left ventricular mass in the *mature heart* is the result of hypertrophy (an increase in cell size) of terminally differentiated cardiomyocytes.[59] The afterloaded immature heart is capable of capillary replication that is proportional to cardiomyocyte replication, so capillary density remains normal and coronary flow reserve remains normal.[59,60] The increase in left ventricular mass characterized by myocyte hyperplasia with proportionate growth in the microvascular bed sets the stage for low left ventricular systolic wall stress and supernormal ejection performance.[59] The left ventricle thickens concentrically and the cavity size is normal or small,[59] so distensibility decreases. A greater force of left atrial contraction generates the end-diastolic fiber length necessary for left ventricular performance appropriate for the increased afterload without an increase in end-diastolic volume or left atrial mean pressure. The normal trileaflet aortic valve and its annulus increase in anatomic cross-sectional area with age even after maturity.[61] The normal trileaflet physiologic orifice, which is the cross-sectional area defined by the leaflets in systole, is flow-dependent, varying directly with the volume and rate of left ventricular ejection. In the resting state, less than half the cross-sectional area of a normal trileaflet aortic valve is used during ejection, so a large reserve is available during high-flow states.

The physiologic consequences of congenital aortic stenosis take into account the morphology of the obstruction, the degree of obstruction, the age of onset, and whether or not the obstruction is progressive. A functionally normal bicuspid aortic valve awaits adulthood to become stenotic as its leaflets thicken and calcify. An stenotic aortic valve in infants and young children tends to generate an increasingly higher gradient in response to the progressive increase in transaortic flow that accompanies the normal age-related increase in body mass.[62] In Williams syndrome, progressive supravalvular aortic stenosis results from inadequate growth of the sinotubular junction.[63] Fixed *subaortic stenosis* is not present *in utero* but usually begins after the first year of life and undergoes a progressive decrease in cross-sectional area (see previous discussion).[41,46] The time course in adults is much slower.

The subendocardium of the left ventricle in aortic stenosis is vulnerable to ischemia because of a selective decrease in perfusion.[49] In neonates and infants with severe aortic stenosis, subendocardial ischemia is responsible for papillary muscle infarction with mitral regurgitation[49] and for endocardial fibrosis and reduced cavity size that depress left ventricular contractility.[64] A progressive rise in left ventricular filling pressure, in left atrial mean pressure, and in pulmonary arterial pressure provokes right ventricular failure.[65] *Supravalvular* aortic stenosis incurs the additional impediment of compromised coronary perfusion (see previous discussion).

The physiologic response of the neonate to severe aortic stenosis is best understood in light of the fetal circulation. Intrauterine left ventricular volume is low because pulmonary blood flow is virtually nil. When lungs expand at birth, pulmonary blood flow commences and a severely obstructed, thick-walled left ventricle with reduced cavity size suddenly receives a sizable increment in volume. Left ventricular filling pressure rises steeply, left atrial pressure rises in parallel, and a left-to-right shunt is established across a stretched valve-incompetent foramen ovale. If a small left ventricular cavity is beset with endocardial fibrosis or fibroelastosis, the hemodynamic consequences are correspondingly worse.[64] Vasoreactive pulmonary arterioles constrict, pulmonary artery pressure rises, and pressure overload is imposed on an already volume-overloaded right ventricle. Temporary patency of the ductus arteriosus diverts right ventricular blood into the aorta and delays the onset of symptoms, but when the ductus closes, that advantage is lost because the entire right ventricular output enters the pulmonary circulation and the left side of the heart.

The response to dynamic exercise mild aortic stenosis is normal, but when stenosis is severe, left ventricular stroke volume is blunted at each level of graded isotonic stress.[66-68] In congenital aortic *valve* stenosis, the augmented flow and increased left ventricular systolic pressure induced by exercise result in a larger computed aortic valve area, which implies that the stenotic valve is sufficiently mobile to open more widely when stressed.[66] Activation of canine left ventricular baroreceptors in response to an increase in left ventricular pressure or stretch induces hypotension from skeletal muscle vasodilation. Reflex vasodilation and bradycardia induced by activation of left ventricular baroreceptors during isotonic exercise are responsible for hypotension and exertional syncope.[69]

History

Congenital aortic valve stenosis is considerably more common in males, with a gender ratio of approximately 4:1.[4,39,70] Male prevalence is less common in supravalvular aortic stenosis, depending in part on genetic transmission. Discrete and tunnel subaortic stenosis both have a distinct female prevalence.[38] In the Newfoundland dog, genetically transmitted subaortic stenosis has an equal gender ratio.[44]

When congenital aortic stenosis is present at birth, the murmur is also present because the anatomic and physiologic conditions required to generate the murmur exist.[41,46] An exception is fixed subaortic stenosis, which is *not* present at birth, and an additional qualification relates to specific types of congenitally malformed aortic valves.[5] As a rule, the fewer the cusps and commissures, the greater the likelihood of an intrinsically stenotic valve and of a

murmur in the newborn.[6] Intrinsically stenotic valves are usually unicuspid unicommissural or bicuspid,[6] but when a bicuspid aortic valve is functionally normal,[4,6] the onset of the murmur awaits the development of fibrocalcific thickening in adulthood.[1,4,6,39] Stenosis of a unicommissural aortic valve occasionally follows a protracted course similar to that of a bicuspid aortic valve.[2,14]

An impression of murmur intensity (loudness) can be inferred in the history with determination of how readily a murmur was heard during follow-up examinations. A loud murmur is likely to be heard even in uncooperative infants, whereas the soft murmur of mild obstruction is likely to be overlooked or mistaken for a normal murmur, even in cooperative infants and older children (see Chapter 2).

Growth and development are affected in patients with Williams syndrome (see subsequent discussion). Symptoms associated with aortic stenosis, especially in children, may be absent even in the presence of severe obstruction,[39] and progression from mild to severe is not necessarily accompanied by symptomatic deterioration.[71] Effort dyspnea and fatigue reflect an inadequate increment in cardiac output and an increase in left ventricular end-diastolic pressure. *Effort syncope* arouses suspicion of aortic stenosis in an acyanotic patient with a prominent cardiac murmur dating from infancy or childhood. Syncope depends on the degree of obstruction, not on its morphologic type,[70] and is the result of reflex vasodilation and bradycardia induced by activation of left ventricular baroreceptors during isotonic exercise (see previous discussion).[69] Syncope can be recurrent,[39] and sudden death looms as a threat,[70] although the risk in children is small compared with adults. Subtle cerebral symptoms consist of mild giddiness, faintness, or lightheadedness with effort. Syncope-induced hypotension may provoke electrical ventricular instability in adults with atherosclerotic coronary artery disease but not in young patients with aortic stenosis and normal coronary arteries.[49,72]

A potential disparity exists between the oxygen requirements of an hypertrophied left ventricle and coronary blood flow and flow reserve. The disparity is aggravated by acquired coronary artery disease in adults with fibrocalcific bicuspid aortic stenosis and in children with coronary artery abnormalities that accompany supravalvular aortic stenosis.[73] *Angina pectoris* in young patients is a symptom of congenital aortic stenosis that arrests attention.

Inappropriate diaphoresis increases with the onset of congestive heart failure, especially in neonates.[64,74] In infants with severe aortic stenosis, mitral regurgitation from papillary muscle infarction adds to the hemodynamic burden.[72]

Bicuspid aortic stenosis and subaortic stenosis are genetically transmitted (see previous discussion).[44,75-77] Familial and nonfamilial types of *supravalvular* aortic stenosis are the basis of the following classification: (1) *familial* with normal facies and normal intelligence; (2) *nonfamilial* with normal facies and normal intelligence; and (3) *nonfamilial* with Williams syndrome,[51,78] which results from mutation or deletion of the elastin gene located at chromosome 7q11.23.[79-82] Pulmonary artery stenosis in Williams syndrome tends to improve with time, and the supravalvular aortic stenosis is progressive because of growth failure of the sinotubular junction, which may be associated with obstruction of coronary artery ostia.[63] Supravalvular aortic stenosis has been experimentally produced in newborn rabbits with administration of maternal vitamin D during gestation[83] and has occurred in human offspring when infantile hypercalcemia resulted from administration of vitamin D during pregnancy. The history should therefore include questions regarding maternal vitamin D ingestion.

Infective endocarditis is a potential risk in all types of congenital aortic stenosis,[6,39] but the *bicuspid aortic valve* is especially vulnerable, whether functionally normal, stenotic, or incompetent, an observation made by William Osler[84] more than a century ago. *Dissecting aneurysm* of the ascending aorta may dramatically interrupt the clinical course of bicuspid aortic stenosis (see Figure 7-5).[85] Gastrointestinal bleeding associated with aortic stenosis, sometimes called Heyde's syndrome, occurs in older adults.[86] *Angiodysplasia* has been used to designate the offending lesions that tend to be present in the ascending colon but may be distributed throughout the gastrointestinal tract.[86] Aortic stenosis is not thought to cause the lesions but is thought to increase the likelihood that the lesions will bleed.

Physical Appearance

Williams syndrome (nonfamilial supravalvular aortic stenosis) is characterized by peculiar facies, short stature, and mental retardation.[3,51,52] The chin is small (hypoplastic mandible), the mouth is large, the lips are patulous, the nose is blunt and upturned, the eyes are widely set with occasional internal strabismus, the cheeks are baggy (Figure 7-9), the teeth are malformed, and the bite is abnormal (malocclusion; Figure 7-10). Flat molar regions accentuate the prominence of a wide mouth with full lips, small jaw, and long philtrum.[54] The brow is broad with prominent supraorbital ridges. The nasal tip is broad, and the nacres are anteverted. Adults with Williams syndrome are relatively short and tend to have lordosis, kyphoscoliosis, and joint abnormalities of the lower limbs that result in a stiff awkward gait.[54] Friendly temperaments and deep, somewhat metallic voices further emphasize the similarities. XO *Turner's syndrome* (see Chapter 8) represents another distinctive physical appearance that coexists with a bicuspid aortic valve.[87] Congenital heart disease with Turner's syndrome has been known since the initial description by Morgagni, and is coupled with different patterns of X monosomies.[88] Abnormal karyotypes consist of 45 X mosaicism and X structural abnormalities.[89] Patients with severe dysmorphic features have a significantly higher prevalence rate of congenital heart disease,[89] and patients with 45 X Turner's syndrome have the highest prevalence rate.[89] X structural abnormalities are associated with an increased prevalence rate of bicuspid aortic valve,[89] but with X deletion, the incidence rate of congenital heart disease is not increased.[88] In Noonan's syndrome (Turner's phenotype with normal genotype), obstruction

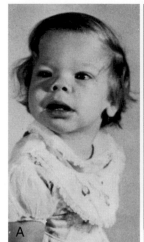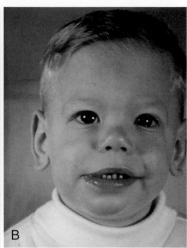

FIGURE 7-9 Characteristic facial appearance of a 20-month-old girl (**A**) and a 24-month-old boy (**B**) with nonfamilial supravalvular aortic stenosis and pulmonary artery stenosis (Williams syndrome). The children closely resemble each other. Both were mentally retarded and had large mouths, patulous lips, small chins, baggy cheeks, blunt upturned noses, wide-set eyes, left internal strabismus, and malformed teeth.

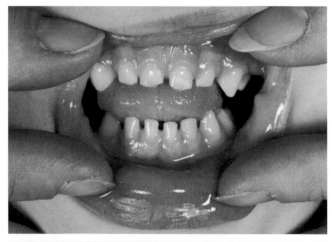

FIGURE 7-10 Small widely spaced malformed teeth from the 2-year-old boy referred to in Figure 7-9.

to left ventricular outflow is the result of hypertrophic obstructive cardiomyopathy (Figure 7-11).

Arterial Pulse

The object of the following paragraphs is to consider the aid in the diagnosis of aortic stenosis that may be supplied by a study of the pulse (Graham Steell, The Lancet, November 1894). Fixed obstruction to left ventricular outflow distinctively alters the arterial pulse.[3,90] The pulse pressure is small, the rate of rise is slow, the peak is sustained, and the decline is gentle (Figures 7-12 and 7-13). This typical configuration is not as frequent in children as

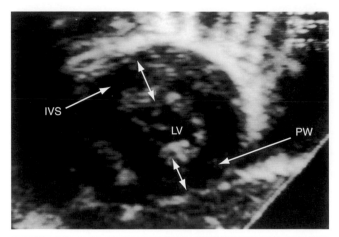

FIGURE 7-11 Echocardiogram (subzyphoid short axis) from a 1-month-old boy with Noonan's syndrome and hypertrophic obstructive cardiomyopathy. The interventricular septum (IVS) is thicker than the posterior wall (PW). (LV = left ventricle.)

the aorta and the Coanda effect (affinity of a jet stream for adherence to a wall) carries the jet into the innominate artery.[93–95] Experimental observations with an aortic arch model showed that kinetic energy developed in a jet stream under conditions simulating supravalvular aortic stenosis is sufficient to account for the clinically observed differences in arterial pressure.[93] Selective narrowing of the origins of the left carotid and left subclavian arteries (see Figure 7-8B) is an uncommon cause of asymmetric pulses.[95] In healthy adults, the systolic pressure in the *right arm* is 10 to 15 mm Hg higher than in the left arm.[90] *Simultaneous* determination of blood pressure in both arms minimizes these differences, and the technique of palpation shown in Figure 7-14 is useful in the clinical comparison of the right and left brachial pulses.[3,90]

In valvular and fixed subaortic aortic stenosis, *arterial thrills* or *shudders* are common in the suprasternal notch and over the carotid and subclavian arteries.[3,90,92] In *supravalvular* aortic stenosis, the thrill is distinctly more pronounced over the *right* carotid artery, which exhibits an increased pulsation.

in adults with equivalent aortic stenosis.[90,91] Children with severe obstruction may have a brachial arterial pulse that is interpreted as normal, although palpation of the carotid artery improves accuracy.[91,92] A bisferiens pulse (twin peaked) implies coexisting aortic regurgitation.[90]

The right and left brachial and carotid arterial pulses are symmetric in valvular or fixed subvalvular aortic stenosis, but in supravalvular aortic stenosis, the rate of rise, the systolic pressure, and the pulse pressure are greater in the *right* brachial artery and in the *right* carotid artery (see Figure 7-13)[93,94] because the hourglass deformity directs the high-velocity jet toward the right wall of

Jugular Venous Pulse

Directing attention to the amplitude of the *jugular venous A wave* in subjects with isolated obstruction to *left* ventricular outflow is seemingly paradoxical.[3,90] However, *left* ventricular hypertrophy serves to decrease *right* ventricular distensibility, so the right atrium contracts with greater force and the amplitude of the jugular venous A wave increases in the absence of pulmonary hypertension (Figure 7-15).[3,90,96]

BRACHIAL ARTERY

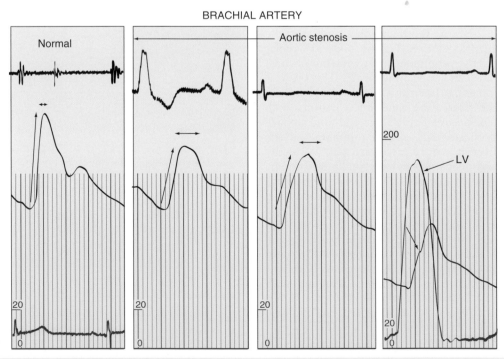

FIGURE 7-12 Brachial arterial pulses from a healthy (normal) young adult and from three patients with aortic valve stenosis. The aortic stenotic pulses (two central panels) exhibit a slow rate of rise, a small pulse pressure, a sustained peak, and a gentle decline. In the fourth panel, an anacrotic notch *(left oblique arrow)* is seen midway along the ascending limb of the arterial pulse. (LV = left ventricle.)

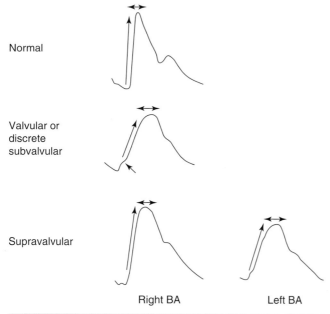

Normal

Valvular or discrete subvalvular

Supravalvular

Right BA   Left BA

FIGURE 7-13 Wave forms of brachial arterial (BA) pulses in various types of congenital aortic stenosis (compare with the normal). With valvular stenosis or discrete subaortic stenosis, there is a slow rate of rise *(oblique arrow)*, a reduced pulse pressure, a single sustained peak *(horizontal arrows)*, and a gradual decline. The lower unmarked arrow identifies a small anacrotic notch. With supravalvular aortic stenosis, the pulse pressure *right* brachial artery is increased, and the rate of rise is brisker than in the left brachial pulse.

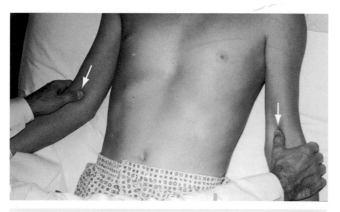

FIGURE 7-14 Recommended method for simultaneous palpation of right and left brachial arterial pulses. The examiner sits or stands on the patient's right.

Precordial Movement and Palpation

Neonates with severe aortic valve stenosis have a prominent right ventricular impulse because of pulmonary hypertension and a left-to-right shunt at the atrial level.[97] With these exceptions, the characteristic precordial impulse is *left ventricular*, varying from normal in mild aortic stenosis to the strong sustained impulse generated by an hypertrophied left ventricle of severe aortic stenosis.[3,90] Presystolic distention is in response to the increased force of left atrial contraction (Figure 7-16), which is evidence that the aortic stenosis is

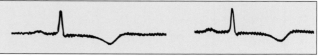

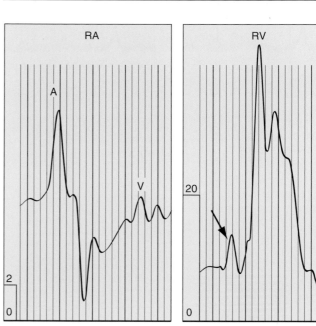

RA

RV

A

V

20

2

0

0

FIGURE 7-15 Pressure pulses from a 68-year-old man with severe calcific bicuspid aortic stenosis. The A wave in the right atrium (RA) is elevated to 12 mm Hg (first panel) with equivalent presystolic distention *(arrow)* of the right ventricle (RV) (second panel).

hemodynamically appreciable.[98] Dilation of the ascending aorta rarely transmits an impulse because the rate of ejection is blunted by the stenotic aortic valve. If an ascending aortic impulse occurs at all, it is likely to do so in patients with mild obstruction and an aortic aneurysm (see Figure 7-4).[85]

Systolic thrills are trivial or absent when aortic stenosis is mild or when severe aortic stenosis occurs with left ventricular failure. The thrill radiates upward and to the right, is maximal in the second right intercostal space, and is detected in the suprasternal notch and over both carotid arteries.[90] The thrill in infants is sometimes maximal to the *left* of the sternum, inviting a mistaken diagnosis of ventricular septal defect. Even in older children, the thrill is occasionally more pronounced in the second or third left interspace, although radiation is still upward and to the right.[90] In *supravalvular* aortic stenosis, the thrill is especially prominent below the right clavicle and on the right side of the neck.

Auscultation

Normal splitting of the first heart sound must be distinguished from a first heart sound followed by an aortic ejection sound, which has considerable diagnostic significance.[3,90] The ejection sound is separated from the first heart sound by a distinct interval, is louder and higher

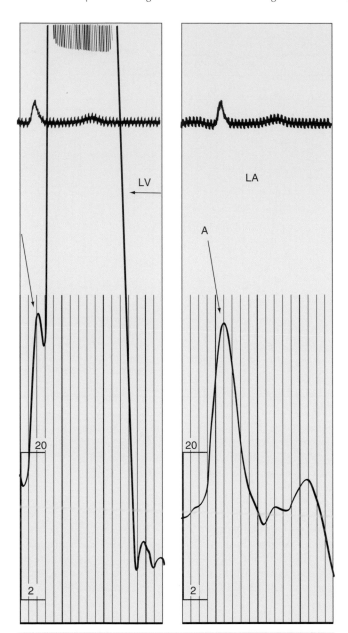

FIGURE 7-16 Left ventricular (LV) and left atrial (LA) pressure pulses from a 15-year-old boy with severe bicuspid aortic stenosis. Presystolic distention of the left ventricle *(oblique arrow)* was in response to the increased force of left atrial contraction reflected in the large left atrial A wave.

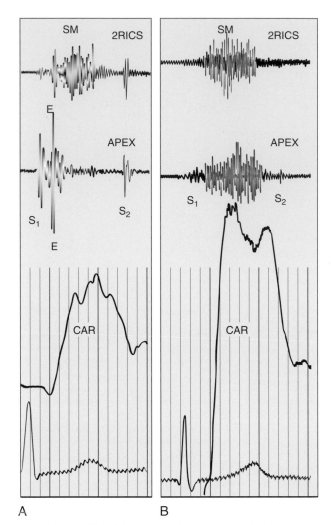

FIGURE 7-17 A, Recordings from a 12-year-old boy with bicuspid aortic stenosis. The phonocardiogram from the second right intercostal space (2RICS) shows a loud aortic ejection sound (E) followed by a midsystolic murmur (SM) that ends before a prominent aortic component of the second heart sound (S_2). The ejection sound selectively transmitted to the apex. **B,** Recordings from a 9-year-old boy with fixed subaortic stenosis of the same severity as in panel **A.** An aortic ejection sound was conspicuous by its absence, and the aortic component of the second sound (S_2) was soft. The midsystolic murmur was transmitted to the apex. (CAR = carotid pulse; S_1 = first heart sound.)

pitched than the first sound, and is heard best at the cardiac apex (Figure 7-17A). An aortic ejection sound is a valuable auscultatory sign of the level but not the degree of aortic stenosis.[99] The sound coincides with abrupt cephalad movement of a mobile dome-shaped stenotic valve (see Figure 7-3B).[17,99] The ejection sound may be difficult to hear in infants and disappears in adults when fibrocalcific changes impair valve mobility (see Figure 7-2C). Because the ejection sound is valvular in origin, it does not occur in fixed subaortic stenosis (Figure 7-17B) or in supravalvular aortic stenosis (Figure 7-18).

The aortic stenotic murmur is the prototype of the left-sided midsystolic murmur, beginning after the first

heart sound or with the ejection sound, rising in crescendo to a systolic peak, and then declining in decrescendo to end before the aortic component of the second sound (Figures 7-17 through 7-19).[3,90] The murmur is harsh, rough, and grunting, especially when loud, and may have an early systolic peak and a short duration, a relatively late peak and a prolonged duration, or all gradations in between, but *the shape remains symmetric* (see Figure 7-19).[3,90] Intensity varies from bare audibility to grade 6/6, decreases in the presence of left ventricular failure, and may alternate in a fashion analogous to pulsus alternans.[59,90] Although configuration, length, and loudness do not necessarily correspond to the degree of obstruction, some conclusions can be drawn (see Figure 7-19).[100] The longer and louder the murmur,

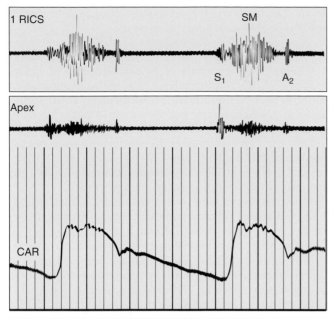

FIGURE 7-18 Phonocardiogram from a 7-year-old boy with supravalvular aortic stenosis and a gradient of 55 mm Hg. The midsystolic murmur (SM) was maximal in the first right intercostal space (1 RICS). There is no aortic ejection sound, and the aortic component of the second sound (A_2) is normal.

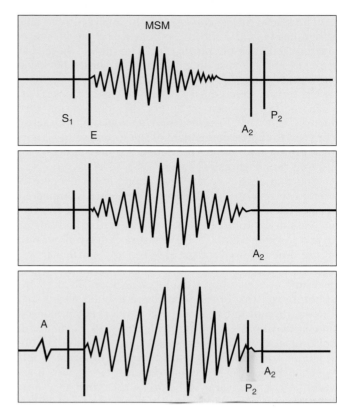

FIGURE 7-19 Schematic illustrations of auscultatory and phonocardiographic signs of mild, moderate, and severe bicuspid aortic stenosis. *Mild aortic stenosis* (upper): An ejection sound (E) introduces a short symmetric midsystolic murmur (MSM) that peaks early in systole. The second sound splits normally, and the aortic component (A_2) is prominent. *Moderate aortic stenosis* (middle): The ejection sound introduces a longer but still symmetric midsystolic murmur with a later systolic peak. The second sound (A_2) is single. *Severe aortic stenosis* (lower): A fourth heart sound (A) precedes a normal first heart sound. An aortic ejection sound introduces a long but still symmetric midsystolic murmur. The second heart sound is paradoxically split (A_2 follows P_2). (P_2 = pulmonary component.)

and the later its symmetric systolic peak, the greater the likelihood of severe stenosis. The shorter and softer the murmur and the *earlier* its symmetric peak, the greater the likelihood of mild stenosis or of a functionally normal bicuspid aortic valve. Irrespective of length, the murmur remains symmetric. A late symmetric peak reflects prolonged ejection and increased severity (see Figure 7-19), but severity does not change the *shape* of the aortic stenotic murmur, as in congenital *pulmonary* valve stenosis in which the murmur becomes progressively *asymmetric* as severity increases (see Chapter 11).

The typical murmur of congenital aortic valve stenosis is maximal in the second right interspace with radiation upward, to the right, and into the neck, reflecting the upward and rightward direction of the high velocity jet within the ascending aorta. Very loud murmurs are occasionally transmitted to the shoulders and elbows. In infants with aortic valve stenosis, the murmur may be maximal to the *left* of the sternum and mistaken for the murmur of ventricular septal defect, but with the passage of time, maximum intensity shifts to the right base.[3] Maximum intensity in *tubular* subaortic stenosis is likely to be at the mid left sternal edge.[45]

When aortic stenosis is *supravalvular*, the jet may be as distal as the innominate artery, so the murmur is most prominent in the *first* right intercostal space (see Figure 7-18) and in the *right* side of the neck.[90] A saccular aneurysm near the orifice of the innominate artery was ascribed to the jet impact. Systolic murmurs in the axillae and back are likely to be caused by coexisting stenosis of the pulmonary artery and its branches.[52,90] Normal supraclavicular systolic murmurs in children can be mistaken for aortic stenosis,[90] but supraclavicular murmurs

are softer *below* the clavicles and decrease or vanish with hyperextension of the shoulders (see Chapter 2).[90,101]

An aortic stenotic midsystolic murmur at the apex must be distinguished from the holosystolic murmur of mitral regurgitation. Clear audibility of the aortic component of the second heart sound in the presence of a prominent apical murmur generally means that the murmur ends before aortic closure and is therefore midsystolic.[90] An apical holosystolic murmur is likely to envelope the aortic component second sound, which is then inaudible. When the aortic valve is fibrocalcific and immobile, the closure sound is soft or inaudible at the base *and* at the apex, so an accurate auscultatory assessment of murmur length is difficult or impossible. However, an aortic stenotic murmur is louder in the beat *after* the compensatory pause that follows a premature ventricular contraction, whereas the murmur of mitral regurgitation does *not* amplify in the postpremature beat.[102]

The *second heart sound* should be analyzed regarding the intensity of the aortic component and the presence, degree, and type of splitting.[3,90] The mobile valve that generates an ejection sound during its abrupt cephalad movement generates a well-preserved aortic component of the second sound during its abrupt caudal movement, even in the presence of appreciable obstruction (see Figure 7-17A).[103] In *subvalvular* or *supravalvular* aortic stenosis, the aortic component of the second sound is normal, diminished, or absent, depending on the degree of stenosis (see Figures 7-17 and 7-18).

Splitting of the second heart sound is not necessarily related to severity.[3,90] A delay in the aortic component results from prolonged left ventricular ejection from an increase in duration of left ventricular systole and a delay in the aortic incisura.[104] The incisura is delayed because of the time required for the elevated left ventricular systolic pressure to fall below the level of the low aortic root pressure, at which point the incisura is inscribed.[104] Inspiratory splitting of the second heart sound means that the duration of left ventricular ejection is not prolonged and aortic stenosis is mild (see Figure 7-19). *Paradoxical* splitting or reversed sequence of semilunar valve closure (Figures 7-19 and 7-20) means that the duration of left ventricular ejection is prolonged and aortic stenosis is severe. Left ventricular systolic pressure is then at or near its maximum of 250 mm Hg in older children and adults, so the approximate gradient is the difference between 250 mm Hg and the cuff brachial arterial systolic blood pressure.[3,90] Reversed splitting may appear after exercise. Because paradoxical splitting is difficult to detect and because prominent inspiratory splitting is confined to mild obstruction, it follows that most patients with

aortic stenosis have a second sound that is single or closely split through a wide range of severity.

A soft early diastolic murmur of aortic regurgitation occurs in approximately 50% of cases of fixed *subvalvular* stenosis because of the high incidence rate of abnormalities of the aortic valve.[6] An aortic regurgitation murmur may be present with mild bicuspid aortic stenosis or with a functionally normal bicuspid aortic valve because the free edges of the bicuspid leaflets must be greater than the diameter if the aortic annulus to permit unobstructed flow (see Figure 7-1A). Aortic regurgitation is least likely to accompany *supravalvular* aortic stenosis but may do so when the cusps are malformed.[6]

A fourth heart sound (see Figure 7-19) is the auscultatory counterpart of presystolic distention of the left ventricle (see Figure 7-16), although the low frequency sound may be soft or absent despite the presence of a presystolic impulse. These signs imply an increased force of left atrial contraction required by the hypertrophied left ventricle to achieve an end-diastolic fiber length appropriate for greater contractile force (see Figure 7-16). Potain recognized this tendency in left ventricular hypertrophy when he wrote that the wall of the ventricle *is placed under tension precisely at the moment that this (the added sound) occurs.*[98] Accordingly, the fourth heart sound is a feature of hemodynamically significant aortic stenosis.[98] However, after age 40 years, the fourth heart sound is not a reliable sign of severity because it is heard in healthy adults.[98]

A third heart sound appears with the advent of left ventricular failure and usually coexists with a fourth heart sound. With an increase in heart rate and an increase in PR interval, these two sounds occur in close

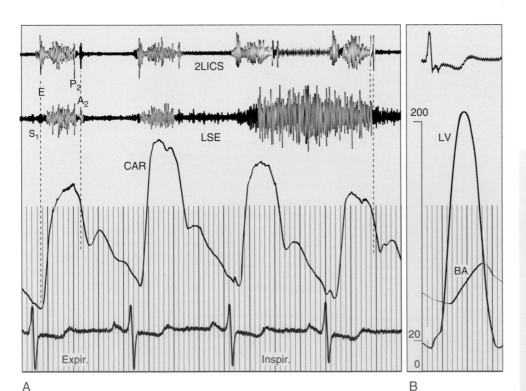

FIGURE 7-20 Recordings from a 62-year-old man with severe bicuspid aortic stenosis (see gradient in panel **B**). **A,** Phonocardiogram from the second left intercostal space (2LICS) recorded an aortic ejection sound (E), a midsystolic murmur (SM), and paradoxical splitting of the second heart sound. The ejection sound and the prominent aortic component of the second sound (A_2) indicate that the bicuspid aortic valve was mobile. **B,** Left ventricular (LV) and brachial arterial (BA) pressure pulses display the large gradient.

proximity or summate and generate a short low-frequency mid-diastolic murmur.

Electrocardiogram

Left ventricular hypertrophy in the electrocardiogram can occur with no more than mild to moderate congenital aortic stenosis (Figure 7-21),[105,106] and sudden death occasionally occurs, with severe aortic stenosis and a normal or near normal electrocardiogram.[107] Severity can progress without a change in the electrocardiogram, which if initially normal, remains so. Although these points are noteworthy, they should not detract from the value derived from careful interpretation of the scalar tracing.[108]

P waves are usually normal (Figures 7-21 and 7-22). Broad notched P waves are exceptional and are likely to indicate significant coexisting mitral regurgitation.[106] The QRS axis is usually normal irrespective of severity (see Figures 7-21 and 7-22).[106] Depolarization is clockwise, so Q waves appear in leads 3 and aVF (see Figures 7-21 and 7-22). In severe congenital aortic stenosis, electrocardiographic evidence of subendocardial ischemia or infarction can occur even in infants (Figure 7-23).[109] The electrocardiogram in supravalvular aortic stenosis can reflect the ischemia of coronary ostial obstruction.

Left ventricular hypertrophy is manifested by tall R waves in leads 2 and aVF, deep S waves in lead V_1, tall

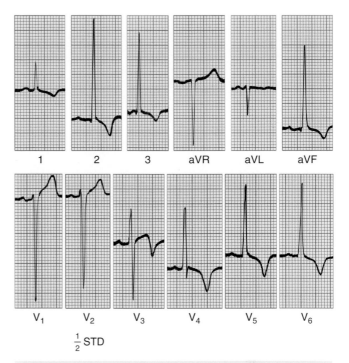

FIGURE 7-22 Electrocardiogram from an 18-year-old man with severe bicuspid aortic stenosis. The P waves and the QRS axis are normal. Left ventricular hypertrophy is reflected in the tall R waves and deeply inverted T waves in leads 2, 3, aVF, and V_{4-6} and the deep S waves in right precordial leads.

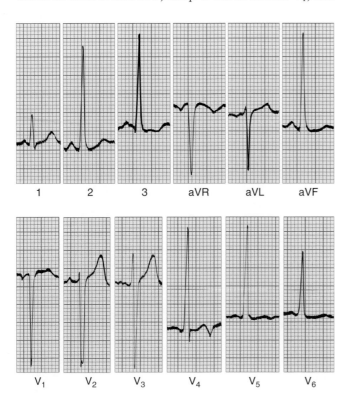

FIGURE 7-21 Electrocardiogram from a 19-year-old man with bicuspid aortic stenosis and a gradient of 35 mm Hg. The P waves and the QRS axis are normal. Left ventricular hypertrophy is reflected in the tall R waves in leads 2, 3, and aVF; the deep S waves in leads V_{1-3}; and the tall R waves with biphasic or inverted T waves in leads V_{4-5}.

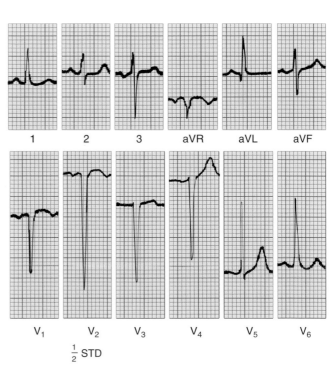

FIGURE 7-23 Electrocardiogram from a 13-year-old boy with severe fixed subaortic stenosis and moderate regurgitation. The P waves are normal, and the QRS axis is horizontal. The r waves in leads V_{1-4} are small to absent. Deep S waves of left ventricular hypertrophy appear in right and mid precordial leads.

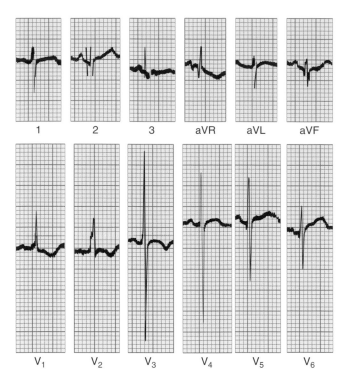

FIGURE 7-24 Electrocardiogram from a 5-day-old boy with severe unicuspid unicommissural aortic valve stenosis. The QRS axis is normal for age. Except for biphasic RS complexes in leads V_{3-4}, pure right ventricular hypertrophy is reflected in the dominant R waves in leads aVR and V_1 and the deep S waves in leads V_{5-6}.

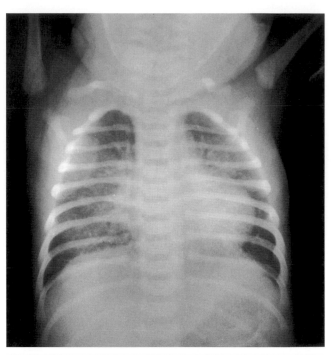

FIGURE 7-25 X-ray from a 48-hour-old male with severe unicuspid unicommissural aortic valve stenosis. The ascending aorta is not border forming, the apex is occupied by a convex left ventricle, and there is pulmonary venous congestion.

R waves in V_{5-6}, and deeply inverted asymmetric T waves (see Figures 7-21 through 7-23).[106] The T waves usually point in a direction opposite the QRS complex (wide QRS-T angle; see Figure 7-22). Exercise stress tests can provoke ST-T wave abnormalities when the resting electrocardiogram is normal,[68] and digitalis glycosides induce or exaggerate the ST-T patterns of left ventricular hypertrophy. Electrocardiographic evidence of *right* ventricular hypertrophy is reserved for neonates with pinpoint aortic valve stenosis, pulmonary hypertension, a small left ventricular cavity, and a left-to-right shunt through a patent foramen ovale (Figure 7-24). Right ventricular hypertrophy occurs when mild to moderate *supravalvular* aortic stenosis is accompanied by severe pulmonary artery stenosis.[52]

X-Ray

In neonates with severe aortic stenosis, pulmonary venous congestion coincides with an increase in left ventricular filling pressure (Figure 7-25). Dilation of the ascending aorta is an important radiologic sign of bicuspid aortic stenosis, but not of its severity, and may be the only abnormality in the x-ray when the stenosis is mild (Figure 7-26).[110] The ascending aorta is normal in fixed subvalvular aortic stenosis (Figure 7-27),[45] is normal to small in supravalvular aortic stenosis (Figure 7-28), and is distinctly undersized with hypoplasia of the ascending aorta (see Figure 7-8B) or with a hypoplastic aortic

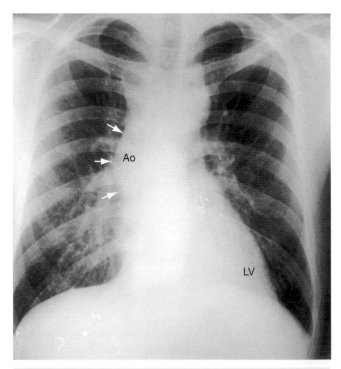

FIGURE 7-26 X-ray from a 28-year-old man with mild bicuspid aortic stenosis. The x-ray is normal except for conspicuous dilation of the ascending aortic (Ao). (LV = left ventricle.)

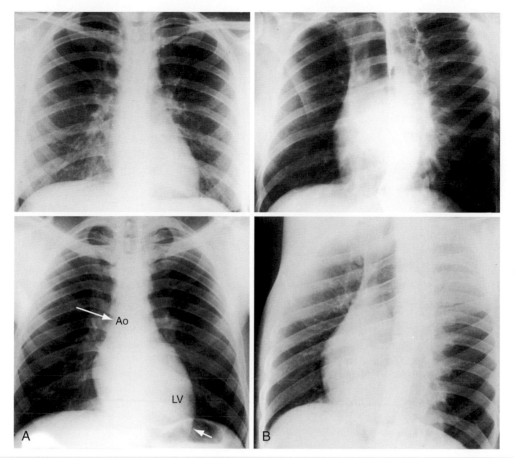

FIGURE 7-27 A, X-rays from a 21-year-old woman with fixed subaortic stenosis and a gradient of 30 mm Hg. The cardiac silhouette is normal in both views, and the ascending aorta is not dilated. **B,** X-rays from a 22-year-old man with fixed subaortic stenosis and a gradient of 100 mm Hg. The ascending aorta *(arrow)* is not dilated in either view. An elongated left ventricular (LV) silhouette extends below the left hemidiaphragm. (Ao = aorta.)

annulus and a miniature valve.[45] Dilation of the ascending aorta in XO Turner's syndrome reflects a medial abnormality that is present whether or not the aortic valve is bicuspid (see Chapter 8, Figure 8-6).[87]

Calcification is presumptive evidence that the stenosis is valvular, and dense calcium is evidence of severity.[1,39,110] A calcified *bicuspid* aortic valve can be recognized by the bulbous club-like configuration of a calcified raphe or by a circle or semicircle of calcium with the bulbous raphe pointing toward its center (see Figure 7-2C).[111]

The left ventricle attracts attention because of its shape rather than its size (Figures 7-27 through 7-29) and can remain normal-sized through a wide range of severity because the adaptive response is concentric hypertrophy with a normal or reduced cavity. The left ventricle enlarges downward and to the left and posterior so that in the frontal view the apex extends below the left hemidiaphragm (see Figures 7-27B and 7-29) and, in the left lateral projection, extends behind the inferior vena cava (see Figure 7-27B). Significant left ventricular enlargement is reserved for infants with severe aortic stenosis and congestive heart failure and for adults with chronic congestive heart failure, whether or not the aortic stenosis is severe. An increase in left atrial size in the lateral projection is a sign of severity.[110]

Echocardiogram

Echocardiography is used to identify the level, morphologic type, and severity of congenital aortic stenosis.[112] The gradient is determined with continuous-wave Doppler scan (Figure 7-30), the aortic orifice size can be calculated, and the two-dimensionally targeted M mode can be used to measure septal/free wall thickness and left ventricular cavity size. Real-time imaging is used to determine the ejection fraction.

The parasternal long axis view is used to identify doming of a bicuspid aortic valve, and the parasternal short axis is used to identify a single diastolic closure line (Figure 7-31 and Video 7-1). The bicuspid valve can appear trileaflet when the false raphe is prominent, but error is avoided with imaging of the open valve that shows doming of two unequal leaflets with an elliptical orifice (see Figure 7-31) and an M mode that shows an eccentric diastolic closure line. The suprasternal notch view visualizes the dilated ascending aorta (Figure 7-32 and Video 7-2). Transesophageal echocardiography is used to confirm the bicuspid aortic valve (see Figure 7-31) and the aortic root size and to detect a dissecting aneurysm (see Figure 7-5). Infants with severe aortic valve stenosis usually have a unicommissural unicuspid valve that is less mobile and

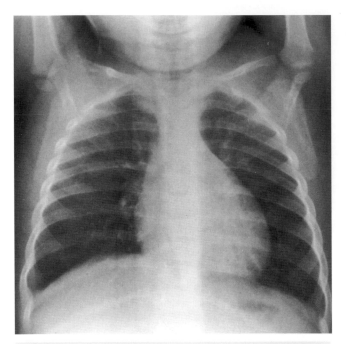

FIGURE 7-28 X-ray from a 4-year-old boy with supravalvular aortic stenosis, a gradient of 90 mm Hg, and mild pulmonary artery stenosis (gradient, 10 mm Hg). The ascending aorta is not border forming. A convex left ventricle occupies the apex. Pulmonary vascularity is normal.

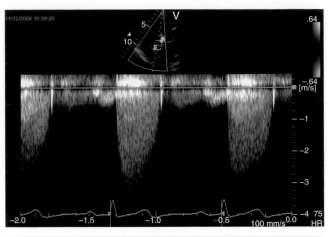

FIGURE 7-30 Continuous wave Doppler scan from a 16-year-old boy with bicuspid aortic stenosis. Peak velocity is 4.5 m/sec, which indicates a peak instantaneous gradient of 80 mm Hg.

more echodense than a bicuspid valve and may be accompanied by increased reflectivity of an infarcted fibrotic mitral papillary muscle.

In the parasternal long-axis view, a subaortic membrane is imaged immediately beneath the aortic valve attached to the ventricular septum and anterior mitral leaflet (Figure 7-33 and Video 7-3). A subaortic fibromuscular collar or tunnel produces a long dense ridge of echoes that attach to the ventricular septum and extend onto the anterior mitral leaflet. The M mode in fixed subaortic stenosis reveals distinctive brisk early systolic closure of the aortic valve followed by marked fluttering.[113]

The hourglass deformity of *supravalvular* aortic stenosis is identified in the parasternal long-axis view just above the sinuses of Valsalva (Figure 7-34 and Video 7-4). Continuous-wave Doppler scan establishes the gradient.

Summary

Congenital aortic stenosis irrespective of level is much more common in males. A murmur is typically present at birth. Most patients are asymptomatic during childhood. The neonate with severe aortic stenosis and congestive failure is an exception. Deferred onset of a murmur is likely to mean progressive fibrocalcific obstruction of a functionally normal bicuspid aortic valve or delayed development of fixed subaortic stenosis. Symptoms reflect cardiac failure, myocardial ischemia (angina pectoris), and cerebral ischemia (giddiness, lightheadedness, and syncope). Congenital aortic stenosis can be suspected when angina pectoris or syncope occurs in a young acyanotic male with a cardiac murmur that dates from birth or

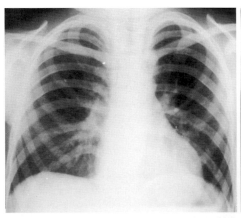

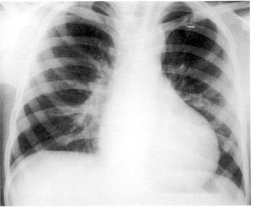

FIGURE 7-29 X-rays at 6 and 10 years of age from the same patient with bicuspid aortic stenosis and a gradient of 110 mm Hg. At age 10 years, the apex-forming left ventricle is more convex and extends below the left hemidiaphragm.

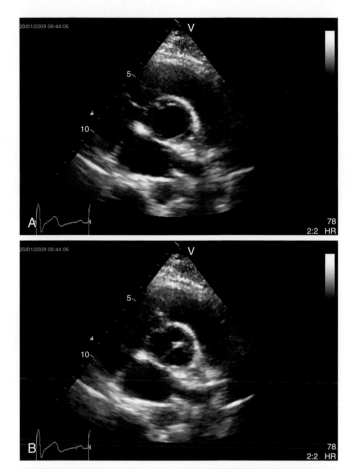

FIGURE 7-31 Transesophageal echocardiograms of a functionally normal bicuspid aortic valve. **A,** The valve is in its open systolic position. **B,** The valve is in its closed diastolic position (Video 7-1).

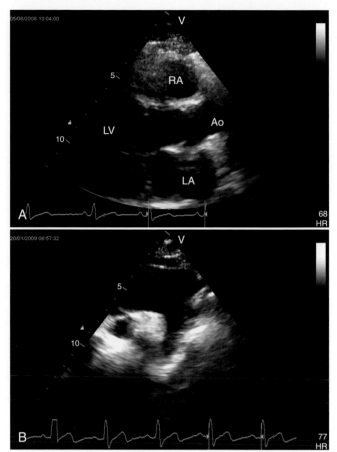

FIGURE 7-32 **A,** Echocardiogram (parasternal long axis) from a 5-year-old boy with bicuspid aortic stenosis and a gradient of 90 mm Hg. **B,** Suprasternal notch view shows a dilated ascending aorta (Video 7-2). (Ao = aorta; LA = left atrium.)

early childhood. The risk of sudden death in children and adolescents with congenital aortic stenosis and normal coronary arteries is appreciably less than in adults with calcific bicuspid aortic stenosis and acquired coronary artery disease. Inappropriate diaphoresis increases with the advent of congestive heart failure. Dissecting aneurysm of the ascending aorta is a distinctive and dramatic feature of a bicuspid aortic valve, which is a highly susceptible substrate for infective endocarditis. Familial recurrence weighs in favor of supravalvular aortic stenosis.

The following points summarize features of the physical examination, the electrocardiogram, the chest x-ray, and the echocardiocardiogram in valvular, subvalvular, and supravalvular congenital aortic stenosis.

Congenital Aortic Valve Stenosis

The right and left brachial and carotid pulses are symmetric, and the pulse pressure is small, with a slow rate of rise, a sustained peak, and a gentle decline. Jugular venous A waves are increased when an hypertrophied ventricular septum decreases the diastolic distensibility of the right ventricle. A systolic thrill is maximal in the second right intercostal space, with radiation to the suprasternal notch

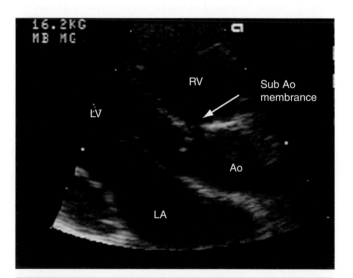

FIGURE 7-33 Echocardiogram (parasternal long axis) with fixed subaortic stenosis and a gradient of 55 mm Hg. Single arrow identifies a subaortic membrane. (LV = left ventricle; LA = left atrium) (Video 7-3).

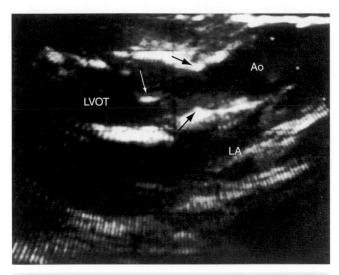

FIGURE 7-34 Parasternal long-axis view from an 8-year-old boy with supravalvular aortic stenosis and a gradient of 50 mm Hg. Paired black arrow tips point to the hourglass narrowing. The small white vertical arrow identifies an echo from the aortic valve (Video 7-4). (Ao = ascending aorta; LA = left atrium; LVO = left ventricular outflow tract.)

and to both sides of the neck. Severe aortic stenosis is accompanied by a prominent sustained left ventricular impulse with presystolic distension. An aortic ejection sound is most evident at the apex and is a characteristic feature of a mobile bicuspid aortic valve. The murmur is midsystolic, harsh, rough, noisy, and maximal in the second right intercostal space with radiation into the neck. The second heart sound is usually single but may split normally or paradoxically. When a bicuspid valve is mobile, the aortic component is preserved or accentuated and may be followed by an early diastolic murmur of aortic regurgitation. The electrocardiogram exhibits normal sinus rhythm, a normal or vertical QRS axis, and varying degrees of left ventricular hypertrophy. A dilated ascending aorta is a distinctive radiologic feature of a bicuspid aortic valve. The apex is occupied by the convex silhouette of concentric left ventricular hypertrophy. Cardiac enlargement is reserved for infants or adults with severe aortic stenosis and congestive heart failure. Calcification establishes the level of aortic stenosis in the valve, and the pattern of calcification can be used to identify a bicuspid aortic valve. Echocardiography shows systolic doming of a mobile stenotic bicuspid valve, is used to identify its morphology, and with Doppler interrogation, establishes the gradient and permits calculation of the orifice size. Unicommisural unicuspid aortic valves in symptomatic infants are less mobile and relatively echo dense.

Congenital Fixed Subaortic Stenosis

The right and left brachial and carotid arterial pulses are symmetric and exhibit a slow rate of rise, a small pulse pressure, a sustained peak, and a gentle decline. A systolic thrill is maximal in the second right intercostal space with radiation into the neck, but with tunnel subaortic stenosis, the thrill is usually maximal at the mid left sternal border. The left ventricular impulse is sustained and may be accompanied by presystolic distention and a fourth heart sound. An aortic ejection sound is absent. The stenotic murmur is coarse and rough, with a location and radiation that corresponds to the thrill. The aortic component of the second heart sound is normal or reduced. Aortic regurgitation occurs in at least 50% of cases. The electrocardiogram is indistinguishable from that of aortic valve stenosis. The x-ray discloses a nondilated ascending aorta. Echocardiography is used to identify the morphologic variations of fixed subaortic stenosis.

Congenital Supravalvular Aortic Stenosis

The Williams syndrome phenotype permits a correct diagnosis at a glance. The facial appearance is characterized by small chin, large mouth, patulous lips, blunt upturned nose, wide-set eyes, broad forehead, baggy cheeks, malformed teeth and abnormal bite (malocclusion). Growth can be retarded irrespective of the degree of obstruction and in the absence of heart failure. Brachial and carotid arterial pulses are *asymmetric*, with the pulse pressure and rate of rise greater on the right. The left ventricular impulse is sustained with presystolic distention accompanied by a fourth heart sound. An aortic ejection sound is conspicuous by its absence, and the aortic component of the second heart sound is normal. A midsystolic stenotic murmur is prominent in the *first* right intercostal space, with disproportionate radiation into the *right* side of the neck. Aortic regurgitation is uncommon if not rare. The electrocardiogram of isolated supravalvular aortic stenosis with normal coronary arteries is identical with that of congenital aortic valve stenosis. The x-ray shows a nondilated ascending aorta. Echocardiography is used to identify the presence and severity of the supravalvular obstruction.

CONGENITAL AORTIC REGURGITATION

The classic features of chronic severe aortic regurgitation have been familiar to clinicians since Corrigan's[114]1832 treatise, *On Permanent Patency of the Mouth of the Aorta, or Inadequacy of the Aortic Valves.* The remainder of this chapter deals with pure congenital aortic regurgitation when the regurgitant flow is through an incompetent aortic valve directly into the left ventricle (Boxes 7-2 and 7-3). Regurgitant flow that reaches the left ventricle through channels other than the aortic valve is dealt with briefly (see Boxes 7-2 and 7-3).

The causes of pure aortic regurgitation include abnormalities of the aortic valve, abnormalities of the aortic wall, and abnormalities that affect neither the valve nor the aortic wall.[115,116] Abnormalities that primarily affect the aortic valve are the most common causes of pure aortic regurgitation.

Pure *congenital aortic regurgitation* occurs with valves that are unicuspid unicommissural,[2] bicuspid,[117] tricuspid,

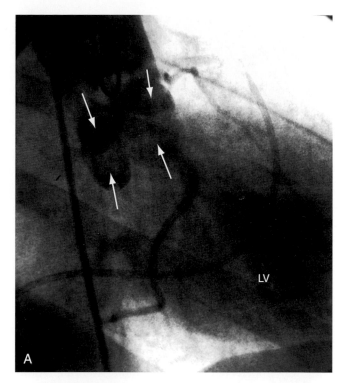

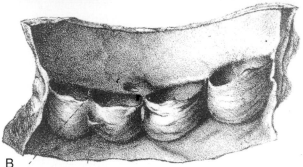

FIGURE 7-35 **A,** Aortogram from a 21-year-old man with a quadricuspid aortic valve *(four arrows)* and pure severe aortic regurgitation. **B,** Four leaflets at the aortic orifice from a preparation in St. Thomas's Hospital Museum. (LV = left ventricle). *(From Thomas B. Peacock. On malformations of the human heart. London: John Churchill; 1858.)*

or quadricuspid[41,118] or that are devoid of one or more cusps[119–121] and occurs with ventricular septal defect (see Chapter 17), aortic–left ventricular tunnel,[122,123] and coronary artery to left ventricular fistula.[124] The most common cause of pure congenital aortic valve regurgitation is the *bicuspid* aortic valve.[4] Tricuspid aortic valves with cuspal inequality are seldom incompetent in the young but become incompetent in older patients in whom minor degrees of fibrocalcification exaggerate inherent cuspal inequality and interfere with leaflet coaptation.[90] Isolated *quadricuspid aortic valves* are rare (Figure 7-35) and usually function normally in early life despite cuspal inequality.[125,126] When quadricuspid aortic valves function abnormally, the physiologic derangement is almost always expressed as pure regurgitation (see Figure 7-35A).[118,125,127] Unicuspid unicommissural valves rarely have sufficient redundancy of the free edge of the single leaflet to render the mechanism incompetent.[2]

The foregoing types of congenital aortic regurgitation are characterized by regurgitant flow that is *mild or absent* in infancy and early childhood. However, three types of *severe* aortic regurgitation begin in the young. One or more cusps or the entire aortic valve mechanism can be congenitally absent,[119,121,128–130] with deleterious effects that begin *in utero* and continue in neonates and infants.[119–121,130] A second form of severe aortic regurgitation that originates in infancy is an aortic–left ventricular tunnel, a rare malformation characterized by a vascular channel that originates immediately above the right sinus of Valsalva, tunnels through the ventricular septum, terminates in the paramembranous or infundibular septum, and enters the left ventricle immediately below the right and noncoronary cusps.[122] The aortic end of the tunnel is separated from the right coronary ostium

(Figure 7-36 and Video 7-5). A third and also rare form of severe aortic regurgitation that begins in infancy is a large coronary artery to left ventricular fistula, fewer than 10% of which terminate in the left ventricle (see Chapter 22). Although congestive heart failure can develop in the neonate, the magnitude of flow is usually limited, so adult survival is the rule.[131]

A functionally normal bicuspid aortic valve[4] is associated with mild aortic regurgitation (Figure 7-37) because the free edges of bicuspid leaflets are longer than the diameter of the aortic ring to permit unobstructed systolic flow (see Figure 7-1A, left panel). Regurgitation may remain mild or gradually or acutely increase (Figure 7-38).[4,132,133] Chronic severe bicuspid aortic regurgitation is caused by gradually increasing prolapse of the

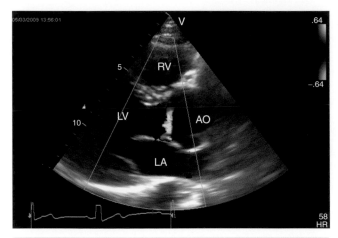

FIGURE 7-36 Echocardiogram, parasternal long-axis, from a 13-year-old boy with a functionally normal bicuspid aortic valve and mild aortic regurgitation (Video 7-5). (LV = left ventricle; AO = aortic root; LA = left atrium; RV = right ventricle.)

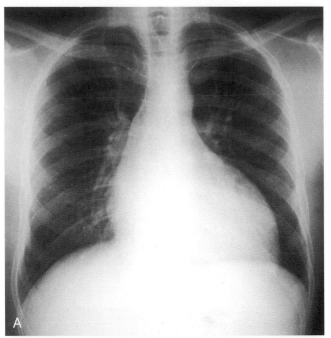

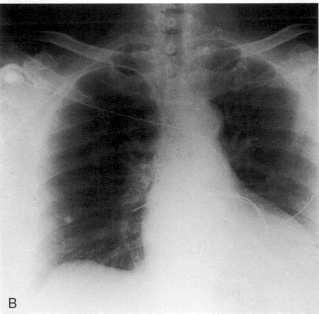

FIGURE 7-37 **A,** X-ray from a 22-year-old man with chronic severe bicuspid aortic regurgitation. The ascending aorta is dilated, and a large convex left ventricle extends below the left hemidiaphragm. **B,** Portable x-ray (anteroposterior projection) from a 62-year-old woman with acute severe aortic regurgitation caused by infective endocarditis on a previously unrecognized bicuspid aortic valve. The left ventricle is moderately dilated. There is pulmonary venous congestion.

relatively redundant edge of the larger of the two bicuspid leaflets.[132] Regurgitation is insidious, with the fully developed hemodynamic fault awaiting adulthood.[117] However, infective endocarditis can convert a functionally normal congenital bicuspid aortic valve into the catastrophic hemodynamic fault of acute severe aortic regurgitation (see Figure 7-38B).[4,132,133] Bicuspid aortic regurgitation is augmented by dilation and dissection of the aortic root caused by an inherent medial abnormality of the ascending aorta above a bicuspid aortic valve (see previous discussion and Figure 7-4).[28,85,127]

The *physiologic consequences* of aortic regurgitation depend on the magnitude of regurgitant flow, its rate development, and the adaptive response of the left ventricle to volume overload. Fundamental differences between *gradual* progression culminate decades later in severe aortic regurgitation and the development of *acute severe* aortic regurgitation.[133,134] Adaptation of the left ventricle to gradual chronic aortic regurgitation was addressed in 1858 by Peacock[22]: "This process is often so slow in its progress, that the ventricle accommodates itself to the additional exertion required; the disease becomes a source of manifest evil only after the lapse of many years." *Gradual* development of severe aortic regurgitation permits an adaptive response of the left ventricle that is precluded if equivalent aortic regurgitation is suddenly incurred.[133]

The response of the left ventricle to a gradual increase in volume is typified by chronic severe aortic regurgitation incurred before the onset of depressed myocardial contractility (Table 7-1). The volume-overloaded ventricle achieves an adaptive increase in mass by increasing its internal dimensions (radius and base to apex) with a proportionate increase in septal/free wall thickness. The result is a magnified normal heart that is geometrically ideal for ejecting an augmented stroke volume against normal or reduced systemic resistance.[59] The increase in ventricular mass is initially a desirable adaptive response that permits the heart to function normally at greater workloads.[59] Left ventricular end-diastolic volume and fiber length increase; end-diastolic pressure remains normal. Stroke volume and ejection fraction increase, so effective cardiac output is maintained. The velocity of ejection increases, left ventricular and aortic systolic pressures rise, and aortic diastolic pressure falls, so the pulse pressure widens. Despite a considerable increase in stroke volume, the duration of left ventricular contraction remains

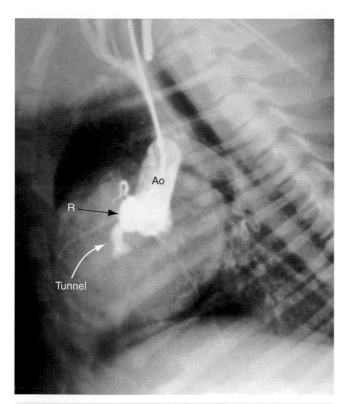

FIGURE 7-38 Contrast material injected into the ascending aorta (Ao) of a mixed-breed dog. The *arrow* points to a blind aortic to left ventricular tunnel. The right aortic sinus (R) is enlarged. *(Courtesy Dr. N. Sidney Moise, Cornell University College of Veterinary Medicine, Ithaca, New York.)*

Table 7-1 Major Hemodynamic Features of Chronic and Acute Severe Aortic Regurgitation

	Chronic	Acute
LV compliance	Increased	Not increased
Regurgitant volume	Increased	Increased
LV end-diastolic pressure	Normal	Markedly increased
LV ejection velocity (dp/dt)	Markedly increased	Not significantly increased
Aortic systolic pressure	Increased	Not increased
Aortic diastolic pressure	Markedly decreased	Not significantly decreased
Systemic arterial pulse pressure	Markedly increased	Not significantly increased
Ejection fraction	Increased	Not increased
Effective stroke volume	Normal	Decreased
Effective cardiac output	Normal	Decreased
Heart rate	Normal	Increased
Peripheral vascular resistance	Normal	Increased

LV, Left ventricular; *dp/dt.*

normal because the velocity of ejection is increased and the pre-ejection period is shortened. With isotonic exercise, systemic systolic pressure rises, peripheral resistance falls, diastole shortens as heart rate increases, and regurgitant fraction per beat decreases. An appropriate increment in effective cardiac output is achieved without an increase in end-diastolic volume or end-diastolic pressure.[135] Despite these favorable adaptations, left ventricular response to isotonic or isometric exercise is not necessarily normal, even in young asymptomatic patients.[135,136]

Acute severe aortic regurgitation is characterized by a dramatic rise in left ventricular end-diastolic pressure in response to the sudden increase in volume imposed on a ventricle that is operating on the less compliant portion of its pressure-volume curve.[134] As stroke volume falls, heart rate accelerates in a vain attempt to maintain cardiac output. Peripheral resistance rises in an equally vain attempt to maintain systemic arterial pressure.[134] The velocity of ejection does not significantly increase, left ventricular and aortic systolic pressures are not significantly elevated, and aortic diastolic pressure cannot fall below the relatively high left ventricular end-diastolic pressure, so the systemic arterial pulse pressure remains normal or nearly so. The steep rise in left ventricular end-diastolic pressure exceeds left atrial pressure, prematurely closing the mitral valve before inscription of the P wave in the electrocardiogram.[133] The mitral valve opens later than normal because of prolonged ejection from the acutely volume-loaded left ventricle.[133] Premature closure and delayed opening of the mitral valve, together with obligatory tachycardia, reduce the time during which the mitral valve is open. The pulmonary arterial pressure rises in tandem with left atrial mean pressure, but competence of the mitral valve protects the left atrium from linear transmission of the high left ventricular end-diastolic pressure into the pulmonary venous bed.[134] This protection is lost with the advent of mitral regurgitation, so left atrial pressure rises further and cardiac output reciprocally falls.[134]

History

Congenital aortic valve regurgitation predominates in males, a gender distribution that reflects the prevalence of bicuspid aortic valves.[4] In asymptomatic infants and children, the soft diastolic murmur of bicuspid aortic regurgitation usually goes undetected. Patients with moderate to severe aortic regurgitation are often asymptomatic except for awareness of neck pulsations or awareness of left ventricular premature contractions when lying in the left lateral decubitus position.[135] Vascular wall pain is occasionally experienced in the carotid and subclavian arteries and in the thoracic or abdominal aorta. The retrosternal chest pain of myocardial ischemia occasionally accompanies acute severe aortic regurgitation.[137] Inappropriate diaphoresis sometimes begins long before the onset of congestive heart failure. When bicuspid valve infective endocarditis causes acute severe aortic regurgitation, cardiac failure is sudden and intractable.[133]

When aortic regurgitation is caused by an aortic–left ventricular tunnel, severe regurgitant flow and congestive heart failure develop early, but exceptional asymptomatic survivals have been reported in children and young adults.[123] Congenital absence of one or more aortic cusps with severe regurgitation is manifest by *in utero* heart failure with nonimmune fetal hydrops.[128] Exceptional childhood or postadolescent survivals have been reported.[121]

Physical Signs

In 1832, Dominic Corrigan[114] described the visible arterial pulse associated with inadequacy of the aortic valve:

> *When a patient affected by the disease is stripped, the arterial trunks of the head, neck, and superior extremities immediately catch the eye by their singular pulsation. At each diastole the subclavian, carotid, temporal, brachial, and in some cases even the palmar arteries, are suddenly thrown from their bed, bounding up under the skin ... though a moment before unmarked, they are at each pulsation thrown out on the surface in the strongest relief. From its singular and striking appearance, the name visible pulsation is given to this beating of the arteries.*

The arterial pulse in *chronic* severe aortic regurgitation is characterized by a rapid rate of rise, an increased pulse pressure (high systolic/low diastolic), a single or double peak (bisferiens), and a brisk collapse.[90] The Quincke's pulse (flushing and blanching of the digital capillary bed), palpable pulsations in the fingertips, and posteroanterior head movements are synchronous with systole and diastole.[90] The arterial pulse in *acute* severe aortic regurgitation is characterized by an unimpressive rate of rise, a moderately increased pulse pressure (systolic normal, diastolic normal or slightly diminished), a single peak, and the pulsus alternans of left ventricular failure.[133]

Precordial palpation in *chronic* severe aortic regurgitation reveals a laterally displaced hyperdynamic left ventricular impulse that imparts a rocking motion to the chest. A systolic thrill and murmur are present in the suprasternal notch and over the carotid and subclavian arteries (Corrigan's *bruit de soufflet*)[114] because of high-velocity ejection. In *acute* severe aortic regurgitation, the location of the left ventricular impulse is normal or moderately displaced and is not hyperdynamic.

In chronic severe aortic regurgitation, the first heart sound is normal, the aortic component of the second sound is soft, and there is neither a third nor a fourth heart sound.[138] There is a grade 3/6 right basal aortic midsystolic murmur, a long high-pitched aortic diastolic murmur at the mid left sternal border, and a presystolic Austin Flint murmur at the apex.[90] An aortic ejection sound is absent because a severely incompetent bicuspid aortic valve does not dome.[138] Peripheral arterial auscultatory signs include Traube's *pistol shot* sounds and the systolic/diastolic Duroziez's murmur over a partially compressed femoral artery.

In *acute* severe aortic regurgitation,[133] the first heart sound is soft or absent and a fourth heart sound is precluded because of premature closure of the mitral valve. A third heart sound reflects left ventricular failure. The pulmonary component of the second sound is increased in response to elevated pulmonary artery pressure.

A midsystolic aortic flow murmur is less than grade 3 and is followed by an aortic diastolic murmur that is short, medium-pitched, and disarmingly soft because of the relatively low velocity of regurgitant flow. Distinguishing systole from diastole is difficult because the first heart sound is soft or absent and the heart rate is rapid. A presystolic Austin Flint murmur is precluded because of premature closure of the mitral valve. No auscultatory signs are found over peripheral arteries.[133]

An *aortic–left ventricular tunnel* is accompanied by a systolic/diastolic to-and-fro murmur analogous to midsystolic/early diastolic murmur of chronic severe aortic regurgitation.[123] Doppler scan interrogation of flow patterns within the ascending aorta and within the tunnel are used to identify diastolic flow from the tunnel into the left ventricle and systolic flow from left ventricle into the tunnel.[139] The phasic flow is predominantly diastolic, which is consistent with the auscultatory observation that the diastolic murmur is loud and the systolic murmur is soft.[123] Occasionally, only the diastolic murmur is audible.

Electrocardiogram

The typical electrocardiogram of *chronic* severe aortic regurgitation displays the voltage and repolarization criteria of left ventricular hypertrophy with prominent left precordial Q waves of chronic volume overload. Isotonic exercise, even in children and young adults, sometimes provokes or exaggerates ST segment depressions. In *acute* severe aortic regurgitation, left ventricular hypertrophy is absent, the QRS voltage is normal, repolarization abnormalities are minor, and left precordial Q waves are inconspicuous.

X-Ray

In *chronic* severe bicuspid aortic regurgitation, the x-ray shows an enlarged convex left ventricle and a conspicuously dilated ascending aorta because pulsatile regurgitant flow aggregates the dilatory effect of an inherent medial abnormality (see Figure 7-38A).[28] Pulmonary venous vascularity is normal because left ventricular filling pressure is not increased. In *acute* severe aortic regurgitation, the left ventricular silhouette is nearly normal, and pulmonary venous vascularity is increased because left ventricular filling pressure is elevated (see Figure 7-38B). In aortic regurgitation associated with *aortic–left ventricular tunnel*, the ascending aorta is consistently dilated and is sometimes aneurysmal.[123,139]

Echocardiogram

Echocardiography with Doppler scan interrogation and color flow imaging establishes the presence and degree of aortic regurgitation, determines aortic valve morphology, and defines the physiologic consequences of regurgitant flow. Mild aortic regurgitation of a functionally normal bicuspid aortic valve is identified with color flow imaging (see Figure 7-37B). The regurgitant jet of bicuspid aortic regurgitation is eccentric in the left ventricular outflow tract (Figure 7-39 and Video 7-6). Continuous-wave Doppler

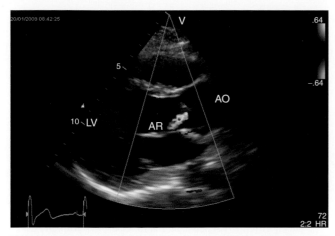

FIGURE 7-39 Echocardiogram from a 32-year-old man with a functionally normal bicuspid aortic valve. The eccentric jet of mild to moderate aortic regurgitation (AR) is directed toward the anterior mitral leaflet (Video 7-6). (AO = dilated aorta root; LV = left ventricle.)

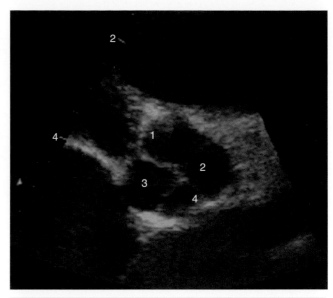

FIGURE 7-41 Echocardiogram (short axis) from a 66-year-old man with a quadricuspid aortic valve (1, 2, 3, 4 cusps) (Video 7-7).

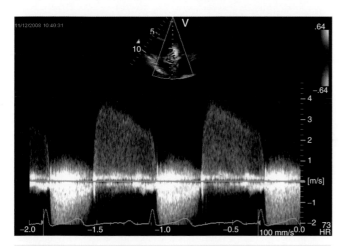

FIGURE 7-40 Continuous wave Doppler across a bicuspid aortic valve showing regurgitation in diastole.

Summary

The most common cause of congenital aortic regurgitation is a bicuspid aortic valve. The degree of regurgitation varies from mild to severe. Most patients are males with no history of a cardiac murmur in infancy and childhood. Bicuspid aortic regurgitation progresses insidiously and usually presents in young adults who have few or no symptoms despite appreciable regurgitant flow. Severe regurgitation presents in neonates or infants with absence of one or more aortic cusps, an aortic–left ventricular tunnel, and a large coronary artery to left ventricular fistula. Patients are subjectively and sometimes unpleasantly aware of neck pulsations and of forceful left ventricular contractions, especially with premature beats, and may experience inappropriate diaphoresis or vascular pain over carotid arteries or over the thoracic and abdominal aorta. The systemic arterial pulse pressure is wide, and the rate of rise is rapid, with a bisferiens peak and a brisk collapse. The dilated hyperdynamic left ventricle generates a rocking precordial motion. A systolic thrill is often present at the right base and in the suprasternal notch and neck despite the absence of aortic stenosis. A short prominent right basal midsystolic murmur radiates into the neck. The first heart sound is normal or soft. Third and fourth heart sounds are absent. An early diastolic murmur is loud and long, and Duroziez's murmur and Traube's pistol shot sounds are heard over peripheral arteries. The electrocardiogram exhibits voltage and repolarization criteria of left ventricular hypertrophy. The x-ray reveals an enlarged left ventricle, a dilated ascending aorta, and normal pulmonary venous vascularity. The clinical course of a bicuspid aortic valve, whether functionally normal, stenotic, or incompetent, may suddenly be punctuated by a dissecting aortic aneurysm and an increase in regurgitant flow. An unrecognized functionally normal bicuspid aortic valve can announce itself when infective endocarditis causes acute severe aortic regurgitation with

scan records the profile of regurgitant flow and is used to determine whether aortic stenosis coexists (Figure 7-40). The four cusps of a congenitally quadricuspid aortic valve are best recognized in a transesophageal echocardiogram (Figure 7-41 and Video 7-7).

Two-dimensionally targeted M-mode echocardiography establishes end-diastolic and end-systolic left ventricular dimensions and septal/free wall thickness. Left ventricular ejection fraction is determined from two-dimensional real-time imaging.

An aortic–left ventricular tunnel can be identified as the cause of aortic regurgitation, and Doppler interrogation with color flow imaging permits study of phasic directional flow within the tunnel.[122,124,139] An aortic–left ventricular tunnel arising from the *left* aortic sinus was diagnosed with echocardiography.

sudden intractable heart failure. Systemic arterial pulse pressure is only moderately increased, the rate of rise is not brisk, pulsus alternant is common, and peripheral arterial signs of chronic severe aortic regurgitation are absent. The left ventricular impulse is only moderately displaced and is not hyperdynamic. The first heart sound is soft or inaudible despite tachycardia. A fourth heart sound is absent, but a third sound is prominent. The aortic midsystolic murmur is grade 3 or less, and the murmur of aortic regurgitation is short, medium-pitched, and relatively soft. An Austin Flint murmur cannot be presystolic. The electrocardiogram does not show left ventricular hypertrophy. The x-ray exhibits a near normal or only moderately enlarged left ventricle and a conspicuous increase in pulmonary venous vascularity.

REFERENCES

1. Campbell M. Calcific aortic stenosis and congenital bicuspid aortic valves. *Br Heart J.* 1968;30:606–616.
2. Falcone MW, Roberts WC, Morrow AG, Perloff JK. Congenital aortic stenosis resulting from a unicommisssural valve. Clinical and anatomic features in twenty-one adult patients. *Circulation.* 1971;44:272–280.
3. Perloff J. Clinical recognition of aortic stenosis the physical signs and differential diagnosis of the various forms of obstruction to left ventricular outflow. *Prog Cardiovasc Dis.* 1968;10: 323–352.
4. Roberts WC. The congenitally bicuspid aortic valve. A study of 85 autopsy cases. *Am J Cardiol.* 1970;26:72–83.
5. Roberts WC. The structure of the aortic valve in clinically isolated aortic stenosis: an autopsy study of 162 patients over 15 years of age. *Circulation.* 1970;42:91–97.
6. Roberts WC. Valvular, subvalvular and supravalvular aortic stenosis: morphologic features. *Cardiovasc Clin.* 1973;5:97–126.
7. Roberts WC, Ko JM. Clinical and morphologic features of the congenitally unicuspid acommissural stenotic and regurgitant aortic valve. *Cardiology.* 2007;108:79–81.
8. Tzemos N, Therrien J, Yip J, et al. Outcomes in adults with bicuspid aortic valves. *JAMA.* 2008;300:1317–1325.
9. Movahed M-R, Hepner AD, Ahmadi-Kashani M. Echocardiographic prevalence of bicuspid aortic valve in the population. *Heart Lung Circ.* 2006;15:297–299.
10. Lewin MB, Otto CM. The bicuspid aortic valve: adverse outcomes from infancy to old age. *Circulation.* 2005;111:832–834.
11. Sabet HY, Edwards WD, Tazelaar HD, Daly RC. Congenitally bicuspid aortic valves: a surgical pathology study of 542 cases (1991 through 1996) and a literature review of 2,715 additional cases. *Mayo Clin Proc.* 1999;74:14–26.
12. Biner S, Rafique AM, Ray I, Cuk O, Siegel RJ, Tolstrup K. Aortopathy is prevalent in relatives of bicuspid aortic valve patients. *J Am Coll Cardiol.* 2009;53:2288–2295.
13. Khan W, Milsevic M, Salciccioli L, Lazar J. Low prevalence of bicuspid aortic valve in African Americans. *Am Heart J.* 2008; 156:e25.
14. Subramanian R, Olson LJ, Edwards WD. Surgical pathology of pure aortic stenosis: a study of 374 cases. *Mayo Clin Proc.* 1984;59:683–690.
15. Chan KL, Ghani M, Woodend K, Burwash IG. Case-controlled study to assess risk factors for aortic stenosis in congenitally bicuspid aortic valve. *Am J Cardiol.* 2001;88:690–693.
16. Da Vinci L. *Leonardo on the human body.* Mineola, NY: Dover Publications; 1983.
17. Waider W, Craige E. First heart sound and ejection sounds. Echocardiographic and phonocardiographic correlation with valvular events. *Am J Cardiol.* 1975;35:346–356.
18. Fernandes SM, Sanders SP, Khairy P, et al. Morphology of bicuspid aortic valve in children and adolescents. *J Am Coll Cardiol.* 2004;44:1648–1651.
19. Beppu S, Suzuki S, Matsuda H, Ohmori F, Nagata S, Miyatake K. Rapidity of progression of aortic stenosis in patients with congenital bicuspid aortic valves. *Am J Cardiol.* 1993;71:322–327.
20. Davis GL, Mcalister WH, Friedenberg MJ. Congenital aortic stenosis due to failure of histogenesis of the aortic valve (myxoid dysplasia). *Am J Roentgenol Radium Ther Nucl Med.* 1965;95: 621–628.
21. Sans-Coma V, Cardo M, Thiene G, Fernandez B, Arque JM, Duran AC. Bicuspid aortic and pulmonary valves in the Syrian hamster. *Int J Cardiol.* 1992;34:249–254.
22. Peacock T. *On malformations of the human heart.* London: John Churchill; 1858.
23. Song Z-Z. Valve calcification and patients with bicuspid aortic valves. *JAMA.* 2009;301:935–936; author reply 936.
24. Kalan JM, Mcintosh CL, Bonow RO, Roberts WC. Development of severe stenosis in a previously purely regurgitant, congenitally bicuspid aortic valve. *Am J Cardiol.* 1988;62:988–989.
25. Bonow RO. Bicuspid aortic valves and dilated aortas: a critical review of the ACC/AHA practice guidelines recommendations. *Am J Cardiol.* 2008;102:111–114.
26. Basso C, Boschello M, Perrone C, et al. An echocardiographic survey of primary school children for bicuspid aortic valve. *Am J Cardiol.* 2004;93:661–663.
27. Beroukhim RS, Kruzick TL, Taylor AL, Gao D, Yetman AT. Progression of aortic dilation in children with a functionally normal bicuspid aortic valve. *Am J Cardiol.* 2006;98:828–830.
28. Niwa K, Perloff JK, Bhuta SM, et al. Structural abnormalities of great arterial walls in congenital heart disease: light and electron microscopic analyses. *Circulation.* 2001;103:393–400.
29. Silberbach M. Bicuspid aortic valve and thoracic aortic aneurysm: toward a unified theory. *J Am Coll Cardiol.* 2009;53: 2296–2297.
30. Novaro GM, Griffin BP. Congenital bicuspid aortic valve and rate of ascending aortic dilatation. *Am J Cardiol.* 2004;93:525–526.
31. Novaro GM, Tiong IY, Pearce GL, Grimm RA, Smedira N, Griffin BP. Features and predictors of ascending aortic dilatation in association with a congenital bicuspid aortic valve. *Am J Cardiol.* 2003;92:99–101.
32. Gurvitz M, Chang R-K, Drant S, Allada V. Frequency of aortic root dilation in children with a bicuspid aortic valve. *Am J Cardiol.* 2004;94:1337–1340.
33. Nistri S, Grande-Allen J, Noale M, et al. Aortic elasticity and size in bicuspid aortic valve syndrome. *Eur Heart J.* 2008;29:472–479.
34. Nemes A, Soliman OI, Csanady M, Forster T. Aortic distensibility in patients with bicuspid aortic valves. *Am J Cardiol.* 2008;102: 370.
35. Reeve Jr R, Robinson SJ. Hypoplastic annulus—an unusual type of aortic stenosis: a report of three cases in children. *Dis Chest.* 1964; 45:99–102.
36. Vollebergh FE, Becker AE. Minor congenital variations of cusp size in tricuspid aortic valves. Possible link with isolated aortic stenosis. *Br Heart J.* 1977;39:1006–1011.
37. Fratellone P, Berger M, Khan M, Bassiri-Tehrani M. Quadricuspid aortic valve diagnosed by echocardiography in two cases identical twins. *Am J Cardiol.* 2007;100:1490–1491.
38. Tentolouris K, Kontozoglou T, Trikas A, et al. Fixed subaortic stenosis revisited. congenital abnormalities in 72 new cases and review of the literature. *Cardiology.* 1999;92:4–10.
39. Campbell M. The natural history of congenital aortic stenosis. *Br Heart J.* 1968;30:514–526.
40. Choi JY, Sullivan ID. Fixed subaortic stenosis: anatomical spectrum and nature of progression. *Br Heart J.* 1991;65:280–286.
41. Firpo C, Maitre Azcarate MJ, Quero Jimenez M, Saravalli O. Discrete subaortic stenosis (DSS) in childhood: a congenital or acquired disease? Follow-up in 65 patients. *Eur Heart J.* 1990;11:1033–1040.
42. Laskey WK, Kussmaul WG. Subvalvular gradients in patients with valvular aortic stenosis: prevalence, magnitude, and physiological importance. *Circulation.* 2001;104:1019–1022.
43. El Habbal MH, Suliman RF. The aortic root in subaortic stenosis. *Am Heart J.* 1989;117:1127–1132.
44. Pyle RL, Patterson DF, Chacko S. The genetics and pathology of discrete subaortic stenosis in the Newfoundland dog. *Am Heart J.* 1976;92:324–334.
45. Maron BJ, Redwood DR, Roberts WC, Henry WL, Morrow AG, Epstein SE. Tunnel subaortic stenosis. left ventricular outflow tract obstruction produced by fibromuscular tubular narrowing. *Circulation.* 1976;54:404–416.

46. Freedom RM, Fowler RS, Duncan WJ. Rapid evolution from "normal" left ventricular outflow tract to fatal subaortic stenosis in infancy. *Br Heart J.* 1981;45:605–609.

47. Stamm C, Li J, Ho SY, Redington AN, Anderson RH. The aortic root in supravalvular aortic stenosis: the potential surgical relevance of morphologic findings. *J Thorac Cardiovasc Surg.* 1997; 114:16–24.

48. Vaideeswar P, Shankar V, Deshpande JR, Sivaraman A, Jain N. Pathology of the diffuse variant of supravalvar aortic stenosis. *Cardiovasc Pathol.* 2001;10:33–37.

49. Vincent WR, Buckberg GD, Hoffman JI. Left ventricular subendocardial ischemia in severe valvar and supravalvar aortic stenosis. A common mechanism. *Circulation.* 1974;49:326–333.

50. Yilmaz AT, Arslan M, Ozal E, Byngol H, Tatar H, Ozturk OY. Coronary artery aneurysm associated with adult supravalvular aortic stenosis. *Ann Thorac Surg.* 1996;62:1205–1207.

51. Williams JC, Barratt-Boyes BG, Lowe JB. Supravalvular aortic stenosis. *Circulation.* 1961;24:1311–1318.

52. Beuren AJ, Apitz J, Harmjanz D. Supravalvular aortic stenosis in association with mental retardation and a certain facial appearance. *Circulation.* 1962;26:1235–1240.

53. Ingelfinger JR, Newburger JW. Spectrum of renal anomalies in patients with Williams syndrome. *J Pediatr.* 1991;119: 771–773.

54. Morris CA, Leonard CO, Dilts C, Demsey SA. Adults with Williams syndrome. *Am J Med Genet Suppl.* 1990;6:102–107.

55. Pober BR, Lacro RV, Rice C, Mandell V, Teele RL. Renal findings in 40 individuals with Williams syndrome. *Am J Med Genet.* 1993; 46:271–274.

56. Daniels SR, Loggie JM, Schwartz DC, Strife JL, Kaplan S. Systemic hypertension secondary to peripheral vascular anomalies in patients with Williams syndrome. *J Pediatr.* 1985;106: 249–251.

57. Salaymeh KJ, Banerjee A. Evaluation of arterial stiffness in children with Williams syndrome: Does it play a role in evolving hypertension? *Am Heart J.* 2001;142:549–555.

58. Rein AJ, Preminger TJ, Perry SB, Lock JE, Sanders SP. Generalized arteriopathy in Williams syndrome: an intravascular ultrasound study. *J Am Coll Cardiol.* 1993;21:1727–1730.

59. Perloff JK. Normal myocardial growth and the development and regression of increased ventricular mass. In: Perloff JK, Child JS, eds. *Congenital heart disease in adults.* 2nd ed. Philadelphia: W.B. Saunders; 1998:346.

60. Rakusan K, Flanagan MF, Geva T, Southern J, Van Praagh R. Morphometry of human coronary capillaries during normal growth and the effect of age in left ventricular pressure-overload hypertrophy. *Circulation.* 1992;86:38–46.

61. Krovetz LJ, Kurlinski JP. Subendocardial blood flow in children with congenital aortic stenosis. *Circulation.* 1976;54:961–965.

62. El-Said G, Galioto Jr FM, Mullins CE, Mcnamara DG. Natural hemodynamic history of congenital aortic stenosis in childhood. *Am J Cardiol.* 1972;30:6–12.

63. Kim YM, Yoo SJ, Choi JY, Kim SH, Bae EJ, Lee YT. Natural course of supravalvar aortic stenosis and peripheral pulmonary arterial stenosis in Williams' syndrome. *Cardiol Young.* 1999;9: 37–41.

64. Mocellin R, Sauer U, Simon B, Comazzi M, Sebening F, Buhlmeyer K. Reduced left ventricular size and endocardial fibroelastosis as corrclates of mortality in newborns and young infants with severe aortic valve stenosis. *Pediatr Cardiol.* 1983;4: 265–272.

65. Gould L, Venkataraman K, Goswami M, Demartino A, Gomprecht RF. Right-sided heart failure in aortic stenosis. *Am J Cardiol.* 1973;31:381–383.

66. Bache RJ, Wang Y, Jorgensen CR. Hemodynamic effects of exercise in isolated valvular aortic stenosis. *Circulation.* 1971;44: 1003–1013.

67. Cyran SE, James FW, Daniels S, Mays W, Shukla R, Kaplan S. Comparison of the cardiac output and stroke volume response to upright exercise in children with valvular and subvalvular aortic stenosis. *J Am Coll Cardiol.* 1988;11:651–658.

68. Kveselis DA, Rocchini AP, Rosenthal A, et al. Hemodynamic determinants of exercise-induced ST-segment depression in children with valvar aortic stenosis. *Am J Cardiol.* 1985;55: 1133–1139.

69. Mark AL, Kioschos JM, Abboud FM, Heistad DD, Schmid PG. Abnormal vascular responses to exercise in patients with aortic stenosis. *J Clin Invest.* 1973;52:1138–1146.

70. Keane JF, Driscoll DJ, Gersony WM, et al. Second natural history study of congenital heart defects. Results of treatment of patients with aortic valvar stenosis. *Circulation.* 1993;87:I16–I27.

71. Friedman WF, Modlinger J, Morgan JR. Serial hemodynamic observations in asymptomatic children with valvar aortic stenosis. *Circulation.* 1971;43:91–97.

72. Moller JH, Nakib A, Edwards JE. Infarction of papillary muscles and mitral insufficiency associated with congenital aortic stenosis. *Circulation.* 1966;34:87–91.

73. Conway Jr EE, Noonan J, Marion RW, Steeg CN. Myocardial infarction leading to sudden death in the Williams syndrome: report of three cases. *J Pediatr.* 1990;117:593–595.

74. Morgan C, Nadas A. Sweating and congestive heart failure. *N Engl J Med.* 1963;268:580–585.

75. Gale AW, Cartmill TB, Bernstein L. Familial subaortic membranous stenosis. *Aust N Z J Med.* 1974;4:576–581.

76. Richardson ME, Menahem S, Wilkinson JL. Familial fixed subaortic stenosis. *Int J Cardiol.* 1991;30:351–353.

77. Ensing GJ, Schmidt MA, Hagler DJ, Michels VV, Carter GA, Feldt RH. Spectrum of findings in a family with nonsyndromic autosomal dominant supravalvular aortic stenosis: A Doppler echocardiographic study. *J Am Coll Cardiol.* 1989; 13:413–419.

78. Eisenberg R, Young D, Jacobson B, Boito A. Familial supravalvular aortic stenosis. *Am J Dis Child.* 1964;108:341–347.

79. Dridi SM, Ghomrasseni S, Bonnet D, et al. Skin elastic fibers in Williams syndrome. *Am J Med Genet.* 1999;87:134–138.

80. Morris CA. Genetic aspects of supravalvular aortic stenosis. *Curr Opin Cardiol.* 1998;13:214–219.

81. Urban Z, Michels VV, Thibodeau SN, et al. Isolated supravalvular aortic stenosis: functional haploinsufficiency of the elastin gene as a result of nonsense-mediated decay. *Hum Genet.* 2000;106: 577–588.

82. Von Dadelszen P, Chitayat D, Winsor EJ, et al. De novo 46,XX, t(6;7)(q27;q11;23) associated with severe cardiovascular manifestations characteristic of supravalvular aortic stenosis and Williams syndrome. *Am J Med Genet.* 2000;90:270–275.

83. Friedman WF, Roberts WC. Vitamin D and the supravalvar aortic stenosis syndrome. The transplacental effects of vitamin D on the aorta of the rabbit. *Circulation.* 1966;34:77–86.

84. Osler W. The bicuspid condition of the aortic valves. *Trans Assoc Am Physicians.* 1886;1:185–192.

85. Larson EW, Edwards WD. Risk factors for aortic dissection: a necropsy study of 161 cases. *Am J Cardiol.* 1984;53:849–855.

86. Scheffer SM, Leatherman LL. Resolution of Heyde's syndrome of aortic stenosis and gastrointestinal bleeding after aortic valve replacement. *Ann Thorac Surg.* 1986;42:477–480.

87. Miller MJ, Geffner ME, Lippe BM, et al. Echocardiography reveals a high incidence of bicuspid aortic valve in Turner syndrome. *J Pediatr.* 1983;102:47–50.

88. Prandstraller D, Mazzanti L, Picchio FM, et al. Turner's syndrome: cardiologic profile according to the different chromosomal patterns and long-term clinical follow-Up of 136 nonpreselected patients. *Pediatr Cardiol.* 1999;20:108–112.

89. Mazzanti L, Cacciari E. Congenital heart disease in patients with Turner's syndrome. Italian Study Group for Turner Syndrome (ISGTS). *J Pediatr.* 1998;133:688–692.

90. Perloff JK. *Physical examination of the heart and circulation.* 4th ed. Shelton, Connecticut: People's Medical Publishing House; 2009.

91. Farrar JF, Gray RE. The pulse of aortic stenosis during childhood. *Br Heart J.* 1965;27:199–204.

92. Alpert JS, Vieweg WV, Hagan AD. Incidence and morphology of carotid shudders in aortic valve disease. *Am Heart J.* 1976;92: 435–440.

93. Goldstein RE, Epstein SE. Mechanism of elevated innominate artery pressures in supravalvular aortic stenosis. *Circulation.* 1970;42:23–29.

94. Lurie P, Mendelbaum I. Mechanism of brachial pulse asymmetry in congenital aortic stenotic lesions. *Circulation.* 1963;28:760.

95. Franch R, Oran E. Asymmetric arm and neck pulses: A clue to supravalvular aortic stenosis. *Circulation.* 1963;28:722.

96. Braunwald E, Goldblatt A, Aygen MM, Rockoff SD, Morrow AG. Congenital aortic stenosis. I. Clinical and hemodynamic findings in 100 patients. II. Surgical treatment and the results of operation. *Circulation*. 1963;27:426–462.

97. Lakier JB, Lewis AB, Heymann MA, Stanger P, Hoffman JI, Rudolph AM. Isolated aortic stenosis in the neonate. Natural history and hemodynamic considerations. *Circulation*. 1974;50: 801–808.

98. Caulfield WH, De Leon Jr AC, Perloff JK, Steelman RB. The clinical significance of the fourth heart sound in aortic stenosis. *Am J Cardiol*. 1971;28:179–182.

99. Epstein EJ, Criley JM, Raftery EB, Humphries JO, Ross RS. Cineradiographic studies of the early systolic click in aortic valve stenosis. *Circulation*. 1965;31:842–853.

100. Gamboa R, Hugenholtz PG, Nadas AS. Accuracy of the phonocardiogram in assessing severity of aortic and pulmonic stenosis. *Circulation*. 1964;30:35–46.

101. Nelson WP, Hall RJ. The innocent supraclavicular arterial bruit—utility of shoulder maneuvers in its recognition. *N Engl J Med*. 1968;278:778.

102. Perloff JK, Roberts WC. The mitral apparatus. Functional anatomy of mitral regurgitation. *Circulation*. 1972;46:227–239.

103. Hirschfeld S, Liebman J, Borkat G, Bormuth C. Intracardiac pressure-sound correlates of echographic aortic valve closure. *Circulation*. 1977;55:602–604.

104. Kumar S, Luisada AA. Mechanism of changes in the second heart sound in aortic stenosis. *Am J Cardiol*. 1971;28:162–167.

105. Cripps T, Leech G, Leatham A. Inappropriate left ventricular hypertrophy in minor aortic valve disease: a source of error in clinical assessment. *Eur Heart J*. 1987;8:895–901.

106. Hugenholtz PG, Lees MM, Nadas AS. The scalar electrocardiogram, vectorcardiogram, and exercise electrocardiogram in the assessment of congenital aortic stenosis. *Circulation*. 1962;26: 79–91.

107. Braverman IB, Gibson S. The outlook for children with congenital aortic stenosis. *Am Heart J*. 1957;53:487–493.

108. Griep AH. Pitfalls in the electrocardiographic diagnosis of left ventricular hypertrophy; a correlative study of 200 autopsied patients. *Circulation*. 1959;20:30–34.

109. Kangos JJ, Ferrer MI, Franciosi RA, Blanc WA, Blumenthal S. Electrocardiographic changes associated with papillary muscle infarction in congenital heart disease. *Am J Cardiol*. 1969;23: 801–809.

110. Rockoff SD, Levine ND, Austen WG. Roentgenographic clues to the cardiac hemodynamics of aortic stenosis. *Radiology*. 1964;83: 58–62.

111. Spindola-Franco H, Fish BG, Dachman A, Grose R, Attai L. Recognition of bicuspid aortic valve by plain film calcification. *AJR Am J Roentgenol*. 1982;139:867–872.

112. Child J. Transthoracic and transesophageal echocardiographic imaging: anatomic and hemodynamic assessment. In: *Congenital heart disease in adults*. WB Saunders Company; 1998:91.

113. Sabbah HN, Stein PD. Mechanism of early systolic closure of the aortic valve in discrete membranous subaortic stenosis. *Circulation*. 1982;65:399–402.

114. Corrigan D. On permanent patency of the mouth of the aorta, or inadequacy of the aortic valves. In: Willus RA, ed. *Classics of cardiology: a collection of classic works on the heart and circulation with comprehensive biographic accounts of the authors*. Malabar, FL: Robert E. Krieger Pub. Co; 1983.

115. Waller B, Howard J, Fess S. Pathology of aortic valve stenosis and pure aortic regurgitation. A clinical morphologic assessment—Part I. *Clin Cardiol*. 1994;17:85–92.

116. Waller BF, Howard J, Fess S. Pathology of aortic valve stenosis and pure aortic regurgitation: a clinical morphologic assessment—Part II. *Clin Cardiol*. 1994;17:150–156.

117. Sadee AS, Becker AE, Verheul HA, Bouma B, Hoedemaker G. Aortic valve regurgitation and the congenitally bicuspid aortic valve: a clinico-pathological correlation. *Br Heart J*. 1992;67: 439–441.

118. Waller BF, Taliercio CP, Dickos DK, Howard J, Adlam JH, Jolly W. Rare or unusual causes of chronic, isolated, pure aortic regurgitation. *Clin Cardiol*. 1990;13:577–581.

119. Carvalho AC, Andrade JL, Lima VC, Leal SB, Martinez EE, Buffolo E. Absence of an aortic valve cusp, a cause of severe aortic regurgitation in infancy. *Pediatr Cardiol*. 1992;13:122–124.

120. Issenberg HJ, Mathew R, Kim ES, Bharati S. Congenital absence of the noncoronary aortic cusp. *Am Heart J*. 1987;113: 400–402.

121. Lin AE, Chin AJ. Absent aortic valve: a complex anomaly. *Pediatr Cardiol*. 1990;11:195–198.

122. Humes RA, Hagler DJ, Julsrud PR, Levy JM, Feldt RH, Schaff HV. Aortico-left ventricular tunnel: Diagnosis based on two-dimensional echocardiography, color flow Doppler imaging, and magnetic resonance imaging. *Mayo Clin Proc*. 1986;61: 901–907.

123. Levy MJ, Schachner A, Blieden LC. Aortico-left ventricular tunnel: Collective review. *J Thorac Cardiovasc Surg*. 1982;84: 102–109.

124. Wu JR, Huang TY, Chen YF, Lin YT, Roan HR. Aortico-left ventricular tunnel: Two-dimensional echocardiographic and angiocardiographic features. *Am Heart J*. 1989;117:697–699.

125. Fernicola DJ, Mann JM, Roberts WC. Congenitally quadricuspid aortic valve: Analysis of six necropsy patients. *Am J Cardiol*. 1989; 63:136–138.

126. Hurwitz LE, Roberts WC. Quadricuspid semilunar valve. *Am J Cardiol*. 1973;31:623–626.

127. Olson LJ, Subramanian R, Edwards WD. Surgical pathology of pure aortic insufficiency: A study of 225 cases. *Mayo Clin Proc*. 1984;59:835–841.

128. Bicoff JP, Thompson W, Arbeiter HI, Weinberg Jr M, Agustsson MH. Severe aortic stenosis in infancy. *J Pediatr*. 1963; 63:161–164.

129. Hashimoto R, Miyamura H, Eguchi S. Congenital aortic regurgitation in a child with a tricuspid non-stenotic aortic valve. *Br Heart J*. 1984;51:358–360.

130. Tran Quang H, Smolinsky A, Neufeld HN, Goor DA. Dysplastic aortic valve with absence of aortic valve cusp: An unreported cause of congenital aortic insufficiency. *J Thorac Cardiovasc Surg*. 1986; 91:471–472.

131. Starc TJ, Bowman FO, Hordof AJ. Congestive heart failure in a newborn secondary to coronary artery-left ventricular fistula. *Am J Cardiol*. 1986;58:366–367.

132. Carter JB, Sethi S, Lee GB, Edwards JE. Prolapse of semilunar cusps as causes of aortic insufficiency. *Circulation*. 1971;43:922–932.

133. Morganroth J, Perloff JK, Zeldis SM, Dunkman WB. Acute severe aortic regurgitation. Pathophysiology, clinical recognition, and management. *Ann Intern Med*. 1977;87:223–232.

134. Welch Jr GH, Braunwald E, Sarnoff SJ. Hemodynamic effects of quantitatively varied experimental aortic regurgitation. *Circ Res*. 1957;5:546–551.

135. Bonow RO, Rosing DR, Mcintosh CL, et al. The natural history of asymptomatic patients with aortic regurgitation and normal left ventricular function. *Circulation*. 1983;68:509–517.

136. Goforth D, James FW, Kaplan S, Donner R, Mays W. Maximal exercise in children with aortic regurgitation: An adjunct to non-invasive assessment of disease severity. *Am Heart J*. 1984;108: 1306–1311.

137. Saito S, Naik MJ, Westaby S. Ischemic pain in aortic regurgitation. *Circulation*. 2001;104:1984.

138. Sabbah HN, Khaja F, Anbe DT, Stein PD. The aortic closure sound in pure aortic insufficiency. *Circulation*. 1977;56:859–863.

139. Fripp RR, Werner JC, Whitman V, Nordenberg A, Waldhausen JA. Pulsed Doppler and two-dimensional echocardiographic findings in aortico-left ventricular tunnel. *J Am Coll Cardiol*. 1984;4: 1012–1014.

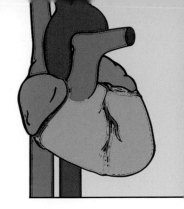

Chapter 8

Coarctation of the Aorta and Interrupted Aortic Arch

In 1760, the Prussian anatomist, Johann Friedreich Meckel, characterized coarctation of the aorta as an "extraordinary dilatation of the heart which came from the fact that the aortic conduit was too narrow."[1] Saul Jarcho's[1–5] historic papers underscored the accuracy of early accounts of this congenital malformation.

Coarctation of the aorta is typically located near the aortic attachment of the ligamentum arteriosum or patent ductus arteriosus (Figures 8-1A and 8-2). An obtuse indentation in the posterolateral wall of the aorta corresponds to the location of an internal ridge or shelf that eccentrically narrows the aortic lumen, hence the term *coarctatus* (Latin, *contracted* or *tightened*). The ridge that forms the coarctation consists of smooth muscle, fibrous tissue, and elastic tissue similar in composition to a muscular arterial ductus (see Chapter 20).[6] Intimal proliferation distal to the ridge narrows the lumen.[6] The junction between the ductus and the elastic aorta is clearly defined, with extension of ductal tissue into the aortic wall not exceeding 30% of the aortic circumference. In preductal coarctation, however, ductal tissue forms a circumferential sling that extends around the aorta.[7] In juxtaductal coarctation, ductal tissue is not a significant part of the aortic wall.[7] The coarctation ridge is thought to represent the original wall of the distal left sixth aortic arch. The neural crest is thought to play a role in the pathogenesis of some types of coarctation.[7]

The common form of aortic coarctation is represented by a localized constriction that contains the ridge or shelf as just described.[6] Less commonly, a relatively long segment of constriction extends beyond the left subclavian artery. Rarely, congenital coarctation is in the mid thoracic aorta.[8] *Tubular hypoplasia* refers to uniform narrowing within the aortic arch.[6] Localized coarctation and tubular hypoplasia sometimes coexist.

The mechanisms that account for the typical location of coarctation take into account a number of variables: (1) the quantitative morphology and growth of the aortic arch in the normal fetus[9–11]; (2) the site of the aortic orifice of the ductus arteriosus; (3) the presence of ductal tissue in the coarctation[6]; (4) constriction of ductal tissue immediately after birth; and (5) coarctation in the presence of a widely patent ductus in the fetus[12,13] and after birth.[6] Current consensus favors an interplay between aortic growth and blood flow.[9–11] High-resolution echocardiographic imaging in the healthy fetus has disclosed progressive tapering of the diameter of the aortic arch at all gestational ages, with the smallest diameter at the isthmus.[9] Tapering is thought to reflect the relative proportion of fetal cardiac output traversing each aortic segment. The smallest proportion traverses the isthmus, which maintains its smaller dimension relative to the remainder of the aortic arch well into postnatal life, especially in premature infants.[9] Neonatal coarctation is characterized by hypoplasia of the transverse aorta in the presence of a relatively large pulmonary trunk, a combination that is thought to reflect an *in utero* decrease in aortic arch flow together with an increase in flow through the main pulmonary artery and ductus.[11]

The coarctation ridge is located either immediately *proximal* to the aortic insertion of the ductus, *opposite* the aortic insertion (juxtaductal), or immediately *distal* to the aortic insertion.[6,14,15] Infants with a juxtaductal coarctation show no signs of aortic obstruction as long as the ductus is widely patent, assuring unobstructed pulmonary trunk/ductus/descending aortic continuity. When the ductus closes, the coarctation becomes apparent immediately and dramatically and the femoral pulses disappear. The left subclavian artery is dilated because coarctation is usually located immediately distal to its origin (Figure 8-1A, 8-3D, and 8-4A). However, coarctation may lie at or proximal to the left subclavian orifice, compromising its lumen (Figure 8-1B). Exceptionally, the *right* subclavian artery arises *distal* to the coarctation (Figure 8-1C) or the coarctation is in a right aortic arch.[16]

Coarctation of the abdominal aorta can be part of a noncongenital systemic vascular disorder, such as Takayasu's arteritis or von Recklinghausen's disease, but can also be congenital and is therefore appropriate for inclusion here.[17–20] Abdominal coarctation is rare, accounting for 0.5% to 2% of all varieties of aortic coarctation,[18] and can be suprarenal, infrarenal, or interrenal.[18] Systemic hypertension is believed to result from involvement of the renal artery.[20] A congenital etiology is based on the combination of a localized hourglass deformity with an intraluminal membrane, occurrence at a young age, absence of a systemic vascular disorder, and slow progression with development of extensive collaterals.[20]

Pseudocoarctation refers to a rare anomaly characterized by buckling or kinking of the aorta in the vicinity of the ligamentum arteriosus that results in elongation, tortuosity, and dilation of the distal aortic arch and the proximal descending aorta.[21–25] Occasionally, pseudocoarctation involves the abdominal aorta (Figure 8-5).[26] *Pseudo* signifies absence of a gradient at the site of the

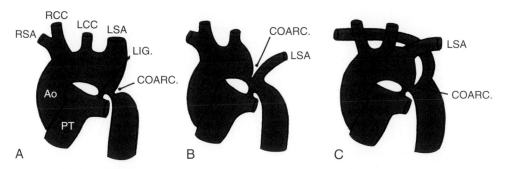

FIGURE 8-1 A, Typical coarctation of the aorta immediately *distal* to the left subclavian artery (LSA). **B,** Coarctation immediately *proximal* to the left subclavian artery. **C,** The *right* subclavian artery (RSA) arises anomalously *distal* to the coarctation. (RSA = right subclavian artery; RCC and LCC = right and left common carotid arteries; LIG = ligamentum arteriosum; Ao = ascending aorta; PT = pulmonary trunk.)

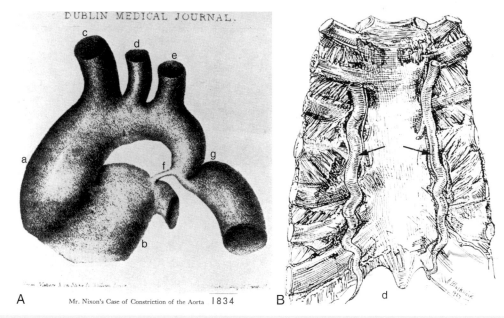

FIGURE 8-2 A, Anatomic drawing of coarctation of the aorta published in 1834 (Nixon RL. *Chemical Science* 5:386, 1834). **B,** Anatomic drawing of retrosternal internal mammary arterial collaterals *(oblique black arrows)* in coarctation of the aorta. *(**A,** Courtesy Dr. Saul Jarcho. **B,** From Maude Abbott's* Atlas of congenital cardiac disease. *Montreal: Osler Library, McGill University; 1936. Reproduced with permission.)*

localized external deformity, absence of collaterals, and absence of systemic hypertension, although refractory hypertension has been reported.[27] Occasionally, transformation from *pseudo*coarctation to true coarctation occurs.[28] The femoral pulses are sometimes reduced because of the damping effect of sharp angulation of the aortic arch (see Figure 8-5).[22] Thin-walled saccular aneurysms may form in the distal segment,[21] spontaneous rupture and dissection have been reported in the proximal descending thoracic aorta[29] and in the ascending aorta,[30] and bicuspid aortic valve may coexist.[31]

Coarctation of the aorta is usually and simplistically regarded as isolated obstruction of the aortic isthmus[32] but in fact is a widespread disorder in which isthmic obstruction is only one of a cluster of abnormalities that include the proximal and distal paracoarctation aorta, the ascending and transverse aorta, the coronary arteries, conduit arteries (radial, brachial, carotid), the retinal vascular bed, dissecting aneurysm, cerebral aneurysms, vascular rings, and systemic hypertension. The strongest association is with a functionally normal, stenotic, or incompetent bicuspid aortic valve (Figure 8-6B; see Chapter 7)[33,34] characterized by fusion of the right and left coronary cusps.[34,35] A decrease in left ventricular interpapillary muscle distance is common[36] and culminates in the single papillary muscle of a parachute mitral valve (see Chapter 9).[37,38] Coarctation in the fetus tends to be associated with a left superior vena cava.[39] Endocardial fibroelastosis is patchy rather than confluent.[40] Two shunts accompany coarctation (patent ductus arteriosus[41] and ventricular septal defect[41–44]), which is usually characterized by leftward malalignment that curtails the amount of blood that reaches the aortic isthmus.[42–44] Dissecting aneurysm with hemopericardium was reported in 1830.[45]

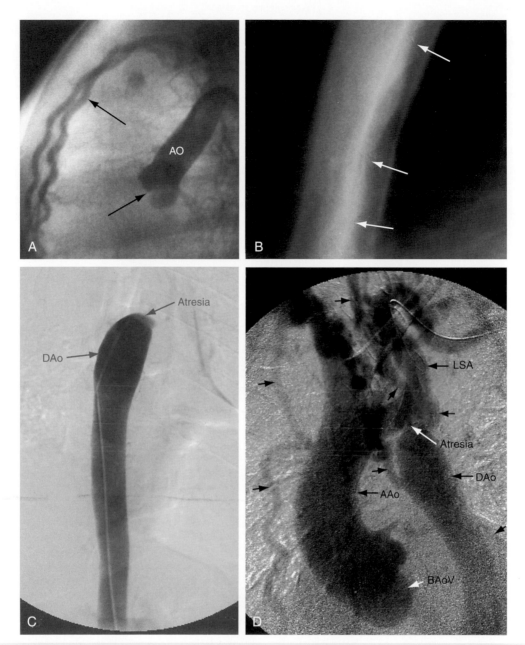

FIGURE 8-3 A, Lateral view of a large retrosternal internal mammary collateral artery in a 9-year-old boy with coarctation of the aorta. **B,** Close-up of the lateral view showing retrosternal notching *(arrows).* **C,** Retrograde descending aortogram (DAo) in a 65-year-old man with coarctation of the aorta and atresia at the coarctation site. **D,** Lateral ascending aortogram showing the coarctation atresia *(curved white arrow),* proximal to which the left subclavian artery (LSA) is dilated. The descending aorta (DAo) opacified through abundant collaterals *(unmarked arrows).* Internal mammary collaterals *(two small left arrows)* were responsible for retrosternal notching. The ascending aorta (AAo) is dilated above a bicuspid aortic valve (BAoV).

Aneurysmal dilation, which can be large, saccular, and calcified, occurs in the low-pressure high-velocity distal paracoarctation segment.[46] The substrate for aneurysm formation is an inherent abnormality of medial smooth muscle and extracellular matrix that is a consistent feature of the proximal and distal paracoarctation aorta.[47,48] Aneurysms of the circle of Willis set the stage for intracranial

hemorrhage (Figure 8-7). Relatively benign aneurysms occasionally develop in intercostal arteries.[49] A large aneurysm of the left subclavian artery was acutely dissected.[50] The retinal arterioles are characteristically U shaped (see subsequent discussion).[51]

Arterial collaterals are important vascular sequelae of coarctation and depend on subclavian artery patency for

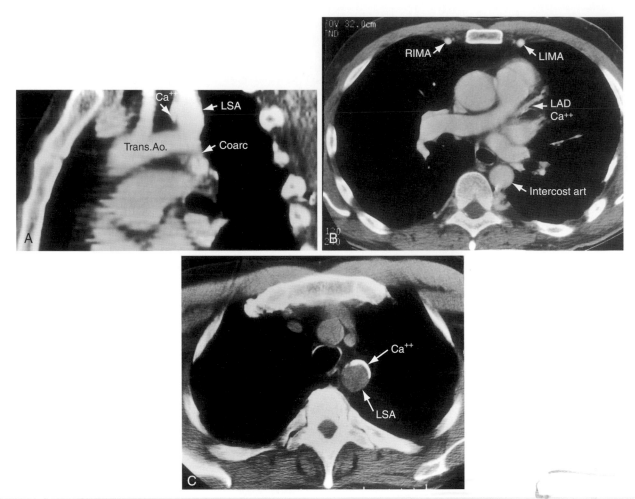

FIGURE 8-4 Magnetic resonance images from a 62-year-old woman. **A,** Sagittal plane showing the site of coarctation (Coarc) distal to a dilated left subclavian artery (LSA) that is calcified (Ca⁺⁺). **B,** Transverse plane shows right internal mammary and left internal mammary artery collaterals (RIMA and LIMA), a large intercostal collateral (Intercost Art), and calcium in the left anterior descending coronary artery (LAD Ca⁺⁺). **C,** Calcified dilated left subclavian artery (LSA). (Trans Ao = transverse aorta.)

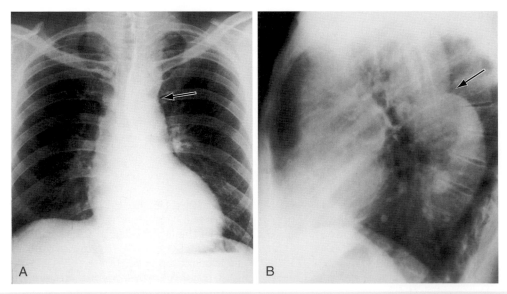

FIGURE 8-5 A, Anteroposterior x-ray from a 62-year-old man with *pseudocoarctation* characterized by buckling of the aorta *(arrow)* in the vicinity of the ligamentum arteriosum. The aortic lumen is not narrowed at the site of the external deformity. **B,** Lateral x-ray from a 68-year-old woman with pseudocoarctation and a buckled aorta *(arrow).*

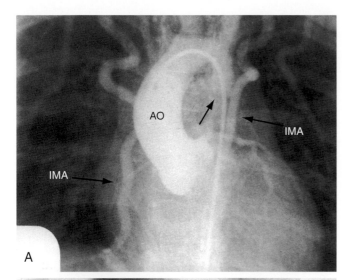

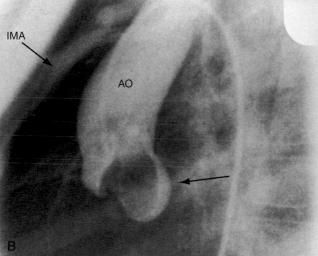

their development (see Figures 8-3 and 8-6A). When coarctation obstructs the orifice of the left subclavian artery, ipsilateral collaterals fail to develop (see Figure 8-27). A subclavian steal may result from retrograde flow down the ipsilateral vertebral artery.[52] Systemic-to-pulmonary collaterals normally present after birth gradually disappear.[53]

Retinal arterioles are the site of a distinctive vascular pattern.[51,54] In 1948, at the annual meeting of the Swedish Ophthalmological Society, Professor K.O. Granstrom[55] stated, "As in other cases of hypertension, these patients are sent as a matter of routine for examination to the eye department. As soon as I had seen a few such cases, it became evident that the retinal picture in coarctation of the aorta is often somewhat characteristic, the principal feature being pronounced tortuosity of the arteries." The U-shaped tortuous retinal arterioles (Figure 8-8) may be accompanied by serpentine pulsations synchronous with

FIGURE 8-6 Aortograms from a 9-year-old boy with coarctation of the aorta and a bicuspid aortic valve. **A,** The *thick black arrow* points to the coarctation. The two *thin arrows* identify internal mammary artery collaterals (IMA). **B,** Lateral aortogram showing the bicupid aortic valve *(unmarked arrow)* above which the aorta (AO) is dilated. There is a large retrosternal internal mammary artery (IMA) collateral.

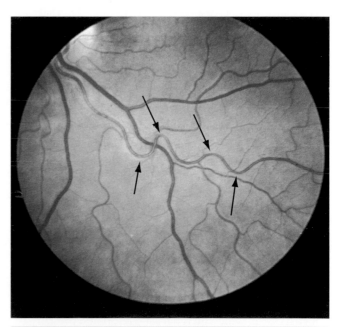

FIGURE 8-8 Typical U-shaped corkscrew retinal arterioles *(arrows)* in a 22-year-old woman with coarctation of the aorta.

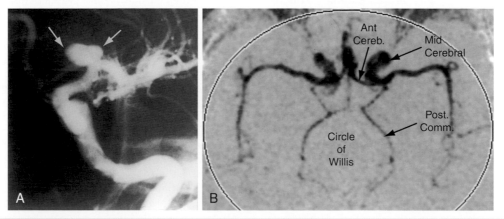

FIGURE 8-7 A, Cerebral arteriogram from a 28-year-old woman. There is an 11-mm aneurysm *(paired arrows)* of the circle of Willis. **B,** Normal circle of Willis showing the delicate posterior communicating artery (Post Comm). The middle cerebral artery and anterior cerebral artery are not parts of the circle of Willis.

the arterial pulse.[54] Granstrom[55] correctly concluded that the distinctive retinal abnormality in coarctation was benign and that hypertensive retinopathy was conspicuous by its absence.

Coarctation of the aorta can contribute to a *vascular ring* that consists of a double aortic arch or a right aortic arch, a left ligamentum arteriosum, and an aberrant subclavian artery.[56–58] An anomalous retroesophageal right subclavian artery occasionally accompanies coarctation of the aorta (see Figure 8-1C) but does not cause tracheoesophageal compression.

The *pathogenesis of systemic hypertension* in coarctation of the aorta has been the subject of three theories. The *mechanical theory* focuses on resistance at the site of obstruction. This theory in itself cannot be sustained but is central to the *neural theory* that involves the sensitivity of carotid sinus baroreceptors and the distensibility characteristics of the precoarctation aorta.[59] The proximal aortic segment of coarctation has an increase in collagen and a decrease in smooth muscle that are responsible for an increase in stiffness and a decrease in distensibility.[60] The poorly compliant precoarctation aorta is responsible for the elevation of systolic blood pressure at rest, the disproportionate rise during isotonic exercise,[61,62] and the resetting of carotid sinus baroreceptors to operate at higher pressures.[59,61] The *renal theory* of pathogenesis takes into account a unique feature of coarctation hypertension, namely, that the *elevated blood pressure is confined to the upper extremities.* Accordingly, the renal arteries are exposed to the *neurohumeral* effects of hypertension but not the *hydraulic* effects. The coarctation gradient increases during isotonic exercise, which is accompanied by a disproportionate increase in *systolic* pressure,[63] an exaggeration of the inherent disproportionate systolic hypertension related to rigidity of the precoarctation aortic wall. The response of the *mean* blood pressure to exercise is approximately the same as in control subjects.[64] Experimental hypertension has been produced by aortic constriction that assigns the renal arteries to the distal low pressure zone.[65] When the constriction is *below* the renal arteries, blood pressure remains normal.[65,66] Toxemia of pregnancy is not a feature of coarctation hypertension. Eye grounds do not exhibit hypertensive retinopathy but instead exhibit distinctive serpentine retinal arterioles (see Figure 8-8).[51,54]

The increase in left ventricular mass induced by the afterload of coarctation is characterized as *myocyte replication* rather than myocyte hypertrophy,[67] which is thought to account for reduced end-systolic wall stress and enhanced left ventricular ejection performance.[68]

History

The male:female ratio of coarctation is from 1.4:1 to 3:1.[69] Familial recurrence has occurred in siblings, in monozygotic twins, and in parent and child[70–75] and as autosomal dominant in four generations.[76] True coarctation and pseudocoarctation have been reported in siblings.[77] Turner's syndrome (see section Physical Appearance) cannot be transmitted because of sterility, but seven women in three generations of one family had Turner's syndrome attributed to loss of the short arm of one

X chromosome that permitted transmission from phenotypically normal female carriers with a balanced X-1 translocation.[78] A peak seasonal incidence of coarctation is found from September through November and from January through March.[79] The reported rarity of coarctation in African Americans is open to question.[80,81]

Coarctation of the aorta usually produces significant symptoms in early infancy[69,82,83] and after age 20 to 30 years.[84] Neonates with severe coarctation become acutely symptomatic when the ductus closes. Most who survive the hazards of infancy reach adulthood, although more than a quarter die by age 20 years, half by age 30 years, and more than three quarters by age 50 years.[33,84,85] Figures 8-24 and 8-26 are from patients aged 54 years, 62 years, and 70 years. Survival has been reported at age 74 years and 76 years.[86] Isolated atresia of the aortic arch was surgically repaired at age 65 years.[87] The longest recorded survival was Reynaud's account (1828) of a 92-year-old man with coarctation.[3] The anatomic illustrations in this report are noteworthy. However, examples of exceptional longevity should not obscure the inherent risk of coarctation that results in death at an average age of 33 years.

Mild coarctation is not always benign, and severe coarctation is not always asymptomatic. A case in point, albeit rare, is a 20-year-old woman with severe coarctation, borderline hypertension, and no symptoms.[88] Except for symptomatic infants, patients tend to be clinically well when the diagnosis is first made. Initial suspicion requires little more than attention to upper and lower extremity arterial pulses and blood pressure (see section The Arterial Pulse). Nevertheless, delayed recognition is not uncommon,[89,90] and diagnoses have been made by chance in the fifth decade.[91] *Minor symptoms* include epistaxis and leg fatigue. When coarctation compromises the orifice of the left subclavian artery in left-handed patients, muscular fatigue involves the left arm. Leg fatigue occurs in about half of patients, but claudication is reserved for abdominal coarctation. Patients are sometimes subjectively aware of amplified arterial pulsations in the neck, especially after effort or excitement. Dysphagia occurs when a retroesophageal right subclavian artery originates distal to the coarctation and passes behind the esophagus (see Figure 8-1C)[92] or when coarctation is a component of a vascular ring.

Major symptoms are features of four eventualities: (1) congestive heart failure; (2) rupture or dissection of the aorta; (3) infective endarteritis or endocarditis; and (4) cerebral hemorrhage.[83,84,93–95] Hypertension is chiefly responsible for morbidity and mortality with advancing age.[83] The incidence rate of cardiac failure is highest in infants[69,96] and is high again after the fourth decade.[97] In a review of 234 patients with coarctation of the aorta aged 1 day to 72 years, congestive heart failure occurred in two thirds of patients less than 1 year of age and more than age 40 years but in only 4% of patients between 1 year and 40 years of age.[83] Many, if not most, neonates and infants with congestive heart failure have a coexisting ventricular septal defect or patent ductus arteriosus.[98,99] In brief, more than 90% of infants and children with *uncomplicated* coarctation experience little or no difficulty.[100]

When coarctation is juxtaductal or proximal to the neonatal ductus, continuity between the pulmonary trunk and descending aorta is maintained, so the femoral arterial pulses remain palpable.[6,96] When the ductus closes, the femoral pulses disappear, pulmonary blood flow is diverted into the lungs, the left ventricle is suddenly volume overloaded, and blood pressure and blood flow proximal to the coarctation suddenly increase. A high left atrial pressure opens the pliant valve of the foramen ovale, initiating a left-to-right shunt that imposes a volume load on the right ventricle that is already pressure overloaded because of pulmonary hypertension.[101] Initial closure of the pulmonary arterial end of the ductus can leave the aortic end sufficiently patent to permit the proximal aorta to decompress.[15] When the aortic end of the ductus closes, the isthmus is suddenly obstructed. Distal aortic pressure and flow fall, renal perfusion falls, and the renin-angiotensin system is activated.[65,102]

Rupture or dissection of the aorta is a dramatic complication with peak incidence in the third and fourth decades.[83,85,94,97] The rupture originates either in a paracoarctation aneurysm[47,48,94] or above a coexisting bicuspid aortic valve because of an inherent medial abnormality of the ascending aorta (see Chapter 7).[48,94,97] Rupture of a postcoarctation aneurysm may be accompanied by bleeding into the esophagus that is announced by hematemesis and melena. In XO Turner's syndrome (see section Physical Appearance), rupture or dissection of an ascending aortic aneurysm occurs because of an inherent medial abnormality,[48] whether or not a coexisting coarctation or a bicuspid aortic valve exists (Figure 8-9).[103–105] Aneurysms of intercostal arteries are almost always

occult and relatively benign.[49] Pseudocoarctation has been regarded as a disorder that incurs little or no risk, but the malformation is not necessarily benign and is not necessarily *pseudo* (see previous discussion). Pseudocoarctation has been reported with Turner's syndrome.[106] Cerebral arterial aneurysms are discussed in the section on cerebrovascular accidents (see subsequent discussion).

Infective endarteritis or endocarditis is a major complication of coarctation of the aorta, although the more susceptible site is a coexisting bicuspid aortic valve (see Chapter 7).[83,97] Saccular septic aneurysms are occasional sequelae of infective endarteritis.[94]

Cerebrovascular accidents are the fourth major eventuality in coarctation of the aorta.[83,93,107] Hypertension is not a necessary precondition because cerebral complications can occur with normotensive conditions long after successful repair. An aneurysm of the circle of Willis, first described in 1927,[108] is the chief offender (see Figure 8-7) and sets the stage for rupture and cerebral hemorrhage.[109] Less common, but not less important, are aneurysms in other cerebral arteries.[93] Infective endocarditis on a bicuspid aortic valve can give rise to septic cerebral aneurysms that rupture. Rarely and oddly, an unruptured intracranial aneurysm triggers *musical hallucinations*.[110]

Coarctation hypertension is a risk factor for premature atherosclerotic coronary artery disease (see Figure 8-4B; see previous discussion).[83,111,112] Evidence also exists of structural abnormalities of terminal intramural coronary arteries.[111] Gonadal dysgenesis of Turner's syndrome reportedly increases atherosclerotic cardiovascular risk.[113]

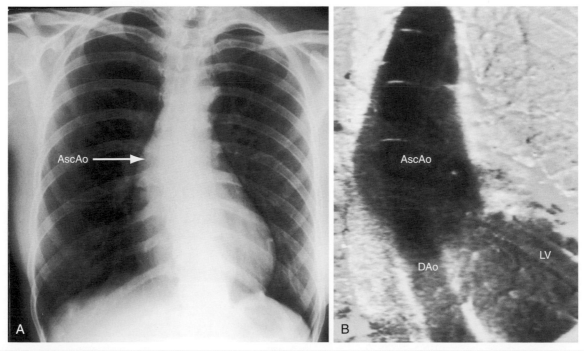

FIGURE 8-9 A, X-ray from a 28-year-old woman with 45 XO Turner's syndrome, an aneurysm of the ascending aorta (Asc Ao), and a bicuspid aortic valve. **B,** Digital vascular image angiogram after injection of contrast material into the superior vena cava. The ascending aortic aneurysm ruptured 8 weeks later. (LV = left ventricle; DAo = descending aorta.)

Physical Appearance

An athletic appearance of chest and shoulders contrasts with narrow hips and thin legs. When coarctation compromises the origin of the left subclavian artery, the left arm tends to be small. General growth and development are impaired in infants with congestive heart failure.

XO Turner's syndrome with its distinctive physical appearance (Figure 8-10) arouses suspicion of coarctation of the aorta.[114,115] Chromosomal patterns 45 XO and X-mosaicism are coupled with additional cardiac expressions.[116–119] Aortic rupture or dissection in Turner's syndrome was mentioned previously (see Figure 8-9).[103,104,120] The typical XO Turner's phenotypic female (Figure 8-11) is of short stature with webbing of the neck, absent or scanty auxiliary and pubic hair (ovarian dysgenesis), broad chest with widely spaced hypoplastic or inverted nipples, low anterior and posterior hairlines, small chin, prominent ears because of large auricles, cubitus valgus, short fourth metacarpals and metatarsals, distal palmar triaxial radii, narrow hyperconvex nails, and pigmented cutaneous nevi.[115] Infants with Turner's syndrome exhibit lymphedema of the neck with loose skin, puffiness of the dorsum of the hands and feet, and low hairlines.[115,121] Congenital heart disease is much more frequent in Turner's syndrome with webbing of the neck than in Turner's syndrome without webbing,[116,121] and coarctation of the aorta is eight times as frequent when Turner's syndrome is accompanied by webbing of the neck.[121] Noonan's syndrome (Turner's phenotype with normal genotype; see Figure 8-10) is only occasionally accompanied by coarctation of the aorta[122] and rarely by ascending aortic aneurysm.[95,115,123] Systemic hypertension in Turner's syndrome occurs without

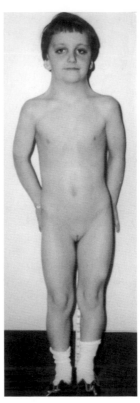

FIGURE 8-11 Thirteen-year-old girl with 45 XO Turner's syndrome and coarctation of the aorta. Physical appearance is characterized by short stature, webbing of the neck, absent pubic hair, wide-set nipples, and small chin. Bangs obscure a low anterior hairline.

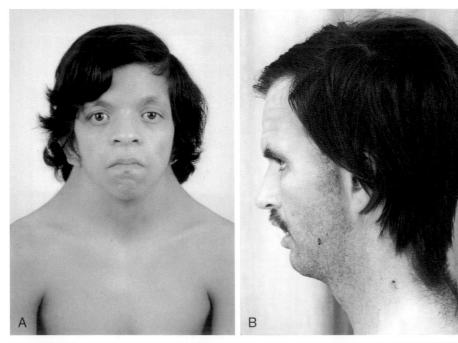

FIGURE 8-10 A, An 18-year-old man with Noonan's syndrome (Turner's phenotype with normal genotype). There is typical webbing of the neck. Long hair obscures low anterior and posterior hair lines. **B,** A 24-year-old man with Noonan's syndrome and a dissecting aneurysm of the ascending aorta. There is a low posterior hairline, webbing of the neck, low-set auricles, and micrognathia.

coarctation. Another distinctive physical appearance associated with coarctation of the aorta is the PHACE syndrome[124]: *P,* posterior fossa brain malformations; *H,* hemangioma of the head or neck; *A,* arterial abnormalities of the head or neck; *C,* cardiac abnormalities, including coarctation of the aorta; *E,* eye abnormalities.

Arterial Pulse

Abnormal differences in upper and lower extremity arterial pulses and blood pressure are hallmarks of coarctation of the aorta. If proper attention were paid to these pulses, few or no diagnoses would be missed.[90,125] Two methods have been advocated for comparison of upper and lower extremity arterial pulsations. One method compares femoral and *radial* pulses; the other method compares femoral and *brachial* pulses. Normally, radial and femoral pulses are sensed as synchronous, so that *any* femoral delay is considered abnormal. Positioning the patient's wrist next to the groin is believed to facilitate comparison. In infants and newborns, the *brachial* artery is more readily palpated than the tiny radial artery, which is surrounded by subcutaneous fat pads (Figure 8-12B). The author's preference is comparative palpation of *brachial* and femoral pulses, which is accomplished with placing a thumb on each (Figure 8-12A).[125] The slight delay in perceived arrival time of the normal femoral pulse (15 msec in adults, less in infants and children) is easily sensed as a norm against which even slight deviations can be judged. With palpation of the femoral pulse in an infant, the patient must be allowed to relax the legs voluntarily because forceful restraint can decrease or abolish a normal femoral pulse.

What is perceived as an abnormal delay of the femoral pulse in coarctation is not a delay in *arrival* time but instead a slow rate of rise to a delayed peak (Figure 8-13). The presence of a normal femoral pulse effectively eliminates all but mild coarctation, provided the aortic valve is functioning normally (see subsequent discussion). Palpation begins with applying to the brachial and femoral arterial pulses the amount of digital pressure necessary to elicit the maximal systolic impact.[125] Stiffness of the precoarctation aortic wall results in disproportionate systolic hypertension and forceful carotid and suprasternal notch pulsations, which are sensed by the patient and become increasingly apparent with age and exercise (see previous discussion).[59,61,62]

Bicuspid aortic regurgitation reinforces the femoral pulse, which can be misjudged unless properly compared with the brachial pulse (Figure 8-14A).[126] Bicuspid aortic stenosis may not dampen the brachial arterial pulse because coarctation amplifies the ascending aortic and brachial arterial systolic pressures (Figure 8-14B).[126] Conversely, if aortic stenosis dampens the ascending aortic systolic pressure, evidence of coarctation is obscured (Figure 8-14C).[126]

The right and left brachial arteries should be compared with palpation and with cuff blood pressure (see Figure 8-12B). A decreased or absent left brachial arterial pulse indicates that the coarctation has compromised the lumen of the left subclavian artery (see Figure 8-1B) or is proximal to its origin (see previous discussion).

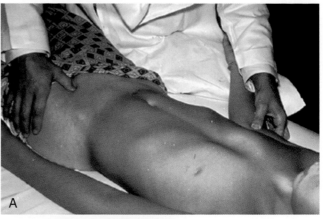

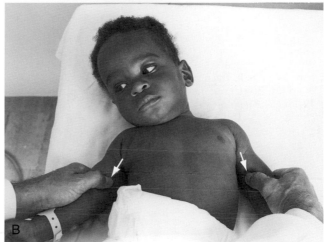

FIGURE 8-12 **A,** Palpation of brachial and femoral arteries as shown here is a useful way of comparing upper and lower extremity pulses. Application of the thumbs allows simultaneous or sequential palpation, which permits detection of subtle differences in amplitude and timing. **B,** Recommended method of simultaneous palpation of right and left brachial arterial pulses *(arrows).*

In comparison of the two brachial pulses, account must be taken of normal systolic pressure differences of 10 to 15 mm Hg lower in the left arm.[125] Diminution or absence of the *right* brachial pulse implies that the right subclavian artery originates *distal* to the coarctation (see Figure 8-1C). Absence of *both* brachial arterial pulses signifies that coarctation is compromising the lumen of the *left* subclavian artery and that the *right* subclavian artery arises distal to the coarctation.[127] At birth, femoral arterial pulses are temporarily palpable if the coarctation is juxtaductal, if the ductus is distal to the coarctation, or if the aortic end of the ductus is patent.[6] The abdominal aorta is readily palpable proximal to *abdominal* coarctation but is not palpable when coarctation is in the aortic isthmus. *Pseudocoarctation* leaves the arterial pulses normal because there is no aortic obstruction, although angulation at the level of the ligamentum arteriosum occasionally dampens the femoral pulses (see Figure 8-5).[22]

Collateral arterial pulsations are specifically sought with patients who are old enough standing and bending forward with arms hanging at the sides while the

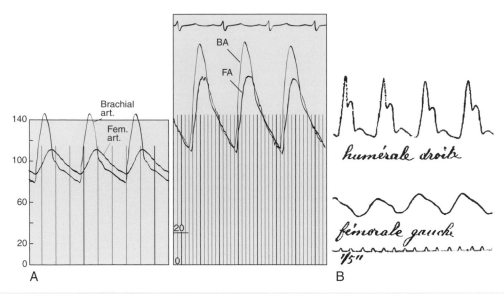

FIGURE 8-13 A, Simultaneous direct brachial and femoral arterial pressure pulses from a 10-year-old boy and a 4-year-old boy with coarctation of the aorta. The femoral arterial pulses (Fem. art.) were palpable but smaller than the brachial arterial pulses (Brachial art.). The diastolic pressures virtually coincide. The important differences are systolic not diastolic. There is no delay in *arrival* time of the femoral pulse. **B,** The right brachial arterial pulse *(humerale droite)* and the left femoral arterial pulse *(femoral gauche)* are characteristic of aortic coarctation. *(From Maude Abbott's Atlas of congenital cardiac disease. Montreal: Osler Library, McGill University; 1936. Reproduced with permission.)*

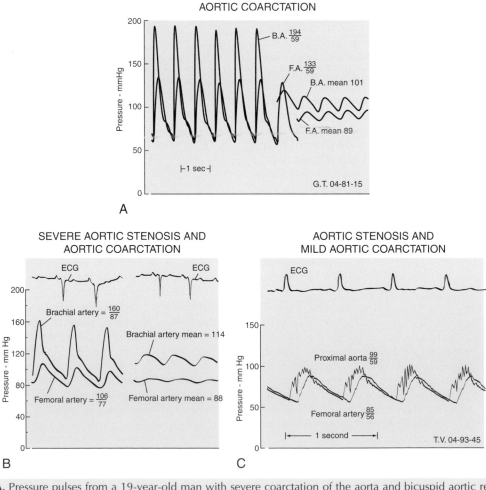

FIGURE 8-14 A, Pressure pulses from a 19-year-old man with severe coarctation of the aorta and bicuspid aortic regurgitation. The brachial arterial pressure (B.A.) is higher than the femoral arterial pressure (F.A.) because of the coarctation, although the femoral arterial pulse pressure is wide because of aortic regurgitation. **B,** A 38-year-old man with coarctation of the aorta and severe bicuspid aortic stenosis. The brachial pulse is amplified by the coarctation despite aortic stenosis. **C,** A 5-year-old boy with moderately severe bicuspid aortic stenosis and mild coarctation of the aorta. The proximal aortic, and therefore brachial arterial systolic pressure, is damped by aortic stenosis, but the femoral arterial systolic pressure is preserved because the coarctation was mild. *(From Glancy DL, Morrow AG, Simon AL, Roberts WC. American Journal of Cardiology 1983;51:537. With permission.)*

examiner scrutinizes the patient's back, especially around and between the scapulae.[128] A tangential light in a darkened room highlights subcutaneous collaterals in shadowed relief. Collateral arteries occasionally appear around the shoulders, along the right and left sternal borders, and rarely over the upper abdominal wall.

Cuff blood pressure is an important supplement to palpation of the arterial pulses. Blood pressure should be taken in the right arm, left arm, and leg. Correct cuff size is essential because improper size results in inaccurate readings.[125,129–133] An undersized cuff overestimates and an oversized cuff underestimates intraarterial blood pressure by as much as 10 to 30 mm Hg.[133] The American Heart Association recommendations for cuff size[130] are shown in Table 8-1. References to cuff size apply to the width and length of the inner inflatable bladder, not to the cloth covering. Cuff size is determined by limb circumference, not by patient age. The width of the inflatable bladder within the cuff should be 40% of the circumference of the midpoint of the limb. The length of the inflatable bladder must be sufficient to encircle the limb without overlapping.[129,130]

The examining room should be quiet, and the patient must be comfortable and reassured. Sufficient time should elapse for recovery from recent activity and tension. When an infant is quieted with a bottle or a pacifier, blood pressure can be obtained with the usual auscultatory method. An alternative is the flush technique, which requires two examiners.[129] An uninflated cuff is applied to the infant's forearm, which is elevated while the limb distal to the cuff is massaged to induce blanching. The cuff is inflated above anticipated systolic pressure while the arm remains elevated and blanched. The arm is then slowly lowered into a horizontal position while the cuff is slowly deflated. The point at which the blanched hand becomes flushed is an estimate of the *mean* arterial pressure. Doppler ultrasound or oscillometric techniques can be used by a single examiner and accurately determine systolic and diastolic blood pressure.[90,129]

Upper extremity blood pressure in infants and adults is usually recorded in the supine position, but a comfortable sitting position in a parent's lap is acceptable for relaxation of infants and young children. Lower extremity blood pressure is best determined from the popliteal artery with the patient prone.[125] While the popliteal artery is palpated, a thigh cuff is applied and must be inflated slowly to avoid discomfort. The cuff is inflated to a level just above the brachial arterial systolic pressure until the popliteal pulse vanishes. Systolic and diastolic pressures are then estimated with auscultation of popliteal Korotkoff's sounds. Diagnostic differences in arm and leg blood pressures are based on *systolic* levels when only *systolic* Korotkoff's sounds are heard. However, the diastolic pressures are important in confirmation of accuracy because they are not significantly different in the upper and lower extremities (see Figure 8-13). When *intraarterial* systolic, diastolic, and mean brachial and femoral pressures are compared in healthy persons, no significant difference is found, although the femoral *auscultatory* systolic pressure is about 10 mm Hg higher than the direct femoral arterial pressure.[133] Differences between arm and leg systolic pressures in coarctation are exaggerated by exercise, which causes an increase in brachial arterial pressure, with no change or a reduction in femoral arterial pressure.[134]

Measurements of blood pressure should be a routine part of the physical examination after infancy and are desirable in infants at least once.[90,135] *Normal* arterial pressure is based on age and gender.[129,136,137] The average systolic blood pressure in females rises to a plateau at around age 14 years and remains almost constant during the early reproductive years.[136] The average systolic blood pressure in males may not plateau until around age 20 years.[129,136,137] Diastolic pressure differences are in the same direction but smaller in degree.

From birth to 6 months, normal upper extremity blood pressure averages 80/45 mm Hg. From 2 years to puberty, the average upper extremity blood pressure is 90/60 to 100/60 mm Hg,[129,136] with the diastolic pressure more consistent than the systolic pressure. Coarctation of the aorta is accompanied by a progressive age-related increase in blood pressure, especially systolic, so the pulse pressure widens.[61,73]

In pregnant females with coarctation, blood pressure fluctuations are similar in direction to fluctuations in uncomplicated pregnancy but occur from a higher baseline.[138] Coarctation is not a resistance vessel disease, so the incidence rate of toxemia is lower than in pregnant women with other forms of hypertension.[138,139] Gestational hypertension is related to a significant coarctation gradient.[140] Pregnancy increases the risk of aortic rupture and intracranial hemorrhage because gestational changes in connective tissue reinforce the medial abnormalities inherent in the arterial walls of coarctation.[48,138] In abdominal coarctation, hypertension is likely to be caused by renal artery stenosis rather than by the coarctation.[20]

Table 8-1 **Recommended Bladder Dimensions for Blood Pressure Cuff**		
Arm Circumference at Midpoint* (cm)	**Bladder Width (cm)**	**Bladder Length (cm)**
5-7.5 Newborn	3	5
7.5-13 Infant	5	8
13-20 Child	8	13
17-26 Small adult	11	17
24-32 Average adult	13	24
32-42 Large adult	17	32
42-50 Thigh	20	42

From Kirkendall WM, Feinleib M, Freis ED, Mark AL. AHA committee report: recommendations for human blood pressure determinations by sphygmomanometers. *Circulation* 1980;62:1146A. Reprinted with permission of the American Heart Association.
*Midpoint is defined as half the distance from the acromion to the olecranon.

Jugular Venous Pulse

Prominent arterial pulsations can make assessment of the jugular venous pulse difficult; pulse is normal except in patients with coarctation and biventricular failure.

Precordial Movement and Palpation

The left ventricular impulse varies from normal to the sustained heaving impulse of pressure overload hypertrophy.[125] In symptomatic infants with biventricular failure, the right ventricular impulse is dynamic because the pressure overload of pulmonary hypertension is coupled with volume overload of a right-to-left shunt through the foramen ovale. *Suprasternal* notch systolic thrills are frequent in uncomplicated coarctation, but *precordial* thrills are generated by coexisting bicuspid aortic stenosis.

Auscultation

Coarctation of the aorta is associated with systolic, diastolic, and continuous murmurs (Figure 8-15). An ejection sound is an auscultatory sign of a coexisting bicuspid aortic valve (Figures 8-15 and 8-16). Systolic murmurs originate from three sources (see Figure 8-15): (1) arterial collaterals; (2) the coarctation itself; and (3) the brachiocephalic arteries. That murmurs can originate in collateral arteries is based on observations that localized superficial collateral murmurs are abolished by compression and that murmurs have been recorded from the surfaces of surgically exposed collateral arteries.[141] A murmur cannot be generated across coarctation when obstruction is complete (see Figure 8-3B), but murmurs are prominent because arterial collaterals are well developed (see Figure 8-3A,C).[141] The widespread *anatomic* distribution of the collateral arterial circulation accounts for the widespread *thoracic* distribution of accompanying murmurs.[142] Collateral murmurs are crescendo-decrescendo and are delayed in onset and termination because they originate at a distance from the heart (Figures 8-15, 8-17, and 8-18).[141] Widely distributed thoracic murmurs constitute presumptive evidence of collateral circulation, but in young children, collaterals may be well-developed without generating murmurs and in

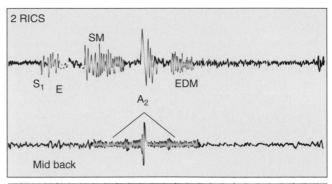
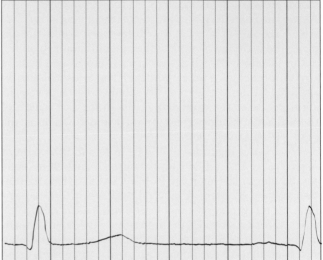

FIGURE 8-16 Phonocardiograms from a 10-year-old boy with coarctation of the aorta and a bicuspid aortic valve. In the second right intercostal space (2 RICS), there is an aortic ejection sound (E), a short midsystolic murmur (SM), and an early diastolic murmur (EDM) of bicuspid aortic regurgitation. The tracing from the mid back was recorded over the site of coarctation and shows a continuous murmur that is delayed in onset and extends into diastole *(paired arrows)*.

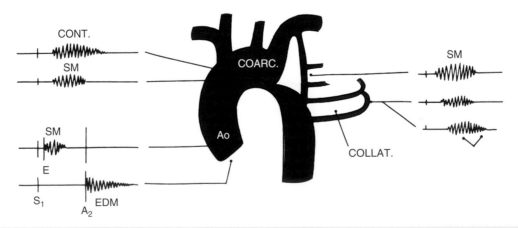

FIGURE 8-15 Illustration of the principal murmurs that accompany coarctation of the aorta (COARC, Ao). At the lower left are auscultatory events associated with a bicuspid aortic valve: namely, an aortic ejection sound (E), a short midsystolic murmur (SM), and an early diastolic murmur (EDM) of aortic regurgitation. At the upper left are the continuous murmur (CONT) and the delayed systolic murmur (SM) that originate at the coarctation site and are heard posteriorly over the thoracic spine. On the right are collateral arterial murmurs (COLLAT) that are crescendo decrescendo and delayed in onset and termination because their origins are at a distance from the heart. Collateral murmurs are shown on one side only as a matter of convenience. (S₁ = first heart sound; A₂ = aortic second sound.)

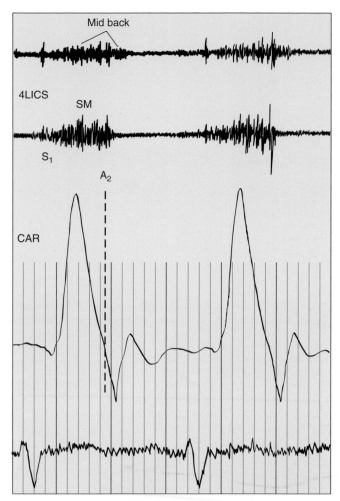

FIGURE 8-17 Tracings from a 22-year-old man with coarctation of the aorta. The phonocardiogram from the mid back over the site of coarctation shows a systolic murmur that is delayed in onset and continues into diastole (paired arrows). The systolic murmur in the fourth left intercostal space (4LICS) originated in a left internal mammary collateral (see Figure 8-3). (CAR = carotid.)

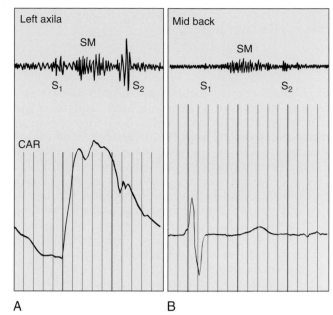

FIGURE 8-18 Tracings from a 6-year-old boy with coarctation of the aorta. **A,** The phonocardiogram in the left axila shows a delayed systolic murmur (SM) that originated in arterial collaterals. **B,** The phonocardiogram in the mid back over the vertebral column shows a delayed systolic murmur at the coarctation site. (CAR = carotid pulse; S_1 = first heart sound; S_2 = second heart sound.)

occasional adults with abundant collaterals, murmurs are inconspicuous.

The coarctation itself is responsible for a systolic murmur[141] that correlates with the *size* of the coarctation, and the localized posterior position over the thoracic spine correlates with the coarctation *site* (see Figures 8-15 and 8-18B). Typical isthmic coarctation generates a posterior murmur at the level of the fourth or fifth thoracic spinous process (see Figures 8-15 through 8-18).[141] In infants, murmurs are typically absent, except in this posterior location. Heart failure causes the coarctation murmur to decrease or disappear.

Infants are best examined prone, and older patients are examined prone or in a relaxed sitting position that minimizes muscle tremor. Posterior auscultation begins in the midline at the upper thoracic spine and descends to the midthoracic and lumbar spine. The murmur overlying a coarctation is soft and high-frequency, so detection is best achieved with the stethoscopic diaphragm or firm pressure of the bell. As severity increases, the short posterior thoracic systolic murmur lenthens (see Figures 8-15 and 8-18B) and continues into diastole (see Figures 8-15 through 8-17). When the coarctation diameter decreases to 2.5 mm, the murmur occupies all of the cardiac cycle.[141] The continuous murmur is soft and high-frequency, so assessment requires a quiet room and a cooperative patient. Rarely, the coarctation murmur is loud enough to radiate to the anterior chest.[141] A loud brachiocephalic systolic murmur accompanied by a thrill is heard in the suprasternal notch, and prominent systolic murmurs are heard over the right and left subclavian arteries. A short low-frequency to medium-frequency *diastolic murmur* over the left ventricular impulse is caused by a decrease in interpapillary distance, which culminates in the single papillary muscle of a parachute mitral valve (see previous discussion; see Chapter 9).[37] The murmur of abdominal coarctation is heard anteriorly in the epigastrium or just below and posteriorly over the lower thoracic or lumbar spine.[20] *Pseudocoarctation* generates a systolic murmur posteriorly over the site of the aortic kink (see Figure 8-5).[23,143]

The *second heart sound in coarctation of the aorta* is either single or normally split with increased intensity of the aortic component. A loud single second sound in the second left interspace is the result of augmented aortic valve closure (see Figure 8-16). In symptomatic infants with pulmonary hypertension, the loud single second sound is the summation of aortic and pulmonary components.

Fourth heart sounds reflect the afterload-induced left ventricular hypertrophy of coarctation. Third heart sounds or summation sounds occur in infants with heart failure and a rapid heart rate.

Electrocardiogram

Electrocardiographic patterns are related to two age-groups: namely, symptomatic neonatal coarctation and coarctation after childhood. Left atrial P wave abnormalities occur in adults (Figure 18-19), and right atrial P wave abnormalities occur in symptomatic infants (Figure 8-20). The mean QRS axis in adults is normal, although axis is occasionally leftward in older patients (Figure 8-21). Right axis deviation with right ventricular hypertrophy is typical of the electrocardiogram in symptomatic infants with right ventricular pressure and volume overload (see previous discussion). Right ventricular hypertrophy that persists beyond infancy is rare in uncomplicated coarctation.

Left ventricular hypertrophy is characterized by tall R waves and low, flat, or inverted T waves in left precordial leads (see Figure 8-19). Prominent coved ST segment depressions with deeply inverted T waves are exceptional (see Figure 8-21) and imply coexisting bicuspid aortic stenosis. Prominent left precordial Q waves suggest the volume overload of bicuspid aortic regurgitation.

X-Ray

In asymptomatic infants and young children, the x-ray is normal. The descending thoracic aorta is a straight line that runs parallel to the left edge of the vertebral column,

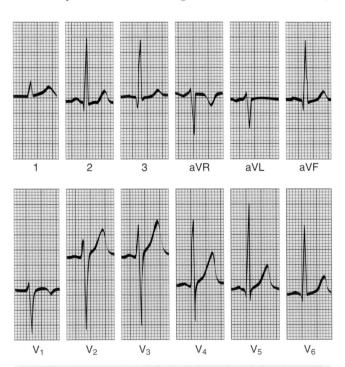

FIGURE 8-19 Electrocardiogram from a 23-year-old man with coarctation of the aorta. The QRS axis is normal. There is a broad left atrial P wave in lead 2. Left ventricular hypertrophy is suggested by the sum of the S wave in V_1 and the R wave in V_5.

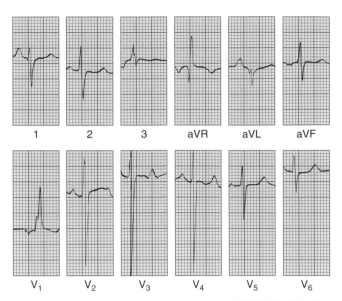

FIGURE 8-20 Electrocardiogram from a 6-year old-boy with coarctation of the aorta and congestive heart failure in infancy (see Figure 8-18). The QRS axis is rightward. There is a tall right atrial P wave in lead 1. Right ventricular hypertrophy is manifested by a tall monophasic R wave in led V_1 and deep S waves in left precordial leads.

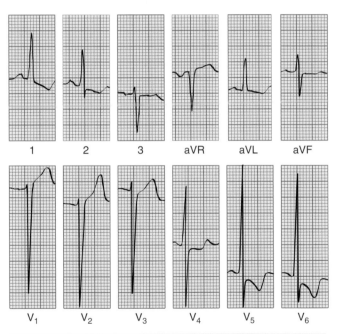

FIGURE 8-21 Electrocardiogram from a 41-year-old man with coarctation of the aorta. The QRS axis is horizontal. There are broad left atrial P waves in leads 1 and 2. Left ventricular hypertrophy is manifested by deep S waves in right precordial leads and tall R waves with ST segment depressions and T wave inversions in left precordial leads.

but in children and young adults, the postcoarctation descending thoracic aorta has a distinctive leftward convexity that is accompanied by dilation of the left subclavian artery (Figure 8-22).[144] The x-ray in symptomatic infants discloses pulmonary venous congestion with

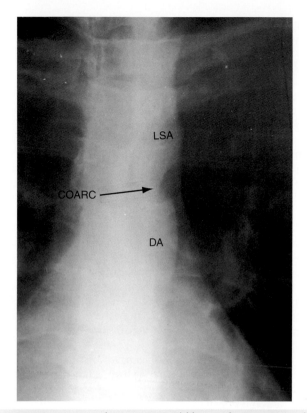

FIGURE 8-22 X-ray from a 3-year-old boy with coarctation of the aorta (COARC). The child was too young to have development of rib notching, but the radiologic diagnosis can be suspected because the descending aorta (DA) is convex to the left and the left subclavian artery (LSA) is dilated—the *figure 3 sign.*

dilation of the right ventricle and the right and left atria (Figure 8-23). Left ventricular size remains normal or nearly so.

Notching of the ribs is a classic radiologic sign of coarctation caused by collateral flow through dilated, tortuous, pulsatile *posterior* intercostal arteries (Figures 8-3, 8-24, and 8-25). Notches vary from rib to rib and from patient to patient and may be single, multiple, shallow, deep, broad, or narrow.[41,135] Notching originates in *posterior* intercostal arteries that run in intercostal grooves (see Figure 8-24), so the anterior ribs are spared because anterior intercostal arteries do not run in intercostal grooves.[135,145] Rarely, the *superior* margin of a rib is notched because of contact with an overhanging intercostal artery.[146] Rib notching seldom appears before age 6 years, although exceptional examples have been described as early as 2 years of age.[41,145,147]

Typical coarctation distal to the left subclavian artery results in *bilateral* notching between the third and the eighth posterior ribs, but rarely above the third or below the ninth rib (Figures 8-25 and 8-26A).[135] Anatomic variations of the coarctation site are accompanied by variations in the radiologic patterns. The development of arterial collaterals depends on patency of the ipsilateral subclavian artery; so when the left subclavian lumen is compromised, ipsilateral collaterals fail to develop, and *unilateral* rib notching is confined to the *right* hemithorax (Figure 8-27).[135,145] Anomalous origin of the *right* subclavian artery *distal* to the coarctation (see Figure 8-1C) results in failure of collateral development in the *right* hemithorax, so unilateral notching is confined to the *left* hemithorax.[92,145] Lateral x-rays show *retrosternal* notching or scalloping caused by dilated tortuous internal

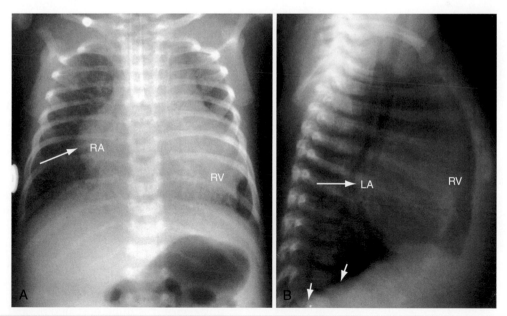

FIGURE 8-23 A, X-ray from a 1-month-old male with coarctation of the aorta, congestive heart failure, and a left-to-right shunt through a patent foramen ovale. There is pulmonary venous congestion. An enlarged right ventricle (RV) occupies the apex, and a dilated right atrium (RA) forms the right lower cardiac border. **B,** Lateral chest x-ray from a 4-month-old female with 45 XO Turner's syndrome, coarctation of the aorta, congestive heart failure, and a left-to-right shunt through a foramen ovale. The left atrium (LA) is enlarged. The retrosternal space is occupied by a dilated right ventricle (RV), but the left ventricle is not enlarged. The crural portions of the diaphragm are flat *(curved white arrows)* because the lungs were hyperinflated.

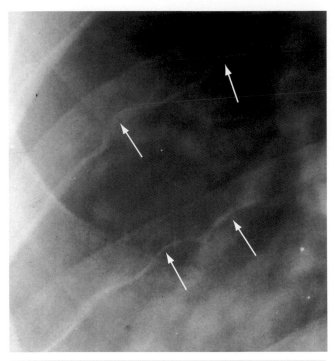

FIGURE 8-24 Close-up showing irregular scalloped notching of the inferior margins of posterior ribs in a 54-year-old man with coarctation of the aorta.

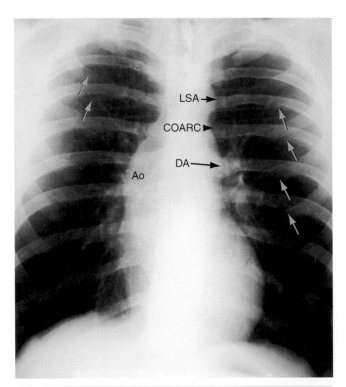

FIGURE 8-25 X-ray from a 23-year-old man with coarctation of the aorta (COARC). Arrows point to notching on the undersurfaces of the posterior ribs. The ascending aorta (Ao) is dilated. The left subclavian artery (LSA) dilated above the coarctation, and the descending aorta (DA) is dilated below the coarctation, forming a *figure 3*.

mammary arteries (see Figure 8-3A,B).[41,147] When coarctation is in the *abdominal* aorta, notching, if present at all, is confined to the *lower* ribs.[148]

In older children and adults with coarctation, the ascending aorta is moderately to markedly dilated (see Figure 8-25).[147] In XO Turner's syndrome, the ascending aorta may be aneurysmal (see Figure 8-9). The proximal and distal paracoarctation aorta are typically dilated (see Figure 8-2).[41,48,144] Postcoarctation aortic dilation is sometimes aneurysmal, and calcification is occasionally visible in the wall of the aneurysm. The combination of a dilated left subclavian artery proximal to the coarctation and a dilated aorta distal to the coarctation produces a *figure 3* silhouette in the x-ray (see Figures 8-22 and 8-25).[41,144] The mirror image of the figure three sign is seen when the left subclavian artery and descending aorta indent a barium esophagram (Figure 8-28).[41,147] The left subclavian cannot dilate when its lumen is compromised by the coarctation, so dilation of the distal paracoarctation aorta exists alone (see Figure 8-27). A retroesophageal aberrant right subclavian artery is sometimes identified as a posterior indentation of the barium esophagram.[135]

The kinked aorta of *pseudocoarctation* has a transverse arch and a descending aorta that form a large *3 sign* above and below the kink (see Figure 8-5).[24,77,143,149] Pseudocoarctation is conspicuous, but rib notching is conspicuous by its absence (see Figure 8-5).

Echocardiogram

Transthoracic and transesophageal echocardiography with Doppler scan interrogation and color flow imaging (Figures 8-29 [and Video 8-1], 8-30, and 8-31) permit segment-by-segment analysis of the ascending aorta, the aortic arch, the brachiocephalic arteries, the aortic isthmus, and the proximal descending aorta from birth to maturity.[150,151] A long segment of luminal narrowing can be identified. The suprasternal notch window with color flow imaging is identifies the coarctation by a zone of localized accelerated flow and by providing the target through which the continuous wave Doppler beam can be aligned to determine the gradient (see Figures 8-29A,B, 8-30, and 8-31).[150,151] Peak *systolic* velocity reflects the maximal systolic gradient, and persistent high-velocity *diastolic* forward flow indicates severity (see Figures 8-29B and 8-31B).[150–152] The Doppler pattern across the coarctation is affected by reduced proximal aortic compliance.[153] Color flow identifies the level at which laminar flow becomes turbulent (see Figure 8-29C). An echocardiographic diagnosis of coarctation can be made *in utero*.[12] In the fetus and neonate, normal tapering of the aortic isthmus[9] can be mistaken for isthmic obstruction, and artifacts from the ductus insertion sometimes make interpretation difficult.[151] The relationship between the site of coarctation and the aortic insertion of the ligamentum arteriosum establishes preductal, juxtaductal, or postductal location.[151]

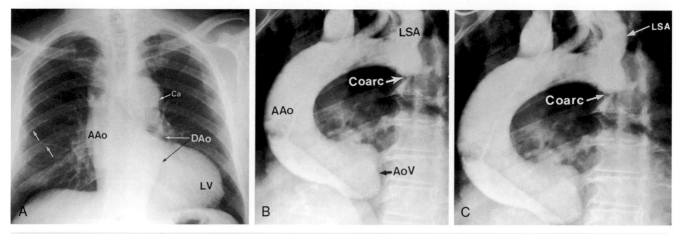

FIGURE 8-26 A, X-ray from a 62-year-old man with coarctation of the aorta distal to the left subclavian artery. *Unmarked arrows* in the right hemithorax identify subtle rib notching. The ascending aorta (AAo) is dilated, and calcium (Ca) appears in the aortic knuckle. The descending thoracic aorta (DAo) is convex to the left, which in part is age-related. An enlarged convex left ventricle (LV) occupies the apex. **B,** Thoracic aortogram shows a dilated and elongated ascending aorta (AAo) and complete obstruction at the coarctation site (CoARC). The aortic valve (AoV) is trileaflet. **C,** Lateral aortogram from a 70-year-old woman with complete obstruction at the coarctation site (Coarc). The left subclavian artery (LSA) is dilated.

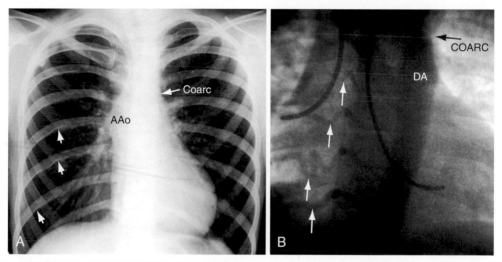

FIGURE 8-27 A, X-ray from a 14-year-old boy with coarctation of the aorta (Coarc) that obstructed the orifice of the left subclavian artery, which is therefore not dilated above the coarctation site. The ascending aorta (AAo) is dilated. *Arrows* point to *unilateral* notching of the ribs on the right. **B,** The aortogram opacified unilateral collateral arteries on the right *(arrows)*. *Black arrow* identifies the coarctation site. The descending aorta (DA) is convex to the left.

Summary

Coarctation of the aorta is not overlooked if attention is paid to upper and lower extremity arterial pulses and blood pressure during routine physical examination. The diagnosis is evident when systemic hypertension is accompanied by reduced femoral pulses. Aortic coarctation is a widespread disorder in which isthmic obstruction is only one of an array of abnormalities that include abnormalities of the proximal and distal paracoarcration aorta, the ascending and transverse aorta, the coronary arteries, the conduit arteries (radial, brachial, carotid), and the retinal vascular bed, in addition to systemic hypertension, dissecting aneurysm, cerebral aneurysms, and vascular rings. Minor symptoms include headache, epistaxis, and leg fatigue. Major complications are congestive heart failure, especially in infants; rupture or dissection of the paracoarctation aorta; infective endarteritis; and rupture of an aneurysm of the circle of Willis. The physical appearance of XO Turner's syndrome increases the probability of coarctation. Pulse pressure proximal to the coarctation increases with age, resulting in conspicuous carotid and suprasternal notch pulsations. Collateral arterial pulsations should be sought beneath the skin, especially around the scapulae. Tortuous U-shaped retinal arterioles are distinctive. A left ventricular impulse occupies the apex. A right ventricular impulse is reserved for symptomatic infants with heart failure, pulmonary hypertension, and a right-to-left shunt across a patent foramen ovale. Auscultatory signs include

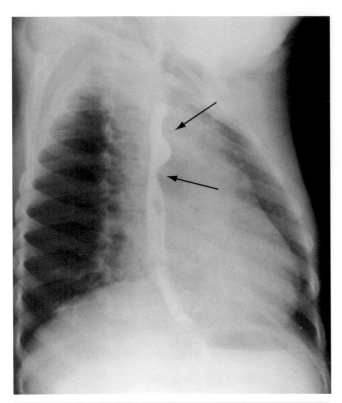

FIGURE 8-28 Right anterior oblique view from a 6-year-old boy with coarctation of the aorta. The barium esophagram exhibits the *E sign (arrows)* caused by compression from the dilated left subclavian artery above and the dilated descending aorta below. The *E sign* is the mirror image of the *3 sign* (see Figure 8-25).

widespread thoracic systolic murmurs through arterial collaterals and a posterior systolic or continuous murmur over the coarctation site. Systolic murmurs are especially prominent in the suprasternal notch and along the left sternal border over internal mammary collaterals. Auscultatory signs in infants are limited to the posterior interscapular murmur over the coarctation. Electrocardiographic criteria for left ventricular hypertrophy reflect increased afterload. Right ventricular hypertrophy characterizes the electrocardiogram of symptomatic infants. Notching of the third to eighth posterior ribs is a radiologic feature of major diagnostic importance but is seldom present before age 6 years. Dilation of the left subclavian artery and the proximal descending aorta is a useful radiologic sign in children too young to have rib notching. Transthoracic and transesophageal echocardiograms with Doppler scan interrogation and color flow imaging are used to identify the coarctation and determine its severity.

INTERRUPTION OF THE AORTIC ARCH

The thoracic aorta lends itself to segmental analysis of its ascending portion, arch, isthmus, and descending portion. Atresia or interruption of the aortic arch is the ultimate expression of obstructive thoracic aortic anomalies that begin with isthmic coarctation. The embryogenesis of these anomalies is similar if not identical.

Interruption of the aortic arch was first described in the 18th century by Raphael Steidele[154] of the University of Vienna. *Steidele's complex* is occasionally applied as an eponym to this rare malformation,[155,156] which is characterized by complete anatomic discontinuity or by an atretic fibrous strand between the aortic arch and the descending aorta (Figure 8-32).[157–160] The classification of complete interruption by Celoria and Patton[158] refers to one of three sites,[155,156,160,161] two of which were described in 1927 by Maude Abbott.[162] Interruption between the left common carotid and left subclavian arteries (type B; Figures 8-32 and 8-33) is more common than interruption distal to the left subclavian artery (type A). The least common site is between the innominate artery and the left carotid artery (type C; Figure 8-34).[158,163,164] Subtypes are based on anomalous origin of the right subclavian artery.[127,163,165] Rarely, interruption is in a right aortic arch.[166]

Interruption of the aortic arch seldom occurs as an isolated anomaly.[167–170] Patent ductus arteriosus and ventricular septal defect are coexisting malformations on which tenuous neonatal survival depends. The clinical picture in infants is largely determined by patency of the ductus arteriosus, which provides nonrestrictive flow from the pulmonary trunk into the descending aorta (see Figure 8-32).[155,159,160] In most patients with interrupted aortic arch, the ductus is histologically mature with prominent intimal cushions that prefigure constriction. In a minority of patients, an immature ductus is devoid of intimal cushions and has marked elastification that set the stage for persistent patency. A ventricular septal defect almost invariably coexists when interruption is between the left carotid and left subclavian arteries (type B) and also coexists in about 50% of interruptions distal to the left subclavian artery (type A).[42,155,159–161,163,168] A posterior malaligned ventricular septal defect is the rule when the interrupted arch is between the left carotid and left subclavian arteries (type B).[157,161,171] Defects in the perimembranous and muscular septum are uncommon.[42] Posterior deviation of the infundibular septum encroaches on the left ventricular outflow tract and causes subaortic obstruction.[42,161] When the ventricular septum is intact, a physiologically equivalent aortopulmonary window is almost always present,[172] and the interrupted arch is distal to the left subclavian artery (type A).[172]

Theories on *pathogenesis* have focused on the role of reduced aortic flow during early morphogenesis, analogous to theories proposed for the pathogenesis of coarctation (see previous discussion).[165,172] The malaligned ventricular septal defect in type B interruption encroaches on the left ventricular outflow tract, reducing aortic blood flow[165] and favoring pulmonary blood flow.[161,165] These anatomic arrangements are in keeping with the small caliber of the ascending aorta because of the paucity of aortic blood flow during fetal development.[42] Unique vascular morphology of the fourth aortic arches has been implicated in the pathogenesis of type B interruption with anomalous right subclavian artery.[173] An unresolved morphogenic point is the relatively rare

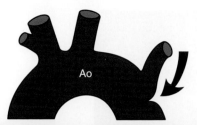

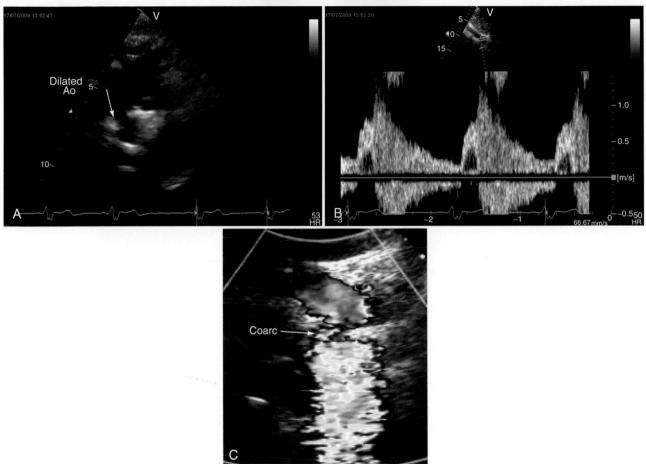

FIGURE 8-29 Schematic illustration of aortic coarctation with corresponding echocardiograms: **A,** Images from a 5-year-old boy with coarctation of the aorta. The two-dimensional echocardiogram identifies the coarctation. **B,** Continuous wave Doppler scan shows systolic turbulence across the coarctation that continued through most of diastole. **C,** Color flow image from a 3-year-old boy showing an abrupt change from laminar flow to turbulent flow at the coarctation site (Coarc) (Video 8-1). (Ao = aorta.)

occurrence of interruption between the innominate artery and the left common carotid artery (type C, 4% of cases), which implies that this segment of the arch is less vulnerable to decreased flow or depends on a separate developmental defect. Aortic arch interruption distal to the left subclavian artery (type A) and coarctation of the aorta are believed to be morphogenetically related.

The *physiologic consequences* of interrupted aortic arch with patent ductus arteriosus and ventricular septal defect consist of *ascending* aortic blood flow from the left ventricle and *descending* aortic blood from the pulmonary trunk through the ductus (see Figure 8-32).[159,168] The left-to-right interventricular shunt is reinforced by resistance to left ventricular outflow

caused by the malaligned ventricular septal defect. The magnitude of the right-to-left shunt through the ductus depends on the relative resistances in the pulmonary and systemic vascular beds. Constriction of the ductus is catastrophic, suddenly abolishing flow into the descending aorta and diverting virtually all pulmonary blood flow into the already overloaded lungs.[174] Nevertheless, interruption or atresia of the aortic arch *without* a patent ductus is compatible with life,[164,175] even adult survival,[87,174,176,177] provided that both subclavian arteries arise from the descending aorta, an arrangement that potentially permits retrograde flow to the entire body except for the head.[164,175,176] A variation on this theme is the congenital subclavian

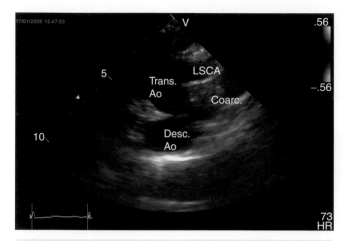

FIGURE 8-30 Echocardiogram (suprasternal notch) from a 10-month-old male with coarctation of the aorta (Coarc), localized distal to the left subclavian artery (LSCA). (Trans Ao = transverse aorta; Desc Ao = descending aorta.)

steal that occurs when both subclavian arteries arise distal to the interruption.[52,178] Constriction of the ductus prompts a fall in pressure in the subclavian arteries and a steal *into* those arteries through collateral channels from ascending to descending aorta via the circle of Willis and the vertebral arteries.[178]

History

Complete interruption of the aortic arch is estimated to occur in 19 per million live births according to the New England Regional Infant Cardiac Program.[179] Males and females are equally represented.[155,156,160] Recurrence has been reported in siblings,[180–183] and a 2.5% recurrence rate of congenital heart disease has been reported in siblings of patients with type B interruption.[184]

The typical clinical picture is represented by a neonate who becomes acutely ill as the ductus closes, prompting a

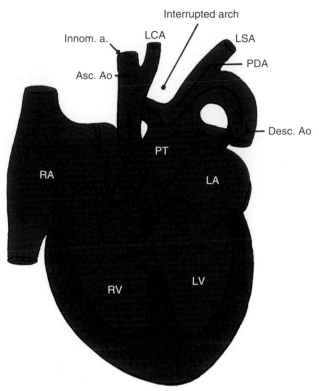

FIGURE 8-32 Illustration of the anatomic and circulatory derangements in the most common type of complete interruption of the aortic arch (type B). The ascending aorta (Asc. Ao) gives rise to the innominate artery (Innom. a.) and to the left carotid artery (LCA). The left subclavian artery (LSA) arises from the descending aorta (Desc. Ao), which is continuous with the pulmonary trunk (PT) via a nonrestrictive patent ductus arteriosus (PDA). A large ventricular septal defect provides the left ventricle with access to the descending aorta via pulmonary trunk/ductus/descending aortic continuity. (RA/LA = right atrium and left atrium; RV/LV = right ventricle and left ventricle.)

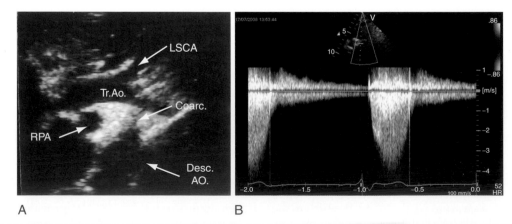

FIGURE 8-31 **A,** Echocardiogram from a 12-year-old boy with coarctation of the aorta (Coarc.) distal to the left subclavian artery (LSCA). The transverse aorta (Tr. Ao.) tapers toward the isthmus. Distal to the coarctation, the descending aorta (Desc. Ao.) is dilated. **B,** Continuous wave Doppler scan from a 27-year-old man with coarctation of the aorta.

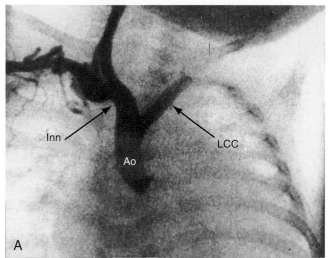

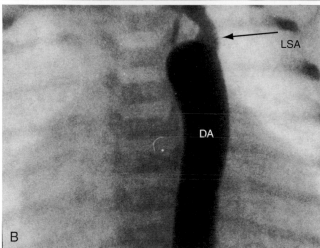

FIGURE 8-33 **A,** Aortogram from a female neonate with complete interruption of the aortic arch distal to the left common carotid artery (LCC). The innominate artery (Inn) gives rise to the right common carotid artery and to the right subclavian artery. **B,** Aortogram from a 3-day-old male with complete interruption of the aortic arch distal to the left common carotid artery. The left subclavian artery (LSA) originates from the descending aorta (DA). Compare with Figure 8-32. (Ao = ascending aorta.)

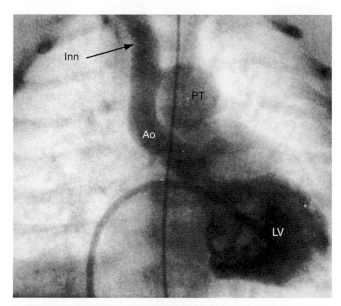

FIGURE 8-34 Left ventriculogram (LV) from a female neonate with complete interruption of the aortic arch distal to the innominate artery (Inn). The ascending aorta (Ao) ascends vertically and is small compared with the dilated pulmonary trunk (PT). The left common carotid artery and left subclavian artery originated from the descending aorta. Compare with Figure 8-32.

Physical Appearance

Cyanosis is inconspicuous until the acute advent of congestive heart failure. *Differential* cyanosis caused by right-to-left ductal flow into the descending aorta is, with rare exception, canceled by the left-to-right shunt through the ventricular septal defect (see Figure 8-32),[155,159,160,168] a mechanism that was recognized in 1852 by Greig,[191] who wrote:

> *The additional complication . . . of such a large aperture between the ventricles must have established complete admixture of the blood of the two sides of the heart before it was sent into the aorta and pulmonary artery, so that, independent of subsequent abnormalities of the vessels, all parts of the body would be supplied with blood of the same quality.*

A 22q 11.2 deletion and the DiGeorge syndrome (see Chapter 28, Figure 28-6), which consists of hypoplastic mandible, defective ears, short philtrum, and aplasia or hypoplasia of the thymus and parathyroid glands, are associated with type A or type B interruption.[108,170,192–195]

Arterial Pulse

Femoral arterial pulses are maintained because of continuity between the pulmonary trunk, ductus, and descending aorta (see Figure 8-32).[160,168,186] A reduction in femoral pulses signifies ductal constriction, which initially may be intermittent.[168] When the left subclavian artery originates from the descending aorta (type B), ductal constriction reduces the *left brachial pulse* in addition

sudden *increase* in pulmonary blood flow and a sudden *decrease* in circulation to the trunk and lower limbs.[156,160,167] The result is shock, acidosis, renal failure, intracranial hemorrhage,[174] and a mean survival time of 4 to 10 days.[156,160,161] Three quarters of infants who do not undergo operation are dead within a month, with only 10% reaching their first birthday.[155,160,185] Occasional survivals into childhood, adolescence, and young adulthood have been reported,[168,175,176,184,186,187] with three patients surviving to their early or mid thirties.[156,177,188] Interruption of the aortic arch or aortic arch atresia without patent ductus arteriosus or ventricular septal defect resembles severe coarctation.[87,167,176] Rupture of an intracranial aneurysm was reported in a teenager[189] and in an adult.[190]

to the femoral pulse. Anomalous origin of the *right* sub-clavian artery places the right brachial pulse in the distal low pressure zone.[165] On the rare occasion of interruption of the aortic arch or arch atresia *without* patent ductus or ventricular septal defect, palpation of the systemic arterial pulses is analogous to palpation in coarctation of the aorta.[127,167–169,175,176] When interruption occurs proximal to *both* subclavian arteries (anomalous origin of the right subclavian), the carotid pulses are bounding, but the brachial and femoral pulses are diminished or absent.[127,169,176] If either or both subclavian arteries originate *proximal* to the interruption, the arms are hypertensive, the carotid pulses are bounding, and the femoral pulses are weak or absent.[167,176]

Precordial Movement and Palpation

An isolated *right ventricular impulse* is palpated in infants with interruption of the aortic arch because of obligatory pulmonary hypertension and is associated with a nonrestrictive patent ductus arteriosus and ventricular septal defect. A left ventricular impulse is absent despite the left-to-right shunt at ventricular level because blood entering the pulmonary trunk is diverted through the ductus into the descending aorta rather than through the pulmonary circulation into the left side of the heart (see Figure 8-32). Interruption of the aortic arch without patent ductus or ventricular septal defect results in a left ventricular impulse analogous to coarctation of the aorta.[176]

Auscultation

Murmurs are negligible or absent.[160] The ductus is silent because the shunt is entirely right-to-left through a single nonrestrictive arterial conduit formed by continuity of the pulmonary trunk, ductus, and descending aorta. Murmurs originating through the ventricular septal defect are early systolic, decrescendo, and grade 3/6 or less.[186,196] A continuous murmur has been attributed to collateral circulation that connects the ascending and descending aortas.[186] Diastolic murmurs from pulmonary hypertensive pulmonary regurgitation[160] are introduced by a loud pulmonary component of the second heart sound. Interruption of the aortic arch without a ductus or ventricular septal defect presents with auscultatory signs similar to those of imperforate coarctation, with widespread collateral murmurs that include the head, especially behind the ears.[167,176,197]

Electrocardiogram

Peaked right atrial P waves and right ventricular hypertrophy are electrocardiographic features in the neonate with interruption of the aortic arch, ventricular septal defect, and patent ductus arteriosus (Figure 8-35).[196] Biventricular hypertrophy is in response to left ventricular volume overload and persistent right ventricular pressure overload (Figure 8-36).[160] Interruption *without* patent ductus or ventricular septal defect results in right ventricular hypertrophy in infants[127] but left ventricular hypertrophy in older patients.

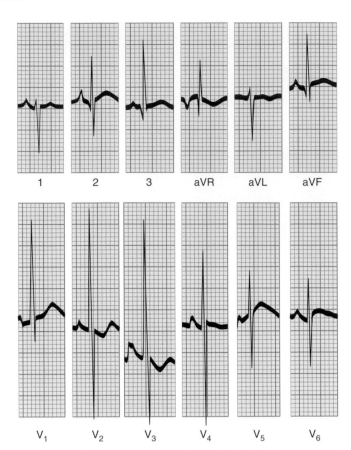

FIGURE 8-35 Electrocardiogram from a 3-day-old male with complete interruption of the aortic arch. There is a tall peaked right atrial P wave in lead 2. Right ventricular hypertrophy is represented by the tall monophasic R wave in lead V_1 and the deep S wave in lead V_6. Biventricular hypertrophy is represented by the large biphasic RS complexes in the mid precordial leads.

X-Ray

The cardiac silhouette enlarges and pulmonary venous congestion develops rapidly when closure of the ductus arteriosus suddenly causes an increase in pulmonary blood flow and volume overload of the left ventricle. The aortic knuckle is absent because the ascending aorta is small and ascends vertically (Figures 8-37 and 8-38).[163] The trachea is not deviated by an aortic arch and is therefore midline.[163] The x-ray shows increased pulmonary venous and pulmonary arterial vascularity with enlargement of the left ventricle (Figures 8-37 and 8-39).[186,196] Isolated interruption of the aortic arch *without* a ductus or a ventricular septal defect is radiologically similar to coarctation of the aorta, including rib notching.[164,167,197] Whether the notching is bilateral or unilateral depends on the site of interruption, the origin of the subclavian arteries, and the length of survival.[163,164]

Echocardiogram

Echocardiography with Doppler scan interrogation and color flow imaging is used to identify the major segments of the thoracic aorta, visualize the patent ductus and the

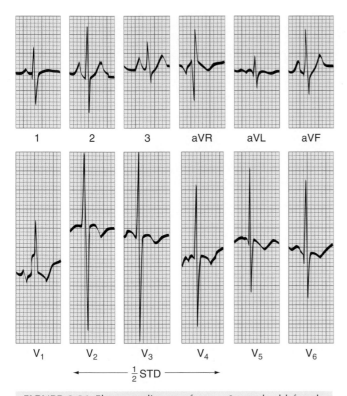

FIGURE 8-36 Electrocardiogram from a 6-month-old female with complete interruption of the aortic arch. There are tall peaked right atrial P waves in leads 2, 3, and aVF. Right ventricular hypertrophy is represented by the tall notched R wave in lead V_1 and the deep S wave in lead V_6. The prominent Q wave and well-developed R wave in lead V_6 are evidence of left ventricular volume overload. Biventricular hypertrophy is represented by large equidiphasic RS complexes in leads V_{2-4}, which are half standardized.

ventricular septal defect, and distinguish interruption of the aortic arch from coarctation with tubular hypoplasia. In type C interruption, echocardiography is used to identify antegrade flow in the right carotid and basilar arteries and retrograde flow in the left carotid artery.[198] Echocardiography is used to identify type B interruption of a *right* aortic arch.[199]

A normal aorta exhibits a continuous smooth curvature from its ascending to its descending portion, but when the *arch is interrupted* distal to the left carotid artery (type B), the ascending aorta rises vertically, exhibits little curvature, and bifurcates into the innominate and left carotid arteries,[170] with the carotid appearing as an index finger pointing upward (see Figure 8-38). When the arch is interrupted distal to the left subclavian artery (type A), the ascending aorta exhibits a slight curvature and gives off three branches (the innominate, the left carotid, and the left subclavian arteries)[170] because the right subclavian artery is prone to anomalous origin (Figure 8-40). A useful echocardiographic observation is the discrepancy between the small caliber of the ascending aorta and conspicuous dilation of the pulmonary trunk. The image created by continuity of pulmonary trunk, ductus, and descending aorta superficially resembles an *uninterrupted* aortic arch, but identification of the origins of the right and left pulmonary arterial branches, together with absence of brachiocephalic branches, prevents error (see Figure 8-40).[170] Characterization of a ventricular septal defect is an important part of the echocardiographic examination. An *intact* ventricular septum with an interrupted aortic arch prompts search for an aortopulmonary window.[170] A malaligned ventricular septal defect is associated with posterior and leftward deviation of the conal septum and varying degrees of subaortic narrowing.[170,171,200]

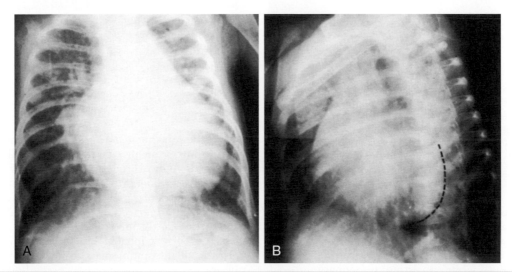

FIGURE 8-37 X-rays from the 6-month-old female whose electrocardiogram is shown in Figure 8-36. **A,** Prominent pulmonary soft tissue densities represent venous congestion in addition to increased pulmonary arterial vascularity. The pulmonary trunk is dilated in contrast to the inconspicuous ascending aorta, and the right atrium is markedly enlarged. **B,** In the left anterior oblique projection, the right and left ventricles are both enlarged.

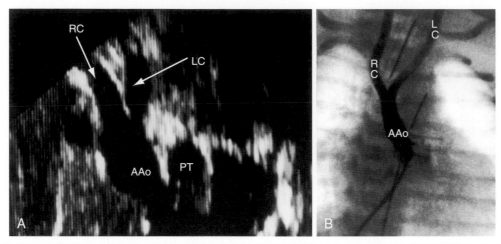

FIGURE 8-38 **A,** Echocardiogram from a neonate with complete interruption of the aortic arch distal to the left carotid artery. The ascending aorta (AAo) rises vertically, exhibits no curvature, and branches as the right carotid (RC) and left carotid artery (LC). **B,** The aortogram shows a small ascending aorta that rises vertically and exhibits no curvature. The right carotid artery (RC) and the left carotid artery (LC) are as in the echocardiogram. (PT = pulmonary trunk.)

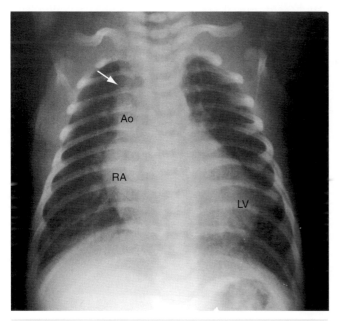

FIGURE 8-39 X-ray from a 2-day-old male with complete interruption of the aortic arch. The lungs show pulmonary venous congestion. The patient is slightly rotated to the left, increasing the prominence of the ascending aorta (Ao) and right atrium (RA) and decreasing the prominence of the left ventricle (LV). The density at the right thoracic inlet is thymus *(arrow)*.

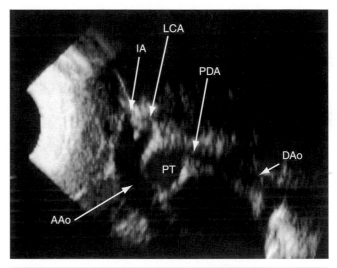

FIGURE 8-40 Echocardiogram from a 7-month-old female with complete interruption of the aortic arch. The ascending aorta (AAo) gives rise to the innominate artery (IA) and to the left carotid artery (LCA) distal to which the arch was interrupted. The pulmonary trunk (PT) is continuous with the descending aorta (DAo) via a patent ductus arteriosus (PDA).

Summary

The typical clinical picture of interruption of the aortic arch is an acyanotic neonate who initially appears well but who suddenly becomes ill when the ductus arteriosus constricts and deprives the trunk and lower limbs of arterial circulation, while diverting pulmonary arterial blood into the lungs and into the left side of the heart. Tachypnea and symmetric cyanosis develop, the femoral pulses disappear, and the chest x-ray exhibits pulmonary venous congestion with progressive cardiac enlargement. When the interruption is proximal to the left subclavian artery, the left brachial arterial pulse disappears as well. No murmur or inconspicuous early systolic decrescendo murmur is found through the ventricular septal defect. The electrocardiogram shows peaked right atrial P waves and right ventricular hypertrophy, but if survival permits, biventricular hypertrophy emerges. Echocardiography is used to identify the interrupted arch. The ascending aorta takes a straight cephalad course and is small compared with the dilated pulmonary trunk. Continuity between pulmonary trunk, ductus, and descending aorta create a smooth unbroken contour. A leftward and posterior malaligned ventricular septal defect is the rule when interruption is between the left carotid and left subclavian arteries. An aortopulmonary window is likely if the ventricular septum is intact.

REFERENCES

1. Jarcho S. Coarctation of the aorta (Meckel, 1750; Paris, 1791). *Am J Cardiol.* 1961;7:844–852.
2. Jarcho S. Coarctation of the aorta (Otto, 1824; Bertin, 1824). *Am J Cardiol.* 1961;8:843–845.
3. Jarcho S. Coarctation of the aorta (Reynaud, 1828). *Am J Cardiol.* 1962;9:591–597.
4. Jarcho S. Coarctation of the aorta (Legrand, 1833). *Am J Cardiol.* 1962;10:266–271.
5. Jarcho S. Aortic coarctation and aortic stenosis (Nixon 1834). *Am J Cardiol.* 1963;11:238–245.
6. Elzenga NJ, Gittenberger-De Groot AC. Localised coarctation of the aorta. An age dependent spectrum. *Br Heart J.* 1983;49:317–323.
7. Kappetein AP, Gittenberger-De Groot AC, Zwinderman AH, Rohmer J, Poelmann RE, Huysmans HA. The neural crest as a possible pathogenetic factor in coarctation of the aorta and bicuspid aortic valve. *J Thorac Cardiovasc Surg.* 1991;102:830–836.
8. Park HK, Cho SH, Park Y-H. Atypical coarctation of the aorta: congenital stenosis of the mid-thoracic aorta. *J Am Coll Cardiol.* 2009;53:2098.
9. Hornberger LK, Weintraub RG, Pesonen E, et al. Echocardiographic study of the morphology and growth of the aortic arch in the human fetus. Observations related to the prenatal diagnosis of coarctation. *Circulation.* 1992;86:741–747.
10. Langille BL, Brownlee RD, Adamson SL. Perinatal aortic growth in lambs: relation to blood flow changes at birth. *Am J Physiol.* 1990;259:H1247–H1253.
11. Morrow WR, Huhta JC, Murphy Jr DJ, Mcnamara DG. Quantitative morphology of the aortic arch in neonatal coarctation. *J Am Coll Cardiol.* 1986;8:616–620.
12. Allan LD, Chita SK, Anderson RH, Fagg N, Crawford DC, Tynan MJ. Coarctation of the aorta in prenatal life: an echocardiographic, anatomical, and functional study. *Br Heart J.* 1988;59:356–360.
13. Allan LD, Crawford DC, Tynan M. Evolution of coarctation of the aorta in intrauterine life. *Br Heart J.* 1984;52:471–473.
14. Rudolph AM, Heymann MA, Spitznas U. Hemodynamic considerations in the development of narrowing of the aorta. *Am J Cardiol.* 1972;30:514–525.
15. Talner NS, Berman MA. Postnatal development of obstruction in coarctation of the aorta: role of the ductus arteriosus. *Pediatrics.* 1975;56:562–569.
16. Mcmahon CJ, Vick 3rd GW, Nihill MR. Right aortic arch and coarctation: delineation by three dimensional magnetic resonance angiogram. *Heart.* 2001;85:492.
17. Bahabozorgui S, Nemir Jr P. Coarctation of the abdominal aorta. *Am J Surg.* 1966;111:224–229.
18. Bergamini TM, Bernard JD, Mavroudis C, Backer CL, Muster AJ, Richardson JD. Coarctation of the abdominal aorta. *Ann Vasc Surg.* 1995;9:352–356.
19. Riemenschneider TA, Emmanouilides GC, Hirose F, Linde LM. Coarctation of the abdominal aorta in children: report of three cases and review of the literature. *Pediatrics.* 1969;44:716–726.
20. Roques X, Bourdeaud'hui A, Choussat A, et al. Coarctation of the abdominal aorta. *Ann Vasc Surg.* 1988;2:138–144.
21. Bahabozorgui S, Bernstein RG, Frater RW. Pseudocoarctation of aorta associated with aneurysm formation. *Chest.* 1971;60:616–617.
22. Bilgic A, Ozer S, Atalay S. Pseudocoarctation of the aorta. *Jpn Heart J.* 1990;31:875–879.
23. Griffin JF. Congenital kinking of the aorta (pseudocoarctation). *N Engl J Med.* 1964;271:726–728.
24. Smyth PT, Edwards JE. Pseudocoarctation, kinking or buckling of the aorta. *Circulation.* 1972;46:1027–1032.
25. Wang W-B, Lin G-M. Pseudocoarctation and coarctation. *Int J Cardiol.* 2009;133:e62–e64.
26. Schellhammer F, Von Den Driesch P, Gaitzsch A. Pseudocoarctation of the abdominal aorta. *Vasa.* 1997;26:308–310.
27. Joseph M, Leclerc Y, Hutchison SJ. Aortic pseudocoarctation causing refractory hypertension. *N Engl J Med.* 2002;346:784–785.
28. Yamada M, Horigome H, Ishii S. Pseudocoarctation of the aorta coexistent with coarctation. *Eur J Pediatr.* 1996;155:993.
29. Ikonomidis JS, Robbins RC. Cervical aortic arch with pseudocoarctation: presentation with spontaneous rupture. *Ann Thorac Surg.* 1999;67:248–250.
30. Safir J, Kerr A, Morehouse H, Frost A, Berman H. Magnetic resonance imaging of dissection in pseudocoarctation of the aorta. *Cardiovasc Intervent Radiol.* 1993;16:180–182.
31. Angelini GD, Kulatilake EN, Hayward M, Ruttley MS. Pseudocoarctation of the aortic arch associated with bicuspid aortic valve lesion: is it a surgical entity? *Thorac Cardiovasc Surg.* 1985;33:36–37.
32. Mulder BJM, Van Der Wall EE. Optimal imaging protocol for evaluation of aortic coarctation; time for a reappraisal. *Int J Cardiovasc Imaging.* 2006;22:695–697.
33. Abbott ME. Coarctation of the aorta of adult type; statistical study and historical retrospect of 200 recorded cases with autopsy; of stenosis or obliteration of descending arch in subjects above age of two years. *Am Heart J.* 1928;3:574.
34. Folger Jr GM, Stein PD. Bicuspid aortic valve morphology when associated with coarctation of the aorta. *Cathet Cardiovasc Diagn.* 1984;10:17–25.
35. Fernandes SM, Sanders SP, Khairy P, et al. Morphology of bicuspid aortic valve in children and adolescents. *J Am Coll Cardiol.* 2004;44:1648–1651.
36. Freed MD, Keane JF, Van Praagh R, Castaneda AR, Bernhard WF, Nadas AS. Coarctation of the aorta with congenital mitral regurgitation. *Circulation.* 1974;49:1175–1184.
37. Celano V, Pieroni DR, Morera JA, Roland JM, Gingell RL. Two-dimensional echocardiographic examination of mitral valve abnormalities associated with coarctation of the aorta. *Circulation.* 1984;69:924–932.
38. Rosenquist GC. Congenital mitral valve disease associated with coarctation of the aorta: a spectrum that includes parachute deformity of the mitral valve. *Circulation.* 1974;49:985–993.
39. Pasquini L, Fichera A, Tan T, Ho SY, Gardiner H. Left superior caval vein: a powerful indicator of fetal coarctation. *Heart.* 2005;91:539–540.
40. Oppenheimer EH. The association of adult-type coarctation of the aorta with endocardial fibroelastosis in infancy. *Bull Johns Hopkins Hosp.* 1953;93:309–319.
41. Baron MG. Radiologic notes in cardiology: obscuration of the aortic knob in coarctation of the aorta. *Circulation.* 1971;43:311–316.
42. Anderson RH, Lenox CC, Zuberbuhler JR. Morphology of ventricular septal defect associated with coarctation of aorta. *Br Heart J.* 1983;50:176–181.
43. Moene RJ, Gittenberger-De Groot AC, Oppenheimer-Dekker A, Bartelings MM. Anatomic characteristics of ventricular septal defect associated with coarctation of the aorta. *Am J Cardiol.* 1987;59:952–955.
44. Smallhorn JF, Anderson RH, Macartney FJ. Morphological characterisation of ventricular septal defects associated with coarctation of aorta by cross-sectional echocardiography. *Br Heart J.* 1983;49:485–494.
45. Doyle L. Coarctation of the aorta with dissecting aneurysm and haemopericardium: an account by Joseph Jordan, Manchester, 1830. *Thorax.* 1991;46:268–269.
46. Celik T, Iyisoy A, Kursaklioglu H, et al. A large calcified saccular aneurysm in a patient with aortic coarctation. *Int J Cardiovasc Imaging.* 2006;22:93–95.
47. Isner JM, Donaldson RF, Fulton D, Bhan I, Payne DD, Cleveland RJ. Cystic medial necrosis in coarctation of the aorta: a potential factor contributing to adverse consequences observed after percutaneous balloon angioplasty of coarctation sites. *Circulation.* 1987;75:689–695.
48. Niwa K, Perloff JK, Bhuta SM, et al. Structural abnormalities of great arterial walls in congenital heart disease: light and electron microscopic analyses. *Circulation.* 2001;103:393–400.
49. Wallace RB, Nast EP. Postcoarctation mycotic intercostal arterial pseudoaneurysm. *Am J Cardiol.* 1987;59:1014–1015.
50. Henderson RA, Ward C, Campbell C. Dissecting left subclavian artery aneurysm: an unusual presentation of coarctation of the aorta. *Int J Cardiol.* 1993;40:69–70.
51. Shamsa K, Perloff JK, Lee E, Wirthlin RS, Tsui I, Schwartz SD. Retinal vascular patterns after operative repair of aortic isthmic coarctation. *Am J Cardiol.* 2010;105:408–410.
52. Deeg KH, Singer H. Dopplersonographic diagnosis of subclavian steal in infants with coarctation of the aorta and interrupted aortic arch. *Pediatr Radiol.* 1989;19:163–166.
53. Yu C-H, Chen M-R. Clinical investigation of systemic-pulmonary collateral arteries. *Pediatr Cardiol.* 2008;29:334–338.

54. Johns KJ, Johns JA, Feman SS. Retinal vascular abnormalities in patients with coarctation of the aorta. *Arch Ophthal.* 1991;109:1266–1268.
55. Granstrom KO. Retinal changes in coarctation of the aorta. *Br J Ophthalmol.* 1951;35:143–148.
56. Chun K, Colombani PM, Dudgeon DL, Haller Jr JA. Diagnosis and management of congenital vascular rings: a 22-year experience. *Ann Thorac Surg.* 1992;53:597–602; discussion 602–593.
57. Ettedgui JA, Lorber A, Anderson D. Double aortic arch associated with coarctation. *Int J Cardiol.* 1986;12:258–260.
58. Brockmeier K, Demirakca S, Metzner R, Floemer F. Images in cardiovascular medicine. Double aortic arch. *Circulation.* 2000;102:E93–E94.
59. Sehested J, Baandrup U, Mikkelsen E. Different reactivity and structure of the prestenotic and poststenotic aorta in human coarctation. Implications for baroreceptor function. *Circulation.* 1982;65:1060–1065.
60. Brili S, Dernellis J, Aggeli C, et al. Aortic elastic properties in patients with repaired coarctation of aorta. *Am J Cardiol.* 1998;82:1140–1143, A1110.
61. Igler FO, Boerboom LE, Werner PH, et al. Coarctation of the aorta and baroreceptor resetting. A study of carotid baroreceptor stimulus-response characteristics before and after surgical repair in the dog. *Circ Res.* 1981;48:365–371.
62. O'rourke MF, Cartmill TB. Influence of aortic coarctation on pulsatile hemodynamics in the proximal aorta. *Circulation.* 1971;44:281–292.
63. Cumming GR, Mir GH. Exercise haemodynamics of coarctation of the aorta. Acute effects of propranolol. *Br Heart J.* 1970;32:365–369.
64. Earley A, Joseph MC, Shinebourne EA, De Swiet M. Blood pressure and effect of exercise in children before and after surgical correction of coarctation of aorta. *Br Heart J.* 1980;44:411–415.
65. Alpert BS, Bain HH, Balfe JW, Kidd BS, Olley PM. Role of the renin-angiotensin-aldosterone system in hypertensive children with coarctation of the aorta. *Am J Cardiol.* 1979;43:828–834.
66. Warren DJ, Smith RS, Naik RB. Inappropriate renin secretion and abnormal cardiovascular reflexes in coarctation of the aorta. *Br Heart J.* 1981;45:733–736.
67. Perloff JK. Normal myocardial growth and the development and regression of increased ventricular mass. In: Perloff JK, Child JS, Aboulhosn J, eds. *Congenital heart disease in adults.* 3rd ed. Philadelphia: W.B. Saunders; 2009.
68. Borow KM, Colan SD, Neumann A. Altered left ventricular mechanics in patients with valvular aortic stenosis and coarction of the aorta: effects on systolic performance and late outcome. *Circulation.* 1985;72:515–522.
69. Gutgesell HP, Barton DM, Elgin KM. Coarctation of the aorta in the neonate: associated conditions, management, and early outcome. *Am J Cardiol.* 2001;88:457–459.
70. Gough JH. Coarctation of the aorta in father and son. *Br J Radiol.* 1961;34:670–672.
71. Moss AJ. Coarctation of the aorta in siblings. *J Pediatr.* 1955;46:707–709.
72. Rowen MJ. Coarctation of the aorta in father and son. *Am J Cardiol.* 1959;4:540–542.
73. Sehested J. Coarctation of the aorta in monozygotic twins. *Br Heart J.* 1982;47:619–620.
74. Simon AB, Zloto AE, Perry BL, Sigmann JM. Familial aspects of coarctation of the aorta. *Chest.* 1974;66:687–689.
75. Taylor RR, Pollock BE. Coarctation of the aorta in three members of a family. *Am Heart J.* 1953;45:470–475.
76. Beekman RH, Robinow M. Coarctation of the aorta inherited as an autosomal dominant trait. *Am J Cardiol.* 1985;56:818–819.
77. Keller HI, Cheitlin MD. The occurrence of mild coarctation of the aorta (pseudocoarctation) and coarctation in one family. *Am Heart J.* 1965;70:115–118.
78. Leichtman DA, Schmickel RD, Gelehrter TD, Judd WJ, Woodbury MC, Meilinger KL. Familial Turner syndrome. *Ann Intern Med.* 1978;89:473–476.
79. Miettinen OS, Reiner ML, Nadas AS. Seasonal incidence of coarctation of the aorta. *Br Heart J.* 1970;32:103–107.
80. Hernandez FA, Miller RH, Schiebler GL. Rarity of coarctation of the aorta in the American Negro. *J Pediatr.* 1969;74:623–625.
81. Van Der Horst RL, Gotsman MS. Racial incidence of coarctation of aorta. *Br Heart J.* 1972;34:289–294.
82. Becker AE, Becker MJ, Edwards JE. Anomalies associated with co-arctation of aorta: particular reference to infancy. *Circulation.* 1970;41:1067–1075.
83. Liberthson RR, Pennington DG, Jacobs ML, Daggett WM. Coarctation of the aorta: review of 234 patients and clarification of management problems. *Am J Cardiol.* 1979;43:835–840.
84. Campbell M. Natural history of coarctation of the aorta. *Br Heart J.* 1970;32:633–640.
85. Reifenstein GH, Levine SA, Gross RE. Coarctation of the aorta; a review of 104 autopsied cases of the adult type, 2 years of age or older. *Am Heart J.* 1947;33:146–168.
86. Miro O, Jimenez S, Gonzalez J, De Caralt TM, Ordi J. Highly effective compensatory mechanisms in a 76-year-old man with a coarctation of the aorta. *Cardiology.* 1999;92:284–286.
87. Milo S, Massini C, Goor DA. Isolated atresia of the aortic arch in a 65-year-old man. Surgical treatment and review of published reports. *Br Heart J.* 1982;47:294–297.
88. Barili F, Biglioli P, Polvani G. A case of asymptomatic high-grade aortic coarctation. *Heart.* 2008;94:82.
89. Strafford MA, Griffiths SP, Gersony WM. Coarctation of the aorta: a study in delayed detection. *Pediatrics.* 1982;69:159–163.
90. Ward KE, Pryor RW, Matson JR, Razook JD, Thompson WM, Elkins RC. Delayed detection of coarctation in infancy: implications for timing of newborn follow-up. *Pediatrics.* 1990;86:972–976.
91. Braimbridge MV, Yen A. Coarctation in the elderly. *Circulation.* 1965;31:209–218.
92. Silander T. Anomalous origin of the right subclavian artery and its relation to coarctation of the aorta. *Acta Chir Scand.* 1962;124:412–418.
93. Schievink WI, Mokri B, Piepgras DG, Gittenberger-De Groot AC. Intracranial aneurysms and cervicocephalic arterial dissections associated with congenital heart disease. *Neurosurgery.* 1996;39:685–689; discussion 689–690.
94. Edwards JE. Aneurysms of the thoracic aorta complicating coarctation. *Circulation.* 1973;48:195–201.
95. Shachter N, Perloff JK, Mulder DG. Aortic dissection in Noonan's syndrome (46 XY turner). *Am J Cardiol.* 1984;54:464–465.
96. Graham Jr TP, Atwood GF, Boerth RC, Boucek Jr RJ, Smith CW. Right and left heart size and function in infants with symptomatic coarctation. *Circulation.* 1977;56:641–647.
97. Baylis JH, Campbell M. The course and prognosis of coarctation of the aorta. *Br Heart J.* 1956;18:475–495.
98. Graham Jr TP, Burger J, Boucek Jr RJ, et al. Absence of left ventricular volume loading in infants with coarctation of the aorta and a large ventricular septal defect. *J Am Coll Cardiol.* 1989;14:1545–1552.
99. Shinebourne EA, Tam AS, Elseed AM, Paneth M, Lennox SC, Cleland WP. Coarctation of the aorta in infancy and childhood. *Br Heart J.* 1976;38:375–380.
100. Hesslein PS, Gutgesell HP, Mcnamara DG. Prognosis of symptomatic coarctation of the aorta in infancy. *Am J Cardiol.* 1983;51:299–303.
101. Jentsch E, Liersch R, Bourgeois M. Prolapsed valve of the foramen ovale in newborns and infants with coarctation of the aorta. *Pediatr Cardiol.* 1988;9:29–32.
102. Bailie MD, Donoso VS, Gonzalez NC. Role of the renin-angiotensin system in hypertension after coarctation of the aorta. *J Lab Clin Med.* 1984;104:553–562.
103. Anabtawi IN, Ellison RG, Yeh TJ, Hall DP. Dissecting aneurysm of aorta associated with Turner's syndrome. *J Thorac Cardiovasc Surg.* 1964;47:750–754.
104. Lie JT. Aortic dissection in Turner's syndrome. *Am Heart J.* 1982;103:1077–1080.
105. Lin AE, Lippe BM, Geffner ME, et al. Aortic dilation, dissection, and rupture in patients with Turner syndrome. *J Pediatr.* 1986;109:820–826.
106. Klein LW, Levin JL, Weintraub WS, Agarwal JB, Helfant RH. Pseudocoarctation of the aortic arch in a patient with Turner's syndrome. *Clin Cardiol.* 1984;7:621–623.
107. Shearer WT, Rutman JY, Weinberg WA, Goldring D. Coarctation of the aorta and cerebrovascular accident: a proposal for early corrective surgery. *J Pediatr.* 1970;77:1004–1009.

108. Woltman HW, Shelden WD. Neurologic complications associated with congenital stenosis of the isthmus of the aorta: a case of cerebral aneurysm with rupture and a case of intermittent lameness presumably related to stenosis of the isthmus. *Arch Neurol Psychiatry.* 1927;17:303.

109. Hodes HL, Steinfeld L, Blumenthal S. Congenital cerebral aneurysms and coarctation of the aorta. *Arch Pediatr.* 1959;76: 28–43.

110. Roberts DL, Tatini U, Zimmerman RS, Bortz JJ, Sirven JI. Musical hallucinations associated with seizures originating from an intracranial aneurysm. *Mayo Clin Proc.* 2001;76:423–426.

111. Schneeweiss A, Sherf L, Lehrer E, Lieberman Y, Neufeld HN. Segmental study of the terminal coronary vessels in coarctation of the aorta: a natural model for study of the effect of coronary hypertension on human coronary circulation. *Am J Cardiol.* 1982;49:1996–2002.

112. Vlodaver Z, Neufeld HN. The coronary arteries in coarctation of the aorta. *Circulation.* 1968;37:449–454.

113. Cracowski JL, Vanzetto G, Douchin S, Atger O, Bost M, Machecourt J. Myocardial infarction and Turner's syndrome. *Clin Cardiol.* 1999;22:245–247.

114. Goldberg MB, Scully AL, Solomon IL, Steinbach HL. Gonadal dysgenesis in phenotypic female subjects. A review of eighty-seven cases, with cytogenetic studies in fifty-three. *Am J Med.* 1968;45:529–543.

115. Nora JJ, Torres FG, Sinha AK, Mcnamara DG. Characteristic cardiovascular anomalies of XO Turner syndrome, XX and XY phenotype and XO-XX Turner mosaic. *Am J Cardiol.* 1970;25: 639–641.

116. Mazzanti L, Cacciari E. Congenital heart disease in patients with Turner's syndrome. Italian Study Group for Turner Syndrome (ISGTS). *J Pediatr.* 1998;133:688 692.

117. Prandstraller D, Mazzanti L, Picchio FM, et al. Turner's syndrome: cardiologic profile according to the different chromosomal patterns and long-term clinical follow-up of 136 nonpreselected patients. *Pediatr Cardiol.* 1999;20:108–112.

118. Mccrindle BW. Coarctation of the aorta. *Curr Opin Cardiol.* 1999;14:448–452.

119. Miller MJ, Geffner ME, Lippe BM, et al. Echocardiography reveals a high incidence of bicuspid aortic valve in Turner syndrome. *J Pediatr.* 1983;102:47–50.

120. Edwards WD, Leaf DS, Edwards JE. Dissecting aortic aneurysm associated with congenital bicuspid aortic valve. *Circulation.* 1978;57:1022–1025.

121. Lin AE, Garver KL. Monozygotic Turner syndrome twins—correlation of phenotype severity and heart defect. *Am J Med Genet.* 1988;29:529–531.

122. Digilio MC, Marino B, Picchio F, et al. Noonan syndrome and aortic coarctation. *Am J Med Genet.* 1998;80:160–162.

123. Siggers DC, Polani PE. Congenital heart disease in male and female subjects with somatic features of Turner's syndrome and normal sex chromosomes (Ullrich's and related syndromes). *Br Heart J.* 1972;34:41–46.

124. Bijulal S, Sivasankaran S, Krishnamoorthy KM, Titus T, Tharakan JA, Krishnamanohar SR. Unusual coarctation-the PHACE syndrome: report of three cases. *Congenital Heart Disease.* 2008;3:205–208.

125. Perloff JK. *Physical examination of the heart and circulation.* 3rd ed. Philadelphia: W.B. Saunders; 1998.

126. Glancy DL, Morrow AG, Simon AL, Roberts WC. Juxtaductal aortic coarctation. Analysis of 84 patients studied hemodynamically, angiographically, and morphologically after age 1 year. *Am J Cardiol.* 1983;51:537–551.

127. Subramanian AR. Coarctation or interruption of aorta proximal to origin of both subclavian arteries. Report of three cases presenting in infancy. *Br Heart J.* 1972;34:1225–1226.

128. Campbell M, Suzman S. Coarctation of the aorta. *Br Heart J.* 1947;9:185–212.

129. Blumenthal S, Epps RP, Heavenrich R, et al. Report of the task force on blood pressure control in children. *Pediatrics.* 1977;59: I–II, 797–820.

130. Kirkendall WM, Feinleib M, Freis ED, Mark AL. Recommendations for human blood pressure determination by sphygmomanometers. Subcommittee of the AHA Postgraduate Education Committee. *Circulation.* 1980;62:1146A–1155A.

131. Manning DM, Kuchirka C, Kaminski J. Miscuffing: inappropriate blood pressure cuff application. *Circulation.* 1983;68:763–766.

132. Falkner B (Chair). Update on the 1987 Task Force Report on High Blood Pressure in Children and Adolescents: a working group report from the National High Blood Pressure Education Program. National High Blood Pressure Education Program Working Group on Hypertension Control in Children and Adolescents. *Pediatrics.* 1996;98:649–658.

133. Park MK, Guntheroth WG. Direct blood pressure measurements in brachial and femoral arteries in children. *Circulation.* 1970;41: 231–237.

134. Dahlbaeck O, Dahn I, Westling H. Hemodynamic observations in coarctation of the aorta, with special reference to the blood pressure above and below the stenosis at rest and during exercise. *Scand J Clin Lab Invest.* 1964;16:339–346.

135. Boone ML, Swenson BE, Felson B. Rib notching: its many causes. *Am J Roentgenol Radium Ther Nucl Med.* 1964;91:1075–1088.

136. De Man SA, Andre JL, Bachmann H, et al. Blood pressure in childhood: pooled findings of six European studies. *J Hypertens.* 1991; 9:109–114.

137. Miller RA, Shekelle RB. Blood pressure in tenth-grade students: results from the Chicago Heart Association Pediatric Heart Screening Project. *Circulation.* 1976;54:993–1000.

138. Perloff JK. Pregnancy in congenital heart disease: the mother and the fetus. In: Perloff JK, Child JS, eds. *Congenital heart disease in adults.* 3rd ed. Philadelphia: W.B. Saunders; 2009:144.

139. Vriend JW, Drenthen W, Pieper PG, et al. Outcome of pregnancy in patients after repair of aortic coarctation. *Eur Heart J.* 2005;26: 2173–2178.

140. Beauchesne LM, Connolly HM, Ammash NM, Warnes CA. Coarctation of the aorta: outcome of pregnancy. *J Am Coll Cardiol.* 2001;38:1728–1733.

141. Spencer MP, Johnston FR, Meredith JH. The origin and interpretation of murmurs in coarctation of the aorta. *Am Heart J.* 1958; 56:722–736.

142. Kirks DR, Currarino G, Chen JT. Mediastinal collateral arteries: important vessels in coarctation of the aorta. *AJR Am J Roentgenol.* 1986;146:757–762.

143. Nasser WK, Helmen C. Kinking of the aortic arch (pseudocoarctation). Clinical, radiographic, hemodynamic, and angiographic findings in eight cases. *Ann Intern Med.* 1966;64:971–978.

144. Garman JE, Hinson RE, Eyler WR. Coarctation of the aorta in infancy: detection on chest radiographs. *Radiology.* 1965;85: 418–422.

145. Drexler CJ, Stewart JR, Kincaid OW. Diagnostic implications of rib notching. *Am J Roentgenol Radium Ther Nucl Med.* 1964;91: 1064–1074.

146. Sloan RD, Cooley RN. Coarctation of the aorta; the roentgenologic aspects of one hundred and twenty-five surgically confirmed cases. *Radiology.* 1953;61:701–721.

147. Bjork L, Friedman R. Routine roentgenographic diagnosis of coarctation of the aorta in the child. *Am J Roentgenol Radium Ther Nucl Med.* 1965;95:636–641.

148. Ben-Shoshan M, Rossi NP, Korns ME. Coarctation of the abdominal aorta. *Arch Pathol.* 1973;95:221–225.

149. Kavanagh-Gray D, Chiu P. Kinking of the aorta (pseudocoarctation): report of six cases. *Can Med Assoc J.* 1970;103:717–720.

150. Child JS. Transthoracic and transesophageal echocardiographic imaging: anatomic and hemodynamic assessment. In: Perloff JK, Child JS, eds. *Congenital heart disease in adults.* Philadelphia: W.B. Saunders; 1998.

151. Simpson IA, Sahn DJ, Valdes-Cruz LM, Chung KJ, Sherman FS, Swensson RE. Color Doppler flow mapping in patients with coarctation of the aorta: new observations and improved evaluation with color flow diameter and proximal acceleration as predictors of severity. *Circulation.* 1988;77:736–744.

152. Carvalho JS, Redington AN, Shinebourne EA, Rigby ML, Gibson D. Continuous wave Doppler echocardiography and coarctation of the aorta: gradients and flow patterns in the assessment of severity. *Br Heart J.* 1990;64:133–137.

153. Tacy TA, Baba K, Cape EG. Effect of aortic compliance on Doppler diastolic flow pattern in coarctation of the aorta. *J Am Soc Echocardiogr.* 1999;12:636–642.

154. Steidele R.J. Sammlung Verschiedener in der chirurgisch Praktik: *Lehrschule Germachten Beobb.* 1777;2:114.

155. Lie JT. The malformation complex of the absence of the arch of the aorta—Steidele's complex. *Am Heart J.* 1967;73:615–625.

156. Takashina T, Ishikura Y, Yamane K, Yorifuji S, Iwasaki T. The congenital cardiovascular anomalies of the interruption of the aorta—Steidele's complex. *Am Heart J.* 1972;83:93–99.

157. Blake HA, Manion WC, Spencer FC. Atresia or absence of the aortic isthmus. *J Thorac Cardiovasc Surg.* 1962;43:607–614.

158. Celoria GC, Patton RB. Congenital absence of the aortic arch. *Am Heart J.* 1959;58:407–413.

159. Moller JH, Edwards JE. Interruption of aortic arch; anatomic patterns and associated cardiac malformations. *Am J Roentgenol Radium Ther Nucl Med.* 1965;95:557–572.

160. Roberts WC, Morrow AG, Braunwald E. Complete interruption of the aortic arch. *Circulation.* 1962;26:39–59.

161. Freedom RM, Bain HH, Esplugas E, Dische R, Rowe RD. Ventricular septal defect in interruption of aortic arch. *Am J Cardiol.* 1977;39:572–582.

162. Abbott ME. Congenital cardiac disease. In: *Osler's modern medicine.* Philadelphia: Lea & Febiger; 1927.

163. Jaffe RB. Complete interruption of the aortic arch. 1. Characteristic radiographic findings in 21 patients. *Circulation.* 1975;52:714–721.

164. Jaffe RB. Complete interruption of the aortic arch. 2. Characteristic angiographic features with emphasis on collateral circulation to the descending aorta. *Circulation.* 1976;53:161–168.

165. Kutsche LM, Van Mierop LH. Cervical origin of the right subclavian artery in aortic arch interruption: pathogenesis and significance. *Am J Cardiol.* 1984;53:892–895.

166. Mishaly D, Birk E, Katz J, Vidne BA. Interruption of right sided aortic arch. Case report and review of the literature. *J Cardiovasc Surg.* 1995;36:277–279.

167. Dische MR, Tsai M, Baltaxe HA. Solitary interruption of the arch of the aorta. Clinicopathologic review of eight cases. *Am J Cardiol.* 1975;35:271–277.

168. Higgins CB, French JW, Silverman JF, Wexler L. Interruption of the aortic arch: preoperative and postoperative clinical, hemodynamic and angiographic features. *Am J Cardiol.* 1977;39:563–571.

169. Judez VM, Maitre MJ, De Artaza M, De Miguel JM, Valles F, Marquez J. Interruption of aortic arch without associated cardiac abnormalities. *Br Heart J.* 1974;36:313–317.

170. Riggs TW, Berry TE, Aziz KU, Paul MH. Two-dimensional echocardiographic features of interruption of the aortic arch. *Am J Cardiol.* 1982;50:1385–1390.

171. Al-Marsafawy HM, Ho SY, Redington AN, Anderson RH. The relationship of the outlet septum to the aortic outflow tract in hearts with interruption of the aortic arch. *J Thorac Cardiovasc Surg.* 1995;109:1225–1236.

172. Braunlin E, Peoples WM, Freedom RM, Fyler DC, Goldblatt A, Edwards JE. Interruption of the aortic arch with aorticopulmonary septal defect. An anatomic review. *Pediatr Cardiol.* 1982;3:329–335.

173. Bergwerff M, Deruiter MC, Hall S, Poelmann RE, Gittenberger-De Groot AC. Unique vascular morphology of the fourth aortic arches: possible implications for pathogenesis of type-B aortic arch interruption and anomalous right subclavian artery. *Cardiovasc Res.* 1999;44:185–196.

174. Schumacher G, Schreiber R, Meisner H, Lorenz HP, Sebening F, Buhlmeyer K. Interrupted aortic arch: natural history and operative results. *Pediatr Cardiol.* 1986;7:89–93.

175. Morgan JR, Forker AD, Fosburg RG, Neugebauer MK, Rogers AK, Bemiller CR. Interruption of the aortic arch without a patent ductus arteriosus. *Circulation.* 1970;42:961–965.

176. Sharratt GP, Carson P, Sanderson JM. Complete interruption of aortic arch, without persistent ductus arteriosus, in an adult. *Br Heart J.* 1975;37:221–224.

177. Wong CK, Cheng CH, Lau CP, Leung WH, Chan FL. Interrupted aortic arch in an asymptomatic adult. *Chest.* 1989;96:678–679.

178. Garcia OL, Hernandez FA, Tamer D, Poole C, Gelband H, Castellanos AW. Congenital bilateral subclavian steal: ductus-dependent symptoms in interrupted aortic arch associated with ventricular septal defect. *Am J Cardiol.* 1979;44:101–104.

179. Flyer DC, Buckley LP, Hellenbrand WE, Cohn HE. Report of the New England Regional Infant Cardiac Program. *Pediatrics.* 1980;65:375–461.

180. Buch J, Wennevold A, Efsen F, Andersen GE. Interrupted aortic arch in two siblings. *Acta Paediatr Scand.* 1980;69:783–785.

181. Pankau R, Funda J, Wessel A. Interrupted aortic arch type B1 in a brother and sister: suggestion of a recessive gene. *Am J Med Genet.* 1990;36:175–177.

182. Gobel JW, Pierpont ME, Moller JH, Singh A, Edwards JE. Familial interruption of the aortic arch. *Pediatr Cardiol.* 1993;14:110–115.

183. Nakada T, Yonesaka S. Interruption of aortic arch type A in two siblings. *Acta Paediatr Jpn.* 1996;38:63–65.

184. Pierpont ME, Gobel JW, Moller JH, Edwards JE. Cardiac malformations in relatives of children with truncus arteriosus or interruption of the aortic arch. *Am J Cardiol.* 1988;61:423–427.

185. Gokcebay TM, Batillas J, Pinck RL. Complete interruption of the aorta at the arch. *Am J Roentgenol Radium Ther Nucl Med.* 1972;114:362–370.

186. Merrill DL, Webster CA, Samson PC. Congenital absence of the aortic isthmus; report of a case with successful surgical repair. *J Thorac Surg.* 1957;33:311–320.

187. Rangel A, Chavez E, Espinosa I. Interruption of the aortic arch in adults. *Arch Inst Cardiol Mex.* 1999;69:144–148.

188. Kerkar P, Dalvi B, Kale P. Interruption of the aortic arch with associated cardiac anomalies. Survival to adulthood. *Chest.* 1993;103:279–280.

189. Baysal T, Kutlu R, Sarac K, Karaman I. Ruptured intracranial aneurysm associated with isolated aortic arch interruption. *Neuroradiology.* 2000;42:842–844.

190. Hu WY, Sevick RJ, Tranmer BI, Maitland A, Gray RR. Aortic arch interruption associated with ruptured cerebral aneurysm. *Can Assoc Radiol J.* 1996;47:20–23.

191. Greig D. Case of malformation of the heart and blood vessels of the foetus; pulmonary artery giving off the descending aorta and left subclavian. *Monthly Journal of Medical Science.* 1852;15:28–30.

192. Jonas RA. Interrupted aortic arch. *Curr Opin Cardiol.* 1988;3(September/October):776–780.

193. Van Mierop LH, Kutsche LM. Cardiovascular anomalies in DiGeorge syndrome and importance of neural crest as a possible pathogenetic factor. *Am J Cardiol.* 1986;58:133–137.

194. Moerman P, Dumoulin M, Lauweryns J, Van Der Hauwaert LG. Interrupted right aortic arch in DiGeorge syndrome. *Br Heart J.* 1987;58:274–278.

195. Takahashi K, Kuwahara T, Nagatsu M. Interruption of the aortic arch at the isthmus with DiGeorge syndrome and 22q11.2 deletion. *Cardiol Young.* 1999;9:516–518.

196. Tabakin BS, Hanson JS. Congenital absence of the aortic arch associated with patent ductus arteriosus and ventricular septal defect. *Am J Cardiol.* 1960;6:689–696.

197. Starreveld JS, Van Rossum AC, Hruda J. Rapid formation of collateral arteries in a neonate with interruption of the aortic arch. *Cardiol Young.* 2001;11:464–467.

198. Thomson PS, Teele RL. Reversal of left carotid arterial flow as a sign of type C interruption of the aortic arch. *Pediatr Radiol.* 1994;24:300–301.

199. Geva T, Gajarski RJ. Echocardiographic diagnosis of type B interruption of a right aortic arch. *Am Heart J.* 1995;129:1042–1045.

200. Kreutzer J, Van Praagh R. Comparison of left ventricular outflow tract obstruction in interruption of the aortic arch and in coarctation of the aorta, with diagnostic, developmental, and surgical implications. *Am J Cardiol.* 2000;86:856–862.

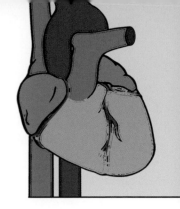

Chapter 9

Congenital Obstruction to Left Atrial Flow: Mitral Stenosis, Cor Triatriatum, Pulmonary Vein Stenosis

Congenital obstruction to left atrial flow can originate at or near the junction of the pulmonary veins and the left atrium (pulmonary vein stenosis), within the left atrium (cor triatriatum), immediately above the mitral valve (supravalvular stenosing ring), or within the mitral apparatus (mitral stenosis; Figure 9-1; Box 9-1). Pure or relatively pure forms of each defect are emphasized in this chapter, although a variety of anomalies often coexist.[1–3] Pulmonary veno-occlusive disease is covered in Chapter 14, total anomalous pulmonary venous connection with obstruction is covered in Chapter 15, and hypoplastic left heart with a hypoplastic mitral orifice is covered in Chapter 31.

CONGENITAL MITRAL STENOSIS

Congenital mitral stenosis involves the annulus, the zone immediately above and contiguous with the annulus, the leaflets, the chordae tendineae, and the papillary muscles. The physiologic consequences of congenital mitral stenosis are analogous to acquired mitral stenosis.

The incidence rate has been estimated at 0.6% of necropsy cases of congenital heart disease and 0.21% to 0.42% of clinical cases.[4] Congenital mitral stenosis with a functionally adequate left ventricle includes the following malformations in approximate order of frequency (see Box 9-1):[5–9]

1. Short chordae tendineae with reduction in or obliteration of interchordal spaces and a decrease in interpapillary muscle distance (Figure 9-2A).[1]
2. Parachute mitral valve, which consists of a single eccentric papillary muscle (absence of one papillary muscle or fusion of the two papillary muscles) into which all chordae tendineae from both leaflets insert (Figures 9-2B and 9-3 and Video 9-1).[1,2,10]
3. Anomalous mitral arcade characterized by a band of fibrous tissue that runs adjacent to the free margins of the mitral leaflets with short or absent chordae tendineae and multiple contiguous papillary muscles.[11] The arcade can permit normal function[12] or can render the valve mechanism incompetent when the chordae tendineae are well formed.[13,14] Rarely, an anomalous mitral arcade coexists with a tricuspid arcade and incompetence of both atrioventricular valves. A supravalvular stenosing ring consists of a circumferential diaphragm at the base of the atrial surfaces of the mitral leaflets (Figure

9-2C).[6,8–10,15] Rarely, a supravalvular ring occurs with an isolated obstructive lesion[16] or coexists with mitral regurgitation.[17]
4. Accessory mitral valve tissue.[18]
5. Anomalous left ventricular muscle bundles or anomalous obstructing papillary muscles.[18,19]
6. Double orifice mitral valve, which can be stenotic, incompetent, or functionally normal.

Flow across a normal mitral orifice is between the leaflets (interleaflet) and the chordae tendineae (interchordal). In a parachute mitral valve, all chordae tendineae insert into a single papillary muscle and the interchordal spaces are reduced or obliterated,[10] so flow cannot be interchordal (see Figures 9-2B and 9-3).

A parachute mitral valve is usually one of the components of Shone's complex, a developmental combination of four obstructive lesions: namely, supravalvular stenosing ring, parachute mitral valve, subaortic stenosis, and coarctation of the aorta (Figures 9-3 and 9-10).[1,2,15,16] All four lesions are not always present; if they are present, they may not be functionally significant.[2,10,20] The supravalvular mitral ring can be rudimentary (see Figure 9-3C), or can bridge the mitral orifice as a stenosing diaphragm (see Figure 9-3B).[8,9,18]

History

There is a male predilection in congenital mitral stenosis,[1] in contrast to rheumatic mitral stenosis, which has a female predilection. Familial recurrence has not been reported. If stenosis is severe, symptoms begin shortly after birth when pulmonary blood flow commences and suddenly enters the obstructed left atrium. Fifty percent of symptomatic infants die within 6 months, but an occasional infant is asymptomatic and a few remain relatively free of symptoms for years.[21] With a parachute mitral valve or a supravalvular mitral ring, longevity is better (median, 10 years and 5.5 years, respectively), but short chordae tendineae and obliterated interchordal spaces result in death at a median age of 6 months.[6,10] Anomalous mitral arcade or double-orifice mitral valve permits adult survival when the mitral apparatus functions normally or is purely regurgitant.[5,14]

Orthopnea, dyspnea, tachypnea, and paroxysmal cough are results of pulmonary edema that is punctuated by lower respiratory infections.[1,21–23] Congenital mitral stenosis is occasionally associated with syncope[21] but seldom with hemoptysis.[23] Aphonia has been

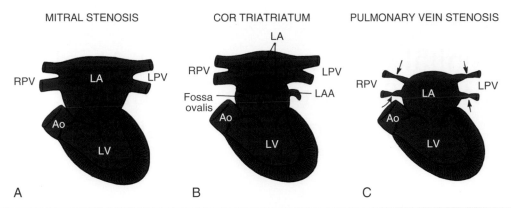

FIGURE 9-1 A, Illustration of congenital obstruction to left atrial flow involving the mitral apparatus or immediately above or contiguous with the mitral annulus. **B,** Illustration of typical cor triatriatum. A fibrous or fibromuscular diaphragm partitions the left atrium. The proximal compartment receives the pulmonary veins and is a high-pressure zone. The distal compartment contains the fossa ovalis and the left atrial appendage (LAA) and is a low-pressure zone. **C,** Illustration of pulmonary vein stenosis in which one or more pulmonary veins are narrowed near their left atrial junction. (Ao = aorta; LA = left atrium; LV = left ventricle; LPV = left pulmonary veins; RPV = right pulmonary veins.)

BOX 9-1 CONGENITAL OBSTRUCTION TO LEFT ATRIAL FLOW WITH A FUNCTIONALLY ADEQUATE LEFT VENTRICLE

Congenital Mitral Stenosis

Obstruction within the mitral apparatus: short chordae tendineae with decreased interpapillary muscle distance and reduced or obliterated interchordal spaces

Parachute mitral valve

Anomalous mitral arcade

Accessory mitral valve tissue

Anomalous left ventricular muscle bundles or obstructing papillary muscles

Double-orifice mitral valve

Supravalvular stenosing ring

Cor Triatriatum

Pulmonary Vein Stenosis

---

attributed to compression of the recurrent laryngeal nerve by a dilated hypertensive pulmonary trunk, analogous to hoarseness in adults with pulmonary hypertension and rheumatic mitral stenosis. Infective endocarditis is rare.[1]

Physical Appearance

Mild cyanosis coincides with congestive heart failure.[21,22] Recurrent lower respiratory infections and the catabolic effects of heart failure account for physical underdevelopment.[21,23]

Arterial Pulse, Jugular Venous Pulse, Precordial Movement, and Palpation

The arterial pulse is normal and confirms normal sinus rhythm, which is the rule in congenital mitral stenosis.[21] The jugular venous pulse has an increased A wave because of pulmonary hypertension (Figure 9-4). A precordial bulge is common,[23] and a right ventricular impulse is palpable at the lower left sternal border and subxiphoid area.[21,23]

Auscultation

Neither a loud first heart sound nor an opening snap are heard; the necessary preconditions of these two auscultatory signs—abrupt opening and closing movements of the belly of a mobile anterior mitral leaflet—are not features of congenital mitral stenosis (Figures 9-5 and 9-6).[1,10,11,23]

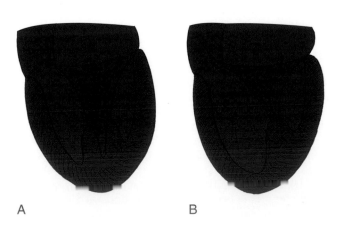

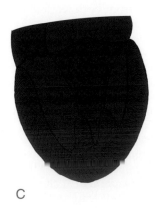

FIGURE 9-2 Illustrations of three anatomic types of congenital mitral stenosis involving the mitral apparatus. **A,** The typical form is characterized by decreased interpapillary muscle distance and a reduction in interchordal spaces. **B,** Parachute mitral valve with a single eccentric papillary muscle. **C,** Supravalvular stenosing mitral ring.

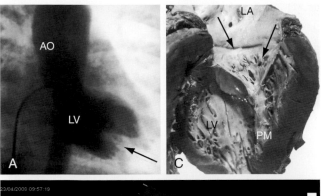

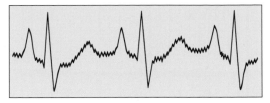

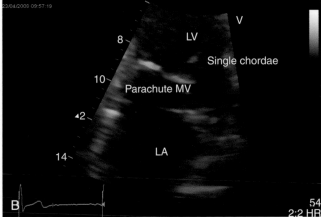

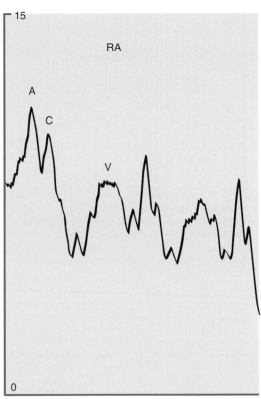

FIGURE 9-3 **A,** Left ventriculogram from an 8-year-old girl with a parachute mitral valve identified by the single papillary muscle (wedge of negative contrast, *arrow*). **B,** Echocardiogram (apical four-chamber) from a 10-year-old boy with Shone's complex consisting of a supravalvular stenosing ring, seen between LA and parachute mitral valve (MV). The parachute mitral valve and single chordae are shown. **C,** Necropsy specimen from a 14-year-old boy with a parachute mitral valve *(thick arrow)*, obstructing interchordal slits, and insertion into a single eccentric papillary muscle (PM). A supravalvular ring is identified by the *thin arrow*. Compare with the echocardiogram in part **B** (Video 9-1). (AO = ascending aorta; LA = left atrium; LV = left ventricle.)

FIGURE 9-4 Right atrial pressure pulse (RA) showing a prominent A wave in a 3-year-old girl with congenital mitral stenosis.

In the presence of a parachute mitral valve or a supravalvular ring,[17] a holosystolic murmur at the apex or lower left sternal edge is the result of mitral regurgitation or pulmonary hypertensive tricuspid regurgitation.[22] An apical mid-diastolic murmur with presystolic accentuation (see Figures 9-5 and 9-6) is exceptional because the rapid heart rate in infants shortens diastole[1,23] and because a dilated hypertensive right ventricle displaces the left ventricle from the apex.[24,25] The pulmonary component of the second heart sound is loud because of pulmonary hypertension that sets the stage for the Graham Steell murmur of high-pressure pulmonary regurgitation.[1,18]

Electrocardiogram

Atrial fibrillation is exceptional in contrast to rheumatic mitral regurgitation.[1] Pulmonary hypertension results in right atrial P wave abnormalities,[1] right axis deviation,[1] and right ventricular hypertrophy (Figure 9-7).[1]

X-Ray

Pulmonary venous congestion includes Kerley's lines (Figure 9-8).[1,23] Mild to moderate left atrial enlargement is recognized in the lateral projection (see Figure 9-8B). Straightening of the left cardiac border (Figure 9-9) by an enlarged left atrial appendage is much less common than in rheumatic mitral stenosis.[1] Calcification of the mitral valve is absent in the x-ray and absent histologically.[26] The pulmonary trunk, right ventricle, and right atrium are enlarged because of pulmonary hypertension (see Figures 9-8 and 9-9).

Echocardiogram

Congenital mitral stenosis is characterized by two well-formed papillary muscles with a reduced interpapillary distance.[10] A parachute mitral valve is characterized by a single papillary muscle into which all chordae tendineae converge (Figures 9-3B,C and 9-10).[16,27–29] The effective orifice size cannot be determined with two-dimensional echocardiography because flow is interchordal and the

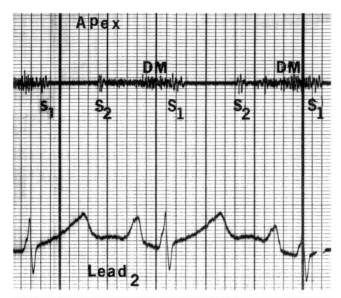

FIGURE 9-5 Phonocardiogram from a 2-year-old girl with Shone's complex (supravalvular stenosing ring, parachute mitral valve, coarctation of the aorta) and a patent ductus arteriosus with pulmonary vascular disease and reversed shunt. The first heart sound (S_1) is soft, and there is no opening snap. There is a soft mid-diastolic murmur (DM). (S_2 = second heart sound.)

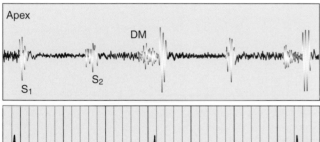

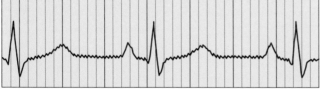

FIGURE 9-6 Phonocardiogram from the 3-year-old girl with congenital mitral stenosis referred to in Figure 9-4. The first heart sound (S_1) is loud, but there is no opening snap. A soft mid-diastolic murmur (DM) is followed by presystolic accentuation.

valve is eccentric (see Figure 9-10B), but Doppler scan interrogation can determine the gradient and the functional orifice size (see Figure 9-10C,D). A supravalvular ring is more readily identified when it is not attached to the mitral leaflets (see Figures 9-3B and 9-10A).[6] Otherwise, the ring is imaged only in diastole.[6] An anomalous mitral arcade has multiple papillary muscles with few or no chordae tendineae interposed between the arcade and the leaflets.[27] The relative sizes of the two orifices of a double-orifice mitral valve can be determined, the chordal insertions can be characterized, and the functional state of the valve can be established as normal, stenotic, or incompetent.[7]

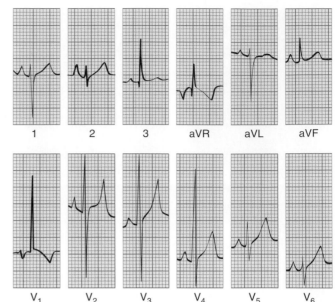

FIGURE 9-7 Electrocardiogram from the 2-year-old girl with Shone's complex and pulmonary vascular disease referred to in Figure 9-5. Tall peaked right atrial P waves are present in leads 1, 2, and V_2. There is marked right axis deviation. Right ventricular hypertrophy is manifested by the tall monophasic R wave in lead V_1 and the deep S wave in lead V_6. Large RS complexes in lead V_2 and V_3 suggest biventricular hypertrophy because of coarctation of the aorta.

Summary

Congenital mitral stenosis is a rare form of obstruction to left atrial flow that becomes manifest in infancy. Symptoms typically begin shortly after the newborn lungs inflate and pulmonary blood flow commences. Dyspnea, tachypnea, and cough are provoked by pulmonary venous congestion. The physical signs of pulmonary hypertension and right ventricular failure are overt, but the auscultatory signs of mitral stenosis are muted. The electrocardiogram exhibits right atrial P waves, right axis deviation, and right ventricular hypertrophy. The x-ray shows pulmonary venous congestion, left atrial enlargement, and dilation of the pulmonary trunk, right ventricle, and right atrium. Echocardiography establishes the anatomic type of congenital mitral stenosis and the degree of obstruction.

COR TRIATRIATUM

Partition of the left atrium into two compartments was recognized by Andral[30] in 1829. Four decades later, Church[31] published the first detailed pathologic description of the malformation that Borst[32] (1905) called cor triatriatum. The anomaly is rare, with a prevalence rate of about 0.1% of cases of congenital heart disease.[33] Cor triatriatum occurs typically as an isolated defect or atypically in association with other congenital cardiac anomalies.[3] The anomaly is characterized by a membrane that partitions the left atrium into a proximal accessory

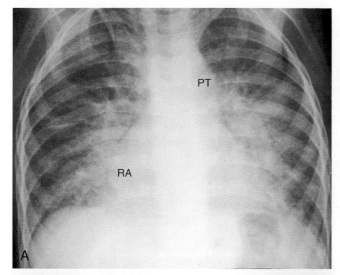

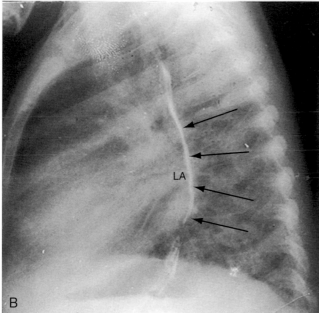

FIGURE 9-8 X-rays from the 2-year-old girl with Shone's complex whose phonocardiogram is shown in Figure 9-5. **A,** Pulmonary venous congestion is striking. The pulmonary trunk (PT) and right atrium (RA) are dilated. **B,** The lateral film shows displacement of the barium esophagram by an enlarged left atrium (LA).

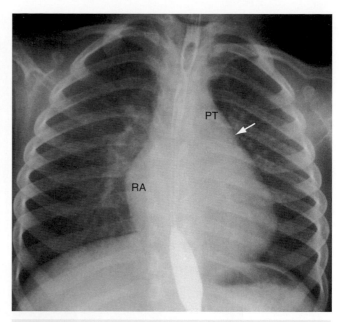

FIGURE 9-9 X-ray from the 3-year-old girl with congenital mitral stenosis referred to in Figures 9-4 and 9-6. There is bilateral hilar pulmonary venous congestion. The right atrium (RA) and pulmonary trunk (PT) are dilated, and the left cardiac border is straightened by an enlarged left atrial appendage *(arrow)*.

chamber that receives the pulmonary veins and by a distal true left atrial chamber that contains the left atrial appendage and the fossa ovalis (Figures 9-1B and 9-11).[4,33–37]

The pathogenesis of cor triatriatum is persistence of the right valve of the embryonic sinus venosus,[38] which results in failure of incorporation of the common pulmonary vein into the left atrium, a process that begins at about the fifth week of gestation and proceeds through subsequent stages of embryogenesis.[36,38] The proximal accessory chamber represents persistence of the common pulmonary vein of the embryo and cannot be identified externally.[35]

The three anatomic varieties of cor triatriatum are referred to as diaphragmatic, hourglass, and tubular.[33,35] In the diaphragmatic type, which is the most representative, the proximal accessory chamber and the distal true left atrial chamber are separated by a fibrous or fibromuscular diaphragm (see Figure 9-11) that contains either a single opening or multiple openings, the sizes of which determine the degree of obstruction.[35,39] Functionally insignificant ridges of tissue go unrecognized or appear as incidental findings at necropsy.[39,40] At the other extreme, no communication exists between the accessory chamber and the true left atrium—atresia of the common pulmonary vein.[41]

Tubular cor triatriatum is the most primitive and least common variety.[35] The proximal chamber retains the shape of the common pulmonary vein, which is the anatomic basis of the tubular configuration, the distal end of which joins the left atrium directly without an intervening membrane.[35]

The hourglass type of cor triatriatum is developmentally intermediate between the diaphragmatic and tubular types. The constriction projects inward as an obstructing shelf, which is seen externally as an hourglass deformity at the junction of the accessory chamber and the true left atrium.[35]

An interatrial communication usually takes the form of a valve-incompetent foramen ovale positioned between the right atrium and the distal true left atrium.[35] Alternatively, an ostium secundum atrial septal defect communicates with the true left atrium or, exceptionally, with the accessory chamber.[35]

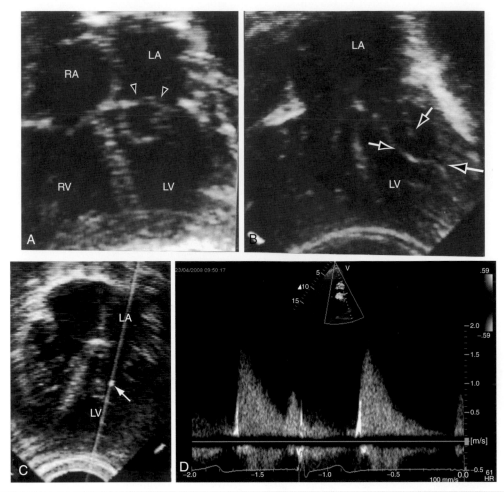

FIGURE 9-10 Echocardiograms (apical four-chamber) with Doppler scan interrogation from a 3-year-old boy with Shone's complex. **A,** *Unmarked paired arrowheads* point to a supravalvular stenosing ring. **B,** *Paired oblique arrows* identify a parachute mitral valve with chordae tendineae that insert into a single eccentric papillary muscle *(large right unmarked arrowhead)*. **C,** The Doppler sample volume within the parachute mitral valve *(arrow)*. **D,** Doppler signal in diastole across the parachute mitral valve. (LA = left atrium; LV = left ventricle; RA = right atrium; RV = right ventricle.)

Cor triatriatum dexter is a rare type of triatrial heart (Figure 9-12).[42–45] During early cardiogenesis, the right horn of the sinus venosus is guarded by two valves. The smaller left valve becomes incorporated into the septum secundum. The larger right valve initially divides the right atrium into two chambers and then regresses between the ninth and the 15th week of gestation.[42] In cor triatriatum dexter, a persistent embryonic right valve of the sinus venosus becomes a septating membrane. The venae cavae and the coronary sinus are on one side of the membrane, and the right atrial appendage and tricuspid orifice are on the other side. One or more perforations in the membrane permit communication from one side to the other. Septation ranges from partial to complete.

The physiologic consequences of cor triatriatum are analogous to other forms of congenital obstruction to left atrial flow with the following unique qualification.[35,46] In cor triatriatum, the pressure is elevated in the accessory chamber that is proximal to the obstruction and is normal in true left atrium that is distal to the obstruction. Accordingly, the stenotic orifice remains open throughout the cardiac cycle, so blood flow across the obstructing partition is continuous.

History

Mild asymptomatic cor triatriatum is diagnosed incidentally during routine echocardiography or is discovered incidentally at necropsy. An echocardiographic diagnosis was made in a 70-year-old woman during routine investigation of a murmur,[46] and the condition was inadvertently discovered in an elderly asymptomatic patient.[47] Severe cor triatriatum announces itself in neonates and young children because of dyspnea, tachypnea, paroxysmal cough, irritability, poor feeding, and failure to thrive.[34] However, symptoms may be delayed until adolescence or adulthood, and severe obstruction occasionally remains virtually asymptomatic until announced by acute pulmonary edema.[35,46] Sudden deterioration may follow years of good health. Massive recurrent hemoptysis can be the precipitating cause of death,[46] in contrast to congenital mitral stenosis, in which hemoptysis is uncommon (see previous discussion).

Physical Appearance

Physical appearance is normal except for failure to thrive in chronically ill infants and young children.

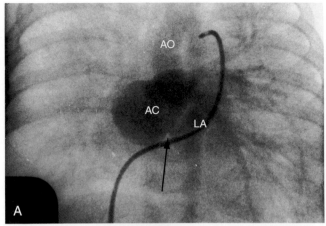

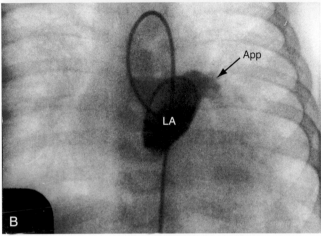

FIGURE 9-11 **A,** Levophase angiocardiogram after injection of contrast material into the pulmonary trunk in the typical diaphragmatic type of cor triatriatum. *Arrow* points to a linear zone of negative contrast that represents the diaphragm separating the proximal accessory chamber (AC) from the left atrium proper (LA). **B,** Contrast material outlines the distal compartment (LA), the upper margin of which is sharply delineated by the diaphragm. The left atrial appendage (App) lies within the distal chamber. (AO = ascending aorta.)

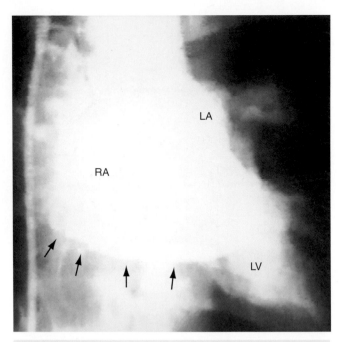

FIGURE 9-12 Angiocardiogram from a 22-year-old woman with cor triatriatum dexter. Contrast material filled an enlarged proximal right atrial chamber (RA; *arrows*) and opacified the left atrium (LA) through a sinus venosus atrial septal defect. The superior vena cava drained anomalously into the left atrium through the sinus venosus atrial septal defect. (LV = left ventricle.) *(Courtesy Dr. Irving R. Tessler, St. Vincent's Medical Center, Los Angeles, California.)*

Arterial Pulse, Jugular Venous Pulse, Precordial Movement, and Palpation

Atrial fibrillation is uncommon if not rare.[48] The jugular venous pulse reflects pulmonary hypertension and an increased A wave. With the advent of tricuspid regurgitation and right ventricular failure, a large V wave appears. Pulmonary hypertension is responsible for a palpable right ventricle and a palpable pulmonary component of the second sound.

Auscultation

The first heart sound is not increased because diastolic pressure is not exerted against the belly of the anterior mitral leaflet, so its systolic excursion is not brisk (Figure 9-13). The second heart sound is closely split or single with a loud pulmonary component that reflects pulmonary hypertension (see Figure 9-13). An opening snap is rare for the same reason that the first sound is not loud.[48]

The stenosing diaphragm of cor triatriatum is responsible for systolic, diastolic, or continuous murmurs or may be accompanied by no murmur at all (Figures 9-13 and 9-14).[48,49] The undulating membrane moves toward the mitral valve during diastole, reflecting a diastolic gradient, and moves away from the mitral valve during systole, reflecting reversal of the gradient as left ventricular contraction exerts pressure on the membrane through the closed mitral valve.[48] Systolic and diastolic thrills over the left atrium at surgery are in accord with these pressure/flow relationships and coincide with the systolic/diastolic murmurs heard at the bedside.[50] A continuous murmur reflects continuous flow across the partitioning diaphragm and is the result of a systolic murmur that continues into diastole and is reinforced as left ventricular pressure falls below the pressure in the true left atrium. Pulmonary hypertension is responsible for the high-frequency holosystolic murmur of tricuspid regurgitation (see Figure 9-14). When the enlarged right ventricle occupies the apex, the tricuspid systolic murmur is heard at the apex and is mistaken for mitral regurgitation. A high-frequency early diastolic murmur at the mid-left sternal edge is a Graham Steell murmur.

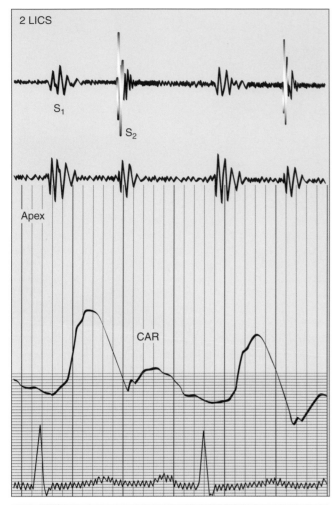

FIGURE 9-13 Tracings from an 18-year-old man with cor triatriatum and suprasystemic pulmonary vascular resistance. The single second heart sound (S$_2$) was the loud pulmonary component. There were no murmurs. (CAR = carotid; 2 LICS = second left intercostal space.)

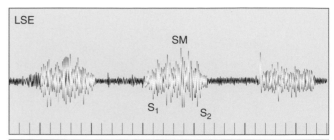

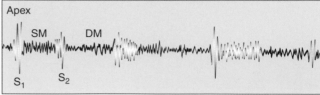

FIGURE 9-14 Phonocardiogram from a 17-month-old boy with cor triatriatum. The pulmonary artery systolic pressure was 115 mm Hg, and the systemic systolic pressure was 90 mm Hg. A high-frequency holosystolic murmur (SM) of pulmonary hypertensive tricuspid regurgitation was loudest at the lower left sternal edge (LSE) with radiation to the apex where a mid-diastolic/presystolic murmur (DM) and a prominent first heart sound (S$_1$) were recorded. (S$_2$ = second heart sound.)

Electrocardiogram

Peaked right atrial P waves are common (Figure 9-15). Broad notched left atrial P waves have been ascribed to prolonged conduction in the proximal accessory chamber.[50] Right axis deviation and right ventricular hypertrophy are typical features of the electrocardiogram (see Figure 9-15).

X-Ray

The lung fields exhibit pulmonary venous congestion with a diffuse ground-glass appearance (Figures 9-16 through 9-18), and Kerley's lines (see Figure 9-17). Radiologic hemosiderosis has been verified at necropsy and is in accord with a history of hemoptysis (see previous discussion).[51] The configuration of the heart varies from normal or nearly so to conspicuous enlargement of the right ventricle, right atrium, and pulmonary trunk in response to pulmonary hypertension (see Figures 9-16 through 9-18). The radiologic appearance of the left

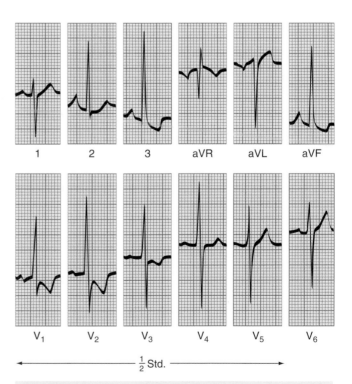

FIGURE 9-15 Electrocardiogram from an 18-year-old man with cor triatriatum and suprasystemic pulmonary vascular resistance (see Figure 9-13). Pulmonary hypertension is reflected in the tall peaked right atrial P wave in lead 2, right axis deviation, and striking evidence of right ventricular hypertrophy with tall R waves and ST-T wave abnormalities in right precordial leads and deep S waves in the left precordium.

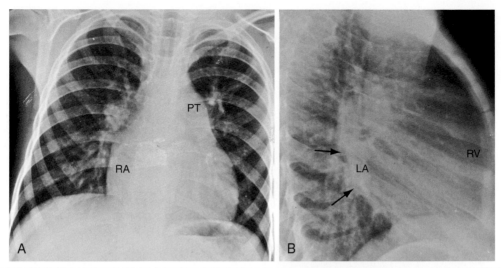

FIGURE 9-16 X-rays from a 6-year-old boy with cor triatriatum and a severely obstructing membrane. **A,** Pulmonary venous congestion is conspicuous. The pulmonary trunk (PT) and the right atrium (RA) are dilated, but the left atrial appendage is not visible. **B,** The proximal accessory left atrial compartment (LA) is dilated. An enlarged right ventricle (RV) occupies the retrosternal space.

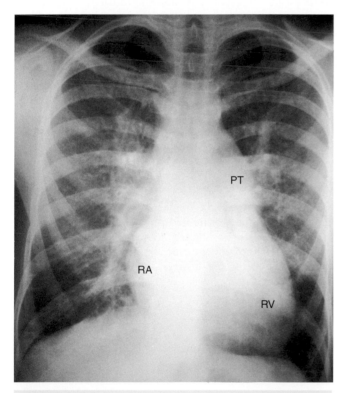

FIGURE 9-17 X-ray from an 18-year-old man with cor triatriatum and suprasystemic pulmonary vascular resistance. The phonocardiogram is shown in Figure 9-13. Pulmonary venous congestion, especially hilar, is striking. The pulmonary trunk (PT), right atrium (RA), and right ventricle (RV) are enlarged. The left atrial appendage is conspicuous by its absence.

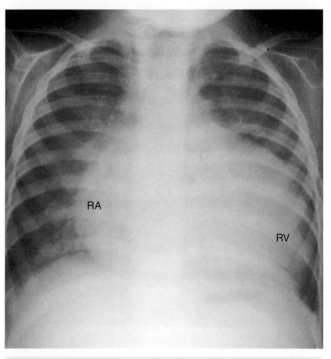

FIGURE 9-18 X-ray from a 17-month-old boy with cor triatriatum and suprasystemic vascular resistance (phonocardiogram is shown in Figure 9-14). There is moderate pulmonary venous congestion. The right atrium (RA) is huge. The pulmonary trunk is obscured by the dilated outflow tract of a huge right ventricle (RV). A left atrial appendage is not seen.

atrium is of special interest because the size of the true distal left atrial chamber is normal. The combination of pulmonary venous congestion *without* left atrial enlargement is therefore an important radiologic feature of cor triatriatum. Slight enlargement of the proximal accessory compartment should not be mistaken for enlargement of the left atrium proper (see Figure 9-16).[46] Because the left atrial appendage resides in the distal low-pressure compartment, it is not seen in the x-ray (see Figures 9-11, 9-16, and 9-17).[46] Calcium has been found in specimens of the stenosing diaphragm but not in the x-ray.[46]

Echocardiogram

Echocardiography is used to identify an essential anatomic feature of cor triatriatum: the thin undulating intra-atrial membrane, which is characterized by diastolic movement toward the mitral funnel and systolic movement away (Figures 9-19 and 9-20 and Videos 9-2 and 9-3).[48,49,52]

The left atrial appendage lies within the distal compartment (see Figure 9-20), thus distinguishing cor triatriatum from a supravalvular mitral ring.[28,48] The position of the left atrial appendage is best determined during ventricular systole when the membrane moves away from the mitral orifice (see Figure 9-20). The mitral valve itself is normal in cor triatriatum, except for high-frequency diastolic oscillations,[49] in contrast to a supravalvular stenosing ring, which is accompanied by a deformed mitral valve (see previous discussion). Color flow imaging and continuous wave Doppler scan interrogation disclose continuous flow across the membrane with peak flow during diastole.[53] The true distal left atrium is normal, but the proximal accessory chamber may be slightly dilated (see Figure 9-19).

Echocardiography is used to diagnose cor triatriatum dexter, together with the location, size, and attachment site of the anomalous remnant of the valve of the right sinus venosus (see Figure 9-12).[42,43,45]

Summary

Cor triatriatum is characterized by obstruction to left atrial flow and pulmonary hypertension. Murmurs that originate at the site of obstruction are systolic, diastolic, or continuous, but more often than not, there is no murmur at all. When obstruction is mild or moderate, symptoms await adolescence or adulthood, or remain absent altogether. Severe obstruction comes to light in infants and young children because of dyspnea, tachypnea, paroxysmal cough, and hemoptysis. The physical signs are typical of pulmonary hypertension. The electrocardiogram exhibits right atrial P waves with right ventricular hypertrophy. The x-ray shows pulmonary venous congestion without enlargement of the left atrium but with enlargement of the right atrium, right ventricle, and pulmonary trunk. The proximal accessory chamber may dilate slightly and reveal itself on the lateral chest x-ray. The left atrial appendage is in the distal low-pressure compartment, so it does not enlarge and does not reveal itself on the x-ray. Echocardiography with color flow imaging and Doppler scan interrogation is used to identify the anatomic and physiologic features of cor triatriatum. The undulating membrane is proximal to the left atrial appendage and the mitral valve, a feature that distinguishes cor triatriatum from a supravalvular stenosing ring.

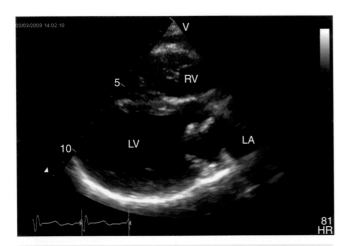

FIGURE 9-19 Echocardiogram (parasternal long axis) from a 21-year-old woman with cor triatriatum. The membrane is seen between the left atrium and mitral valve (Video 9-2). (LV = left ventricle; LA = left atrium; RA = right atrium.)

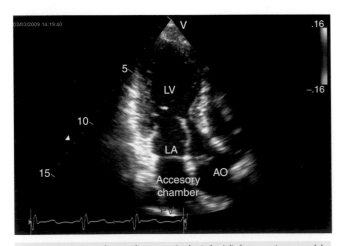

FIGURE 9-20 Echocardiogram (subxiphoid) from a 1-year-old boy with cor triatriatum. The accessory chamber is seen between the pulmonary veins (PV) and the membrane which inserts proximal to the left atrial appendage (Video 9-3). (LA = left atrium; LV = left ventricle.)

CONGENITAL PULMONARY VEIN STENOSIS

The incidence rate of congenital pulmonary vein stenosis is estimated at 0.4% to 0.6% of pediatric cardiac necropsies.[54] Isolated pulmonary vein stenosis is far more rare.[55] The abnormality is characterized by hypoplasia of one or more pulmonary veins or by focal narrowing at or near their left atrial junction (see Figure 9-1C).[39,54–56] Hypoplasia varies from slight narrowing to atresia of individual pulmonary veins or of a common pulmonary vein.[41,57,58] Focal narrowing is caused by a circumferential collar of fibrous intimal thickening or by a membranous diaphragm.[59,60] Focal stenosis, hypoplasia, and atresia may coexist with involvement of most or all of the pulmonary veins.[61] Congenital pulmonary vein stenosis is believed to be a developmental fault of the common pulmonary vein, a structure that is normally incorporated into the left atrium as four separate venous channels (see previous discussion).[57,58]

The following discussion deals with pulmonary vein stenosis as an isolated cause of congenital obstruction to left atrial inflow, although the disorder usually coexists with a number of other congenital malformations.[55,56,59] The physiology of the circulation resembles congenital mitral stenosis or cor triatriatum, but left atrial pressure is normal. Except for stenosis or atresia of the common pulmonary vein,[57] high pulmonary venous pressure is not distributed uniformly within the lungs because of variation in the location and severity of individual sites of stenosis.[39]

Clinical Features

Pulmonary vein stenosis causes dyspnea, orthopnea, cough, hemoptysis, and lower respiratory infections.[54,56,59,60] Lifespan occasionally extends into the middle or late teens, but only a minority of patients survive childhood.[56] Precordial palpation detects a right ventricular and pulmonary trunk impulse and a loud pulmonary component of the second heart sound.[54] Murmurs are absent except for a Graham Steell murmur or tricuspid regurgitation.[59,60] The electrocardiogram reflects pulmonary hypertension with right atrial P wave abnormalities, right axis deviation, and right ventricular hypertrophy.[54,60] Left atrial P wave abnormalities are absent. Pulmonary vascular patterns in the x-rays are determined by which of the four pulmonary veins are stenosed and by the degree of stenosis.[58] Regional differences are characterized by asymmetry between the right and left lungs and by nonuniform distribution within each lung.[58] Left atrial size remains normal because pulmonary vein stenosis is proximal to the left atrium.[39,60] The heart tends to shift toward the side of major involvement, which is usually the left hemithorax.[62] The echocardiogram excludes congenital mitral stenosis or cor triatriatum as the cause of obstruction to left atrial flow. Color flow imaging and Doppler scan interrogation disclose continuous turbulent flow with normal velocities in the involved pulmonary veins.[55] Interrogation of each pulmonary vein is required because focal and long-segment stenoses are associated with different flow patterns.[55] Atresia of the common pulmonary vein has been diagnosed with fetal echocardiography.[63]

Summary

The clinical manifestations of congenital pulmonary vein stenosis resemble congenital mitral stenosis and cor triatriatum, but with important differences. In congenital pulmonary vein stenosis, electrocardiographic and radiologic signs of left atrial enlargement are absent. Pulmonary venous congestion is not uniformly distributed in the x-ray because pulmonary vein stenosis varies among the four pulmonary veins. The echocardiogram rules out congenital mitral stenosis or cor triatriatum and focuses on abnormal flow patterns in the pulmonary veins as the cause of obstruction to left atrial inflow.

REFERENCES

1. Collins-Nakai RL, Rosenthal A, Castaneda AR, Bernhard WF, Nadas AS. Congenital mitral stenosis. A review of 20 years' experience. *Circulation.* 1977;56:1039–1047.
2. Tandon R, Moller JH, Edwards JE. Anomalies associated with the parachute mitral valve: a pathologic analysis of 52 cases. *Can J Cardiol.* 1986;2:278–281.
3. Alphonso N, Norgaard MA, Newcomb A, D'udekem Y, Brizard CP, Cochrane A. Cor triatriatum: presentation, diagnosis and long-term surgical results. *Ann Thorac Surg.* 2005;80:1666–1671.
4. Godoy I, Tantibhedhyangkul W, Karp R, Lang R. Images in cardiovascular medicine. Cor triatriatum. *Circulation.* 1998;98:2781.
5. Bano-Rodrigo A, Van Praagh S, Trowitzsch E, Van Praagh R. Double-orifice mitral valve: a study of 27 postmortem cases with developmental, diagnostic and surgical considerations. *Am J Cardiol.* 1988;61:152–160.
6. Sullivan ID, Robinson PJ, De Leval M, Graham Jr TP. Membranous supravalvular mitral stenosis: a treatable form of congenital heart disease. *J Am Coll Cardiol.* 1986;8:159–164.
7. Trowitzsch E, Bano-Rodrigo A, Burger BM, Colan SD, Sanders SP. Two-dimensional echocardiographic findings in double orifice mitral valve. *J Am Coll Cardiol.* 1985;6:383–387.
8. Collison SP, Kaushal SK, Dagar KS, et al. Supramitral ring: good prognosis in a subset of patients with congenital mitral stenosis. *Ann Thorac Surg.* 2006;81:997–1001.
9. Mychaskiw 2nd G, Sachdev V, Braden DA, Heath BJ. Supramitral ring: an unusual cause of congenital mitral stenosis. Case series and review. *J Cardiovasc Surg.* 2002;43:199–202.
10. Ruckman RN, Van Praagh R. Anatomic types of congenital mitral stenosis: report of 49 autopsy cases with consideration of diagnosis and surgical implications. *Am J Cardiol.* 19/8;42:592–601.
11. Castaneda AR, Anderson RC, Edwards JE. Congenital mitral stenosis resulting from anomalous arcade and obstructing papillary muscles. Report of correction by use of ball valve prosthesis. *Am J Cardiol.* 1969;24:237–240.
12. Parr GV, Fripp RR, Whitman V, Bharati S, Lev M. Anomalous mitral arcade: echocardiographic and angiographic recognition. *Pediatr Cardiol.* 1983;4:163–165.
13. Layman TE, Edwards JE. Anomalous mitral arcade. A type of congenital mitral insufficiency. *Circulation.* 1967;35:389–395.
14. Perez JA, Herzberg AJ, Reimer KA, Bashore TM. Congenital mitral insufficiency secondary to anomalous mitral arcade in an adult. *Am Heart J.* 1987;114:894–895.
15. Shone JD, Sellers RD, Anderson RC, Adams Jr P, Lillehei CW, Edwards JE. The developmental complex of "parachute mitral valve," supravalvular ring of left atrium, subaortic stenosis, and coarctation of aorta. *Am J Cardiol.* 1963;11:714–725.
16. Smallhorn J, Tommasini G, Deanfield J, Douglas J, Gibson D, Macartney F. Congenital mitral stenosis. Anatomical and functional assessment by echocardiography. *Br Heart J.* 1981;45:527–534.
17. Isner JM, Salem DN, Seaver PR, Payne DD, Cleveland RJ. Supravalvular stenosing ring of the left atrium associated with bilateral atrioventricular valvular regurgitation. *Am Heart J.* 1983;106:1150–1152.
18. Davachi F, Moller JH, Edwards JE. Diseases of the mitral valve in infancy. An anatomic analysis of 55 cases. *Circulation.* 1971;43:565–579.
19. Shrivastava S, Moller JH, Tadavarthy M, Fukuda T, Edwards JE. Clinical pathologic conference. *Am Heart J.* 1976;91:513–519.
20. Rosenquist GC. Congenital mitral valve disease associated with coarctation of the aorta: a spectrum that includes parachute deformity of the mitral valve. *Circulation.* 1974;49:985–993.
21. Daoud G, Kaplan S, Perrin EV, Dorst JP, Edwards FK. Congenital mitral stenosis. *Circulation.* 1963;27:185–196.
22. Elliott LP, Anderson RC, Amplatz K, Lillehei CW, Edwards JE. Congenital mitral stenosis. *Pediatrics.* 1962;30:552–562.
23. Singh SP, Gotsman MS, Abrams LD, Astley R, Parsons CG, Roberts KD. Congenital mitral stenosis. *Br Heart J.* 1967;29:83–90.
24. Perloff JK. Auscultatory and phonocardiographic manifestations of pulmonary hypertension. *Prog Cardiovasc Dis.* 1967;9:303–340.
25. Perloff JK. *Physical examination of the heart and circulation.* 4th ed. Shelton, Connecticut: People's Medical Publishing House; 2009.

26. Rodan BA, Chen JT, Kirks DR, Benson Jr DW. Mitral valve calcification in congenital mitral stenosis. *Am Heart J*. 1983;105: 514–515.

27. Grenadier E, Sahn DJ, Valdes-Cruz LM, Allen HD, Oliveira Lima C, Goldberg SJ. Two-dimensional echo Doppler study of congenital disorders of the mitral valve. *Am Heart J*. 1984;107: 319–325.

28. Snider AR, Roge CL, Schiller NB, Silverman NH. Congenital left ventricular inflow obstruction evaluated by two-dimensional echocardiography. *Circulation*. 1980;61:848–855.

29. Vitarelli A, Landolina G, Gentile R, Caleffi T, Sciomer S. Echocardiographic assessment of congenital mitral stenosis. *Am Heart J*. 1984;108:523–531.

30. Andral G. *Precis d'anatomie pathologique*. Paris: Gabon; 1829.

31. Church WS. Congenital malformation of the heart: abnormal septum in the left auricle. *Transactions of the Pathology Society of London*. 1868;19:188–190.

32. Borst M. Ein cor triatriatum. *Zentralbl f Path*. 1905;16:812.

33. Thilenius OG, Bharati S, Lev M. Subdivided left atrium: an expanded concept of cor triatriatum sinistrum. *Am J Cardiol*. 1976;37:743–752.

34. Gheissari A, Malm JR, Bowman Jr FO, Bierman FZ. Cor triatriatum sinistrum: one institution's 28-year experience. *Pediatr Cardiol*. 1992;13:85–88.

35. Marin-Garcia J, Tandon R, Lucas Jr RV, Edwards JE. Cor triatriatum: study of 20 cases. *Am J Cardiol*. 1975;35:59–66.

36. Van Praagh R, Corsini I. Cor triatriatum: pathologic anatomy and a consideration of morphogenesis based on 13 postmortem cases and a study of normal development of the pulmonary vein and atrial septum in 83 human embryos. *Am Heart J*. 1969;78: 379–405.

37. Gahide G, Barde S, Francis-Sicre N. Cor triatriatum sinister: a comprehensive anatomical study on computed tomography scan. *J Am Coll Cardiol*. 2009;54:487.

38. Lee Y-S, Kim K-S, Lee J-B, Kean-Ryu J, Choi J-Y, Chang S-G. Cor triatriatum dexter assessed by three-dimensional echocardiography reconstruction in two adult patients. *Echocardiography*. 2007;24: 991–994.

39. Nakib A, Moller JH, Kanjuh VI, Edwards JE. Anomalies of the pulmonary veins. *Am J Cardiol*. 1967;20:77–90.

40. Patel AK, Ninneman RW, Rahko PS. Surgical resection of cor triatriatum in a 74-year-old man. Review of echocardiographic findings with emphasis on Doppler and transesophageal echocardiography. *J Am Soc Echocardiogr*. 1990;3:402–407.

41. Lucas Jr RV, Woolfrey BF, Andersonrc LRG, Edwards JE. Atresia of the common pulmonary vein. *Pediatrics*. 1962;29:729–739.

42. Alboliras ET, Edwards WD, Driscoll DJ, Seward JB. Cor triatriatum dexter: two-dimensional echocardiographic diagnosis. *J Am Coll Cardiol*. 1987;9:334–337.

43. Burton DA, Chin A, Weinberg PM, Pigott JD. Identification of cor triatriatum dexter by two-dimensional echocardiography. *Am J Cardiol*. 1987;60:409–410.

44. Hansing CE, Young WP, Rowe GG. Cor triatriatum dexter. Persistent right sinus venosus valve. *Am J Cardiol*. 1972;30: 559–564.

45. Trakhtenbroit A, Majid P, Rokey R. Cor triatriatum dexter: antemortem diagnosis in an adult by cross sectional echocardiography. *Br Heart J*. 1990;63:314–316.

46. Mcguire LB, Nolan TB, Reeve R, Dammann Jr JF. Cor triatriatum as a problem of adult heart disease. *Circulation*. 1965;31:263–272.

47. Almendro-Delia M, Trujillo-Berraquero F, Araji O, De Vinuesa PG-G, Fernandez JMC. Cor triatriatum sinistrum in an elderly man. *Int J Cardiol*. 2008;125:e27–e29.

48. Schluter M, Langenstein BA, Thier W, et al. Transesophageal two-dimensional echocardiography in the diagnosis of cor triatriatum in the adult. *J Am Coll Cardiol*. 1983;2:1011–1015.

49. Ludomirsky A, Erickson C, Vick 3rd GW, Cooley DA. Transesophageal color flow Doppler evaluation of cor triatriatum in an adult. *Am Heart J*. 1990;120:451–455.

50. Ehrich DA, Vieweg WV, Alpert JS, Folkerth TL, Hagan AD. Cor triatriatum: report of a case in a young adult with special reference to the echocardiographic features and etiology of the systolic murmur. *Am Heart J*. 1977;94:217–221.

51. Darke CS, Emery JL, Lorber J. Triatrial heart. *Br Heart J*. 1961;23: 329–332.

52. Vuocolo LM, Stoddard MF, Longaker RA. Transesophageal two-dimensional and Doppler echocardiographic diagnosis of cor triatriatum in the adult. *Am Heart J*. 1992;124:791–793.

53. Alwi M, Hamid ZA, Zambahari R. A characteristic continuous wave Doppler signal in cor triatriatum? *Br Heart J*. 1992;68:6–8.

54. Geggel RL, Fried R, Tuuri DT, Fyler DC, Reid LM. Congenital pulmonary vein stenosis: structural changes in a patient with normal pulmonary artery wedge pressure. *J Am Coll Cardiol*. 1984;3: 193–199.

55. Webber SA, De Souza E, Patterson MW. Pulsed wave and color Doppler findings in congenital pulmonary vein stenosis. *Pediatr Cardiol*. 1992;13:112–115.

56. Driscoll DJ, Hesslein PS, Mullins CE. Congenital stenosis of individual pulmonary veins: clinical spectrum and unsuccessful treatment by transvenous balloon dilation. *Am J Cardiol*. 1982;49: 1767–1772.

57. Hawker RE, Celermajer JM, Gengos DC, Cartmill TB, Bowdler JD. Common pulmonary vein atresia. Premortem diagnosis in two infants. *Circulation*. 1972;46:368–374.

58. Nasrallah AT, Mullins CE, Singer D, Harrison G, Mcnamara DG. Unilateral pulmonary vein atresia: diagnosis and treatment. *Am J Cardiol*. 1975;36:969–973.

59. Mortensson W, Lundstrom NR. Congenital obstruction of the pulmonary veins at their atrial junctions. Review of the literature and a case report. *Am Heart J*. 1974;87:359–362.

60. Shone JD, Amplatz K, Anderson RC, Adams Jr P, Edwards JE. Congenital stenosis of individual pulmonary veins. *Circulation*. 1962; 26:574–581.

61. Mori K, Dohi T. Mitral and pulmonary vein blood flow patterns in cor triatriatum. *Am Heart J*. 1989;117:1167–1169.

62. Cullen S, Deasy PF, Tempany E, Duff DF. Isolated pulmonary vein atresia. *Br Heart J*. 1990;63:350–354.

63. Samuel N, Sirotta L, Bar-Ziv J, Dicker D, Feldberg D, Goldman JA. The ultrasonic appearance of common pulmonary vein atresia in utero. *J Ultrasound Med*. 1988;7:25–28.

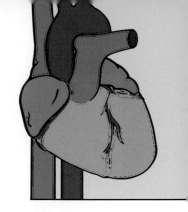

Chapter 10

Endocardial Fibroelastosis

Endocardial fibroelastosis, a self-defining term introduced in 1943,[1] is characterized by an opaque, pearly-white thickening that results from proliferation of collagen and elastic fibers (Figure 10-1).[2,3] Isolated endocardial fibroelastosis involves the endocardium of a dilated hypertrophied left ventricle,[2,3] hence the term *primary endocardial fibroelastosis of the dilated type.* Conversely, albeit rarely, the left ventricular cavity is small, hence the term *endocardial fibroelastosis of the contracted* type.[2,3] Another form of endocardial fibroelastosis is considered *secondary* because it accompanies certain congenital malformations of the heart,[3] especially aortic stenosis,[4] coarctation of the aorta,[5] anomalous origin of the left coronary artery from the pulmonary trunk,[6] and hypoplastic left heart.[7] Endocardial fibrosis is a substrate for mural thrombosis, which sets the stage for systemic emboli.[8,9] The endocardium occasionally calcifies.

Pathogenesis takes into account the gross and histologic endocardial abnormalities and ventricular hypertrophy that characterize primary endocardial fibroelastosis of the dilated type. Fibroelastosis *per se* is a response to a variety of endocardial stimuli, with intrauterine endocardial injury as the common denominator.[10–14] The disorder has been reported with or without complete heart block in fetuses and children of mothers who are positive for anti-Ro or anti-La antibodies.[15,16] Fibroelastosis occurs in infants and adults after myocardial infarction,[9,17] underscoring the endocardial response to injury.

Primary dilated endocardial fibroelastosis is the type that occurs in infants.[18,19] Beyond infancy, the endocardial lesion tends to be patchy and is associated with myocardial fibrosis. The relationship between the infantile, the adolescent, and the adult form of the disease is unclear,[18–21] and the relationship between the dilated and nondilated types has not been established.[3,10,22]

Primary endocardial fibroelastosis of the dilated type principally involves the left ventricle.[3,23,24] The left atrium, right atrium, and right ventricle are only occasionally affected.[25,26] Mitral regurgitation coexists with the dilated type[3,27] because the papillary muscles originate high on the left ventricular wall (i.e., from the upper third) and accordingly exert undesirable lateral axes of tension on the chordae tendineae and mitral cusps, resulting in faulty leaflet apposition.[3] In addition to being laterally aligned, the chordae tendineae are short and thick,[26,27] and the papillary muscles tend to be small with histologic changes that resemble infarction.[27]

The *physiologic consequences* of primary endocardial fibroelastosis of the dilated type reflect the basic disorder of left ventricular endocardium, in concert with mitral regurgitation (Figures 10-2 and 10-3). Endocardial thickening restricts contraction of the dilated left ventricle and is responsible for global hypokinesis (see Figures 10-1 and 10-2).[23] Elevated pressure in the left atrium, pulmonary veins, and pulmonary artery result in high left ventricular filling pressure and mitral regurgitation.[23] Pulmonary hypertension is more pronounced in the nondilated form of the disease because the filling pressure in the small left ventricle is especially high.[22,28]

HISTORY

Primary endocardial fibroelastosis of the dilated type is equally distributed between the genders.[29] It has been reported in siblings, in identical twins,[30–32] and in more than one generation.[20,33,34] The disease manifests itself in the first 6 to 12 months of life.[3,29] Most affected children do not live beyond their second birthday.[2] Prognosis is especially poor in neonates.[14] Symptoms can run a protracted course and can begin suddenly, and death can be sudden and unexpected.[2,35,36] Systemic emboli from left ventricular mural thrombi result in serious neurologic sequelae.[2,8]

PHYSICAL APPEARANCE

The catabolic effects of chronic congestive heart failure are responsible for poor growth and development. Arterial oxygen unsaturation is related to cardiac failure.

ARTERIAL PULSE

The slow rate of rise is because of impaired left ventricular contractility. Sinus tachycardia and pulsus alternans are reflections of heart failure.[2]

JUGULAR VENOUS PULSE

The jugular pulse cannot be analyzed in symptomatic infants. A high systemic venous pressure provokes hepatomegaly and a liver pulse.

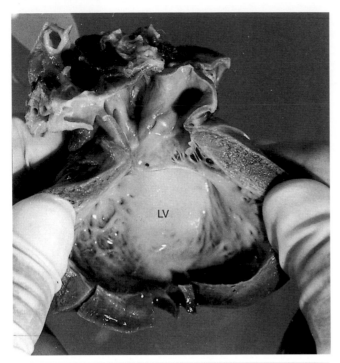

FIGURE 10-1 Necropsy specimen from a 2-month-old male. The left ventricle (LV) is markedly dilated, the walls are hypertrophied, and the endocardium exhibits the typical diffuse pearly-white, opaque thickening of endocardial fibroelastosis.

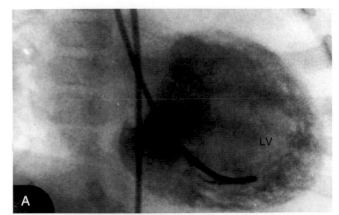

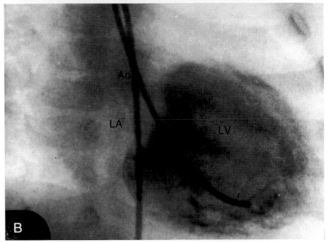

FIGURE 10-2 Angiocardiogram from a 15-month-old male with primary endocardial fibroelastosis of the dilated type. **A,** The diastolic frame shows the typical spherically dilated left ventricle (LV). **B,** The systolic frame shows a trivial decrease in left ventricular size reflecting striking global hypokinesis. Visualization of the aorta (Ao) was faint because of the low stroke volume. (LA = left atrium.)

PRECORDIAL MOVEMENT AND PALPATION

The impulse of the dilated left ventricle is hypodynamic because endocardial restriction impairs contractility. Mid-diastolic distention represents a palpable third heart sound or a summation sound generated by rapid flow into a poorly compliant left ventricle. Mid-diastolic distention is more pronounced when mitral regurgitation coexists. Mitral regurgitation causes systolic expansion of an enlarged left atrium and systolic anterior movement of the precordium that can be mistaken for an intrinsic right ventricle. The relatively dynamic impulse of a dilated failing *right* ventricle may obscure the hypokinetic left ventricular impulse.

AUSCULTATION

Hypokinetic left ventricular contraction diminishes the murmur of mitral incompetence despite appreciable regurgitant flow (Figure 10-4).[2,29] Elevated pulmonary artery pressure augments the pulmonary component of the second heart sound and narrows the splitting. A third heart sound reflects the decrease in left ventricular distensibility[2,23,29] and is especially prominent when mitral regurgitation coexists. Third and fourth heart sounds can summate to produce a triple rhythm or a short mid-diastolic murmur (see Figure 10-4).

ELECTROCARDIOGRAM

The electrocardiogram records a variety of disturbances in rhythm and conduction, including paroxysmal atrial, junctional or ventricular tachycardia, and neonatal atrial fibrillation.[3,32,37] Complete heart block has been detected in utero[2,32,38] and raises the question of a relationship between maternal antibodies, congenital complete heart block, and endocardial fibroelastosis (see previous discussion[15,16] and Chapter 4).[13] P waves show left atrial, biatrial, or right atrial abnormalities (Figure 10-5), especially in the presence of mitral regurgitation and elevated pulmonary arterial pressure.[3,29,37] The PR interval is normal or slightly increased,[3,29,37] except in sporadic cases with Wolff-Parkinson-White accessory pathways.[37]

The QRS axis is normal, although rightward or leftward axes occasionally occur.[29,37] Left ventricular hypertrophy is an important electrocardiographic feature of primary endocardial fibroelastosis of the dilated type (Figures 10-5 and 10-6).[39] Right ventricular or biventricular hypertrophy is reserved for infants with left

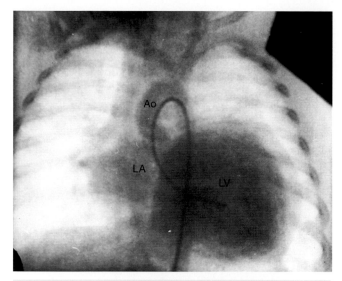

FIGURE 10-3 Angiocardiogram in a 4-month-old male with primary endocardial fibroelastosis of the dilated type. The spherical left ventricle (LV) is strikingly dilated. Mitral regurgitation opacified the left atrium (LA). Visualization of the aorta (Ao) was faint because of the low stroke volume.

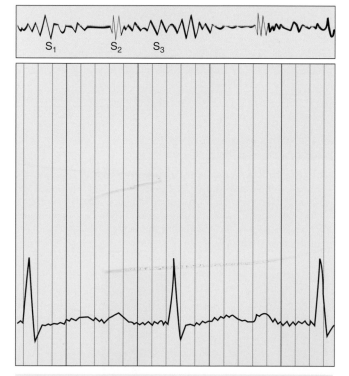

FIGURE 10-4 Phonocardiogram from the cardiac apex of a 6-month-old female with primary endocardial fibroelastosis of the dilated type. The third heart sound (S_3) is followed by a short mid-diastolic murmur. A systolic murmur was absent despite angiographic mitral regurgitation because the dilated left ventricle was hypokinetic. (S_1 = first heart sound; S_2 = second heart sound.)

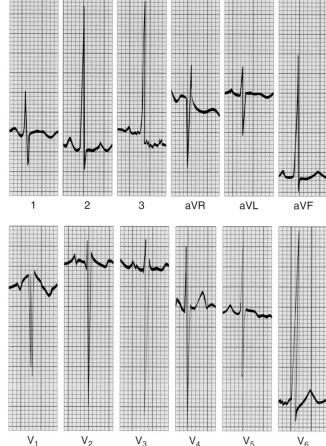

FIGURE 10-5 Electrocardiogram from a 2-month-old male with primary endocardial fibroelastosis of the dilated type. Notched P waves in leads V_{2-5} are the result of an enlarged left atrium. Left ventricular hypertrophy is indicated by tall R waves in leads 2, 3, and aVF and in lead V_6.

ventricular failure and reactive pulmonary hypertension.[3,23,37] Isolated right ventricular hypertrophy occurs in the nondilated form of the disorder.[23,29,40] Q waves are common in left precordial leads in the dilated form because of the volume overload of mitral regurgitation (see Figure 10-6).[29] An infarct pattern is a feature of endocardial fibroelastosis associated with anomalous origin of the left coronary artery from the pulmonary trunk (see Chapter 21).[41] If an infarct pattern occurs in primary endocardial fibroelastosis, the Q waves are in *right precordial* leads,[41] not in leads 1 and aVL (see Chapter 21).

X-RAY

In the dilated form, cardiomegaly is the result of enlargement of the left ventricle and left atrium, which can be massive (Figures 10-7 and 10-8).[3,29,39] Calcification of the thickened endocardium is occasionally identified at necropsy but rarely in the x-ray.[29] The ascending aorta and pulmonary trunk are inconspicuous compared with the striking increase in heart size (see Figures 10-7 and 10-8).

ECHOCARDIOGRAM

The dilated type of primary endocardial fibroelastosis appears as spherical left ventricular enlargement with striking global hypokinesis.[11] Septal and free wall thicknesses are increased because of left ventricular hypertrophy

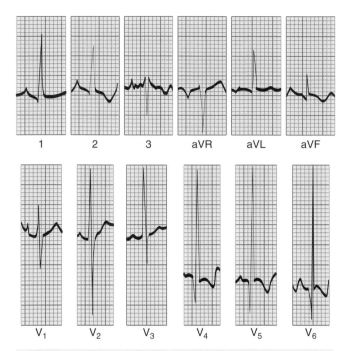

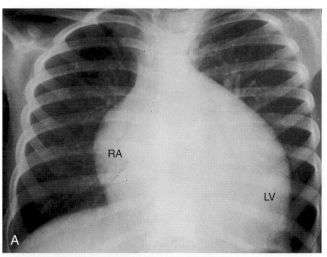

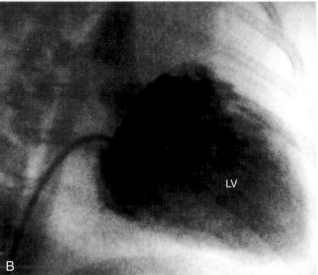

FIGURE 10-6 Electrocardiogram recorded the day before death of a 4-month-old female with endocardial fibroelastosis of the dilated type. Left precordial leads exhibit the tall R waves and inverted T waves of left ventricular hypertrophy. Q waves are prominent in leads V_{4-6} despite absence of the volume overload of mitral regurgitation.

(Figure 10-9). The left atrium is dilated, sometimes massively so. Color flow imaging is used to determine the degree of mitral regurgitation. The echocardiogram permits intrauterine detection.[10] The diagnosis of primary endocardial fibroelastosis can be difficult to establish with echocardiography, even though bright echoes appear in the thickened endocardium (see Figures 10-1 and 10-9). Magnetic resonance imaging with perfusion and myocardial delayed enhancement[42] and multidetector computed tomography[43] can be useful.

FIGURE 10-8 A, X-ray from the 6-month-old female whose phonocardiogram is shown in Figure 10-4. The left ventricle (LV) and the right atrium (RA) are strikingly enlarged in contrast with the inconspicuous great arteries. There is pulmonary venous congestion. **B,** Angiogram showing the dilated hypokinetic left ventricle (LV).

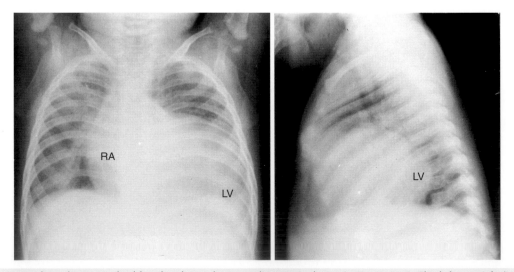

FIGURE 10-7 X-rays from the 2-month-old male whose electrocardiogram is shown in Figure 10-5. The left ventricle (LV) is strikingly dilated in both projections, and the right atrium (RA) is considerably enlarged. The great arteries are inconspicuous. The lung fields exhibit pulmonary venous congestion.

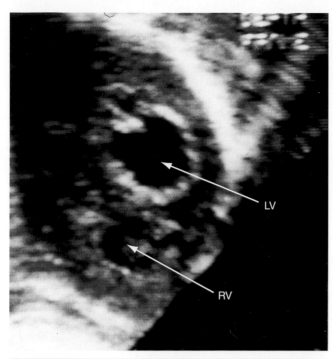

FIGURE 10-9 Echocardiogram (short axis) from a 1-day-old male with critical aortic valve stenosis. The endocardial thickening of the hypertrophied left ventricle (LV) is highly echogenic. (RV = right ventricle.)

SUMMARY

Endocardial fibroelastosis is classified as dilated, contracted, or secondary to certain types of congenital malformations of the heart, notably aortic stenosis, coarctation of the aorta, anomalous origin of the left coronary artery from the pulmonary trunk, and hypoplastic left heart. Fibroelastosis *per se* is a response to a variety of endocardial provocations, with intrauterine endocardial injury as the common denominator. In fetuses and children of mothers positive for anti-Ro or anti-La antibodies, the disorder has been reported with or without complete heart block.

Primary endocardial fibroelastosis of the dilated type is characterized by: (1) congestive heart failure and mitral regurgitation; (2) hypokinesis of the dilated left ventricle despite its hypertrophied wall; (3) absent or inconspicuous cardiac murmurs despite mitral regurgitation; (4) electrocardiographic signs of left ventricular hypertrophy; (5) radiologic left ventricular and left atrial dilation that are sometimes striking; and (6) an echocardiogram that images a spherically dilated hypertrophied but hypokinetic left ventricle with bright echoes arising from the thickened endocardium. Magnetic resonance imaging and computed tomography can be diagnostically useful.

REFERENCES

1. Weinberg T, Himelfarb AJ. Endocardial fibroelastosis (so-called fetal endocarditis). *Bulletin of the Johns Hopkins Hospital.* 1943; 72:299.
2. Andersen DH, Kelly J. Congenital endocardial fibro-elastosis. II. A clinical and pathologic investigation of those cases without associated cardiac malformations including report of two familial instances. *Pediatrics.* 1956;18:539–555.
3. Moller JH, Lucas Jr RV, Adams Jr P, Anderson RC, Jorgens J, Edwards JE. Endocardial fibroelastosis. A clinical and anatomic study of 47 patients with emphasis on its relationship to mitral insufficiency. *Circulation.* 1964;30:759–782.
4. Dushane JW, Edwards JE. Cardiac clinics. CXLII. Congenital aortic stenosis in association with endocardial sclerosis of the left ventricle. *Proceedings of the Staff Meetings Mayo Clinic.* 1954; 29:102–108.
5. Oppenheimer EH. The association of adult-type coarctation of the aorta with endocardial fibroelastosis in infancy. *Bulletin of the Johns Hopkins Hospital.* 1953;93:309–319.
6. Noren GR, Raghib G, Moller JH, Amplatz K, Adams Jr P, Edwards JE. Anomalous origin of the left coronary artery from the pulmonary trunk with special reference to the occurrence of mitral insufficiency. *Circulation.* 1964;30:171–178.
7. Noonan JA, Nadas AS. The hypoplastic left heart syndrome; an analysis of 101 cases. *Pediatr Clin North Am.* 1958;5:1029–1056.
8. Branch GL, Castle RF. Thromboembolic complications in primary endocardial fibroelastosis. *J Pediatr.* 1966;69:250–258.
9. Lee KT, Mcgavran MH, Rabin ER, Thomas WA. Endocardial fibroelastosis in infants associated with thrombosis and calcification of arteries and myocardial infarcts. *N Engl J Med.* 1956;255: 464–468.
10. Carceller AM, Maroto E, Fouron JC. Dilated and contracted forms of primary endocardial fibroelastosis: a single fetal disease with two stages of development. *Br Heart J.* 1990;63:311–313.
11. Schryer MJ, Karnauchow PN. Endocardial fibroelastosis; etiologic and pathogenetic considerations in children. *Am Heart J.* 1974; 88:557–565.
12. Shone JD, Munoz Armas S, Manning JA, Keith JD. The mumps antigen skin test in endocardial fibroelastosis. *Pediatrics.* 1966; 37:423–429.
13. Singsen BH, Akhter JE, Weinstein MM, Sharp GC. Congenital complete heart block and SSA antibodies: obstetric implications. *Am J Obstet Gynecol.* 1985;152:655–658.
14. Westwood M, Harris R, Burn JL, Barson AJ. Heredity in primary endocardial fibroelastosis. *Br Heart J.* 1975;37:1077–1084.
15. Nield LE, Silverman ED, Smallhorn JF, et al. Endocardial fibroelastosis associated with maternal anti-Ro and anti-La antibodies in the absence of atrioventricular block. *J Am Coll Cardiol.* 2002;40: 796–802.
16. Nield LE, Silverman ED, Taylor GP, et al. Maternal anti-Ro and anti-La antibody-associated endocardial fibroelastosis. *Circulation.* 2002;105:843–848.
17. Hutchins GM, Bannayan GA. Development of endocardial fibroelastosis following myocardial infarction. *Arch Pathol.* 1971;91: 113–118.
18. Rafinski T, Golenia A, Wozniewicz B, Wlad S. Familial endocardial fibroelastosis. *J Pediatr.* 1967;70:574–576.
19. Thomas WA, Randall RV, Bland EF, Castleman B. Endocardial fibroelastosis; a factor in heart disease of obscure etiology: a study of 20 autopsied cases in children and adults. *N Engl J Med.* 1954; 251:327–338.
20. Hanukoglu A, Fried D, Somekh E. Inheritance of familial primary endocardial fibroelastosis. *Clin Pediatr (Phila).* 1986;25: 272–275.
21. Hoffman FG. Adult endocardial fibroelastosis associated with dextrocardia and situs inversus. *Circulation.* 1960;22:437–447.
22. Ursell PC, Neill CA, Anderson RH, Ho SY, Becker AE, Gerlis LM. Endocardial fibroelastosis and hypoplasia of the left ventricle in neonates without significant aortic stenosis. *Br Heart J.* 1984;51: 492–497.
23. Lynfield J, Gasul BM, Luan LL, Dillon RF. Right and left heart catheterization and angiocardiographic findings in idiopathic cardiac hypertrophy with endocardial fibroelastosis. *Circulation.* 1960;21: 386–400.
24. Manning JA, Keith JD. Fibroelastosis in children. *Prog Cardiovasc Dis.* 1964;7:172–178.
25. Bjorkhem G, Lundstrom NR, Wallentin I, Carlgren LE. Endocardial fibroelastosis with predominant involvement of left atrium. Possibility of diagnosis by non-invasive methods. *Br Heart J.* 1981;46: 331–337.
26. Burke EC. Pediatric clinicopathologic conference. *Mayo Clin Proc.* 1970;45:467.
27. Davachi F, Moller JH, Edwards JE. Diseases of the mitral valve in infancy. An anatomic analysis of 55 cases. *Circulation.* 1971;43: 565–579.

28. Fixler DE, Cole RB, Paul MH, Lev M, Girod DA. Familial occurrence of the contracted form of endocardial fibroelastosis. *Am J Cardiol.* 1970;26:208–213.
29. Sellers FJ, Keith JD, Manning JA. The diagnosis of primary endocardial fibroelastosis. *Circulation.* 1964;29:49–59.
30. Greaves JL, Wilkins PS, Pearson S. Endocardial fibro-elastosis in identical twins. *Arch Dis Child.* 1954;29:447–450.
31. Lee MH, Liebman J, Steinberg AG, Perrin EV, Whitman V. Familial occurrence of endocardial fibroelastosis in three siblings, including identical twins. *Pediatrics.* 1973;52: 402–411.
32. Rios B, Duff J, Simpson JW. Endocardial fibroelastosis with congenital complete heart block in identical twins. *Am Heart J.* 1984;107: 1290–1293.
33. Nielsen JS. Primary endocardial fibroelastosis in three siblings. *Acta Med Scand.* 1965;177:145–151.
34. Vestermark S. Primary endocardial fibroelastosis in siblings. *Acta Paediatr.* 1962;51:94–96.
35. Alter BP, Czapek EE, Rowe RD. Sweating in congenital heart disease. *Pediatrics.* 1968;41:123–129.
36. Vestermark S. Primary endocardial fibroelastosis. *Cardiologia.* 1966;48:520–531.
37. Vlad P, Rowe RD, Keith JD. The electrocardiogram in primary endocardial fibroelastosis. *Br Heart J.* 1955;17:189–197.
38. Hung W, Walsh BJ. Congenital auricular fibrillation in a newborn infant with endocardial fibroelastosis. Report of a case with necropsy. *J Pediatr.* 1962;61:65–69.
39. Freundlich E, Munk J, Griffel B, Steinlauf J. Primary myocardial disease in infancy. *Am J Cardiol.* 1964;13:721–733.
40. Tingelstad JB, Shiel FO, Mccue CM. The elctrocardiogram in the contracted type of primary endocardial fibroelastosis. *Am J Cardiol.* 1971;27:304–308.
41. Lintermans JP, Kaplan EL, Morgan BC, Baum D, Guntheroth WG. Infarction patterns in endocardial fibroelastosis. *Circulation.* 1966; 33:202.
42. Stranzinger E, Ensing GJ, Hernandez RJ. MR findings of endocardial fibroelastosis in children. *Pediatr Radiol.* 2008;38:292–296.
43. Suh SY, Kim EJ, Yong HS, et al. Endocardial fibroelastosis demonstrated on multidetector computed tomography. *Int J Cardiol.* 2008;124:e51–e52.

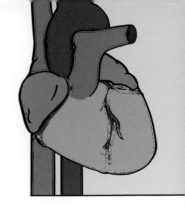

Chapter 11

Congenital Pulmonary Stenosis

Congenital obstruction to right ventricular outflow in hearts with two noninverted ventricles originates in, below, or above the pulmonary valve. Three morphologic types of pulmonary stenosis involve the pulmonary valve: (1) typical mobile dome-shaped; (2) dysplastic; and (3) bicuspid. *Dome-shaped pulmonary valve stenosis* was described in 1761 by John Baptist Morgagni[1] and is characterized by a thin mobile valve mechanism with a narrow central opening at its apex (Figure 11-1). Three rudimentary raphes extend from the central opening to the wall of the pulmonary artery, but separate leaflets and separate commissures cannot be identified. Pinpoint dome-shaped pulmonary valve stenosis in neonates is sometimes referred to as functional pulmonary atresia (see Figure 11-1A,B, lower). The pulmonary trunk is consistently dilated because of an inherent medial abnormality[2] that is coupled with the mobile dome-shaped valve but not with its functional state (see Figure 11-1). The jet from the stenotic valve breaks up on striking the apex of the pulmonary trunk. The pressure component of total energy increases with a proportionate increase in pressure in the left branch (see Figure 11-35A).[3] The physics of jet dispersion is believed to account for the larger size of the left branch. Calcification of a dome-shaped stenotic pulmonary valve is exceptional and is reserved for older patients (see section X-Ray).[4] *Dysplastic pulmonary valve stenosis* is much less common and is characterized by myomatous thickening of three separate but poorly mobile leaflets without commissural fusion (Figure 11-2; Box 11-1).[5,6] *Bicuspid pulmonary valve stenosis* is a feature of Fallot's tetralogy (see Chapter 18). Isolated bicuspid pulmonary valves are rare and are of little or no functional significance.

Subvalvular pulmonary stenosis can be *infundibular* or *subinfundibular*. The *infundibular* variety is caused by anterior and rightward deviation (malalignment) of the infundibular septum and is dealt with in Chapter 18. *Secondary hypertrophic infundibular pulmonary stenosis* accompanies—is secondary to—severe pulmonary valve stenosis (Figure 11-3 and see also Figure 11-38). *Stenosis of the ostium of the infundibulum* is a rare form of fixed obstruction to right ventricular outflow (see Figures 11-32 and 11-37). *Subinfundibular stenosis* or *double-chambered right ventricle*, described by Thomas Peacock[7] in 1858, is a rare form of congenital obstruction to right ventricular outflow. Obstructing muscle bundles within the right ventricular cavity were the subject of Sir Arthur Keith's[8] Hunterian lecture in 1909. The double-chambered right ventricle is divided into a high-pressure inlet portion and a low-pressure outlet portion by normal or anomalous muscle bundles[9,10] or by apical trabecular muscle sequestered from the rest of the right ventricle.[11] The degree of obstruction varies from nil to severe to virtually complete.[10] Double-chambered right ventricle usually coexists with a ventricular septal defect.[9,10]

Pulmonary artery stenosis (supravalvular), described by Oppenheimer[12] in 1938, is caused by narrowing of the pulmonary trunk, its bifurcation, or its primary or intrapulmonary branches (Figures 11-4 and 11-5).[13] Stenosis of the pulmonary artery and its branches usually occurs as an isolated malformation[13] and can be unilateral or bilateral, single or multiple, and segmental or tubular (see Figures 11-4 and 11-5).[13] Intrapulmonary arteries distal to the stenoses tend to be dilated (see Figures 11-4 and 11-5). Rarely, a membranous form of obstruction occurs immediately above the valve.[13]

Neonates, especially premature, normally exhibit a disparity in size between the pulmonary trunk and its proximal branches. Angulations at the origins of the branches cause a drop in systolic pressure in the absence of morphologic pulmonary artery stenosis (see Chapter 2, Figure 2-4).[14,15] The small pulmonary trunk and small proximal branches in Fallot's tetralogy are discussed in Chapter 18. In Williams syndrome, bilateral stenosis of pulmonary artery branches is associated with supravalvular aortic stenosis (see Chapter 7).[16] Experimental constriction of the pulmonary trunk in fetal lambs results in thin-walled intrapulmonary resistance vessels.[17]

In 1941, McAlister Gregg,[18] an Australian ophthalmologist, described a relationship between maternal rubella and congenital abnormalities in offspring. What came to be known as the *rubella syndrome* consists of stenosis of the pulmonary artery and its branches with patent ductus arteriosis.[19,20] Maternal rubella can have serious noncardiac effects that include spontaneous abortion, stillbirth, mental retardation, cataracts, and deafness. Viremia with placental and fetal infection during initial exposure is a prerequisite for the rubella syndrome. Fetal risk is small when infection occurs later than the 16th week of gestation.[20] A worldwide rubella epidemic in 1962 was followed in 1964 and 1965 by an epidemic in the United States that affected approximately 12.5 million patients and caused 11,000 fetal deaths.[19] Of an estimated 20,000 infants born with the rubella syndrome, approximately 2,100 died as neonates.[19]

The *physiologic consequences* of pulmonary stenosis result from increased resistance to right ventricular

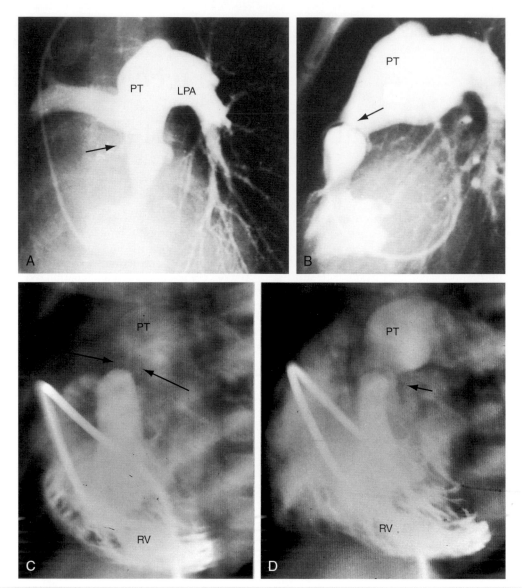

FIGURE 11-1 A and **B,** Angiocardiograms with contrast material injected into the right ventricle of a 47-year-old woman with pulmonary valve stenosis (gradient, 106 mm Hg). **A,** *Arrow* points to the level of the stenotic pulmonary valve. The dilated pulmonary trunk (PT) continues as a dilated left branch (LPA). **B,** Lateral projection. The stenotic pulmonary valve is mobile and domed *(arrow)*, and the pulmonary trunk (PT) is conspicuously dilated. There is an hourglass narrowing of the ostium of the infundibulum. **C** and **D,** Angiocardiograms with contrast material injected into the right ventricle (RV) of a 10-month-old female with pinpoint pulmonary valve stenosis. **C,** A wisp of contrast crosses the valve *(arrow)* and faintly visualizes the dilated pulmonary trunk (PT). **D,** The mobile stenotic valve is dome-shaped *(arrow)*, and the pulmonary trunk (PT) is conspicuously dilated.

discharge. Systolic pressure is elevated proximal to the obstruction and is normal or reduced distally. *Pulmonary artery stenosis* causes an increase in systolic pressure in the pulmonary trunk, which is proximal to the obstruction (see Figure 11-19). Valvular and subvalvular pulmonary stenosis increase the systolic pressure in the right ventricle, which is proximal to the obstruction. The gross morphologic response of the right ventricle to pressure overload is new sarcomeres in parallel, hence an increase in thickness of the free wall and ventricular septum, adaptive responses appropriate for developing power.[21] Cavity size remains normal.[22] In neonates with pinpoint pulmonary stenosis, cavity size is reduced.

The ultrastructural response to mechanical stress depends on myocyte maturity or immaturity at the time the inciting stimulus of overload becomes operative.[21] In pulmonary stenosis, the inciting stimulus is present at birth when cardiomyocytes are *immature* and capable of replication, which is accompanied by capillary angiogenesis. Accordingly, each replicated normal-sized myocyte is paired with its own capillary, so the myocyte:capillary ratio (capillary density) is normal. However, a morphologic right ventricle is perfused by a morphologic right coronary artery, which imposes an inherent limitation

Children and young adults with mild to moderate pulmonary valve stenosis have normal or near normal right

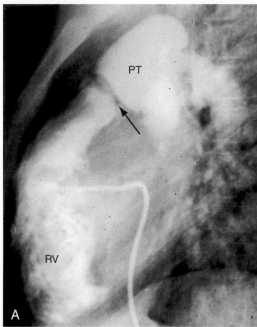

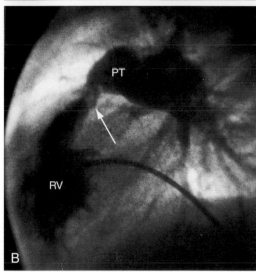

FIGURE 11-2 **A,** Right ventriculogram (RV) from a 6-year-old girl with a thickened immobile dysplastic pulmonary valve *(arrow).* The pulmonary trunk (PT) is only moderately dilated. **B,** Right ventriculogram (lateral projection) from a 3-year-old boy with a thickened dysplastic pulmonary valve *(arrow).* The pulmonary trunk (PT) and its left branch are moderately dilated.

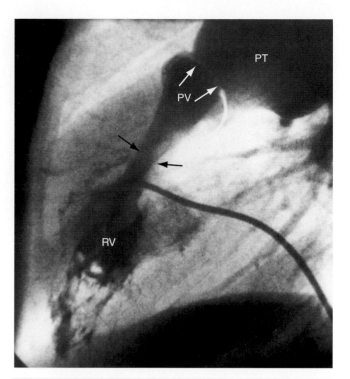

FIGURE 11-3 Right ventriculogram (RV), lateral projection, from a 37-year-old man with severe stenosis of a mobile dome pulmonary valve (PV) and secondary hypertrophic subpulmonary stenosis *(paired black arrows).* The pulmonary trunk (PT) is conspicuously dilated.

BOX 11-1 **CONGENITALLY DYSPLASTIC PULMONARY VALVE**

Three immobile cusps without commissural fusion
Noonan's syndrome
Family history
Absent ejection sound
Absent pulmonary component of the second heart sound
Nondilated pulmonary trunk

ventricular function and can increase cardiac output with exercise.[23] In *severe* pulmonary valve stenosis, however, stroke volume and cardiac output are fixed.[24] Systolic contraction of hypertrophied infundibular muscle (see Figure 11-3) is reinforced by exercise.[23]

Pressure overload of the *right* ventricular can result in systolic and diastolic dysfunction of the *left* ventricle.[25,26] *Systolic* dysfunction has been ascribed to chronic underfilling of the left ventricle, and diastolic dysfunction has been ascribed to displacement of the hypertrophied septum into the left ventricular cavity.

HISTORY

Typical mobile dome-shaped pulmonary valve stenosis is relatively common, with a prevalence rate as high as 10% of cases of congenital heart disease.[27,28] Gender distribution is equal or with female prevalence.[28] This is also the case in dysplastic pulmonary valve stenosis.[29]

The murmur of pulmonary stenosis is usually discovered at birth because the anatomic and physiologic conditions necessary for its production are present at birth. Parents are told that their newborn has congenital heart disease before discharge. However, the murmur of pinpoint pulmonary stenosis (see Figure 11-1, lower) is disarmingly soft. Murmurs at nonprecordial thoracic sites accompany pulmonary artery stenosis and in neonates and infants are easily overlooked or lost in the rapid

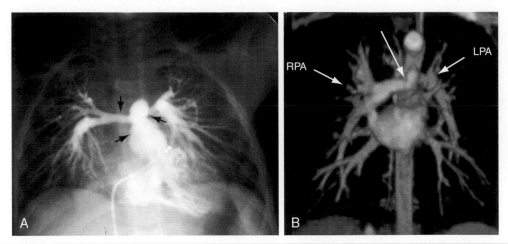

FIGURE 11-4 A, Angiocardiogram from a 2-year-old girl with stenosis of the pulmonary artery and its branches (gradient, 46 mm Hg). *Left lower arrow* points to a normal pulmonary valve. *Left upper vertical arrow* points to tubular hypoplasia of the proximal right pulmonary artery. The *right middle arrow* identifies stenosis of the pulmonary trunk. The intrapulmonary arteries are dilated distal to the stenoses. Tubular hypoplasia of the proximal left pulmonary artery is not shown. **B,** Gadolinium-enhanced magnetic resonance angiogram from a 32-year-old woman with rubella syndrome and status postductal ligation. There is moderate segmental stenosis *(large arrow)* of the proximal left pulmonary artery (LPA). (RPA = right pulmonary artery.)

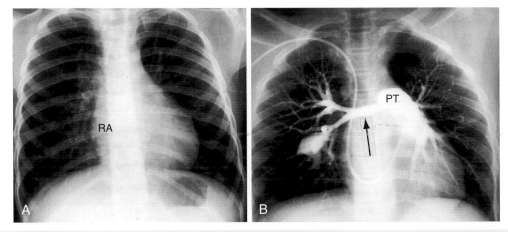

FIGURE 11-5 A, X-ray from a 7-year-old boy with stenosis of the pulmonary arterial branches. The pulmonary trunk (PT) is not dilated. The right atrium (RA) is prominent, and a convex right ventricle occupies the apex above the left hemidiaphragm. **B,** Pulmonary angiogram discloses tubular hypoplasia of the right pulmonary artery *(arrow)* with distal dilation. Tubular hypoplasia of the left pulmonary artery is not shown.

breath sounds. A history of first trimester maternal rubella arouses suspicion of pulmonary artery stenosis.

Familial recurrence of isolated pulmonary valve stenosis is uncommon if not rare (Figure 11-6).[30–33] In dysplastic pulmonary valve stenosis, the converse is the case.[5] Some family members have a dysplastic valve, and others have a mobile dome-shaped valve.[5] Similar observations have been made in the hereditary canine pulmonary valve dysplasia of beagles,[34] in whom dysplastic pulmonary stenosis and dome-shaped pulmonary stenosis occur in litter mates.[34] Familial Noonan's syndrome frequently occurs with dysplastic pulmonary valve stenosis and has appeared in three generations.[35,36] Successful pregnancy is possible in females with Noonan's syndrome.[37]

Familial *pulmonary artery stenosis* occurs as an isolated anomaly or with coexisting supravalvular aortic stenosis. Members of the same family may have either or both anomalies.

Normal birth weights and normal growth and development are characteristic of mobile dome-shaped pulmonary valve stenosis. However, in Noonan's syndrome with dysplastic pulmonary valve stenosis, growth and development are poor.[5,29,38] *Pulmonary artery stenosis* is associated with low birth weights and retarded physical and mental development in the rubella syndrome and in Williams syndrome (see Chapter 7).[19,39]

Neonates with pinpoint pulmonary valve stenosis experience rapidly progressive cardiac failure and early

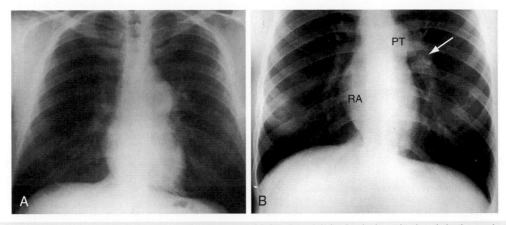

FIGURE 11-6 X-ray from a 39-year-old father **(A)** and his 14-year-old daughter **(B)**, both of whom had mobile dome-shaped pulmonary valve stenosis with gradients of 22 mm Hg and 67 mm Hg, respectively. Both x-rays show conspicuous dilation of the pulmonary trunk (PT) and its left branch (arrow) and mild convexity of the right atrium (RA).

death. However, most patients with mobile dome-shaped pulmonary valve stenosis experience little or no difficulty in infancy and childhood.[40] In a review of 69 cases, the average age at death was 26 years; seven patients survived to age 50 years, and three survived to 70 and 75 years. In 21 adults, the average follow-up period was 50 years.[41] Examples are found of survival into the sixth, seventh, and eighth decades,[42-46] with one patient reaching 78 years.[42] Longevity depends on three variables: 1, the initial severity of stenosis; 2, whether a given degree of stenosis remains constant or progresses; and 3, whether the function of the afterloaded right ventricle is preserved.[24,40,47]

The normal pulmonary valve orifice increases linearly with age and body surface area.[48] The orifice of a stenotic mobile dome-shaped pulmonary valve increases with age, but not necessarily at the rate of somatic growth.[40,48-50] Mild pulmonary valve stenosis in infancy usually remains mild,[51] but moderate to severe pulmonary stenosis tends to progress.[44] Stenosis of the pulmonary artery and its branches is not progressive. Fibrous thickening and occasionally calcification are responsible for increasing the degree of stenosis in older adults.

Equivalent degrees of pulmonary stenosis may handicap one patient in childhood but leave another relatively free of symptoms in adulthood. That mild pulmonary stenosis is asymptomatic is not surprising, but it is surprising that an appreciable number of patients with *moderate to severe* pulmonary stenosis claim to be virtually asymptomatic. Patients with right ventricular systolic pressures between 50 and 100 mm Hg include a New Zealand long-distance swimmer, a long-distance runner, and an English hockey captain.[52] The author's patients have included a 17-year-old boy who played baseball despite a right ventricular systolic pressure of nearly 200 mm Hg, a 32-year-old man who had run the quarter mile in high school despite a right ventricular systolic pressure of 75 mm Hg, and a woman with a right ventricular pressure of nearly 200 mm Hg who worked fulltime and had recurrent ascites for

7 years before death at age 60 years. Dyspnea and fatigue are mild as long as the right ventricle maintains a normal stroke volume at rest and augments its stroke volume with exercise.[24,47] However, relatively asymptomatic patients can have rapid deterioration. Cardiac output is inadequate even at rest when the hemodynamic burden imposed on the right ventricle leads to right ventricular failure, which is the commonest cause of death.[43]

Giddiness and light-headedness with effort prefigure syncope.[52] Children and adults occasionally experience the chest pain of right ventricular myocardial ischemia.[46,53] A 3-year-old with severe pulmonary artery stenosis died during an episode of chest pain and at necropsy had infarction of the right ventricular free wall and interventricular septum.[53] Sudden death has been associated with right ventricular infarction and an abnormal right coronary artery.[54] Dilated thin-walled intrapulmonary artery aneurysms distal to the stenoses of pulmonary artery branches (see Figure 11-5B) are sources of hemoptyses that can be intermittent and mild or recurrent and brisk.[13]

Severe pulmonary stenosis is accompanied by giant jugular venous A waves (Figure 11-7) of which patients are subjectively aware, especially during effort or excitement. These neck pulsations can be seen in the mirror when a young man shaves or when a young woman sits at her vanity. A 13-year-old girl with pulmonary valve stenosis and congenital complete heart block was aware of *intermittent* amplification of A waves as her right atrium randomly contracted against a closed tricuspid valve, and a 15-year-old boy was unpleasantly aware of intermittent amplification of jugular venous A waves caused by premature ventricular beats.

Mobile dome-shaped pulmonary valve stenosis is a substrate for *infective endocarditis*[44] that can induce a *medical valvotomy* when tissue is interrupted and orifice size increases.[52] Jet lesions in *pulmonary artery stenosis* can serve as substrates for infective endarteritis.[13]

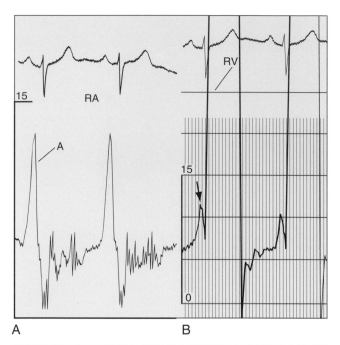

FIGURE 11-7 Pressure pulses from the 47-year-old woman with severe pulmonary valve stenosis referred to in Figure 11-1. **A,** Large right atrial (RA) A wave. **B,** Presystolic distention *(arrow)* of the right ventricle (RV) coincided with the large right atrial A wave.

PHYSICAL APPEARANCE

The following six types of physical appearance are relevant in patients with congenital pulmonary stenosis: (1) round bloated facies in infants with mobile dome-shaped pulmonary valve stenosis; (2) Noonan's syndrome; (3) rubella syndrome; (4) Williams syndrome; (5) Alagille syndrome; and (6) Cornelia de Lange's syndrome.

Infants with *mobile dome-shaped pulmonary valve stenosis* occasionally have chubby, round, bloated facies with highly colored cheeks (Figure 11-8A) and well-developed fat deposits.[52] The digits may be erythematous or frankly red in response to a small or intermittent right-to-left shunt through a patent foramen ovale (see Chapter 16).[36,55]

Noonan's syndrome (Figure 11-8C)[37,55,56] is characterized by short stature, webbed neck, pterygium colli, ptosis, hypertelorism, lymphedema, low-set ears, low anterior and posterior hairlines, flat or shield chest, pectus excavatum or carinatum, hyperelastic skin, inguinal hernia, nevi, dystrophic nails, micrognathia, hypospadias, and small undescended or cryptorchid testes.

About one third of patients with Noonan's syndrome are mentally retarded, and approximately two thirds have congenital heart disease, especially dysplastic pulmonary valve stenosis (60%) and hypertrophic cardiomyopathy (20%).[36,55,57–59]

The *rubella syndrome* is characterized by cataracts, retinopathy, deafness, hypotonia, dermatoglyphic abnormalities, and mental retardation.[60] Height and weight are

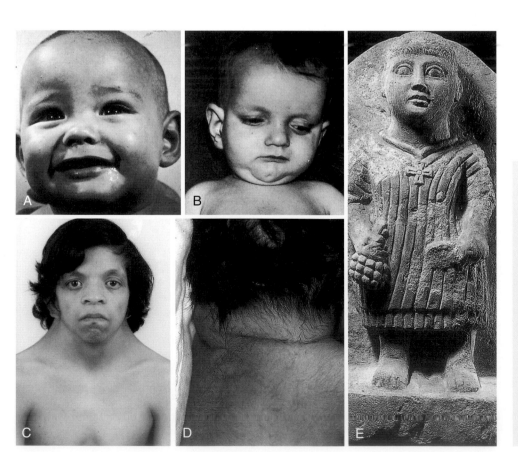

FIGURE 11-8 A, The chubby, round, bloated face of an infant with typical mobile dome-shaped pulmonary valve stenosis. **B,** Facial appearance of arteriohepatic dysplasia (Alagille syndrome) characterized by deeply set eyes, overhanging forehead, and small pointed chin. **C,** Noonan's syndrome in an 18-year-old man phenotype with webbing of the neck, low-set ears, abnormal auricles, hypertelorism, and small chin. **D,** Low posterior hairline of a neonate with Noonan's syndrome. **E,** Fourth century AD stele of a phenotypic male with the short stature and broad webbed neck suggesting Noonan's syndrome.

usually normal for age despite intrauterine growth retardation. Stenosis of the pulmonary artery and its branches and patent ductus arteriosis (see Chapter 20) are the most frequent types of coexisting congenital heart disease.[60]

Williams syndrome includes a small chin, large mouth, patulous lips, blunt upturned nose, wide-set eyes, broad forehead, baggy cheeks, and malformed teeth (see Chapter 7). The most frequent coexisting congenital heart disease is pulmonary artery stenosis with supravalvular aortic stenosis (see Chapter 7).

Alagille syndrome, also called arteriohepatic dysplasia or the Alagille-Watson syndrome, is an autosomal dominant disorder with abnormalities of liver, eyes, kidneys, and skeleton.[61,62] Facial appearance is characterized by a prominent overhanging forehead, deep-set eyes, and a small pointed chin (Figure 11-8B).[61-63] The most frequent coexisting congenital heart disease is stenosis of the pulmonary artery and its branches.[62]

Cornelia de Lange's syndrome expresses itself with low birth weight, slow growth, small stature, microcephaly, thin eyebrows that meet at midline, long eyelashes, short upturned nose, thin downturned lips, hirsutism, small hands and feet, incurved fifth fingers, cleft palate, and missing limbs or portions of limbs. The incidence rate of pulmonary valve stenosis is reportedly 39%.[64]

Pulmonary stenosis also occurs in LEOPARD syndrome, which is characterized by multiple lentigines and café-au-lait spots.[65]

ARTERIAL PULSE

When severe pulmonary stenosis is accompanied by right ventricular failure, especially with coexisting left ventricular dysfunction, the arterial pulse is reduced. *Asymmetry* of right and left brachial and carotid arterial pulses (right greater than left) is a feature of supravalvular aortic stenosis that may accompany stenosis of the pulmonary artery and its branches (see Chapter 7).

JUGULAR VENOUS PULSE

The jugular venous A wave is distinctive and increases progressively as the stenosis increases (Figures 11-8A and 11-9), culminating in a giant A wave that *leaps to the eye, towering above and dwarfing the other waves of the venous* pulse.[27] Powerful right atrial contraction generates a giant A wave via the superior vena cava and a presystolic liver pulse via the inferior cava. With the advent of right ventricular failure and tricuspid regurgitation, the large A wave is accompanied by an increase in the V wave. The liver then manifests presystolic *and* systolic pulsations.

PRECORDIAL MOVEMENT AND PALPATION

The thrill associated with pulmonary *valve stenosis* is maximal in the second left intercostal space, with radiation upward and to the left because the intrapulmonary

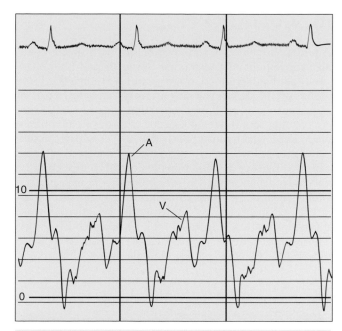

FIGURE 11-9 Prominent right atrial A wave in a 4-year-old girl with pulmonary valve stenosis and a systolic gradient of 50 mm Hg.

jet is directed upward and toward the left pulmonary artery (see Figure 11-35A).[3] When secondary hypertrophic subpulmonary stenosis coexists, the thrill is maximal in the third or fourth left intercostal space (see Figure 11-3).

Palpation of the right ventricular impulse is best achieved with applying the fingertips between the ribs along the left sternal edge during full held exhalation or with applying a single fingertip against the diaphragm in the subzyphoid area.[66,67] The subzyphoid technique is especially useful in infants because rapid respiratory excursions interfere with parasternal palpation.

The gentle right ventricular impulse of mild pulmonary valve stenosis is more readily palpated after exercise or in infants after the stress of feeding or crying. In severe pulmonary valve stenosis, the right ventricular impulse is forceful and sustained and is detected up to and including the third intercostal space.[66-68] *Infundibular* pulmonary stenosis relegates the high-pressure zone to the inflow portion of the right ventricle, so the accompanying impulse is assigned to the fourth and fifth left intercostal spaces. *Subinfundibular* stenosis is accompanied by a deceptively unimpressive right ventricular impulse confined to the fifth interspace or subxyphoid area. The pulmonary trunk is necessarily distal to the stenosis and cannot be palpated despite conspicuous dilation.

A *presystolic* impulse along the lower left sternal border and in the subxyphoid area (see Figure 11-7B) indicates presystolic distention of the right ventricle in response to the increased force of right atrial contraction that is also responsible for the large jugular venous A wave (see Figure 11-7A). A prominent pulmonary ejection sound is occasionally palpable in the second left intercostal space during held exhalation.

AUSCULTATION

A pulmonary ejection sound coincides with abrupt cephalad movement of the mobile dome-shaped pulmonary valve (see Figures 11-1B, upper, and 11-3) and is therefore an important sign in the auscultatory characterization of right ventricular outflow obstruction (Figure 11-10).[67,69] An ejection sound does not occur with dysplastic pulmonary valves, which move poorly if at all,[5] or with fixed subvalvular or pulmonary artery stenosis.[67] An ejection sound can also originate in a functionally normal bicuspid pulmonary valve.[70] The sound is recognized by its high-pitched clicking quality, by its maximal intensity in the second left intercostal space, and by its distinctive selective decrease during inspiration (Figures 11-11 through 11-13).[67,71,72] The inspiratory decrease is related to the reduced cephalad movement available to the mobile valve as the right

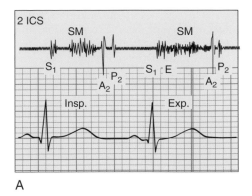

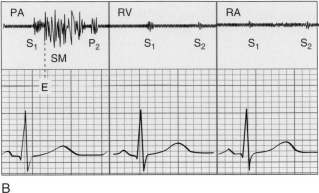

B

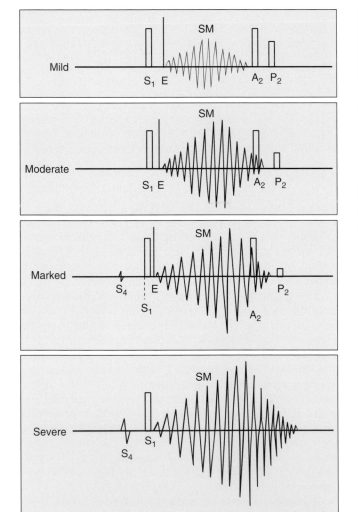

FIGURE 11-10 Schematic phonocardiograms illustrating the auscultatory signs of mild to severe mobile dome-shaped pulmonary valve stenosis. (S₁ = first heart sound; E = pulmonary ejection sound; SM = systolic murmur; A₂ = aortic component of the second sound; P₂ = pulmonary component of the second sound; S₄ = fourth heart sound.)

FIGURE 11-11 Phonocardiograms from a 9-year-old girl with mild mobile dome-shaped pulmonary valve stenosis (gradient, 25 mm Hg). **A,** In the second left intercostal space (2 ICS), the pulmonary ejection sound (E) is absent during inspiration (Insp) and present during expiration (Exp). A systolic murmur (SM) diminishes before the aortic component of the second heart sound (A₂). The pulmonary component of the second sound (P₂) is clearly evident and delayed. The split widened further during inspiration and narrowed but persisted during expiration. **B,** A phonocardiogram from within the main pulmonary artery (PA) showed an amplified midsystolic murmur (SM) that promptly vanished when the catheter tip microphone was withdrawn into the right ventricle (RV). (RA = right atrium.)

ventricle contracts.[71] The inspiratory increase in right atrial contractile force is transmitted into the right ventricle and onto the undersurface of the mobile pulmonary valve, which moves into a relatively cephalad position.[73] Additional cephalad movement is necessarily reduced, so the ejection sound is reduced or vanishes altogether.[71] Conversely, right atrial contractile force decreases during expiration, leaving the mobile pulmonary valve in a slack position, so right ventricular contraction induces maximal cephalad movement and maximal intensity of the ejection sound.[71]

The interval between the first heart sound and the ejection sound varies inversely with the degree of stenosis (see Figure 11-10).[69,74] As severity increases, the velocity of right ventricular contraction increases, the pulmonary valve opens earlier, and the ejection sound occurs earlier and merges with the first heart sound (see Figure 11-10) but retains its distinctive respiratory variation that

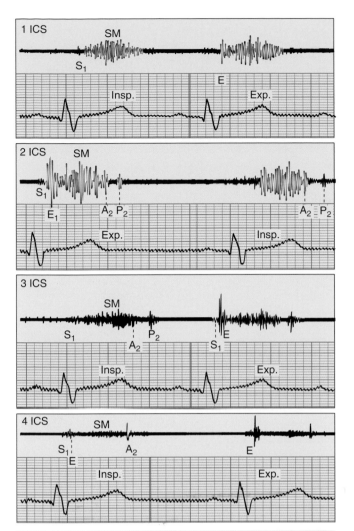

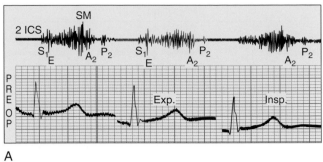

A

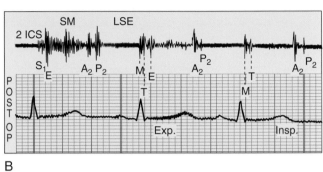

B

FIGURE 11-13 Phonocardiograms from a 21-year-old woman with mobile dome-shaped pulmonary valve stenosis and a gradient of 80 mm Hg. **A,** Before pulmonary valvotomy (PRE OP), the systolic murmur (SM) peaked late and enveloped the aortic component of the second sound (A_2). The pulmonary component (P_2) was soft and delayed. A pulmonary ejection sound (E) was recorded during expiration (Exp) but was absent during inspiration (Insp). **B,** After valvotomy (POST OP), the gradient fell to 20 mm Hg, and the phonocardiogram resembled mild pulmonary valve stenosis (see Figures 11-10 and 11-11). (M = mitral component of the first sound; T = tricuspid component.)

FIGURE 11-12 Phonocardiograms from the first through the fourth left intercostal spaces (1 ICS through 4 ICS) of a 12-year-old boy with mobile dome-shaped pulmonary valve stenosis and a gradient of 50 mm Hg. The midsystolic murmur goes up to the aortic component of the second sound (A_2) and is maximal in the second intercostal space with radiation upward and to the left. The pulmonary ejection sound vanishes during inspiration and is prominent during expiration. The second sound is widely split because a soft pulmonary component (P_2) is delayed. The splitting increased further during inspiration.

distinguishes it from a loud first heart sound.[74,75] Accordingly, a pulmonary ejection sound that occurs at a well-defined interval after the first heart sound is a sign of mild pulmonary valve stenosis and an ejection sound that merges with the first heart sound is a sign of severe pulmonary stenosis. Fibrosis and calcification in older patients impair mobility, so the ejection sound decreases or disappears altogether.

The murmur of pulmonary valve stenosis was recognized in 1858 by Peacock.[7] The maximum precordial site is the second left intercostal space (see Figures 11-11 through 11-13), which topographically overlies the pulmonary trunk and coincides with the location of the murmur recorded with intracardiac phonocardiography (see

Figure 11-11B).[67] Prominence of the murmur in the *third* left intercostal space occurs with secondary hypertrophic subpulmonary stenosis (Figures 11-3 and 11-14B). The murmur radiates upward and to the left (see Figure 11-12) because the intrapulmonary jet is directed upward and to the left (see Figure 11-35A). Loud systolic murmurs radiate into the suprasternal notch and the base of the neck, especially the left side. Intensity varies directly with the degree of obstruction, but intensity *per se* is not necessarily an index of severity. In neonates with *pinpoint pulmonary stenosis*, the murmur is deceptively soft (see Figure 11-1A,B, lower). Grade 3/6 murmurs are features of mild pulmonary stenosis (see Figure 11-11), and grade 3/6 to 6/6 murmurs are features of moderate to severe pulmonary stenosis (see Figures 11-12 through 11-14).

The severity determines the duration of right ventricular ejection, which in turn determines the duration of the systolic murmur. The length of the murmur relative to the aortic component of the second heart sound permits comparison of the duration of right and left ventricular ejection (see Figure 11-10). When pulmonary stenosis is mild, right ventricular remains normal, so a symmetric systolic murmur ends before the aortic component of the second sound (see Figures 11-10 and

INFUNDIBULAR

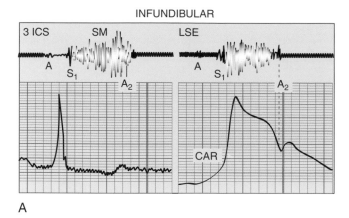

A

VALVULAR

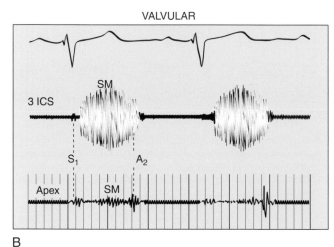

B

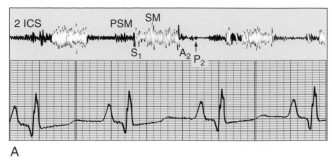

A

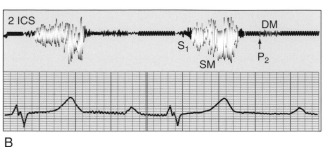

B

FIGURE 11-15 **A,** Phonocardiogram from a 10-month-old female with mobile dome-shaped pulmonary valve stenosis and a 95–mm Hg gradient. The right atrial A wave of 17 to 20 mm Hg coincided with a presystolic murmur (PSM). A long systolic murmur (SM) encroached on the aortic component of the second heart sound (A_2). The faint pulmonary component (P_2) was considerably delayed. **B,** Phonocardiogram in the second intercostal space (2 ICS) of a 6-year-old boy with mobile dome-shaped pulmonary valve stenosis and a gradient of 100 mm Hg. A faint diastolic murmur (DM) began with a markedly delayed pulmonary component of the second heart sound (P_2). The long kite-shaped systolic murmur enveloped the aortic component of the second heart sound.

FIGURE 11-14 **A,** Phonocardiogram from a 34-year-old man with severe infundibular pulmonary stenosis (gradient, 140 mm Hg). A long systolic murmur (SM) enveloped the aortic component of the second heart sound (A_2) and was equally prominent in the third intercostal space (3 ICS) and at the lower left sternal edge (LSE). **B,** Phonocardiogram from a 14-year-old boy with mobile dome-shaped pulmonary valve stenosis and a gradient of 115 mm Hg. The systolic murmur enveloped the aortic component of the second sound (A_2) and was prominent in the third left intercostal space (3 ICS) because of secondary hypertrophic subpulmonary stenosis. (S_4 = fourth heart sound; CAR = carotid pulse.)

11-11).[75] When stenosis is moderate, the murmur ends at or slightly after the aortic component of the second sound, which remains audible (see Figures 11-10 and 11-12).[75] When stenosis is severe, the murmur extends *beyond* the aortic component, which is partially or completely obscured (see Figures 11-10, 11-13 and 11-14).[75] With a still greater increase in severity, the murmur lengthens further, peaks later in systole, and assumes an asymmetric kite shape.[74,75] Figure 11-10 illustrates the relationship between the duration and configuration of the systolic murmur and the degree of pulmonary stenosis. The holosystolic murmur of tricuspid regurgitation accompanying right ventricular failure is distinguished by its high frequency, its location along the lower left or right sternal edge, and its selective increase during inspiration.

Stenosis of the ostium of the infundibulum (see Figures 11-32 and 11-37) is accompanied by a murmur that is maximal in the third and fourth left intercostal spaces (see Figure 11-14).[27,75] *Subinfundibular* stenosis assigns the murmur still lower—to the *fourth* or *fifth* left intercostal space.[76]

Several types of *diastolic murmurs* occur, although rarely, in pulmonary valve stenosis. A low-intensity *atrial systolic murmur* is attributed to presystolic flow across the pulmonary valve (Figure 11-15A).[69] Powerful right atrial contraction generates a giant A wave that exceeds the diastolic pressure in the pulmonary trunk, so the pulmonary valve opens before the onset of ventricular contraction, permitting presystolic flow and a presystolic murmur (see Figure 11-38).[67,69,75] Presystolic murmurs are occasionally generated by prolonged vibrations of a fourth heart sound,[67] and soft diastolic murmurs have been attributed to low-pressure pulmonary regurgitation (Figures 11-15B, 11-35B, and 11-38).[69,75] Dysplastic or calcific pulmonary valves[77] are rarely incompetent.

Murmurs associated with *pulmonary artery stenosis* are typically confined to systole (Figures 11-16 and 11-17) but exceptionally continue into diastole.[13,78] The racic distribution is determined by the locations of the stenotic pulmonary artery segments, which are usually

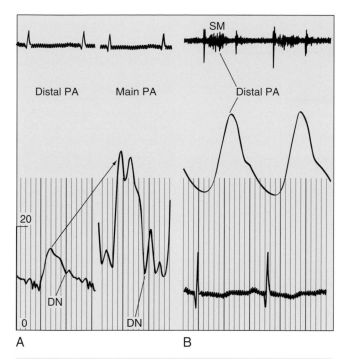

FIGURE 11-16 Tracings from a 4-year-old girl with stenosis of the pulmonary artery and its branches. **A,** Pressure pulses from within the distal pulmonary artery (PA) and main pulmonary artery (PA) established the systolic gradient and illustrated the distinctive contour of the main pulmonary arterial pressure pulse, which was characterized by a rapid rise, a rapid descent, and a low dicrotic notch (DN). **B,** Phonocardiogram from within a distal pulmonary artery (PA) recorded a crescendo-decrescendo systolic murmur (SM).

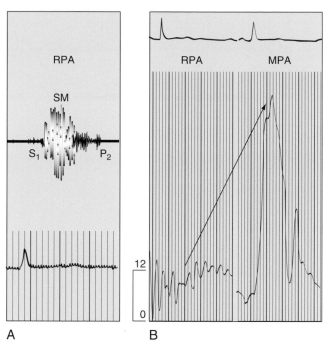

FIGURE 11-17 Tracings from a 19-year-old man with pulmonary artery stenosis. **A,** Intracardiac phonocardiogram from the distal right pulmonary artery (RPA) recorded a delayed crescendo decrescendo systolic murmur (SM). **B,** As the catheter was withdrawn from the distal right pulmonary artery (RPA) into the main pulmonary artery (MPA), a gradient was recorded *(oblique arrow)* together with the distinctive contour of the main pulmonary artery pressure pulse (see Figure 11-16A). The systolic gradient did not continue into diastole, so the murmur was confined to systole.

multiple and involve the pulmonary trunk and the proximal and distal branches (see Figures 11-4 and 11-5B). The accompanying murmurs are heard *anteriorly* in the vicinity of the second left and right intercostal spaces and are heard *peripherally* in the axillae and back (Figure 11-18).[13] An attempt should be made to distinguish murmurs that originate peripherally from a loud central murmur that radiates widely. Peripheral pulmonary systolic murmurs from high flow accompany uncomplicated atrial septal defect and are difficult to distinguish from murmurs of coexisting pulmonary artery stenosis.[78] Healthy neonates, especially when premature, experience a physiologic drop in systolic pressure from pulmonary trunk to proximal branches. This pressure drop is accompanied by peripheral pulmonary systolic murmurs that vanish as the lungs mature (see Chapter 2).[14,15]

Systolic murmurs of *pulmonary artery stenosis* are crescendo-decrescendo (see Figures 11-16 and 11-17) with delayed onset because of their relatively distal origins (see Figure 11-17). Stenoses that originate at or near the bifurcation of the pulmonary trunk generate murmurs that occasionally reach grade 4/6 in the second left intercostal space, but as a rule, the central precordial murmur is grade 3/6 and the peripheral murmurs are softer. When the intensities of precordial and nonprecordial murmurs are equal, one can assume that the widespread nonprecordial murmurs originate peripherally. Intrapulmonary

phonocardiograms confirm that systolic murmurs originate distal to stenoses in the pulmonary trunk and proximal pulmonary arterial branches (see Figures 11-16 through 11-18). Peripheral pulmonary systolic murmurs are overlooked because of their low intensity and because auscultation is not routinely conducted at nonprecordial sites. The difficulty is compounded in infants because of rapid respiratory rates and because the frequency composition of breath sounds is close to the frequency of composition of peripheral pulmonary systolic murmurs. The diaphragm of the stethoscope should be applied during held respiration with the patient supine, prone, and sitting comfortably.

Continuous murmurs imply continuous gradients across the stenotic sites, but recordings of pressure pulses proximal and distal to the zones of stenosis show that systolic gradients seldom continue into diastole.[79] The central pulmonary arterial pulse is characterized by an elevated *systolic* pressure and a rapid fall to diastolic levels that are normal or nearly so (Figures 11-17 and 11-19). Gradients are confined to *systolic*, so the accompanying murmur is confined to systole (see Figures 11-17 and 11-19).[79] Why, then, do continuous murmurs occur at all? It has been postulated that systolic expansion of the high-pressure pulmonary trunk proximal to the stenosis sets the stage for brisk diastolic flow across the distal

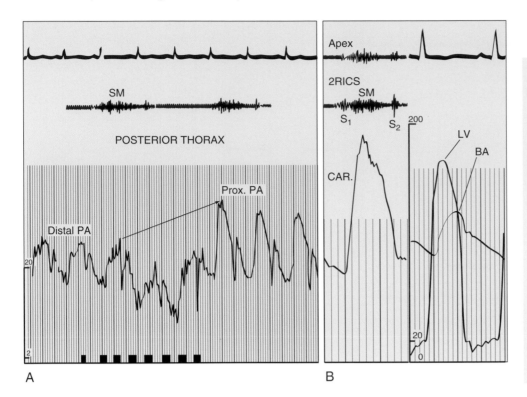

FIGURE 11-18 Recordings from a 7-year-old boy with pulmonary artery stenosis and supravalvular aortic stenosis. **A,** Phonocardiogram from the posterior thorax shows the peripheral pulmonary stenotic murmur (SM). As the catheter was withdrawn from distal to proximal pulmonary artery (PA), a systolic gradient was recorded *(oblique arrow)* together with the distinctive contour of the proximal pulmonary artery pressure pulse. **B,** Phonocardiogram in the second right intercostal space (2RICS) recorded the supravalvular aortic stenotic murmur (SM). The left ventricular (LV) and brachial arterial (BA) pressure pulses reflect the supravalvular gradient. (CAR = carotid pulse.)

segments as the expanded proximal segments recoil.[79] Modest diastolic flow following a large systolic gradient explains the occasional occurrence of a soft low-frequency diastolic murmur that precedes a prominent systolic murmur. Pulmonary artery stenosis may also give rise to increased flow through bronchial arterial collaterals.[80] Angiographically demonstrated bronchial collaterals are believed to be responsible for continuous murmurs.[81]

Splitting of the second heart sound and the intensity of the pulmonary component are important signs in the auscultatory characterization of obstruction to right ventricular outflow. In typical mobile dome-shaped pulmonary valve stenosis, the intensity of the pulmonary component varies from normal to inaudible as severity increases (see Figures 11-10 through 11-15). However, timing is more important than intensity in assessment of severity.[69,74] The more severe the stenosis, the longer the duration of right ventricular ejection, the later the timing of pulmonary valve closure, and the wider the split (see Figure 11-10). With mild stenosis, splitting is mild (see Figure 11-11).[82] With severe stenosis, splitting may be as great as 120 to 140 msec (see Figure 11-15) and, if heard at all, is fixed because right ventricular stroke volume is fixed.[82] The long systolic murmur of severe pulmonary stenosis obscures the aortic component of the second sound, and the soft pulmonary component may be inaudible (see Figures 11-10 and 11-14).[69,82,83] When stenosis is mild, the pulmonary component may be delayed by the increased capacitance of the pulmonary vascular bed associated with dilation of the pulmonary trunk and its proximal branches.[75,82–84] These qualifications notwithstanding, a slight increase in splitting with normal intensity of the pulmonary component favors mild stenosis (see Figure 11-11) and a marked increase in

splitting with a faint or inaudible pulmonary component favors severe stenosis (see Figures 11-14 and 11-15).

In *pulmonary artery stenosis*, factors that influence the behavior of the second heart sound differ from those that influence the second sound in valvular or subvalvular stenosis.[78] Stenosis of the pulmonary artery and its branches is unique among causes of pulmonary hypertension because it elevates systolic but not diastolic pressure in the pulmonary trunk. Accordingly, the valve closes at a normal or near normal pressure, so the intensity of the pulmonary component of the second sound is normal (Figures 11-19 through 11-21).[13,78,85] The abruptness with which the leaflets seat affects the intensity of the pulmonary component of the second heart sound. The cusps might bulge abruptly toward the right ventricle during isometric relaxation, suddenly increasing the volume capacity of the pulmonary trunk. In pulmonary artery stenosis, the intensity of the pulmonary second sound remains unchanged as severity increases[78] in contrast to mobile dome-shaped pulmonary valve stenosis or fixed subvalvular stenosis in which the intensity of the pulmonary component varies inversely with the degree of stenosis. The timing of pulmonary valve closure cannot be judged with criteria that apply to valvular or fixed subvalvular pulmonary stenosis, both of which prolong right ventricular ejection. Potential prolongation of right ventricular ejection in pulmonary artery stenosis is countered by the rapidity with which the pulmonary artery pressure falls from its systolic peak (see Figure 11-17). The second heart sound is therefore normally split even in the presence of appreciable obstruction[10]; the degree of splitting varies appropriately with respiration (see Figures 11-20 and 11-21).[78]

Abrahams and Wood[27] drew attention to the significance of fourth heart sounds in pulmonary stenosis,

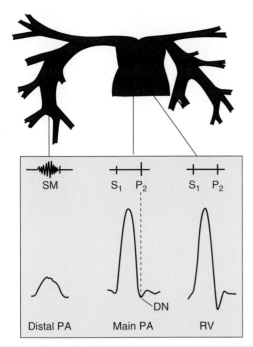

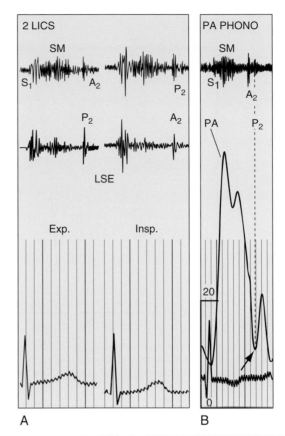

FIGURE 11-19 Illustrations of the anatomic, phonocardiographic (intracardiac), and hemodynamic features of pulmonary artery stenosis. A systolic murmur (SM) originates in the pulmonary artery segment distal to the stenosis. In the main pulmonary artery (PA), the pressure pulse is characterized by a rapid rise, an elevated peak, and a rapid descent to a low dicrotic notch (DN). The gradient does not continue into diastole, so the accompanying murmur is systolic. The pulmonary component of the second heart sound (P_2) is not increased because the pulmonary valve closes at a low pressure. (DN = dicrotic notch; S_1 = first heart sound; P_2 = pulmonary component of the second heart sound.)

FIGURE 11-20 Recordings from a 4-year-old girl with pulmonary artery stenosis. **A,** Phonocardiogram in the second left intercostal space (2 LICS) recorded a midsystolic murmur (SM) followed by normal splitting of the second heart sound with normal intensity of the pulmonary component. **B,** Phonocardiogram (PHONO) and pressure pulse from within the proximal pulmonary artery (PA). The pulmonary component of the second heart sound (P_2) is soft because the valve closed at a low pressure despite systolic hypertension. A short systolic murmur (SM) was recorded in the pulmonary trunk. (A_2, P_2 = aortic and pulmonary components of the second sound; LSE = left sternal edge; Exp = expiration; Insp = inspiration.)

reasoning that "strong right atrial contraction in presystole helps the hypertrophied right ventricle generate a high systolic pressure." This was considered "an example of Starling's law of the heart, strong atrial systole augmenting late diastolic distention of the right ventricle so that the chamber contracts more forceably."[27] Presystolic distension of the right ventricle and fourth heart sounds are features of severe pulmonary stenosis because these physiologic conditions prevail when obstruction to right ventricular outflow is severe (Figures 11-7B, 11-10, and 11-22).[69]

ELECTROCARDIOGRAM

As severity increases, P waves become tall and peaked (Figure 11-23).[86] Giant P waves occasionally appear especially in lead 2 (Figure 11-24). The P wave in lead V_1 may be entirely negative because the P terminal force is written by a dilated right atrium (see Figure 11-24).[87] PR interval prolongation has been attributed to an increase in right atrial size that prolongs the transit time from sinus node to atrioventricular node (Figure 11-25).[22] Right axis deviation tends to vary with right ventricular systolic pressure (Figures 11-23 through 11-26).[49] Superior orientation of the QRS axis occurs in infants with pulmonary artery stenosis and the rubella syndrome.[88]

R wave amplitude in lead V_1 and R/S ratio in leads V_1 and V_6 are closely coupled with severity (Figures 11-23 through 11-27).[49,89] After infancy, the R wave in lead V_1 is normally less than 8 mm; and in children, an R wave amplitude greater than 10 mm is exceptional. With severe pulmonary stenosis, the R wave in lead V_1 is tall and monophasic, and lead V_6 exhibits a reciprocally deep S wave (see Figures 11-23 and 11-24). Children tend to generate higher R waves in lead V_1 than adults with similar gradients.

The configuration of the QRS in lead V_1 varies (see Figure 11-27). In mild pulmonary stenosis, an rSr′ is difficult to distinguish from normal.[80,90,91] With greater degrees of stenosis, the terminal R wave becomes taller, writing an rsR pattern (see Figure 11-26),[80] or a small r wave appears as a notch on the upstroke of a tall R prime (see Figures 11-26 and 11-27). In severe pulmonary stenosis, the pattern in lead V_1 is either a monophasic R wave (see Figures 11-23 and 11-24) or a qR, with the q wave reflecting right

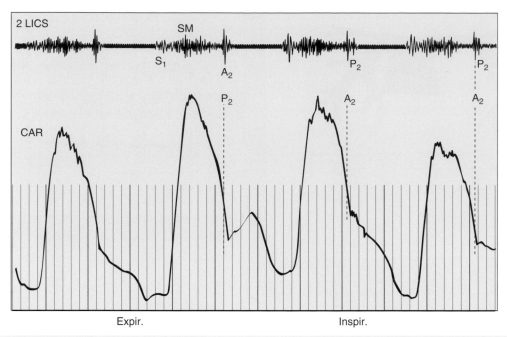

FIGURE 11-21 Phonocardiogram from a 5-year-old boy with pulmonary artery stenosis and 63–mm Hg gradient. A midsystolic murmur (SM) was recorded in the second left intercostal space (2 LICS). The second sound split normally. The pulmonary component (P₂) was neither increased nor delayed. (CAR = carotid pulse; Expir = expiration; Inspir = inspiration.)

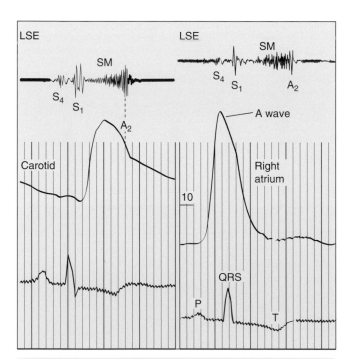

FIGURE 11-22 Recordings from a 23-year-old woman with severe mobile dome-shaped pulmonary valve stenosis and a gradient of 118 mm Hg. The fourth heart sound (S₄) at the lower left sternal edge (LSE) coincided with a large A wave in the right atrium. The soft systolic murmur (SM) at the lower sternal edge increased to grade 4 in the second left interspace (not shown).

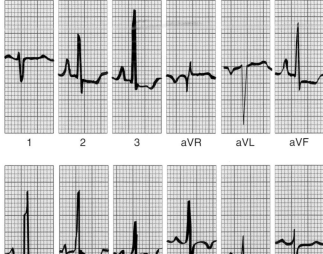

FIGURE 11-23 Electrocardiogram from a 43-year-old woman with mobile dome-shaped pulmonary valve stenosis and a gradient of 135 mm Hg. Tall peaked right atrial P waves appear in leads 2, 3, and aVF. Right ventricular hypertrophy is manifested by right axis deviation, tall monophasic R waves in right precordial leads that indicate suprasystemic right ventricular systolic pressure, coved ST segments with inverted T waves in right/mid precordial leads, and deep S waves in the left precordium.

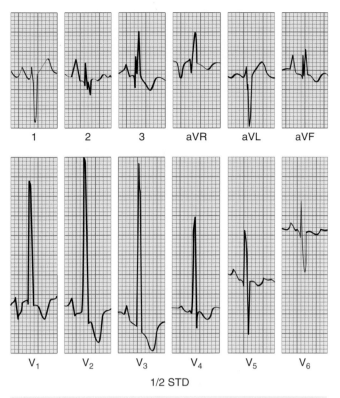

1/2 STD

FIGURE 11-24 Electrocardiogram from an 8-month-old female with mobile dome-shaped pulmonary valve stenosis and suprasystemic right ventricular pressure. A tall peaked right atrial P wave is present in lead 2. The right atrial P wave abnormality in lead V_1 is characterized by negativity (compare with lead aVR). Right ventricular hypertrophy is manifested by right axis deviation, striking monophasic R waves, and deeply inverted T waves in right precordial leads and deep S waves in left precordial leads, patterns that are typical of suprasystemic right ventricular systolic pressure.

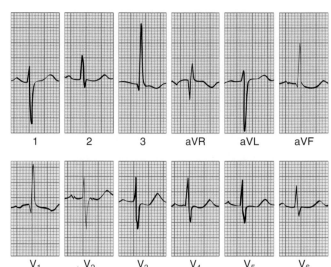

FIGURE 11-25 Electrocardiogram from a 16-year-old girl with mobile dome-shaped pulmonary valve stenosis and a gradient of 70 mm Hg. The PR interval is 200 msec. Right ventricular hypertrophy is manifested by right axis deviation and a monophasic R wave in lead V_1. The qR complex in lead V_1 is similar to the qR complex in lead aVR, which is evidence of right atrial enlargement.

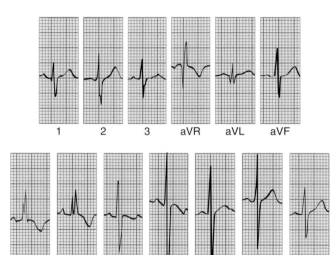

FIGURE 11-26 Electrocardiogram from a 2-year-old girl with stenosis of the main pulmonary artery and a gradient of 46 mm Hg. Right ventricular hypertrophy is indicated by the rightward, superior, and anterior direction of the QRS axis; the tall R wave in lead aVR; the rR prime in lead V_3R; and deep S waves in mid and left precordial leads.

atrial enlargement (see Figure 11-25). The neonate with pinpoint pulmonary stenosis and a small right ventricular cavity has an electrocardiogram that resembles pulmonary atresia with intact ventricular septum, namely a normal QRS axis and adult progression in precordial leads (Figure 11-28).[92] In *subinfundibular* pulmonary stenosis (double-chambered right ventricle), a smaller portion of right ventricle is in the high-pressure compartment, so the degree of right ventricular hypertrophy in leads V_{1-3} is appreciably less than expected based on the severity of stenosis alone.[76]

In healthy neonates, upright right precordial T waves become inverted by 4 days of age. In infants and children with *mild* pulmonary stenosis, upright right precordial T waves may persist as the *only* electrocardiographic sign of elevated right ventricular systolic pressure (Figure 11-29).[93] In severe pulmonary stenosis, the T wave direction shifts leftward, superiorly and posteriorly, as the QRS axis shifts to the right and anteriorly. The QRS-T angle widens, so inverted T waves appear in leads 2, 3, and aVF and in right precordial leads (see Figures 11-23 and 11-24). Deeply inverted T waves that cove upward on their descending limbs and are accompanied by ST segment depressions extending beyond

lead V_2 are features of severe pulmonary stenosis (see Figures 11-23 and 11-24).

Noonan's syndrome with dysplastic pulmonary valve stenosis has an electrocardiogram that differs from the patterns just described. Axis deviation may be extreme,[5,94] the QRS tends to be splintered and prolonged, and a QS pattern appears in inferior and left precordial leads.[29] However, the pattern of left axis deviation,

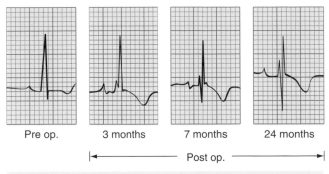

Pre op.	3 months	7 months	24 months
	|←	Post op.	→|

FIGURE 11-27 Preoperative and postoperative lead V_1 in a 6-year-old girl with mobile dome-shaped pulmonary valve stenosis and a prevalvotomy gradient of 100 mm Hg. The postoperative sequence is electrocardiographic evidence of regression of right ventricular hypertrophy. The tall monophasic preoperative R wave sequentially became an rR prime, an rsR prime, and 24 months later, an rSr prime, where it remained.

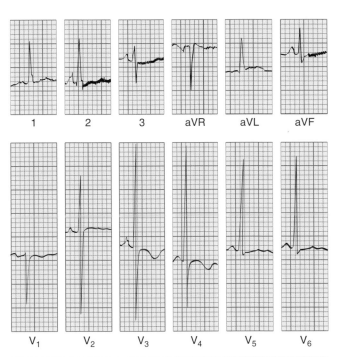

FIGURE 11-28 Electrocardiogram from a 9-day-old male with pinpoint pulmonary valve stenosis and a thick-walled right ventricle with small cavity size. Peaked right atrial P waves appear in leads 2 and V_3. The QRS axis and the r wave in lead V_1 are normal because of the small cavity size of the right ventricle.

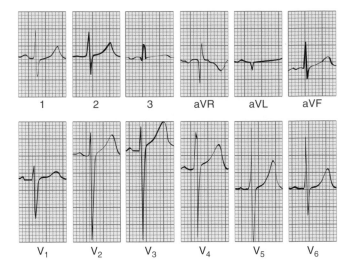

FIGURE 11-29 Electrocardiogram from a 5-year-old boy with mild mobile dome-shaped pulmonary valve stenosis (gradient, 25 mm Hg). The tracing is normal except for upright right precordial T waves.

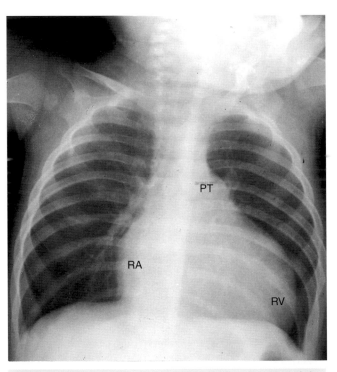

FIGURE 11-30 X-ray from a 10-month-old female with mobile dome-shaped pulmonary valve stenosis and suprasystemic right ventricular systolic pressure. Pulmonary vascularity is reduced, the pulmonary trunk (PT) is dilated, the right atrium (RA) is enlarged, and a dilated convex right ventricle (RV) occupies the apex.

abnormal R/S ratio over the left precordium with abnormal Q waves is related to the syndrome *per se* and not to a specific accompanying cardiac defect.[95]

X-RAY

Pulmonary vascularity remains normal, even in severe pulmonary stenosis, until the right ventricle fails and blood flow to the lungs declines (Figure 11-30). Flow to the right lung is occasionally less than flow to the left lung (unequal distribution).[96] Radiologic signs of *pulmonary artery stenosis* include zones of segmental hypovascularity that correspond to locations of the arterial obstructions and areas of fusiform intrapulmonary dilation beyond the zones of stenosis (Figures 11-4, 11-5B, and 11-31).[13]

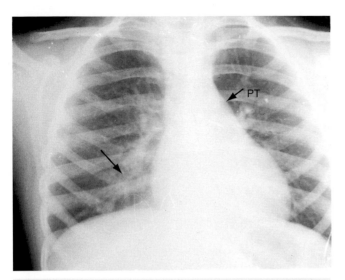

FIGURE 11-31 X-ray from a 5-year-old girl with pulmonary artery stenosis and a gradient of 40 mm Hg. Vascular densities (arrow) adjacent to the right lower cardiac border are dilated intrapulmonary arteries distal to the zones of stenosis. The pulmonary trunk (PT) is virtually normal.

Conspicuous increases in right atrial and right ventricular size are radiologic signs of severity, especially when the enlargement appears at an early age (see Figure 11-30). The dilated right ventricle is rounded rather than boot-shaped, and its apex lies *above* the left hemidiaphragm (see Figure 11-30). The aortic arch is left-sided, with rare exceptions (Figure 11-32).[97] In Noonan's syndrome, in contrast to Turner's syndrome, ascending aortic dilation is rare (see Chapter 7).[98]

Typical mobile dome-shaped pulmonary valve stenosis is accompanied by conspicuous dilation of the pulmonary trunk (Figures 11-1, 11-3, 11-6, 11-30, and 11-33).[27] Dilation is present at an early age (see Figures 11-1

and 11-30) and may reach aneurysmal proportions (Figure 11-34) but without risk of rupture.[27,99,100] Dilation of the pulmonary trunk above a mobile dome-shaped pulmonary valve is related to intrinsic abnormalities of the media associated with the specific dome-shaped congenital valve morphology, not with its functional state.[2] Disproportionate dilation of the *left branch* often accompanies dilation of the pulmonary trunk (see Figure 11-1, upper).[101] The jet from the stenotic valve breaks up as it strikes the dome of the pulmonary trunk (Figure 11-35A and Video 11-1) whose left branch is a geometric continuation of the dilated trunk.[3] Calcification of a dome-shaped stenotic pulmonary valve is rare and is reserved for older adults,[4,102] although calcific deposits can be sequelae of infective endocarditis.[77] *Dysplastic* pulmonary valve stenosis is accompanied by comparatively little dilation of the pulmonary trunk (Figure 11-36), an observation that discounts turbulent flow as an cause of dilation.[2,5,6] Localized stenosis of the *ostium of the infundibulum* is characterized by slight indentation at that site, above which the infundibular chamber is moderately dilated (Figure 11-37).

ECHOCARDIOGRAM

Color flow imaging in typical mobile dome-shaped pulmonary valve stenosis discloses a high-velocity jet directed toward the left pulmonary artery (see Figure 11-35A).[103] Continuous wave Doppler scan establishes the velocity across the stenotic pulmonary valve from which the peak instantaneous gradient can be estimated (see Figure 11-35B).[103]

During right ventricular systole, the mobile pulmonary valve domes briskly cephalad as a single unit. A bicuspid pulmonary valve can occasionally be identified.[104] In severe pulmonary stenosis, the increased force of right atrial contraction is transmitted into the right ventricle

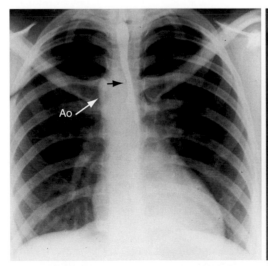
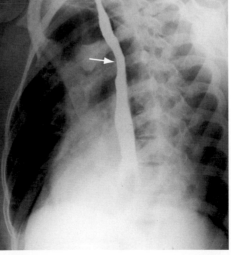

FIGURE 11-32 Posteroanterior and left anterior oblique x-rays from a 22-year-old woman with isolated stenosis of the ostium of the infundibulum and a gradient of 40 mm Hg. The pulmonary trunk is not border-forming. A right aortic arch (Ao) displaced the barium-filled esophagus to the left *(arrow)*, then descended along the right vertebral border. The left anterior oblique view shows posterior displacement of the barium-filled esophagus by the right aortic arch *(arrow)*.

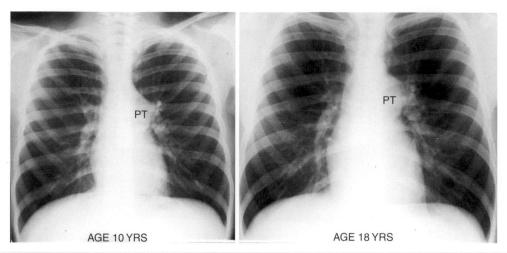

FIGURE 11-33 Identical cardiac silhouettes at 10 years and 18 years of age in a male with mild mobile dome-shaped pulmonary valve stenosis. The x-rays are normal except for conspicuous dilation of the pulmonary trunk (PT) and proximal branches. A 25–mm Hg gradient was unchanged.

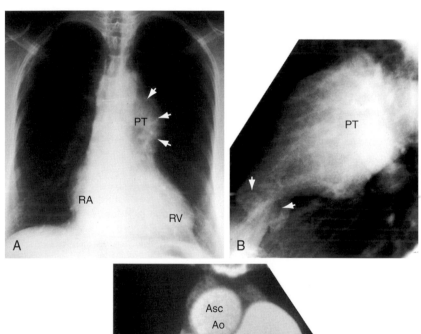

FIGURE 11-34 A, X-ray from a 61-year-old woman with mobile dome-shaped pulmonary valve stenosis and a gradient of 35 mm Hg. The pulmonary trunk (PT) is aneurysmal. A somewhat convex right atrium (RA) forms the lower right cardiac border. An enlarged right ventricle (RV) occupied the apex. **B,** Lateral angiogram visualizes the aneurysmal pulmonary trunk (PT) and the mobile dome-shaped pulmonary valve *(paired arrows).* **C,** Computed tomographic angiogram showing the aneurysmal pulmonary trunk (PT) and dilated right and left pulmonary artery branches (RPA, LPA). (Asc Ao = ascending aorta; RV = right ventricle; SVC = superior vena cava.)

onto the under surface of the mobile pulmonary valve, which opens in presystole, generating a Doppler signal (Figure 11-38; see previous discussion). Secondary hypertrophic subpulmonary stenosis is recognized as an envelope within the major continuous wave Doppler signal (see Figure 11-38). Mild pulmonary regurgitation is occasionally detected in the presence of pulmonary valve stenosis (see Figures 11-35B and 11-38).

The position of the atrial septum is imaged as concave to the left, reflecting the high pressure in the right atrium. Color flow detects a right-to-left interatrial shunt across a patent foramen ovale. Right atrial size can be estimated,

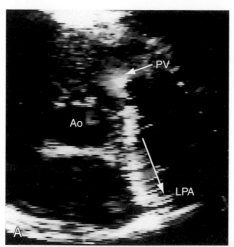

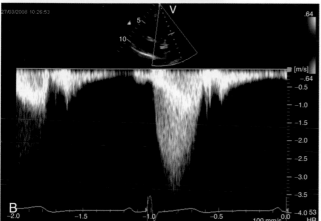

FIGURE 11-35 Echocardiogram with color flow imaging and Doppler scan interrogation from a 39-year-old woman with a dome-shaped pulmonary valve. **A,** Black- and-white rendition of a color flow image in the short axis shows a high-velocity jet originating at the stenotic pulmonary valve (PV) and entering the left pulmonary artery (LPA). **B,** Continuous wave Doppler scan across the stenotic pulmonary valve (Video 11-1). (Ao = aorta.)

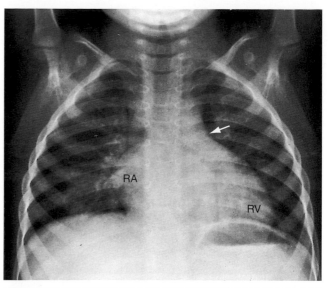

FIGURE 11-36 X-ray from a 3-year-old boy with dysplastic pulmonary valve stenosis (see Figure 11-2B). The pulmonary trunk is conspicuous by its absence *(arrow)*. A convex right atrium (RA) occupies the right lower cardiac border, and an enlarged right ventricle (RV) occupies the apex.

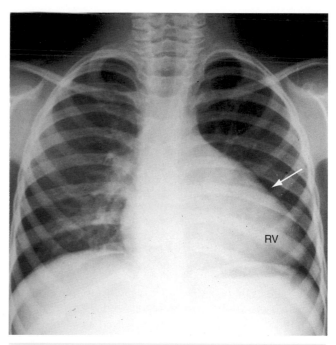

FIGURE 11-37 X-ray from a 5-year-old girl with severe fixed stenosis of the ostium of the infundibulum *(arrow)*, distal to which the infundibulum is moderately convex. An enlarged right ventricle (RV) occupies the apex. Hypovascularity of the upper lobe of the left lung was the result of isolated stenosis of the left pulmonary artery.

and the size, function, and degree of right ventricular hypertrophy can be established.[103] When pulmonary stenosis is severe, the ventricular septum thickens and flattens.[103] Color flow imaging determines the presence and degree of tricuspid regurgitation from which right ventricular systolic pressure can be estimated by the velocity of the regurgitant jet. Systolic and diastolic function of the *left ventricle* can and should be assessed because right ventricular pressure overload influences the function of the left ventricle (see previous discussion).[25,26]

Dysplastic pulmonary valve stenosis is imaged as thickened immobile leaflets. The pulmonary trunk is not significantly dilated. Stenosis of the *ostium of the infundibulum* and *subinfundibular stenosis* (double-chambered right ventricle) can be identified and physiologically assessed. *Pulmonary artery stenosis* is accompanied by a normal-sized pulmonary trunk and small proximal

pulmonary arteries. Doppler scan interrogation records the velocities across the sites of branch stenosis and distinguishes congenital pulmonary artery stenosis from the normal neonatal physiologic drop in systolic pressure between the pulmonary trunk and its proximal branches.[15]

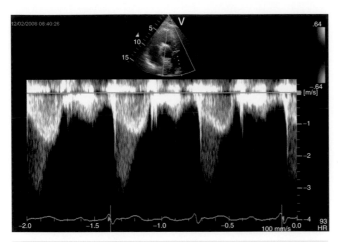

FIGURE 11-38 Continuous wave Doppler scan from a 32-year-old man with severe mobile dome-shaped pulmonary valve stenosis (PS) and secondary hypertrophic subpulmonary stenosis (compare with Figure 11-3). The asymmetric profile within the envelope of the continuous wave Doppler signal represents the gradient across the zone of secondary hypertrophic subpulmonary stenosis.

SUMMARY

The murmur of *mobile dome-shaped pulmonary valve stenosis* dates from birth. The physical appearance in infancy is sometimes represented by round bloated faces and well-developed fat pads. The jugular venous A wave is prominent, even giant; the right ventricular impulse is as high as the third left intercostal space. Auscultation detects a pulmonary ejection sound, a midsystolic systolic murmur that radiates upward and to the left, and a delayed soft pulmonary component of the second heart sound. A thrill is maximal in the second left intercostal space. The electrocardiogram shows right atrial P wave abnormalities and varying degrees of right ventricular hypertrophy. The chest x-ray discloses normal blood flow with dilation of the pulmonary trunk and its left branch. The echocardiogram is used to identify the mobile dome-shaped pulmonary valve, and continuous-wave Doppler scan is used to estimate the right ventricular systolic pressure and the gradient.

Dysplastic pulmonary valve stenosis is a feature of Noonan's syndrome that is recognized by a distinctive phenotype. Echocardiography is used to identify the thickened dysplastic cusps that exhibit little or no motion. Because of the limited mobility of the thickened dysplastic valve, a pulmonary ejection sound and the pulmonary component of the second heart sound are absent.

Stenosis of the ostium of the infundibulum is represented by a right ventricular impulse *below* the third left intercostal space, by absence of a pulmonary ejection sound, and by a midsystolic murmur that is maximal in the third left intercostal space. The x-ray shows a slight indentation at the site of the ostium above which the infundibular chamber is slightly convex. The pulmonary trunk is not dilated.

Subinfundibular stenosis (double-chambered right ventricle) is represented by a right ventricular impulse confined to the lower left sternal border or subxyphoid area, a midsystolic murmur below the third left intercostal space, absence of an ejection sound, a nondilated pulmonary trunk, an electrocardiogram that shows less right ventricular hypertrophy than anticipated for the estimated degree of stenosis, and an echocardiogram that images obstructing muscle bundles within the right ventricular cavity. A Doppler flow disturbance is within the right ventricle.

Pulmonary artery stenosis is accompanied by a murmur that may not be identified at birth. The history may disclose familial recurrence and hemoptysis from rupture of thin-walled intrapulmonary aneurysms distal to the sites of stenoses. The physical appearance of rubella syndrome or Williams syndrome constitutes important evidence. A pulmonary ejection sound is absent, there is normal intensity and splitting of the second heart sound, and widespread systolic murmurs are heard in the axillae and back. The x-ray shows no dilation of the pulmonary trunk but instead areas of segmental hypovascularity that correspond to locations of the arterial obstructions and areas of fusiform intrapulmonary dilation beyond the zones of stenosis.

REFERENCES

1. Morgagni GB. *The seats and causes of diseases investigated by anatomy.* London: Millar, Cadell, Johnson and Payne; 1769.
2. Niwa K, Perloff JK, Bhuta SM, et al. Structural abnormalities of great arterial walls in congenital heart disease: light and electron microscopic analyses. *Circulation.* 2001;103:393–400.
3. Muster AJ, Van Grondelle A, Paul MH. Unequal pressures in the central pulmonary arterial branches in patients with pulmonary stenosis. The influence of blood velocity and anatomy. *Pediatr Cardiol.* 1982;2:7–14.
4. Roberts WC, Mason DT, Morrow AG, Braunwald E. Calcific pulmonic stenosis. *Circulation.* 1968;37:973–978.
5. Koretzky ED, Moller JH, Korns ME, Schwartz CJ, Edwards JE. Congenital pulmonary stenosis resulting from dysplasia of valve. *Circulation.* 1969;40:43–53.
6. Schneeweiss A, Blieden LC, Shem-Tov A, Goor D, Milo S, Neufeld HN. Diagnostic angiocardiographic criteria in dysplastic stenotic pulmonic valve. *Am Heart J.* 1983;106:761–762.
7. Peacock TB. *On malformations of the human heart.* London: J. Churchill and Sons; 1866.
8. Keith A. The Hunterian lectures on malformations of the heart. *Lancet.* 1909;174:359–363.
9. Lucas Jr RV, Varco RL, Lillehei CW, Adams Jr P, Anderson RC, Edwards JE. Anomalous muscle bundle of the right ventricle. Hemodynamic consequences and surgical considerations. *Circulation.* 1962;25:443–455.
10. Perloff JK, Ronan Jr JA, De Leon Jr AC. Ventricular septal defect with the "two-chambered right ventricle" *Am J Cardiol.* 1965;16:894–900.
11. Yoo SJ, Kim YM, Bae EJ, Sohn S, Ko JK, Park IS. Rare variants of divided right ventricle with sequestered apical trabecular component. *Int J Cardiol.* 1997;60:249–255.
12. Oppenheimer EH. Partial atresia of the main branches of the pulmonary artery occurring in infancy and accompanied by calcification of the pulmonary artery and aorta. *Bulletin of the Johns Hopkins Hospital.* 1938;63:261.
13. Franch RH, Gay Jr BB. Congenital stenosis of the pulmonary artery branches. A classification, with postmortem findings in two cases. *Am J Med.* 1963;35:512–529.
14. Danilowicz DA, Rudolph AM, Hoffman JI, Heymann M. Physiologic pressure differences between main and branch pulmonary arteries in infants. *Circulation.* 1972;45:410–419.

15. Rodriguez RJ, Riggs TW. Physiologic peripheral pulmonic stenosis in infancy. *Am J Cardiol.* 1990;66:1478–1481.
16. Beuren AJ, Schulze C, Eberle P, Harmjanz D, Apitz J. The syndrome of supravalvular aortic stenosis, peripheral pulmonary stenosis, mental retardation and similar facial appearance. *Am J Cardiol.* 1964;13:471–483.
17. Levin DL, Heymann MA, Rudolph AM. Morphological development of the pulmonary vascular bed in experimental pulmonic stenosis. *Circulation.* 1979;59:179–182.
18. Gregg NM. Congenital cataract following German measles in the mother. *Trans Ophthalmol Soc Aust.* 1941;3:35–46.
19. Cochi SL, Edmonds LE, Dyer K, et al. Congenital rubella syndrome in the United States, 1970–1985. On the verge of elimination. *Am J Epidemiol.* 1989;129:349–361.
20. Munro ND, Sheppard S, Smithells RW, Holzel H, Jones G. Temporal relations between maternal rubella and congenital defects. *Lancet.* 1987;2:201–204.
21. Perloff JK. Myocardial growth and the development and regression of increased ventricular mass. In: Perloff JK, Child JS, Aboulhosn J, eds. *Congenital heart disease in adults.* 3rd ed. Philadelphia: Saunders/Elsevier; 2009.
22. Nakazawa M, Marks RA, Isabel-Jones J, Jarmakani JM. Right and left ventricular volume characteristics in children with pulmonary stenosis and intact ventricular septum. *Circulation.* 1976;53: 884–890.
23. Truccone NJ, Steeg CN, Dell R, Gersony WM. Comparison of the cardiocirculatory effects of exercise and isoproterenol in children with pulmonary or aortic valve stenosis. *Circulation.* 1977; 56:79–82.
24. Moller JH, Rao S, Lucas Jr RV. Exercise hemodynamics of pulmonary valvular stenosis. Study of 64 children. *Circulation.* 1972;46: 1018–1026.
25. Kelly DT, Spotnitz I IM, Beiser GD, Pierce JE, Epstein SE. Effects of chronic right ventricular volume and pressure loading on left ventricular performance. *Circulation.* 1971;44:403–412.
26. Stenberg RG, Fixler DE, Taylor AL, Corbett JR, Firth BG. Left ventricular dysfunction due to chronic right ventricular pressure overload. Resolution following percutaneous balloon valvuloplasty for pulmonic stenosis. *Am J Med.* 1988;84:157–161.
27. Abrahams DG, Wood P. Pulmonary stenosis with normal aortic root. *Br Heart J.* 1951;13:519–548.
28. Grech V. History, diagnosis, surgery and epidemiology of pulmonary stenosis in Malta. *Cardiol Young.* 1998;8:337–343.
29. Sanchez-Cascos A. The Noonan syndrome. *Eur Heart J.* 1983; 4:223–229.
30. Campbell M. Factors in the aetiology of pulmonary stenosis. *Br Heart J.* 1962;24:625–632.
31. Hsu J-H, Dai Z-K, Wu J-R, et al. Critical pulmonary stenosis in two successive siblings. *Int J Cardiol.* 2003;87:297–299.
32. Klinge T, Laursen HB. Familial pulmonary stenosis with underdeveloped or normal right ventricle. *Br Heart J.* 1975;37: 60–64.
33. Mccarron WE, Perloff JK. Familial congenital valvular pulmonic stenosis. *Am Heart J.* 1974;88:357–359.
34. Patterson DF, Haskins ME, Schnarr WR. Hereditary dysplasia of the pulmonary valve in beagle dogs. Pathologic and genetic studies. *Am J Cardiol.* 1981;47:631–641.
35. Baird PA, De Jong BP. Noonan's syndrome (XX and XY Turner phenotype) in three generations of a family. *J Pediatr.* 1972;80: 110–114.
36. Mendez HM, Opitz JM. Noonan syndrome: a review. *Am J Med Genet.* 1985;21:493–506.
37. Cullimore AJ, Smedstad KG, Brennan BG. Pregnancy in women with Noonan syndrome: report of two cases. *Obstet Gynecol.* 1999;93:813–816.
38. Noonan JA. Hypertelorism with Turner phenotype. A new syndrome with associated congenital heart disease. *Am J Dis Child.* 1968;116:373–380.
39. Wasserman MP, Varghese PJ, Rowe RD. The evolution of pulmonary arterial stenosis associated with congenital rubella. *Am Heart J.* 1968;76:638–644.
40. Hayes CJ, Gersony WM, Driscoll DJ, et al. Second natural history study of congenital heart defects. Results of treatment of patients with pulmonary valvar stenosis. *Circulation.* 1993; 87:128–137.
41. Johnson LW, Grossman W, Dalen JE, Dexter L. Pulmonic stenosis in the adult. Long-term follow-up results. *N Engl J Med.* 1972;287: 1159–1163.
42. Genovese PD, Rosenbaum D. Pulmonary stenosis with survival to the age of 78 years. *Am Heart J.* 1951;41:755–761.
43. Geraci JE, Burchell HB, Edwards JE. Cardiac clinics. 140. Congenital pulmonary stenosis with intact ventricular septum in persons more than 50 years of age: report of 2 cases. *Proc Staff Meet Mayo Clin.* 1953;28:346–352.
44. Mody MR. The natural history of uncomplicated valvular pulmonic stenosis. *Am Heart J.* 1975;90:317–321.
45. White PD, Hurst JW, Fennell RH. Survival to the age of seventy-five years with congenital pulmonary stenosis and patent foramen ovale. *Circulation.* 1950;2:558–564.
46. Wild JB, Eckstein JW, Van Epps EF, Culbertson JW. Three patients with congenital pulmonic valvular stenosis surviving for more than fifty-seven years; medical histories and physiologic data. *Am Heart J.* 1957;53:393–403.
47. Stone FM, Bessinger Jr FB, Lucas Jr RV, Moller JH. Pre- and postoperative rest and exercise hemodynamics in children with pulmonary stenosis. *Circulation.* 1974;49:1102–1106.
48. Lueker RD, Vogel JH, Blount Jr SG. Regression of valvular pulmonary stenosis. *Br Heart J.* 1970;32:779–782.
49. Danilowicz D, Hoffman JI, Rudolph AM. Serial studies of pulmonary stenosis in infancy and childhood. *Br Heart J.* 1975;37: 808–818.
50. Moller JH, Adams Jr P. The natural history of pulmonary valvular stenosis. Serial cardiac catheterizations in 21 children. *Am J Cardiol.* 1965;16:654–664.
51. Ardura J, Gonzalez C, Andres J. Does mild pulmonary stenosis progress during childhood? A study of its natural course. *Clin Cardiol.* 2004;27:519–522.
52. Wood P. *Diseases of the heart and circulation.* 2nd ed. Philadelphia: J.B. Lippincott; 1956.
53. Genkins G, Lasser RP. Chest pain in patients with isolated pulmonic stenosis. *Circulation.* 1957;15:258–266.
54. Shirani J, Zafari AM, Roberts WC. Sudden death, right ventricular infarction, and abnormal right ventricular intramural coronary arteries in isolated congenital valvular pulmonic stenosis. *Am J Cardiol.* 1993;72:368–370.
55. Burch M, Sharland M, Shinebourne E, Smith G, Patton M, Mckenna W. Cardiologic abnormalities in Noonan syndrome: phenotypic diagnosis and echocardiographic assessment of 118 patients. *J Am Coll Cardiol.* 1993;22:1189–1192.
56. Noonan JA, Ehmke DA. Associated noncardiac malformations in children with congenital heart disease. *J Pediatr.* 1963;63: 468–470.
57. Ucar T, Atalay S, Tekin M, Tutar E. Bilateral coronary artery dilatation and supravalvular pulmonary stenosis in a child with Noonan syndrome. *Pediatr Cardiol.* 2005;26:848–850.
58. Collins E, Turner G. The Noonan syndrome—a review of the clinical and genetic features of 27 cases. *J Pediatr.* 1973;83: 941–950.
59. Wong CK, Cheng CH, Lau CP, Leung WH. Congenital coronary artery anomalies in Noonan's syndrome. *Am Heart J.* 1990;119: 396–400.
60. Freij BJ, South MA, Sever JL. Maternal rubella and the congenital rubella syndrome. *Clin Perinatol.* 1988;15:247–257.
61. Berrocal T, Gamo E, Navalon J, et al. Syndrome of Alagille: radiological and sonographic findings. A review of 37 cases. *Eur Radiol.* 1997;7:115–118.
62. Krantz ID, Piccoli DA, Spinner NB. Alagille syndrome. *J Med Genet.* 1997;34:152–157.
63. Levin SE, Zarvos P, Milner S, Schmaman A. Arteriohepatic dysplasia: association of liver disease with pulmonary arterial stenosis as well as facial and skeletal abnormalities. *Pediatrics.* 1980;66: 876–883.
64. Selicorni A, Colli AM, Passarini A, et al. Analysis of congenital heart defects in 87 consecutive patients with Brachmann-de Lange syndrome. *Am J Med Genet.* 2009;Part A. 149A:1268–1272.
65. Digilio MC, Sarkozy A, De Zorzi A, et al. LEOPARD syndrome: clinical diagnosis in the first year of life. *Am J Med Genet.* 2006; Part A. 140:740–746.
66. Holt Jr JH, Eddleman Jr EE. The precordial movements in adults with pulmonic stenosis. *Circulation.* 1967;35:492–500.

67. Perloff JK. *Physical examination of the heart and circulation*. 4th ed. Shelton, Connecticut: People's Medical Publishing House; 2009.

68. Nagle RE, Tamara FA. Left parasternal impulse in pulmonary stenosis and atrial septal defect. *Br Heart J*. 1967;29:735–741.

69. Leatham A, Weitzman D. Auscultatory and phonocardiographic signs of pulmonary stenosis. *Br Heart J*. 1957;19:303–317.

70. Mehlman DJ, Troncoso P, Hay R, Glagov S. Midsystolic click accompanying isolated bicuspid pulmonic valve. *Am Heart J*. 1982;103:145–147.

71. Hultgren HN, Reeve R, Cohn K, Mcleod R. The ejection click of valvular pulmonic stenosis. *Circulation*. 1969;40:631–640.

72. Leatham A, Vogelpoel L. The early systolic sound in dilatation of the pulmonary artery. *Br Heart J*. 1954;16:21–33.

73. Riggs TW, Weinhouse E. Respiratory influence on Doppler estimation of valvar gradients in congenital pulmonic stenosis. *Am J Cardiol*. 1992;70:956–958.

74. Gamboa R, Hugenholtz PG, Nadas AS. Accuracy of the phonocardiogram in assessing severity of aortic and pulmonic stenosis. *Circulation*. 1964;30:35–46.

75. Vogelpoel L, Schrire V. Auscultatory and phonocardiographic assessment of pulmonary stenosis with intact ventricular septum. *Circulation*. 1960;22:55.

76. Patel R, Astley R. Right ventricular obstruction due to anomalous muscle bands. *Br Heart J*. 1973;35:890–893.

77. Alday LE, Moreyra E. Calcific pulmonary stenosis. *Br Heart J*. 1973;35:887–889.

78. Perloff JK, Lebauer EJ. Auscultatory and phonocardiographic manifestations of isolated stenosis of the pulmonary artery and its branches. *Br Heart J*. 1969;31:314–321.

79. Eldridge F, Selzer A, Hultgren H. Stenosis of a branch of the pulmonary artery; an additional cause of continuous murmurs over the chest. *Circulation*. 1957;15:865–874.

80. Ellison RC, Miettinen OS. Interpretation of RSR' in pulmonic stenosis. *Am Heart J*. 1974;88:7–10.

81. Lees MH, Dotter CT. Bronchial circulation in severe multiple peripheral pulmonary artery stenosis; case report illustrating the origin of continuous murmur. *Circulation*. 1965;31:759–761.

82. Singh SP. Unusual splitting of the second heart sound in pulmonary stenosis. *Am J Cardiol*. 1970;25:28–33.

83. Shaver JA, Nadolny RA, O'toole JD, et al. Sound pressure correlates of the second heart sound. An intracardiac sound study. *Circulation*. 1974;49:316–325.

84. Schrire V, Vogelpoel L. The role of the dilated pulmonary artery in abnormal splitting of the second heart sound. *Am Heart J*. 1962;63:501–507.

85. Perloff JK. Auscultatory and phonocardiographic manifestations of pulmonary hypertension. *Prog Cardiovasc Dis*. 1967;9:303–340.

86. Deverall PB, Roberts NK, Stark J. Arrhythmias in children with pulmonary stenosis. *Br Heart J*. 1970;32:472–476.

87. Macruz R, Perloff JK, Case RB. A method for the electrocardiographic recognition of atrial enlargement. *Circulation*. 1958;17:882–889.

88. Halloran KH, Sanyal SK, Gardner TH. Superiorly oriented electrocardiographic axis in infants with the rubella syndrome. *Am Heart J*. 1966;72:600–606.

89. Rasmussen K, Sorland SJ. Prediction of right ventricular systolic pressure in pulmonary stenosis from combined vectorcardiographic data. *Am Heart J*. 1973;86:318–328.

90. Camerini F, Davies LG. Secondary R waves in right chest leads. *Br Heart J*. 1955;17:28–32.

91. Fowler RS. Terminal QRS conduction delay in pulmonary stenosis in children. *Am J Cardiol*. 1968;21:669–672.

92. Miller GA, Restifo M, Shinebourne EA, et al. Pulmonary atresia with intact ventricular septum and critical pulmonary stenosis presenting in first month of life. Investigation and surgical results. *Br Heart J*. 1973;35:9–16.

93. Celermajer JM, Izukawa T, Varghese PJ, Rowe RD. Upright T wave in V1: a useful diagnostic sign of mild pulmonic valve stenosis in children. *J Pediatr*. 1969;74:413–415.

94. Rasmussen K, Sorland SJ. Electrocardiogram and vectorcardiogram in Turner phenotype with normal chromosomes and pulmonary stenosis. *Br Heart J*. 1973;35:937–945.

95. Raaijmakers R, Noordam C, Noonan JA, Croonen EA, Van Der Burgt CJAM, Draaisma JMT. Are ECG abnormalities in Noonan syndrome characteristic for the syndrome? *Eur J Pediatr*. 2008; 167:1363–1367.

96. Chen JT, Robinson AE, Goodrich JK, Lester RG. Uneven distribution of pulmonary blood flow between left and right lungs in isolated valvular pulmonary stenosis. *Am J Roentgenol Radium Ther Nucl Med*. 1969;107:343–350.

97. Bressie JL. Pulmonary valvular stenosis with intact ventricular septum and right aortic arch. *Br Heart J*. 1964;26:154–156.

98. Shachter N, Perloff JK, Mulder DG. Aortic dissection in Noonan's syndrome (46 XY turner). *Am J Cardiol*. 1984;54: 464–465.

99. Shindo T, Kuroda T, Watanabe S, Hojo Y, Sekiguchi H, Shimada K. Aneurysmal dilatation of the pulmonary trunk with mild pulmonic stenosis. *Intern Med*. 1995;34:199–202.

100. Tami LF, Mcelderry MW. Pulmonary artery aneurysm due to severe congenital pulmonic stenosis. Case report and literature review. *Angiology*. 1994;45:383–390.

101. Gay Jr BB, Franch RH. Pulsations in the pulmonary arteries as observed with roentgenoscopic image amplification. Observations in patients with isolated pulmonary valvular stenosis. *Am J Roentgenol Radium Ther Nucl Med*. 1960;83:335–344.

102. Gabriele OF, Scatliff JH. Pulmonary valve calcification. *Am Heart J*. 1970;80:299–302.

103. Nishimura RA, Pieroni DR, Bierman FZ, et al. Second natural history study of congenital heart defects. Pulmonary stenosis: echocardiography. *Circulation*. 1993;87:I73–I79.

104. Mcaleer E, Kort S, Rosenzweig BP, et al. Unusual echocardiographic views of bicuspid and tricuspid pulmonic valves. *J Am Soc Echocardiogr*. 2001;14:1036–1038.

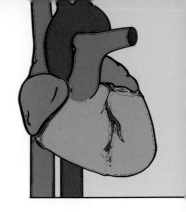

Chapter 12

Congenital Pulmonary Valve Regurgitation

William Osler[1] described pulmonary regurgitation in *The Principles and Practice of Medicine* (1892): "This rare affection is occasionally due to a congenital malformation, particularly fusion of the two segments.... The condition is extremely rare and of little practical significance." The distinctive diastolic murmur of low-pressure pulmonary regurgitation was characterized in 1910[2]; and in 1936, isolated congenital pulmonary valve regurgitation was reported with a review of the literature.[3] Maude Abbott's[4] necropsy study of 1000 cases of congenital heart disease included two examples of isolated congenital pulmonary valve regurgitation. In 1955, the first clinical diagnosis was made in an asymptomatic 24-year-old medical student.[5]

The morphology of the congenitally malformed valve is variable.[6–8] One, two, or three cusps may undergo faulty development[9,10]; all three cusps may be rudimentary[9]; one cusp may be absent[11] and the other two rudimentary[8]; very rarely, the pulmonary cusps are dysplastic[12]; or no valve tissue may be found at all—congenital absence of the pulmonary valve[13,14]—as reported by Chevers[15] in 1846. The anomaly seldom occurs in isolation[16–20] but instead coexists with Fallot's tetralogy[21] (see Chapter 18) and sporadically with other malformations.[8,22,23]

A *bicuspid* pulmonary valve is rare as an isolated anomaly and is only occasionally incompetent. A *quadricuspid* pulmonary valve typically occurs with truncus arteriosus (see Chapter 28) and only rarely in isolation.[24,25] If the four cusps are equal, the quadricuspid valve functions normally; but with cuspal inequality or a supernumerary cusp, the valve is rendered incompetent, especially if the pulmonary artery pressure is elevated.[24]

This chapter is concerned with pulmonary valve regurgitation as an isolated congenital malformation. Regurgitation associated with pulmonary hypertension and a structurally normal pulmonary valve is dealt with in Chapter 14 on primary pulmonary hypertension.

Significance of the diagnosis of pulmonary valve regurgitation must take into account the relatively high incidence of trivial to mild pulmonary regurgitation identified incidentally with color flow imaging and Doppler interrogation in individuals whose hearts are structurally normal.[26,27] Prevalence rate from birth to age 14 years is nil under 1 year of age, with a peak incidence rate of 42% between 6 and 11 years of age.[26]

The mature right ventricle is a low-pressure low-resistance pump that readily adapts to augmented volume, although the degree and duration of regurgitant flow are important determinants of this response.[7] The physiologic consequences of pulmonary regurgitation are especially dramatic *in utero* because systemic pressure in the pulmonary trunk augments regurgitant flow, more so with agenesis of the fetal ductus.[9,19] Acquired elevation of pulmonary arterial pressure in adults with bronchopulmonary disease or left ventricular failure is analogous but less dramatic.[28]

HISTORY

Isolated congenital pulmonary valve regurgitation usually comes to light because of a murmur or because of a dilated pulmonary arterial trunk in a routine chest x-ray. The diagnosis tends to be delayed, however, because the murmur is not detected at birth[9] and routine chest x-rays are seldom done before adulthood. Gender distribution is about equal.[29]

Clinical manifestations of isolated congenital pulmonary valve regurgitation fall into three categories. The first and largest category consists of asymptomatic children, adolescents, and young adults,[6,29] who tolerate the anomaly through middle age[30] and occasionally into the sixth or even eighth decade.[31] Isolated congenital *absence* of the pulmonary valve has been reported at age 69 years[32] and 73 years.[18]

The second and much smaller category consists of adults in whom right ventricular failure occurs after decades of stability.[28,29] *Severe* pulmonary valve regurgitation *per se* can cause the right ventricle to fail,[33] but *moderate* regurgitation produces little or no ill effect until the degree of regurgitant flow is increased by adult-acquired elevation in pulmonary artery pressure associated with bronchopulmonary disease[33] or left ventricular failure.[28] Infective endocarditis is a low-probability cause of increased regurgitation.

A third and rare category of congenital pulmonary valve regurgitation occurs in the fetus[19] or neonate[9,29] when elevated pulmonary arterial pressure augments the volume of regurgitant flow across a congenitally malformed or absent pulmonary valve.[19,29] *In utero* patency of the ductus is desirable because ductal agenesis increases resistance to right ventricular discharge and increases regurgitant flow. The converse is the case with ductal patency *after* birth, which adds to the burden of the right ventricle by allowing diastolic flow to proceed from the aorta through the ductus into the pulmonary artery and across the incompetent pulmonary valve into the right ventricle.[17,19,29,34]

PHYSICAL APPEARANCE, ARTERIAL PULSE, AND JUGULAR VENOUS PULSE

Physical appearance and the arterial pulse are normal. The A wave, V wave, and mean jugular venous pressure rise with the advent of right ventricular failure.

PRECORDIAL MOVEMENT AND PALPATION

When pulmonary regurgitation is mild to moderate, the right ventricular impulse is gentle and is detected only in the sub-zyphoid area during held inspiration. Severe regurgitation that accompanies congenital absence of the pulmonary valve generates a hyperdynamic impulse at the left sternal border and subzyphoid area, in addition to an impulse in the second left intercostal space caused by systolic expansion of the dilated pulmonary trunk (see Figure 12-7).[29,31]

AUSCULTATION

A normal first heart sound is occasionally followed by an ejection sound into the dilated pulmonary trunk. The pulmonary component of the second heart sound is absent when the leaflets are absent or rudimentary[29,35] and soft when the cusps are present but defective, although audibility *per se* indicates the presence of valve tissue.[36] The split tends to be wide because of a delay in the pulmonary component caused by increased capacitance of the pulmonary vascular bed and slow elastic recoil.[36–38] The occasional occurrence of complete right bundle branch block also delays the pulmonary component of the second sound (Figure 12-1). Inspiration increases the degree of splitting unless the right ventricle has failed.[36] Narrow splitting sometimes occurs because rapid right ventricular ejection coupled with brisk decline in the descending limb of the pulmonary artery pressure pulse cancels a potential delay in pulmonary valve closure.

The hallmark of congenital pulmonary valve regurgitation is the distinctive diastolic murmur. The murmur of low-pressure low-velocity regurgitant flow is maximal in the second or third left intercostal space, medium-pitched to low-pitched, crescendo-decrescendo, delayed in onset, and short in duration; and it ends well before the subsequent first heart sound (Figures 12-1 and 12-2).[29,30,33,39] The murmur begins immediately after the right ventricular and pulmonary arterial pressure pulses diverge in early diastole, and is loudest at the timing of an early diastolic dip when the diastolic gradient is maximal (Figure 12-3A).[33,39] If the pulmonary component of the second heart sound is soft or absent, a silent interval exists between the aortic component and the onset of the diastolic murmur (see Figure 12-2).[39] Equilibration of pulmonary arterial and right ventricular pressures in latter diastole reduces or eliminates the regurgitant gradient and eliminates the murmur (Figures 12-3A, 12-4, and 12-5).[39] The normally low

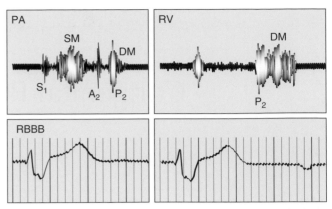

FIGURE 12-1 Intracardiac phonocardiograms from a 17-year-old boy with congenital pulmonary valve regurgitation. A prominent midsystolic murmur (SM) was recorded in the main pulmonary artery (PA), and a short diastolic murmur (DM) issued from the delayed pulmonary component of the second sound (P_2). The second sound is widely split because of complete right bundle branch block (RBBB). The diastolic murmur (DM) was most prominent in the right ventricle (RV) just beneath the pulmonary valve. (S_1 = first heart sound; A_2 = aortic component of the second sound.)

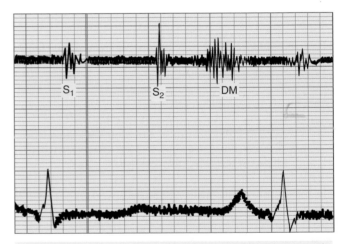

FIGURE 12-2 Phonocardiogram from the third left intercostal space of a 36-year-old woman with congenital pulmonary valve regurgitation. A short medium-frequency mid-diastolic murmur (DM) begins well after the aortic component of the second sound (S_2) and ends well before the subsequent first sound (S_1).

diastolic pressure in the pulmonary trunk is responsible for the low rate of regurgitant flow and the correspondingly low to medium pitch of the murmur.[39] Conversely, maximal instantaneous diastolic flow velocity in pulmonary hypertensive pulmonary regurgitation is maintained at about the same signal strength throughout diastole, which is appropriate for the high-frequency holodiastolic Graham Steell murmur (Figure 12-3B).[40] The velocity of low-pressure pulmonary regurgitation peaks in early diastole and is followed by a gradual decline toward end-diastole. Accordingly, the low-frequency to medium frequency diastolic murmur ends well before the subsequent first heart sound (see Figure 12-3A). Mild congenital pulmonary regurgitation permits the

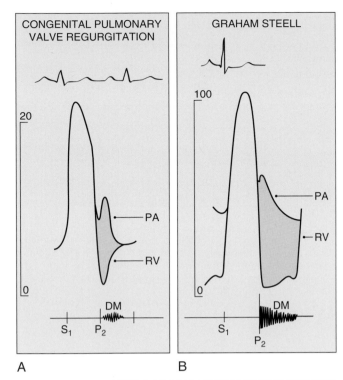

A   **B**

FIGURE 12-3 Line drawings from actual pressure pulses and phonocardiograms in **(A)** congenital pulmonary valve regurgitation and **(B)** hypertensive pulmonary regurgitation (Graham Steele). **A,** The diastolic murmur (DM) begins shortly after the right ventricular (RV) and pulmonary artery (PA) pressure pulses diverge and is loudest when the diastolic gradient (shaded area) is maximal at the timing of the early diastolic dip in the right ventricular pulse (RV). Equilibration of the pulmonary arterial and right ventricular pressures later in diastole abolishes the regurgitant gradient and eliminates the murmur. **B,** When high pulmonary arterial diastolic pressure is exerted against an incompetent pulmonary valve, the regurgitant gradient (shaded area) persists throughout diastole because the PA and RV pressure pulses do not equilibrate. The accompanying murmur begins in early diastole and is holodiastolic, decrescendo, and high frequency (Graham Steell).

diastolic pressure in the pulmonary trunk to remain higher than the diastolic pressure in the right ventricle, so the low-frequency to medium-frequency murmur extends throughout diastole (see Figure 12-5).

Intensity of the diastolic murmur varies from grade 1/6 to 3/6, but exceptionally it is loud and rough enough to generate a thrill.[30,31] During inspiration, the early diastolic dip in the right ventricular pressure pulse falls more rapidly than the diastolic pressure in the pulmonary trunk, so the regurgitant gradient transiently increases and the murmur becomes correspondingly louder.[19]

A midsystolic murmur with congenital pulmonary valve regurgitation is the result of rapid ejection of an increased right ventricular stroke volume into a dilated pulmonary trunk (see Figure 12-1).[29] The systolic murmur is short and crescendo-decrescendo and ends well before both components of the second heart sound (see Figure 12-1). Rarely, a low-frequency *presystolic* murmur assigned to vibrations of the tricuspid valve is thought to represent a *right-sided* Austin Flint.[29]

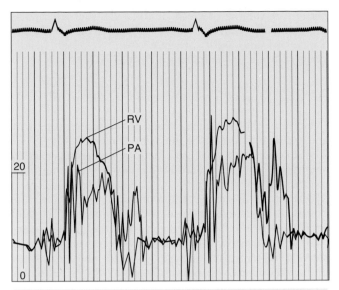

FIGURE 12-4 Right ventricular (RV) and pulmonary artery (PA) pressure pulses from an 18-year-old man with appreciable congenital pulmonary valve regurgitation. The regurgitant gradient appears immediately after the pressure pulses diverge and is rapidly abolished as the pressure pulses equilibrate (compare with Figure 12-3A).

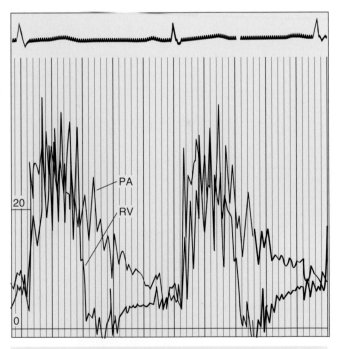

FIGURE 12-5 Pulmonary artery (PA) and right ventricular (RV) pressure pulses from a 23-year-old man with congenital pulmonary valve regurgitation. The diastolic pressures in the pulmonary artery (PA) and right ventricle (RV) do not equilibrate until the end of diastole because the regurgitation was mild.

ELECTROCARDIOGRAM

The electrocardiogram is normal when congenital pulmonary regurgitation is mild to moderate.[18,30,31] Atrial fibrillation is exceptional even with congenital absence of the pulmonary valve.[32] The most common change in the QRS reflects the pattern of volume overload of the right ventricle and is represented by terminal r waves in leads V_1 and aVR, and S waves in leads 1 and V_{5-6} (Figure 12-6).[29,32,41] Right bundle branch block is uncommon (see Figure 12-1).[6,32]

X-RAY

Dilation of the pulmonary trunk is the most prominent and consistent feature of the x-ray (Figure 12-7).[30,31,41] The dilation has been ascribed to coexisting medial abnormalities[42] and varies considerably in size, sometimes reaching aneurysmal proportions (see Figure 12-7).[13] Vigorous pulsations of the pulmonary trunk and its proximal branches are seen with fluoroscopy[29,30] and with real-time echocardiography (see subsequent section). Occasionally, the chest x-ray fortuitously records striking intermittent changes in size of the dilated pulmonary trunk (Figures 12-7 and 12-8).[31] Right ventricular enlargement corresponds to the degree of volume overload.

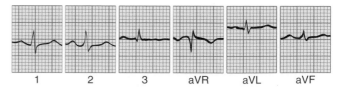

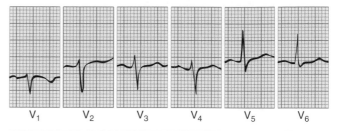

FIGURE 12-6 Electrocardiogram from a 34-year-old woman with mild to moderate congenital pulmonary valve regurgitation. The terminal force of the QRS points to the right and superior, writing a terminal r in lead aVR and small S waves in leads 1, 2, aVL, aVF, and V_6.

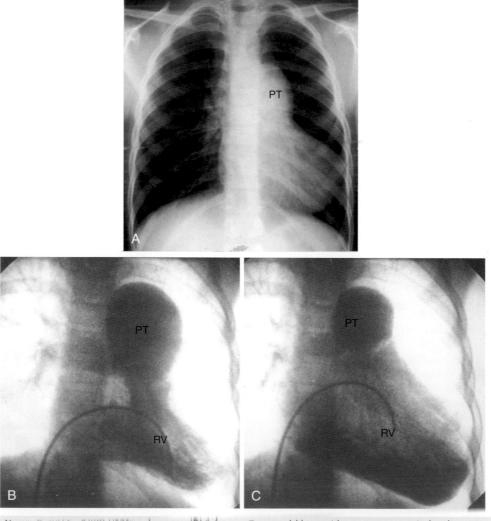

FIGURE 12-7 **A,** X-ray. **B** and **C,** Right ventriculograms (RV) from a 7-year-old boy with severe congenital pulmonary valve regurgitation. There is striking systolic expansion of the dilated pulmonary trunk (PT). (**B,** Systole; **C,** diastole.)

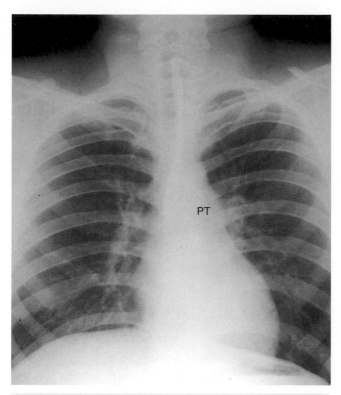

FIGURE 12-8 X-ray from a 10-year-old boy with congenital pulmonary valve regurgitation. The pulmonary trunk (PT) is moderately dilated. The x-ray is otherwise normal.

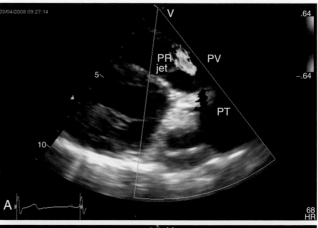

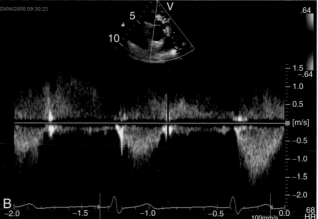

FIGURE 12-9 A, Color flow image (short axis view) from an 11-year-old boy with moderate congenital pulmonary valve regurgitation (PR jet) that begins at the pulmonary valve (PV). The pulmonary trunk (PT) is moderately dilated. **B,** Continuous-wave Doppler scan across the right ventricular outflow tract shows low-pressure, low-velocity pulmonary regurgitation. The systolic signal is low velocity because there was no gradient across the pulmonary valve.

ECHOCARDIOGRAM

Color flow imaging and Doppler interrogation are used to establish the diagnosis of congenital pulmonary valve regurgitation and to establish the depth, width, duration, and peak velocity of the diastolic jet (Figure 12-9), which differs from pulmonary hypertensive pulmonary regurgitation (Figure 12-10 and Video 12-1). Mild pulmonary regurgitation detected in healthy subjects is not accompanied by a diastolic murmur.[26,27]

Echocardiography defines the size of the pulmonary trunk and its proximal branches and the vigor of pulsations in response to rapid ejection of the regurgitant volume. The physiologic consequences of congenital pulmonary valve regurgitation are reflected in the size and contractility of the right ventricle and in paradoxic motion of the ventricular septum.

SUMMARY

Congenital pulmonary valve regurgitation comes to light in healthy asymptomatic individuals with dilation of the pulmonary trunk in a routine chest x-ray or with diastolic/systolic murmurs that are discovered on routine physical examination. An exception is the neonate with severe isolated congenital pulmonary valve regurgitation or complete absence of the pulmonary valve. Precordial palpation is used to detect a right ventricular impulse that corresponds to the degree of regurgitation. Systolic expansion of the pulmonary trunk imparts an impulse in the second left intercostal space. Auscultation reveals a distinctive diastolic murmur that is maximal in the second or third left interspace, low frequency to medium frequency, crescendo-decrescendo, delayed in onset, short in duration, and occasionally louder during inspiration. A pulmonary midsystolic murmur is usually present. The second heart sound is normal or widely split, the pulmonary component is soft or inaudible, and the split tends to be persistent but not fixed. The electrocardiogram is either normal or exhibits signs of volume overload of the right ventricle with an rSr prime in lead V_1. The x-ray shows dilation of the pulmonary trunk that is occasionally aneurysmal together with dilation of the right ventricle. Color flow imaging and Doppler interrogation establish the presence and degree of pulmonary regurgitation and its physiologic consequences.

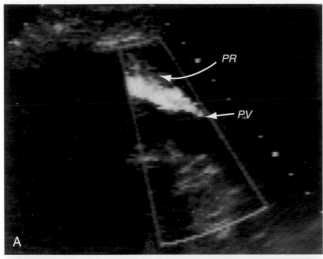

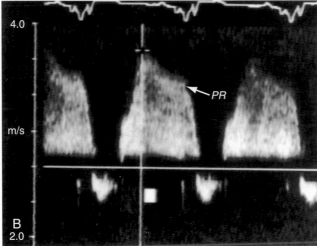

FIGURE 12-10 Echocardiograms from an 18-year-old woman with primary (idiopathic) pulmonary hypertension. **A,** Short axis shows the high-velocity jet of pulmonary hypertensive pulmonary regurgitation (PR) beginning at the pulmonary valve (PV). **B,** Continuous-wave Doppler scan across the right ventricular outflow tract shows high-pressure, high-velocity pulmonary regurgitation (PR) with a peak velocity just over 3 m/sec. Compare with Figure 12-9 (Video 12-1).

REFERENCES

1. Osler W. *The principles and practice of medicine.* New York: D. Appleton And Company; 1892.
2. Hirschfelder A. *Diseases of the heart and aorta.* Philadelphia: J.B. Lippincott Company; 1910.
3. Kissin M. Pulmonary insufficiency with supernumerary cusp in pulmonary valve; report of a case and review of the literature. *Am Heart J.* 1936;12:206.
4. Abbott ME. *Atlas of congenital cardiac disease.* New York: American Heart Association; 1936.
5. Kezdi P, Priest WS, Smith JM. Pulmonic regurgitation. *Q Bull Northwest Univ Med Sch.* 1955;29:368–373.
6. Cortes FM, Jacoby WJ. Isolated congenital pulmonary valvular insufficiency. *Am J Cardiol.* 1962;10:287–290.
7. Lau KC, Cheung HH, Mok CK. Congenital absence of the pulmonary valve, intact interventricular septum, and patent ductus arteriosus. management in a newborn infant. *Am Heart J.* 1990;120:711–714.
8. Wennevold A, Jacobsen JR, Efsen F. Spontaneous change from pulmonic stenosis to pulmonic regurgitation. *Am Heart J.* 1984;108:608–609.
9. Berman Jr W, Fripp RR, Rowe SA, Yabek SM. Congenital isolated pulmonary valve incompetence: neonatal presentation and early natural history. *Am Heart J.* 1992;124:248–251.
10. Tanabe Y, Takahashi M, Kuwano H, et al. Long-term fate of isolated congenital absent pulmonary valve. *Am Heart J.* 1992;124:526–529.
11. Sayger P, Lewis M, Arcilla R, Ilbawi M. Isolated congenital absence of a single pulmonary valve cusp. *Pediatr Cardiol.* 2000;21:487–489.
12. Mori K, Hayabuchi Y, Kuroda Y. Diagnosis and natural history of isolated congenital pulmonary regurgitation in fetal life. *Cardiol Young.* 2000;10:162–165.
13. Attie F, Rijlaarsdam M, Chuquiure E. Images in cardiovascular medicine. isolated congenital absence of the pulmonary valve. *Circulation.* 1999;99:455–456.
14. Pouget JM, Kelly CE, Pilz CG. Congenital absence of the pulmonic valve. report of a case in a seventy-three-year-old man. *Am J Cardiol.* 1967;19:732–740.
15. Chevers N. A collection of facts illustrative of the morbid conditions of the pulmonary artery, as bearing upon the treatment of cardiac and pulmonary diseases. *London Medical Gazette.* 1846;38:828–835.
16. Laneve SA, Uesu CT, Taguchi JT. Isolated pulmonic valvular regurgitation. *Am J Med Sci.* 1962;244:446–458.
17. Lendrum BL, Shaffer AB. Isolated congenital pulmonic valvular regurgitation. *Am Heart J.* 1959;57:298–308.
18. Price BO. Isolated incompetence of the pulmonic valve. *Circulation.* 1961;23:596–602.
19. Takao S, Miyatake K, Izumi S, et al. Clinical implications of pulmonary regurgitation in healthy individuals: detection by cross sectional pulsed doppler echocardiography. *Br Heart J.* 1988;59:542–550.
20. Venables AW. Absence of the pulmonary valve with ventricular septal defect. *Br Heart J.* 1962;24:293–296.
21. Chaturvedi RR, Redington AN. Pulmonary regurgitation in congenital heart disease. *Heart.* 2007;93:880–889.
22. Baker WP, Kelminson LL, Turner Jr WM, Blount SG. Absence of pulmonic valve associated with double-outlet right ventricle. *Circulation.* 1967;36:452–455.
23. Vlad P. Congenital pulmonary regurgitation: a report of 6 autopsied cases. *Am J Dis Child.* 1960;100:640.
24. Becker AE. Quadricuspid pulmonary valve. Anatomical observations in 20 hearts. *Acta Morphol Neerl Scand.* 1972;10:299–309.
25. Fernandez-Armenta J, Villagomez D, Fernandez-Vivancos C, Vazquez R, Pastor L. Quadricuspid pulmonary valve identified by transthoracic echocardiography. *Echocardiography.* 2009;26:288–290.
26. Brand A, Dollberg S, Keren A. The prevalence of valvular regurgitation in children with structurally normal hearts: a color Doppler echocardiographic study. *Am Heart J.* 1992;123:177–180.
27. Choong CY, Abascal VM, Weyman J, et al. Prevalence of valvular regurgitation by Doppler echocardiography in patients with structurally normal hearts by two-dimensional echocardiography. *Am Heart J.* 1989;117:636–642.
28. Fish RG, Takaro T, Crymes T. Prognostic considerations in primary isolated insufficiency of the pulmonic valve. *N Engl J Med.* 1959;261:739–742.
29. Ansari A. Isolated pulmonary valvular regurgitation: current perspectives. *Prog Cardiovasc Dis.* 1991;33:329–344.
30. Collins NP, Braunwald E, Morrow AG. Isolated congenital pulmonic valvular regurgitation. Diagnosis by cardiac catheterization and angiocardiography. *Am J Med.* 1960;28:159–164.
31. Goldberg E, Katz I. Isolated pulmonic regurgitation with intermittent pulmonary artery dilatation. *Am J Cardiol.* 1962;9:619–625.
32. Thanopoulos BD, Fisher EA, Hastreiter AR. Large ductus arteriosus and intact ventricular septum associated with congenital absence of the pulmonary valve. *Br Heart J.* 1986;55:602–604.
33. Hamby RI, Gulotta SJ. Pulmonic valvular insufficiency: etiology, recognition, and management. *Am Heart J.* 1967;74:110–125.
34. Ettedgui JA, Sharland GK, Chita SK, Cook A, Fagg N, Allan LD. Absent pulmonary valve syndrome with ventricular septal defect: role of the arterial duct. *Am J Cardiol.* 1990;66:233–234.

35. Sanyal SK, Hipona FA, Browne MJ, Talner NS. Congenital insufficiency of the pulmonary valve. *J Pediatr*. 1964;64:728–734.

36. Jacoby Jr WJ, Tucker DH, Sumner RG. The second heart sound in congenital pulmonary valvular insufficiency. *Am Heart J*. 1965;69: 603–609.

37. Shaver JA, Nadolny RA, O'toole JD, et al. Sound pressure correlates of the second heart sound. An intracardiac sound study. *Circulation*. 1974;49:316–325.

38. Sloman G, Wee KP. Isolated congenital pulmonary valve incompetence. *Am Heart J*. 1963;66:532–537.

39. Maciel BC, Simpson IA, Valdes-Cruz LM, et al. Color flow Doppler mapping studies of "physiologic" pulmonary and tricuspid regurgitation: evidence for true regurgitation as opposed to a valve closing volume. *J Am Soc Echocardiogr*. 1991;4:589–597.

40. Perloff JK. *Physical examination of the heart and circulation*. 4th ed. Shelton, Connecticut: People's Medical Publishing House; 2009.

41. Schrire V, Vogelpoel L. The role of the dilated pulmonary artery in abnormal splitting of the second heart sound. *Am Heart J*. 1962;63: 501–507.

42. Niwa K, Perloff JK, Bhuta SM, et al. Structural abnormalities of great arterial walls in congenital heart disease: light and electron microscopic analyses. *Circulation*. 2001;103:393–400.

that leaves the atrioventricular orifice unguarded (see Figure 13-32). Congenital *dysplasia* of the tricuspid valve refers to nodular thickening and rolling of the edges of the leaflets without downward displacement.[25]

Idiopathic dilation of the right atrium has been reported in children without Ebstein's anomaly.[26,27] Transient tricuspid regurgitation of the newborn has no definable anatomic basis and resolves within a few weeks.[28] Uhl's anomaly is discussed at the end of this chapter.

Abnormalities of the left side of the heart have been reported in 39% of patients with Ebstein's anomaly[17,29] and consist of derangements in left ventricular geometry, impairment of systolic and diastolic function,[29,30] and noncompaction.[17,31] Superior systolic displacement of the mitral valve (prolapse) occurs because mitral leaflets with normal areas and chordal lengths are housed in a left ventricular cavity that is geometrically altered and reduced in size (see Figure 13-31).[19,29,32,33] Depressed systolic function is the result of a combination of abnormal shape, impaired diastolic filling, and increased fibrous content of the free wall and the ventricular septum.[19]

The *physiologic consequences* of Ebstein's anomaly are determined by the morphologic derangement of the tricuspid leaflets, by the hemodynamic burden imposed on an inherently flawed the right ventricle, by left ventricular function, and by atrial rhythm. The tricuspid orifice is typically incompetent, occasionally stenotic, and rarely imperforate. Functional impairment of the right ventricle depends on the severity of tricuspid regurgitation and on the size of the right atrium and atrialized right ventricle relative to the size of the functional right ventricle. The thin-walled atrialized right ventricle is either passive during the cardiac cycle or functions as an aneurysm that expands paradoxically during systole and therefore acts a physiologic impediment (see previous discussion). Exercise intolerance has been ascribed to an inadequate increment in pulmonary blood flow and a fall in systemic arterial oxygen saturation.[34,35] Atrial tachyarrhythmias have serious physiologic implications, especially the rapid heart rates associated with accessory pathways (see sections The Electrocardiogram and The History).

The functionally inadequate right ventricle is especially vulnerable *in utero* and at birth. High neonatal pulmonary vascular resistance increases right ventricular afterload and augments tricuspid regurgitation. Right atrial pressure increases, and a right-to-left shunt is established across a patent foramen ovale or an atrial septal defect. The process is reversed as neonatal pulmonary vascular resistance falls and right ventricular afterload normalizes. The enlarging right atrium becomes sufficiently commodious to accommodate a large volume of regurgitant flow with little or no increase in pressure (Figure 13-5). In older patients, right ventricular filling pressure may increase, provoking a rise in right atrial pressure with reestablishment of the right-to-left interatrial shunt.

Ebstein's original case was an example of obstruction at the tricuspid orifice (see Figure 13-1).[1] He wrote, "The membrane divided the right ventricle into two halves. These halves communicated with each other in two ways: one through the oval opening which leads into the right conus arteriosus, and two through the already described multiple openings in the fenestrated membrane."[1] When the tricuspid orifice is stenotic or imperforate, the elevation of right atrial pressure reflects the degree of obstruction. The A wave is often giant, and a right-to-left interatrial shunt persists after the fall in neonatal pulmonary vascular resistance.

The *electromechanical properties* of the right atrium, atrialized right ventricle, and functional right ventricle provided the first secure basis for the clinical diagnosis of Ebstein's anomaly (Figures 13-2 and 13-3).[36,37] The

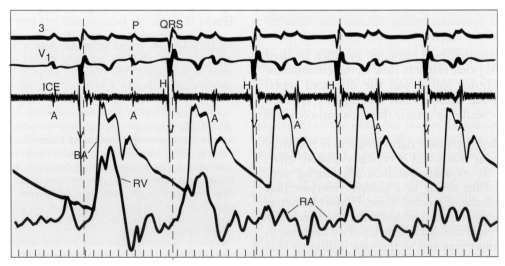

FIGURE 13-3 The electrophysiologic abnormalities in Ebstein's anomaly identified with a filtered bipolar system. Lead 3, lead V₁, and an intracardiac electrogram (ICE) are shown with a right ventricular (RV) and a right atrial (RA) pressure pulse. In the intracardiac electrogram (ICE), atrial depolarization (A) coincides with P waves in lead 3 and lead V₁, and ventricular depolarization (V) coincides with the QRS complex in lead 3 and V₁. In the first two cycles, the intracardiac electrogram recorded right ventricular depolarization with a right ventricular pressure pulse (RV). In the subsequent three cycles, the intracardiac electrogram continued to record right ventricular depolarization, but the pressure pulse was right atrial (RA) because the recording was over the atrialized right ventricle. (BA = brachial arterial pulse.)

right atrium proper generates a *right atrial pressure pulse* and an *intracavitary atrial electrogram*. The *functional right ventricle* generates a *right ventricular pressure pulse* and a *right ventricular intracavitary electrogram*. The *atrialized right ventricle* generates a *right ventricular intracavitary electrogram* but an *atrial pressure pulse* (see Figures 13-2 and 13-3). Mechanical stimulation of the atrialized right ventricle provokes a right ventricular electrogram and incurs the risk of triggering ventricular tachycardia.[38,39] Clusters of ventricular cardiomyocytes are isolated within a fibrous matrix that prevents spiral/scroll reentrant waves from anchoring.[40] When spiral/scroll waves do not anchor, they meander erratically as polymorphic ventricular tachycardia. Accordingly, mechanical stimulation of the atrialized right ventricle does not provoke monomorphic ventricular tachycardia that depends on slow conduction, unidirectional block, and a substrate that permits reentry but instead results in polymorphic ventricular tachycardia.[38,40]

The geometric configuration and function of the right and left ventricles are closely coupled in Ebstein's anomaly.[29] Leftward displacement of the ventricular septum (see Figure 13-31) reduces the volume of left ventricular diastolic filling and, accordingly, reduces the ejection fraction. Exercise provokes an increase in left ventricular ejection fraction because end-systolic volume decreases with little or no change in end-diastolic volume. The right ventricular free wall contributes feebly if at all to forward flow, which is materially assisted by paradoxical motion of the ventricular septum that functions as part of the right ventricle as in Uhl's anomaly (see subsequent). In brief, left ventricular function is adversely affected by the diastolic position of the ventricular septum, geometric distortion of the ventricle (see Figure 13-31), reduced end-diastolic volume, paradoxical motion of the ventricular septum, an increase in fibrous tissue, and a decrease in cardiomyocytes in the free wall and septum.[19]

HISTORY

Males and females are equally affected.[41–44] Familial Ebstein's anomaly has been reported,[41,43,45–51] and a patient with Ebstein's anomaly of a right-sided tricuspid valve had a cousin with congenitally corrected transposition of the great arteries and Ebstein's anomaly of an inverted *left-sided atrioventricular* valve.[41] A novel mutation is held responsible for the genetic syndrome of ventricular preexcitation and conduction system disease of childhood onset,[52] but these observations cannot be extrapolated to the general population of patients with preexicationor to patients with Ebstein's anomaly in the absence of preexcitation.

The Danish Registry estimates that the relative risk of Ebstein's anomaly is increased by 500-fold in offspring exposed to *in utero* lithium carbonate, which is used for treatment of bipolar disorders.[12,53,54]

The probability of occurrence of Ebstein's anomaly in the general population is 1:20,000, so the likelihood of the malformation occurring *spontaneously* in a pregnant woman taking lithium is 1:20 million.[54] Estimates now show that the increased risk incurred with lithium does

not exceed 28-fold, which is considerably less than estimates from the Danish Registry.[12,53]

The clinical course of Ebstein's anomaly ranges from intrauterine death to asymptomatic survival to late adulthood.[43,55–58] The most common presentations are: 1, detection of the anomaly in a routine fetal echocardiogram; 2, neonatal cyanosis; 3, heart failure in infancy; 4, murmur in childhood; and 5, arrhythmias in adolescents and adults.[41,57] The outlook for fetal Ebstein's anomaly has aptly been characterized as *appalling*.[57] Of neonates with Ebstein's anomaly, 20% to 40% do not survive 1 month, and less than 50% survive to 5 years.[17] Fetal hydrops is almost invariably fatal with rare exception.[59,60] Neonates not only have high mortality rates but also a significant ongoing risk of morbidity and death.[43,57,58] Even if symptoms resolve in the first month of life, the infant may then die suddenly. *Transient neonatal cyanosis* that recurs a decade or more later is an uncommon but distinctive and usually benign feature of Ebstein's anomaly.[57] A neonatal right-to-left interatrial shunt disappears as pulmonary vascular resistance normalizes; the shunt subsequently reappears as filling pressure rises in the functionally abnormal right ventricle. Tachyarrhythmic sudden death looms as a threat regardless of severity of the anomaly[56,61] and is responsible for the decline in survival rate in the fifth decade.[56] Wolff-Parkinson-White syndrome in otherwise healthy individuals carries an estimated sudden cardiac death risk of 0.02%,[62] but in Ebstein's anomaly, atrial flutter or fibrillation with accelerated conduction is accompanied by a major increase in the risk of sudden death. Stimulation of the arrhythmogenic atrialized right ventricle initiates polymorphic ventricular tachycardia that promptly degenerates into ventricular fibrillation (Figure 13-4; see previous discussion), and spontaneous ventricular tachycardia/fibrillation looms as a threat. The degree of cyanosis does not necessarily correspond with symptoms, but once cyanosis and symptoms develop, disability tends to be progressive, even in patients who were relatively asymptomatic before adulthood. The onset of chronic atrial fibrillation prefigures death within 5 years.[56]

Despite qualifications, legendary accounts are found of astonishing longevity in Ebstein's anomaly, with survivals into the eighth and ninth decades.[13,41,43,63,64] Ebstein's

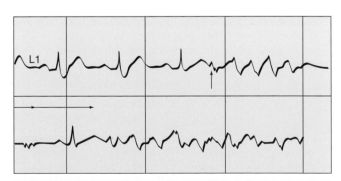

FIGURE 13-4 Continuous tracing of lead 1 (L1). A catheter tip in the atrialized right ventricle induced ventricular fibrillation (vertical arrow) that abated and then recurred (horizontal arrow) without ventricular tachycardia.

anomaly was discovered at necropsy in a 75-year-old man who as a youth had been a lumberjack working on log booms.[65] He was reportedly asymptomatic until his fifties when he was obliged to outrun an irate female bear.[65] At necropsy 25 years later, his right atrium was thin-walled and greatly dilated, and the tricuspid valve was characteristically malformed.[65] The oldest recorded patient with Ebstein's anomaly lived to age 85 years and was devoid of cardiac symptoms until age 79 years.[66]

The chest pain that occasionally occurs with Ebstein's anomaly is an enigma.[41] The pain is retrosternal, epigastric or in the right or left anterior chest, and is sharp, stabbing, or shooting, features that suggest serous surface origin. A fibrinous pericardium has been found at necropsy over the atrialized right ventricle (see section on Auscultation).

Important although less frequent manifestations result from paradoxical emboli or brain abscess. Infective endocarditis is uncommon because regurgitant flow across the malformed tricuspid valve is low velocity with low turbulence. Prophylaxis for the low risk of infective endocarditis is open to question.[17] Pregnancy incurs the risks inherent in a functionally inadequate volume-overloaded right ventricle that copes poorly with the additional hemodynamic burden of gestation.[67] Paroxysmal atrial tachyarrhythmias are potential hazards during pregnancy, especially the rapid rates associated with accessory pathways. Cyanosis may first become manifest during pregnancy because of a rise in filling pressure in the volume-overloaded right ventricle. Hypoxemia increases the risk of fetal wastage,[68] and a right-to-left interatrial shunt incurs a puerperal risk of paradoxical embolization.

PHYSICAL APPEARANCE

Growth and development are normal in patients who were asymptomatic as neonates and infants. Persistent cyanosis or intermittent exercise-induced cyanosis occurs in more than 50% of cases.[41]

Precordial asymmetry is usually *left* parasternal prominence, but occasionally the *right* anterior chest is prominent, presumably because of the enlarged right atrium.

ARTERIAL PULSE

The arterial pulse is normal but diminishes as left ventricular stroke volume falls.

JUGULAR VENOUS PULSE

The jugular pulse is normal except for a prominent C wave that coincides with mobility of the anterior tricuspid leaflet (Figures 13-5 and 13-6, first panel). The interval between the jugular A wave and the carotid pulse is often prolonged, reflecting prolongation of the PR interval (see section on The Electrocardiogram). Prominent A waves are seldom seen in the jugular pulse, but atrial contraction sometimes generates presystolic

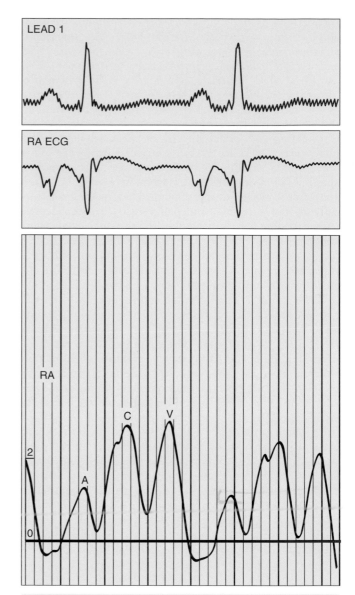

FIGURE 13-5 Tracings from a 14-year-old boy with Ebstein's anomaly. The electrode catheter in the right atrium recorded an intracardiac atrial electrogram (RA ECG) and a right atrial (RA) pressure pulse. A and V waves in the right atrial pressure pulse are normal, and the X descent is preserved despite severe tricuspid regurgitation. The C wave is prominent because of a large mobile anterior tricuspid leaflet.

waves in the pulmonary arterial pressure pulse. A stenotic or imperforate tricuspid orifice is accompanied by A waves that may be giant. An attenuated X descent and a systolic venous V wave of tricuspid regurgitation seldom appear in the jugular pulse despite severe regurgitant flow because of the damping effect of the commodious right atrium and the thin-walled toneless atrialized right ventricle and because tricuspid regurgitation is low-pressure and hypokinetic (see Figures 13-5 and 13-6). Right ventricular failure induces a rise in mean jugular venous pressure and a rise in A and V wave crests, but systolic pulsations of the liver are inconspicuous because the right ventricle is hypokinetic.

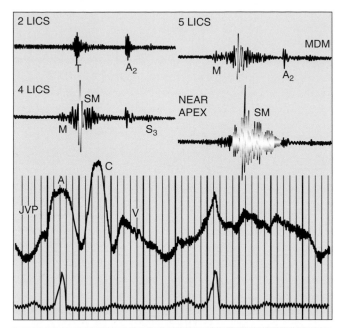

FIGURE 13-6 Phonocardiograms and jugular venous pulse (JVP) from a 17-year-old acyanotic boy with Ebstein's anomaly. The A and V waves are normal despite severe tricuspid regurgitation, but the C wave is prominent because of a large mobile anterior tricuspid leaflet. The loud sound labeled T was generated by the mobile anterior tricuspid leaflet. The soft preceding sound (M) is mitral. A decrescendo systolic murmur (SM) is loudest near the cardiac apex over the displaced tricuspid valve. The second heart sound is single (A_2 = aortic component). A third heart sound (S_3) is found in the fourth left intercostal space (4 LICS) and a short mid-diastolic murmur (MDM) in the fifth left intercostal space (5 LICS). (2 LICS = second left intercostal space.)

PRECORDIAL MOVEMENT AND PALPATION

A right ventricular impulse and a tricuspid systolic thrill are reserved for neonates before normalization of pulmonary vascular resistance.[41] With this exception, *absence* of a systolic impulse over the inflow portion of the right ventricle is an important negative sign in the clinical diagnosis of Ebstein's anomaly.[41,69] An undulating rippling motion over the atrialized right ventricle is sometimes seen in older patients. Enlargement of the infundibular portion of the right ventricle is accompanied by a systolic impulse in the third left intercostal space.[70] Ebstein described a gentle *left* ventricular impulse, stating, "... the cardiac apex was visible under the sixth rib somewhat outside the mammary line."[1] Ebstein also percussed the enlarged right atrium: "... the cardiac dullness extended for two centimeters beyond the right border of the sternum at the level of the fourth rib and for three centimeters at the level of the sixth rib, where it merged with the liver dullness which was normal in extent."[1]

The initial component of a widely split first heart sound coincides with mitral valve closure, and the second

component, which is delayed, coincides with closure of the large anterior tricuspid leaflet (Figures 13-6 through 13-9).[69–72] The delay in tricuspid valve closure is not simply the result of complete right bundle branch block and a hypokinetic right ventricle but instead is the result of the large size and increased excursion of the anterior leaflet, which requires longer to reach its fully tensed closed position.[72] The increased tension developed by the large anterior leaflet as it reaches the limits of its systolic excursion accounts for the loudness of the tricuspid component of the first heart sound—*the sail sound*—which is an important auscultatory sign of anterior leaflet mobility (see Figure 13-30).[68,71] When a long PR interval softens the mitral component, the first heart sound is then represented by a loud single tricuspid component. Preexcitation of the right ventricle buries the mitral component of the first sound in an early loud tricuspid component (Figure 13-10).[73]

The systolic murmur of tricuspid regurgitation is typically grade 2/6 or 3/6, maximal over the displaced tricuspid valve, and therefore most prominent in a relatively leftward location toward the apex (see Figures 13-6 and 13-9). Intensity of the murmur does not increase during

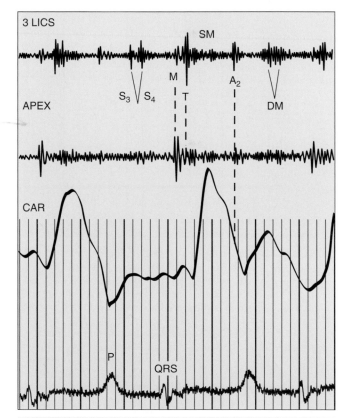

FIGURE 13-7 Phonocardiograms and carotid pulse (CAR) from an acyanotic 22-year-old woman with Ebstein's anomaly. The first heart sound is widely split. The tricuspid component (T) is prominent in the third left intercostal space (3 LICS) rather than at the apex. There is a soft decrescendo tricuspid systolic murmur (SM). A third heart sound (S_3) and a fourth sound with duration (S_4) were recorded in the first cycle. In the second cycle, the third and fourth heart sounds fuse to form a short mid-diastolic murmur (DM). (M = mitral component.)

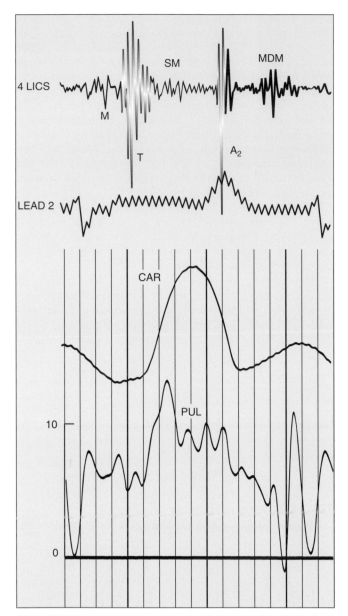

FIGURE 13-8 Phonocardiogram (4 LICS = fourth left intercostal space), electrocardiogram (LEAD 2), carotid pulse (CAR), and pulmonary arterial pulse (PUL) from an 18-year-old cyanotic man with Ebstein's anomaly. The first heart sound is widely split with a loud tricuspid component (T) caused by a large mobile anterior tricuspid leaflet. The tricuspid systolic murmur (SM) is soft and decrescendo. A short mid-diastolic murmur (MDM) represents fusion of a third and fourth heart sound. (A₂ = aortic component of the second heart sound; M = mitral component of the first heart sound.)

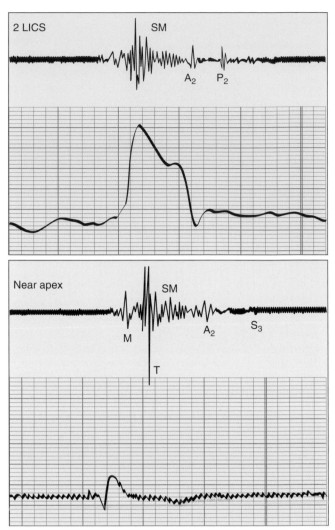

FIGURE 13-9 Phonocardiograms from a 37-year-old acyanotic woman with Ebstein's anomaly. The first heart sound is widely split. The tricuspid component (T) is prominent in the second left intercostal space (2 LICS) and near the apex. The tricuspid systolic murmur (SM) is decrescendo. The second heart sound is widely split (A₂ = aortic component; P₂ = pulmonary component). A soft third heart sound (S₃) was recorded near the apex. (M = mitral component.)

inspiration because the functionally inadequate right ventricle cannot increase its stroke volume and regurgitant flow. An early systole decrescendo murmur is a recognized feature of low-pressure tricuspid regurgitation because flow diminishes in latter systole as the large right atrial V wave reaches the height of normal right ventricular systolic pressure.[74] The systolic murmur in Ebstein's anomaly is medium-frequency and decrescendo because regurgitant flow is low-velocity from a hypokinetic low-pressure right ventricle (see Figures 13-7 through 13-10).[69] However, in neonates with Ebstein's anomaly, the tricuspid regurgitant murmur is holosystolic because right ventricular systolic pressure is elevated.

Wide splitting of the second heart sound is the result of delay in the pulmonary component caused by complete right bundle branch block (see Figure 13-9).[69] However, the second sound is often single because pulmonary closure is inaudible from low pressure in the pulmonary trunk (see Figures 13-6 and 13-7).[41,69] The split changes little if at all with respiration[69] but is paradoxical when an accessory pathway prematurely activates the right side of the ventricular septum.[70]

Third and fourth heart sounds produce a distinctive triple or quadruple rhythm (see Figures 13-6, 13-7, and 13-9),[69] often summate because of PR interval prolongation, and may increase during inspiration because of

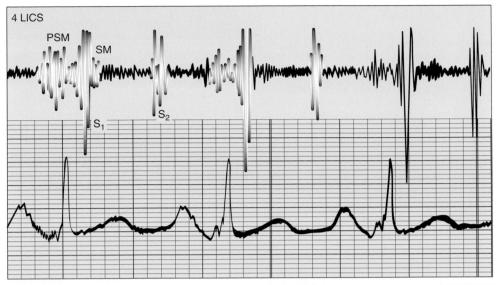

FIGURE 13-10 Tracings from an acyanotic 21-year-old man with Ebstein's anomaly. The phonocardiogram in the fourth left intercostal space (4 LICS) shows a prominent presystolic murmur (PSM), a prominent first heart sound (S_1), and a soft tricuspid early systolic murmur (SM). The loud tricuspid component of the first heart sound occurred early because of a short PR interval associated with preexcitation of the right ventricle. The electrocardiogram (lead 2) shows the short PR interval and the delta wave of type B Wolff-Parkinson-White preexcitation. (S_2 = second heart sound.)

origin in the right side of the heart. Third and fourth heart sounds are sometimes sufficiently prolonged to produce short diastolic murmurs (Figures 13-8, 13-10, and 13-11), especially when the sounds occur in close proximity or when they summate (see Figure 13-7). Early diastolic sounds with the timing of opening snaps have been described in Ebstein's anomaly and attributed to opening movements of the large mobile anterior tricuspid leaflet.[69] The timing and quality of systolic and diastolic murmurs occasionally create the impression of a pericardial friction rub (Figure 13-12). A fibrinous pericardium has been found at necropsy over the atrialized right ventricle.

A rublike systolic murmur, a rublike mid-diastolic murmur, and a rublike presystolic murmur create a distinctive cadence that resembles the rhythmic chugging of a locomotive engine as it gathers speed (see Figure 13-12).

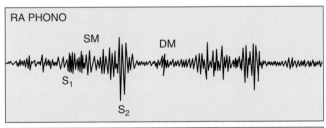

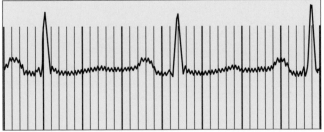

FIGURE 13-11 Right atrial intracardiac phonocardiogram (RA PHONO) from the 17-year-old boy with Ebstein's anomaly. The tricuspid murmur (SM) was holosystolic when recorded with an intracardiac microphone but decrescendo when recorded on the thoracic wall (see Figure 13-6). DM is a short tricuspid mid-diastolic murmur.

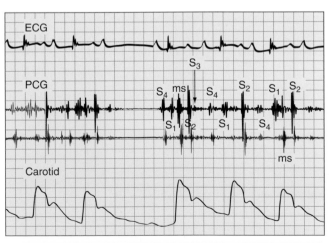

FIGURE 13-12 Phonocardiogram (PCG) from a 20-year-old man with Ebstein's anomaly. Auscultation suggested a three-component friction rub because prolonged impure third and fourth heart sounds (S_3, S_4) were accompanied by an impure short midsystolic murmur (ms) and because these auscultatory events were brought closer to the chest wall by the dilated atrialized right ventricle.

ELECTROCARDIOGRAM

A confident diagnosis of Ebstein's anomaly can often be made based on the electrocardiogram *per se*.[36,75] The tracing is seldom normal even when the anomaly is mild (Figure 13-13), but rarely and oddly, the electrocardiogram can be normal even when the anomaly is severe (Figure 13-14).[36] The major electrophysiologic features of Ebstein's anomaly are summarized in Table 13-1.

P waves are abnormal in height, duration, and configuration (Figures 13-15 through 13-17).[41,75,76] Taussig aptly characterized the tall peaked P waves as *Himalayan*,[41,77] patterns that have been ascribed to prolonged aberrant conduction in the enlarged right atrium.[75,76] Permanent atrial standstill, which has been reported in

Table 13-1 **Major Electrophysiologic Abnormalities in Ebstein's Anomaly**
1. Intraatrial conduction disturbance: right atrial P wave abnormalities, PR interval prolongation
2. Atrioventricular nodal conduction: PR interval prolongation
3. Infranodal conduction
a. Intra-His or infra-His conduction abnormalities
b. Right bundle branch block
c. Bizarre *second* QRS attached to preceding normal QRS
4. Type B Wolff-Parkinson-White preexcitation
5. Supraventricular tachycardia
6. Atrial fibrillation or flutter
7. Arrhythmogenic atrialized right ventricle
8. Deep Q waves in leads V_{1-4} and in inferior leads

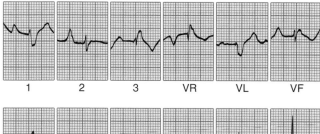
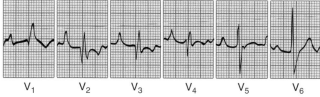

FIGURE 13-13 Electrocardiogram from an 18-year-old acyanotic man with Ebstein's anomaly. The typical electrocardiogram includes PR interval prolongation, tall peaked right atrial P waves in lead 2 and V_{2-5}, complete right bundle branch block, and QR complexes in leads V_{1-4}.

familial Ebstein's anomaly, is a rare and distinctive electrophysiologic abnormality in which atrial myocardium is unresponsive to electrical or mechanical stimuli, and P waves are absent in scalar and transesophageal electrocardiograms.[49]

The PR interval is prolonged (Figures 13-13, 13-15, and 13-18), sometimes markedly so (see Figure 13-18).[75] The duration of the PR interval and the width of the P wave correlate with prolonged conduction in the large right atrium.[64,76] In the presence of preexcitation, the PR interval is usually (Figure 13-19) but not invariably short (see Figure 13-18) because of early inscription of the delta wave. However, a short PR interval occasionally occurs *without* a delta wave and without a history of paroxysmal rapid heart action (see Figure 13-14).

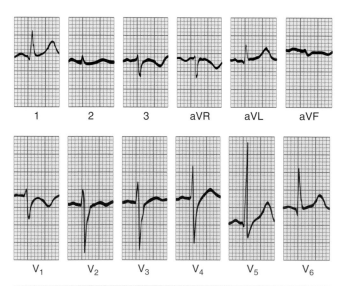

FIGURE 13-14 Electrocardiogram from an 11-year-old girl with mild Ebstein's anomaly. The tracing is normal except for a short PR interval (120 msec) and a horizontal QRS axis. The diagnosis was confirmed with transesophageal echocardiography.

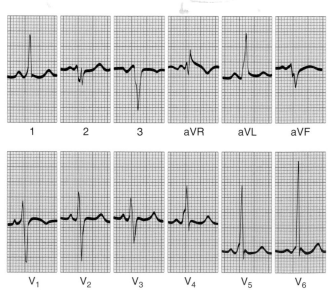

FIGURE 13-15 Electrocardiogram from a 17-year-old boy with Ebstein's anomaly. Low-amplitude P waves are peaked in leads V_{1-2} but are otherwise normal. A short PR interval is followed by delta waves that are positive in leads 1, aVL, and V_{4-6} and are negative in leads 2, 3, and aVF. These patterns suggest a right posterior atrial directory pathway. The delta wave is isoelectric in leads V_1 and V_2, which is presumptive evidence that the accessory pathway is in the right posterolateral free wall.

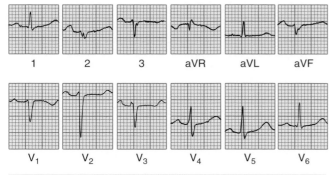

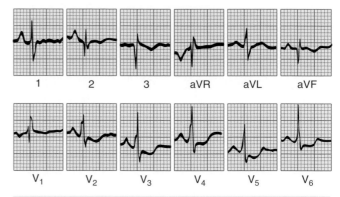

FIGURE 13-16 Electrocardiogram from a 39-year-old woman with a mild form of Ebstein's anomaly and a patent foramen ovale confirmed with transesophageal echocardiography. She came to attention because of a cerebral ischemic event caused by a paradoxical embolus. Her x-ray is shown in Figure 13-21. The P waves are normal, the PR interval is 200 msec, and there is left axis deviation but without delta waves. The terminal R wave in aVR is slightly prolonged.

FIGURE 13-18 Electrocardiogram from an 11-month-old female with Ebstein's anomaly and recurrent supraventricular tachycardia. Tall peaked right atrial P waves appear in leads 1, 2, and V_{2-4}. The PR interval is prolonged for age. Delta waves are positive in lead aVL and in leads V_{2-6} and are negative in leads 2, 3, and aVF. These limb lead patterns together with an abrupt transition from an isoelectric delta wave in lead V_1 (rsR) to a positive delta wave in lead V_2 (slurred rS) suggest a right posterior septal accessory pathway. The prolonged terminal force of the QRS points to the right, superior and anterior because of a right ventricular conduction defect.

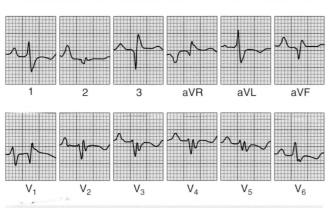

FIGURE 13-17 Electrocardiogram from a 58-year-old woman with acyanotic Ebstein's anomaly. The PR interval is 220 msec. There are tall peaked right atrial P waves in leads 1, 2, and aVF and in leads V_{2-5}. Recurrent Mobitz II atrioventricular block progressed to complete heart block that required a pacemaker, which was implanted onto the left ventricular *epicardium*.

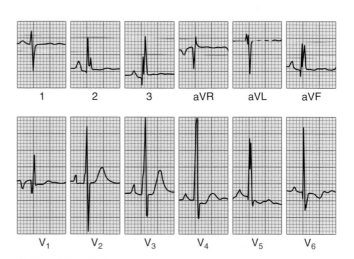

FIGURE 13-19 Electrocardiogram from a moderately cyanotic female neonate with Ebstein's anomaly. The PR interval is prolonged for age. A right atrial abnormality is indicated with tall peaked P waves in lead 2 and V_{2-3}, a deep P terminal force in lead V_1, and a Q wave in lead V_1 that is similar to the Q wave pattern in aVR. The QRS is splintered, and the terminal force is prolonged. The relatively tall R wave in lead V_1 suggests unanticipated right ventricular hypertrophy.

Electrophysiologic studies have identified intra-His and infra-His delay in Ebstein's anomaly.[76] Prolonged HV intervals have been ascribed to lengthened and impaired conduction within the atrialized right ventricle,[76,78] conclusions that are in accord with the observation that complete heart block is rare despite prolongation of the PR interval and HV interval (see Figure 13-17).[79]

In 75% to 95% of cases, the QRS is characterized by a right ventricular conduction defect of the right bundle branch type (see Figures 13-16 and 13-17).[76,80] QRS prolongation is largely if not exclusively the result of prolonged activation of the atrialized right ventricle and is less fully manifest in infants (see Figure 13-15). The conduction defect is therefore *distal* to the right bundle branch[76] and is sometimes present despite a septal accessory pathway (see Figure 13-18). A distinctive *second QRS complex* attached to the preceding *normal QRS complex* originates in the atrialized right ventricle according to intracardiac mapping (Figure 13-20).[76]

The QRS axis is inferior, although a splintered polyphasic QRS makes the axis difficult to determine. *Left*

axis deviation represents type B preexcitation (see Figure 13-19), but a horizontal QRS axis occasionally occurs in the absence of accessory pathways (see Figure 13-13).[81] Initial force abnormalities apart from delta waves are important features of the electrocardiogram. Deep Q waves appear in leads 2, 3, and aVF (see Figure 13-17),[80,81] but most important are *right precordial Q waves* in lead V_1 (see Figure 13-15) or in leads V_{1-4} (see Figures 13-16 and 13-17).[80] This distinctive Q wave pattern occurs because the precordial surface

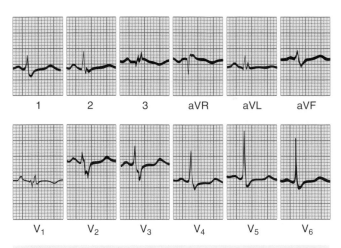

FIGURE 13-20 Electrocardiogram from an acyanotic 30-year-old woman with Ebstein's anomaly. A bizarre *second* QRS complex is attached to the preceding normal QRS complex. The PR interval and the P waves and are normal.

leads record right ventricular intracavitary potentials unusually far leftward as a result of the large size of the right atrium.[80] For the same reason, QRS patterns are similar, if not identical, in lead V_1 and lead aVR (see Figures 13-16 and 13-17). Prominent Q waves in right precordial leads can be misleading when adults with Ebstein's anomaly present with chest pain (see section History).

Supraventricular tachycardia, atrial fibrillation, and atrial flutter occur in 25% to 30% of cases.[36,41,61,75,76,82] Ebstein[1] reported that his patient "has always been troubled with palpitations." Wide QRS tachycardia via bypass tracts must be distinguished from ventricular tachycardia, which is uncommon if not as rare as a spontaneous tachyarrhythmia (see Figure 13-4).[39,82] Right bundle branch block is a feature of Brugada's syndrome, which occurs with ST segment elevation in leads V_{1-2} and ventricular fibrillation, but without structural heart disease.[83–85]

Wolff-Parkinson-White preexcitation, which was described in 1930[86] and characterized electrophysiologically in 1967,[87] occurs in 5% to 25% of the electrocardiograms in Ebstein's anomaly (see Figures 13-18 and 13-19).[41,43,76,80] Downward displacement of the septal tricuspid leaflet is accompanied by discontinuity between the central fibrous body and the septal atrioventricular ring, which creates a substrate for preexcitation (see previous discussion). Recurrent tachyarrhythmias have been known to occur in Ebstein's anomaly for more than six decades. *Ebstein's anomaly is the only cyanotic congenital cardiac malformation consistently associated with preexcitation*, which is uniformly via a right bypass tract (i.e., type B Wolff-Parkinson-White; see Figures 13-18 and 13-19). Patients with preexcitation may not experience atrial tachyarrhythmias, and atrial tachyarrhythmias are not confined to patients with accessory atrioventricular conduction. Nevertheless, *the combination of type B preexcitation and cyanosis constitutes presumptive evidence of Ebstein's anomaly.* Accessory pathway conduction can be permanent or intermittent and can occur without delta waves; and delta waves can occur with a short or normal PR interval (see Figure 13-14).[81] The type B bypass conduction of Ebstein's anomaly is associated with a left superior QRS axis (see Figures 13-18 and 13-19), but a left superior axis is not always associated with delta waves (see Figure 13-16). The QRS configuration and the direction of the delta wave vector assign the accessory atrioventricular pathway to the right posterolateral free wall or to the right posterior septum (see Figures 13-18 and 13-19).[82] When accessory pathways are multiple, as they are in more than a third of patients with Ebstein's anomaly, conduction tends to be via the septal pathway.[82] Mahaim nodoventricular fibers are likely to be present when a left bundle branch block pattern occurs during sinus rhythm or during an episode of tachycardia.[82]

X-RAY

The cardiac silhouette varies from near normal (Figures 13-21 and 13-22) to diagnostic (Figures 13-23 through 13-27).[41,88] Heart size in symptomatic infants is immense (Figures 13-28 and 13-29). Pulmonary vascularity is normal in mild acyanotic Ebstein's anomaly (see Figures 13-21 and 13-22) and is reduced when the anomaly is severe and cyanotic (see Figures 13-25, 13-26, and 13-27).[88] Cyanosis with normal or reduced pulmonary blood flow and a dominant left ventricle is a useful combination in the clinical diagnosis of Ebstein's anomaly. The infundibulum either straightens the left cardiac border (see Figures 13-22, 13-23, and 13-24) or forms a conspicuous convex shoulder (see Figures 13-25, 13-26, and 13-27). The most consistent and dramatic radiologic feature is the right atrial silhouette, which is almost always enlarged (see Figures 13-23 through 13-25), sometimes dramatically so (see Figures 13-26 through 13-29), and is seldom normal even when the cardiac silhouette is otherwise normal (see Figures 13-21 and 13-22A). Marked rightward convexity of the enlarged right atrium together with marked leftward convexity of the enlarged infundibulum account for a boxlike configuration (see Figures 13-26 and 13-27).[41] The vascular pedicle is narrow because the pulmonary trunk is not border forming and the ascending aortic shadow is inconspicuous or absent (see Figures 13-22 through 13-27), with rare exception (see Figure 13-21).

ECHOCARDIOGRAM

Echocardiography with color flow imaging and Doppler interrogation is the diagnostic test of choice and is used to establish the diagnosis and severity of Ebstein's anomaly.[17,25,89,90] The diagnosis can be made in utero.[51,59,60] Apical displacement of the septal tricuspid leaflet in the anomaly exceeds 15 mm in children and 20 mm in adults (Figure 13-30).[89] The right atrium proper lies proximal to the anatomic tricuspid annulus, and the atrialized right ventricle occupies the interval between the anatomic tricuspid annulus and the distally displaced septal tricuspid leaflet (see Figure 13-30). The

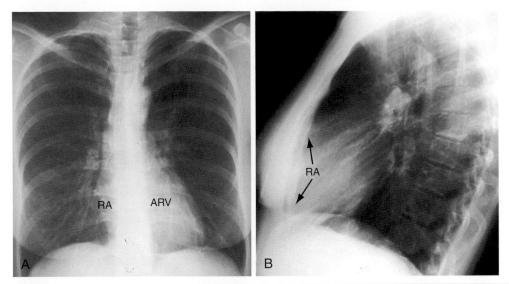

FIGURE 13-21 X-rays from the 39-year-old woman with mild Ebstein's anomaly whose electrocardiogram is shown in Figure 13-16. **A,** The size and configuration of the heart are normal, but the ascending and transverse aortas are relatively prominent for age and gender. **B,** In the lateral projection, the retrosternal right atrium (RA) reveals itself. (RA = right atrium; ARV = atrialized right ventricle.)

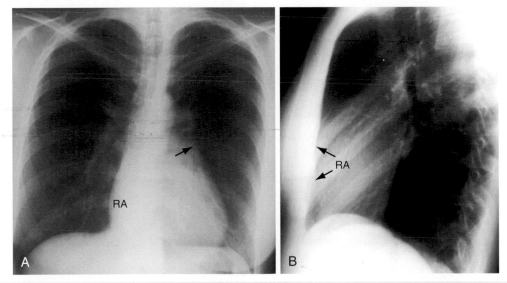

FIGURE 13-22 X-rays from a 33-year-old woman with mild Ebstein's anomaly. **A,** The left cardiac border is straightened by the infundibulum (arrow). The right atrial contour is only slightly prominent (RA). **B,** Retrosternal right atrial enlargement is more apparent in the lateral projection.

displaced tethered septal tricuspid leaflet moves little if at all in contrast to the large elongated anterior leaflet, which may exhibit brisk sail-like movements in real-time imaging (Figures 13-30 and 13-31). Rarely, a broad echogenic band separates the atrialized right ventricle from the distal functional right ventricle, and the proximal annulus is unguarded by tricuspid leaflet tissue (Figure 13-32).

Echocardiography defines left ventricular geometry and cavity size, and real-time imaging identifies displacement of the ventricular septum into the left ventricular cavity with paradoxical septal motion (see Figure 13-31).[29]

Superior systolic displacement (mitral prolapse) occurs because normal-sized leaflets and chordae tendinae are housed in a left ventricular cavity that is reduced in size and altered in shape (see Figure 13-31).[29] The right ventricular outflow tract in the short axis is dilated in contrast to the adjacent normal or small aortic root. Color flow imaging and Doppler interrogation quantify tricuspid regurgitation and establish the relatively low velocity of regurgitant flow, which begins at the level of the displaced septal and posterior leaflets and courses through the atrialized right ventricle into the right atrium proper (Figure 13-33, Video 13-1, and Figure 13-34).

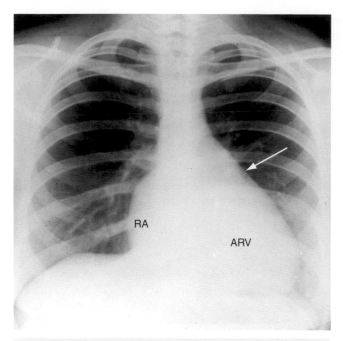

FIGURE 13-23 X-ray from an acyanotic 23-year-old woman with Ebstein's anomaly who came to attention because of recurrent paroxysmal rapid heart action without electrocardiographic evidence of an accessory pathway. The infundibulum is border-forming (arrow), the right atrium (RA) is prominent, and the vascular pedicle is narrow. (ARV = atrialized right ventricle.)

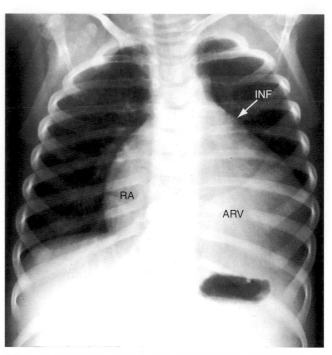

FIGURE 13-25 X-ray from a 19-month-old acyanotic female with Ebstein's anomaly. The lung fields are oligemic. The infundibulum (INF) is prominent. Neither the pulmonary trunk nor the ascending aorta is border-forming. Cardiac enlargement is from a huge right atrium (RA) and an atrialized right ventricle (ARV).

Echocardiography identifies a patent foramen ovale or an ostium secundum atrial septal defect. Color flow imaging with Doppler interrogation confirms the presence of the interatrial communication and determines whether a right-to-left shunt coexists.

Three-dimensional echocardiography[58] and magnetic resonance imaging allow precise anatomic and functional assessment of the tricuspid valve and right ventricle.[58]

SUMMARY

Cyanosis with normal or reduced pulmonary blood flow and a dominant left ventricle is a useful combination in the clinical diagnosis of Ebstein's anomaly. When these features are associated with type B Wolff-Parkinson-White preexcitation, the diagnosis is virtually secure. Outlook is poorest in symptomatic newborns, but

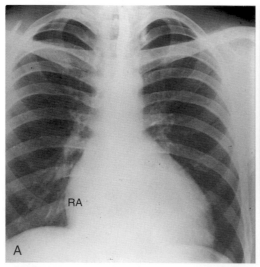
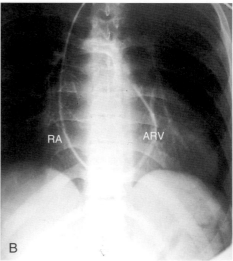

FIGURE 13-24 X-rays from an 18-year-old cyanotic man with Ebstein's anomaly. **A,** The increase in heart size is the result of enlargement of the right atrium and contiguous atrialized right ventricle. The vascular pedicle is narrow. **B,** The loop of the catheter outlines the right atrium (RA) and contiguous atrialized right ventricle (ARV).

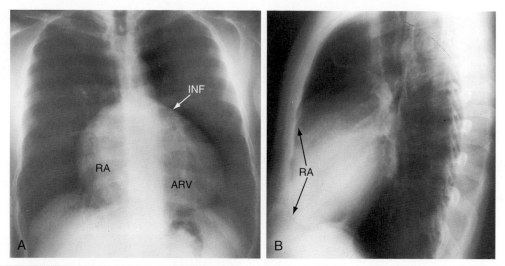

FIGURE 13-26 X-rays from an acyanotic 41-year-old man with Ebstein's anomaly and exercise-induced hypoxemia. **A,** The lung fields are oligemic, although the film is overpenetrated. The infundibulum (INF) is prominent, but the vascular pedicle is narrow because neither the ascending aorta nor the pulmonary trunk is border-forming. Cardiac enlargement is the result of a huge right atrium (RA) and an atrialized right ventricle (ARV). The x-ray bears a striking resemblance to Figure 13-25 from the 19-month-old acyanotic female with Ebstein's anomaly. **B,** The retrosternal space is occupied by the enlarged right atrium (RA, arrows).

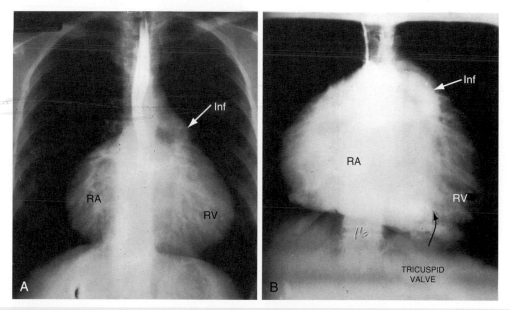

FIGURE 13-27 X-ray and angiocardiogram from a 32-year-old acyanotic woman with Ebstein's anomaly. **A,** The infundubulum (Inf) is prominent, but the vascular pedicle is narrow because neither the ascending aorta nor the pulmonary trunk is border-forming. Cardiomegaly is the result of enlargement of the right atrium (RA) and atrialized right ventricle. The lung fields are remarkably clear, although the x-ray is overpenetrated. **B,** Angiocardiogram shows the huge right atrium and contiguous atrialized right ventricle with the displaced tricuspid valve (arrow). The cardiac silhouette is boxlike because of the prominent infundibulum and the large right atrium. (RV = functional right ventricle.)

neonatal cyanosis occasionally regresses only to recur years later. The crests of the A and V waves and the mean jugular venous pressure are normal. An enlarged infundibulum is palpable in the third left intercostal space, but a right ventricular inflow impulse is conspicuously absent. The first heart sound is widely split, and the tricuspid component is loud and delayed. The low-pressure low-velocity murmur of tricuspid regurgitation is early systolic, decrescendo, medium-frequency, and maximal toward the apex over the displaced tricuspid valve. Triple or quadruple rhythms are caused by third and fourth heart sounds that may fuse to form short

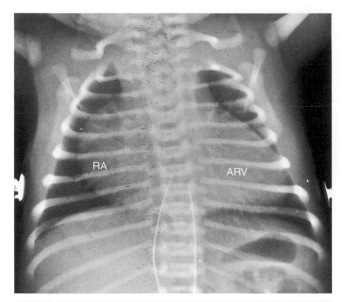

FIGURE 13-28 X-ray from a symptomatic cyanotic female neonate with Ebstein's anomaly. The huge cardiac silhouette covers all but a fraction of the oligemic lung fields. Cardiomegaly is from a huge right atrium (RA) and an atrialized right ventricle (ARV). Diagnosis was confirmed at necropsy.

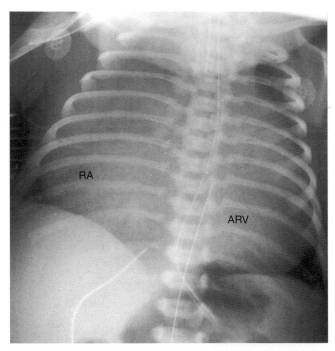

FIGURE 13-29 X-ray from a symptomatic cyanotic male neonate with Ebstein's anomaly. Striking cardiomegaly was the result of a huge right atrium (RA) and an atrialized right ventricle (ARV). Thymus occupies the thoracic inlet. Compare with Figure 13-28. Diagnosis was confirmed at necropsy.

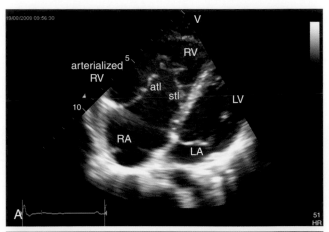

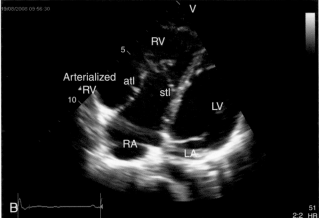

FIGURE 13-30 Echocardiograms (apical four-chamber) from a 5-year-old girl with acyanotic Ebstein's anomaly. The septal tricuspid leaflet (stl) is displaced into the right ventricle and tethered to the septum. The large anterior tricuspid leaflet (atl) was highly mobile in real-time imaging and is shown here in diastole (A) and in systole (B). A, The atrialized right ventricle (ARV) lies between the displaced septal tricuspid leaflet and the anatomic tricuspid anulus. The functional right ventricle (RV) lies distally, and the anatomic right atrium (RA) lies proximally. (LV = left ventricle; LA = left atrium.)

mid-diastolic or presystolic murmurs, especially when the PR interval is prolonged. The electrocardiogram is characterized by tall broad right atrial P waves, a prolonged PR interval, right bundle branch block, and deep Q waves in right precordial leads. The x-ray shows normal or decreased pulmonary vascularity, a narrow vascular pedicle, a prominent infundibulum, and a large right atrium. In symptomatic neonates, the cardiac silhouette may occupy virtually the entire chest. Echocardiography, color flow imaging, and Doppler interrogation identify abnormalities of the three tricuspid leaflets and identify the atrialized right ventricle, paradoxical motion of the ventricular septum, the size and shape of the left ventricle, the degree of tricuspid regurgitation, and the presence of a patent foramen ovale or an atrial septal defect.

UHL'S ANOMALY

The *parchment heart* was so designated by Osler[91] in 1905 and was redescribed in 1950.[92] Two years later, Uhl[93] reported "almost total absence of myocardium of

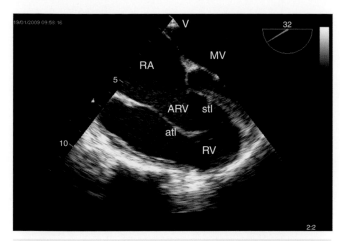

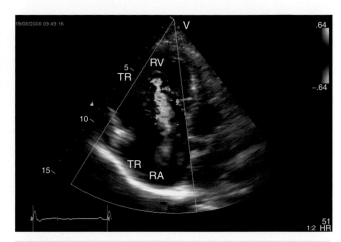

FIGURE 13-31 Transesophageal echocardiogram from the 41-year-old man. An immobile septal tricuspid leaflet (stl) is apically displaced. The large nondisplaced anterior tricuspid leaflet (atl) was highly mobile on real-time imaging. The size and configuration of the left ventricle (LV) are abnormal because of encroachment by the ventricular septum. (ARV = atrialized right ventricle; MV = mitral valve.)

FIGURE 13-33 Echocardiograms from a patient with Ebstein's anomaly. Color flow shows the jet of tricuspid regurgitation (TR) originating at the junction of the functional right ventricle (RV) and the atrialized right ventricle (Video 13-1). (RA = right atrium.)

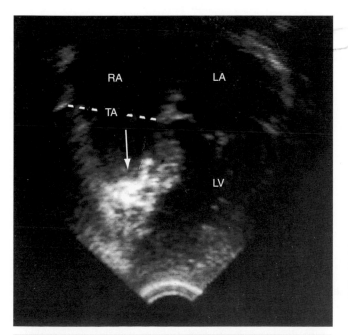

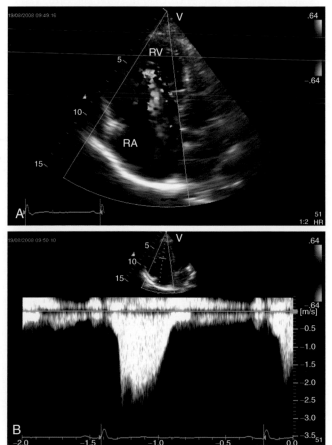

FIGURE 13-32 Echocardiogram (four-chamber view) from an 8-week-old female with cyanotic Ebstein's anomaly. Unmarked arrow points to a broad echogenic band that completely divided the atrialized right ventricle from the functional right ventricle. At necropsy, the thick muscular partition was partially calcified. The tricuspid annulus (TA) above the partition was devoid of tricuspid leaflet tissue. (RA = right atrium; LA = left atrium; LV = left ventricle.)

FIGURE 13-34 A, Color flow imaging from a 19-year-old man with acyanotic Ebstein's anomaly. The jet of tricuspid regurgitation (TR) originated within the right ventricular cavity at the junction of the functional right ventricle (RV) and the atrialized right ventricle. **B,** Continuous wave Doppler shows the low-velocity tricuspid regurgitant jet (TR). (RA = right atrium.)

the right ventricle." Aplasia or hypoplasia of most if not all of the myocardium in the trabecular portions of the right ventricle occurs with a structurally normal and functionally competent tricuspid valve.[94,95] The parchment right ventricle of Uhl's anomaly has been characterized as *inexcitable* in contrast to the arrhythmogenic atrialized right ventricle of Ebstein's anomaly.[96] Uhl's anomaly has been reported in identical twins and has been diagnosed *in utero*.[97]

The essential hemodynamic fault in Uhl's anomaly is lack of right ventricular contraction. The chamber functions as a passive conduit through which right atrial blood is channeled on its way into the pulmonary trunk. The thin-walled right ventricle balloons aneurysmally with each systole. The morphologically uninvolved ventricular septum exhibits vigorous paradoxical systolic motion and functions as part of the right ventricle, contributing materially to forward flow. Survival into adulthood is expected despite the functionally inadequate right ventricle. The jugular venous pulse is normal because the tricuspid valve is competent and because the force of right atrial contraction is not increased despite the parchment right ventricle. An elevation in right ventricular end-diastolic pressure and mean right atrial pressure rarely causes a right-to-left shunt interatrial shunt. A left ventricular impulse occupies the apex. A right ventricular impulse is absent by definition. A right ventricular third heart sound is generated by passive flow into the poorly compliant parchment right ventricle. The second heart sound is widely split even though the right ventricular conduction defect is thought to be peripheral (Figure 13-35). The electrocardiogram exhibits right atrial P waves (see Figure 13-35) because the right atrium tends to be larger than normal despite a competent tricuspid valve (Figure 13-36). The PR interval is normal, and preexcitation is unknown. The x-ray shows normal pulmonary vascularity and an increase in heart size chiefly from the dilated parchment ventricle (see Figure 13-36). The right atrial silhouette is rounded but unimpressive compared with Ebstein's anomaly (see Figure 13-36).

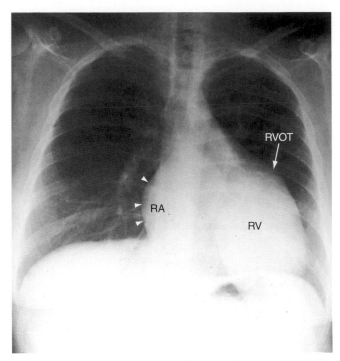

FIGURE 13-36 X-ray from a 25-year-old woman with Uhl's anomaly. The cardiac silhouette is enlarged because of dilation of the right ventricle (RV) and right atrium (RA). The right ventricular outflow tract (RVOT) is hump-shaped. The ascending aorta is inconspicuous.

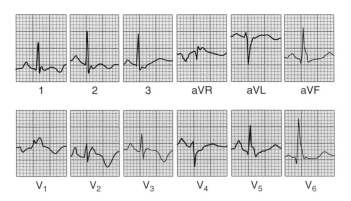

FIGURE 13-35 Electrocardiogram from a 25-year-old woman with Uhl's anomaly. A right atrial abnormality is indicated by the deep broad P terminal force in lead V_1 and the tall peaked P wave in lead V_2. The QRS duration is prolonged because of a right ventricular conduction defect.

The morphologically spared infundibulum presents as a hump-shaped convexity at the upper the left cardiac border (see Figure 13-36). Echocardiography identifies a large right ventricle with an akinetic free wall, brisk paradoxical motion of the ventricular septum, and normal tricuspid leaflets (Figure 13-37). Doppler echocardiography with color flow imaging confirms that the tricuspid valve is competent.

Arrhythomegenic right ventricular dysplasia varies from mild focal lesions detected histologically to widespread segmental transmural involvement of the free wall of the right ventricle and infundibulum.[95,98–101] Biventricular involvement is infrequent.[102,103] Prevalence rate has been estimated at 1/5000.[84] Dysplasia is represented by focal replacement of myocardium with fibrous and adipose tissue, not by focal congenital absence of the myocardium.[99,100] The lesions can be detected with magnetic resonance imaging and with low-amplitude endocardial electrograms that identify replaced myocardium.[104] Familial recurrence of right ventricular dysplasia was confirmed in a study of nine families.[99,100] The echocardiogram discloses segmental and generalized abnormalities of right ventricular wall motion, abnormal trabecular architecture, and areas of saccular dilation.[100,105] Isolated noncompaction of *left ventricular* myocardium, or *Barth's syndrome*, is arrhythmogenic and is characterized morphologically by numerous prominent trabeculations and conspicuous intertrabecular recesses that penetrate deeply into the left ventricular myocardium.[106,107]

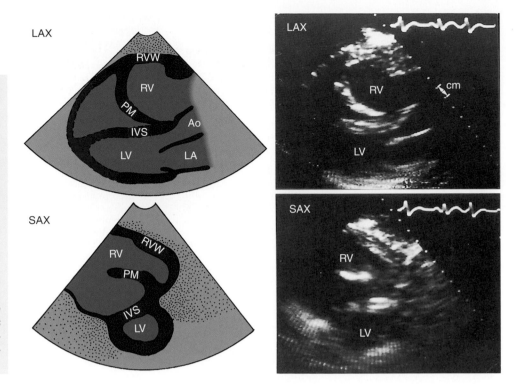

FIGURE 13-37 Echocardiograms (parasternal long-axis [LAX] and short-axis [SAX]) from the 25-year-old woman with Uhl's anomaly whose x-ray is shown in Figure 13-36. The right ventricle (RV) is dilated, and its cavity contains a large refractile papillary muscle (PM) shown in the short axis sketch (SAX). The interventricular septum (IVS labeled in the sketches) exhibited brisk paradoxical systolic motion in real time, whereas the right ventricular wall (RVW labeled in the sketch) was akinetic. (Ao = aorta; LA = left atrium.) *(From Child JS, Perloff JK, et al. Uhl's anomaly (parchment right ventricle). American Journal of Cardiology 53:635, 1984.)*

REFERENCES

1. Ebstein W. On a very rare case of insufficiency of the tricuspid valve caused by a severe congenital malformation of the same. *Am J Cardiol.* 1968;22:867.
2. Konstantinov IE. History of cardiology: Wilhelm Ebstein, MD. Interview by Mark Nicholls. *Circulation.* 2007;116:f101–f102.
3. Mann RJ, Lie JT. The life story of Wilhelm Ebstein (1836-1912) and his almost overlooked description of a congenital heart disease. *Mayo Clin Proc.* 1979;54:197–204.
4. Sekelj P, Benfey BG. Fundamentals of clinical cardiology: historical landmarks: Ebstein's anomaly of the tricuspid valve. *Am Heart J.* 1974;88:108–114.
5. Van Son JA, Konstantinov IE, Zimmermann V. Wilhelm Ebstein and Ebstein's malformation. *Eur J Cardiothorac Surg.* 2001;20:1082–1085.
6. Yater WM, Shapiro MJ. Congenital displacement of the tricuspid valve (Ebstein's disease): review and report of a case with electrocardiographic abnormalities and detailed histologic study of the conduction system. *Ann Intern Med.* 1937;11:1043.
7. Tourniaire M, Tourniaire F, Tartulier M. Maladie d'Epstein. *Arch Mal Cœur Vaiss.* 1949;42:1211.
8. Engle MA, Payne TP, Bruins C, Taussig HB. Ebstein's anomaly of the tricuspid valve; report of three cases and analysis of clinical syndrome. *Circulation.* 1950;1:1246–1260.
9. Reynolds G. Ebstein's disease a case diagnosed clinically. *Guys Hospital Reports.* 1950;99:275–283.
10. Soloff LA, Stauffer HM, Zatuchni J. Ebstein's disease: report of the first case diagnosed during life. *Am J Med Sci.* 1951;222:554–561.
11. Soloff LA, Stauffer HM, Zatuchni J. Ebstein's disease: description of the heart of the first case diagnosed during life. *Am J Med Sci.* 1957;233:23–27.
12. Nora JJ, Nora AH, Toews WH. Letter: Lithium, Ebstein's anomaly, and other congenital heart defects. *Lancet.* 1974;2:594–595.
13. Patane S, Marte F, Di Bella G, Chiribiri A. Ebstein's anomaly in adult. *Int J Cardiol.* 2009;136:e6–e7.
14. Hauck AJ, Freeman DP, Ackermann DM, Danielson GK, Edwards WD. Surgical pathology of the tricuspid valve: a study of 363 cases spanning 25 years. *Mayo Clin Proc.* 1988;63:851–863.
15. Silver MD, Lam JH, Ranganathan N, Wigle ED. Morphology of the human tricuspid valve. *Circulation.* 1971;43:333–348.
16. Gussenhoven EJ, Stewart PA, Becker AE, Essed CE, Ligtvoet KM, De Villeneuve VH. "Offsetting" of the septal tricuspid leaflet in normal hearts and in hearts with Ebstein's anomaly. Anatomic and echographic correlation. *Am J Cardiol.* 1984;54:172–176.
17. Attenhofer Jost CH, Connolly HM, Dearani JA, Edwards WD, Danielson GK. Ebstein's anomaly. *Circulation.* 2007;115:277–285.
18. Dearani JA, Danielson GK. Congenital Heart Surgery Nomenclature and Database Project: Ebstein's anomaly and tricuspid valve disease. *Ann Thorac Surg.* 2000;69:S106–S117.
19. Celermajer DS, Dodd SM, Greenwald SE, Wyse RK, Deanfield JE. Morbid anatomy in neonates with Ebstein's anomaly of the tricuspid valve: pathophysiologic and clinical implications. *J Am Coll Cardiol.* 1992;19:1049–1053.
20. Zuberbuhler JR, Becker AE, Anderson RH, Lenox CC. Ebstein's malformation and the embryological development of the tricuspid valve. With a note on the nature of "clefts" in the atrioventricular valves. *Pediatr Cardiol.* 1984;5:289–295.
21. Tabatabaei N, Katanyuwong P, Breen JF, et al. Images in cardiovascular medicine. Uncommon variant of Ebstein anomaly with tricuspid stenosis. *Circulation.* 2009;120:e1–e2.
22. Anderson KR, Lie JT. The right ventricular myocardium in Ebstein's anomaly: a morphometric histopathologic study. *Mayo Clin Proc.* 1979;54:181–184.
23. Frescura C, Angelini A, Daliento L, Thiene G. Morphological aspects of Ebstein's anomaly in adults. *Thorac Cardiovasc Surg.* 2000;48:203–208.
24. Anderson RH, Silverman NH, Zuberbuhler JR. Congenitally unguarded tricuspid orifice: its differentiation from Ebstein's malformation in association with pulmonary atresia and intact ventricular septum. *Pediatr Cardiol.* 1990;11:86–90.
25. Lang D, Oberhoffer R, Cook A, et al. Pathologic spectrum of malformations of the tricuspid valve in prenatal and neonatal life. *J Am Coll Cardiol.* 1991;17:1161–1167.
26. Beder SD, Nihill MR, Mcnamara DG. Idiopathic dilation of the right atrium in a child. *Am Heart J.* 1982;103:134–137.
27. Sheldon WC, Johnson CD, Favaloro RG. Idiopathic enlargement of the right atrium. Report of four cases. *Am J Cardiol.* 1969;23:278–284.

28. Gewillig M, Dumoulin M, Van Der Hauwaert LG. Transient neonatal tricuspid regurgitation: a Doppler echocardiographic study of three cases. *Br Heart J.* 1988;60:446–451.

29. Benson LN, Child JS, Schwaiger M, Perloff JK, Schelbert HR. Left ventricular geometry and function in adults with Ebstein's anomaly of the tricuspid valve. *Circulation.* 1987;75:353–359.

30. Inai K, Nakanishi T, Mori Y, Tomimatsu H, Nakazawa M. Left ventricular diastolic dysfunction in Ebstein's anomaly. *Am J Cardiol.* 2004;93:255–258.

31. Stollberger C, Kopsa W, Finsterer J. Non-compaction of the right atrium and left ventricle in Ebstein's malformation. *J Heart Valve Dis.* 2006;15:719–720.

32. Cabin HS, Roberts WC. Ebstein's anomaly of the tricuspid valve and prolapse of the mitral valve. *Am Heart J.* 1981;101:177–180.

33. Roberts WC, Glancy DL, Seningen RP, Maron BJ, Epstein SE. Prolapse of the mitral valve is described in two patients with the Ebstein's anomaly of the tricuspid. *Am J Cardiol.* 1976;38: 377–382.

34. Barber G, Danielson GK, Heise CT, Driscoll DJ. Cardiorespiratory response to exercise in Ebstein's anomaly. *Am J Cardiol.* 1985;56:509–514.

35. Driscoll DJ, Mottram CD, Danielson GK. Spectrum of exercise intolerance in 45 patients with Ebstein's anomaly and observations on exercise tolerance in 11 patients after surgical repair. *J Am Coll Cardiol.* 1988;11:831–836.

36. Lowe KG, Emslie-Smith D, Robertson PG, Watson H. Scalar, vector, and intracardiac electrocardiograms in Ebstein's anomaly. *Br Heart J.* 1968;30:617–629.

37. Watson H. Electrode catheters and the diagnosis of Ebstein's anomaly of the tricuspid valve. *Br Heart J.* 1966;28:161–171.

38. Obioha-Ngwu O, Milliez P, Richardson A, Pittaro M, Josephson ME. Ventricular tachycardia in Ebstein's anomaly. *Circulation.* 2001;104:E92–E94.

39. Lo HM, Lin FY, Jong YS, Tseng YZ, Wu TL. Ebstein's anomaly with ventricular tachycardia: evidence for the arrhythmogenic role of the atrialized ventricle. *Am Heart J.* 1989;117:959–962.

40. Tede NH, Shivkumar K, Perloff JK, et al. Signal-averaged electrocardiogram in Ebstein's anomaly. *Am J Cardiol.* 2004;93:432–436.

41. Bialostozky D, Horwitz S, Espino-Vela J. Ebstein's malformation of the tricuspid valve. A review of 65 cases. *Am J Cardiol.* 1972; 29:826–836.

42. Samanek M. Boy:girl ratio in children born with different forms of cardiac malformation: a population-based study. *Pediatr Cardiol.* 1994;15:53–57.

43. Watson H. Natural history of Ebstein's anomaly of tricuspid valve in childhood and adolescence. An international co-operative study of 505 cases. *Br Heart J.* 1974;36:417–427.

44. Flores Arizmendi A, Fernandez Pineda L, Quero Jimenez C, et al. The clinical profile of Ebstein's malformation as seen from the fetus to the adult in 52 patients. *Cardiol Young.* 2004;14:55–63.

45. Balaji S, Dennis NR, Keeton BR. Familial Ebstein's anomaly: a report of six cases in two generations associated with mild skeletal abnormalities. *Br Heart J.* 1991;66:26–28.

46. Donegan Jr CC, Moore MM, Wiley Jr TM, Hernandez FA, Green Jr JR, Schiebler GL. Familial Ebstein's anomaly of the tricuspid valve. *Am Heart J.* 1968;75:375–379.

47. Lo KS, Loventhal JP, Walton Jr JA. Familial Ebstein's anomaly. *Cardiology.* 1979;64:246–255.

48. Mcintosh N, Chitayat D, Bardanis M, Fouron JC. Ebstein anomaly: report of a familial occurrence and prenatal diagnosis. *Am J Med Genet.* 1992;42:307–309.

49. Pierard LA, Henrard L, Demoulin JC. Persistent atrial standstill in familial Ebstein's anomaly. *Br Heart J.* 1985;53:594–597.

50. Emanuel R, O'brien K, Ng R. Ebstein's anomaly. Genetic study of 26 families. *Br Heart J.* 1976;38:5–7.

51. Uyan C, Yazici M, Uyan AP, Akdemir R, Imirzalioglu N, Dokumaci B. Ebstein's anomaly in siblings: an original observation. *Int J Cardiovasc Imaging.* 2002;18:435–438.

52. Gollob MH, Seger JJ, Gollob TN, et al. Novel PRKAG2 mutation responsible for the genetic syndrome of ventricular preexcitation and conduction system disease with childhood onset and absence of cardiac hypertrophy. *Circulation.* 2001;104:3030–3033.

53. Park JM, Sridaromont S, Ledbetter EO, Terry WM. Ebstein's anomaly of the tricuspid valve associated with prenatal exposure to lithium carbonate. *Am J Dis Child.* 1980;134:703–704.

54. Zalzstein E, Koren G, Einarson T, Freedom RM. A case-control study on the association between first trimester exposure to lithium and Ebstein's anomaly. *Am J Cardiol.* 1990;65:817–818.

55. Hong YM, Moller JH. Ebstein's anomaly: a long-term study of survival. *Am Heart J.* 1993;125:1419–1424.

56. Gentles TL, Calder AL, Clarkson PM, Neutze JM. Predictors of long-term survival with Ebstein's anomaly of the tricuspid valve. *Am J Cardiol.* 1992;69:377–381.

57. Celermajer DS, Bull C, Till JA, et al. Ebstein's anomaly: presentation and outcome from fetus to adult. *J Am Coll Cardiol.* 1994;23: 170–176.

58. Paranon S, Acar P. Ebstein's anomaly of the tricuspid valve: from fetus to adult: congenital heart disease. *Heart.* 2008;94:237–243.

59. Hsieh YY, Lee CC, Chang CC, Tsai HD, Yeh LS, Tsai CH. Successful prenatal digoxin therapy for Ebstein's anomaly with hydrops fetalis. A case report. *J Reprod Med.* 1998;43:710–712.

60. Pavlova M, Fouron JC, Drblik SP, et al. Factors affecting the prognosis of Ebstein's anomaly during fetal life. *Am Heart J.* 1998;135: 1081–1085.

61. Rossi L, Thiene G. Mild Ebstein's anomaly associated with supraventricular tachycardia and sudden death: clinicomorphologic features in 3 patients. *Am J Cardiol.* 1984;53:332–334.

62. Fitzsimmons PJ, Mcwhirter PD, Peterson DW, Kruyer WB. The natural history of Wolff-Parkinson-White syndrome in 228 military aviators: a long-term follow-up of 22 years. *Am Heart J.* 2001;142:530–536.

63. Cabin HS, Wood TP, Smith JO, Roberts WC. Structure–function correlations in cardiovascular and pulmonary diseases (CPC): Ebstein's anomaly in the elderly. *Chest.* 1981;80:212–214.

64. Makous N, Vander Veer JB. Ebstein's anomaly and life expectancy. Report of a survival to over age 79. *Am J Cardiol.* 1966; 18:100–104.

65. Harris RH. Ebstein's anomaly: discovered in a 75-year-old subject in the dissecting laboratory. *Can Med Assoc J.* 1960;83:653–655.

66. Seward JB, Tajik AJ, Feist DJ, Smith HC. Ebstein's anomaly in an 85-year-old man. *Mayo Clin Proc.* 1979;54:193–196.

67. Donnelly JE, Brown JM, Radford DJ. Pregnancy outcome and Ebstein's anomaly. *Br Heart J.* 1991;66:368–371.

68. Oki T, Fukuda N, Tabata T, et al. The 'sail sound' and tricuspid regurgitation in Ebstein's anomaly: the value of echocardiography in evaluating their mechanisms. *J Heart Valve Dis.* 1997;6: 189–192.

69. Crews TL, Pridie RB, Benham R, Leatham A. Auscultatory and phonocardiographic findings in Ebstein's anomaly. Correlation of first heart sound with ultrasonic records of tricuspid valve movement. *Br Heart J.* 1972;34:681–687.

70. Pocock WA, Tucker RB, Barlow JB. Mild Ebstein's anomaly. *Br Heart J.* 1969;31:327–336.

71. Fontana ME, Wooley CF. Sail sound in Ebstein's anomaly of the tricuspid valve. *Circulation.* 1972;46:155–164.

72. Willis PWT, Craige E. First heart sound in Ebstein's anomaly: observations on the cause of wide splitting by echophonocardiographic studies before and after operative repair. *J Am Coll Cardiol.* 1983;2:1165–1168.

73. Koiwaya Y, Narabayashi H, Koyanagi S, et al. Early closure of the tricuspid valve in a case of Ebstein's anomaly with type B Wolff-Parkinson-White Syndrome. *Circulation.* 1979;60:446–450.

74. Perloff JK. *Physical examination of the heart and circulation.* 4th ed. Shelton, Connecticut: People's Medical Publishing House; 2009.

75. Macruz R, Tranchesi J, Ebaid M, Pileggi F, Romero A, Decourt LV. Ebstein's disease. Electrovectorcardiographic and radiologic correlations. *Am J Cardiol.* 1968;21:653–660.

76. Kastor JA, Goldreyer BN, Josephson ME, et al. Electrophysiologic characteristics of Ebstein's anomaly of the tricuspid valve. *Circulation.* 1975;52:987–995.

77. Kaushik ML, Sharma M, Kashyap R. 'Himalayan' p wave. *J Assoc Physicians India.* 2007;55:856.

78. Ho SY, Goltz D, Mccarthy K, et al. The atrioventricular junctions in Ebstein malformation. *Heart.* 2000;83:444–449.

79. Price JE, Amsterdam EA, Vera Z, Swenson R, Mason DT. Ebstein's disease associated with complete atrioventricular block. *Chest.* 1978;73:542–544.

80. Bialostozky D, Medrano GA, Munoz L, Contreras R. Vectorcardiographic study and anatomic observations in 21 cases of

Ebstein's malformation of the tricuspid valve. *Am J Cardiol.* 1972; 30:354–361.

81. Follath F, Hallidie-Smith KA. Unusual electrocardiographic changes in Ebstein's anomaly. *Br Heart J.* 1972;34:513–519.

82. Smith WM, Gallagher JJ, Kerr CR, et al. The electrophysiologic basis and management of symptomatic recurrent tachycardia in patients with Ebstein's anomaly of the tricuspid valve. *Am J Cardiol.* 1982;49:1223–1234.

83. Surawicz B. Brugada syndrome: manifest, concealed, "asymptomatic," suspected and simulated. *J Am Coll Cardiol.* 2001;38: 775–777.

84. Wichter T, Matheja P, Eckardt L, et al. Cardiac autonomic dysfunction in Brugada syndrome. *Circulation.* 2002;105:702–706.

85. Priori SG, Napolitano C, Gasparini M, et al. Natural history of Brugada syndrome: insights for risk stratification and management. *Circulation.* 2002;105:1342–1347.

86. Wolff L, Parkinson J, White PD. Bundle-branch block with short P-R interval in healthy young people prone to paroxysmal tachycardia. 1930. *Ann Noninvasive Electrocardiol.* 2006;11:340–353.

87. Durrer D, Roos JP. Epicardial excitation of the ventricles in a patient with Wolff-Parkinson-White syndrome (type B). *Circulation.* 1967;35:15–21.

88. Tao MS, Partridge J, Radford D. The plain chest radiograph in uncomplicated Ebstein's disease. *Clin Radiol.* 1986;37:551–553.

89. Ammash NM, Warnes CA, Connolly HM, Danielson GK, Seward JB. Mimics of Ebstein's anomaly. *Am Heart J.* 1997; 134:508–513.

90. Ahmed S, Nanda NC, Nekkanti R, Pacifico AD. Transesophageal three-dimensional echocardiographic demonstration of Ebstein's anomaly. *Echocardiography.* 2003;20:305–307.

91. Osler W. *The principles and practice of medicine.* 6th ed. New York: Appleton-Century-Crofts; 1905.

92. Segall HN. Parchment heart (Osler). *Am Heart J.* 1950;40: 948–950.

93. Uhl HS. A previously undescribed congenital malformation of the heart: almost total absence of the myocardium of the right ventricle. *Bull Johns Hopkins Hosp.* 1952;91:197–209.

94. Reeve R, Macdonald D. Partial absence of the right ventricular musculature—partial parchment heart. *Am J Cardiol.* 1964;14: 415–419.

95. Vecht RJ, Carmichael DJ, Gopal R, Philip G. Uhl's anomaly. *Br Heart J.* 1979;41:676–682.

96. Bharati S, Ciraulo DA, Bilitch M, Rosen KM, Lev M. Inexcitable right ventricle and bilateral bundle branch block in Uhl's disease. *Circulation.* 1978;57:636–644.

97. Hoback J, Adicoff A, From AH, Smith M, Shafer R, Chesler E. A report of Uhl's disease in identical adult twins: evaluation of right ventricular dysfunction with echocardiography and nuclear angiography. *Chest.* 1981;79:306–310.

98. Ouyang F, Fotuhi P, Goya M, et al. Ventricular tachycardia around the tricuspid annulus in right ventricular dysplasia. *Circulation.* 2001;103:913–914.

99. Marcus FI, Fontaine GH, Guiraudon G, et al. Right ventricular dysplasia: a report of 24 adult cases. *Circulation.* 1982;65:384–398.

100. Nava A, Thiene G, Canciani B, et al. Familial occurrence of right ventricular dysplasia: a study involving nine families. *J Am Coll Cardiol.* 1988;12:1222–1228.

101. Virmani R, Robinowitz M, Clark MA, Mcallister Jr HA. Sudden death and partial absence of the right ventricular myocardium: a report of three cases and a review of the literature. *Arch Pathol Lab Med.* 1982;106:163–167.

102. Pinamonti B, Pagnan L, Bussani R, Ricci C, Silvestri F, Camerini F. Right ventricular dysplasia with biventricular involvement. *Circulation.* 1998;98:1943–1945.

103. Mccrohon JA, John AS, Lorenz CH, Davies SW, Pennell DJ. Images in cardiovascular medicine. Left ventricular involvement in arrhythmogenic right ventricular cardiomyopathy. *Circulation.* 2002;105:1394.

104. Boulos M, Lashevsky I, Reisner S, Gepstein L. Electroanatomic mapping of arrhythmogenic right ventricular dysplasia. *J Am Coll Cardiol.* 2001;38:2020–2027.

105. Baran A, Nanda NC, Falkoff M, Barold SS, Gallagher JJ. Two-dimensional echocardiographic detection of arrhythmogenic right ventricular dysplasia. *Am Heart J.* 1982;103:1066–1067.

106. Chin TK, Perloff JK, Williams RG, Jue K, Mohrmann R. Isolated noncompaction of left ventricular myocardium. A study of eight cases. *Circulation.* 1990;82:507–513.

107. Ichida F, Tsubata S, Bowles KR, et al. Novel gene mutations in patients with left ventricular noncompaction or Barth syndrome. *Circulation.* 2001;103:1256–1263.

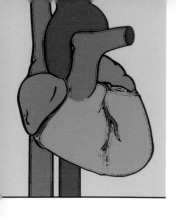

Chapter 14

Primary Pulmonary Hypertension

Pulmonary arterial pressure was measured in 1852,[1] but a century elapsed before cardiac catheterization provided the means for studying the physiology of the lesser circulation. *Elevated* pulmonary arterial pressure—*pulmonary hypertension*—results from disorders of the pulmonary vascular bed, the pulmonary parenchyma, the respiratory system, and the pulmonary venous bed and from chronic thromboembolic disease (Box 14-1).[2] This chapter focuses on the pulmonary vascular bed, specifically on *primary (idiopathic) pulmonary hypertension*, a disorder that originates in the terminal muscular pulmonary arteries and arterioles.[3,4]

The earliest description of idiopathic pulmonary hypertension was a report in 1891 of the cardiac pathology in a patient with pulmonary artery sclerosis and right ventricular hypertrophy of unknown cause.[5] *Primary pulmonary hypertension*, a term coined by Dresdale in 1951, referred to an idiopathic disorder residing in the terminal pulmonary arteries and arterioles. The prevalence rate of primary pulmonary hypertension is estimated at one or two cases per million in the general population.[3] Shortly after Dresdale's report, Wood[6] characterized the clinical manifestations of primary pulmonary hypertension. Two decades later, the World Health Organization (WHO) proposed a classification based on three histopathologic patterns: plexogenic pulmonary arteriopathy, microthrombotic pulmonary arteriopathy, and pulmonary venoocclusive disease.[7] In 1975, WHO defined primary pulmonary hypertension as a disorder with no identifiable cause in which resting mean pulmonary artery pressure in adults at sea level is above 25 mm Hg and above 30 mm Hg with exercise. Pulmonary vascular resistance does not exceed three Wood units, and pulmonary capillary wedge pressure is normal.[3,4,7] In 1981, the National Heart, Lung, and Blood Institute established a *Registry* to collect information on *primary pulmonary hypertension* in accordance with a uniform database.[8] Enlightening histopathologic studies abound.[8–13]

The pulmonary vascular bed consists of an elaborately branched system of arteries, arterioles, capillaries, venules, and veins that accommodate the cardiac output at low pressures. Approximately 17 gradations of arterial vascular channels separate the main pulmonary artery from the pulmonary arterioles. In the fetus, the pulmonary arteriole is structurally analogous to the systemic arteriole and is therefore equipped to meet the full force of systemic pressure the moment the neonatal lungs expand and pulmonary blood flow commences. The thick-walled neonatal pulmonary arterioles rapidly involute, and the pulmonary vascular bed remodels, establishing the low-resistance lesser circulation. Remodeling continues for 1 or 2 months as the lungs adapt to extrauterine life and then proceeds slowly throughout childhood as the pulmonary vascular bed matures.[14]

The essential role of the *pulmonary* circulation is to receive oxygen passively and to eliminate carbon dioxide passively, in contrast to the *systemic* circulation, which is designed to deliver oxygen selectively (actively) to metabolizing tissues and therefore requires vasoreactive arterioles that regulate regional blood flow in accordance with local metabolic needs.

The major airways and the major pulmonary arterial branches are formed by 16 weeks of gestation. An understanding of the density per unit area of small peripheral pulmonary arteries relative to alveolar density is necessary to understand normal and abnormal fetal and postnatal pulmonary arterial development.[15] The number of peripheral acinar units increases in proportion to the number of intraacinar arteries until lung growth is completed at 8 to 10 years of age. Two thirds of the normal number of intraacinar arteries are formed by 18 months, and most of the remainder are formed by 5 years of age.[15] Also important is the normal age-related distal extension of medial smooth muscle.[15] At birth, the vascular channels beyond the terminal bronchioles are devoid of medial smooth muscle, but within 2 to 3 years, medial smooth muscle extends to the junction of respiratory bronchioles and alveolar ducts and, by the mid-teens, extends among alveoli into precapillary vessels.

The histologic findings in primary pulmonary hypertension (see previous discussion) include luminal hyperplasia, medial hypertrophy, adventitial proliferation and fibrosis, occlusion of small arteries, *in situ* thrombosis, and infiltration of inflammatory and progenitor cells.[4] In 1958, Heath and Edwards[16] published elegant descriptions of the histology of pulmonary vascular disease together with a comprehensive classification.[17] The earliest abnormality was muscular thickening of small pulmonary arteries from medial hyperplasia, followed by intimal thickening (hyperplasia) that ranged from minimal to virtual luminal occlusion. The end stage was the angioproliferative plexiform lesion that corresponds to one of the three major histopathologic types of primary pulmonary hypertension in the WHO classification.[7] Originally, plexiform lesions were thought to be unique to primary pulmonary hypertension,[4] but now the belief is that plexogenic pulmonary arteriopathy is a nonspecific response of the pulmonary vasculature to hemodynamic injury.[3] The progression of lesion severity from medial hypertrophy to plexiform arteriopathy and the functional relevance of plexiform lesions remain uncertain.[4]

Plexogenic pulmonary arteriopathy resides in small muscular arteries 100 to 200 μm in diameter and is a complex process that involves intimal cell proliferation, migration of medial smooth muscle cells, recruitment of inflammatory cells, and deposition of extracellular matrix proteins.[8,12,18] Intimal proliferation is disproportionate to medial hypertrophy and culminates in complete luminal obliteration. Plexiform lesions are found in 70% to 85% of patients with primary pulmonary hypertension in whom lung tissue is available.[3,12]

Microthrombotic pulmonary arteriopathy occurs in 20% to 50% of cases of primary pulmonary hypertension[12] and is represented by recanalized *in situ* microthrombi that consist of fibrous webs with eccentric intimal fibrosis together with medial hypertrophy but without plexiform lesions.[8,12,18]

Pulmonary venoocclusive disease is found in less than 7% of cases of primary pulmonary hypertension[12] and is characterized by fibrosis and intimal proliferation of intrapulmonary venules, culminating in complete obliteration of venous channels that tend to recanalize.[8,12,18,19] Studies with use of light and electron microscopy have confirmed and extended these observations of pulmonary vascular pathophysiology (Box 14-2).[20] The clinical manifestations of primary pulmonary hypertension do not distinguish among the histopathologic types of pulmonary vascular disease. Early vasoreactivity ultimately becomes fixed,[11] but once the disorder is established, it rarely regresses.[12,16,17,21,22]

Advances in pulmonary vascular biology continue to shed light on the pathogenesis of primary pulmonary

(Modified from Ye and Rabinovich. See reference 20.)

hypertension.[23-25] Endothelial abnormalities have been identified (vasoconstrictor endothlin-1 homeostasis),[26-28] together with defects in voltage-gated potassium channels,[4] abnormalities in metalloproteinase and elastase activity,[4,29] transforming growth factor beta,[30,31] and bone morphogenetic protein.[32] Mediators of inflammation can cause pulmonary vasoconstriction, but the role of inflammation in *chronic* pulmonary hypertension is less clear. Genetic mechanisms are generally accepted to play a pathogenetic role in familial and sporadic cases of primary pulmonary hypertension (see section The History).[4,32-36] *Persistent fetal circulation* or persistent pulmonary hypertension of the newborn, a disorder of unknown etiology that was described in 1969,[37] is characterized by muscularization of small pulmonary arteries in the fetal lung, high neonatal pulmonary vascular resistance that fails to regress, and persistent right-to-left shunts through the ductus arteriosus and foramen ovale.[37-40] A relationship between persistent fetal circulation and primary pulmonary hypertension is tenuous.[41] *Portal hypertension* can be associated with pulmonary hypertension presumably because the pulmonary vascular bed is exposed to vasoreactive substances normally metabolized by the liver.[42,43] An association between *human immunodeficiency infection* and hypertensive pulmonary arteriopathy has been reported.[44] *Alveolar hypoventilation* and *sleep apnea* caused by chronic upper airway obstruction of hypertrophied tonsils and adenoids in children result in an increase in pulmonary vascular resistance (see Box 14-1).[45-48] *High-altitude pulmonary hypertension* clinically and histologically resembles primary pulmonary hypertension, which is more common at high altitudes and which is aggravated by the low partial pressure of oxygen (see section The History).[49-51]

The *physiologic consequences* of primary pulmonary hypertension are direct reflections of the increased resistance to blood flow through the lesser circulation. The pressure in the pulmonary arteries can exceed systemic pressure (Figure 14-1). Pulmonary vasoreactivity can be present initially but diminishes and is ultimately lost. Resting pulmonary blood flow and cardiac output fall and either fail to increase during exercise or fall still further.[52] Asymptomatic gene carriers for primary pulmonary hypertension have been identified with abnormal responses to exercise.[53]

Forceful right atrial contraction generates a large A wave and an increase in right ventricular end-diastolic segment length. Right ventricular end-diastolic pressure rises in response, right atrial mean pressure rises, and a right-to-left shunt is established through a stretched patent foramen ovale. Tricuspid regurgitation increases mean right atrial pressure still further.[54] Systemic venous pressure can be sufficiently elevated to cause venous stasis retinopathy.[55,56]

The *atrial natriuretic peptide* system is activated in primary pulmonary hypertension in response to increased right atrial pressure.[57] The polypeptide hormone is secreted by atrial myocytes; is involved in the homeostatic control of body water, sodium, and potassium; and correlates significantly with right ventricular preload and afterload.[57] *Brain natriuretic peptide* levels increase in proportion to right ventricular dysfunction.[58]

A mild albeit significant reduction in total lung capacity occurs in females with primary pulmonary hypertension,

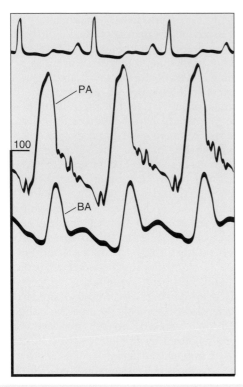

FIGURE 14-1 Pressure pulses from an 18-year-old man with primary pulmonary hypertension. Pulmonary arterial (PA) pressure exceeds brachial arterial (BA) pressure. The low systemic arterial pressure and the narrow pulse pressure are the result of low systemic stroke volume.

and a reduction in forced vital capacity occurs in both males and females.[8] Hypoxemia and hypocapnia are almost invariable because of a ventilation-perfusion mismatch, not because of a right-to-left shunt across a patent foramen ovale.[8] The diffusing capacity for carbon monoxide is significantly less than predicted.[8]

The ventricular septum encroaches on the left ventricular cavity, sometimes appreciably.[59] End-systolic and early diastolic deformations of the left ventricular cavity result in impaired filling in early diastole and in redistribution of filling in late diastole.[59–61] Early diastolic filling of the *right ventricle* is also encroached upon because high pulmonary vascular resistance prolongs the duration of right ventricular systole and prolongs isovolumetric relaxation.[61]

The time course of pulmonary hypertension can be established from the histology of the pulmonary trunk compared with the histology of the aortic root.[17,62,63] When pulmonary hypertension begins at birth, the histology of the pulmonary trunk and the histology of the aortic root are virtually identical (Figures 14-2C and 14-2D). When pulmonary hypertension begins after birth, the histology of the pulmonary trunk and aortic root differ significantly (Figures 14-2A and 14-2B). Primary pulmonary hypertension is rarely present at birth,[17,62,63] but when that is the case, it serves as a model of isolated pure pulmonary hypertension with which pulmonary hypertension with congenital heart disease can be compared.

HISTORY

The frequency of primary pulmonary hypertension in young females was cited as early as 1927,[64] with a female:male ratio subsequently reported as high as 3:1.[9] In the National Institutes of Health (NIH) registry, however, the gender incidence rate in *children* was equal; and in *adults*, the female:male ratio was 1.7:1, with a relatively constant incidence rate decade by decade.[8] Oral contraceptives are a consideration in light of evidence that birth control pills can aggravate if not initiate pulmonary vascular disease.[65]

Variations in gender incidence may in part reflect differences among the three histopathologic subgroups. *Plexogenic pulmonary arteriopathy*, the most frequent of the three histopathologic subgroups of primary pulmonary hypertension,[8,18] has a female:male ratio of 3:1. In the less common *microthrombotic* pulmonary hypertension, the female:male ratio is approximately equal,[18] and in the *venoocclusive* subgroup, which accounts for less than 7% of cases, a slight male predominance is seen.[12]

Familial primary pulmonary hypertension is well recognized (see Figure 14-12A) and occasionally recurs in more than one generation.[66–71] In the NIH registry, 6% of patients with primary pulmonary hypertension had a first-degree relative with primary pulmonary hypertension.[3] Inheritance is autosomal dominant with incomplete penetrance.[53] The genetic basis has been assigned to mutations in the bone morphogenetic protein receptor.[72–74]

Mean patient age in three large studies of primary pulmonary hypertension was 21 to 30 years, with a range of 2 to 56 years.[75] In the NIH registry, only 8% of patients reached the seventh decade,[8] although primary pulmonary hypertension of long duration has been reported. Regression has been suspected, albeit rarely.[21,22] Short-term survival is related to the severity of endothelial dysfunction.[27] Median survival after diagnosis is approximately 2.8 years,[3,76] with right ventricular failure the most common cause of death.[76–78] Longevity and morbidity are significantly influenced by lifestyle. Abrupt, strenuous, or isometric exercise should be avoided, and isotonic exercise should cease at the very onset of dyspnea, light-headedness, dizziness, or chest pain. Exposure to high altitude is an avoidable risk, and certain constraints are appropriate for air travel. A commercial jetliner flying at 33,000 to 36,000 ft has a cabin atmosphere equivalent to approximately 6000 to 8000 ft, which is comparable with breathing 15% oxygen at sea level.[17,79] Airline passengers experience a significant decrease in arterial PO_2, but only a mild decrease in arterial oxygen saturation.[79] Low humidity causes dehydration and an undesirable fall in systemic blood pressure. Just as important are the risks incurred by non–flight-related stress and travel fatigue. Rushing at the last minute, carrying heavy baggage, and transferring from one terminal to another at large airports are recognized risks.

The most common symptoms associated with primary pulmonary hypertension are effort dyspnea, fatigue, light-headedness, and chest pain. An increase in ventilatory response to exercise—hyperventilatory

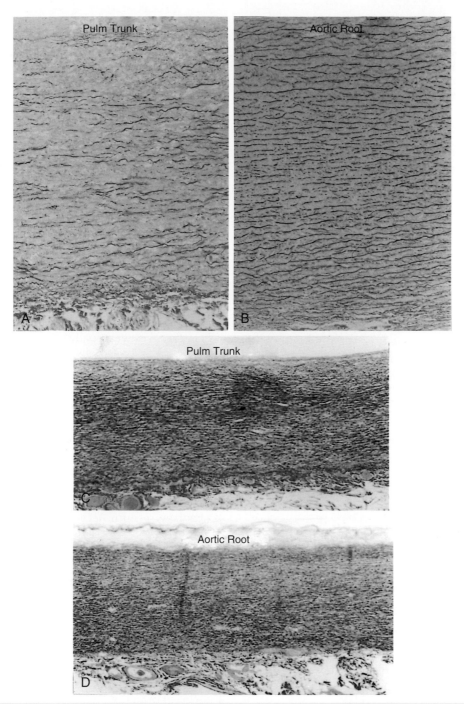

FIGURE 14-2 *Upper panels:* Histology of the pulmonary trunk and aortic root in an 11-year-old girl with primary pulmonary hypertension. **A,** Elastic fibers in the media of the pulmonary trunk are widely spaced, short, irregular, sparse, and branched. **B,** Elastic fibers in the media of the aortic root are long, uniform, and parallel. These differences in media between the pulmonary trunk and aortic root indicate that pulmonary hypertension was not present at birth. *Lower panels:* Histology of the pulmonary trunk **(C)** and aortic root **(D)** in a 46-year-old woman with a nonrestrictive ventricular septal defect and Eisenmenger's syndrome. The media of the pulmonary trunk and aortic root are identical, which indicates that pulmonary hypertension was present at birth.

dyspnea—is attributed chiefly to a ventilation/perfusion mismatch.[12,52]

Muscle fatigue is attributed to a reduction in the rate of aerobic regeneration of adenosine triphosphate (ATP).[52] Hypothyroidism is surprisingly prevalent in primary pulmonary hypertension[80] and should be considered in patients with inappropriate fatigue. Stress-related or exercise-related light-headedness, giddiness, dizziness, or faintness reflects an inability to achieve sufficient cardiac output and systemic blood pressure to maintain cerebral blood flow. The chest pain of myocardial ischemic originates in the hypertrophied hypoperfused right ventricle.[81] Histologic evidence of right ventricular infarction occurs in patients with primary pulmonary hypertension and normal coronary arteries. Myocardial ischemia has also been attributed to compression of the left main coronary artery by a dilated hypertensive pulmonary trunk.[82,83] Syncope, which is usually provoked by effort or excitement, is ominous and heralds sudden death.[8,12,84] Sudden death can also follow relatively innocuous stress, such as bone marrow aspiration and cardiac catheterization, especially in children.[77,85] Surgery, anesthesia, and even sedatives are poorly tolerated. Symptoms may first appear during pregnancy, which warrants special emphasis.[86–90] Fixed pulmonary vascular resistance blunts or precludes adaptive responses to the hemodynamic fluctuations of labor, delivery, and the puerperium. Maternal mortality rate is as high as 50%.[88] A hypercoagulable state in the third trimester reinforces the propensity for *in situ* thromboses in small terminal pulmonary arteries (see previous discussion).

Hemoptysis is a feature of Eisenmenger's syndrome (see Chapter 17) but not primary pulmonary hypertension. Raynaud's phenomenon is occasionally associated with primary pulmonary hypertension and calls attention to autoimmunity (see previous discussion).[24] Hoarseness, Ortner's syndrome, results from compression of the left recurrent laryngeal nerve by a dilated hypertensive pulmonary trunk.[12,69] Patients are sometimes unpleasantly aware of visible neck pulsations caused by giant jugular A waves (Figure 14-3; see previous discussion).

PHYSICAL APPEARANCE

Mild dusky hues of the face, nose, ears, and extremities are related to low cardiac output and reduced skin blood flow. Central cyanosis with a decrease in systemic arterial oxygen saturation reflects a right-to-left shunt through a patent foramen ovale.

ARTERIAL PULSE AND JUGULAR VENOUS PULSE

The systemic arterial pulse is small with a narrow pulse pressure (see Figure 14-1) because left ventricular stroke volume is reduced.[6] The small arterial pulse is in striking contrast to the large if not giant jugular venous A wave (Figures 14-3 and 14-4A), which Paul Wood aptly described: "This presystolic venous pulse is abrupt and collapsing in quality; is little influenced by change in posture and may be more noticeable on inspiration. Thus it is best seen when the patient sits bolt upright or stands up, when the V wave usually disappears altogether."[6] An increase in V wave awaits the advent of tricuspid

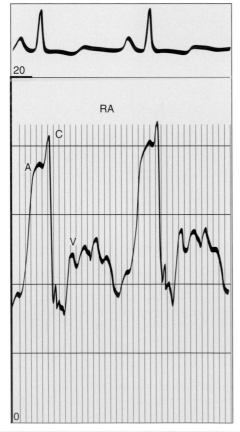

FIGURE 14-3 Right atrial pressure pulse from the 18-year-old man referred to in Figure 14-1 shows A waves of 14 to 16 mm Hg.

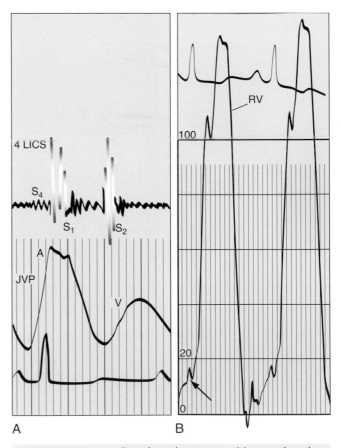

FIGURE 14-4 Recordings from the 18-year-old man referred to in Figure 14-1. **A,** Fourth heart sound (S_4) was present in the fourth left intercostal space (4 LICS). The jugular venous pulse (JVP) exhibits a correspondingly prominent A wave. **B,** Increased force of right atrial contraction resulted in presystolic distention of the right ventricle (arrow, lower left). (RV = right ventricle; S_1 = first heart sound; S_2 = second heart sound.)

regurgitation,[54] which attenuates the X descent and exaggerates the Y trough. Giant V waves reach the mandible when tricuspid regurgitation is accompanied by a ruptured tricuspid papillary muscle.[91]

PRECORDIAL MOVEMENT AND PALPATION

The right ventricular impulse varies in prominence with the severity and duration of pulmonary hypertension and with the size and function of the right ventricle. An enlarged right ventricle displaces the left ventricle from the apex. An increased force of right atrial contraction causes presystolic distention, which is palpated at the lower left sternal edge and subxyphoid area (Figures 14-4 and 14-5). Palpation in the second left intercostal space detects the systolic impulse of a dilated

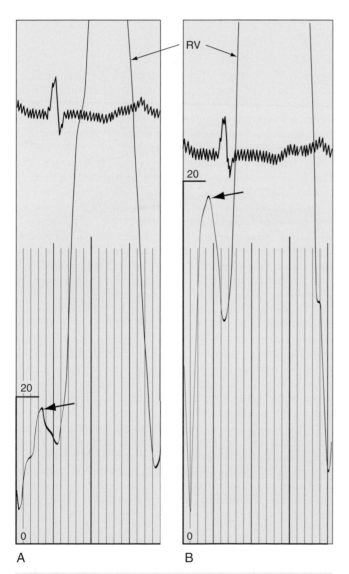

A   **B**

FIGURE 14-5 Presystolic distention of the right ventricle (RV) recorded at different sensitivities (**A** and **B**) in a 29-year-old woman with primary pulmonary hypertension.

hypertensive pulmonary trunk together with a loud pulmonary ejection sound and, as Graham Steell wrote in 1888, "... the closure of the semilunar valve being generally perceptible to the hand placed over the pulmonary area as a sharp thud."[92]

AUSCULTATION

The eight auscultatory signs are reflections of pure pulmonary hypertension:[93,94] the pulmonary ejection sound, the pulmonary midsystolic murmur, the tricuspid holosystolic murmur, the second heart sound, the Graham Steell murmur, third and fourth heart sounds, and a mid-diastolic–presystolic murmur (Figure 14-6).[94] The *pulmonary ejection sound* is identified by its high-pitched sharp clicking quality, by its maximal intensity in the second left intercostal space, and occasionally but distinctively by its selective decrease during inspiration (Figures 14-6, 14-7, and 14-8A). The timing of the ejection sound coincides with the interval between the onset of right ventricular systole and the opening of the pulmonary valve (isovolumetric contraction). The slower the rate of right ventricular contraction and the higher the pulmonary arterial diastolic pressure, the later the ejection sound (see Figures 14-7 and 14-8A).[93] A loud ejection sound radiates to the lower left sternal edge and apex, especially when the right ventricle occupies the apex. A *pulmonary midsystolic murmur* results from ejection into the dilated hypertensive pulmonary trunk (see Figures 14-6 and 14-7). The murmur is confined to the second left intercostal space, is introduced by the pulmonary ejection sound, and is symmetric, short, impure, and grade 1/6 or 2/6. The *tricuspid regurgitation* murmur is maximal at the lower left sternal edge (see Figures 14-6, 14-7 and 14-8B); but when the right ventricle occupies the apex, the murmur is well heard at the apex, and when the right atrium is enlarged, the murmur is heard to the right of the sternum. The tricuspid murmur is holosystolic and high-pitched because regurgitant flow is holosystolic and high velocity.[94] Intensity can be sufficient to generate a thrill or barely sufficient to achieve audibility. An increase in intensity during active inspiration, Rivero-Carvallo sign, is diagnostically important (see Figure 14-6).[93–95] The murmur is sometimes audible *only* during deep inspiration. Amplification during inspiration depends on a right ventricle that is functionally capable of converting an inspiratory increase in venous return into an increase in stroke volume and regurgitant flow.[93] This capacity is lost with right ventricular failure, so Carvallo's sign disappears.[94]

The pulmonary component of the second heart sound is altered in its timing, intensity, and precordial location.[93,94] The degree of splitting is the net effect of two variables: 1, the decreased capacitance and increased resistance in the pulmonary vascular bed that serves to narrow the split; and 2, prolongation of right ventricular systole that serves to increase the split.[96–98] When right ventricular function is normal, inspiratory splitting is normal or close (see Figure 14-6).[98] A functionally depressed right ventricle cannot increase its stroke volume with inspiration, so the split becomes fixed.[96,98] A loud

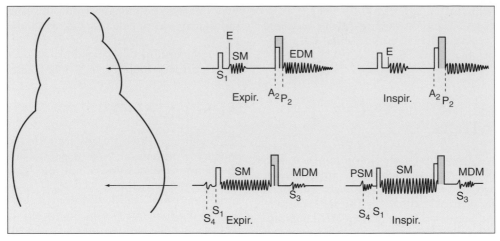

FIGURE 14-6 Composite drawing of the auscultatory features of pulmonary hypertension. (S_1 = first heart sound; E = pulmonary ejection sound; A_2/P_2 = aortic and pulmonary components of the second heart sound; S_3 = third heart sound; S_4 = fourth heart sound; SM = systolic murmur; PSM = presystolic murmur; EDM = early diastolic murmur; MDM = mid-diastolic murmur; Expir. = expiration; Inspir. = inspiration.)

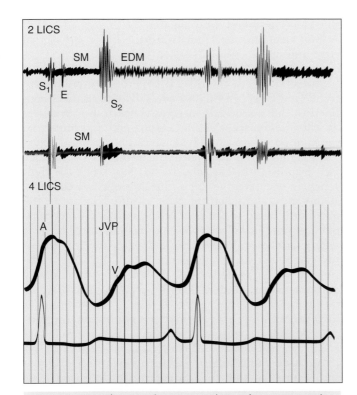

FIGURE 14-7 Phonocardiograms with jugular venous pulse (JVP) from the 18-year-old man with primary pulmonary hypertension referred to in Figure 14-1. In the second left intercostal space (2 LICS), a pulmonary ejection sound (E) begins at a long interval after the first heart sound and introduces a soft, short, midsystolic murmur (SM). The single second heart sound (S_2) is prolonged and loud because the pulmonary component was of great amplitude. A soft early diastolic murmur (EDM) issues from the loud second sound. A high-frequency holosystolic murmur of tricuspid regurgitation appears in the fourth left intercostal space (4 LICS). The A wave in the jugular venous pulse is prominent.

pulmonary component in the second left interspace obscures a closely preceding aortic component (see Figures 14-7 and 14-8), but auscultation at the right base, lower left sternal edge, or apex permits analysis of the transmitted but attenuated pulmonary component and allows detection of splitting (Figures 14-8B and 14-9).[93] Of all the auscultatory signs of pulmonary hypertension, the loud pulmonary component of the second sound is the most consistent (Figures 14-6 through 14-10). Graham Steell wrote that "accentuation of the pulmonary second sound is always present, the closure of the semilunar valves being generally perceptible to the hand placed over the pulmonary area as a sharp thud"[92] (see section Precordial Palpation). Detection of the loud pulmonary component transmitted to the apex is a useful sign of elevated pressure in the pulmonary artery.[93]

"There is occasionally heard over the pulmonary area ... and below this region for the distance of an inch or two along the left border of the sternum, and rarely over the lowest part of the bone itself, a soft blowing diastolic murmur immediately following or more exactly running off the accentuated second sound, while the usual indications of aortic regurgitation afforded by the pulse, etc., are absent. When the second sound is reduplicated, the murmur proceeds from its latter part. That such a murmur as I have described does exist, there can, I think, be no doubt."[92] Graham Steell made this auscultatory observation with a light boxwood monaural stethoscope.[99] The *Graham Steell murmur* is typically located in the second and third left intercostal spaces adjacent to the sternum (see Figures 14-6 and 14-7), but when it is loud, it is heard at the lower left sternal edge or even to the right of the sternum. Elevated diastolic pressure is exerted on the incompetent pulmonary valve at the inscription of the dichotic notch when the right ventricular and pulmonary arterial pressure pulses diverge, so the murmur begins with or immediately after the accentuated pulmonary component of the second

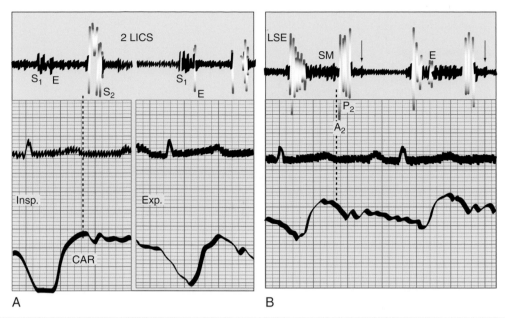

FIGURE 14-8 Phonocardiograms from a 21-year-old woman with primary pulmonary hypertension. **A,** The first heart sound (S_1) in the second left intercostal space (2 LICS) is followed by a pulmonary ejection sound (E) that selectively decreased with inspiration (Insp.) and was transmitted to the lower left sternal edge (LSE). The second heart sound (S_2) is loud and prolonged because of increased intensity of the pulmonary component (CAR = carotid). **B,** The holosystolic murmur of tricuspid regurgitation (SM) is present at the lower left sternal edge (LSE). The loud transmitted pulmonary component of the second heart sound (P_2) permitted identification of both components at the left sternal edge (LSE). A low amplitude early diastolic sound with the timing of an opening snap was recorded but not heard (thin vertical arrows). (A_2 = aortic component.)

sound (Figures 14-10 and 14-11). The marked difference between the diastolic pressure in the pulmonary artery and right ventricle exists from the beginning to the end of diastole, so the accompanying murmur is prolonged and high frequency (see Figures 14-10 and 14-11). The configuration is decrescendo (see Figures 14-7 and 14-11), but vibrations can be almost equal throughout diastole, or the murmur is sometimes crescendo-decrescendo (see Figure 14-10). Intensity can be sufficient to generate a thrill or soft and variable to the point of inaudibility. Steell was adept at detecting these murmurs despite his monaural boxwood stethoscope because of the "absolute quiet which prevailed during his lengthy round."[100]

Fourth heart sounds accompany presystolic distention of the right ventricle (see Figures 14-4 and 14-6) and are best detected with the bell of the stethoscope applied lightly at the lower left sternal edge, but they are heard at the apex when the apex is formed by the right ventricle. Fourth heart sounds are distinguished from split first heart sounds or pulmonary ejection sounds by their quality, precordial location, and response to respiration.[93,94] The low-frequency fourth sound can be more readily palpated than heard, a feature recognized by Potain who stated that "if one applies the ear to the chest, it affects the tactile sensation more than the auditory sense."[101] Right-sided fourth sounds become louder and occur earlier during inspiration (see Figure 14-6) because the greater force of right atrial contraction is translated into earlier and more vigorous presystolic filling of the right ventricle.

Third heart sounds occur during the rapid filling phase of the cardiac cycle and are signs of right ventricular failure (see Figure 14-6).[94] With the advent of tricuspid

regurgitation, third sounds intensify because high right atrial V waves are followed by accelerated atrioventricular flow. Third heart sounds are low-frequency events best detected with the bell of the stethoscope applied over the body of the right ventricle, but they are audible at the apex when the apex is occupied by the right ventricle.

In 1931, MacCallum reported a mid-diastolic rumbling murmur in a young woman with pulmonary hypertension.[102] The occasional occurrence of mid-diastolic/presystolic murmurs (Figures 14-6 and 14-12) represents prolonged vibrations of third or fourth heart sounds (see Figure 14-6).[93,94] Mid-diastolic murmurs increase during inspiration and are more apt to occur when the tricuspid valve is incompetent and the rate of atrioventricular flow is rapid (see Figure 14-12A). Right-sided Austin Flint mid-diastolic/presystolic murmurs have been described with pulmonary hypertensive pulmonary regurgitation.[103]

In a 1957 article on solitary pulmonary hypertension, Bedford, Evans, and Short[104] wrote that "a sound that resembles a mitral opening snap was heard in early diastole." McKusick recorded an "early diastolic snap" in a patient with necropsy-confirmed primary pulmonary hypertension and assigned the sound to the tricuspid valve. On one occasion, a soft early diastolic sound was recorded but not heard (see Figure 14-8B).[93]

ELECTROCARDIOGRAM

The electrocardiogram plays a useful role in the clinical assessment of primary pulmonary hypertension (Figure 14-13).[12,105] Abnormal P waves display pure right

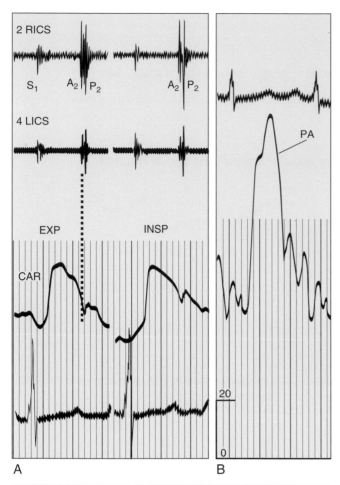

A

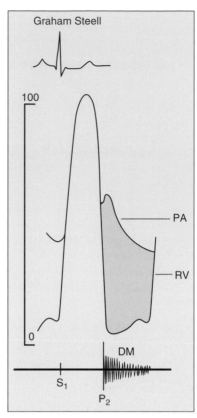

FIGURE 14-11 Drawings from pulmonary arterial (PA) and right ventricular (RV) pressure pulses with phonocardiogram illustrating an early diastolic Graham Steell murmur (DM). High pressure is exerted against the incompetent pulmonary valve throughout diastole (cross-hatched area). The high-velocity regurgitant flow is associated with a high-frequency holodiastolic murmur.

FIGURE 14-9 Recordings from a 21-year-old woman with primary pulmonary hypertension. **A,** The upper phonocardiograms show a loud pulmonary component of the second heart sound (P₂) that was transmitted to the second *right* intercostal space (2 RICS). The second sound was closely split during expiration (INSP). **B,** The pulmonary arterial (PA) pressure was at systemic level (120 mm Hg). (4 LICS = fourth left intercostal space.)

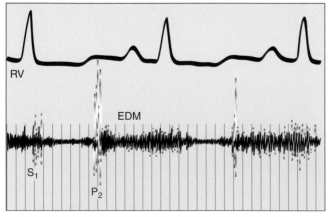

FIGURE 14-10 Intracardiac phonocardiogram from the right ventricular (RV) outflow tract of the 18-year-old man with primary pulmonary hypertension referred to in Figure 14-1. A high-frequency early diastolic Graham Steell murmur (EDM) begins with the loud pulmonary component of the second sound (P₂). The murmur lasts throughout diastole. The configuration varies from beat to beat.

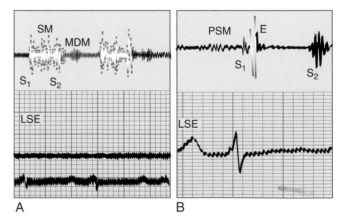

A　　　　　　　　B

FIGURE 14-12 A, Phonocardiogram from a 20-year-old man with primary pulmonary hypertension. His younger sister also had primary pulmonary hypertension. The tracing at the lower left sternal edge (LSE) shows a holosystolic murmur of tricuspid regurgitation and a short middiastolic murmur (MDM). **B,** Phonocardiogram from the 29-year-old woman referred to in Figure 14-5. A short presystolic murmur (PSM) and a prominent pulmonary ejection sound (E) are shown at the lower left sternal edge. (S₂ = second heart sound.)

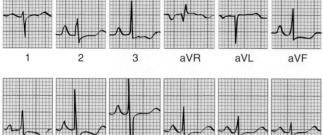

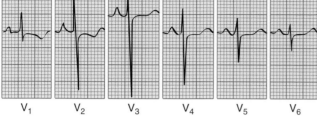

FIGURE 14-13 Electrocardiogram from a 27-year-old woman with primary pulmonary hypertension. Tall peaked right atrial P waves appear in leads 2 and aVF and in the midprecordium. Right ventricular hypertrophy is manifested by right axis deviation, a monophasic R wave in lead V₁, and a prominent S wave in lead V₆.

atrial configurations (see Figure 14-13). The PR interval is normal or slightly prolonged. Atrial fibrillation is exceptional.[12] The QRS axis varies from normal to right axis deviation, and the QRS duration is normal or slightly increased (see Figure 14-13). The degree of right ventricular hypertrophy reflects the severity and duration of right ventricular (pulmonary) hypertension. At one end of the spectrum, the electrocardiogram shows little more than a rightward QRS axis. At the other end of the spectrum, there is marked right axis deviation, right precordial leads that exhibit tall monophasic R waves with ST segment depressions and asymmetric T wave inversions, and left precordial that exhibit deep S waves (see Figure 14-13).

X-RAY

Enlargement of the pulmonary trunk and its proximal branches is characteristic in primary pulmonary hypertension and varies from moderate to marked but is seldom aneurismal (Figures 14-14 through 14-16).[12] The lucent pruned appearance of the peripheral lung fields stands out in sharp contrast to the prominence of the pulmonary trunk and its central branches (see Figures 14-15 and 14-16). Pulmonary venous congestion is reserved for the occasional patient with venoocclusive pulmonary hypertension.[12] The ascending aorta is inconspicuous, especially when compared with the dilated pulmonary trunk (see Figures 14-14 and 14-15). Enlargement of the right ventricle reflects the degree and chronicity of right ventricular failure (see Figure 14-15). The size of the right atrium varies from a slight convexity at the right lower cardiac border (see Figure 14-14) to striking enlargement provoked by right ventricular failure with tricuspid regurgitation (Figures 14-15, 14-16, and 14-17).

ECHOCARDIOGRAM

Transthoracic and transesophageal echocardiography with Doppler interrogation and color flow imaging exclude congenital or acquired heart disease as causes

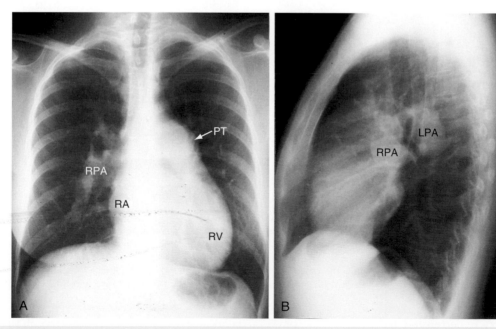

FIGURE 14-14 X-rays from a 31-year-old woman with primary pulmonary hypertension. **A,** Pulmonary vascularity is reduced. The pulmonary trunk (PT) and right pulmonary artery (RPA) are dilated, but the ascending aorta is not border-forming. A convex right ventricle (RV) occupies the apex, but the right atrial (RA) silhouette is not increased. **B,** The right pulmonary artery (RPA) and left pulmonary artery (LPA) are dilated. The right ventricle and right atrial appendage do not encroach on the retrosternal space.

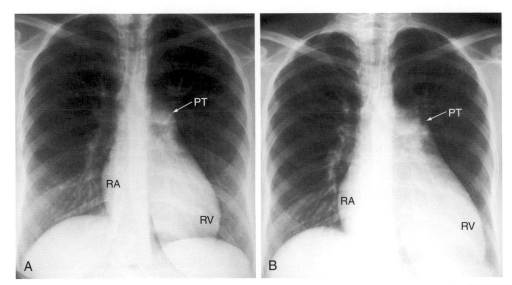

FIGURE 14-15 A, X-ray from a 24-year-old woman with primary pulmonary hypertension. Pulmonary vascularity is reduced. The pulmonary trunk (PT) is dilated. The ascending aorta is not border-forming. A convex right ventricle (RV) occupies the apex, and the right atrium (RA) is moderately enlarged. **B,** X-ray from the same patient 28 months later after the onset of right ventricular failure and tricuspid regurgitation. The pulmonary trunk, right atrium, and right ventricle have considerably increased in size.

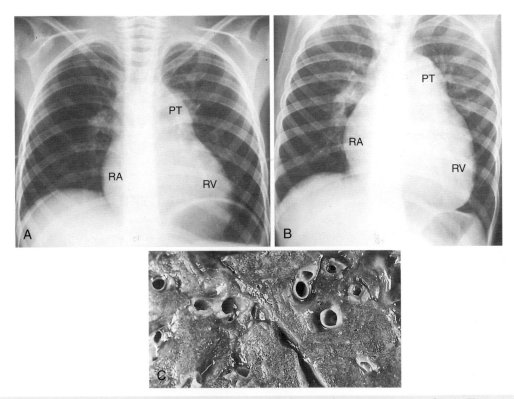

FIGURE 14-16 A, X-ray at age 6 years from the patient with primary pulmonary hypertension referred to in Figure 14-2. Pulmonary vascularity is reduced. The pulmonary trunk (PT) is dilated, the right atrial silhouette (RA) is increased, and a dilated convex right ventricle (RV) occupies the apex and extends below the left hemidiaphragm. **B,** X-ray at age 10 years after the onset of right ventricular failure. There is a striking increase in size of the pulmonary trunk, right atrium, and right ventricle. **C,** The patient died at age 11 years. Cross section of the lung at necropsy shows thick-walled intrapulmonary arteries that rise well above the surface. See also Figure 14-2.

of the pulmonary hypertension and establish the physiologic and morphologic consequences of elevated pressure in the lesser circulation.[54,106–110] Intravascular ultrasound scan is another method of assessing the pulmonary circulation in pulmonary hypertension.[111]

Echocardiography defines the size of the right atrium and right ventricle, characterizes right ventricular free wall motion, provides an estimate of right ventricular ejection fraction, establishes the position and motion of the ventricular septum, and determines the effect of

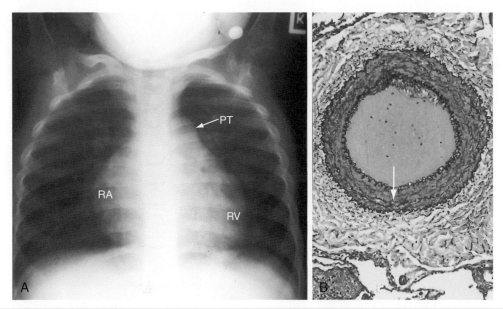

FIGURE 14-17 A, X-ray from a 3-year-old girl with primary pulmonary hypertension. Pulmonary vascularity is reduced. The pulmonary trunk (PT), right atrium (RA), and right ventricle (RV) are considerably enlarged. **B,** Histology of an intrapulmonary artery at necropsy shows medial hypertrophy (arrow).

ventricular septal position on the diastolic size and shape of the left ventricle (Figure 14-18).[59] The ventricular septum flattens toward the left ventricular cavity at end systole and in early diastole,[60] resulting in deformation of the left ventricular cavity, underfilling of the left ventricle in early diastole, and redistribution of filling into late diastole (Figures 14-18 and 14-19).[60,61] Color flow imaging establishes the presence and degree of pulmonary and tricuspid regurgitation (Figures 14-19 through 14-21). Continuous-wave Doppler scan across the right ventricular outflow tract and tricuspid valve permits estimates of the pulmonary arterial diastolic pressure and the right ventricular systolic pressure (see Figures 14-19 through 14-21).

SUMMARY

The typical patient with primary pulmonary hypertension is an otherwise healthy young acyanotic female with effort dyspnea, fatigue, light-headedness, and chest pain but no history of heart disease. Physical signs include a small arterial pulse, a large jugular venous A wave, a palpable right ventricle and pulmonary trunk, presystolic distention of the right ventricle that coincides with a right ventricular fourth heart sound, a pulmonary ejection sound, a short pulmonary midsystolic murmur, a loud pulmonary component of the second heart sound, a murmur of tricuspid regurgitation, and a Graham Steell murmur of hypertensive pulmonary regurgitation. The electrocardiogram is characterized by a right atrial P wave abnormality, right axis deviation, and pure right ventricular hypertrophy. The chest x-ray discloses dilation of the pulmonary trunk and its proximal branches, clear

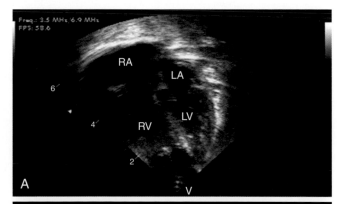

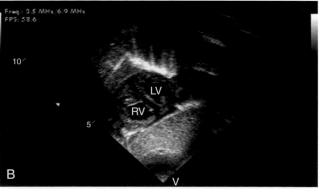

FIGURE 14-18 Echocardiogram of a patient with pulmonary hypertension. **A,** The four-chamber view shows striking dilation of the right atrium (RA) and right ventricle (RV). The left ventricular cavity size (LV) is reduced. **B,** Short-axis view shows the flat interventricular septum consistent with pulmonary hypertension.

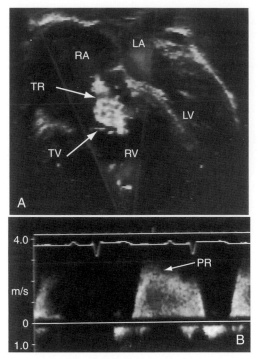

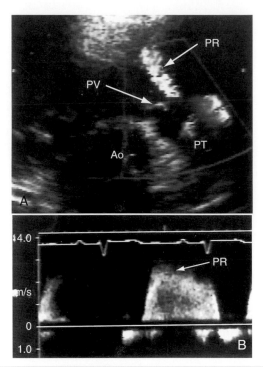

FIGURE 14-19 A, Black and white print of a color flow image from the 11-year-old girl referred to in Figures 14-2, 14-16, and 14-18. A high-velocity regurgitant jet (TR) originates at the tricuspid valve (TV) and enters an enlarged right atrium (RA). A dilated right ventricle (RV) encroaches on the left ventricular cavity (LV). **B,** Continuous-wave Doppler scan across the pulmonary valve records a peak velocity of pulmonary regurgitation (PR) that indicates a diastolic pressure of 45 mm Hg. Peak velocity across the tricuspid valve (not shown) indicated a right ventricular systolic pressure of 100 mm Hg. (LA = left atrium.)

FIGURE 14-20 Black and white print of a color flow image from an 18-year-old woman with primary pulmonary hypertension. **A,** High-velocity diastolic jet of pulmonary regurgitation (PR) originates at the pulmonary valve (PV). The pulmonary trunk (PT) is dilated. **B,** Continuous wave Doppler scan across the pulmonary valve records a peak regurgitant velocity (PR) that indicates a pulmonary artery diastolic pressure of 40 mm Hg. (Ao = aorta.)

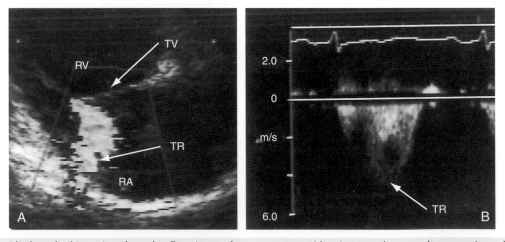

FIGURE 14-21 Black and white print of a color flow image from a woman with primary pulmonary hypertension who died at age 21 years. **A,** The high-velocity regurgitant jet (TR) originates at the tricuspid valve (TV) and enters an enlarged right atrium (RA). The right ventricle is dilated (RV). **B,** Continuous-wave Doppler scan across the tricuspid valve records a peak velocity that indicates a right ventricular systolic pressure of 75 mm Hg.

peripheral lung fields, and enlargement of the right ventricle and right atrium. Echocardiography with color flow imaging and Doppler interrogation exclude congenital or acquired heart disease as causes of pulmonary hypertension, establish the anatomic and physiologic consequences of elevated pressure in the lesser circulation, establish the size of the right atrium and right ventricle, assess right ventricular free wall motion, estimate the right ventricular ejection fraction, and define the abnormal position and movement of the ventricular septum and the abnormal size and shape of the left ventricular cavity. Color flow imaging determines the presence and degree of tricuspid and pulmonary regurgitation, and continuous wave Doppler scan permits an estimate of right ventricular systolic pressure and pulmonary artery diastolic pressure. Pulsed Doppler scan characterizes the physiologic abnormalities of left ventricular inflow.

REFERENCES

1. Beutner A. ZF rat. *Medicine*. 1852;2:97.
2. Gaine S. Pulmonary hypertension. *JAMA*. 2000;284:3160–3168.
3. Helmersen DS, Ford GT, Viner SM, Auger WR. POEMS syndrome: a clue to understanding primary pulmonary hypertension? A review of current insights into the pathogenesis of primary pulmonary hypertension. *Can J Cardiol*. 2000;16:975–981.
4. Archer S, Rich S. Primary pulmonary hypertension: a vascular biology and translational research "Work in progress." *Circulation*. 2000;102:2781–2791.
5. Romberg E. Ueber sklerose der lungen arterie. *Dtsch Arch Klin Med*. 1891;48:197–206.
6. Wood P. Pulmonary hypertension. *Br Med Bull*. 1952;8:348–353.
7. Hatano S, Strasser T. *Primary pulmonary hypertension: report on a WHO meeting, Geneva, 15–17 October 1973*. World Health Organization; 1975.
8. Rich S, Dantzker DR, Ayres SM, et al. Primary pulmonary hypertension. A national prospective study. *Ann Intern Med*. 1987;107:216–223.
9. Bjornsson J, Edwards WD. Primary pulmonary hypertension: a histopathologic study of 80 cases. *Mayo Clin Proc*. 1985;60:16–25.
10. Heath D, Smith P, Gosney J, et al. The pathology of the early and late stages of primary pulmonary hypertension. *Br Heart J*. 1987;58:204–213.
11. Palevsky HI, Schloo BL, Pietra GG, et al. Primary pulmonary hypertension. Vascular structure, morphometry, and responsiveness to vasodilator agents. *Circulation*. 1989;80:1207–1221.
12. Rich S. Primary pulmonary hypertension. *Prog Cardiovasc Dis*. 1988;31:205–238.
13. Yamaki S, Wagenvoort CA. Plexogenic pulmonary arteriopathy: significance of medial thickness with respect to advanced pulmonary vascular lesions. *Am J Pathol*. 1981;105:70–75.
14. Haworth SG. Pulmonary vascular remodeling in neonatal pulmonary hypertension. State of the art. *Chest*. 1988;93:133S–138S.
15. Hislop A, Reid L. Pulmonary arterial development during childhood: branching pattern and structure. *Thorax*. 1973;28:129–135.
16. Heath D, Edwards JE. The pathology of hypertensive pulmonary vascular disease; a description of six grades of structural changes in the pulmonary arteries with special reference to congenital cardiac septal defects. *Circulation*. 1958;18:533–547.
17. Wagenvoort CA. *The pathology of the pulmonary vasculature*. Springfield, Illinois: Charles C Thomas; 1964.
18. Pietra GG, Edwards WD, Kay JM, et al. Histopathology of primary pulmonary hypertension. A qualitative and quantitative study of pulmonary blood vessels from 58 patients in the National Heart, Lung, and Blood Institute, Primary Pulmonary Hypertension Registry. *Circulation*. 1989;80:1198–1206.
19. Resten A, Maitre S, Humbert M, et al. Pulmonary hypertension: CT of the chest in pulmonary venoocclusive disease. *AJR Am J Roentgenol*. 2004;183:65–70.
20. Ye C, Rabinovitch M. New developments in the pulmonary circulation in children. *Curr Opin Cardiol*. 1992;7:124–133.
21. Bourdillon PD, Oakley CM. Regression of primary pulmonary hypertension. *Br Heart J*. 1976;38:264–270.
22. Fujii A, Rabinovitch M, Matthews EC. A case of spontaneous resolution of idiopathic pulmonary hypertension. *Br Heart J*. 1981;46:574–577.
23. Rich S, Brundage BH. Pulmonary hypertension: a cellular basis for understanding the pathophysiology and treatment. *J Am Coll Cardiol*. 1989;14:545–550.
24. Rich S, Kieras K, Hart K, Groves BM, Stobo JD, Brundage BH. Antinuclear antibodies in primary pulmonary hypertension. *J Am Coll Cardiol*. 1986;8:1307–1311.
25. Snyder SH. Nitric oxide: first in a new class of neurotransmitters. *Science*. 1992;257:494–496.
26. Chen YF, Oparil S. Endothelin and pulmonary hypertension. *J Cardiovasc Pharmacol*. 2000;35:S49–S53.
27. Lopes AA, Maeda NY, Goncalves RC, Bydlowski SP. Endothelial cell dysfunction correlates differentially with survival in primary and secondary pulmonary hypertension. *Am Heart J*. 2000;139:618–623.
28. Rich S. Clinical insights into the pathogenesis of primary pulmonary hypertension. *Chest*. 1998;114:237S–241S.
29. Lepetit H, Eddahibi S, Fadel E, et al. Smooth muscle cell matrix metalloproteinases in idiopathic pulmonary arterial hypertension. *Eur Respir J*. 2005;25:834–842.
30. Yeager ME, Halley GR, Golpon HA, Voelkel NF, Tuder RM. Microsatellite instability of endothelial cell growth and apoptosis genes within plexiform lesions in primary pulmonary hypertension. *Circ Res*. 2001;88:E2–E11.
31. Morrell NW, Yang X, Upton PD, et al. Altered growth responses of pulmonary artery smooth muscle cells from patients with primary pulmonary hypertension to transforming growth factor-beta(1) and bone morphogenetic proteins. *Circulation*. 2001;104:790–795.
32. Machado RD, Pauciulo MW, Thomson JR, et al. BMPR2 haploinsufficiency as the inherited molecular mechanism for primary pulmonary hypertension. *Am J Hum Genet*. 2001;68:92–102.
33. Geraci MW, Moore M, Gesell T, et al. Gene expression patterns in the lungs of patients with primary pulmonary hypertension: a gene microarray analysis. *Circ Res*. 2001;88:555–562.
34. Thomson JR, Trembath RC. Primary pulmonary hypertension: the pressure rises for a gene. *J Clin Pathol*. 2000;53:899–903.
35. Loscalzo J. Genetic clues to the cause of primary pulmonary hypertension. *N Engl J Med*. 2001;345:367–371.
36. Grunig E, Mereles D, Arnold K, et al. Primary pulmonary hypertension is predominantly a hereditary disease. *Chest*. 2002;121:81S–82S.
37. Gersony WM, Duc GV, Sinclair JC. PFC syndrome (persistence of the fetal circulation). *Circulation*. 1969;40:87.
38. Gersony WM. Neonatal pulmonary hypertension: pathophysiology, classification, and etiology. *Clin Perinatol*. 1984;11:517–524.
39. Hageman JR, Adams MA, Gardner TH. Persistent pulmonary hypertension of the newborn. Trends in incidence, diagnosis, and management. *Am J Dis Child*. 1984;138:592–595.
40. Murphy JD, Rabinovitch M, Goldstein JD, Reid LM. The structural basis of persistent pulmonary hypertension of the newborn infant. *J Pediatr*. 1981;98:962–967.
41. Widlitz A, Barst RJ. Pulmonary arterial hypertension in children. *Eur Respir J*. 2003;21:155–176.
42. Robalino BD, Moodie DS. Association between primary pulmonary hypertension and portal hypertension: analysis of its pathophysiology and clinical, laboratory and hemodynamic manifestations. *J Am Coll Cardiol*. 1991;17:492–498.
43. Ruttner JR, Bartschi JP, Niedermann R, Schneider J. Plexogenic pulmonary arteriopathy and liver cirrhosis. *Thorax*. 1980;35:133–136.
44. Speich R, Jenni R, Opravil M, Pfab M, Russi EW. Primary pulmonary hypertension in HIV infection. *Chest*. 1991;100:1268–1271.
45. Ainger LE. Large tonsils and adenoids in small children with cor pulmonale. *Br Heart J*. 1968;30:356–362.
46. Bland Jr JW, Edwards FK. Pulmonary hypertension and congestive heart failure in children with chronic upper airway obstruction. New concepts of etiologic factors. *Am J Cardiol*. 1969;23:830–837.
47. Brouillette RT, Fernbach SK, Hunt CE. Obstructive sleep apnea in infants and children. *J Pediatr*. 1982;100:31–40.
48. Mauer KW, Staats BA, Olsen KD. Upper airway obstruction and disordered nocturnal breathing in children. *Mayo Clin Proc*. 1983;58:349–353.
49. Khoury GH, Hawes CR. Primary pulmonary hypertension in children living at high altitude. *J Pediatr*. 1963;62:177–185.
50. O'Neill D, Morton R, Kennedy JA. Progressive primary pulmonary hypertension in a patient born at high altitude. *Br Heart J*. 1981;45:725–728.

51. Sime F, Banchero N, Penaloza D, Gamboa R, Cruz J, Marticorena E. Pulmonary hypertension in children born and living at high altitudes. *Am J Cardiol*. 1963;11:143–149.

52. Sun XG, Hansen JE, Oudiz RJ, Wasserman K. Exercise pathophysiology in patients with primary pulmonary hypertension. *Circulation*. 2001;104:429–435.

53. Grunig E, Janssen B, Mereles D, et al. Abnormal pulmonary artery pressure response in asymptomatic carriers of primary pulmonary hypertension gene. *Circulation*. 2000;102:1145–1150.

54. Hinderliter AL, Willis PWT, Long WA, et al. Group PPHS. Frequency and severity of tricuspid regurgitation determined by Doppler echocardiography in primary pulmonary hypertension. *Am J Cardiol*. 2003;91:1033–1037.

55. Bhan A, Rennie IG, Higenbottam TW. Central retinal vein occlusion associated with primary pulmonary hypertension. *Retina*. 2001;21:83–85.

56. Saran BR, Brucker AJ, Bandello F, Verougstraete C. Familial primary pulmonary hypertension and associated ocular findings. *Retina*. 2001;21:34–39.

57. Wiedemann R, Ghofrani HA, Weissmann N, et al. Atrial natriuretic peptide in severe primary and nonprimary pulmonary hypertension: response to iloprost inhalation. *J Am Coll Cardiol*. 2001;38:1130–1136.

58. Nagaya N, Nishikimi T, Uematsu M, et al. Plasma brain natriuretic peptide as a prognostic indicator in patients with primary pulmonary hypertension. *Circulation*. 2000;102:865–870.

59. Marcus JT, Vonk Noordegraaf A, Roeleveld RJ, et al. Impaired left ventricular filling due to right ventricular pressure overload in primary pulmonary hypertension: noninvasive monitoring using MRI. *Chest*. 2001;119:1761–1765.

60. Louie EK, Rich S, Brundage BH. Doppler echocardiographic assessment of impaired left ventricular filling in patients with right ventricular pressure overload due to primary pulmonary hypertension. *J Am Coll Cardiol*. 1986;8:1298–1306.

61. Stojnic BB, Brecker SJ, Xiao HB, Helmy SM, Mbaissouroum M, Gibson DG. Left ventricular filling characteristics in pulmonary hypertension: a new mode of ventricular interaction. *Br Heart J*. 1992;68:16–20.

62. Heath D, Edwards JE. Configuration of elastic tissue of pulmonary trunk in idiopathic pulmonary hypertension. *Circulation*. 1960;21:59–62.

63. Roberts WC. The histologic structure of the pulmonary trunk in patients with "primary" pulmonary hypertension. *Am Heart J*. 1963;65:230–236.

64. Clarke RC, Coombs CF, Hadfield G, Todd AT. On certain abnormalities, congenital and acquired, of the pulmonary artery. *Q J Med*. 1927;21:51–68.

65. Kleiger RE, Boxer M, Ingham RE, Harrison DC. Pulmonary hypertension in patients using oral contraceptives. A report of six cases. *Chest*. 1976;69:143–147.

66. Hood Jr WB, Spencer H, Lass RW, Daley R. Primary pulmonary hypertension: familial occurrence. *Br Heart J*. 1968;30:336–343.

67. Husson GS. Primary pulmonary hypertension in siblings. *Am J Dis Child*. 1956;92:506.

68. Parry WR, Verel D. Familial primary pulmonary hypertension. *Br Heart J*. 1966;28:193–198.

69. Rogge JD, Mishkin ME, Genovese PD. The familial occurrence of primary pulmonary hypertension. *Ann Intern Med*. 1966;65:672–684.

70. Thompson P, Mcrae C. Familial pulmonary hypertension. Evidence of autosomal dominant inheritance. *Br Heart J*. 1970;32:758–760.

71. Eddahibi S, Morrell N, D'Ortho MP, Naeije R, Adnot S. Pathobiology of pulmonary arterial hypertension. *Eur Respir J*. 2002;20:1559–1572.

72. Deng Z, Morse JH, Slager SL, et al. Familial primary pulmonary hypertension (gene PPH1) is caused by mutations in the bone morphogenetic protein receptor-II gene. *Am J Hum Genet*. 2000;67:737–744.

73. Morse JH, Jones AC, Barst RJ, Hodge SE, Wilhelmsen KC, Nygaard TG. Familial primary pulmonary hypertension locus mapped to chromosome 2q31-q32. *Chest*. 1998;114:57S–58S.

74. Newman JH, Wheeler L, Lane KB, et al. Mutation in the gene for bone morphogenetic protein receptor II as a cause of primary pulmonary hypertension in a large kindred. *N Engl J Med*. 2001;345:319–324.

75. Wagenvoort CA. Lung biopsy specimens in the evaluation of pulmonary vascular disease. *Chest*. 1980;77:614–625.

76. D'alonzo GE, Barst RJ, Ayres SM, et al. Survival in patients with primary pulmonary hypertension. Results from a national prospective registry. *Ann Intern Med*. 1991;115:343–349.

77. Rhodes J, Barst RJ, Garofano RP, Thoele DG, Gersony WM. Hemodynamic correlates of exercise function in patients with primary pulmonary hypertension. *J Am Coll Cardiol*. 1991;18:1738–1744.

78. Rozkovec A, Montanes P, Oakley CM. Factors that influence the outcome of primary pulmonary hypertension. *Br Heart J*. 1986;55:449–458.

79. Harinck E, Hutter PA, Hoorntje TM, et al. Air travel and adults with cyanotic congenital heart disease. *Circulation*. 1996;93:272–276.

80. Curnock AL, Dweik RA, Higgins BH, Saadi HF, Arroliga AC. High prevalence of hypothyroidism in patients with primary pulmonary hypertension. *Am J Med Sci*. 1999;318:289–292.

81. Gomez A, Bialostozky D, Zajarias A, et al. Right ventricular ischemia in patients with primary pulmonary hypertension. *J Am Coll Cardiol*. 2001;38:1137–1142.

82. Patrat JF, Jondeau G, Dubourg O, et al. Left main coronary artery compression during primary pulmonary hypertension. *Chest*. 1997;112:842–843.

83. Kawut SM, Silvestry FE, Ferrari VA, et al. Extrinsic compression of the left main coronary artery by the pulmonary artery in patients with long-standing pulmonary hypertension. *Am J Cardiol*. 1999;83:984–986 A910.

84. Mikhail GW, Gibbs JS, Yacoub MH. Pulmonary and systemic arterial pressure changes during syncope in primary pulmonary hypertension. *Circulation*. 2001;104:1326–1327.

85. Taylor CJ, Derrick G, McEwan A, Haworth SG, Sury MRJ. Risk of cardiac catheterization under anaesthesia in children with pulmonary hypertension. *Br J Anaesth*. 2007;98:657–661.

86. Dawkins KD, Burke CM, Billingham ME, Jamieson SW. Primary pulmonary hypertension and pregnancy. *Chest*. 1986;89:383–388.

87. Mccaffrey RM, Dunn LJ. Primary pulmonary hypertension in pregnancy. *Obstet Gynecol Surv*. 1964;19:567–591.

88. Perloff JK. Pregnancy in congenital heart disease: the mother and the fetus. In: Perloff JK, Child JS, Aboulhosn J, eds. *Congenital heart disease in adults*. 3rd ed. Philadelphia: W.B. Saunders; 2009.

89. Roberts NV, Keast PJ. Pulmonary hypertension and pregnancy—a lethal combination. *Anaesth Intensive Care*. 1990;18:366–374.

90. Takeuchi T, Nishii O, Okamura T, Yaginuma T. Primary pulmonary hypertension in pregnancy. *Int J Gynaecol Obstet*. 1988;26:145–150.

91. Kunhali K, Cherian G, Bakthaviziam A, Abraham MT, Krishnaswami S. Rupture of a papillary muscle of the tricuspid valve in primary pulmonary hypertension. *Am Heart J*. 1980;99:225–229.

92. Steell G. The murmur of high pressure in the pulmonary artery. *Medical Chronicle*. 1888;9:182.

93. Perloff JK. Auscultatory and phonocardiographic manifestations of pulmonary hypertension. *Prog Cardiovasc Dis*. 1967;9:303–340.

94. Perloff JK. *The physical examination of the heart and circulation*. 4th ed. Shelton, Connecticut: People's Medical Publishing House; 2009.

95. Rivero-Carvallo JM. New diagnostic sign of tricuspid insufficiency. *Arch Inst Cardiol Mex*. 1946;16:531–540.

96. Perloff JK, Harvey WP. Mechanisms of fixed splitting of the second heart sound. *Circulation*. 1958;18:998–1009.

97. Shapiro S, Clark TJ, Goodwin JF. Delayed closure of the pulmonary valve in obliterative pulmonary hypertension. *Lancet*. 1965;2:1207–1211.

98. Shaver JA, Nadolny RA, O'Toole JD, et al. Sound pressure correlates of the second heart sound. An intracardiac sound study. *Circulation*. 1974;49:316–325.

99. Silverman BD. Graham Steell. *Clin Cardiol*. 1995;18:54–55.

100. Major RH. *Classic descriptions of disease: with biographical sketches of the authors*. 3rd ed. Springfield, Illinois: Charles C Thomas; 1948.

101. Potain PC. Concerning the cardiac rhythm called gallop rhythm. *Bull Mem Soc Med Hop Paris*. 1876;12:137.

102. MacCallum WG. Obliterative pulmonary arteriosclerosis. *Bull Johns Hopkins Hosp*. 1931;49:37.

103. Green EW, Agruss NS, Adolph RJ. Right-sided Austin Flint murmur. Documentation by intracardiac phonocardiography, echocardiography and postmortem findings. *Am J Cardiol.* 1973;32:370–374.

104. Bedford DE, Evans W, Short DS. Solitary pulmonary hypertension. *Br Heart J.* 1957;19:93–116.

105. Bossone E, Paciocco G, Iarussi D, et al. The prognostic role of the ECG in primary pulmonary hypertension. *Chest.* 2002;121:513–518.

106. Bossone E, Duong-Wagner TH, Paciocco G, et al. Echocardiographic features of primary pulmonary hypertension. *J Am Soc Echocardiogr.* 1999;12:655–662.

107. Child JS. Transthoracic and transesophageal imaging: anatomic and hemodynamic assessment. In: Perloff JK, Child JS, eds. *Congenital heart disease in adults.* Philadelphia: W.B. Saunders; 1998:91.

108. Amaki M, Nakatani S, Kanzaki H, et al. Usefulness of three-dimensional echocardiography in assessing right ventricular function in patients with primary pulmonary hypertension. *Hypertens Res Clin Exp.* 2009;32:419–422.

109. Ghio S, Raineri C, Scelsi L, et al. Usefulness and limits of transthoracic echocardiography in the evaluation of patients with primary and chronic thromboembolic pulmonary hypertension. *J Am Soc Echocardiogr.* 2002;15:1374–1380.

110. Raymond RJ, Hinderliter AL, Willis PW, et al. Echocardiographic predictors of adverse outcomes in primary pulmonary hypertension. *J Am Coll Cardiol.* 2002;39:1214–1219.

111. Ivy DD, Neish SR, Knudson OA, et al. Intravascular ultrasonic characteristics and vasoreactivity of the pulmonary vasculature in children with pulmonary hypertension. *Am J Cardiol.* 1998; 81:740–748.

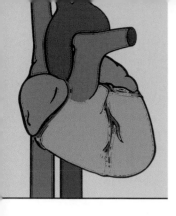

Chapter 15

Atrial Septal Defect: Simple and Complex

Galen was aware of the foramen ovale and its normal postnatal closure.[1] Botallo described a patent foramen ovale after birth without understanding its function in the fetus.[1] Leonardo da Vinci wrote, "I have found from left auricle to right auricle the perforating channel." Leonardo's account of a true atrial septal defect is thought to be the first record of a congenital malformation of the human heart.[2] In 1640, Pierre Gassendi based an entire treatise on observations of a patent foramen ovale in an adult cadaver.[3]

Karl von Rokitansky, in 1875, published superb observations on the pathologic anatomy of atrial septal defects and what he presumed to be their embryologic basis and distinguished septum primum from septum secundum defects. In 1921, Assmann's[4] description of the radiologic features of atrial septal defects paved the way for clinical recognition. In 1934, Roesler[5] analyzed 62 necropsy cases of atrial septal defect, only one of which had been correctly diagnosed during life. In a landmark publication in 1941, Bedford, Papp, and Parkinson[6] described the clinical features of atrial septal defects. Hudson's[7] 1955 description of the normal and abnormal interatrial septum was refined in 1979 by Sweeney and Rosenquist.[8] These early accounts have been extended by studies of the anatomy of the interatrial septum with tranesophageal echocardiography.[9]

The normal atrial septum viewed from its right side is a blade-shaped structure with a superoanterior margin that reflects the curvature of the ascending aorta, an inferior margin that borders the mitral annulus, and a posterior margin that is convex.[8] The left side of the septum has a network of trabeculations that are remnants of the septum primum.

The fossa ovalis occupies about 28% of the septal area, irrespective of age, and is bordered by a limbus and guarded by a valve (see Figure 15-46C).[8] After birth, the patent fetal foramen ovale closes via fusion of its valve with the limbus of the fossa ovalis as left atrial pressure exceeds right atrial pressure. The incidence of persistent patency of the foramen ovale declines from about one third during the first three decades of life to about one quarter during the fourth through eighth decades.[10] The morphogenetic sequence of normal intrauterine formation and closure of the atrial septum is illustrated in Figure 15-1.[7] Redundancy of the valve of the foramen is responsible for an atrial septal aneurysm (see Figure 15-47).[11,12]

The most common type of atrial septal defect is in the *ostium secundum* or fossa ovalis location (Figures 15-2 and 15-3).[13–15] These defects lie in a folded area rather than on a flat plane. Their anatomy is more complex on the right side than on the left side of the septum.[16] Ostium secundum defects result from shortening of the valve of the foramen ovale, excessive resorption of the septum primum, or deficient growth of the septum secundum (see Figures 15-1, 15-2, and Figure 15-46C). Occasionally, the atrial septal perforations resembles Swiss cheese,[17] or the interatrial communication is represented by multiple openings less than 5 mm in diameter.[18]

Next in frequency are *ostium primum* defects, also called *atrioventricular septal defects* because the atrioventricular septum is defective (absent; see Figures 15-1 and 15-2). Oddly and rarely, a communication exists in the atrioventricular septum when septal structures are intact.[19]

Sinus venosus atrial septal defects are uncommon, but not rare, and constitute 2% to 3% of interatrial communications. During normal embryogenesis, the inferior vena cava and the right superior vena cava are incorporated into the right horn of the sinus venosus. Faulty resorption results in a communication near the orifice of the superior or the inferior cava. The right valve of the sinus venosus is a broad membrane that almost partitions the developing right atrium. Both vena cavas are located on the left side of the membrane. The principle type of sinus venosus defect was described in 1868 as a "free communication between the auricles by deficiency of the upper part of the septum auricularum."[20]

Superior vena caval sinus venosus defects are located immediately below the junction of the superior cava and the right atrium (see Figures 15-2 and 15-48) and vary from small to nonrestrictive. The orifice of the superior vena cava may override the defect, which is therefore *biatrial*.[21] *Inferior vena caval sinus venosus defects* are located below the foramen ovale and merge with the floor of the inferior cava (see Figures 15-2 and 15-48).[15,22] As the valve of the inferior vena cava resorbs, its rudiment becomes the *fetal eustachian valve* that directs inferior caval blood across the foramen ovale. Persistence of a large eustachian valve (Figure 15-4 and Videos 15-1A and 15-1B) channels inferior vena caval blood across an ostium secundum atrial septal defect (Figure 15-5 and Video 15-2) or across an inferior vena caval sinus venosus defect (see Figure 15-48).[22,23] Atrial septal defects are usually located in only one of the foregoing locations,

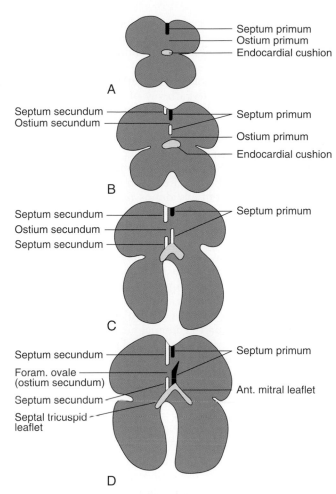

FIGURE 15-1 Schematic illustrations of sequential changes during the formation of the atrial septum. *(Modified from Hudson R. Normal and abnormal interatrial septum. British Heart Journal. 1955;17:489–495; and from Van Mierop LHS. In Feldt RH, editor. Atrioventricular canal defects. Philadelphia: WB Saunders Co; 1976.)*

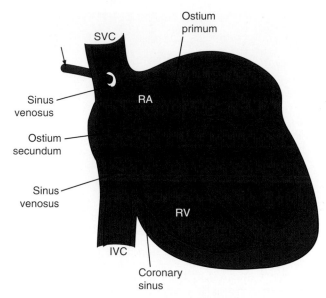

FIGURE 15-2 The locations of an ostium secundum atrial septal defect, an ostium primum atrial septal defect, a superior vena caval (SVC) and an inferior vena caval (IVC) sinus venosus atrial septal defect, and a coronary sinus defect. (RV = right ventricle.) Unmarked arrow at upper left identifies the right superior pulmonary vein.

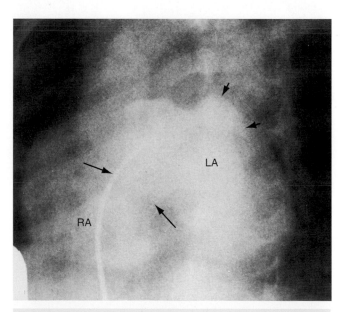

FIGURE 15-3 Angiocardiogram (shallow left oblique) in an 8-year-old boy with an ostium secundum atrial septal defect. Contrast material outlines the left atrium (LA), including its appendage (small paired arrows). Contrast material crossed a nonrestrictive ostium secumdum atrial septal defect (large arrow) and filled the right atrium (RA).

but separate ostium secundum, sinus venosus, and ostium primum defects occasionally coexist.[24]

Coronary sinus atrial septal defects are uncommon but not rare. As the name implies, the defect is located at the site normally occupied by the right atrial ostium of the coronary sinus (see Figure 15-2)[25] and is characterized by an opening in the wall of the distal end of the sinus or by *unroofing* caused by absence of the partition between the coronary sinus and left atrium. A left superior vena cava inserts into the upper left corner of the left atrium. A relatively rare combination consists of absence of the coronary sinus, a defect in the atrial septum in the location of the ostium of the coronary sinus, and a left superior vena cava connected to the left atrium.[25] This combination is necessarily cyanotic because blood from the left superior vena caval enters the left atrium directly.

Spontaneous closure of an ostium secundum atrial septal defect refers to sealing of a true tissue defect, and not to cessation of a left-to-right shunt through a valve-incompetent foramen ovale.[26,27] Ostium secundum atrial septal defects are seldom symptomatic in infants and young children (see Figure 15-46B and Videos 15-3A through 15-3D); but when

they are so manifest, approximately one third close spontaneously between 1 and 2 years of age.[27] The mechanisms responsible for spontaneous closure remain to be established, but multiple small interatrial septal openings (diameters less than 5 mm) in newborns have a strong tendency to close during the first year of life.[18]

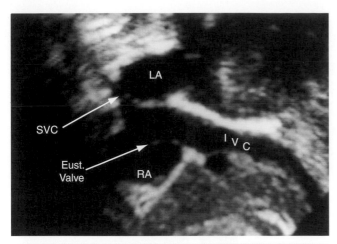

FIGURE 15-4 Echocardiogram (subcostal) showing a eustachian valve (Eust Valve) that extended from the inferior vena cava (IVC) and directed inferior vena caval blood toward the midportion of the atrial septum (Videos 15-1A and 15-1B). (LA = left atrium; RA = right atrium; SVC = superior vena cava.)

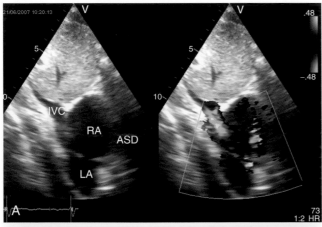

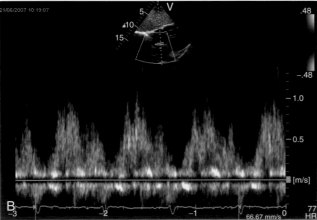

FIGURE 15-5 A, Echocardiogram (subcostal) showing an ostium secundum atrial septal defect in the midportion of the atrial septum (Video 15-2). (RA = right atrium; LA = left atrium; IVC = inferior vena cava.) B, Pulsed Doppler scan within the atrial septal defect shows signals that are positive and maximal in late systole (A) and in early diastole (B).

Anatomic *connections* and physiologic *drainage* of pulmonary veins are important distinctions in atrial septal defects. *Connection* refers to a pulmonary vein that is *anatomically* contiguous—connected—with a morphologic left atrium or a morphologic right atrium.[28,29] *Drainage* refers to the *physiologic* pathway of blood from pulmonary veins into the left or right atrium. Pulmonary veins that connect normally can drain anomalously, but pulmonary veins that connect anomalously drain anomalously. Normal right pulmonary veins connect to the left atrium close to the rim of ostium secundum atrial septal defects,[29,30] so a substantial portion of right pulmonary venous blood preferentially drains into the right atrium even though the veins connect anatomically to the left atrium (Figure 15-6). *Partial* anomalous pulmonary venous connection refers to one or more but not all pulmonary veins that connect anomalously to the right atrium.[28,31] *Total* anomalous pulmonary venous connection exists when *all four* pulmonary veins connect anomalously to the right atrium, directly or indirectly. Ten percent to 15% of ostium secundum atrial septal defects are associated with partial anomalous pulmonary venous connections. Eighty percent to 90% of superior vena caval sinus venosus defects are associated with anomalous connection of the right superior pulmonary vein to the right atrium or superior vena cava (Figures 15-2 and 15-7).[21] About 90% of partial anomalous pulmonary venous connections join the right upper or middle lobe pulmonary veins into the right atrium or superior vena cava.[28,32] Partial anomalous connection of right pulmonary veins is usually associated with ostium secundum atrial septal defects,[33] exceptionally is associated with an intact atrial septum, and may go unrecognized when associated with a restrictive sinus venosus defect (see Figure 15-7). Anomalous connection of *left* pulmonary veins is far less prevalent (incidence rate about 10%) than

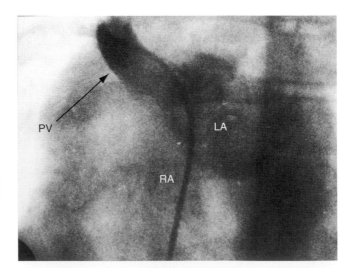

FIGURE 15-6 Angiocardiogram (shallow left oblique) from an 11-year-old girl with an ostium secundum atrial septal defect. Contrast material flows from left atrium (LA) into right atrium (RA) across the nonrestrictive atrial septal defect. The right superior pulmonary vein (PV) connects normally to the left atrium (LA).

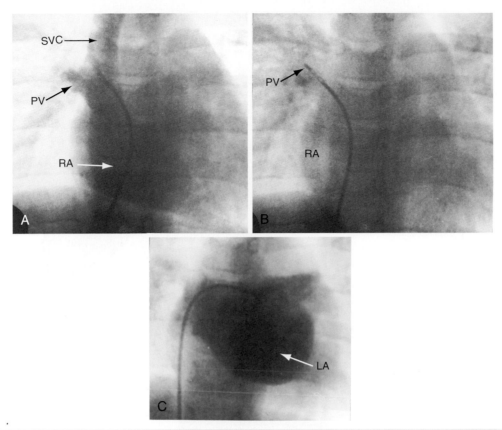

FIGURE 15-7 Angiocardiograms from a 10-year-old boy with a restrictive superior vena caval (SVC) sinus venosus atrial septal defect and anomalous pulmonary venous connection (PV) to the right atrium (RA). **A** and **B,** The catheter tip is in the right superior pulmonary vein (PV) that was entered from the right atrium (RA). **C,** The opacified left atrium (LA) was entered across the sinus venosus atrial septal defect. There was no left-to-right shunt.

anomalous connection of right pulmonary veins and is represented by anomalous connection to the innominate vein or to a persistent left superior vena cava that attaches to the innominate vein. *Bilateral* partial anomalous pulmonary venous connections are rare.

The *scimitar syndrome,* described in 1836 by Chassinat,[34] is a rare anomaly characterized by connection of all of the right pulmonary veins into the inferior vena cava.[35–38] The ipsilateral lung and pulmonary artery are usually hypoplastic (Figures 15-8, 15-9, and 15-10). The syndrome rarely involves the left lung.[39] The term *scimitar* refers to a radiologic shadow that resembles the shape of a Turkish sword (see Figure 15-8C). The lower portion of the right lung is perfused by systemic arteries from the abdominal aorta.[36,37]

In ostium secundum atrial septal defects, anatomic studies of the mitral, tricuspid, and pulmonary valves have disclosed morphologic and architectural modifications.[40] The mitral valve abnormalities consist of thickening and fibrosis of leaflets and chordae tendineae attributed to traumatic cusp movements that result from deformity of the left ventricular cavity. The lesions are thought to be the basis for age-related mitral regurgitation.[41,42] Superior systolic displacement of the mitral leaflets (mitral valve prolapse) occurs because leaflets with normal area and chordal length are housed in a left ventricular cavity that is reduced in size and abnormal in shape

from the leftward position of the ventricular septum (see Figure 15-46B).[41]

In patients with nonrestrictive atrial septal defects and pulmonary vascular disease, the hypertensive proximal pulmonary arteries dilate aneurysmally and contain mural calcification and intraluminal thrombi that can be massive and occlusive (Figure 15-11).[43] Aneurysmal proximal pulmonary arteries may rupture.[44] Abnormalities of medial smooth muscle, elastin, collagen, and ground substance reside in the walls of these pulmonary arteries and are held responsible for dilation that is out of proportion to hemodynamic or morphogenetic expectation.[44]

The *physiologic consequences* of atrial septal defects depend on the magnitude and chronicity of the left-to-right shunt and on the behavior of the pulmonary vascular bed. When the defect is *restrictive*, size *per se* determines the magnitude of the shunt.[45] When the defect is *nonrestrictive*, there is no pressure difference between the right and left atrium, so shunt volume is determined by the relative compliance of the two ventricles.[46] During diastole, all four cardiac chambers are in common communication, so blood can flow from the left atrium through the atrial septal defect into the right atrium and across the tricuspid valve into the right ventricle or can flow directly into the left ventricle across the mitral valve. Alternatively, blood from the *right atrium* can flow across the atrial septal defect into the left atrium across

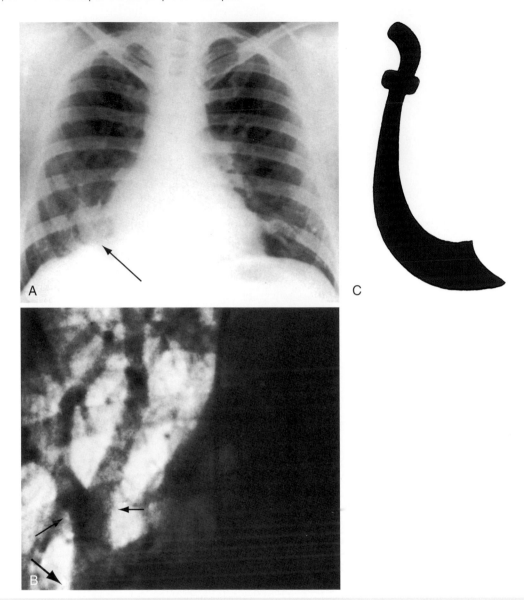

FIGURE 15-8 A, X-ray from a 28-year-old man with anomalous pulmonary venous connection of the entire right lung—*scimitar syndrome*. Right pulmonary veins converge to form a vascular trunk (arrow) that drained into the inferior vena cava. The right lung was not hypoplastic. **B,** Levophase after injection of contrast material into the pulmonary trunk shows the common pulmonary venous channel (scimitar, paired arrows) and the entrance site (left lower arrow). **C,** Turkish sword, or scimitar.

the mitral valve into the left ventricle or directly into the right ventricle across the tricuspid valve. In an ostium secundum atrial septal defect, the right ventricle is thinner and more compliant than the left ventricle, so blood flow is from left atrium through the atrial septal defect across the tricuspid valve into the relatively compliant right ventricle, which thus establishes a left-to-right shunt.[46] The shunt reaches its peak in late systole and early diastole; it diminishes throughout diastole; and in late diastole, it is supplemented by atrial contraction (see Figure 15-5B).[47,48] A small transient right-to-left shunt coincides with the onset of ventricular systole (see Figure 15-5B). Clinical and experimental studies of instantaneous flow across atrial septal defects have confirmed these flow patterns.[47]

The fetal circulation is not altered by an atrial septal defect because *in utero* interatrial flow is normally from right to left through a patent foramen ovale (see Figure 15-46C). At birth, there is little or no shunt in either direction across an atrial septal defect because the compliance of the right and left ventricles is virtually identical.[20,49,50] The right ventricle gradually becomes thinner and more compliant than the left ventricle in response to the fall in neonatal pulmonary vascular resistance, so left atrial blood then flows across the atrial septal defect into the more compliant right ventricle.[51] Pulmonary blood flow that is received by the *right* pulmonary veins is channeled into the right atrium because of proximity of the right pulmonary veins to the rim of the atrial septal defect (see previous; see Figure 15-6). Pulmonary blood flow received by the *left* pulmonary veins is channeled directly into the left atrium and is then shunted across the atrial septal defect. Accordingly, the right ventricle is volume *overloaded* and the left ventricle is volume *underloaded*.

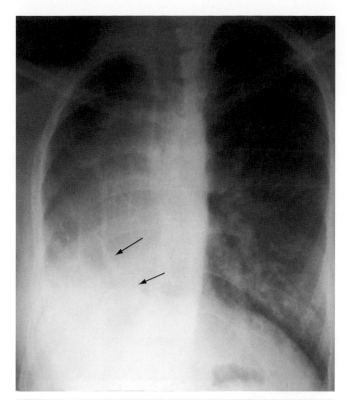

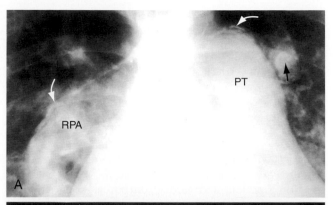

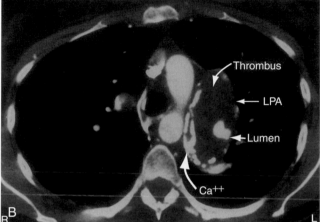

FIGURE 15-9 X-ray from a 16-year-old girl with anomalous pulmonary venous connection of the entire right lung (*scimitar sign*, upper arrow) that drained into the inferior vena cava (lower arrow). The heart was displaced into the right hemithorax, and the right hemidiaphragm was elevated because the right lung was hypoplastic. An ostium secundum atrial septal defect coexisted.

FIGURE 15-11 A, X-ray (close-up) of the central pulmonary arteries of a 38-year-old cyanotic woman with a nonrestrictive ostium secundum atrial septal defect and pulmonary vascular disease. The hypertensive pulmonary trunk (PT) and right pulmonary artery (RPA) are dilated and calcified (curved arrows). The black arrow at the upper right identifies a dilated end-on intrapulmonary artery. **B,** Pulmonary computed tomographic angiogram from a 36-year-old cyanotic woman with a nonrestrictive ostium secundum atrial septal defect and pulmonary vascular disease. The dilated left pulmonary artery (LPA) is extensively calcified (Ca^{++}) and virtually occluded by massive thrombus, leaving a small lumen.

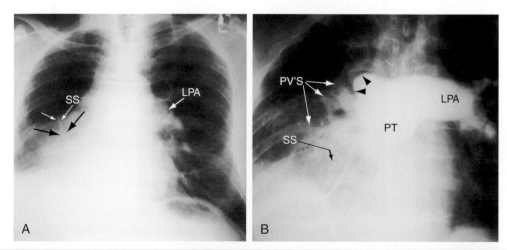

FIGURE 15-10 A, X-ray from a 66-year-old man with anomalous pulmonary venous connection of the entire right lung that drained into the inferior vena cava—*scimitar syndrome* (SS). The right lung was hypoplastic, the heart was displaced into the right hemithorax, the right hemidiaphragm was elevated, and there was proximity of the posterior ribs. The left pulmonary artery (LPA) is prominent because of a left-to-right shunt through an ostium secundum atrial septal defect and elevated pulmonary artery pressure. **B,** Pulmonary arteriogram showing absence of the right pulmonary artery (unmarked black arrow heads). The pulmonary trunk (PT) and left pulmonary artery (LPA) are dilated. The levophase visualizes the right pulmonary veins (PV'S) and faintly visualizes the *scimitar sign* (SS).

The mature right ventricle is a compliant chamber that readily adapts to volume overload and ejects its increased stroke volume into the low-resistance pulmonary vascular bed.[51] Right ventricular function is usually maintained through the fourth decade.[51] Ischemic heart disease and systemic hypertension conspire to reduce left ventricular compliance and thus to increase the left-to-right shunt. The additional volume overload of the right atrium provokes atrial fibrillation and atrial flutter, which further increase the left-to-right shunt and result in heart failure (Figure 15-12).

Left ventricular end-diastolic volume, stroke volume, ejection fraction, and cardiac output are decreased in infants and adults with an atrial septal defect,[52–54] and ejection fraction tends to fall with exercise.[52] Diminished left ventricular functional reserve is related to the mechanical effects of right ventricular volume overload, which displaces the ventricular septum into the left ventricular cavity, reducing its size and changing its shape from ovoid to crescentic (see previous; see Figure 15-46B).[42,52,53] In addition, coronary reserve is compromised in the volume-overloaded right ventricle if the left main coronary artery is compressed by a dilated pulmonary trunk.[55]

An important and poorly understood deviation from the prevailing pattern of an *asymptomatic onset* of the left-to-right shunt across an atrial septal defect is the occasional infant with development of a large shunt and right ventricular failure.[27,56] A left-to-right shunt that begins before the increase in right ventricular compliance has been attributed to more complete emptying of the right ventricle (reduced resistance to discharge). Right ventricular failure ensues because the neonatal right ventricle is volume overloaded before involution of its free wall thickness.[57] Although right ventricular failure is occasionally intractable, there is a propensity for clinical improvement because of spontaneous closure of the atrial septal defect.[18,27]

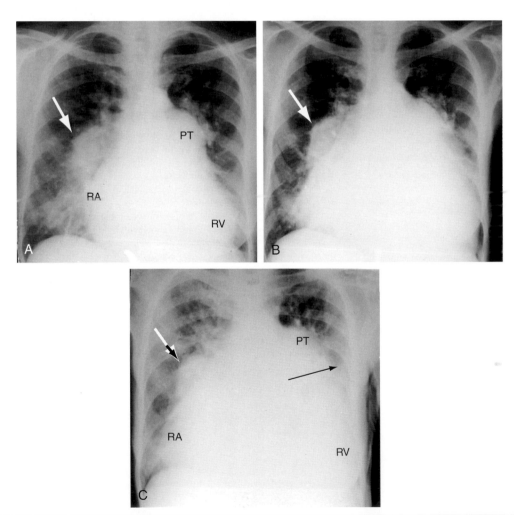

FIGURE 15-12 A, X-rays from a 71-year-old woman in sinus rhythm with a nonrestrictive ostium secundum atrial septal defect. Pulmonary arterial vascularity is increased, the pulmonary trunk (PT) and right branch (arrow) are enlarged, a prominent right atrium (RA) occupies the lower right cardiac border, and a large right ventricle (RV) occupies the apex. **B,** X-ray from the same patient 5 months after the onset of atrial fibrillation. **C,** At age 73 years, the cardiac silhouette was immense because of striking dilation of the right ventricle (RV) and right atrium (RA). An aneurysmal pulmonary trunk (PT) is encroached on by the right ventricular outflow tract (black arrow). The lungs show venous vascularity.

The paucity of pulmonary vascular disease in patients with nonrestrictive atrial septal defects has been ascribed to the onset of the left-to-right shunt *after* pulmonary arterial pressure and pulmonary vascular resistance have normalized. A low-resistance low-pressure pulmonary vascular bed accommodates an appreciable increment in blood flow without a rise in pressure.[58,59] An exception is the propensity for pulmonary hypertension in patients with atrial septal defects who are born at high altitude.[60,61] Pulmonary vascular disease with a right-to-left shunt at sea level occurs in less than 10% of patients with an atrial septal defect and is believed to represent the coincidence in young females of primary pulmonary hypertension and an ostium secundum atrial septal defect (Figure 15-13; see Chapter 14).

Increased resistance to right ventricular discharge can also result from *massive occlusive thrombus* in dilated hypertensive proximal pulmonary arteries (see previous; see Figures 15-11B and 15-42). Older adults experience a moderate rise in pulmonary artery pressure with persistence of the left-to-right shunt. Thus, pulmonary hypertension with a nonrestrictive atrial septal defect at sea level is bimodal and is represented in young females with coexisting *primary pulmonary hypertension* or in older adults, male or female, who have moderate pulmonary hypertension with a persistent left-to-right shunt.

The physiologic consequences of an atrial septal defect with partial anomalous pulmonary venous connection are similar if not identical to those of an isolated atrial septal defect with an equivalent net shunt because the hemodynamic fault remains the left-to-right shunt at atrial level.[21,62] However, flow through anomalous pulmonary veins into the right atrium is obligatory and is therefore established earlier than shunt flow across an atrial septal defect. When partial anomalous pulmonary venous connection occurs with an *intact* atrial septum, flow is increased in the segment of lung with the anomalous pulmonary veins because right atrial pressure is lower than left atrial pressure (intact atrial septum). The pressure gradient across the anomalously draining lung is therefore greater than across the normally draining lung.[32,33]

Anomalous systemic venous drainage from a normally aligned inferior vena cava results in *cyanosis* with *increased* pulmonary blood flow. In an ostium secundum atrial septal defect, small amounts of inferior vena caval blood transiently stream across the defect in early systole, a pattern appropriate for the direction of fetal blood from inferior vena cava across a foramen ovale.[63] A large persistent *eustachian valve* sometimes extends from the orifice of the inferior vena cava to the margin of an ostium secundum atrial septal defect (see Figure 15-4), selectively channeling inferior caval blood into the left atrium and causing cyanosis.[22,64] A large eustachian valve in the presence of an *inferior vena caval sinus venosus* atrial septal defect channels inferior caval blood directly into the left atrium.[22]

History

The female:male ratio is at least 2:1 in patients with an *ostium secundum* atrial septal defect,[57] and the gender ratio in *sinus venosus* defects and in ostium primum defects is approximately equal.[13] Ostium secundum atrial septal defects are sometimes familial, can recur in a several generations,[65,66] and have been found in identical twins.[67] Familial scimitar syndrome has been reported.[68,69] Autosomal dominant inheritance is a feature of atrial septal defect with the Holt-Oram syndrome (see section Physical Appearance).[70] Autosomal dominant inheritance tends to be the mode in inheritance in ostium secundum defects with prolonged atrioventricular conduction.[71-73] In some members of a family, the atrial septal defect occurs with PR interval prolongation; other family members have PR prolongation with an intact atrial septum[71]; and still others experience sudden death. Mutations in the NKX2.5 gene have been associated with familial atrial septal defect and progressive prolongation of atrioventricular conduction.[74] Concordant familial segregation of atrial septal defect has been reported with the Axenfeld-Reiger Anomaly (see section Physical Appearance).[75]

Atrial septal defects may go unrecognized for decades because symptoms are mild or absent and physical signs are subtle.[13] The soft pulmonary midsystolic flow murmur in children and young adults is often dismissed as innocent (see Chapter 2). Conversely, an atrial septal defect may first come to light in a routine chest x-ray.[76] An important exception is the symptomatic infant with an ostium secundum atrial septal defect (see Figure 15-46B) and congestive heart failure followed by spontaneous closure (see previous).[26,27,57]

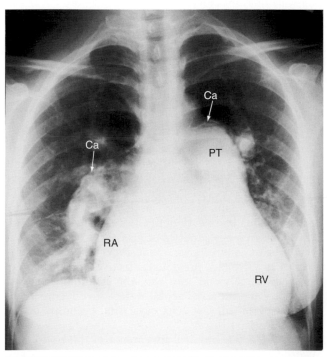

FIGURE 15-13 X-ray from a 32-year-old cyanotic woman with an ostium secundum atrial septal defect, pulmonary vascular disease, and reversed shunt. Pulmonary vascularity above the breast shadows is decreased. The pulmonary trunk (PT) and its right branch are dilated and contain eggshell calcium (Ca). The right atrium (RA) is enlarged, and a dilated right ventricle (RV) occupies the apex.

About half of patients with a *scimitar* syndrome are either asymptomatic or only mildly symptomatic when the diagnosis is made, despite varying degrees of hypoplasia of the right lung (see Figures 15-8, 15-9, and 15-10).[36,38] However, a small but important group of patients with scimitar syndrome consists of symptomatic infants with cyanosis and pulmonary hypertension.[36] Older children and young adults come to light because an x-ray discloses the scimitar sign and the hypoplastic right lung or because of an atrial tachyarrhythmia, recurrent lower respiratory infections, or a murmur.[36,38,77]

Paul Wood remarked, "In any series of geriatric necropsies atrial septal defect is always represented."[78] Ostium secundum atrial septal defects are among the most common congenital cardiac malformations in adults and account for 30% to 40% of patients over 40 years of age who have not undergone an operation.[13,79–81] Patients often survive to advanced age, but life expectancy is not normal. Three quarters of patients are alive through the third decade, but three quarters are dead by age 50 years and 90% are dead by age 60 years.[79] Sporadic survivals have been recorded beyond age 70 years, and rare examples are found of patients in their 80s or 90s (see Figure 15-43B).[80–83] An exceptional case was a patient who died 3 months before his 95th birthday (see Figure 15-43A).[80] Death is often unrelated to the malformation, but when a relationship exists, cardiac failure is the most common cause.

The clinical course of ostium secundum atrial septal defects spans the reproductive years, and most patients are female. It is therefore reassuring that, despite the gestational increase in cardiac output and stroke volume, young gravida with an atrial septal defect generally endure pregnancy, even multiple pregnancies, without tangible ill effects.[84] However, brisk hemorrhage during delivery provokes a rise in systemic vascular resistance and a fall in systemic venous return, a combination that augments the left-to-right shunt, sometimes appreciably.[84] There is also a peripartum risk of paradoxical embolization from leg veins or pelvic veins because emboli carried by the inferior vena cava traverse the atrial septal defect and enter the systemic circulation.[84]

Dyspnea and fatigue are early symptoms of an ostium secundum atrial septal defect. The large left-to-right shunt is responsible for a decrease in pulmonary compliance and an increase in the work of breathing. Orthopnea may be experienced because the supine position increases the work of breathing in patients with reduced lung compliance. Platypnea-orthodeoxia is a rare syndrome characterized by orthostatic provocation of a right-to-left shunt across an atrial septal defect or a patent foramen ovale.[85,86] *Platypnea* (dyspnea induced by the upright position and relieved by recumbency) and *orthodeoxia* (arterial desaturation in the upright position with improvement during recumbency) are features of this rare disorder. Clinical suspicion may originate from the patient who reports that dyspnea is provoked by standing upright.

Recurrent lower respiratory infections are common, especially in children. Although the pulmonary valve is theoretically susceptible to infective endocarditis because of the rapid rate of ejection, only a single case has been reported.[87]

The conditions of older patients deteriorate chiefly on three counts. *First*, a decrease in left ventricular distensibility associated with aging, ischemic heart disease, systemic hypertension, or acquired calcific aortic stenosis augments the left-to-right shunt.[81,88] *Second*, an age-related increase in prevalence of paroxysmal atrial tachycardia, atrial fibrillation, and atrial flutter precipitates congestive heart failure (see Figure 15-45).[89] *Third*, mild to moderate pulmonary hypertension in older adults occurs with a persistent left-to-right shunt, so the aging right ventricle is doubly beset by both pressure and volume overload. Pulmonary vascular disease with reversed shunt is believed to represent the coincidence of primary pulmonary hypertension with an ostium secundum atrial septal in young females who are predisposed to both lesions (see Figure 15-13; see previous).[59] Importantly, the outlook is better when primary pulmonary hypertension occurs with an atrial septal defect or a patent foramen ovale that permits the right heart to decompress (see Chapter 14).

A *patent foramen ovale* is the most common remnant of the fetal circulation (see Figure 15-46C); it occurs in 10% to 15% of healthy adults and in 20% to 30% of normal hearts at postmortem.[10,56,90] The patent foramen varies in anatomic and functional size and is implicated in paradoxical embolization, transient ischemic attacks, venoarterial gas embolism, decompression sickness, and platypnea-orthodeoxia (see previous).[56,91]

Atrial septal aneurysm is characterized by protrusion beyond the plane of the atrial septum and by rapid, dramatic phasic cardiorespiratory oscillations (see Figure 15-47 and Videos 15-4A through 15-4C).[11,12,92] An atrial septal defect may coexist. Cerebral emboli originate from fibrin-platelet aggregates on the left atrial side of the aneurysm and are dislodged by the phasic excursions.[92] Atrial septal aneurysms have been incriminated in atrial arrhythmias in children and adults and in the fetus.

Physical Appearance

Children with an atrial septal defect may have a delicate gracile habitus, with weight more affected than height (Figure 15-14A), and may have a left precordial bulge with Harrison's grooves (Figure 15-14B).[93] Newborns subsequently found to have an atrial septal defect are on average smaller than their healthy siblings.[94] *Symptomatic* infants may be cyanotic because of the effects of congestive heart failure. Cyanosis also occurs when a large eustachian valve (see previous) selectively channels inferior vena caval blood into the left atrium through an ostium secundum atrial septal defect (see Figure 15-4) or through an inferior vena caval sinus venosus defect (see Figure 15-48).[22,63,64]

The distinctive physical appearance of the *Holt-Oram syndrome* heightens suspicion of a coexisting ostium secundum atrial septal defect (Figure 15-15),[70,95,96] less commonly of an ostium primum defect. The thumb is hypoplastic with an accessory phalanx that results in triphalangism, a crooked appearance, and difficulty in apposition of thumb to fingertips. The abnormality becomes more obvious when the palms are supinated (see Figure 15-15B). The thumb may be rudimentary

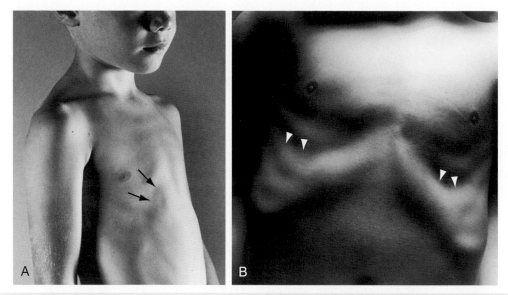

FIGURE 15-14 **A,** Five-year-old boy with a nonrestrictive ostium secundum atrial septal defect and a delicate, gracile appearance, with weight more affected than height. Harrison's grooves caused by chronic dyspnea are identified by the arrows. **B,** Six-year-old girl with a nonrestrictive ostium secundum atrial septal defect and Harrison's grooves (paired arrowheads).

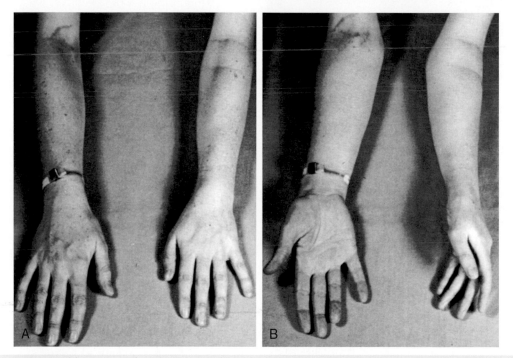

FIGURE 15-15 A 34-year-old woman with Holt-Oram syndrome and an ostium secundum atrial septal defect. **A,** The left thumb is hypoplastic, and the left arm is shorter than the right. **B,** Radial hypoplasia prevented supination, but the crooked hypoplastic triphalangeal thumb became apparent. Fingertips of the supinated right hand are erythematous because of a small right-to-left shunt.

or absent, and the metacarpal bone may be small or absent with hypoplasia extending to the radius (Figure 15-16). The bony anomaly ranges from minor changes identified on x-ray to absence of the arm (abrachia) or absent arms with persistent underdeveloped hands (phocomelia).[97] Other cardiac malformations occur without prevailing patterns.[70] Mutations in a gene on chromosome 12q2 play an important role in skeletal and cardiac development and produce a wide range of partial phenotypes of the Holt-Oram syndrome.[98]

Patau's syndrome (trisomy 13) is characterized by polydactyly, flexion deformities of the fingers, palmar crease, microcephaly, holoproscencephaly, cleft lip, cleft palate, and low-set malformed ears. *Edward's syndrome* (trisomy 18) is characterized by clenched fists, rocker bottom feet, prominent occiput, low-set malformed ears, and micrognathia (see Figures 19-5 and 20-11). The most common congenital cardiac malformations in trisomy 13 and in trisomy 18 are atrial septal defect, ventricular septal defect, and patent ductus arteriosus.[99] An atrial

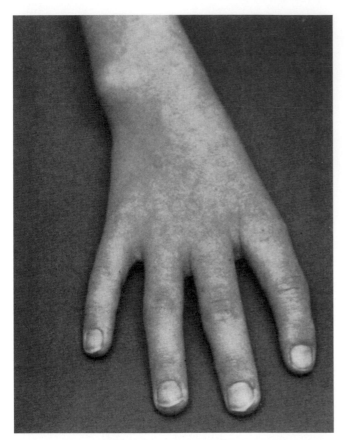

FIGURE 15-16 Photograph from a 26-year-old woman with Holt-Oram syndrome and absent thumb. An ostium secundum atrial septal defect coexisted.

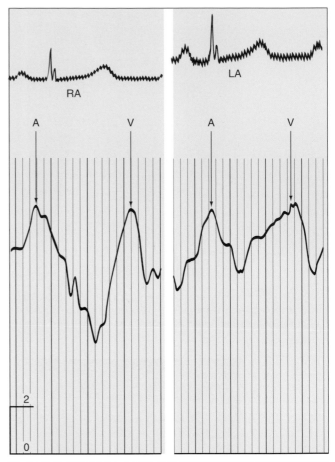

FIGURE 15-17 Sequential pressure pulses recorded as a catheter was withdrawn from right atrium (RA) to left atrium (LA) of an 11-year-old girl with a nonrestrictive ostium secundum atrial septal defect. The crests of A wave and V waves in the right and left atrium are identical because the atrial septal defect was nonrestrictive.

septal defect is associated with the Axenfeld-Rieger anomaly, a genetically heterogeneous autosomal dominant disorder characterized by ocular abnormalities with glaucoma and nonocular abnormalities that include maxillary hypoplasia, dental anomalies, umbilical hernia, and hypospadias.[75]

Arterial Pulse

The arterial pulse is normal even though left ventricular ejection fraction tends to be decreased. Left ventricular output is maintained during the Valsalva's maneuver despite a fall in systemic venous return because of the large volume of blood pooled in the lungs. Tachycardia is less pronounced during the straining phase, and there is a smaller decrease in pulse pressure. Bradycardia less is pronounced after cessation of straining, and the systolic overshoot is smaller. These abnormal responses can be identified with palpation of the brachial arterial pulse.

Jugular Venous Pulse

Most important is *left atrialization of the jugular venous wave form*.[100] The crests of the A and V waves tend to be equal as they are in the left atrium (Figure 15-17) because the two atria are in common communication through a nonrestrictive atrial septal defect. The A wave amplitude varies with heart rate as in healthy subjects.[101]

When left ventricular compliance decreases, left atrial pressure rises, and with it, the right atrial pressure.[100,101] Pulmonary vascular disease results in an increased force of right atrial contraction and a dominant, if not giant, A wave (Figure 15-18).

Precordial Movement and Palpation

In 1934, Roesler[5] called attention to the conspicuous thrust of the right ventricle in atrial septal defect. The impulse is hyperdynamic but not sustained because the volume-overloaded right ventricle contracts vigorously and empties rapidly into a low-resistance pulmonary vascular bed.[102,103] The impulse is especially prominent at the left sternal border during held *exhalation* and in the subxyphoid area during held *inspiration*.[103] Anterior movement at the left sternal border is accompanied by retraction at the apex because the enlarged right ventricle occupies the apex.[6,103] A dilated pulsatile pulmonary trunk is palpable in the second left intercostal space, but a systolic thrill is seldom present despite hyperkinetic right ventricular ejection into a dilated pulmonary trunk.

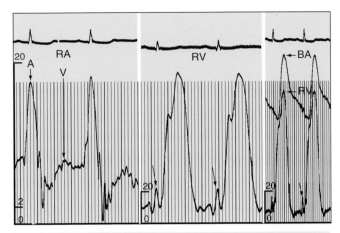

FIGURE 15-18 Pressure pulses from a cyanotic 34-year-old man with a nonrestrictive ostium secundum atrial septal defect and pulmonary vascular disease. Giant A waves in the right atrium (RA; first panel) were transmitted into the right ventricle (RV) as presystolic distention (second panel, arrows). Elevated right ventricular systolic pressure is shown in the third panel. (BA = brachial artery.)

Auscultation

Auscultatory signs are the same in all varieties of isolated nonrestrictive atrial septal defects.[104–106] The first heart sound is split at the lower left sternal edge and apex, and the tricuspid component is loud (Figure 15-19).[103,105,107] Increased diastolic flow across the tricuspid valve depresses the bellies of the leaflets into the right ventricle, and vigorous right ventricular contraction causes abrupt cephalad excursion of the leaflets, generating a loud tricuspid component of the first heart sound.[104,107,108] A pulmonary ejection sound is uncommon, despite dilation of the pulmonary trunk (Figure 15-20).[106,109]

The pulmonary midsystolic flow murmur begins immediately after the first heart sound because right ventricular isovolumetric contraction is short. The murmur is grade 2/6 or 3/6, is maximal in the second left intercostal space over the pulmonary trunk, is impure and superficial because of proximity of the dilated pulmonary trunk to the chest wall, and is crescendo-decrescendo, peaking in early or mid systole and ending well before the second heart sound (Figures 15-21 and 15-22).[6,93,104,105] Origin in the pulmonary trunk has been confirmed with intracardiac phonocardiography (see Figure 15-22)[104] and with phonocardiograms recorded from the surface of the pulmonary trunk during surgery. The murmur radiates to the apex because the right ventricle occupies the apex.[105] A louder murmur is reserved for coexisting pulmonary valve stenosis. Systolic murmurs widely distributed in the right chest, axillae, and back are generated by rapid flow through peripheral pulmonary arteries (see Figure 15-21).[110,111]

The pulmonary component of the second sound is prominent because of proximity of the dilated pulmonary trunk to the chest wall and because of brisk elastic recoil (Figure 15-23).[105] *Wide fixed splitting* is an auscultatory hallmark of atrial septal defect.[105,112,113] The aortic and pulmonary components are widely split during expiration, and the degree of splitting does not change during

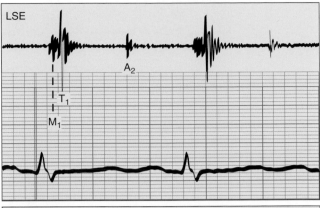

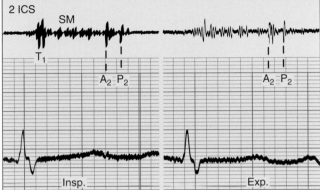

FIGURE 15-19 Phonocardiogram from a 13-year-old girl with a nonrestrictive ostium secundum atrial septal defect and a 2.5 to 1 left-to-right shunt. The loud second component of the split first heart sound (T$_1$) is tricuspid and maximal at the lower left sternal edge (LSE). (M$_1$ = mitral component.) A soft pulmonary midsystolic murmur (SM) in the second left intercostal space (2 ICS) is followed by wide fixed splitting of the second heart sound. (A$_2$ = aortic component; P$_2$ = pulmonary component.)

inspiration (Figures 15-20, 15-21, and 15-24) or during the Valsalva's maneuver (Figure 15-25). Wide splitting is caused by a delay in the pulmonary component associated with an increase in pulmonary vascular capacitance and an increase in "hangout interval" between the descending limbs of the pulmonary arterial and right ventricular pressure pulses.[114–117] With a rise in pulmonary arterial pressure, the hangout interval decreases. The split then becomes a function of the relative duration of right and left ventricular electromechanical systole, which is the same in both ventricles because a potential increase in duration of right ventricular systole from volume overload is countered by accelerated ejection.[116] A healthy child examined in the *supine position* may exhibit relatively wide but not fixed splitting of the second heart sound, but in the sitting position, respiratory splitting is normal.[103,118] The duration of diastole affects the degree of splitting by influencing the relative volumes of the right and left ventricles.[119] As diastole shortens, the split narrows, and as diastole lengthens, the split widens,[119] patterns that are evident in the beat-to-beat variations in cycle length with atrial fibrillation in which splitting tends to vary inversely with the duration of the preceding diastole.

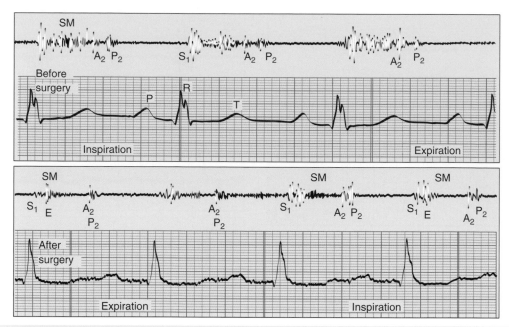

FIGURE 15-20 Phonocardiograms from a 26-year-old woman before and after surgical closure of a nonrestrictive ostium secundum atrial septal defect. *Before surgery,* a grade 3/6 midsystolic pulmonary flow murmur (SM) was followed by wide fixed splitting of the second heart sound. (A_2 = aortic component; P_2 = pulmonary component.) *After surgery,* the pulmonary systolic murmur virtually disappeared, and the second sound split normally. A pulmonary ejection sound (E) was recorded in the postoperative tracing.

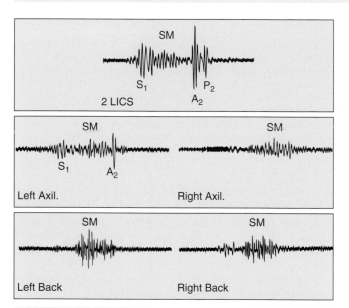

FIGURE 15-21 Phonocardiograms from a 21-year-old man with a nonrestrictive ostium secundum atrial septal defect. A grade 3/6 pulmonary midsystolic murmur (SM) in the second left intercostal space (2 LICS) is followed by wide splitting of second heart sound. (A_2 = aortic component; P_2 = pulmonary component.) Prominent systolic murmurs in the left axilla, right axilla, and right back were the result of rapid flow through peripheral pulmonary arteries. (S_1 = first heart sound.)

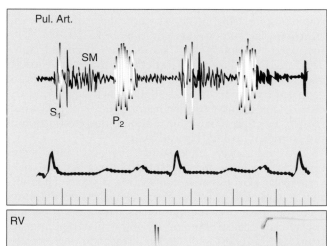

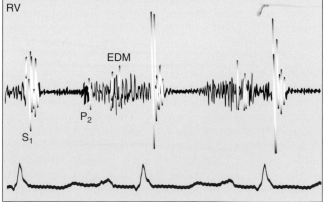

FIGURE 15-22 Intracardiac phonocardiograms from a 14-year-old boy with a nonrestrictive ostium secundum atrial septal defect and a 2.7 to 1 left-to-right shunt. A short midsystolic flow murmur (SM) was recorded in the main pulmonary artery (PUL ART). In the right ventricular outflow tract (RV), an early diastolic murmur of pulmonary regurgitation (EDM) was recorded despite normal pulmonary arterial pressure.

Fixed splitting means that the width of the split remains constant throughout active respiration and during the Valsalva's maneuver. *Persistent splitting* means that the split widens during inspiration and narrows during expiration. Atrial septal defect is characterized

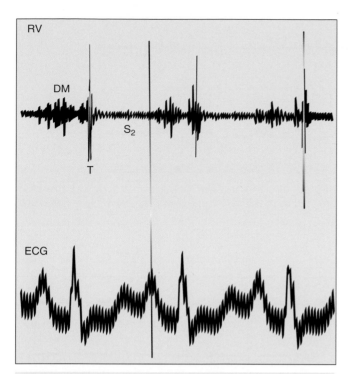

FIGURE 15-23 Intracardiac phonocardiogram from an 8-year-old girl with a nonrestrictive ostium secundum atrial septal defect and 3 to 1 left-to-right shunt. In the *inflow* tract of the right ventricle, just distal to the tricuspid valve, the microphone recorded a mid-diastolic flow murmur (DM) and a loud tricuspid component of the first heart sound (T). (S_2 = second heart sound; RV = right ventricle.)

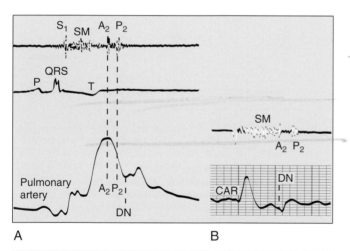

FIGURE 15-24 Tracings from a 28-year-old woman with a nonrestrictive ostium secundum atrial septal defect and a 2.3 to 1 left-to-right shunt. **A,** The grade 2/6 pulmonary midsystolic murmur (SM) is followed by wide splitting of the second heart sound. The pulmonary component (P_2) coincides with the dicrotic notch of the pulmonary artery pressure pulse (DN). **B,** The aortic component of the second sound (A_2) coincides with the dicrotic notch (DN) of the carotid pulse (CAR).

by splitting of the second heart sound that is wide *and* fixed (see Figure 15-20). During inspiration, the aortic and pulmonary components are equally delayed or do not move at all.[120] In the normal heart, inspiratory

splitting is chiefly the result of a delay in the pulmonary component of the second sound because the increase in pulmonary capacitance during inspiration is accompanied by an increase in the hangout interval (Figure 15-26). The high pulmonary capacitance in atrial septal defect precludes an additional increase during inspiration, so there is no inspiratory delay in the pulmonary component of the second sound. Normal phasic changes in systemic venous return during respiration are associated with reciprocal changes in volume of the left-to-right shunt, which minimize the respiratory variations in right and left ventricular filling.[112,113,121] Inspiration is accompanied by an increase in systemic venous return, so right ventricular filling is maintained or increased while the left-to-right shunt decreases reciprocally; thus, left ventricular filling is maintained or is increased by the same amount. An inspiratory decrease in left-to-right shunt has been shown in experimental animals[112] and in human subjects.[122] Wide fixed splitting is unlikely in neonates because there is little or no shunt in either direction.[123]

These patterns of splitting do not apply when partial anomalous pulmonary venous connection occurs with an *intact* atrial septum (Figure 15-27).[113,124] Increased venous return during inspiration is not accompanied by a reciprocal fall in left-to-right shunt because the atrial septum is intact. Accordingly, the aortic component of the second heart sound moves *toward* the first heart sound and the pulmonary component moves *away*, so the split widens with inspiration and narrows with expiration (see Figure 15-27).

Rarely, an opening sound of the tricuspid valve follows the pulmonary component of the second heart sound.[105,107] Echocardiographic timing confirms that the sound coincides with abrupt arrest of the opening movement of the tricuspid valve in early diastole.[107] Mid-diastolic murmurs are the result of augmented tricuspid flow.[104,105,125,126] Origin of the flow murmur at the tricuspid orifice has been shown experimentally in animals and with intracardiac phonocardiography in human subjects (Figure 15-28).[104,127] Tricuspid flow murmurs are medium frequency, impure, soft, short, presystolic or mid-diastolic, and localized at the lower left sternal border and do not increase with inspiration despite their right-sided origin. Intracardiac phonocardiograms identify low-intensity inaudible diastolic murmurs within the atrial septal defect itself.[125–127] The combination of superficial impure presystolic and mid-diastolic murmurs together with a superficial impure midsystolic murmur occasionally creates the impression of a pericardial rub. Occasionally, a rub in fact does occur, and attention has been called to roughened pericardium in patients with an atrial septal defect (Figure 15-29).[128,129] A diastolic murmur of *low-pressure* pulmonary regurgitation is uncommon (see Figure 15-22) and is reserved for aneurysmal dilation of the pulmonary trunk.[130] Continuous murmurs through restrictive atrial septal defects are rare.[131] Atrial septal defects with pulmonary vascular disease and reversed shunts are accompanied by auscultatory signs of pulmonary hypertension (Figures 15-30 and 15-31; see Chapter 14).[105,132,133]

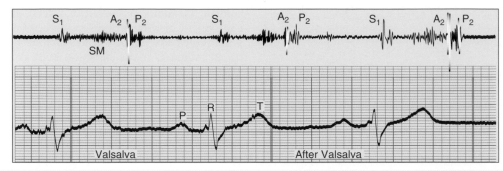

FIGURE 15-25 Phonocardiogram in the second left interspace during and after Valsalva's maneuver in a 17-year-old girl with a nonrestrictive ostium secundum atrial septal defect. Splitting of the second heart sound remained wide and fixed. (S_1 = first heart sound; SM = pulmonary midsystolic murmur.)

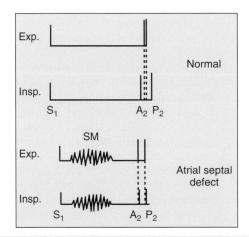

FIGURE 15-26 Respiratory behavior of the second heart sound in the normal heart and in the presence a nonrestrictive atrial septal defect with a left-to-right shunt. *Normal inspiratory splitting* (Insp.) is chiefly the result of a delay in the pulmonary component (P_2), less the result of movement of the aortic component (A_2) in the opposite direction. In an *atrial septal defect*, the second sound is widely split during expiration (Exp.) because the pulmonary component (P_2) is late. The split remains *fixed* during active inspiration and expiration because both components move equally and in the same direction, or do not move at all. (SM = systolic murmur.)

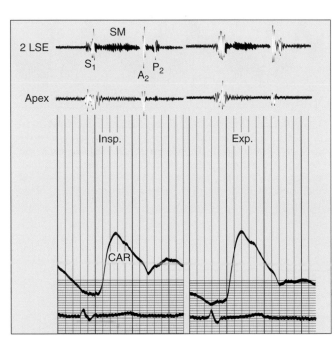

FIGURE 15-27 Phonocardiograms and carotid pulse (CAR) from a 16-year-old girl with anomalous pulmonary venous connection of the entire right lung to the inferior vena cava and an intact atrial septum (see Figure 15-9). The second heart sound is *persistently* split, but the split is not *fixed*. (A_2 = aortic component; P_2 = pulmonary component; SM = systolic murmur; 2 LSE = second intercostal space left sternal edge; Insp./Exp. = inspiration and expiration.)

Electrocardiogram

Sinus node dysfunction has been identified as early as age 2 to 3 years,[134–136] and accelerated atrial rhythms have been recorded on 24-hour ambulatory electrocardiograms in 35% of children with an atrial septal defect.[134] The incidence of atrial fibrillation, atrial flutter, and supraventricular tachycardia increases in the fourth decade (Figures 15-32 and 15-33).[89,136] Interestingly, *sinus arrhythmia* does not occur in adults with an atrial septal defect and is minimal or absent in children (see Figure 15-33). Sinus arrhythmia requires separation of the systemic and pulmonary venous returns. With an atrial septal defect, the two venous returns are by definition not separated.[137]

Atrioventricular conduction defects are intrinsic components of atrial septal defects and are usually age related.[134,136,138] The PR interval tends to be prolonged.[139] Atrioventricular node dysfunction begins in older children and is less frequent than sinus node dysfunction.[135,136] *Advanced* first-degree atrioventricular nodal block occurs with familial or, less commonly, nonfamilial atrial septal defect and occasionally culminates in complete heart block.[71–74] Some family members have an ostium secundum atrial septal defect and first-degree heart block, and others have PR prolongation with an intact atrial septum.[71] In the Holt-Oram syndrome (see Figures 15-15 and 15-16), PR interval prolongation, sinus bradycardia, and ectopic atrial rhythms are relatively common.[70]

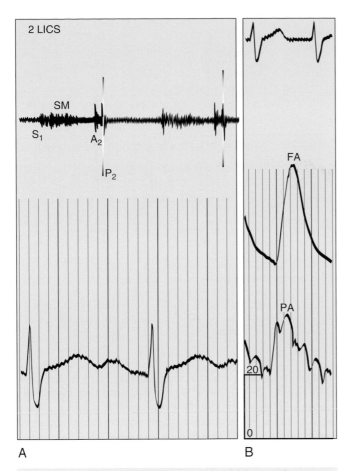

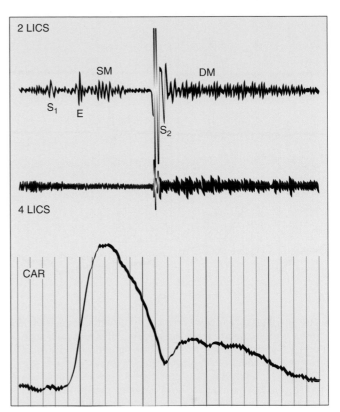

FIGURE 15-28 Tracings from a 4-year-old boy with a nonrestrictive ostium secundum atrial septal defect and a 2.3 to 1 left-to-right shunt. **A,** The pulmonary component (P_2) of the split second sound is loud even though the pulmonary arterial pressure was normal as shown in panel. **B,** (S_1 = first heart sound; A_2 = aortic component of the second sound; SM = systolic murmur; FA = femoral artery pulse; PA = pulmonary artery pulse.)

FIGURE 15-30 Tracings from a 28-year-old cyanotic woman with a nonrestrictive ostium secundum atrial septal defect and pulmonary vascular disease. A pulmonary ejection sound (E) introduced a soft short midsystolic murmur (SM) in the second left intercostal space (2 LICS). The second heart sound (S_2) is loud and single and introduced a decrescendo Graham Steell murmur (DM). (S_1 = first heart sound; 4 LICS = fourth left intercostal space; CAR = carotid pulse.)

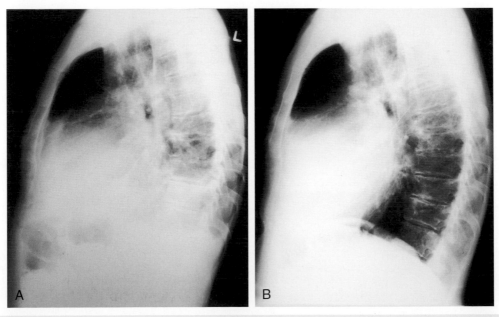

FIGURE 15-29 A, Lateral x-ray from a 65-year-old man with a nonrestrictive ostium secundum atrial septal defect and large pericardial and pleural effusions. **B,** The effusions were benign transudates that decreased appreciably after pericardiocentesis. Thickened pericardium was identified at surgery for closure of the atrial septal defect.

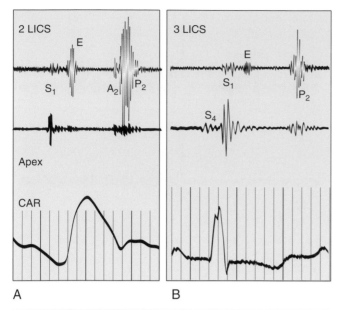

A

B

FIGURE 15-31 Tracings from a 32-year-old woman with a nonrestrictive ostium secundum atrial septal defect, pulmonary vascular disease, a 1.4 to 1 left-to-right shunt, and a small right-to-left shunt. Pulmonary artery systolic pressure was 90 mm Hg, and systemic systolic pressure was 110 mm Hg. **A,** The first heart sound (S_1) is followed by a prominent pulmonary ejection sound (E). (2 LICS = second left intercostal space.) The second heart sound remained split. The loud pulmonary component (P_2) was transmitted to the apex. (A_2 = aortic component.) **B,** The ejection sound and the loud pulmonary component of the second sound transmitted to the third left intercostal space (3 LICS). A prominent fourth heart sound (S_4) was present at the lower left sternal border.

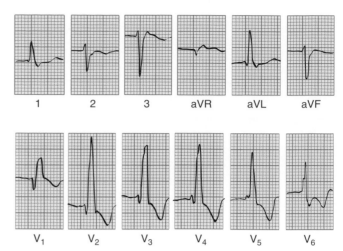

FIGURE 15-32 Electrocardiogram from an acyanotic man with a nonrestrictive ostium secundum atrial septal defect who died 3 months before his 95th birthday. The rhythm was atrial fibrillation. Left axis deviation was the result of acquired left anterior fascicular block. The right ventricular conduction defect was peripheral, not central.

Abnormal right atrial P waves are peaked rather than tall (Figure 15-34), but P wave configurations are usually normal (Figure 15-35).[140] Prolonged P wave duration occurs when the terminal force is written by an enlarged right atrium.[141-143] The P wave axis with an *ostium secundum* atrial septal defect is inferior and to the left with upright P waves in leads 2, 3, and aVF (see Figures 15-34 and 35). With a *superior vena vaval sinus venosus* atrial septal defect, the atrial pacemaker is ectopic because the defect occupies the site of the sinoatrial node. The P wave axis is then leftward, and the P waves are inverted in leads 2, 3, and aVF and upright in lead aVL (Figure 15-36). Superior vana caval sinus venosus

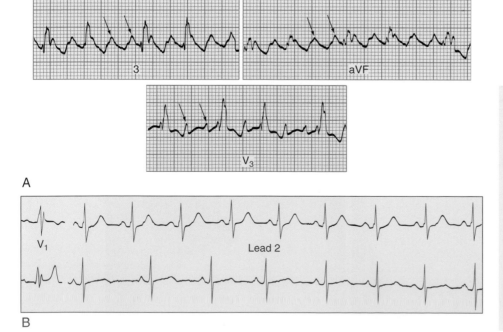

A

B

FIGURE 15-33 A, Leads 3, aVF, and V_3 from a 60-year-old woman with an ostium secundum atrial septal defect and a 2.6 to 1 left-to-right shunt. The rhythm is atrial flutter (paired arrows) with an irregular ventricular response. **B,** The upper rhythm strip (lead 2) illustrates *absence* of sinus arrhythmia in a 19-year-old woman with a nonrestrictive ostium secundum atrial septal defect. The lower rhythm strip illustrates typical sinus arrhythmia that appeared after surgical closure of the atrial septal defect. The rsr prime in lead V1 remained unchanged.

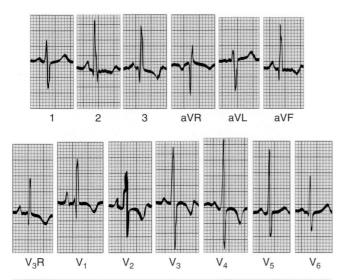

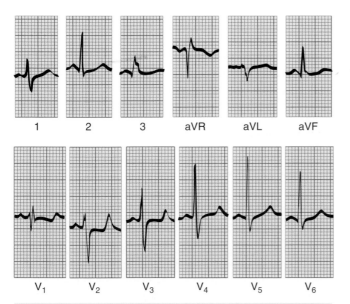

FIGURE 15-34 Electrocardiogram from a 5-year-old boy with a nonrestrictive ostium secundum atrial septal defect and a 3.5 to 1 shunt. P waves are peaked and tall in lead 2 and V_3R and in leads V_{1-2}. The QRS axis is vertical. Depolarization is clockwise, so Q waves appear in leads 2, 3, and aVF. There is an rsR prime pattern in leads V_1 and V_3R.

defects are occasionally accompanied by shifts from sinus rhythm with a normal P axis to an ectopic atrial rhythm with a leftward P axis.

The QRS duration is slightly prolonged in atrial septal defects because of slurring of the terminal force (see Figure 15-35). The duration increases with age and

FIGURE 15-35 Electrocardiogram from a 24-year-old woman with a nonrestrictive ostium secundum atrial septal defect and a 2 to 1 left-to-right shunt. P waves are normal. The QRS axis is vertical with clockwise depolarization and Q waves in leads 2, 3, and aVF. The terminal QRS forces are directed upward, to the right and anterior, and are slightly prolonged, so an rSr prime appears in lead V_1, a slurred terminal R wave appears in lead aVR, and slurred S waves appear in left precordial leads.

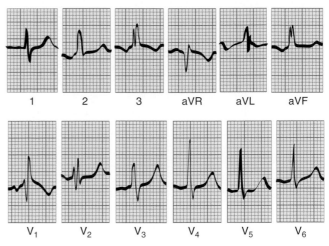

FIGURE 15-36 Electrocardiogram from a 25-year-old woman with a *superior vena caval sinus venosus* atrial septal defect. The P wave axis is leftward and markedly superior, so P waves are inverted in leads 2, 3, and aVF; are isoelectric in lead 1; and are slightly positive in lead aVR. Intracardiac electrophysiologic investigation identified an ectopic left atrial pacemaker. The QRS pattern is typical of a left-to-right shunt at atrial level, namely, a vertical QRS axis and prolonged terminal forces directed to the right, superior and anterior, with an rSR prime in lead V_1 and S waves in left precordial leads.

may culminate in a pattern that resembles complete right bundle branch block (see Figure 15-32). The QRS axis is vertical with clockwise depolarization that writes q waves in leads 2, 3, and aVF (see Figures 15-34 and 15-35). Right axis deviation is reserved for infants with symptomatic pulmonary hypertension or for young females with pulmonary vascular disease. Left axis deviation is exceptional and represents acquired left anterior fascicular block in older adults (see Figure 15-32).[144]

An electrocardiographic hallmark of atrial septal defect is an *rSr prime* or an *rsR prime* in right precordial leads (see Figures 15-34 and 15-35).[6,145,146] The r prime in lead V_1 and aVR is slurred in contrast to thin terminal r waves in 5% of normal electrocardiograms. Q waves are small or absent in left precordial leads because the shunt does not traverse the left ventricle (see Figures 15-34, 15-35, and 15-36). The outflow tract of the right ventricle is the last portion of the heart to depolarize. Enlargement and increased thickness caused by right ventricular volume overload are responsible for the rightward superior and anterior direction of the terminal force of the QRS and for increased QRS duration.[147-149] The term *incomplete right bundle branch block* is a misnomer.[149]

A notch near the apex of the R waves in inferior leads of ostium secundum and sinus venosus atrial septal defects has been called *crochetage*[150] because the notch resembles the work of a crochet needle (Figure 15-37).[151] Crochetage is independent of the terminal force direction of the QRS, but when the rSr prime pattern occurs with crochetage in each of the inferior limb leads, the specificity of the electrocardiographic diagnosis of atrial septal defect is remarkably high.[150] Although crochetage has been correlated with shunt severity, the pattern has also

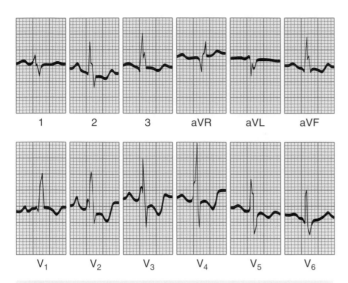

| 1 | 2 | 3 | aVR | aVL | aVF |

| V₁ | V₂ | V₃ | V₄ | V₅ | V₆ |

FIGURE 15-37 Electrocardiogram from a 32-year-old woman with a nonrestrictive ostium secundum atrial septal defect and a 2.6 to1 left-to-right shunt. *Crochetage* is represented by notches on the R waves in leads 2, 3, and aVF.

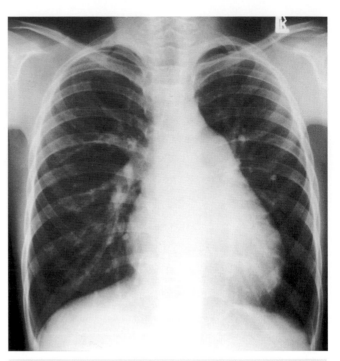

FIGURE 15-38 X-ray from a 5-year-old boy with a non-restrictive ostium secundum atrial septal defect and a 2.5 to 1 left-to-right shunt. Pulmonary vascularity is increased and the pulmonary trunk and its right branch are prominent, but the ascending aorta is inconspicuous. The right atrium occupies the lower right cardiac border, and a dilated right ventricle occupies the apex.

been reported with a patent foramen ovale and has been suggested as an electrocardiographic marker of a patent foramen.[152]

X-Ray

Increased pulmonary arterial vascularity extends to the periphery of the lung fields (Figures 15-38 and 15-39). The pulmonary trunk and its proximal branches are dilated (see Figure 15-39). The left branch is usually obscured by an enlarged pulmonary trunk (see Figure 15-39), but the lateral view discloses dilation of both branches (Figures 15-39 and 15-40). The ascending aorta is seldom border forming because the intracardiac shunt does not traverse the aortic root (see Figures 15-38 and 15-39).[5,153] However, angiographic and echocardiographic assessments indicate that the intrinsic caliber of the ascending aorta is not significantly reduced. A sinus venosus atrial septal defect may be accompanied by localized ampullary dilation of the superior vena cava proximal to its attachment to the right atrium (Figure 15-41).[15] Infants with large left-to-right shunts exhibit both pulmonary arterial and pulmonary venous vascularity with enlargement of all four cardiac chambers.[123] In older adults with moderate pulmonary hypertension and persistent left-to-right shunt, the pulmonary trunk and proximal branches are occasionally aneurysmal (Figure 15-42). In young adults with pulmonary vascular disease and a balanced or reversed shunt, the pulmonary trunk and its branches are strikingly enlarged and calcified (see Figures 15-11 and 15-13).

Right atrial enlargement is characteristic (Figures 15-39A and 15-43), but the left atrium seldom enlarges despite a left-to-right shunt (see Figure 15-39B) because a major portion of pulmonary venous return enters the right atrium directly owing to the proximity of the right pulmonary veins to the rim of the ostium secundum atrial septal defect (see previous).[54,154] Left atrial enlargement is reserved for older adults with atrial fibrillation.[89,155]

Volume elastic properties of the right and left atrium also play a role in determining relative enlargement. For equal increments in volume, the right atrium is more distensible than the left.[154]

An enlarged right ventricle occupies the apex and forms an acute angle with the left hemidiaphragm (see Figure 15-38). Dilation of the outflow tract causes smooth continuity with the enlarged pulmonary trunk above (see Figure 15-38). In the lateral projection, the dilated right ventricle encroaches on the retrosternal space (see Figures 15-39B and 15-40), and displaces the left ventricle posteriorly. The size of the left ventricle is normal because its stroke volume is normal or reduced. The relationship between the inferior vena caval shadow and the left ventricular shadow in the lateral projection distinguishes posterior displacement of the left ventricle from intrinsic dilation (Figure 15-44).[156] The lateral projection in adults often shows disproportionate anterior bowing of the upper third of the sternum (see Figure 15-39B). A progressive and often dramatic increase in heart size is initiated by atrial tachyarrhythmias, especially atrial fibrillation with congestive heart failure (Figures 15-12 and 15-45).[155]

In the *scimitar syndrome*, the confluence of right pulmonary veins forms a distinctive shadow parallel to or behind the right cardiac silhouette as the anomalous venous channels course downward to join the inferior vena cava (see Figures 15-8, 15-9, and 15-10).[28,37,157] The heart is displaced into the right hemithorax because of hypoplasia of the right lung, but the anomalous venous channels usually remain visible (see Figures 15-9 and 15-10).

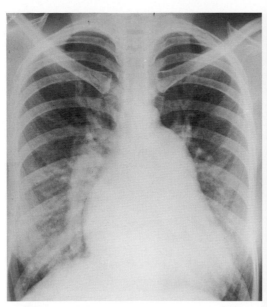
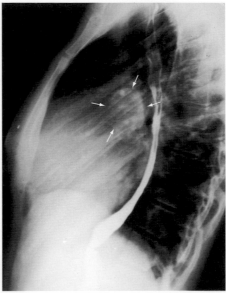

FIGURE 15-39 X-rays from a 31-year-old woman with a nonrestrictive ostium secundum atrial septal defect and a 3.2 to 1 left-to-right shunt. The frontal projection shows increased pulmonary arterial vascularity that extends to the periphery of the lung fields (enhanced by breast tissue). The pulmonary trunk and its right branch are dilated in contrast to the non–border-forming ascending aorta. An enlarged right atrium occupies the lower right cardiac border, and an enlarged right ventricle occupies the apex. In the lateral projection, arrows bracket a dilated right pulmonary artery, which was obscured in the frontal projection by the dilated pulmonary trunk. The retrosternal space is obliterated by enlargement of the right atrium and right ventricle despite an increase in anteroposterior chest dimension caused by bowing of the sternum. In the barium esophagram, the left atrium is not enlarged.

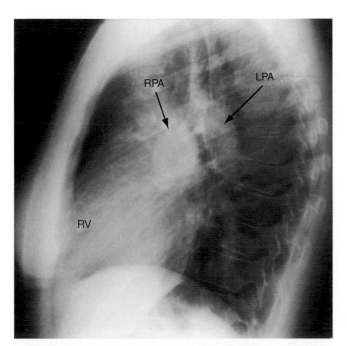

FIGURE 15-40 Lateral x-ray from a 48-year-old man with a nonrestrictive ostium secundum atrial septal defect and a 2.5 to 1 left-to-right shunt. The end-on right pulmonary artery (RPA) is dilated, and the left pulmonary artery (LPA) appears as a large comma-like shadow. The right ventricle (RV) encroaches on the retrosternal space. The left atrium is not enlarged.

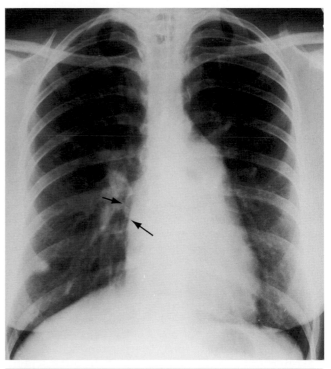

FIGURE 15-41 X-ray from a 26-year-old woman with a superior vena caval sinus venosus atral septal defect and a 2 to 1 left-to-right shunt. Arrows bracket subtle localized dilation of the superior vena cava as it joins the right atrium. The x-ray otherwise resembles an ostium secundum atrial septal defect of equilavent size.

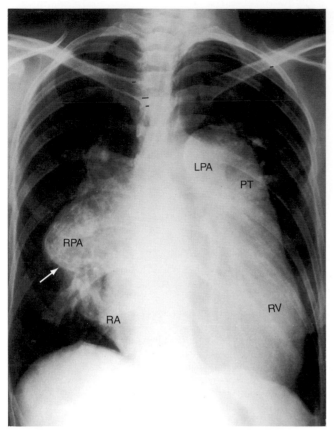

FIGURE 15-42 X-ray from a 64-year-old woman with a nonrestrictive ostium secundum atrial septal defect, pulmonary artery pressure of 60/38 mm Hg, and a 1.8 to 1 left-to-right shunt. Pulmonary vascularity is decreased. The pulmonary trunk (PT) and the right pulmonary artery (RPA) are aneurysmal, the RPA contains a rim of calcium (arrow), and a dilated left pulmonary artery (LPA) lies behind pulmonary trunk. The ascending aorta is not seen. An enlarged right atrium occupies the lower right cardiac border, and an enlarged right ventricle (RV) occupies the apex.

Echocardiogram

Echocardiography with color flow imaging and Doppler interrogation establishes the location and size of an atrial septal defect and its physiologic consequences.[21] Transesophageal echocardiography has refined the anatomic assessment of the interatrial septum[9,158] and identifies partial anomalous pulmonary venous connections.[62,159,160] Pulsed Doppler imaging can identify anomalous pulmonary venous connections in the fetus.[161] Real-time three-dimensional transesophageal echocardiography has optimized assessment of atrial septal defects.[162] An ostium secundum atrial septal defect is represented by an echo-free space in the mid portion of the atrial septum (see Figure 15-5A). Color flow imaging confirms that the echo-free space is a true tissue defect, and pulsed Doppler imaging characterizes instantaneous flow patterns across the defect (see Figure 15-5D). A foramen ovale can be identified (Figure 15-46C and Video 15-3C), and color flow determines its patency.[90,163] An in utero patent

foramen can be distinguished from an ostium secundum atrial septal defect.[27] Transthoracic and transesophageal echocardiography establish the diagnosis of atrial septal aneurysm (Figure 15-47A and Video 15-4A), and color flow imaging or echocontrast determines whether an atrial septal defect coexists (Figure 15-47B and Video 15-4B).[12,164]

Transesophageal echocardiography identifies a *divided* right atrium that consists of a shelf that separates an anterior supratricuspid component from a posterior systemic venous sinus, to which the cava are connected.[165] A rare *double atrial septum* is imaged as a midline chamber between the left and right atrium.[166]

Real-time imaging discloses a dilated hyperkinetic right ventricle with paradoxical motion of the ventricular septum[51,167] and vigorous pulsations of the pulmonary trunk and its branches. The size, shape, and functional reserve of the left ventricle can be determined (see Figure 15-46B).[52,53]

A superior vena caval sinus venosus defect lies near the junction of the superior cava and the right atrium (Figure 15-48A),[21,158] and an inferior vena caval sinus venosus defect lies just beyond the rim of the inferior vena cava.[163] An unroofed coronary sinus is identified by dilation of the sinus and by a defect between the sinus and left atrium.

Summary

Ostium secundum atrial septal defects predominate in females and often come to light in asymptomatic children or young adults. Patients usually reach their fourth decade with little or no handicap. Preadolescents sometimes appear delicate and gracile. Dyspnea, fatigue, and recurrent lower respiratory infections are common. The left-to-right shunt in older adults is augmented by ischemic heart disease, systemic hypertension, and acquired calcific aortic stenosis that decrease left ventricular compliance. Atrial tachyarrhythmias, especially atrial fibrillation, precipitate congestive heart failure. The crests of the jugular venous A and V waves are equal (left atrialization). The right ventricular impulse is hyperdynamic, and a systolic pulsation is palpated over the dilated pulmonary trunk. The first heart sound is split with a loud tricuspid component. A grade 2/6 or 3/6 pulmonary midsystolic murmur is followed by fixed splitting of the second heart sound and a tricuspid mid-diastolic flow murmur.

P waves are peaked but seldom tall. The QRS axis is vertical with clockwise depolarization and q waves in leads 2, 3, and aVF. Terminal forces of the QRS are prolonged and point to the right and anterior, producing an rSr prime in lead V_1. Notching of the R waves in inferior leads results in a distinctive crochetage pattern. The x-ray shows increased pulmonary arterial vascularity, an inconspicuous ascending aorta, dilation of the pulmonary trunk and its proximal branches, and enlargement of the right atrium and right ventricle. The scimitar syndrome is characterized by partial anomalous right pulmonary venous connection with infradiaphragmatic drainage and hypoplasia of the right lung. Echocardiography with color flow imaging and Doppler interrogation establishes the location and size of the atrial septal defect, its physiologic

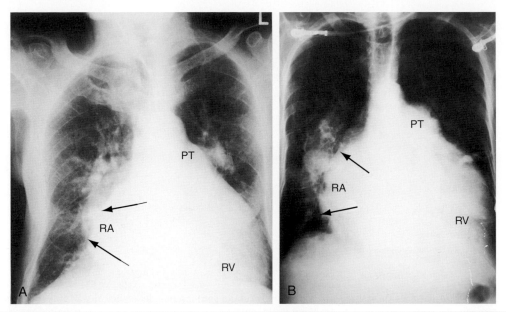

FIGURE 15-43 A, X-ray from the 95-year-old acyanotic man with a nonrestrictive ostium secundum atrial septal defect. The electro-cardiogram (see Figure 15-32) shows atrial fibrillation. Pulmonary arterial and pulmonary venous vascularity are increased. The pulmonary trunk (PT) is dilated, but the ascending aorta is not border-forming. The right atrium (RA) and the right ventricle (RV) are strikingly enlarged. **B,** X-ray from an 87-year-old acyanotic woman with a nonrestrictive ostium secundum atrial septal defect, severe tricuspid regurgitation, and atrial fibrillation. Pulmonary vascularity is decreased. The pulmonary trunk (PT) is dilated, and the enlarged right branch contains eggshell calcification. The ascending aorta is not border-forming. The right atrium (RA) and right ventricle (RV) are strikingly enlarged. At necropsy, there was a large thrombus in the dilated right pulmonary artery and a smaller thrombus in the dilated left pulmonary artery.

consequences, and the presence of partial anomalous pulmonary venous connections. A nonrestrictive ostium secundum atrial septal defect with pulmonary vascular disease is believed to represent the coexistence of primary pulmonary hypertension in young females.

A superior vena caval sinus venosus atrial septal defect is clinically similar to an equivalent ostium secundum defect with two exceptions: first, the atrial pacemaker is ectopic so the P wave axis is leftward and inverted P waves appear in leads 2, 3, and aVF; second, the right hilus may show localized ampullary dilatation of the distal

superior vena cava as it joins the right atrium. Echocardiography confirms the location of the defect.

Ostium secundum atrial septal defects in the young are among the most readily diagnosed congenital malformations of the heart, but these same defects sometimes defy clinical recognition because of diagnostic ambiguities. The diagnosis of *mitral stenosis* is entertained (Box 15-1) because of dyspnea, orthopnea, atrial fibrillation, an increased jugular venous V wave, a right ventricular impulse, a loud first heart sound, a delayed pulmonary component of the second heart sound

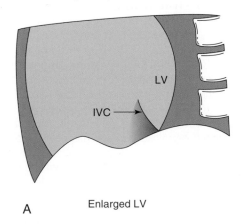
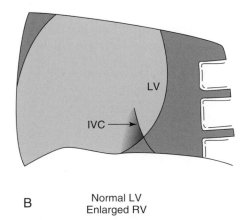

A   Enlarged LV

B   Normal LV
      Enlarged RV

FIGURE 15-44 A, The relationship of the inferior vena cava (IVC) and the posterior silhouette of an *enlarged left ventricle* (LV) when the *right ventricle is normal.* At the level of the diaphragm, the caval shadow lies *within* the left ventricular silhouette. **B,** The relationship of the inferior vena cava to the posterior silhouette of a *normal left ventricle* that is retrodisplaced by an *enlarged right ventricle.* At the level of the diaphragm, the caval shadow lies *behind* the left ventricle. *(Modified from Keats TE, Rudhe U, Foo GW. Inferior vena caval position in the differential diagnosis of atrial and ventricular septal defects. Radiology 83:616, 1964.)*

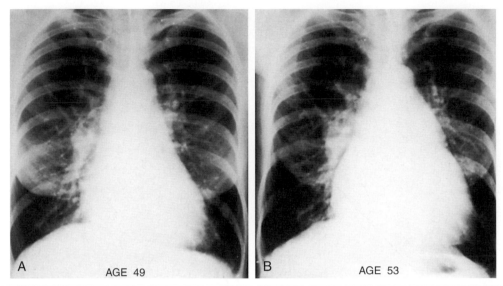

FIGURE 15-45 X-rays from an acyanotic woman with an ostium secundum atrial septal defect before and after the onset of atrial fibrillation. **A,** At age 49 years, the x-ray shows increased pulmonary arterial vascularity, mild prominence of the pulmonary trunk and its right branch, and a moderate increase in right atrial size. **B,** After the onset of atrial fibrillation 4 years later, there is a considerable increase in size of the pulmonary trunk, right atrium, and right ventricle.

mistaken for an opening snap, a tricuspid flow murmur mistaken for a mitral diastolic murmur, shunt vascularity mistaken for pulmonary venous congestion, and dilation of the pulmonary trunk, the right atrium, and occasionally, the left atrium. *Mitral regurgitation* may be misdiagnosed as acquired (Box 15-2) because the holosystolic murmur of tricuspid regurgitation is well heard at the apex, a delayed pulmonary component of the second sound followed by a tricuspid flow murmur is mistaken for an opening snap and the mid-diastolic murmur of mitral stenosis, and a tricuspid flow murmur is mistakenly attributed to flow across the mitral valve. Diagnostic ambiguity in older adults results from atrial arrhythmias, ischemic heart disease, systemic hypertension, and inverted left precordial T waves (Box 15-3).

Symptomatic infants with a large left-to-right shunt through an ostium secundum atrial septal defect pose a diagnostic problem to clinicians who are not accustomed to considering an atrial septal defect in neonates. Splitting of the second heart sound is variable and difficult to assess, the pulmonary component is increased, and a holosystolic murmur of tricuspid regurgitation and a tricuspid diastolic flow murmur are misinterpreted. The diagnosis is established with echocardiography. These infants often experience spontaneous closure of the atrial septal defect.

LUTEMBACHER'S SYNDROME

In 1811, Corvisart[168] described the association of atrial septal defect with mitral stenosis; and in 1916, Lutembacher[169] published the first comprehensive account of these two defects as a combination that has come to be called *Lutembacher's syndrome.* Opinion differs regarding what lesions the syndrome should

include. Lutembacher believed that mitral stenosis was congenital even though his patient was 61 years old. The current consensus is that Lutembacher's syndrome consists of a *congenital defect in the atrial septum* together with *acquired mitral stenosis.*[32,170,171] The syndrome has been broadened to include different anatomic types of congenital interatrial communications and different anatomic types of acquired mitral valve disease.

What then constitutes an acceptable type of left-to-right shunt in Lutembacher's syndrome?

When the interatrial communication is an ostium secundum atrial septal defect, the answer is clear.[32,172] However, a patent foramen ovale is not included in the definition, although Lutembacher stated that the high left atrial pressure of mitral stenosis might stretch the margins of a valve-incompetent foramen ovale and cause a left-to-right shunt.[32,173] An age-related increase in mitral leaflet fibrosis and shortened fibrotic mitral chordae tendineae is found in ostium secundum atrial septal defects,[41,174] the functional consequence of which is mitral regurgitation. But whether pure mitral regurgitation should be included in the definition of Lutembacher's syndrome is debatable. *Congenital* obstruction to left atrial flow that accompanies cor triatriatum or a parachute mitral valve is occasionally associated with an atrial septal defect (see Chapter 9), but by convention, the Lutembacher eponym is not applied. Partial anomalous pulmonary venous connection with intact atrial septum is a left-to-right shunt at atrial level, and cases have been reported with acquired mitral stenosis.[33,170] More recently, *iatrogenic* Lutembacher's syndrome has emerged as a defect in the atrial septal acquired during percutaneous transseptal mitral valvotomy for rheumatic mitral stenosis (Figure 15-49).[175] For the purposes of this chapter, Lutembacher's syndrome is considered as the combination of a *congenital* atrial septal defect and *acquired* rheumatic mitral stenosis.

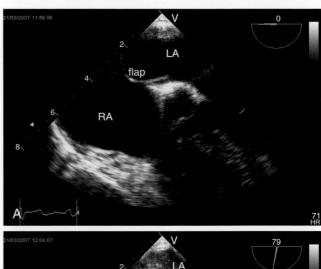

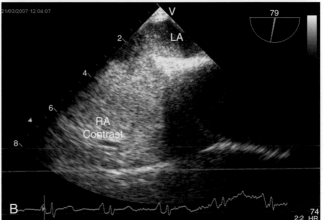

FIGURE 15-47 A, Transesophageal echocardiogram from a 29-year-old woman with transient ischemic attacks attributed to cerebral emboli from an atrial septal aneurysm shown with the flap of the foramen ovale. (RA = right atrium; LA = left atrium.) **B,** Echo contrast in the right atrium with shunt shown from right to left (Videos 15-4A and 15-4B).

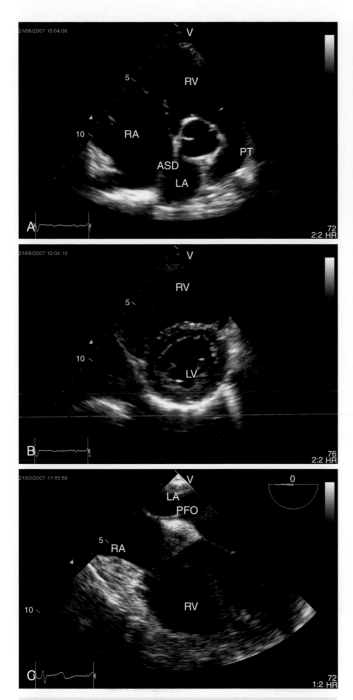

FIGURE 15-46 A, Echocardiogram (subcostal) from a 5-year-old girl with a nonrestrictive ostium secundum atrial septal defect (ASD) and an enlarged right atrium (RA). (LA = left atrium; PT = pulmonary trunk; RV = right ventricle.) **B,** Echocardiogram (short axis) from a patient with a nonrestrictive ostium secundum atrial septal defect, a large left-to-right shunt, and an enlarged right ventricle that flattened the ventricular septum and reduced the size of the left ventricle (LV). **C,** Transesophageal echocardiogram from a 30-year-old woman with transient ischemic attacks and a patent foramen ovale (PFO) guarded by a valve on its left atrial side. (RA = right atrium; RV = right ventricle.) (Videos 15-3A through 15-3C.)

When these disorders coexist, each modifies the hemodynamic and clinical expressions of the other.[176] Let us first examine the physiologic effects that mitral stenosis exerts on an atrial septal defect.[176] The left-to-right shunt across a nonrestrictive atrial septal defect is determined principally by the relative resistances to flow from left atrium into left ventricle and from left atrium through the atrial septum into the right ventricle (see previous). Mitral stenosis increases the resistance to flow from the left atrium into the left ventricle and, in so doing, augments the left-to-right shunt in proportion to the severity of mitral stenosis.[176,177] In the presence of a *restrictive* atrial septal defect, severe mitral stenosis generates a continuous left-to-right shunt because the pressure difference across the restrictive atrial septum exists throughout the cardiac cycle (see Figure 15-49).[178,179]

Now let us examine the effects that an atrial septal defect exerts on mitral stenosis.[176] The idea that an interatrial communication might have a favorable hemodynamic effect was proposed in 1880 by Firkett[180] and formalized in 1949 by Bland and Sweet[181] who surgically treated mitral stenosis by anastomosing a pulmonary vein to the azygos vein, after which the left atrial pressure fell. The mitral valve is normally the only exit from the left atrium. An atrial septal defect constitutes an alternative exit that decompresses the left

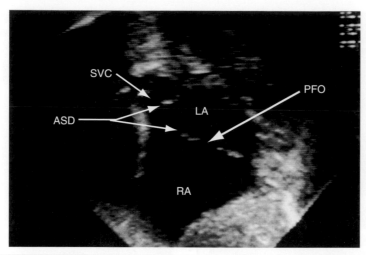

FIGURE 15-48 Echocardiogram from a 4-year-old boy with a nonrestrictive sinus venosus atrial septal defect (ASD) of the superior vena caval type (SVC). The defect is at the junction of the superior vena cava and right atrium (RA) and thus remote from the midportion of the atrial septum as represented by the patent foramen ovale (PFO). (LA = left atrium.)

BOX 15-1   ATRIAL SEPTAL DEFECT SECUNDUM: DIAGNOSTIC AMBIGUITIES IN ADULTS

Mitral Stenosis

Dyspnea, orthopnea

Atrial fibrillation

Increased jugular venous V wave

Right ventricular impulse

Loud first heart sound

Delayed pulmonary component of a widely split second heart sound mistaken for mitral opening snap

Mid-diastolic tricuspid murmur

Increased pulmonary vascularity with ditation of the pulmonary trunk, right ventricle, and left atrium

---

BOX 15-2   ATRIAL SEPTAL DEFECT SECUNDUM: DIAGNOSTIC AMBIGUITIES IN ADULTS

Mitral Regurgitation

Atrial fibrillation

Apical holosystolic murmur

Wide splitting of second heart sound

Mid-diastolic murmur

Third heart sound

BOX 15-3   ATRIAL SEPTAL DEFECT SECUNDUM: DIAGNOSTIC AMBIGUITIES IN ADULTS

Coexisting Acquired Heart Disease

Ischemic heart disease

Inverted left precordial T waves

Atrial tachyarrhythmias

---

atrium and, in so doing, diminishes the transmitral gradient.[171] In brief, mitral stenosis increases the shunt flow across an atrial septal defect, and an atrial septal defect decreases the gradient across a stenotic mitral valve. As the left-to-right shunt increases, left ventricular filling and stroke volume reciprocally fall. Conversely, an increase in pressure in the left atrium and pulmonary artery causes right ventricular hypertrophy that decreases right ventricular distensibility, reduces the left-to-right shunt, and improves left ventricular filling.[171]

History

Lutembacher's syndrome has a predilection for females because ostium secundum atrial septal defect and rheumatic mitral stenosis are both more prevalent in females.[32,176] The incidence rate of mitral stenosis in patients with atrial septal defect has been estimated at 4%.[32,176] The incidence rate of atrial septal defect in patients with mitral stenosis has been estimated at 0.6% to 0.7%.[32,176] Mitral stenosis is rheumatic even when Lutembacher's syndrome is familial because it is the atrial septal defect that is genetically transmitted. The incidence rate of coexisting rheumatic mitral stenosis depends on the geographic prevalence of rheumatic fever.[176] In underdeveloped countries, a history of rheumatic fever has been reported in 40% of patients with Lutembacher's syndrome.[176]

The most important clinical consequence of a nonrestrictive atrial septal defect in Lutembacher's syndrome is its ameliorating effect on the symptoms of mitral stenosis. Orthopnea, paroxysmal nocturnal dyspnea, pulmonary edema, and hemoptysis are infrequent and attenuated and replaced by fatigue from reduced left ventricular filling and low cardiac output.[171] When mitral stenosis is severe and the atrial septal defect *restrictive*, the symptoms and clinical course resemble isolated mitral stenosis of equivalent severity.[32,176]

The ameliorating effects of an atrial septal defect were evident in Lutembacher's original patient, a 61-year-old woman who had had seven pregnancies.[169] Firkett's patient was a 74-year-old woman who experienced 11 pregnancies.[180] An 81-year-old woman had no cardiac symptoms until her 75th year,[182] and survival to advanced age has been reaffirmed.[172,183,184] However,

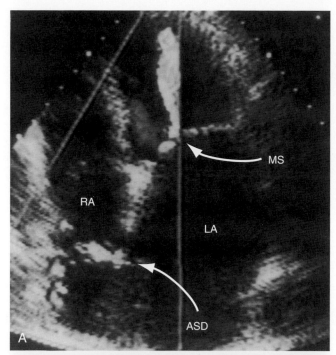

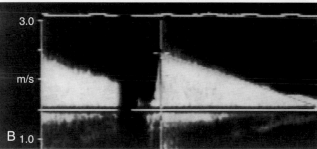

FIGURE 15-49 Echocardiogram from a 63-year-old woman with *iatrogenic* Lutembacher's syndrome consisting of rheumatic mitral stenosis and an acquired interatrial communication produced during percutaneous transseptal mitral valvuloplasty. **A,** Black and white print of a color flow image showing a high-velocity diastolic jet from left atrium (LA) into right atrium (RA) through the acquired interatrial communiction (ASD). Mitral stenosis (MS) produced a high-velocity diastolic jet across the mitral valve. **B,** Continuous-wave Doppler scan across the stenotic mitral valve. The calculated orifice size was 1.8 cm^2.

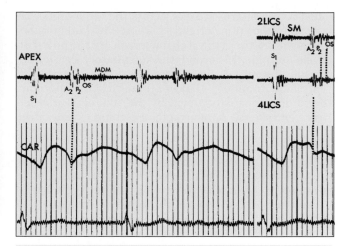

FIGURE 15-50 Tracings from a 42-year-old woman with Lutembacher's syndrome that consisted of rheumatic mitral stenosis and a nonrestrictive superior vena caval sinus venosus atrial septal defect with a left-to-right shunt of 2.5 to 1, a mitral orifice of 1.1 cm^2, and pulmonary artery pressure of 38/18 mm Hg. The carotid pulse (CAR) was small because left ventricular stroke volume was reduced by atrial fibrillation shown in the rhythm strip below. Phonocardiogram at the apex recorded a prominent first heart sound (S$_1$), wide splitting of the second heart sound (A$_2$ = aortic component; P$_2$ = pulmonary component), an opening snap (OS), and a middiastolic murmur (MDM). The pulmonary component of the second sound was transmitted to the apex, which was occupied by the right ventricle. In the second left intercostal space (2 LICS), the phonocardiogram shows a soft pulmonary midsystolic murmur (SM) and wide splitting of the second heart sound followed by an opening snap (OS). (4 LICS = fourth left intercostal space.)

these reports should not discount the unfavorable long-term effect exerted by an atrial septal defect on mitral stenosis that increases the left-to-right shunt and predisposes to atrial fibrillation.[172,176] Susceptibility to infective endocarditis resides in the stenotic mitral valve in contrast to negligible susceptibility in an uncomplicated ostium secundum atrial septal defect.

Arterial Pulse

The arterial pulse is small because left ventricular stroke volume is small. Atrial fibrillation reduces the pulse still further (Figure 15-50).[176]

Jugular Venous Pulse

The right and left atrium function as a common chamber when the atrial septal defect is nonrestrictive, so the height and contour of the *left* atrial pressure pulse are transmitted into the *right* atrium and into the internal jugular vein. Lutembacher's syndrome is therefore responsible for an elevated mean jugular venous pressure in the absence of right ventricular failure and for an elevated jugular venous A wave in the absence of pulmonary hypertension.

Precordial Movement and Palpation

The impulse of the right ventricle and pulmonary trunk are more prominent in Lutembacher's syndrome with a nonrestrictive atrial septal defect than with an uncomplicated atrial septal defect of the same size because mitral stenosis augments the left-to-right shunt. The underfilled left ventricle cannot be palpated. The diastolic thrill of mitral stenosis is exceptional because the velocity of mitral valve flow is comparatively low.

Auscultation

The auscultatory signs of mitral stenosis are attenuated on two counts (see Figure 15-50).[32] First, flow across the stenotic mitral valve is reduced because left atrial blood has an alternative exit across the atrial septal defect, an explanation correctly proposed by Lutembacher to account for the atypical characteristics of the mitral diastolic murmur.[169] Second, the auscultatory signs of uncomplicated mitral stenosis are heard best over the *left* ventricular impulse[103]; but in Lutembacher's syndrome, the cardiac apex is occupied by the volume-overloaded *right* ventricle, so a topographic auscultatory advantage is lost.

When a nonrestrictive atrial septal defect occurs with *mild* mitral stenosis, the auscultatory signs resemble those of the atrial septal defect.[32] The diagnostic yield is improved when the patient turns into a left lateral decubitus position and coughs briskly, while the bell of the stethoscope is applied to the approximate location of the apex.[103] Mitral stenosis increases the left-to-right shunt and augments the midsystolic flow murmur across the pulmonary valve. Right ventricular dilation is accompanied by the holosystolic murmur of tricuspid regurgitation that transmits to the apex, inviting a mistaken diagnosis of mitral regurgitation.[176] Inspiratory augmentation of the tricuspid murmur—Carvallo's sign—should prevent error. When the atrial septal defect is restrictive, mitral stenosis results in a continuous gradient from left atrium to right atrium and a continuous murmur at the lower *right* sternal border because the murmur is generated within the right atrial cavity.[178,179] The continuous murmur may increase with slow deep inspiration because of a delayed inspiratory increase in left atrial volume.[179] During the straining phase of the Valsalva's maneuver, the interatrial gradient is reduced or abolished, and the continuous murmur diminishes.[179]

Electrocardiogram

When the atrial septal defect is restrictive, the electrocardiogram resembles that of mitral stenosis. When the atrial septal defect is nonrestrictive, the electrocardiogram resembles that of an atrial septal defect. P waves show left atrial abnormalities with a broad bifid configuration in lead 2 and a deep prolonged P terminal force in lead V_1 (Figure 15-51).[32,185] However, atrial fibrillation is frequent. Right ventricular hypertrophy is more common than with isolated atrial septal defect.

X-Ray

A *restrictive* atrial septal defect results in an x-ray that resembles mitral stenosis with pulmonary venous congestion and left atrial enlargement. When the atrial septal defect is *nonrestrictive*, the x-ray shows increased pulmonary arterial blood flow but little or no pulmonary venous congestion because the left atrium is decompressed (Figure 15-52). Left atrial enlargement is less than expected for equivalent mitral stenosis but more than expected for an uncomplicated atrial septal defect (see Figure 15-52B).[176,185] Left atrial size increases with the advent of atrial fibrillation.[176] Dilation of the right atrium, right ventricle, and pulmonary trunk exceeds expectations for an uncomplicated atrial septal defect. Whether mitral valve calcification is infrequent or simply overlooked is unclear.

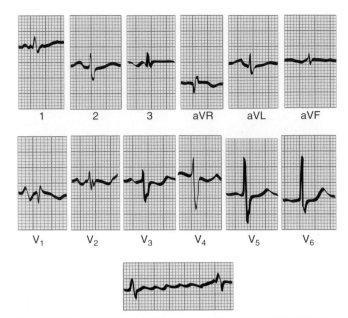

FIGURE 15-51 Electrocardiogram from the 42-year-old woman with Lutembacher's syndrome. The phonocardiogram is shown in Figure 15-50. There are broad notched left atrial P waves in leads 2 and aVL, with a broad deep left atrial P terminal force in leads V_{1-2}. The leftward P wave axis with inverted P waves in leads 3 and aVF was the result of an ectopic atrial pacemaker associated with a superior vena caval sinus venosus atrial septal defect. The QRS pattern resembles an ostium secundum defect with a prolonged terminal force directed to the right, superior, and anterior (rsr prime in lead V_1, a qr in aVR, and a broad S wave in lead V_6). The rhythm strip below shows atrial fibrillation.

Echocardiogram

Echocardiography with color flow imaging and Doppler interrogation is used to establish the diagnosis of Lutembacher's syndrome, identify the location and size of the atrial septal defect, and determine the degree of mitral stenosis (see Figure 15-49).[178,186] A continuous murmur at the right lower sternal border coincides with Doppler flow patterns recorded with transesophageal echocardiography in the presence of a restrictive atrial septal defect.[178]

Summary

Lutembacher's syndrome has a predilection for females because ostium secundum atrial septal defect and rheumatic mitral stenosis are both prevalent in females.* Despite the rheumatic etiology of mitral stenosis, a history of active rheumatic fever in childhood is obtained in less than half the cases.

When the atrial septal defect is *restrictive*, the clinical picture resembles isolated mitral stenosis. A continuous murmur at the right sternal border is generated within

---

Lutembacher is a German name, but Dr Lutembacher spoke French, wrote in French, and preferred a French pronunciation of his name (Loo-tem-bah-share) because he was Alsatian and Alsace-Lorraine was then a part of France. The pronunciation is now anglicized to Loo-tem-bah-ker.

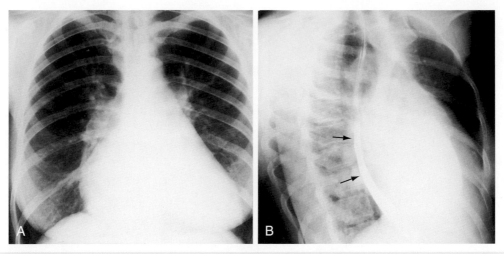

FIGURE 15-52 X-rays from the 42-year-old woman with Lutembacher's syndrome (see Figures 15-50 and 15-51). **A,** The frontal projection shows no signs of pulmonary venous congestion. The pulmonary trunk is moderately prominent and merges with the shadow of the left atrial appendage, resulting in a straight left cardiac border. The ascending aorta is not border-forming. An enlarged right atrium occupies the lower right cardiac border, and an enlarged right ventricle occupies the apex. **B,** The right anterior oblique projection shows retrodisplacement of the barium esophagram by a moderately enlarged left atrium (paired arrows).

the right atrial cavity. The electrocardiogram shows left atrial P wave abnormalities, and the x-ray shows pulmonary venous congestion and left atrial enlargement.

When the atrial septal defect is *nonrestrictive,* the effects of mitral stenosis are attenuated because the left atrium is decompressed, while mitral stenosis augments the left-to-right interatrial shunt. The arterial pulse is small, especially with the advent of atrial fibrillation. The jugular venous pulse exhibits a prominent A wave in the absence of pulmonary hypertension because the left atrial pressure pulse is transmitted into the right atrium through the nonrestrictive atrial septal defect. Auscultatory signs of mitral stenosis are blunted or absent. A pulmonary midsystolic flow murmur is evident because right ventricular stroke volume is increased. The electrocardiogram in sinus rhythm shows left atrial P wave abnormalities. Right ventricular hypertrophy is more common than with an uncomplicated atrial septal defect. The x-ray shows increased pulmonary arterial blood flow with little or no pulmonary venous congestion. The right atrium, right ventricle, and pulmonary trunk are considerably enlarged. Echocardiography with color flow imaging and Doppler interrogation establishes the presence and severity of mitral stenosis, the location and size of the atrial septal defect, and the physiologic consequences of the combination. Mitral stenosis is a substrate for infective endocarditis.

COMMON ATRIUM

Common atrium is a rare variety of interatrial communication characterized by absence or virtual absence of the atrial septum, vestigial remnants of which may remain as diaphanous strands of tissue.[187] The right-sided portion of the common chamber has features of a morphologic

right atrium (crista terminalis, pectinate muscles, right atrial appendage) and receives the superior and inferior vena cavae and coronary sinus.[187] The left-sided portion of the common chamber has features of a morphologic *left* atrium (smooth nontrabeculated walls, a left atrial appendage) and receives the pulmonary veins.[187] Common atrium therefore differs from atrial isomerism with a common atrial chamber that is either a bilateral morphologic right atrium or a bilateral morphologic left atrium (see Chapter 3). Absence of the atrial septum necessarily includes the ostium primum (atrioventricular septal) location, so there is a common atrioventricular valve (Figure 15-53) or a cleft anterior mitral leaflet (Figure 15-54).[188,189] Partial anomalous pulmonary venous connections are frequent.[187] Systemic venous anomalies consist of superior vena caval connection to the left-sided portion of the common atrium, persistent left superior vena cava, and a left hemiazygos vein.[190]

Physiologic consequences of common atrium resemble a nonrestrictive atrial septal defect except for obligatory venoarterial mixing.[187] Common atrium is therefore a *cyanotic* malformation with *increased* pulmonary arterial blood flow.[189] Despite absence of the atrial septum, venoarterial mixing is usually no more than moderate, with systemic arterial oxygen saturations that are often above 90%.[187,191] The relative magnitude of left-to-right and right-to-left components of interatrial mixing are determined chiefly by the distensibility characteristics of the right and left ventricles, as in a nonrestrictive atrial septal defect (see previous).[191] At one end of the spectrum are patients with low pulmonary vascular resistance, a distensible right ventricle, a large left-to-right shunt, and mild or absent cyanosis. At the other end of the spectrum are patients with high pulmonary vascular resistance, poorly distensible right ventricles, a significant right-to-left shunt, and conspicuous cyanosis.

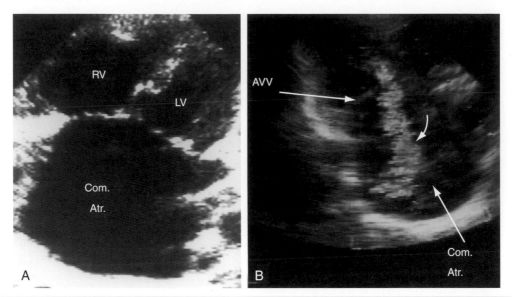

FIGURE 15-53 Echocardiogram with black and white print of a color flow image from the 57-year-old woman with common atrium (see Figures 15-54 and 15-59). **A,** Apical view showing the common atrium (Com. Atr.) and the common atrioventricular valve, whose left and right components lie at the same level. (LV = left ventricle; RV = right ventricle.) **B,** Black-and-white print of a color flow image showing regurgitation (curved arrow) across the left component of the common atrioventricular valve (AVV).

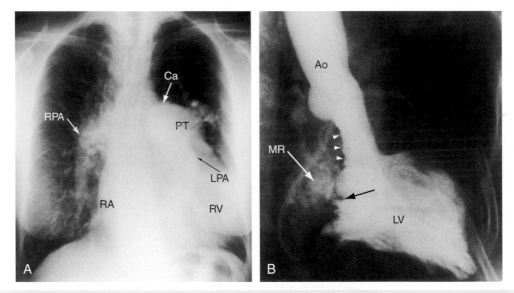

FIGURE 15-54 **A,** X-ray and left ventriculogram from the 57-year-old cyanotic woman with common atrium. The electrocardiogram is shown in Figure 15-59. The lung fields are oligemic. The ascending aorta is not border-forming, in contrast to the huge pulmonary trunk (PT) that contains a rim of calcium (Ca) in its upper margin. The right pulmonary artery (RPA) is dilated and tapers rapidly. A large left pulmonary artery (LPA) lies behind the pulmonary trunk. The right atrium (RA) is dilated, and an enlarged right ventricle (RV) occupies the apex. **B,** Left ventriculogram shows the typical gooseneck deformity (small white arrowheads) and the cleft anterior mitral leaflet (black arrow) of an atrioventricular septal defect. Mitral regurgitation (MR) was only moderate despite a malformed common atrioventricular valve. (Ao = aorta; LV = left vertricle.)

History

Symptoms begin earlier and are more pronounced than with a nonrestrictive atrial septal defect.[187] Most patients experience dyspnea, fatigue, respiratory infections, mild cyanosis, and physical underdevelopment in the first year of life. Occasional patients are relatively well into late childhood or early adolescence[187,191] but are rarely into adulthood (see Figure 15-54).

Physical Appearance

Cyanosis occurs despite insufficient evidence of pulmonary hypertension to account for its presence and may be insignificant at rest but induced by exercise or crying. Small or intermittent right-to-left shunts express themselves as highly colored cheeks or digital erythema. The Down phenotype is not a feature of common atrium, despite the presence of elements of an atrioventricular

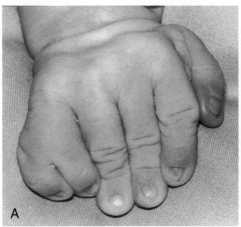 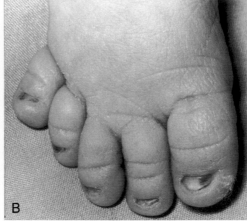

FIGURE 15-55 Photographs from a female neonate with Ellis-van Creveld syndrome and common atrium. **A,** The hand is characterized by a well-formed extra digit on its ulnar aspect (polydactyly), clinodactyly (bent fingers), and syndactyly (interdigital webbing). Hypoplasia of the nails is better seen in the foot **(B)** and in Figure 15-56.

septal defect. However, the Ellis-van Creveld syndrome, chondroectodermal dysplasia, is an important phenotype because 50% of patients with this syndrome have congenital heart disease and half of them have a common atrium.[192–194] Ellis-van Creveld syndrome is autosomal recessive and is characterized by dwarfism with polydactyly of the hands that is invariable (Figures 15-55A), but polydactyly of the feet occurs in only 10% of cases (Figure 15-55B).[194] *Polycarpaly* (a ninth or tenth carpal bone), *clinodactyly* (bent fingers), *syndactyly* (interdigital webbing), and *hypoplasia of the nails*[194,195] are common features (Figures 15-55 and 15-56). Premature eruption of malformed maxillary incisors,

gingival hypertrophy, and multiple frenula are distinctive (Figure 15-57).

Arterial Pulse, Jugular Venous Pulse, Precordial Movement and Palpation, and Auscultation

The arterial pulse, the jugular venous pulse, and precordial palpation are analogous to a nonrestrictive ostium secundum atrial septal defect (see previous). Auscultatory signs are also similar, with the important exception of an apical holosystolic murmur of mitral regurgitation caused by the malformed left atrioventricular valve (see Figure 15-54B). An increase in the jugular A wave and a loud pulmonary component of the second heart sound reflect the early development of pulmonary hypertension.

Electrocardiogram

Absence of the atrial septum assumes deficiency of the superior vena caval sinus venosus location, the ostium primum or atrioventricular septal location, and the ostium secundum location. The electrocardiogram reflects the deficiencies at all of these sites.[188] Leftward deviation of the P wave axis with inverted P waves in the inferior leads is analogous to the ectopic atrial pacemaker in a superior vena caval sinus venous atrial septal defect with an absent sinus node.[188,187,196] Left axis deviation of the QRS with counterclockwise depolarization (Figures 15-58 and 15-59) and splintering of S waves in the inferior leads (see Figure 15-59) is analogous to the electrocardiogram of an atrioventricular septal defect.[21,187,188] The precordial leads are analogous to an ostium secundum atrial septal defect, but early development of pulmonary hypertension results in increased R wave amplitude in right precordial leads (see Figures 15-58 and 15-59). The electrocardiogram therefore reflects the combined absence of the superior, mid, and inferior portions of the atrial septum.

FIGURE 15-56 Close-up view of the fingers of a 53-year-old woman with dwarfism with Ellis-van Creveld syndrome and hypoplasic nails (arrows). *(From Hearst JW. The heart. 4th ed. New York: McGraw-Hill Book Company; 1978, with permission.)*

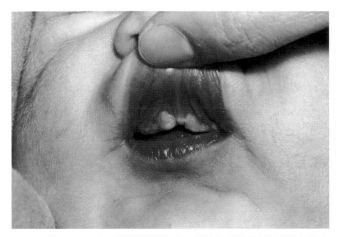

FIGURE 15-57 Female neonate with Ellis-van Creveld syndrome, premature eruption of malformed maxillary incisors, gingival hypertrophy, and multiple frenula.

X-Ray

The chest x-ray is similar to that of a nonrestrictive ostium secundum atrial septal defect (Figures 15-54A and 15-60).[187] Enlargement of the left atrial portion of the common atrium is seldom seen in the x-ray, even in the presence of significant mitral regurgitation.

Echocardiogram

Echocardiography with color flow imaging and Doppler interrogation identifies a common atrial chamber (Figure 15-61), absence of the atrial septum, and a common atrioventricular valve or a cleft anterior mitral leaflet (see Figure 15-53). The right and left components of the

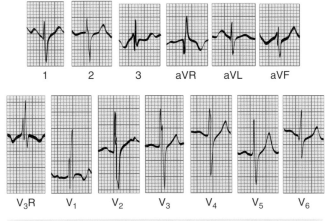

FIGURE 15-58 Electrocardiogram from a 5-year-old boy with common atrium, a cleft anterior mitral leaflet, and a 3.5 to 1 left-to-right shunt. The leftward shift of the P wave axis with inverted P waves in leads 2, 3, and aVF indicates an ectopic pacemaker because of an absent sinus node associated with a superior vena caval sinus venosus atrial septal defect. Left axis deviation with counterclockwise depolarization and splintered S waves in inferior leads indicates that the atrial septum was deficient in the ostium primum location. The terminal force of the QRS points to the right, superior, and anterior as in an ostium secundum atrial septal defect.

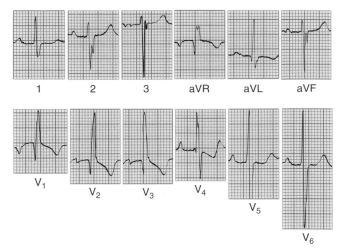

FIGURE 15-59 Electrocardiogram from a 57-year-old cyanotic woman with common atrium, pulmonary hypertension, and moderate incompetence of the left-sided component of a common atrioventricular valve. The PR interval is prolonged. A normal P wave axis implies that the sinus node was functioning despite a superior vena caval sinus venosus artial septal defect. Peaked P waves in leads V_{4-5} together with QS waves in leads V_{1-3} indicate right atrial enlargement, and broad bifid P waves in leads 3, aVL, aVF, and V_6 indicate a left atrial abnormality. Left axis deviation with counterclockwise depolarization and splintered S waves in leads 2, 3, and aVF imply an atrioventricular septal defect with a cleft anterior mitral leaflet. Right ventricular hypertrophy is manifested by tall R waves in right precordial leads and deep S waves in left precordial leads. QRS prolongation is the result of increased duration of the terminal force that is directed to the right, superior, and anterior.

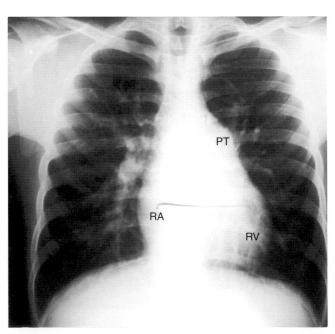

FIGURE 15-60 X-ray from a 5-year-old acyanotic boy with a common atrium. The electrocardiogram is shown in Figure 15-58. The x-ray resembles an ostium secundum atrial septal defect. Pulmonary arterial vascularity is increased, the pulmonary trunk (PT) and its right branch are dilated, the right atrium (RA) is convex, and a prominent right ventricle (RV) occupies the apex.

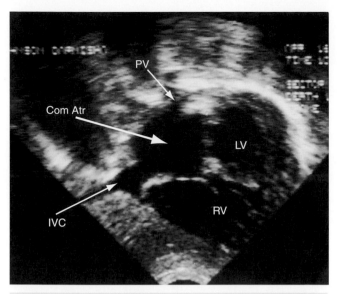

FIGURE 15-61 Echocardiogram (subcostal) from a female neonate with Ellis-van Creveld syndrome and common atrium (Com Atr). The inferior vena cava (IVC) entered the right-sided portion of the common atrium, and the pulmonary veins (PV) entered the left-sided portion. (LV = left ventricle; RV = right ventricle.)

common atrioventricular valve lie at the same level because the atrioventricular septum is absent (see Figure 15-53A). Color flow imaging establishes regurgitation across the left component of the common atrioventricular valve (see Figure 15-53B). The right ventricle is dilated (see Figure 15-53A), the ventricular septum moves paradoxically, and the pulmonary trunk is dilated and pulsatile.

Summary

The clinical features of common atrium resemble a nonrestrictive ostium secundum atrial septal defect with the following qualifications: (1) symptoms begin earlier and are more pronounced; (2) cyanosis occurs with *increased* pulmonary arterial blood flow and with insufficient pulmonary hypertension to account for its presence; (3) the P wave axis indicates that the sinus node is absent, and the atrial pacemaker is ectopic because of the deficiency in the superior vena caval sinus venosus location; (4) the QRS exhibits the left axis deviation and counterclockwise depolarization of an atrioventricular septal defect; and (5) echocardiography identifies absence of the atrial septum, a common atrioventricular valve, or a cleft anterior mitral leaflet.

TOTAL ANOMALOUS PULMONARY VENOUS CONNECTION

In 1798, the *Philosophical Transactions of the Royal Society of London* published "A description of a very unusual formation of the human heart."[197] A 1942 review of 100 cases of anomalous pulmonary venous connections

included 35 examples that were *total*, a term that applies when all four pulmonary veins connect anomalously to a systemic venous tributary of the right atrium or to the right atrium proper but have no connection to the left atrium.[198] The malformation is isolated in approximately two thirds of patients so afflicted,[199,200] occurs in approximately four to six per 100,000 live births,[57] and accounts for about 2% of deaths from congenital heart disease in the first year of life. Total anomalous pulmonary venous connection with atrial isomerism is dealt with in Chapter 3.

Classifications take into account three features: (1) the pathway by which pulmonary venous blood reaches the right atrium; (2) the presence or absence of obstruction along the course of the pathway; and (3) the nature of the interatrial communication. The most widely used clinical classification recognizes *supradiaphragmatic* connections with or without obstruction and *infradiaphragmatic* or *infracardiac* connections that are always obstructed.[31,199]

Supradiaphragmatic varieties constitute more than three quarters of cases.[199,200] Except for mixed connections and connections of all four pulmonary veins directly to the right atrium, all varieties of total anomalous pulmonary venous connections incorporate a *venous confluence* that receives the four pulmonary veins (Figures 15-62 through 15-65). In the *supradiaphragmatic* varieties, the confluence joins the coronary sinus (see Figures 15-63 and 15-64) or a left vertical vein that ascends to join an innominate bridge to the right superior vena cava and right atrium (Figures 15-62, 15-65, and 15-66). Obstruction of the vertical vein is caused by a *hemodynamic vise* formed posteriorly by the left bronchus and anteriorly by the pulmonary trunk (Figures 15-65 and 15-67B).[199] Less commonly, the vertical vein is intrinsically obstructed.[201,202] When the coronary sinus

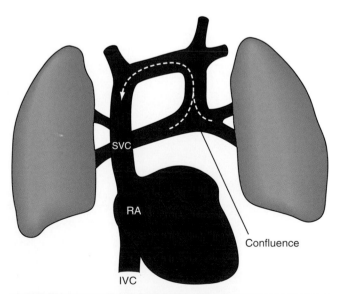

FIGURE 15-62 Illustration of total anomalous pulmonary venous connection. Blood from the confluence reaches the right atrium (RA) through an anomalous left vertical vein, an innominate bridge, and a right superior vena cava (SVC; dashed arrow). (IVC = inferior vena cava.)

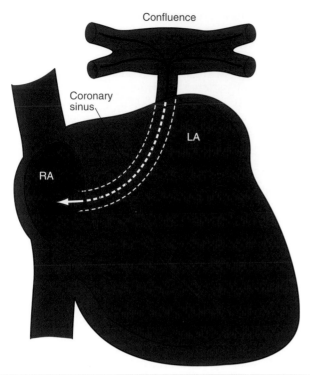

FIGURE 15-63 Illustration of total anomalous pulmonary venous connection in which the venous confluence joined the coronary sinus. (RA = right atrium; LA = left atrium.)

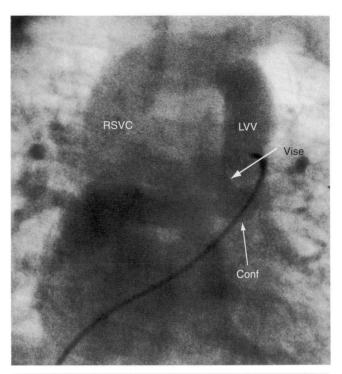

FIGURE 15-65 Levophase after injection of contrast material into the pulmonary trunk of a 3-month-old female with total anomalous pulmonary venous connection and obstruction of a left vertical vein (LVV) by a *hemodynamic vise* that consisted of the dilated anterior pulmonary trunk and the posterior left bronchus (compare with Figure 15-67B). (Conf = confluence; RSVC = right superior vena cava.)

receives the venous confluence (see Figures 15-63 and 15-64), obstruction results from stenosis of the right atrial ostium of the sinus.[201–203] Rarely, the superior vena cava is obstructed at its junction with the right atrium. Uncommon connections include a venous confluence to the right superior vena cava via a right-sided anomalous venous channel (Figure 15-68) or via the azygos venous system (Figure 15-69).

Subdiaphragmatic or *infracardiac* total anomalous pulmonary venous connection refers to a venous

confluence from which a vascular channel originates and descends anterior to the esophagous, penetrates the esophageal hiatus, and terminates in the portal vein, or less commonly in the inferior vena cava or ductus venosus (Figures 15-67A and 15-70).[31,199,200] Obstruction is almost invariable, and is certain when the connection is to

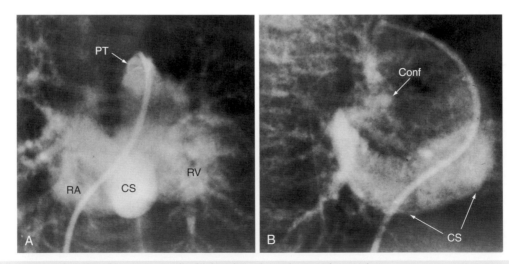

FIGURE 15-64 Angiocardiograms from a 2-month-old female with total anomalous pulmonary venous connection to the coronary sinus. **A,** Levophase after injection of contrast material into the pulmonary trunk (PT). A dilated coronary sinus (CS) is visualized, from which contrast enters the right atrium (RA) and right ventricle (RV). **B,** Lateral projection shows the confluence of pulmonary veins (Conf) entering a strikingly dilated coronary sinus (CS).

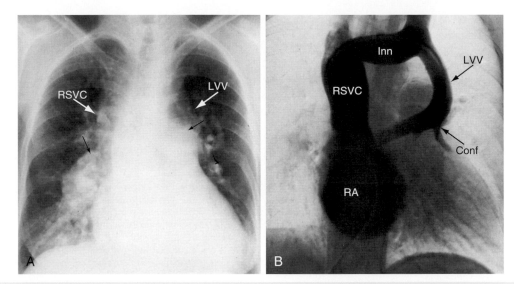

FIGURE 15-66 A, X-ray from a 54-year-old cyanotic woman with total anomalous pulmonary venous connection. The confluence of four pulmonary veins gave rise to a left vertical vein (LVV) that joined an innominate bridge and a right superior vena cava (RSVC). Pulmonary vascular resistance was suprasystemic. The pulmonary trunk and right branch are dilated and contain calcium (small black arrows). **B,** Levophase after injection of contrast material into the pulmonary trunk showing the confluence (Conf), the left vertical vein (LVV), the innominate bridge (Inn), the right superior vena cava (RSVC), and the right atrium (RA).

the portal vein, because blood confronts resistance in the capillary bed of the liver. Alternatively, the descending venous channel is intrinsically obstructed or is compressed as it traverses the esophageal hiatus.[199]

An *interatrial communication* is the only exit from the right atrium and the only access to the left side of the heart. The communication varies from a restrictive patent foramen ovale to a nonrestrictive atrial septal defect.[199,200,202]

The *embryologic fault* responsible for total anomalous pulmonary venous connection is believed to be agenesis of the common pulmonary vein with persistence and enlargement of primitive communications between the pulmonary venous and the systemic venous beds.[199,204] The common pulmonary vein is a temporary outgrowth of the developing left atrium and joins the pulmonary

veins as they arise from lung buds. When the common pulmonary vein fails to develop, the pulmonary venous plexus of lung buds does not join the left atrium but instead communicates with systemic veins via anastomotic channels that represent persistence and enlargement of embryonic vascular channels.

In fetal life, the *physiologic consequences* of total anomalous pulmonary venous connection are negligible because the amount of blood flowing through the lungs and through the pulmonary veins is negligible. When the lungs expand at birth, an obligatory left-to-right shunt is established because pulmonary venous flow is necessarily into the right atrium where it mixes with systemic venous return. Part of this mixture enters the right ventricle, and part crosses the atrial septum to reach the left side of the heart.

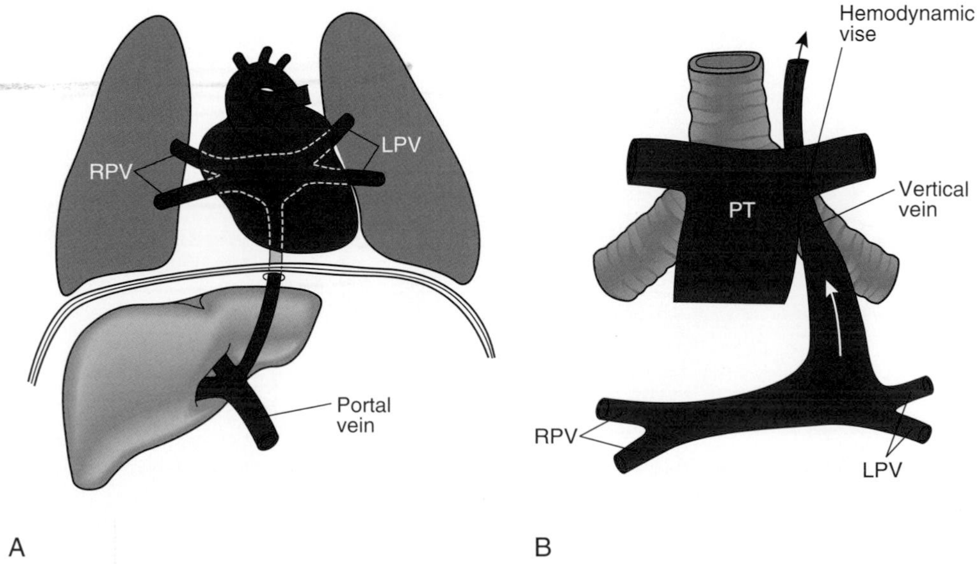

FIGURE 15-67 A, Illustration of the confluence of pulmonary veins giving rise to a vascular channel that enters the abdominal cavity through the diaphragmatic hiatus and terminates in the portal vein. (RPV and LPV = right and left pulmonary veins.) **B,** Illustration of the anomalous left vertical vein compressed in a *hemodynamic vise* consisting of the pulmonary trunk (PT) and the left bronchus.

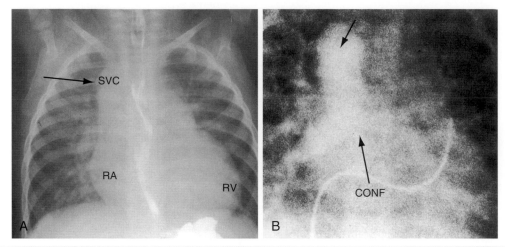

FIGURE 15-68 A, X-ray from a 10-month-old male with total anomalous pulmonary venous connection to a right vertical vein that joined a right superior vena cava (SVC). Arrow points to the shadow formed by the superimposed right vertical vein and superior vena cava. Pulmonary arterial vascularity is increased. The right atrium is prominent, and an enlarged right ventricle (RV) occupies the apex. **B,** Levophase after contrast injection into the pulmonary trunk. The right and left pulmonary veins form a confluence (CONF) that rises as a right-sided anomalous pulmonary venous channel (unmarked arrow) and joins the right superior vena cava. Compare with right SVC shadow in Figure 15-68A.

Once the pulmonary and systemic venous returns converge in the right atrium, the response of the circulation depends on the size of the interatrial communication and the behavior of the pulmonary vascular bed.[199,200] A *restrictive patent foramen ovale* represents an obstruction that results in an increase in right atrial and pulmonary venous pressure, pulmonary hypertension, and a decrease in flow to the left side of the heart. A *nonrestrictive atrial septal defect* provides free access to the left atrium, so the direction taken by right atrial blood becomes a function of the distensibility characteristics

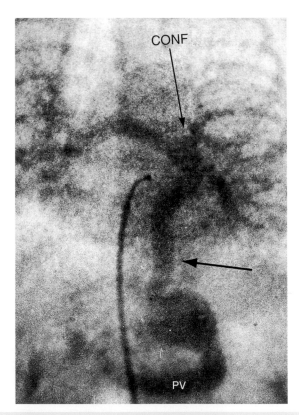

FIGURE 15-70 Levophase after injection of contrast material into the pulmonary trunk of a 4-day-old male with infradiaphragmatic total anomalous pulmonary venous connection. Right and left pulmonary veins form a confluence (CONF) that gives rise to a vascular channel (unmarked horizontal arrow) that enters the abdominal cavity through the diaphragmatic hiatus and terminates in the portal vein (PV). Compare with Figure 15-67A. Obstruction resided in the portal vein and hepatic bed rather than at the diaphragmatic hiatus, accounting for the subdiaphragmatic dilation.

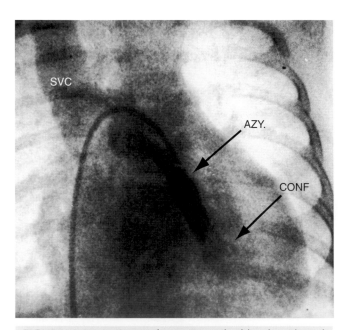

FIGURE 15-69 Angiogram from a 2-month-old male with total anomalous pulmonary venous connection to a confluence (CONF) that joined a prominent right superior vena cava (SVC) via the azygos vein (AZY.).

of the right and left ventricles. Low pulmonary vascular resistance is accompanied by a dilated compliant right ventricle that receives a large volume of blood from the right atrium and ejects the large volume into the pulmonary circulation. Systemic flow is generally maintained despite low left ventricular end-diastolic volume and ejection fraction and the small size of the left atrium and left ventricle. As pulmonary blood flow increases, pulmonary venous return to the right atrium increases, cyanosis is mild, and the systemic oxygen saturation is equal in the right atrium, right ventricle, pulmonary trunk, left atrium, and left ventricle. An increase in pulmonary vascular resistance induces right ventricular hypertrophy, so a smaller fraction of right atrial blood crosses the tricuspid valve into the hypertrophied low-compliant right ventricle. Pulmonary blood flow falls, and cyanosis increases. Elevated pulmonary vascular resistance occurs more frequently with total anomalous pulmonary venous connection than with an isolated nonrestrictive atrial septal defect and an equilavent shunt.[199,200]

Pulmonary venous obstruction, whether supradiaphragmatic or infradiaphragmatic, results in pulmonary hypertension, reduced pulmonary blood flow,[199,200] and a decrease in volume of pulmonary venous blood that reaches the right atrium. Cyanosis increases as oxygen saturation of the right atrial mixture falls. Intrapulmonary and extrapulmonary veins exhibit intimal proliferation, abnormally thick walls, and a reduction in size.[201] More malignant hemodynamic forces come into play when a left vertical venous channel is compressed between the pulmonary trunk and the left bronchus (see Figures 15-65 and 15-67B). A rise in pulmonary venous pressure provokes pulmonary hypertension and further dilation of the pulmonary trunk. The dilated hypertensive pulmonary trunk compresses the vertical venous channel still further, and the vicious cycle continues.

History

Gender ratio with supradiaphragmatic total anomalous pulmonary venous connections is about equal,[200] and infrahepatic connection to the portal vein strongly favors males.[200] These malformations have been reported in first cousins, siblings, and monozygotic and dizygotic twins and in a father and his two children.[200,205,206] Total anomalous pulmonary venous connection with Holt-Oram syndrome has been described in a family with a history of atrial septal defect.[143]

The clinical course is abbreviated even in the absence of pulmonary venous obstruction. Seventy-five percent to 90% of symptomatic infants do not reach their first birthday, and most are dead within 3 to 6 months.[199,200,207] Only 50% of patients who survive to age 3 months are alive at 1 year.[207] The malformation may not be suspected when pulmonary blood flow is increased in the presence of mild cyanosis. Before long, the infant becomes dyspneic and overtly cyanotic, with difficulty feeding and poor growth and development. Those who survive their first year almost always have supradiaphragmatic connections, low pulmonary vascular resistance, and a nonrestrictive atrial septal defect. A 10-year-old boy had an *unobstructed infradiaphragmatic* connection to the inferior vena cava,[208] and a 17-year-old had *obstructed infradiaphragmatic* connection to the hepatic vein. Exceptionally, patients reach their third, fourth, or fifth decade with relatively little disability and a clinical picture that resembles isolated ostium secundum atrial septal defect except for the mild cyanosis.[209,210] A cyanotic woman with suprasystemic pulmonary vascular resistance was 54 years (see Figure 15-66), and a 62-year-old woman came to necropsy.[211] The oldest reported patient underwent surgical repair at age 66 years.[209]

In total anomalous pulmonary venous connection *with obstruction*, lifespan is brief and the clinical course stormy. Tachypnea follows expansion of the lungs because neonatal pulmonary blood flow is obstructed (Figure 15-71).[199,200]

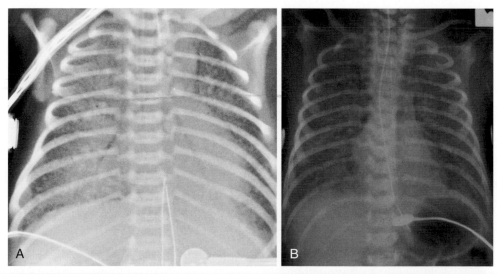

FIGURE 15-71 X-rays from two infants with total anomalous pulmonary venous connection and infradiaphragmatic obstruction. In both x-rays, the lungs show a striking stippled, reticular, ground glass appearance. **A,** Female infant with infradiagphragmatic obstruction. The transverse liver and symmetric bronchi represent right isomerism. **B,** Male neonate with total anomalous pulmonary venous connection and atresia of a left vertical vein distal to the venous confluence. The dramatic appearance of the lungs is in marked contrast to the unimpressive cardiac silhouette.

Cyanosis is conspicuous because only a small fraction of oxygenated pulmonary venous blood reaches the right atrium for mixing. When an infradiaphragmatic venous channel traverses the esophageal hiatus, feeding, crying, and straining induce additional compression that aggravates the dyspnea and increases the cyanosis. Death from pulmonary edema and right ventricular failure comes within days, weeks, or months after birth. Newborns with infradiaphragmatic connections and asplenia have major esophageal varices.[212]

Physical Appearance

In total anomalous pulmonary venous connection without obstruction, mild to moderate cyanosis occurs with *increased pulmonary blood flow*. Infants with congestive heart failure are catabolic.[200] However, a relatively asymptomatic 46-year-old man had been cyanotic since childhood, and a 39-year-old man was never overtly cyanotic. The Holt-Oram syndrome, Klippel-Feil syndrome,[200] and *cat-eye* syndrome sporadically coexist.[213–215]

Arterial Pulse and Jugular Venous Pulse

The arterial pulse is small because left ventricular stroke volume is reduced. When the interatrial communication is nonrestrictive, the jugular venous pulse resembles isolated ostium secundum atrial septal defect. At the inception of right ventricular failure, the right-to-left shunt increases and the jugular venous pressure remains relatively unchanged. Pulmonary hypertension with a restrictive interatrial communication results in a large even giant A wave.

Precordial Movement and Palpation

When the interatrial communication is nonrestrictive, precordial movement and palpation resemble nonrestrictive ostium secundum atrial septal defect, although these precordial signs begin earlier. A rise in pulmonary vascular resistance imposes afterload on the volume-loaded right ventricle, so its impulse becomes more striking (Figure 15-72).[200] A hyperdynamic right ventricle is not a feature in neonates and infants with pulmonary vein obstruction because pulmonary blood flow is reduced.

Auscultation

When the interatrial communication is nonrestrictive, auscultatory signs resemble an ostium secundum atrial septal defect . The tricuspid component of the first heart sound is loud, there is wide fixed splitting of the second heart sound (Figures 15-73 and 15-74), a pulmonary midsystolic murmur is generated by rapid ejection of a large right ventricular stroke volume into a dilated pulmonary trunk (see Figures 15-73 and 15-74), and a tricuspid diastolic flow murmur is common (see Figure 15-73).[200,216] The systolic murmur may have a wide thoracic distribution analogous to the peripheral pulmonary arterial murmurs with ostium secundum atrial septal

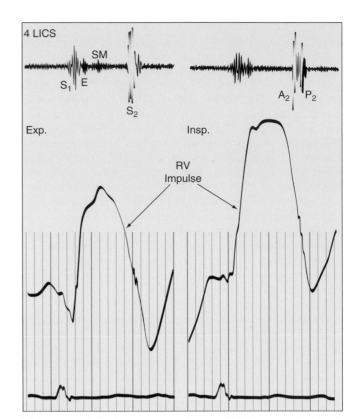

FIGURE 15-72 Tracings from a 13-year-old cyanotic girl with total anomalous pulmonary venous connection, systemic pulmonary arterial pressure, and a confluence of veins that joined the right superior vena cava. The right ventricular (RV) impulse is apparent. The second heart sound (S_2) splits normally during inspiration (Insp.). The prominent pulmonary component (P_2) and the pulmonary ejection sound (E) were transmitted to the fourth left intercostal space (4 LICS). The pulmonary systolic murmur (SM) is attenuated. (A_2 = aortic component of the second sound.)

defect and a hyperkinetic pulmonary circulation.[111] Pulmonary hypertension is accompanied by a pulmonary ejection sound, attenuation of the pulmonary systolic flow murmur, loss of the tricuspid diastolic murmur, inspiratory splitting of the second heart sound (see Figure 15-72),[200] and a high-frequency early diastolic Graham Steell murmur (Figure 15-75). An increased force of right atrial contraction generates a right ventricular fourth heart sound, and right ventricular failure is accompanied by a third heart sound and the holosystolic murmur of tricuspid regurgitation.[200]

A continuous murmur is a noteworthy although uncommon auscultatory sign that originates in continuous flow through the venous confluence, the left vertical vein, and left innominate vein (see Figure 15-62).[217] The continuous murmur has the quality of a soft venous hum and is maximal at the left upper sternal border. Less commonly, a continuous murmur is heard along the *right* upper sternal border where it is believed to originate from flow through a right-sided anomalous pulmonary venous channel into a right superior vena cava (see Figure 15-68).

In infants with pulmonary venous obstruction, auscultatory signs are determined by pulmonary hypertension

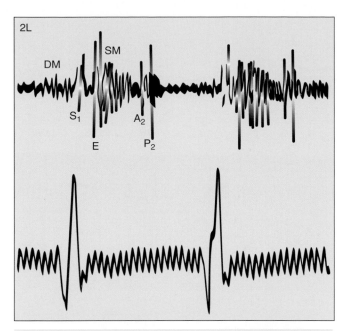

FIGURE 15-73 Phonocardiogram from a 9-month-old male with total anomalous pulmonary venous connection in which the four pulmonary veins joined the right atrium directly. A restrictive foramen ovale constituted a zone of pulmonary venous obstruction. The first heart sound (S_1) is preceded by a tricuspid diastolic flow murmur (DM) and followed by a pulmonary ejection sound (E) that introduced a prominent midsystolic flow murmur (SM). There is wide fixed splitting of the second heart sound. (A_2 = aortic component; P_2 = pulmonary component.)

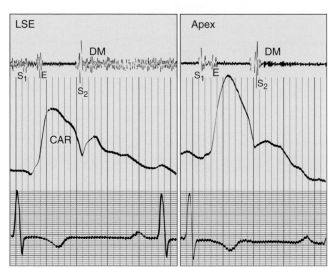

FIGURE 15-75 Tracing from a moderately cyanotic 26-year-old man with total anomalous pulmonary venous connection to the right superior vena cava. Pulmonary artery systolic pressure was 87 mm Hg, and the brachial arterial systolic pressure was 106 mm Hg. Phonocardiogram at the lower left sternal edge (LSE) shows a pulmonary ejection sound (E) and a Graham Steell murmur (DM) issuing from a loud single second heart sound (S_2). The ejection sound and diastolic murmur radiated to the apex because the apex was occupied by the right ventricle. (CAR = carotid pulse.)

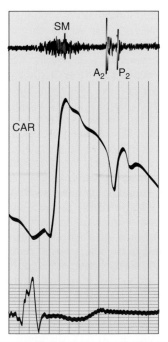

FIGURE 15-74 Tracings from a 9-year-old boy with total anomalous pulmonary venous connection and low pulmonary vascular resistance. A prominent pulmonary systolic flow murmur (SM) ends before both components of a widely split second heart sound. (A_2, P_2 = aortic and pulmonary components; CAR = carotid pulse.)

rather than increased pulmonary blood flow. More than half of these patients have no pulmonary systolic murmur at all because flow across the pulmonary valve is reduced, but an attenuated midsystolic murmur is generated by ejection into the dilated hypertensive pulmonary trunk. The second sound is single or closely split, and the pulmonary component is loud. A high frequency holosystolic murmur of tricuspid regurgitation accompanies pulmonary hypertensive right ventricular failure.

Electrocardiogram

When the interatrial communication is nonrestrictive, the electrocardiogram resembles an ostium secundum atrial septal defect (Figure 15-76). The PR interval tends to be prolonged (see Figure 15-76). Atrial fibrillation occurs in older patients as it does with ostium secundum atrial septal defect. In the presence of pulmonary hypertension, the electrocardiogram exhibits peaked right atrial P waves, right axis deviation, tall right precordial R waves, inverted T waves, and deep left precordial S waves of right ventricular hypertrophy (Figures 15-77 through 15-79).[200]

X-Ray

Cardiac enlargement begins within weeks of birth. Dilation of the right ventricular outflow tract sometimes obscures an enlarged pulmonary trunk (Figure 15-80). When the interatrial communication is nonrestrictive, the x-ray resembles an ostium secundum atrial septal

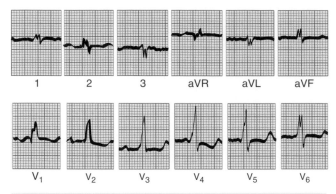

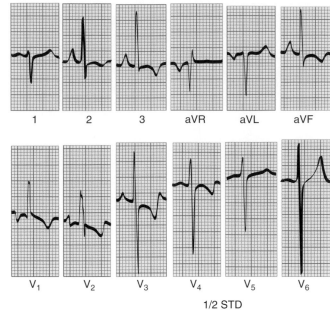

FIGURE 15-76 Electrocardiogram from a 49-year-old man with total anomalous pulmonary venous connection to a left vertical vein, a nonrestrictive ostium secundum atrial septal defect with a 2.5 to 1 shunt, and pulmonary artery pressure of 50/20 mm Hg. The PR interval is prolonged. The right ventricular conduction defect resembles the conduction defect in an adult with an ostium secundum atrial septal defect, but the right precordial R waves are more prominent.

1/2 STD

FIGURE 15-78 Electrocardiogram from a 26-year-old man with total anomalous pulmonary venous connection to the right superior vena cava. Pulmonary artery systolic pressure was 87 mm Hg. Tall peaked right atrial P waves appear in leads 2, 3, and aVF. There is right axis deviation and right ventricular hypertrophy reflected in tall right precordial R waves, deeply inverted T waves, and deep left precordial S waves (half standardized).

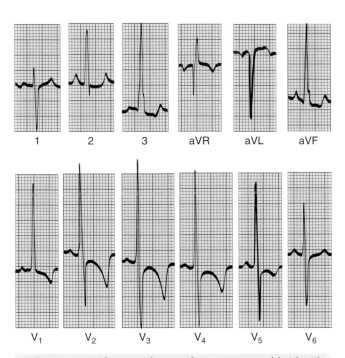

FIGURE 15-77 Electrocardiogram from a 13-year-old girl with total anomalous pulmonary venous connection to the right superior vena cava and systemic pulmonary artery pressure. Peaked right atrial P waves appear in leads 2 and aVF. Right ventricular hypertrophy is accompanied by right axis deviation, tall monophasic R waves, and deeply inverted T waves in leads V$_{1-4}$ and the deep S wave in lead V$_6$.

defect with increased pulmonary blood flow, an enlarged pulmonary trunk and proximal branches, an inconspicuous ascending aorta, a large right atrium, and a large right ventricle (Figure 15-81).

Specific sites of anomalous pulmonary venous connections can be radiologically distinctive.[218] Prominence of the right upper cardiac border represents a right superior vena cava that receives the confluence of pulmonary veins

via a right-sided anomalous venous channel (see Figures 15-67 and 15-80) or via the azygos vein (see Figure 15-69).[200] The coronary sinus dilates when it receives the confluence (see Figure 15-64), and may indent the esophagus. The most distinctive configuration is the *figure-of-eight* or *snowman silhouette* (Figures 15-66 and 15-82A, B).[200,216] The upper portion of the figure is formed by the left vertical vein and the right superior vena cava. The lower portion is formed by the dilated right atrium and right ventricle. The snowman appearance does not reveal itself during the first few months of life because enough time must elapse before the connecting venous channels develop sufficient size and radiodensity to be visible in the x-ray.[200,219]

Rarely, the communicating venous channel is formed within the substance of the lung rather than in the mediastinum and bears a superficial resemblance to the *scimitar sign* of partial anomalous pulmonary venous connection (see previous). However, agenesis of the right lung is rare with total anomalous pulmonary venous connection.[220]

Total anomalous pulmonary venous connection with obstruction results in a very different radiologic picture.[200] Pulmonary edema is striking. The pulmonary veins and lymphatics are distended, and the lung fields exhibit a reticular nodular ground glass appearance (see Figure 15-71)[200,221] and stand out in contrast to the comparatively unimpressive cardiac silhouette (see Figure 15-71B).[200,219]

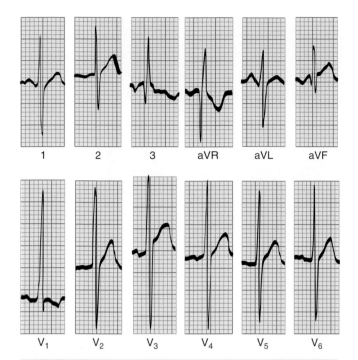

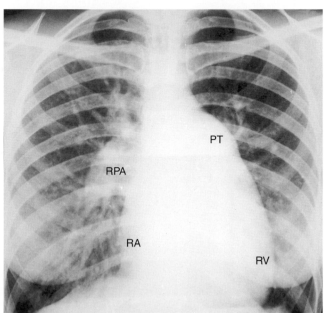

FIGURE 15-79 Electrocardiogram from a 9-month-old male with total anomalous pulmonary venous connection of all four pulmonary veins directly into the right atrium. A restrictive foramen ovale caused pulmonary venous obstruction and severe pulmonary hypertension that promptly decreased after balloon atrial septostomy. The leftward and superior axis of the P wave indicates an ectopic atrial pacemaker. The QRS axis is vertical. Right ventricular hypertrophy is reflected in the tall monophasic R waves in right precordial leads and the deep S waves in left precordial leads.

FIGURE 15-81 X-ray from a mildly cyanotic 21-year-old woman with total anomalous pulmonary venous connection to the coronary sinus. The x-ray resembles an ostium secundum atrial septal defect with increased pulmonary arterial blood flow, dilation of the pulmonary trunk (PT) and right pulmonary atery (RPA), an inconspicuous ascending aorta, and a dilated right ventricle (RV) and right atrium (RA).

Echocardiogram

Echocardiography with color flow imaging and Doppler interrogation locates the four pulmonary veins and their sites of drainage, identifies the venous confluence and its connections, determines whether obstruction is present in the pulmonary venous pathways, and identifies the location and size of the interatrial communication and the physiologic consequences of the malformation (Figures 15-82C, D and 15-83).[32] Color flow imaging establishes the direction and mean velocity of blood flow within the venous channels and permits assessment of the connections of individual pulmonary veins and of the venous confluence (see Figure 15-82D).[32] Doppler interrogation with color flow imaging identifies increased

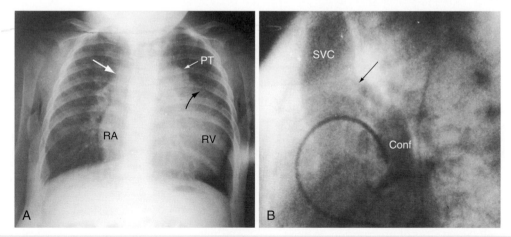

FIGURE 15-80 A, X-ray from a mildly cyanotic 5-month-old female with total anomalous pulmonary venous connection to a right superior vena cava that formed a prominent shadow at the right thoracic inlet (large white arrow). Pulmonary vascularity is increased. A dilated pulmonary trunk (PT) is obscured by the enlarged outflow tract (curved black arrow) of a dilated right ventricle (RV). (RA = right atrium.) **B,** Levophase of a pulmonary arteriogram showing the connection (arrow) of the confluence (Conf) to the right superior vena cava (SVC).

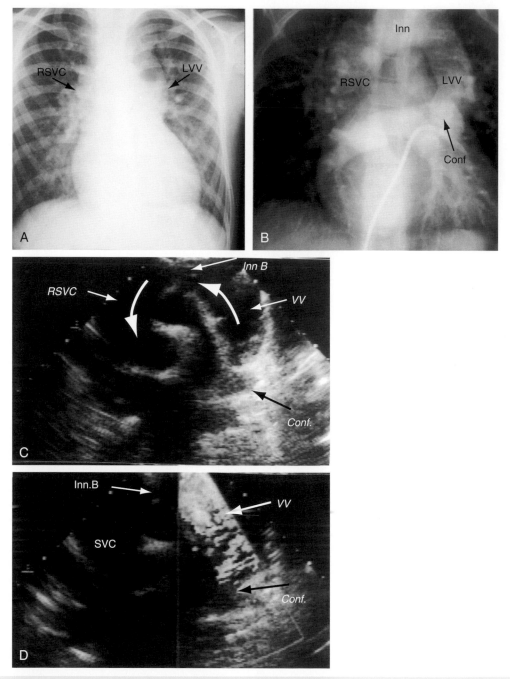

FIGURE 15-82 A, X-ray from a 6-year-old mildly cyanotic boy with total anomalous pulmonary venous connection. Pulmonary arterial vascularity is markedly increased. The cardiac silhouette has a *figure of eight* or *snowman* appearance. **B,** Levophase after injection of contrast material into the pulmonary trunk. Blood from the confluence of pulmonary veins (Conf) flows sequentially through a dilated left vertical vein (LVV), an innominate bridge (Inn), and a dilated right superior vena cava (RSVC), establishing the upper portion of the figure of eight. The lower portion of the figure of eight consisted of the dilated right atrium and the dilated right ventricle. **C,** Echocardiogram from a 12-year-old girl with total anomalous pulmonary venous connection. The four pulmonary veins form a confluence (Conf.) from which a dilated left vertical vein arises (VV, upward curved arrow) and continues as an innominate bridge (Inn B) that joins a dilated right superior vena cava (RSVC, downward curved arrow). **D,** Black-and-white print of a color flow image showing unobstructed flow from the confluence into the vertical vein (VV).

turbulence and velocity at sites of obstruction. When the venous connection is to the coronary sinus, all four pulmonary veins enter a confluence behind the left atrium (see Figures 15-64 and 15-83). Color flow imaging identifies a confluence that joins a left vertical vein and an innominate bridge (see Figure 15-82C, D), and a confluence that joins a right vertical vein and right superior vena cava.[32]

When all four pulmonary veins connect directly to the right atrium, a restrictive interatrial communication causes obstruction to pulmonary venous flow.[32] With infradiaphragmatic connections, color flow imaging and

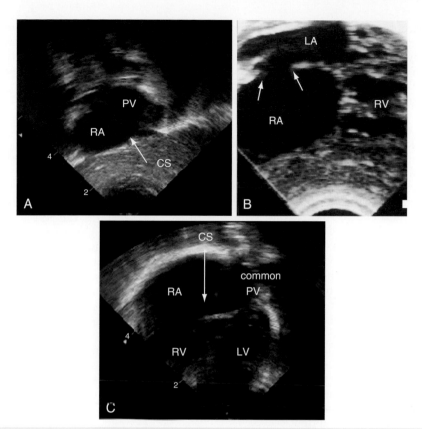

FIGURE 15-83 Echocardiograms (subcostal) from a 5-month-old female with total anomalous pulmonary venous connection to the coronary sinus. **A,** Posterior angulation of the transducer visualized the common pulmonary vein (PV) and coronary sinus (CS). **B,** A change in transducer angulation can help visualize a large ostium secundum atrial septal defect (paired arrows) and a dilated right atrium (RA). (LA = left atrium; RV= right ventricle.) **C,** Four-chamber subcostal views show the anatomy of the anomalous pulmonary venous connection to the coronary sinus without color.

Doppler interrogation identify the inferior vena cava and the anomalous venous channel adjacent to the aorta and determine whether there is a localized site of obstruction as the anomalous channel descends below the diaphragm (Figure 15-84 and Video 15-5).[32] Flow is pulsatile in the aorta but continuous in the anomalous venous channel.

Summary

A large left-to-right shunt is established shortly after birth when total anomalous pulmonary venous connection is accompanied by a nonrestrictive atrial septal defect, low pulmonary vascular resistance, and no obstruction. Dyspnea, cardiac failure, and physical underdevelopment begin shortly thereafter. Most infants do not reach their first birthday. The subsequent clinical picture resembles a nonrestrictive ostium secundum atrial septal defect with the notable exception of mild to moderate cyanosis. Gender distribution is approximately equal in contrast to female preponderence in secundum atrial septal defects. The right ventricular impulse is hyperdynamic. There is a prominent pulmonary midsystolic murmur, fixed splitting of the second heart sound with a loud pulmonary component, and a tricuspid diastolic flow murmur. A soft humlike continuous

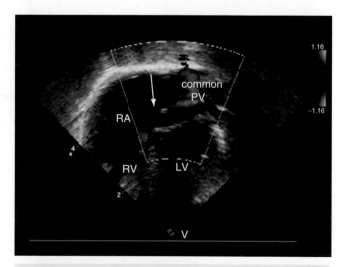

FIGURE 15-84 Color flow Doppler shows flow through the coronary pulmonary vein (Video 15-5).

murmur is occasionally heard along the upper left sternal border when a mildly compressed left vertical vein connects the venous confluence to the left innominate vein. The electrocardiogram shows right atrial P waves and right ventricular hypertrophy or may resemble an ostium secundum atrial septal defect. After the first few months of life, distinctive x-ray features emerge from shadows caused by anomalous venous connections. A prominent shadow at the right base represents the confluence of veins that joins the right superior vena cava via an anomalous right venous channel or via an azygos vein. The figure of eight or snowman appearance is caused by dilation of the left vertical vein and right superior vena cava above and by dilation of the right atrium and right ventricle below.

Total anomalous pulmonary venous connection with obstruction predominates in males, especially when an infradiaphragmatic connection joins the portal vein. Lifespan is short and the clinical course stormy, with symptoms beginning at or shortly after birth. Death from pulmonary edema, congestive heart failure, and hypoxia follows within weeks. Dyspnea and cyanosis are aggravated by crying, feeding, or straining because the anomalous venous channel is further compressed at the esophageal hiatus. Cyanosis is conspicuous, the right ventricular impulse is relatively quiet, the pulmonary midsystolic murmur is attenuated or absent, and the second heart sound is closely split with a loud pulmonary component. The electrocardiogram shows right atrial P waves and right ventricular hypertrophy. The x-ray exhibits dramatic pulmonary venous congestion with a reticulated ground glass appearance in contrast to the unimpressive size of the cardiac silhouette.

Echocardiography with color flow imaging and Doppler interrogation locates the four pulmonary veins, identifies the venous confluence and its connections, determines whether there is obstruction in the pulmonary venous pathway, and establishes the location and size of the interatrial communication and the physiologic consequences of supradiaphragmatic or infradiaphragmatic total anomalous pulmonary venous connection.

ATRIOVENTRICULAR SEPTAL DEFECTS

In the normal heart, the *atrioventricular septum* is a partition that separates the left ventricular outflow tract from the facing right atrium. The malformations discussed here are characterized by complete absence of the atrioventricular septum and are therefore called *atrioventricular septal defects*.[106,222–224] Additional features include a common atrioventricular ring, a five-leaflet valve that guards the common atrioventricular orifice, an unwedged left ventricular outflow tract, an aortic valve that is anterosuperior to the common atrioventricular junction, and a left ventricular mass characterized by a longer distance from apex to aortic valve than from apex to the left atrioventricular valve.

Different types of atrioventricular septal defects result from morphologic variations in the five-leaflet valve that guards the common atrioventricular orifice and from the relationship of the bridging leaflets to contiguous septal structures (Figures 15-85 and 15-86). The two normal

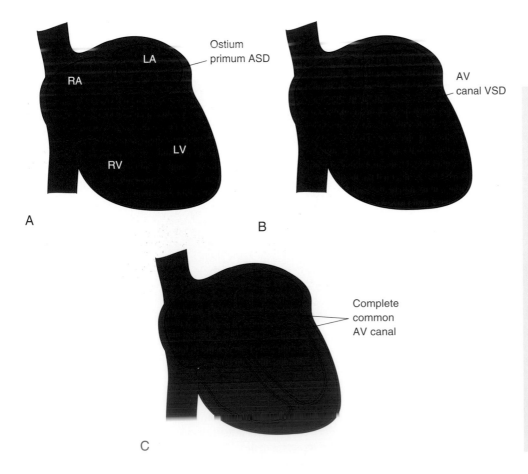

FIGURE 15-85 Schematic illustrations of the shunt levels in atrioventricular septal defects: **A,** The interatrial communication is between the inferior atrial septum and the bridging leaflets, **B,** The interventricular communication is between the bridging leaflets and crest of the ventricular septum. **C,** Interatrial *and* interventricular communications are above and below a freefloating atrioventricular valve (complete common AV canal). (RA = right atrium; LA = left atrium; RV = right ventricle; LV = left ventricle ASD = atrial septal defect; VSD = ventricular septal defect; AV = atrioventricular canal.) *(Modified from Anderson RH, Becker AE, Lucchese FE, Meier MA, Rigby ML, Soto B. Morphology of congenital heart disease. Baltimore: University Park Press; 1983.)*

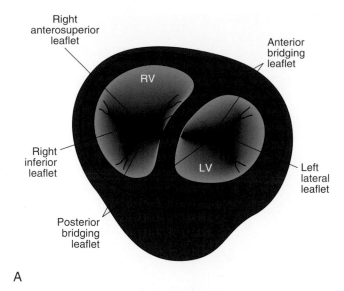

A

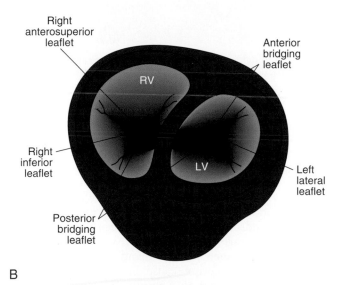

B

FIGURE 15-86 **A,** Illustration of the leaflet patterns in an atrioventricular septal defect with separate right and left atrioventricular orifices. Anterior and posterior bridging leaflets are connected by leaflet tissue that runs in the ventricular septum, an arrangement that results in a *cleft anterior mitral leaflet.* The cleft is more accurately characterized as a functional commissure between the anterior and posterior bridging leaflets. **B,** Illustration of the leaflet patterns in a complete atrioventricular septal defect (complete common atrioventricular canal). The common valve consists of anterior and posterior bridging leaflets that cross the septum, a small left lateral mural leaflet that is housed exclusively in the left ventricle, and small right inferior mural and anterosuperior leaflets that are housed exclusively in the right ventricle. *(Modified from Anderson RH, Becker AE, Lucchese FE, Meier MA, Rigby ML, Soto B. Morphology of congenital heart disease. Baltimore: University Park Press; 1983.)*

atrioventricular valves have *two separate* fibrous rings (annuli) that lie at *different levels* in the ventricular mass. In atrioventricular septal defects, a five-leaflet atrioventricular valve has a *single fibrous ring* (annulus) that lies at one horizontal level in the ventricular mass.[222,223] The five-leaflet valve guards either a common

atrioventricular orifice or separate right and left atrioventricular orifices (see Figure 15-86). A left lateral leaflet is housed exclusively in the left ventricle, and a right inferior leaflet and a right anterosuperior leaflet are housed exclusively in the right ventricle (see Figure 15-86). The other two leaflets are designated anterior and posterior bridging leaflets and have no counterpart in the normal heart.

A common atrioventricular orifice lies within a common atrioventricular annulus when the anterior and posterior bridging leaflets are not divided by connecting leaflet tissue that runs in the ventricular septum (see Figure 15-86B). When the anterior and posterior bridging leaflets are divided by connecting leaflet tissue in the ventricular septum, left and right atrioventricular orifices lie within a common atrioventricular annulus (see Figure 15-86A). What has been called a cleft in the anterior mitral leaflet (Figure 15-87) is in fact a commissure between the left anterior and left posterior bridging leaflets (see Figure 15-86A), the margins of which are supported by chordae tendineae that attach to the ventricular septum, an arrangement that is not represented in normal hearts.[225] The relationship of bridging leaflets to adjacent ventricular septum and to the atrial septum determines the level of shunting through the atrioventricular septal defect (see Figure 15-85). When the bridging leaflets adhere to the crest of the ventricular septum, the shunt is at atrial level (see Figure 15-85A).

The term *ostium primum* atrial septal defect does not accurately characterize this interatrial communication, which is not a defect in the atrial septum but instead is *absence* of the atrioventricular septum (see Figure 85A). When the bridging leaflets are attached to the distal end of the atrial septum, the shunt is at ventricular level (see Figure 15-85B). When the bridging leaflets are free floating and unattached to either atrial or ventricular septum, shunts occur at both atrial and ventricular levels, an arrangement called *complete common atrioventricular canal* (see Figure 15-85C).

The unwedged position of the elongated left ventricular outflow tract together with the anterosuperior position of the aortic valve and the apical position of the deficient inlet septum results in a *gooseneck deformity* (Figures 15-88 and 15-89B). The left ventricular outflow tract is then an elongated anteriorly displaced fibromuscular channel that can develop subaortic obstruction caused by an immobile ridge at the crest of the ventricular septum; by accessory chordal tissue arising from the left anterior atrioventricular valve leaflet, which is fixed to the ventricular septum, or accessory papillary muscle tissue; or by abnormally high insertion of the anterolateral papillary muscle or thickened tissue along the outflow septum and anterior left atrioventricular leaflet.[226–228] The papillary muscles lie in an abnormal fore-aft arrangement that can result in a parachute valve or a double-orifice valve that reinforces left-to-right interatrial shunts.[227,229,230] Left ventricular outflow obstruction augments the left-to-right shunts and augments regurgitation across the left atrioventricular valve.[226,231]

A common atrioventricular annulus is usually shared equally by the right and left ventricles, but either the right-sided or the left-sided component of the annulus

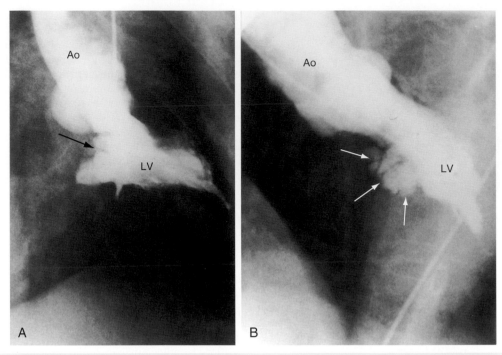

FIGURE 15-87 Left ventriculograms from a 71-year-old woman with a large left-to-right shunt through an ostium primum atrial septal defect. **A,** The left ventriculogram identifies a *cleft in the anterior mitral leaflet* (arrow) that represents the functional commissure between the anterior and posterior bridging leaflets. (Ao = aorta; LV= left ventricle.) **B,** Long-axial view showing saccular herniation of atrioventricular valve tissue into the right ventricular inflow tract (arrows), effectively closing an inlet ventricular septal defect.

can be reduced in size. When the *right-sided* component is small, the right ventricle is hypoplastic, the tricuspid orifice overrides a malaligned inlet ventricular septum, and the right atrioventricular valve has attachments that straddle the ventricular septal defect.[232] When the *left-sided* component is small, the morphologic left ventricle is hypoplastic, but straddling does not occur despite atrioventricular malalignment because straddling is reserved for conoventricular malalignment.[144]

The *physiologic consequences* of an ostium primum atrial septal defect depend on its size and on the functional state of the left atrioventricular valve.[142,233] When the defect is nonrestrictive, the left atrium decompresses as it receives regurgitant flow from the left ventricle. When the atrial septal defect is restrictive, the clinical picture resembles isolated mitral regurgitation.[142,234] A nonrestrictive ventricular septal defect sets the stage for pulmonary vascular disease (see Chapter 17).[235] The physiologic consequences of a complete atrioventricular septal defect are the sum of the nonrestrictive interatrial and interventricular communications and the degree of incompetence of the left and right components of the common atrioventricular valve (see Figures 15-88A and 15-89).

Down syndrome (see section Physical Appearance) is an important independent variable in the propensity for pulmonary vascular disease and does not depend on the size of the ventricular septal defect but is coupled with Down syndrome as an independent variable.[236,237] The proclivity for pulmonary vascular disease in Down syndrome has been explained by morphometric studies that disclose a 35% reduction in the number of alveoli and a reduction in the radial alveolar count, which is an index of alveolar complexity.[238,239] The reduced internal surface area of the lungs implies a comparable reduction in cross-sectional area of the pulmonary vascular bed because the capillary surface area and the alveolar surface area are closely coupled.

Hypoventilation induced by upper airway abnormalities is an additional cause of pulmonary vascular disease in Down syndrome. The midfacial region is small with short nasal passages, small oropharynx, small oral cavity, large tonsils and anenoids, and mandibular and maxillary hypoplasia. Still another cause of pulmonary vascular disease is sleep apnea that results from retrodisplacement of an engorged tongue (Figure 15-90A) and from inspiratory collapse of the hypopharynx because of tracheomalacia.[236–238]

History

The male:female ratio in atrioventricular septal defects is approximately equal. An increased prevalence of trisomy 21 has been reported in offspring of older gravida, but the father has also been incriminated as a source of the extra chromosome 21.[240] The incidence rate of congenital heart disease in the children of females with atrioventricular septal defects has been estimated at 9.6% to 14.3%.[241] Families may have several affected members.[242,243]

Infants with complete atrioventricular septal defects have development of congestive heart failure with fetal hydrops in the first 6 months of life (see Figure 15-90).[244] In nonrestrictive ostium primum atrial septal defects, the chief determinant of symptoms is left AV valve regurgitation, which when severe, results in

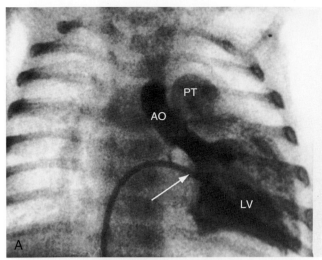

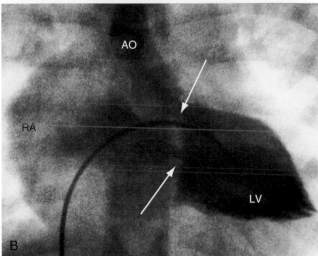

FIGURE 15-88 **A,** Left ventriculogram from an 8-week-old female with a complete atrioventricular septal defect and a virtually competent common atrioventricular valve. Arrow points to the gooseneck deformity of the left ventricular outflow tract. A dilated pulmonary trunk (PT) visualized via the ventricular septal defect. **B,** Left ventriculogram from a 3-year-old girl with a nonrestrictive ostium primum atrial septal defect and left atrioventricular valve regurgitation. A narrow jet (lower arrow) is received by a large right atrium (RA). The gooseneck deformity shown here (upper arrow) was better delineated during diastole. (AO = aorta; LV= left ventricle.)

congestive heart failure[182] and a mortality rate of 33% in the first year.[245] When the left ventricle is hypoplastic, neonatal congestive heart failure is intractable.[231] Long survival is exceptional, although one patient lived to age 46 years[245] and another to age 73 years.[246] Adult survival is expected when a nonrestrictive ostium primum atrial septal defect is associated with a competent left atrioventricular valve.

Twelve percent of patients reach or exceed age 60 years, but those beyond age 45 years are symptomatic. The oldest reported patient was 79 years old,[245] and the patient cited in Figure 15-87 underwent cardiac surgery at age 71 years. Symptomatic deterioration is accelerated by atrial fibrillation or atrial flutter. When a ventricular

septal defect is the only component of an atrioventricular septal defect, the history resembles other forms of isolated ventricular septal defect of equivalent size (see Chapter 17).

Isolated left atrioventricular valve regurgitation generates a murmur that is understandably mistaken for acquired mitral regurgitation. Detection at an early age should arouse suspicion and prevent error. The risk of infective endocarditis coincides with regurgitation rather than with the abnormal structure of a functionally competent valve. Infective endocarditis is rare with complete atrioventricular septal defects.

Paradoxical emboli are rare with ostium primum atrial septal defects because emboli that originate in the *lower extremities* are carried by inferior vena caval blood toward the *mid portion,* not the lower portion of the atrial septum. Superior vena caval streaming targets the lower atrial septum, but emboli rarely originate in the upper extremities.

Spontaneous closure of the ventricular component of an atrioventricular septal defect is uncommon[247,248] and has been attributed to occlusion by tricuspid leaflet tissue derived from the bridging leaflets.[247] This mechanism is believed to have been operative in the 71-year-old woman whose left ventriculogram is shown in Figure 15-87B.

Life expectancy for patients with Down syndrome *without* congenital heart disease is significantly shorter than for comparable patients with mental retardation, implying an adverse effect on life expectancy that is unrelated either to congenital heart disease or mental retardation.[249,250] Morbidity and mortality are adversely effected by respiratory tract infections; congenital anomalies of the gastrointestinal tract; increased risk of hepatitis B virus; hematologic, endocrinologic, and immunologic disorders; and premature Alzheimer's disease.[238] Unique hematologic disorders include transient infantile myelodysplasia, red cell macrocytosis, and increased susceptibility to acute megakaryocytic leukemia.[238]

The gene for amyloid protein in Alzheimer's disease has been cloned and localized to chromosome 21 proximal to the locus that delineates Down syndrome.[238,251,252] Virtually all patients with Down syndrome over age 35 years have the characteristic central nervous system neuropathology and neurochemistry of Alzheimer's syndrome.[251–253] Brain weights are lower in patients with Down syndrome than in patients with senile Alzheimer's disease, with differences most striking in the anterior frontal and anterior temporal regions. Families with autosomal dominant Alzheimer's disease produce a significantly high number of offspring with Down syndrome. Clinical dementia is uncommon, however, and must be distinguished from symptomatic hypothyroidism.[238] An association between autoimmune thyroid dysfunction and Down syndrome is widely recognized.[254]

Physical Appearance

Down syndrome phenotype is the most distinctive appearance associated with an atrioventricular septal defect.[237,255] In 1866, Down[256] wrote, "The face is flat

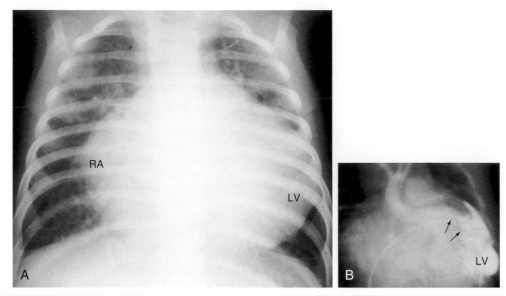

FIGURE 15-89 A, X-ray of a 3-month-old male with a complete atrioventricular septal defect. Pulmonary vascularity is increased. The dramatic increase in heart size reflects enlargement of the right atrium (RA) and right ventricle (RV). **B,** Left ventriculogram visualized the gooseneck deformity (paired arrows) of the outflow tract. (Ao = aorta; LV= left ventricle.)

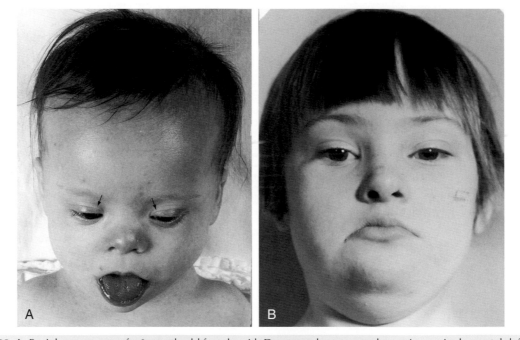

FIGURE 15-90 A, Facial appearance of a 6-month-old female with Down syndrome, complete atrioventricular septal defect, and a bidirectional shunt. The short flat nose is cyanotic, and the nasal bridge is depressed. The tongue is large and protuberant. Two small arrows point to oblique palpebral fissures. **B,** Nine-year-old female with Down syndrome. The corners of the mouth turn downward, creating an expression of sadness. The nose is short and flat with a depressed nasal bridge. The inner epicanthic fold is subtle.

and broad and destitute of prominence. The cheeks are round and extended laterally. The eyes are obliquely placed, and the internal canthi more than normally distant from one another. The palpebral fissure is very narrow. The lips are large and thick with transverse fissures. The tongue is long, thick, and is much roughened. The nose is small." The incidence rate of trisomy 21 in the general population is approximately 1:800 live births, although the frequency is twice as great if based on *all* conceptuses because more than half of trisomy 21 fetuses are spontaneously aborted.[237] The association of congenital heart disease with Down syndrome was recognized in 1894 by Garrod[257] and confirmed by Maude Abbott[258] in 1924. The incidence rate is about 50% compared with an incidence rate of 0.4% for infants with normal chromosomes. Arioventricular septal defects account for two thirds of congenital heart disease in Down syndrome.[237]

The phenotypic features of Down syndrome are well established. The anteroposterior diameter of the skull is shortened. The inner epicanthic skin fold that inserts onto the lower lid may be prominent at birth (Figures 15-90 and 15-91). In Asian children with trisomy 21, the typical Down inner canthal fold is readily identified together with the normal Asian horizontal epicanthic fold above the outer canthus (see Figure 15-91B).[259] Brushfield spots (speckled iris) are distinctive ocular features described by Down as fine white spots at the periphery of the iris readily seen in patients with blue-gray irises (see Figure 15-91A) but not in patients with dark brown irises.[259] The nose is small, the nasal bridge is depressed, and the nares are anteverted and narrow. The ears are low-set with overlapping or folding of the helix. The lips are prominent, thickened, and fissured, and the tongue is large and protuberant (see Figure 15-90A). The corners of the mouth turn down as in a child's drawing of a sad face (see Figure 15-90B). The skin in infants is soft and velvety, but in childhood, the skin is dry, pale, and lax. Neonates have abundant skin and subcutaneous tissue in the posterior neck. The Moro reflex exhibit is absent. The child lies supine with hips externally rotated 90 degrees, prefiguring spontaneous dislocation (Figure 15-92B). The thoracic configuration reflects hyperinflation. The abdomen tends to be protuberant because of reduced muscle tone and diastases recti. The hands are broad and stubby with a short curved fourth finger, a single transverse palmar crease (Figure 15-92A), and a distal axial triradius. Short stubby feet are as common as short stubby hands.

Arterial Pulse and Jugular Venous Pulse

A small water-hammer pulse is the result of rapid ejection of the large left ventricular stroke volume of severe left atrioventricular valve regurgitation. The arterial pulse

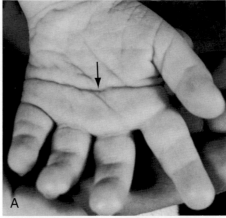
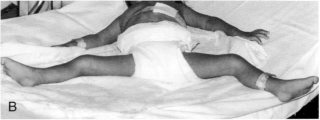

FIGURE 15-92 A, Transverse palmar crease (arrow) in a 6-month-old infant with Down syndrome. **B,** Ninety-degree external rotation of the hips in a 16-month-old child with Down syndrome. At age 3 years, the hips spontaneously dislocated.

is small in infants with an atrioventricular septal defect and congestive heart failure.

The V wave is dominant in the jugular venous pulse (Figure 15-93) because the right atrium receives left ventricular systolic flow across an incompetent left AV valve *directly* through the atrioventricular septal defect or *indirectly* through an ostium primum atrial septal

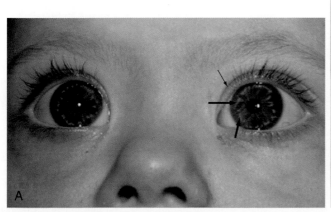
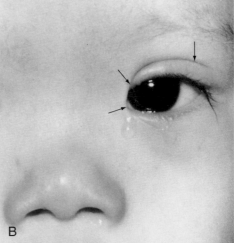

FIGURE 15-91 A, Brushfield spots (speckled iris, large paired arrows) readily seen in a blue-eyed female with Down syndrome. A typical inner eipcanthic fold (thin arrow) inserts onto the lower lid. **B,** A 17-month-old Asian female with Down syndrome. Two arrows on the left identify the typical inner epicanthic fold of Down syndrome. The single vertical arrow on the right identifies the normal horizontal Asian epicanthic fold above the outer canthus. Brushfield spots are not visible because the irises are dark brown.

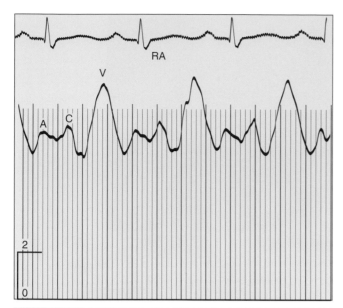

FIGURE 15-93 Right atrial pressure pulse (RA) from a 12-year-old girl with an ostium primum atrial septal defect and moderate left atrioventricular valve regurgitation. The V wave is prominent in the right atrium, despite a competent right atrioventricular valve, because left ventricular blood was ejected into the right atrium via the atrioventricular septal defect.

defect (see Figure 15-88B).[233] Congestive heart failure elevates the mean jugular venous pressure together with the A and V waves.

Precordial Movement and Palpation

An isolated nonrestrictive ostium primum atrial septal defect is associated with precordial movements analogous to an equivalent ostium secundum atrial septal defect. Coexisting left AV valve regurgitation is responsible for a left ventricular impulse and an apical systolic thrill that radiates toward the left sternal border because the right atrium receives the regurgitant flow (see Figure 15-88B). When regurgitation is severe and the interatrial communication is restrictive, systolic expansion of a large left atrium must be distinguished from an intrinsic right ventricular impulse of volume overload.

The right ventricular impulse is tumultuous with complete atrioventricular septal defect because of both volume and pressure overload. A dilated right ventricular outflow tract generates an impulse in the third left intercostal space, an enlarged pulmonary trunk generates an impulse in the second left intercostal space, and a volume overloaded left ventricle occupies the apex (see Figure 15-89). The thrill of left AV valve regurgitation radiates toward the sternum where it is indistinguishable from thrills of ventricular septal defect and tricuspid regurgitation.

Auscultation

An isolated nonrestrictive ostium primum atrial septal defect is accompanied by auscultatory signs analogous to a nonrestrictive ostium secundum atrial septal defect.

Left atrioventricular valve regurgitation adds an apical holosystolic murmur that radiates toward the sternum (Figures 15-94 and 15-95), sometimes as far as the right sternal edge because the right atrium receives regurgitant flow from the left ventricle (see Figure 15-88B). A systolic thrill has been identified over the right atrium at surgery. A pulmonary midsystolic flow murmur in the second left intercostal space is followed by wide fixed splitting of the second heart sound (see Figure 15-95). The delayed pulmonary component is heard at the apex (see Figure 15-94B) and mistaken for an opening snap, which can originate in the incompetent left atrioventricular valve. Mid-diastolic murmurs at the lower left sternal border are caused by augmented flow across the right atrioventricular valve (Figures 15-94, 15-95, and 15-96), and mid-diastolic murmurs at the apex are caused by augmented flow across the left atrioventricular valve.[234] An early to mid-diastolic murmur recorded within the right atrium has been related to the tall left atrial V wave that generates a diastolic pressure gradient across a restrictive atrial septal defect. When left AV valve regurgitation is severe and the interatrial communication is restrictive or absent, auscultatory signs are analogous to isolated mitral regurgitation.[142,234] Wide persistent splitting of the second heart sound then reflects early closure of the aortic valve.[111,234]

When a common atrioventricular orifice is equipped with a common atrioventricular valve, the first heart sound is single and impure. Early vibrations of a

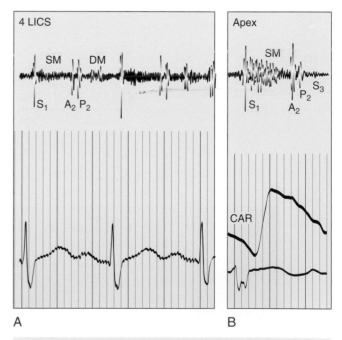

FIGURE 15-94 A, Phonocardiogram (4 LICS = fourth left intercostal space) of a 2-year-old boy with a nonrestrictive ostium primum atrial septal defect and severe left atrioventricular valve regurgitation. A holosystolic murmur (SM) radiates from the apex to the left sternal edge. The murmur is followed by fixed splitting of the second heart sound (A_2/P_2) and a tricuspid mid-diastolic flow murmur (DM). **B,** A prominent apical holosystolic decrescendo murmur ends at the split second heart sound, which is followed by a left ventricular third heart sound (S_3).

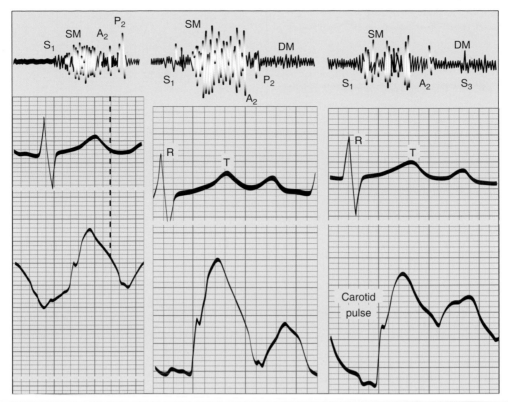

FIGURE 15-95 Tracings from a 13-year-old boy with a nonrestrictive ostium primum atrial septal defect and severe left atrioventricular valve regurgitation. In the first panel (second left intercostal space), a prominent pulmonary midsystolic murmur (SM) ends before a second sound that is widely split with a prominent pulmonary component (P$_2$). The middle panel (lower left sternal border) shows the holosystolic murmur of left atrioventricular regurgitation that radiated from the apex and enveloped the aortic component of the second heart sound (A$_2$). (P$_2$ = pulmonary component; DM = mid-diastolic flow murmur across the right atrioventricular valve.) In the third panel (apex), the systolic regurgitant murmur is softer, and a third heart sound (S$_3$) introduces a short middiastolic flow murmur (DM) across the left atrioventricular valve. (S$_1$ = first heart sound.)

holosystolic murmur obscure the first heart sound that is soft because the PR interval is prolonged. Wide fixed splitting of the second heart sound is difficult to identify because the aortic component is obscured by a holosystolic murmur, leaving an isolated loud pulmonary component. The high-frequency murmur of left AV valve regurgitation preferentially radiates toward the sternum because the right atrium receives systolic flow from the left ventricle through the common atrioventricular canal. The regurgitant murmur radiates to the right of the sternum when the jet reaches the lateral wall of an enlarged right atrium. The ventricular septal defect murmur recorded with an intracardiac phonocardiogram coincides with the murmurs of left and right AV valve regurgitation at the mid to lower left sternal border.[104] Intracardiac phonocardiograms from within the right atrium cannot distinguish the murmurs of left versus right AV valve regurgitation because the regurgitant stream from the left ventricle is directed into the right atrium via the ostium primum atrial septal defect. Similarly, the regurgitant stream from the right ventricle can be directed into the left atrium via the ostium primum defect. An increase in pulmonary vascular resistance diminishes the murmur of ventricular septal defect, reinforces the murmur across the right AV valve, and leaves the murmur across the left AV valve unchanged. A midsystolic

murmur across the gooseneck left ventricular outflow (see Figure 15-88) is seldom recognized.

Electrocardiogram

In 1956, Toscano-Barbosa called attention to three electrocardiographic features of atrioventricular septal defects: the PR interval, the QRS axis, and the sequence of ventricular activation.[260] PR interval prolongation occurs in approximately 50% of cases because of delayed intraatrial and atrioventricular nodal conduction (Figure 15-97).[258,261,262] Complete atrioventricular block occasionally develops. The incidence of atrial fibrillation and atrial flutter increases with age.

Toscano-Barbosa recognized certain distinctive features of the QRS complex, stating, "... the similarity that may exist in the precordial leads may lead one astray from the differences that almost universally exist in the extremity leads which are of real discriminatory value."[260] These features are best illustrated with vectorial analysis (Figure 15-98).[260] Left axis deviation varies from moderate to extreme. The QRS axis is either superior to the left or superior to the right, with a mean that may reach minus 180 degrees.[146,263] Extreme left axis deviation is a feature of Down syndrome (Figure 15-99). Counterclockwise depolarization results

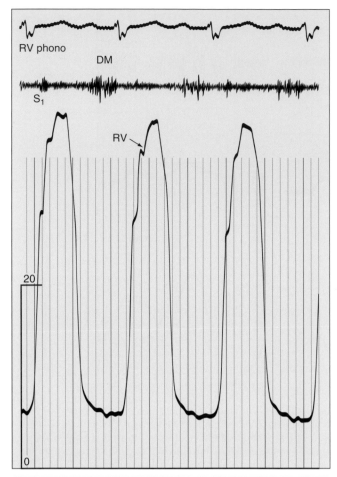

FIGURE 15-96 Recordings from a 5-year-old boy with a nonrestrictive ostium primum atrial septal defect and left atrioventricular valve regurgitation. The right ventricular intracardiac phonocardiogram (RV phono) recorded a mid-diastolic flow murmur (DM) across the right atrioventricular valve. The RV systolic pressure is the slightly elevated.

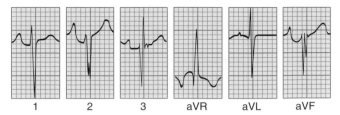

FIGURE 15-97 Limb leads from a symptomatic neonate with Down syndrome and a complete atrioventricular septal defect. Left axis deviation is extreme. Depolarization is counterclockwise with initial r waves in leads 2, 3, and aVF. The S waves in leads 2 and aVF are splintered.

in Q waves in leads 1 and aVL (see Figure 15-97). The S waves in leads 2, 3, and aVF are characteristically notched on their upstrokes (Figures 15-97, 15-99, and 15-100) because of a change in direction of the terminal force of the QRS well illustrated in the vector loop (see Figure 15-98). Occasional examples of ostium secundum atrial septal defects with left axis deviation are likely to represent acquired left anterior fascicular block (see Figure 15-32).[144]

The mechanisms responsible for the characteristic QRS patterns in atrioventricular septal defects stem from congenital alterations of the excitation pathways into the ventricles,[263,264] as Toscano-Barbosa originally proposed.[260] Anatomic studies of the atrioventricular conduction system in human and canine hearts have shed light on these distinctive QRS patterns.[263,265] The atrioventricular conduction axis penetrates only at the crux, and the penetrating bundle is displaced posteriorly, lying on the posteroinferior rim of the ventricular component of the defect. The His bundle is shorter than normal and is posteriorly positioned. The left bundle branch block is displaced posteriorly and arises from the common bundle immediately after it enters the ventricular septum. The left anterior division of the left bundle branch has fewer fibers than normal and is increased in length. The left posterior division is shorter than normal and provides

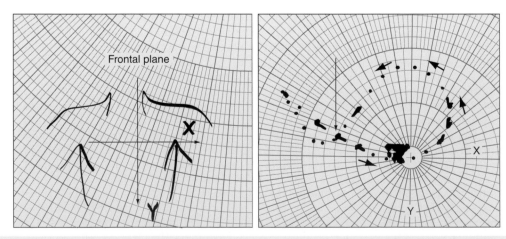

FIGURE 15-98 Vectorcardiogram from a 4-year-old girl with a complete atrioventricular septal defect. Depolarization is counterclockwise (arrowheads). The initial portion of QRS loop is superior and minus 90 degrees. The terminal portion of the loop abruptly changes direction (long vertical arrow) and turns on itself.

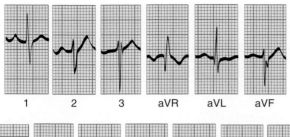

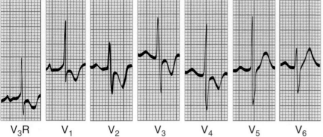

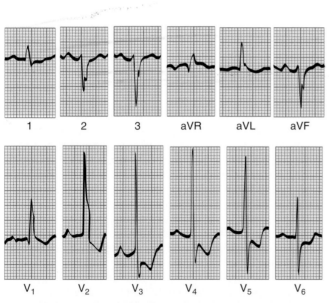

FIGURE 15-99 Electrocardiogram from a 5-year-old boy with a nonrestrictive ostium primum atrial septal defect and severe left atrioventricular valve (see Figure 15-96). The PR interval is prolonged. There is left axis deviation with counterclockwise depolarization and notching of the upstrokes of the S waves in leads 2, 3, and aVF. Right ventricular hypertrophy is indicated by the tall R waves in leads V₃R and V₁ and in the deep S waves in left precordial leads. The terminal tall R wave in lead aVR is slightly prolonged.

small branches to the posterobasal wall of the left ventricle. The right bundle branch is abnormally long.

These anatomic patterns correlate with electrophysiologic observations.[263] Short HV intervals are in accord with elaborate studies that show early activation of the posterobasal left ventricular wall in human and canine atrioventricular septal defects.[263] Early posterobasal activation is consistent with posterior displacement of the left bundle branch and with a short posterior division that sends small branches to the posterobasal wall. Delayed activation of the anterior superior wall is appropriate for hypoplasia and increased length of the left anterior division of the left bundle branch.[263] These anatomic and electrophysiologic observations provide acceptable explanations for left axis deviation and for the depolarization pattern (see Figure 15-98). The delay in right ventricular activation results from increased length of the right bundle branch, not from slowed Purkinje conduction that is incorrectly implied by the terms *partial* or *complete right bundle branch block*.

Right ventricular hypertrophy with an ostium primum atrial septal defect indicates pulmonary hypertension induced by left atrioventricular valve regurgitation (Figure 15-101) or the pulmonary vascular disease of Down syndrome (see previous). Right ventricular hypertrophy with a complete atrioventricular septal defect reflects the pulmonary hypertension accompanying a nonrestrictive defect in the inlet septum (see Figure 15-100), whether or not pulmonary vascular disease coexists. Left precordial leads exhibit prominent Q waves and well-developed R waves of left ventricular volume overload.

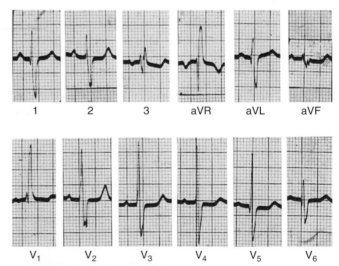

FIGURE 15-100 Electrocardiogram from a pulmonary hypertensive cyanotic 27-year-old man with a complete atrioventricular septal defect but a functionally competent common atrioventricular valve. The PR interval is 200 msec. Peaked right atrial P waves appear in leads V₂₋₃. Right atrial enlargement is indicated by the q wave in lead V₁. There is left axis deviation with counterclockwise depolarization and notching of the upstrokes of the S waves in leads 2, 3, and aVF. The terminal r wave in lead aVR is prolonged. Right ventricular hypertrophy is indicated by tall monophasic R waves, ST segment and T wave changes in right precordial leads, and prominent S waves in left precordial leads.

FIGURE 15-101 Electrocardiogram from a 12-year-old boy with a nonrestrictive ostium primum atrial septal defect, severe left atrioventricular valve regurgitation, and a pulmonary arterial systolic pressure of 45 mm Hg. P waves in leads 1 and 2 are peaked but not tall. Depolarization is counterclockwise with q waves in leads 1 and aVL. The mean electrical axis is minus 90 degrees. The R wave in lead aVR is tall and slightly prolonged. Right ventricular hypertrophy is indicated by the tall R prime in lead V₁ and the deep prolonged S waves in leads V₅₋₆. Volume overload of the left ventricle is reflected in left precordial q waves and well-developed R waves.

X-Ray

In an isolated *ostium primum atrial septal* defect, the x-ray is analogous to an ostium secundum atrial septal defect of equivalent size (Figure 15-102). When *left AV valve regurgitation* coexists, the right atrium is especially enlarged because regurgitant flow is directed into the right atrial cavity (see Figure 15-88B). The left cardiac border is straightened by a prominent right ventricular outflow tract (Figure 15-103). In infants and young children with a complete atrioventricular septal defect, the enlarged cardiac silhouette may obscure all but a small portion of the lung fields (see Figure 15-89). A dilated right atrium occupies the right lower cardiac border, and the left ventricle can occupy the apex despite right ventricular enlargement (see Figure 15-89). A dilated pulmonary trunk may be eclipsed by a prominent right ventricular outflow tract. The ascending aorta is inconspicuous (see Figure 15-89).

The lateral x-ray in Down syndrome may disclose a *double manubrial ossification center* (Figure 15-104A),[265,266] and the posteroanterior projection consistently discloses an *absent or rudimentary 12th rib* (Figure 15-104B). Seckel's syndrome is another phenotype characterized by absence of the 12th rib (i.e., 11 paired ribs).[126] Hyperinflation of the lungs caused by upper airway obstruction in Down syndrome flattens the hemodiaphragms.

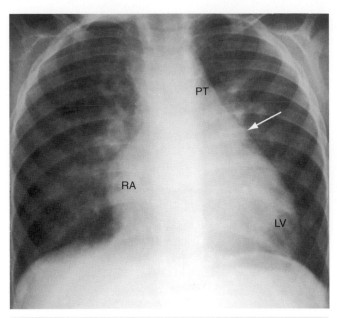

FIGURE 15-103 X-ray from a 19-month-old female with a nonrestrictive ostium primum atrial septal defect, a restrictive inlet ventricular septal defect, a 2 to1 left-to-right shunt, and moderate to marked regurgitation of the left atrioventricular valve. An enlarged left atrial appendage (arrow) straightened the left cardiac border. A prominent right atrium (RA) occupies the right lower cardiac border, and a dilated left ventricle (LV) occupies the apex. Pulmonary vascularity is increased.

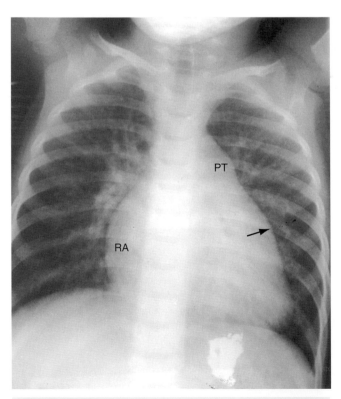

FIGURE 15-102 X-ray from a 3-year-old boy with a nonrestrictive ostium primum atrial septal defect and moderate regurgitation of the left atrioventricular valve. Pulmonary vascularity is increased, the pulmonary trunk (PT) is dilated, the right ventricular outflow tract is prominent (arrow), and the right atrium (RA) is enlarged. The ascending aorta is not seen. It is uncertain which ventricle occupies the apex.

Echocardiogram

Echocardiography with color flow imaging and Doppler interrogation establishes the type of atrioventricular septal defect and its hemodynamic consequences. The diagnosis can be made in the fetus.[267,268] Cross-sectional echocardiographic studies have characterized the pathognomonic morphologic features of atrioventicular septal defects and have defined the relationships between septal structures and the atrioventricular junction.[269] Echocardiography defines the atrioventricular valve attachments, identifies absence of the atrioventricular septum, and determines whether a common annulus is guarded by a common atrioventricular valve or two separate atrioventricular valves. Color flow imaging and Doppler interrogation establish atrial and ventricular level shunts and estimate the degree of atrioventricular valve regurgitation. The gooseneck left ventricular outflow tract is recognized,[227] and the relative size of the left ventricular and right ventricular cavities can be defined.[222,270]

Absence of the atrioventricular septum is verified when the bridging leaflets cross at the same horizontal level above the crest of the ventricular septum and when fused chords are interposed between conjoined atrioventricular leaflets at the crest of the ventricular septum (see Figure 15-86B). An isolated atrial shunt exists when the bridging leaflets attach directly to the crest of the septum or attach indirectly by chordae tendineae (Figure 15-105 and Video 15-5). Doppler interrogation and color flow imaging establish the level of the shunt (Figure 15-106 and Video 15-7) and determine the competence of the right

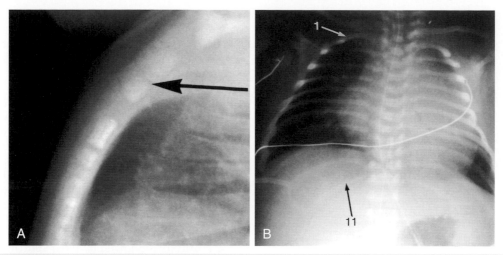

FIGURE 15-104 A, Double manubrial ossification center (arrow) in a 1-year-old male with Down syndrome. **B,** Absence of the 12th rib in a neonate with Down syndrome. Black arrow identifies the 11th rib.

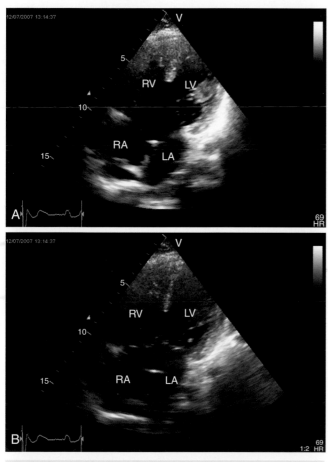

FIGURE 15-105 Echocardiograms (four-chamber) from a 2-year-old girl with a complete atrioventricular septal defect. **A,** The systolic frame shows a common atrioventricular valve with bridging leaflets at the same level because the atrioventricular septum is absent. The bridging leaflets float because they were unattached to either the distal atrial septum above (unmarked paired arrows) or to the crest of the ventricular septum (VS) below. The common atrioventricular canal lies between the crest of the ventricular septum and the distal atrial septum. (RA and LA = right atrium and left atrium; RV and LV = right ventricle and left ventricle.) **B,** The common AV valve is open in diastole (paired oblique arrows) (Videos 15-6A and 15-6B).

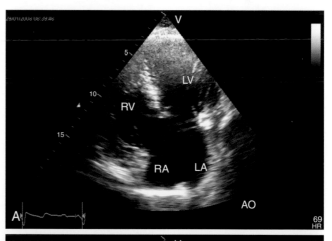

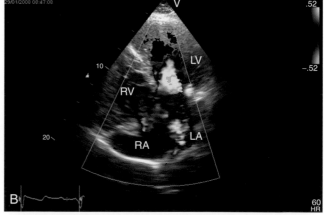

FIGURE 15-106 A, Apical four-chamber view showing a non-restrictive ostium primum atrial septal defect (paired arrows). The right atrium (RA) and right ventricle (RV) are enlarged. **B,** Color flow showing the left-to-right shunt across the ostium primum atrial septal defect with flow continuing across the tricuspid valve into the right ventricle (RV) (Video 15-7). (LV = left ventricle, LA = left atrium.)

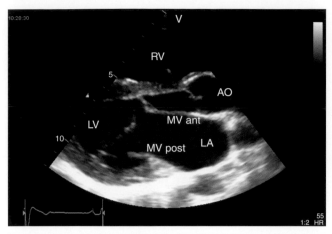

FIGURE 15-107 Echocardiogram (long axis) from a 6-year-old girl with a restrictive ostium primum atrial septal defect and a cleft anterior mitral leaflet that points toward the right ventricle (RV). The cleft represents a functional commissure between the anterior and posterior bridging leaflets. The opened valve has a triangular shape (Videos 15-8A through 15-8C).

and left components of the atrioventricular valve. In the short axis, the left atrioventricular valve assumes a triangular rather than a fish mouth appearance in diastole, and the *cleft* in the anterior leaflet is oriented toward the ventricular septum (Figure 15-107 and Videos 15-8A through 15-8C) because the cleft is in fact a functional commissure between the anterior and posterior bridging leaflets (see Figure 15-86A; see previous). Accessory chordae tendineae originate from the margins of the cleft and insert directly into the ventricular septum.

Continuity between the posterior aortic wall and the left atrioventricular valve is attenuated. Abnormal positions of left ventricular papillary muscles can be identified, and a parachute or double orifice arrangement can be established. Interrogation of the left ventricular outflow tract is achieved from the subcostal view, with the gooseneck deformity sought as shown in the angiocardiogram (see Figure 15-88). Obstruction to left ventricular outflow is represented by a subaortic ridge, thick immobile chordal tissue, thin mobile chordal tissue, or an abnormally high or accessory papillary muscle.[227]

Complete atrioventricular septal defects are represented by bridging leaflets that float below the inferior margin of the atrial septum and above the crest of the ventricular septum (see Figure 15-105A).

During diastole, the floating bridging leaflet moves away from the atrial septum into the ventricles, creating a *complete common atrioventricular canal* (see Figure 15-105B). The anterior bridging leaflet contacts the inferior margin of the atrial septum during systole, so these two structures should be examined in both phases of the cardiac cycle.

Summary

An isolated *ostium primum atrial septal defect* is clinically analogous to an ostium secundum atrial septal defect of equivalent size except for the QSR axis and the sequence of ventricular depolarization. When accompanied by left

atrioventricular valve regurgitation, the clinical expressions are determined by the degree of regurgitation and the magnitude of the shunt. Congestive heart failure begins in childhood when the atrial septal defect is nonrestrictive and left AV valve regurgitation is severe. The incompetent left atrioventricular valve is susceptible to infective endocarditis. The jugular venous pulse displays a dominant V wave because the right atrium receives the regurgitant jet from the left ventricle. Precordial movement and palpitation are similar to ostium secundum atrial septal defect, with the important exception of a left ventricular impulse and an apical systolic thrill. Auscultatory signs resemble those of ostium secundum atrial septal defect with the addition of the apical holosystolic murmur that radiates toward the sternum, occasionally as far as the right sternal border. A pulmonary midsystolic flow murmur is followed by fixed splitting of the second heart sound. The electrocardiogram shows left axis deviation, counterclockwise depolarization, splintered S waves in the inferior leads, and either an rsR prime pattern in right precordial leads or R waves of right ventricular hypertrophy. The x-ray resembles an ostium secundum atrial septal defect. Echocardiography with Doppler interrogation and color flow imaging establishes absence of the atrioventricular septum with the bridging leaflets at the same horizontal level. Color flow imaging identifies the left-to-right interatrial shunt and the degree of left AV valve regurgitation.

Complete atrioventricular septal defect becomes manifest in infancy because of congestive heart failure. Down phenotype is diagnostically important. The right ventricular impulse is hyperdynamic because of combined pressure and volume overload and eclipses the left ventricular impulse. The murmur of left atrioventricular valve regurgitation preferentially radiates toward the sternum, occasionally as far as the right anterior chest, and overlaps with the sites occupied by systolic murmurs of ventricular septal defect and right AV valve regurgitation. A middiastolic flow murmur is generated across the right and left components of the atrioventricular valve. There is fixed splitting of the second heart sound with a prominent pulmonary component. The electrocardiogram shows left axis deviation, counterclockwise depolarization, splintering of the S waves in inferior leads, and right ventricular hypertrophy in precordial leads. The x-ray shows increased pulmonary arterial vascularity and a considerable increase in heart size because of right atrial and right ventricular enlargement. Echocardiography identifies bridging leaflets of the common atrioventricular valve beneath the distal margin of the atrial septum and above the crest of the ventricular septum. Doppler interrogation and color flow imaging establish the levels of the interatrial and interventricular shunts and the degree of left and right AV regurgitation.

REFERENCES

1. Fransson SG. The Botallo mystery. *Clin Cardiol.* 1999;22:434–436.
2. Da Vinci L, O'Malley CD, Saunders JBDC. *Leonardo da Vinci on the human body: the anatomical, physiological and embryological drawings (with his notes) of Leonardo da Vinci.* New York: H. Schuman; 1952.

3. Acierno LJ. *The history of cardiology.* New York: Parthenon Publishing Group; 1994.

4. Assmann H. *Die Roentgendiagnostik der inneren Erkrankungen.* Leipzig: FCW Vogel; 1921.

5. Roesler H. Interatrial septal defect. *Arch Intern Med.* 1934;54: 339–380.

6. Bedford DE, Papp C, Parkinson J. Atrial septal defect. *Br Heart J.* 1941;3:37–68.

7. Hudson R. The normal and abnormal inter-atrial septum. *Br Heart J.* 1955;17:489–495.

8. Sweeney LJ, Rosenquist GC. The normal anatomy of the atrial septum in the human heart. *Am Heart J.* 1979;98:194–199.

9. Schwinger ME, Gindea AJ, Freedberg RS, Kronzon I. The anatomy of the interatrial septum: a transesophageal echocardiographic study. *Am Heart J.* 1990;119:1401–1405.

10. Hagen PT, Scholz DG, Edwards WD. Incidence and size of patent foramen ovale during the first 10 decades of life: an autopsy study of 965 normal hearts. *Mayo Clin Proc.* 1984;59:17–20.

11. Hanley PC, Tajik AJ, Hynes JK, et al. Diagnosis and classification of atrial septal aneurysm by two-dimensional echocardiography: report of 80 consecutive cases. *J Am Coll Cardiol.* 1985;6: 1370–1382.

12. Pearson AC, Nagelhout D, Castello R, Gomez CR, Labovitz AJ. Atrial septal aneurysm and stroke: a transesophageal echocardiographic study. *J Am Coll Cardiol.* 1991;18:1223–1229.

13. Webb G, Gatzoulis MA. Atrial septal defects in the adult: recent progress and overview. *Circulation.* 2006;114:1645–1653.

14. Ullah W, Zeb Q, Heppell R. Secundum atrial septal defect. *J Am Coll Cardiol.* 2009;53:893.

15. Bedford DE. The anatomical types of atrial septal defect. Their incidence and clinical diagnosis. *Am J Cardiol.* 1960;6: 568–574.

16. Dall'agata A, McGhie J, Taams MA, et al. Secundum atrial septal defect is a dynamic three-dimensional entity. *Am Heart J.* 1999; 137:1075–1081.

17. Schwerzmann M, Windecker S, Meier B. Images in cardiovascular medicine. Swiss cheese-like atrial septal defect. *Circulation.* 2008; 117:e490–e492.

18. Ozcelik N, Atalay S, Tutar E, Ekici F, Atasay B. The prevalence of interatrial septal openings in newborns and predictive factors for spontaneous closure. *Int J Cardiol.* 2006;108:207–211.

19. Kaski JP, Wolfenden J, Josen M, Daubeney PEF, Shinebourne EA. Can atrioventricular septal defects exist with intact septal structures? *Heart.* 2006;92:832–835.

20. Waggstaffe W. Two cases of free communication between the auricles, by deficiency of the upper part of the septum auricularum. *Transactions of the Pathological Society of London.* 1868; 19:91–98.

21. Ettedgui JA, Siewers RD, Anderson RH, Park SC, Pahl E, Zuberbuhler JR. Diagnostic echocardiographic features of the sinus venosus defect. *Br Heart J.* 1990;64:329–331.

22. Gallaher ME, Sperling DR, Gwinn JL, Meyer BW, Flyer DC. Functional drainage of the inferior vena cava into the left atrium: three cases. *Am J Cardiol.* 1963;12:561–566.

23. Thomas JD, Tabakin BS, Ittleman FP. Atrial septal defect with right to left shunt despite normal pulmonary artery pressure. *J Am Coll Cardiol.* 1987;9:221–224.

24. Sutherland HD. A case with three atrial septal defects. *Br Heart J.* 1963;25:267–269.

25. Raghib G, Ruttenberg HD, Anderson RC, Amplatz K, Adams Jr. P, Edwards JE. Termination of left superior vena cava in left atrium, atrial septal defect, and absence of coronary sinus; a developmental complex. *Circulation.* 1965;31:906–918.

26. Cayler GG. Spontaneous functional closure of symptomatic atrial septal defects. *N Engl J Med.* 1967;276:65–73.

27. Ghisla RP, Hannon DW, Meyer RA, Kaplan S. Spontaneous closure of isolated secundum atrial septal defects in infants: an echocardiographic study. *Am Heart J.* 1985;109:1327–1333.

28. Mascarenhas E, Javier RP, Samet P. Partial anomalous pulmonary venous connection and drainage. *Am J Cardiol.* 1973;31: 512–518.

29. Swan HJ, Burchell HB, Wood EH. Differential diagnosis at cardiac catheterization of anomalous pulmonary venous drainage related to atrial septal defects or abnormal venous connections. *Proc staff meet Mayo Clin.* 1953;28:452–462.

30. Burchell HB, Hetzel PS, Swan HJ, Wood EH. Relative contribution of blood from each lung to the left-to-right shunt in atrial septal defect; demonstration by indicatordilution technics. *Circulation.* 1956;14:200–211.

31. Nakib A, Moller JH, Kanjuh VI, Edwards JE. Anomalies of the pulmonary veins. *Am J Cardiol.* 1967;20:77–90.

32. Sreeram N, Walsh K. Diagnosis of total anomalous pulmonary venous drainage by Doppler color flow imaging. *J Am Coll Cardiol.* 1992;19:1577–1582.

33. Frye RL, Krebs M, Rahimtoola SH, Ongley PA, Hallermann FJ, Wallace RB. Partial anomalous pulmonary venous connection without atrial septal defect. *Am J Cardiol.* 1968;22:242–250.

34. Chassinat R. Observation d'anomalies anatomiques remarquables de l'appareil circulatoire avec hepatocele cong's enitale a'yant donne'lieu pendant la vie a aucum symptome particulier. *Archives générales de médecine, Paris.* 1836;11:80.

35. Puwanant S, Tumkosit M, Sitthisook S, Buddhari W, Rungpradubvong V, Boonyaratavej S. Scimitar sign in a patient with an atrial septal defect: a comprehensive noninvasive assessment with transthoracic echocardiography and computed tomography. *J Am Coll Cardiol.* 2009;54:1556.

36. Canter CE, Martin TC, Spray TL, Weldon CS, Strauss AW. Scimitar syndrome in childhood. *Am J Cardiol.* 1986;58:652–654.

37. Dupuis C, Charaf LA, Breviere GM, Abou P, Remy-Jardin M, Helmius G. The "adult" form of the scimitar syndrome. *Am J Cardiol.* 1992;70:502–507.

38. Oakley D, Naik D, Verel D, Rajan S. Scimitar vein syndrome: report of nine new cases. *Am Heart J.* 1984;107:596–598.

39. D'cruz IA, Arcilla RA. Anomalous venous drainage of the left lung into the inferior vena cava. A case report. *Am Heart J.* 1964;67: 539–544.

40. Cooksey JD, Parker BM, Weldon CS. Atrial septal defect and calcification of the tricuspid valve. *Br Heart J.* 1970;32:409–411.

41. Davies MJ. Mitral valve in secundum atrial septal defects. *Br Heart J.* 1981;46:126–128.

42. Hynes KM, Frye RL, Brandenburg RO, McGoon DC, Titus JL, Giuliani ER. Atrial septal defect (secundum) associated with mitral regurgitation. *Am J Cardiol.* 1974;34:333–338.

43. Schamroth CL, Sareli P, Pocock WA, et al. Pulmonary arterial thrombosis in secundum atrial septal defect. *Am J Cardiol.* 1987;60:1152–1156.

44. Niwa K, Perloff JK, Bhuta SM, et al. Structural abnormalities of great arterial walls in congenital heart disease: light and electron microscopic analyses. *Circulation.* 2001;103:393–400.

45. Fuse S, Tomita H, Hatakeyama K, Kubo N, Abe N. Effect of size of a secundum atrial septal defect on shunt volume. *Am J Cardiol.* 2001;88:1447–1450, A1449.

46. Rowe GG, Castillo CA, Maxwell GM, Clifford JE, Crumpton CW. Atrial septal defect and the mechanism of shunt. *Am Heart J.* 1961;61:369–374.

47. Alexander JA, Rembert JC, Sealy WC, Greenfield Jr. JC. Shunt dynamics in experimental atrial septal defects. *J Appl Physiol.* 1975;39:281–286.

48. Joffe HS. Effect of age on pressure-flow dynamics in secundum atrial septal defect. *Br Heart J.* 1984;51:469–472.

49. Romero T, Covell J, Friedman WF. A comparison of pressure-volume relations of the fetal, newborn, and adult heart. *Am J Physiol.* 1972;222:1285–1290.

50. Wagenvoort C, Neufeld H, Dushane J, Edwards J, Wagenvoort N. The pulmonary arterial tree in ventricular septal defect: A quantitative study of anatomic features in fetuses, infants, and children. *Circulation.* 1961;23:740.

51. Liberthson RR, Boucher CA, Strauss HW, Dinsmore RE, McKusick KA, Pohost GM. Right ventricular function in adult atrial septal defect. Preoperative and postoperative assessment and clinical implications. *Am J Cardiol.* 1981;47:56–60.

52. Bonow RO, Borer JS, Rosing DR, Bacharach SL, Green MV, Kent KM. Left ventricular functional reserve in adult patients with atrial septal defect: pre- and postoperative studies. *Circulation.* 1981;63:1315–1322.

53. Booth DC, Wisenbaugh T, Smith M, Demaria AN. Left ventricular distensibility and passive elastic stiffness in atrial septal defect. *J Am Coll Cardiol.* 1988;12:1231–1236.

54. Graham Jr. TP, Jarmakani JM, Canent Jr. RV. Left heart volume characteristics with a right ventricular volume overload. Total

anomalous pulmonary venous connection and large atrial septal defect. *Circulation.* 1972;45:389–396.

55. Otani H, Kagaya Y, Yamane Y, et al. Long-term right ventricular volume overload increases myocardial fluorodeoxyglucose uptake in the interventricular septum in patients with atrial septal defect. *Circulation.* 2000;101:1686–1692.

56. Kerut EK, Norfleet WT, Plotnick GD, Giles TD. Patent foramen ovale: a review of associated conditions and the impact of physiological size. *J Am Coll Cardiol.* 2001;38:613–623.

57. Flyer DC, Buckley LP, Hellenbrand WE. Report of the New England Regional Infant Cardiac Program. *Pediatrics.* 1980;65: 375–461.

58. Campbell M, Neill C, Suzman S. The prognosis of atrial septal defect. *Br Med J.* 1957;1:1375–1383.

59. Heath D, Helmholz Jr. HF, Burchell HB, Dushane JW, Edwards JE. Graded pulmonary vascular changes and hemodynamic findings in cases of atrial and ventricular septal defect and patent ductus arteriosus. *Circulation.* 1958;18:1155–1166.

60. Dalen JE, Bruce RA, Cobb LA. Interaction of chronic hypoxia of moderate altitude on pulmonary hypertension complicating defect of the atrial septum. *N Engl J Med.* 1962;266:272–277.

61. Khoury GH, Hawes CR. Atrial septal defect associated with pulmonary hypertension in children living at high altitude. *J Pediatr.* 1967;70:432–435.

62. Klecker RJ, Christoforidis AJ, Sinclair DS. Case 2. Vertical vein (partial anomalous pulmonary venous drainage). *AJR Am J Roentgenol.* 2000;175:867–870.

63. Galve E, Angel J, Evangelista A, Anivarro I, Permanyer-Miralda G, Soler-Soler J. Bidirectional shunt in uncomplicated atrial septal defect. *Br Heart J.* 1984;51:480–484.

64. Bashour T, Kabbani S, Saalouke M, Cheng TO. Persistent Eustachian valve causing severe cyanosis in atrial septal defect with normal right heart pressures. *Angiology.* 1983;34:79–83.

65. Howitt G. Atrial septal defect in three generations. *Br Heart J.* 1961;23:494–496.

66. Nora JJ, McNamara DG, Fraser FC. Hereditary factors in atrial septal defect. *Circulation.* 1967;35:448–456.

67. Macdonald IL, Mcmurtry TJ, Dodek A. Atrial septal defect in adult identical twins: a variation in theme. *Clin Cardiol.* 1983;6: 507–510.

68. Neill CA, Ferencz C, Sabiston DC, Sheldon H. The familial occurrence of hypoplastic right lung with systemic arterial supply and venous drainage "scimitar syndrome." *Bull Johns Hopkins Hosp.* 1960;107:1–21.

69. Ashida K, Itoh A, Naruko T, et al. Familial scimitar syndrome: three-dimensional visualization of anomalous pulmonary vein in young sisters. *Circulation.* 2001;103:E126–E127.

70. Silverman ME, Copeland Jr. AJ, Hurst JW. The Holt-Oram syndrome: the long and the short of it. *Am J Cardiol.* 1970;25: 11–17.

71. Bizarro RO, Callahan JA, Feldt RH, Kurland LT, Gordon H, Brandenburg RO. Familial atrial septal defect with prolonged atrioventricular conduction. A syndrome showing the autosomal dominant pattern of inheritance. *Circulation.* 1970;41:677–683.

72. Bjornstad PG. Secundum type atrial septal defect with prolonged PR interval and autosomal dominant mode of inheritance. *Br Heart J.* 1974;36:1149–1154.

73. Pease WE, Nordenberg A, Ladda RL. Familial atrial septal defect with prolonged atrioventricular conduction. *Circulation.* 1976;53: 759–762.

74. Bjornstad PG, Leren TP. Familial atrial septal defect in the oval fossa with progressive prolongation of the atrioventricular conduction caused by mutations in the NKX2.5 gene. *Cardiol Young.* 2009;19:40–44.

75. Calcagni G, Digilio MC, Capolino R, Dallapiccola B, Marino B. Concordant familial segregation of atrial septal defect and Axenfeld-Rieger anomaly in father and son. *Clin Dysmorphol.* 2006;15:203–206.

76. Seldon WA, Rubinstein C, Fraser AA. The incidence of atrial septal defect in adults. *Br Heart J.* 1962;24:557–560.

77. Ferrari VA, Reilly MP, Axel L, Sutton MG. Images in cardiovascular medicine. Scimitar syndrome. *Circulation.* 1998;98:1583–1584.

78. Dexter L. Atrial septal defect. *Br Heart J.* 1956;18:209–225.

79. Campbell M. Natural history of atrial septal defect. *Br Heart J.* 1970;32:820–826.

80. Perloff JK. Ostium secundum atrial septal defect—survival for 87 and 94 years. *Am J Cardiol.* 1984;53:388–389.

81. Pryor RE, Giannetto L, Bashore TM. Surgical repair of atrial septal defect in an 89-year-old man: progressive shunt due to concomitant aortic stenosis. *Am Heart J.* 1989;118:423–424.

82. Tekin G, Tekin A, Yildirim SV, Yigit F. Long-term survival with partial atrioventricular septal defect. *Int J Cardiol.* 2007;115: e116–e117.

83. Davis MP, Zaidi AN, Orsinelli DA. Sinus venosus atrial septal defect diagnosed at age 82. *Am J Geriatr Cardiol.* 2008;17:114–116.

84. Child JS. Transthoracic and transesophageal echocardiographic imaging: anatomic and hemodynamic assessment. In: Perloff JK, Child JS, eds. *Congenital heart disease in adults.* 2nd ed. Philadelphia: W. B. Saunders Company; 1998.

85. Medina A, De Lezo JS, Caballero E, Ortega JR. Platypnea-orthodeoxia due to aortic elongation. *Circulation.* 2001;104:741.

86. Seward JB, Hayes DL, Smith HC, et al. Platypnea-orthodeoxia: clinical profile, diagnostic workup, management, and report of seven cases. *Mayo Clin Proc.* 1984;59:221–231.

87. Garcia R, Taber RE. Bacterial endocarditis of the pulmonic valve. Association with atrial septal defect of the ostium secundum type. *Am J Cardiol.* 1966;18:275–280.

88. Andersen M, Moller I, Lyngborg K, Wennevold A. The natural history of small atrial septal defects; long-term follow-up with serial heart catheterizations. *Am Heart J.* 1976;92:302–307.

89. Kuzman WJ, Yuskis AS. Atrial septal defects in the older patient simulating acquired valvular heart disease. *Am J Cardiol.* 1965;15: 303–309.

90. Agmon Y, Khandheria BK, Meissner I, et al. Comparison of frequency of patent foramen ovale by transesophageal echocardiography in patients with cerebral ischemic events versus in subjects in the general population. *Am J Cardiol.* 2001;88:330–332.

91. Stollberger C, Schneider B, Abzieher F, Wollner T, Meinertz T, Slany J. Diagnosis of patent foramen ovale by transesophageal contrast echocardiography. *Am J Cardiol.* 1993;71:604–606.

92. Agmon Y, Khandheria BK, Meissner I, et al. Frequency of atrial septal aneurysms in patients with cerebral ischemic events. *Circulation.* 1999;99:1942–1944.

93. Arnfred E. Symptoms, signs, and hemodynamics in one hundred cases of atrial septal defect confirmed by operation. *J Cardiovasc Surg.* 1966;7:349–384.

94. Campbell M, Polani PE. Factors in the aetiology of atrial septal defect. *Br Heart J.* 1961;23:477–493.

95. Brockhoff CJ, Kober H, Tsilimingas N, Dapper F, Munzel T, Meinertz T. Holt-Oram syndrome. *Circulation.* 1999;99:1395–1396.

96. Bohm M. Holt-Oram syndrome. *Circulation.* 1998;98:2636–2637.

97. Lin AE, Perloff JK. Upper limb malformations associated with congenital heart disease. *Am J Cardiol.* 1985;55:1576–1583.

98. Basson CT, Cowley GS, Solomon SD, et al. The clinical and genetic spectrum of the Holt-Oram syndrome (heart-hand syndrome). *N Engl J Med.* 1994;330:885–891.

99. Musewe NN, Alexander DJ, Teshima I, Smallhorn JF, Freedom RM. Echocardiographic evaluation of the spectrum of cardiac anomalies associated with trisomy 13 and trisomy 18. *J Am Coll Cardiol.* 1990;15:673–677.

100. Parikh DN, Fisher J, Moses JW, et al. Determinants and importance of atrial pressure morphology in atrial septal defect. *Br Heart J.* 1984;51:473–479.

101. Thiron JM, Cribier A, Cazor JL, Letac B. Variations in height of jugular "a" wave in relation to heart rate in normal subjects and in patients with atrial septal defect. *Br Heart J.* 1980;44:37–43.

102. Nagle RE, Tamara FA. Left parasternal impulse in pulmonary stenosis and atrial septal defect. *Br Heart J.* 1967;29:735–741.

103. Perloff JK. *Physical examination of the heart and circulation.* 4th ed. Shelton, Connecticut: People's Medical Publishing House; 2009.

104. Feruglio GA, Sreenivasan A. Intracardiac phonocardiogram in thirty cases of atrial septal defect. *Circulation.* 1959;20:1087–1094.

105. Leatham A, Gray I. Auscultatory and phonocardiographic signs of atrial septal defect. *Br Heart J.* 1956;18:193–208.

106. Plass R, Schmidt KH, Guenther KH. Intracardiac sounds and murmurs in atrial septal defect. *Am J Cardiol.* 1971;28:173–178.

107. Tavel ME, Baugh D, Fisch C, Feigenbaum H. Opening snap of the tricuspid valve in atrial septal defect. A phonocardiographic and reflected ultrasound study of sounds in relationship to movement of the tricuspid valve. *Am Heart J.* 1970;80:550–555.

108. Waider W, Craige E. First heart sound and ejection sounds. Echocardiographic and phonocardiographic correlation with valvular events. *Am J Cardiol.* 1975;35:346–356.

109. Barritt DW, Davies DH, Jacob G. Heart sounds and pressures in atrial septal defect. *Br Heart J.* 1965;27:90–98.

110. Mcdonald L, Emanuel R, Towers M. Aspects of pulmonary blood flow in atrial septal defect. *Br Heart J.* 1959;21:279–283.

111. Perloff JK, Caulfield WH, De Leon Jr AC. Peripheral pulmonary artery murmur of atrial septal defect. *Br Heart J.* 1967;29:411–416.

112. Berry WB, Austen WG. Respiratory variations in the magnitude of the left to right shunt in experimental interatrial communications. *Am J Cardiol.* 1964;14:201–203.

113. Leatham A. The 2D heart sound key to auscultation of the heart. *Acta Cardiol.* 1964;19:395–416.

114. Curtiss EI, Matthews RG, Shaver JA. Mechanism of normal splitting of the second heart sound. *Circulation.* 1975;51:157–164.

115. Kumar S, Luisada AA. The second heart sound in atrial septal defect. *Am J Cardiol.* 1971;28:168–172.

116. O'Toole JD, Reddy PS, Curtiss EI, Shaver JA. The mechanism of splitting of the second heart sound in atrial septal defect. *Circulation.* 1977;56:1047–1053.

117. Shaver JA, Nadolny RA, O'Toole JD, et al. Sound pressure correlates of the second heart sound. An intracardiac sound study. Circulation. 1974;49:316–325.

118. Castle RF, Hedden CA, Davis NP. Variables affecting splitting of the second heart sound in normal children. *Pediatrics.* 1969;43:183–191.

119. Fukazawa M, Fukushige J, Ueda Y, Ueda K, Sunagawa K. Effect of increase in heart rate on interatrial shunt in atrial septal defect. *Pediatr Cardiol.* 1992;13:146–151.

120. Shafter HA. Splitting of the second heart sound. *Am J Cardiol.* 1960;6:1013–1022.

121. Ferguson III JJ, Miller MJ, Aroesty JM, Sahagian P, Grossman W, McKay RG. Assessment of right atrial pressure-volume relations in patients with and without an atrial septal defect. *J Am Coll Cardiol.* 1989;13:630–636.

122. Levin AR, Spach MS, Boineau JP, Canent Jr. RV, Capp MP, Jewett PH. Atrial pressure-flow dynamics in atrial septal defects (secundum type). *Circulation.* 1968;37:476–488.

123. Kavanagh-Gray D. Atrial septal defect in infancy. *Can Med Assoc J.* 1963;89:491–499.

124. Morrow AG, Awe WC, Aygen MM. Total unilateral anomalous pulmonary venous connection with intact atrial septum. Diagnostic features and a method of surgical correction. *Am J Cardiol.* 1962;9:933–937.

125. Kambe T, Hibi N, Ito H, Arakawa T, Nishimura K. Clinical study on the flow murmurs at the defect area of atrial septal defect by means of intracardiac phonocardiography. *Am Heart J.* 1976;91:35–42.

126. Seckel H. *Bird-headed dwarfs: studies in developmental anthropology including human proportions.* Basel: Karger; 1960.

127. Wennevold A. The diastolic murmur of atrial septal defects as detected by intracardiac phonocardiography. *Circulation.* 1966;34:132–138.

128. Albers WH, Hugenholtz PG, Nadas AS. Constrictive pericarditis and atrial septal defect, secundum type. With special reference to left ventricular volumes and related hemodynamic findings. *Am J Cardiol.* 1969;23:850–857.

129. Just H, Mattingly TW. Interatrial septal defect and pericardial disease. Coincidence or causal relationship? *Am Heart J.* 1968;76:157–167.

130. Liberthson RR, Buckley MJ, Boucher CA. Pulmonary regurgitation in large atrial shunts without pulmonary hypertension. *Circulation.* 1976;54:966–968.

131. Iga K, Kondo H, Izumi C, Konishi T. Images in cardiology. Continuous murmur through atrial septal defect. *Heart.* 2000;83:613.

132. Perloff JK. Auscultatory and phonocardiographic manifestations of pulmonary hypertension. *Prog Cardiovasc Dis.* 1967;9:303–340.

133. Sutton G, Harris A, Leatham A. Second heart sound in pulmonary hypertension. *Br Heart J.* 1968;30:743–756.

134. Bink-Boelkens MT, Bergstra A, Landsman ML. Functional abnormalities of the conduction system in children with an atrial septal defect. *Int J Cardiol.* 1988;20:263–272.

135. Karpawich PP, Antillon JR, Cappola PR, Agarwal KC. Pre- and postoperative electrophysiologic assessment of children with secundum atrial septal defect. *Am J Cardiol.* 1985;55:519–521.

136. Ruschhaupt DG, Khoury L, Thilenius OG, Replogle RL, Arcilla RA. Electrophysiologic abnormalities of children with ostium secundum atrial septal defect. *Am J Cardiol.* 1984;53:1643–1647.

137. Finley JP, Nugent ST, Hellenbrand W, Craig M, Gillis DA. Sinus arrhythmia in children with atrial septal defect: an analysis of heart rate variability before and after surgical repair. *Br Heart J.* 1989;61:280–284.

138. Greenstein R, Naaz G, Armstrong WF. Usefulness of electrocardiographic abnormalities for the detection of atrial septal defect in adults. *Am J Cardiol.* 2001;88:1054–1056.

139. Anderson PA, Rogers MC, Canent Jr. RV, Spach MS. Atrioventricular conduction in secundum atrial septal defects. *Circulation.* 1973;48:27–31.

140. Carmichael DB, Forrester RH, Inmon TW, Mattingly TW, Pollock BE, Walker WJ. Electrocardiographic and hemodynamic correlation in atrial septal defect. *Am Heart J.* 1956;52:547–561.

141. Guray U, Guray Y, Yylmaz MB, et al. Evaluation of P wave duration and P wave dispersion in adult patients with secundum atrial septal defect during normal sinus rhythm. *Int J Cardiol.* 2003;91:75–79.

142. Macleod CA. Endocardial cushion defects with severe mitral insufficiency and small atrial septal defect. *Circulation.* 1962;26:755.

143. Sanchez-Cascos A, Deuchar D. The P wave in atrial septal defect. *Br Heart J.* 1963;25:202–210.

144. Harrison DC, Morrow AG. Electrocardiographic evidence of left-axis deviation in patients with defects of the atrial septum of the secundum type. *N Engl J Med.* 1963;269:743–745.

145. Blumenschein SD, Barr RC, Spach MS, Gentzler RC. Quantitative Frank vectorcardiograms of normal children and a comparison to those of patients with atrial defects. *Am Heart J.* 1972;83:332–339.

146. Liebman J, Nadas AS. The vectorcardiogram in the differential diagnosis of atrial septal defect in children. *Circulation.* 1960;22:956–975.

147. Boineau JP, Spach MS, Ayers CR. Genesis of the electrocardiogram in atrial septal defect. *Am Heart J.* 1964;68:637–651.

148. Lasser RP, Borun ER, Grishman A. A vectorcardiographic analysis of the RSR complex of the unipolar chest lead electrocardiogram. III. *Am Heart J.* 1951;41:667–686.

149. Moore EN, Boineau JP, Patterson DF. Incomplete right bundle-branch block. An electrocardiographic enigma and possible misnomer. *Circulation.* 1971;44:678–687.

150. Heller J, Hagege AA, Besse B, Desnos M, Marie FN, Guerot C. "Crochetage" (notch) on R wave in inferior limb leads: a new independent electrocardiographic sign of atrial septal defect. *J Am Coll Cardiol.* 1996;27:877–882.

151. Rodriguez-Alvarez A, Martinez De Rodriguez G, Goggans AM, et al. The vectorcardiographic equivalent of the "crochetage" of the QRS of the electrocardiogram in atrial septal defect of the ostium secundum type. Preliminary report. *Am Heart J.* 1959;58:388–394.

152. Ay H, Buonanno FS, Abraham SA, Kistler JP, Koroshetz WJ. An electrocardiographic criterion for diagnosis of patent foramen ovale associated with ischemic stroke. *Stroke.* 1998;29:1393–1397.

153. Chait A, Zucker M. The superior vena cava in the evaluation of atrial septal defect. *Am J Roentgenol Radium Ther Nucl Med.* 1968;103:104–108.

154. Little RC. Volume elastic properties of the right and left atrium. *Am J Physiol.* 1949;158:237–240.

155. Sanders C, Bittner V, Nath PH, Breatnach ES, Soto BS. Atrial septal defect in older adults: atypical radiographic appearances. *Radiology.* 1988;167:123–127.

156. Keats TE, Rudhe U, Foo GW. Inferior vena caval position in the differential diagnosis of atrial and ventricular septal defects. *Radiology.* 1964;83:616–621.

157. Dalith F, Neufeld H. Radiological diagnosis of anomalous pulmonary venous connection: a tomographic study. *Radiology.* 1960;74:1–18.

158. Hausmann D, Daniel WG, Mugge A, Ziemer G, Pearlman AS. Value of transesophageal color Doppler echocardiography for detection of different types of atrial septal defect in adults. *J Am Soc Echocardiogr.* 1992;5:481–488.

159. Miller DS, Schwartz SL, Geggel RL, Smith JJ, Warner K, Pandian NG. Detection of partial anomalous right pulmonary venous return with an intact atrial septum by transesophageal echocardiography. *J Am Soc Echocardiogr*. 1995;8:924–927.

160. Ammash NM, Seward JB, Warnes CA, Connolly HM, O'Leary PW, Danielson GK. Partial anomalous pulmonary venous connection: diagnosis by transesophageal echocardiography. *J Am Coll Cardiol*. 1997;29:1351–1358.

161. Feller PB, Allan LD. Abnormal pulmonary venous return diagnosed prenatally by pulsed Doppler flow imaging. *Ultrasound Obstet Gynecol*. 1997;9:347–349.

162. Skolnick A, Vavas E, Kronzon I. Optimization of ASD assessment using real time three-dimensional transesophageal echocardiography. *Echocardiography*. 2009;26:233–235.

163. Child JS. Echocardiography in anatomic imaging and hemodynamic evaluation of adults with congenital heart disease. In: Perloff JK, Child JS, Aboulhosn J, eds. *Congenital heart disease in adults*. 3rd ed. Philadelphia: Saunders/Elsevier; 2009.

164. Haugland H, Vik-Mo H. Aneurysm of the atrial septum: motion pattern in relation to respiratory and cardiac cycles. *J Clin Ultrasound*. 1986;14:52–54.

165. Schneider A, Razek V, Riede FT. Echocardiographic diagnosis of divided right atrium. *Cardiol Young*. 2009;19:296–297.

166. Roberson DA, Javois AJ, Cui W, Madronero LF, Cuneo BF, Muangmingsuk S. Double atrial septum with persistent interatrial space: echocardiographic features of a rare atrial septal malformation. *J Am Soc Echocardiogr*. 2006;19:1175–1181.

167. Iwasaki Y, Satomi G, Yasukochi S. Analysis of ventricular septal motion by doppler tissue imaging in atrial septal defect and normal heart. *Am J Cardiol*. 1999;83:206–210.

168. Corvisart JN. *Essai sur les maladies et les lésions organiques de coeur et des gros vaisseaux*. 2nd ed. Paris; 1811.

169. Lutembacher R. De la stenose mitrale avec communication interauriculaire. *Arch Mal Coeur*. 1916;9:237–260.

170. Gueron M, Gussarsky J. Lutembacher syndrome obsolete? A new modified concept of mitral disease and left-to-right at the level. *Am Heart J*. 1976;91:535.

171. Sambhi MP, Zimmerman HA. Pathologic physiology of Lutembacher syndrome. *Am J Cardiol*. 1958;2:681–686.

172. Mcginn S, White P. Interauricular septal defect associated with mitral stenosis. *Am Heart J*. 1933;9:1–13.

173. Marshall RJ, Warden HE. Mitral valve disease complicated by left-to-right shunt at atrial level. *Circulation*. 1964;29: 432–439.

174. Liberthson RR, Boucher CA, Fallon JT, Buckley MJ. Severe mitral regurgitation: a common occurrence in the aging patient with secundum atrial septal defect. *Clin Cardiol*. 1981;4: 229–232.

175. Chen CH, Lin SL, Hsu TL, Chen CC, Wang SP, Chang MS. Iatrogenic Lutembacher's syndrome after percutaneous transluminal mitral valvotomy. *Am Heart J*. 1990;119:209–211.

176. Bashi VV, Ravikumar E, Jairaj PS, Krishnaswami S, John S. Coexistent mitral valve disease with left-to-right shunt at the atrial level: clinical profile, hemodynamics, and surgical considerations in 67 consecutive patients. *Am Heart J*. 1987;114:1406–1414.

177. Opdyke DF, Brecher GA. Modifying effects of interatrial septal defect on the cardiodynamics of mitral stenosis. *Am J Physiol*. 1951;164:573–582.

178. Iga K, Tomonaga G, Hori K. Continuous murmur in Lutembacher syndrome analyzed by Doppler echocardiography. *Chest*. 1992; 101:565–566.

179. Ross Jr. J, Braunwald E, Mason DT, Braunwald NS, Morrow AG. Interatrial communications and left atrial hypertension: a cause of continuous murmur. *Circulation*. 1963;28:853–860.

180. Firkett CH. Examen anatomique d'un cas de persistance du trou ovale de botal, avec lésions valvulaires considérables du coeur gauche, chez une femme de 74 ans. *Ann Soc Méd Chir Liège*. 1880; 19:188.

181. Bland EF, Sweet RH. A venous shunt for advanced mitral stenosis. *JAMA*. 1949;140:1259–1265.

182. Rosenthal L. Atrial septal defect with mitral stenosis (Lutembacher's syndrome) in a woman of 81. *Br Med J*. 1956;2:1351.

183. Askey IM, Kahler IE. Longevity in extensive organic heart lesions: a case of Lutembacher's syndrome in a man aged 72. *Ann Intern Med*. 1950;33:1031–1036.

184. Sailer S. Mitral Stenosis with interauricular insufficiency. *Am J Pathol*. 1936;12(253):259–268.

185. Tandon R, Manchanda SC, Roy SB. Mitral stenosis with left-to-right shunt at atrial level. A diagnostic challenge. *Br Heart J*. 1971;33:773–781.

186. Ananthasubramaniam K, Iyer G, Karthikeyan V. Giant left atrium secondary to tight mitral stenosis leading to acquired Lutembacher syndrome: a case report with emphasis on role of echocardiography in assessment of Lutembacher syndrome. *J Am Soc Echocardiogr*. 2001;14:1033–1035.

187. Munoz-Armas S, Gorrin JR, Anselmi G, Hernandez PB, Anselmi A. Single atrium. Embryologic, anatomic, electrocardiographic and other diagnostic features. *Am J Cardiol*. 1968;21: 639–652.

188. Hung JS, Ritter DG, Feldt RH, Kincaid OW. Electrocardiographic and angiographic features of common atrium. *Chest*. 1973;63: 970–975.

189. Rastelli GC, Rahimtoola SH, Ongley PA, Mcgoon DC. Common atrium: anatomy, hemodynamics, and surgery. *J Thorac Cardiovasc Surg*. 1968;55:834–841.

190. De Leval MR, Ritter DG, Mcgoon DC, Danielson GK. Anomalous systemic venous connection. Surgical considerations. *Mayo Clin Proc*. 1975;50:599–610.

191. Shaher RM, Johnson AM. The haemodynamics of common atrium. *Guys Hosp Rep*. 1963;112:166–170.

192. Lynch JI, Perry LW, Takakuwa T, Scott 3rd LP. Congenital heart disease and chondroectodermal dysplasia. Report of two cases, one in a Negro. *Am J Dis Child*. 1968;115:80–87.

193. McKusick VA, Egeland JA, Eldridge R, Krusen DE. Dwarfism in the Amish I. The Ellis-van Creveld syndrome. *Bull Johns Hopkins Hosp*. 1964;115:306–336.

194. Da Silva EO, Janovitz D, De Albuquerque SC. Ellis-van Creveld syndrome: report of 15 cases in an inbred kindred. *J Med Genet*. 1980;17:349–356.

195. Taylor GA, Jordan CE, Dorst SK, Dorst JP. Polycarpaly and other abnormalities of the wrist in chondroectodermal dysplasia: the Ellis-van Creveld syndrome. *Radiology*. 1984;151:393–396.

196. Thomas Jr. HM, Spicer MJ, Nelson WP. Evaluation of P wave axis in distinguishing anatomical site of atrial septal defect. *Br Heart J*. 1973;35:738–742.

197. Wilson J, Baillie M. A description of a very unusual formation of the human heart. *Philosophical Transactions of the Royal Society of London*. 1798;88:346–356.

198. Edwards JE, Helmholz Jr. HF. A classification of total anomalous pulmonary venous connection based on developmental considerations. *Proc staff meet Mayo Clin*. 1956;31:151–160.

199. Delisle G, Ando M, Calder AL, et al. Total anomalous pulmonary venous connection: report of 93 autopsied cases with emphasis on diagnostic and surgical considerations. *Am Heart J*. 1976;91: 99–122.

200. Gathman GE, Nadas AS. Total anomalous pulmonary venous connection: clinical and physiologic observations of 75 pediatric patients. *Circulation*. 1970;42:143–154.

201. Lucas Jr. RV, Lock JE, Tandon R, Edwards JE. Gross and histologic anatomy of total anomalous pulmonary venous connections. *Am J Cardiol*. 1988;62:292–300.

202. Sherman FE, Bauersfeld SR. Total, uncomplicated, anomalous pulmonary venous connection: morphologic observations on 13 necropsy specimens from infants. *Pediatrics*. 1960;25:656–668.

203. Arciniegas E, Henry JG, Green EW. Stenosis of the coronary sinus ostium. An unusual site of obstruction in total anomalous pulmonary venous drainage. *J Thorac Cardiovasc Surg*. 1980;79: 303–305.

204. Becher MW, Rockenmacher S, Marin-Padilla M. Total anomalous pulmonary venous connection: persistence and atresia of the common pulmonary vein. *Pediatr Cardiol*. 1992;13:187–189.

205. Baron P, Gutgesell H, Hawkins E, McNamara D. Infradiaphragmatic total anomalous pulmonary venous connection in siblings. *Am Heart J*. 1982;104:1107–1109.

206. Solymar L, Sabel KG, Zetterqvist P. Total anomalous pulmonary venous connection in siblings. Report on three families. *Acta Paediatr Scand*. 1987;76:124–127.

207. Rodriguez Collado J, Attie F, Zabal C, et al. Total anomalous pulmonary venous connection in adults. Long-term follow-up. *J Thorac Cardiovasc Surg*. 1992;103:877–880.

208. Duff DF, Nihill MR, Vargo TA, Cooley DA. Infradiaphragmatic total anomalous pulmonary venous return. Diagnosis and surgical repair in a 10-year-old child. *Br Heart J.* 1975;37:1093–1096.

209. Mcmullan MH, Fyke 3rd FE. Total anomalous pulmonary venous connection: surgical correction in a 66-year-old man. *Ann Thorac Surg.* 1992;53:520–521, discussion 521–522.

210. Pastore JO, Akins CW, Zir LM, Buckley MJ, Dinsmore RE. Total anomalous pulmonary venous connection and severe pulmonic stenosis in a 52-year-old man. *Circulation.* 1977;55:206–209.

211. Mcmanus BM, Luetzeler J, Roberts WC. Total anomalous pulmonary venous connection: survival for 62 years without surgical intervention. *Am Heart J.* 1982;103:298–301.

212. Chen HY, Chen SJ, Li YW, et al. Esophageal varices in congenital heart disease with total anomalous pulmonary venous connection. *Int J Card Imaging.* 2000;16:405–409.

213. Freedom RM, Gerald PS. Congenital cardiac disease and the "cat eye" syndrome. *Am J Dis Child.* 1973;126:16–18.

214. Mcdermid HE, Duncan AM, Brasch KR, et al. Characterization of the supernumerary chromosome in cat eye syndrome. *Science.* 1986;232:646–648.

215. Schinzel A, Schmid W, Fraccaro M, et al. The "cat eye syndrome": dicentric small marker chromosome probably derived from a no.22 (tetrasomy 22pter to q11) associated with a characteristic phenotype. Report of 11 patients and delineation of the clinical picture. *Hum Genet.* 1981;57:148–158.

216. Whitaker W. Total pulmonary venous drainage through a persistent left superior vena cava. *Br Heart J.* 1954;16:177–188.

217. Chia BL, Tan NC, Tan LK. Total anomalous pulmonary venous drainage. Case presenting with prominent right supraclavicular thrill and loud continuous murmur. *Am J Cardiol.* 1974;34:850–853.

218. Krishnamoorthy KM. Images in cardiology: radiological findings in total anomalous pulmonary venous connection. *Heart.* 1999;82:696.

219. Genz T, Locher D, Genz S, Schumacher G, Buhlmeyer K. Chest x-ray film patterns in children with isolated total anomalous pulmonary vein connection. *Eur J Pediatr.* 1990;150:14–18.

220. Saxena A, Sharma M, Shrivastava S. Right lung agenesis with total anomalous pulmonary venous drainage. *Indian Heart J.* 1994;46:177–178.

221. Robinson AE, Chen JT, Bradford WD, Lester RG. Kerley B lines in total anomalous pulmonary venous connection below the diaphragm (type 3). *Am J Cardiol.* 1969;24:436–440.

222. Minich LA, Snider AR, Bove EL, Lupinetti FM, Vermilion RP. Echocardiographic evaluation of atrioventricular orifice anatomy in children with atrioventricular septal defect. *J Am Coll Cardiol.* 1992;19:149–153.

223. Piccoli GP, Gerlis LM, Wilkinson JL, Lozsadi K, Macartney FJ, Anderson RH. Morphology and classification of atrioventricular defects. *Br Heart J.* 1979;42:621–632.

224. Piccoli GP, Wilkinson JL, Macartney FJ, Gerlis LM, Anderson RH. Morphology and classification of complete atrioventricular defects. *Br Heart J.* 1979;42:633–639.

225. Edwards JE. The problem of mitral insufficiency caused by accessory chordae tendineae in persistent common atrioventricular canal. *Proc staff meet Mayo Clin.* 1960;35:299–305.

226. Gallo P, Formigari R, Hokayem NJ, et al. Left ventricular outflow tract obstruction in atrioventricular septal defects: a pathologic and morphometric evaluation. *Clin Cardiol.* 1991;14:513–521.

227. Sittiwangkul R, Ma RY, McCrindle BW, Coles JG, Smallhorn JF. Echocardiographic assessment of obstructive lesions in atrioventricular septal defects. *J Am Coll Cardiol.* 2001;38:253–261.

228. Mcelhinney DB, Reddy VM, Silverman NH, Hanley FL. Accessory and anomalous atrioventricular valvar tissue causing outflow tract obstruction: surgical implications of a heterogeneous and complex problem. *J Am Coll Cardiol.* 1998;32:1741–1748.

229. Cooke RA, Chambers JB, Curry PV. Doppler echocardiography of double orifice of the left atrioventricular valve in atrioventricular septal defect. *Int J Cardiol.* 1991;32:254–256.

230. Draulans-Noe HA, Wenink AC, Quaegebeur J. Single papillary muscle ("parachute valve") and double-orifice left ventricle in atrioventricular septal defect convergence of chordal attachment: surgical anatomy and results of surgery. *Pediatr Cardiol.* 1990;11:29–35.

231. Freedom RM, Bini M, Rowe RD. Endocardial cushion defect and significant hypoplasia of the left ventricle: a distinct clinical and pathological entity. *Eur J Cardiol.* 1978;7:263–281.

232. Pessotto R, Padalino M, Rubino M, Kadoba K, Buchler JR, Van PR. Straddling tricuspid valve as a sign of ventriculoatrial malalignment: A morphometric study of 19 postmortem cases. *Am Heart J.* 1999;138:1184–1195.

233. Brandenburg RO, Dushane JW. Clinical features of persistent common atrioventricular canal. *Proc staff meet Mayo Clin.* 1956;31:509–513.

234. Perloff JK, Harvey WP. Auscultatory and phonocardiographic manifestations of pure mitral regurgitation. *Prog Cardiovasc Dis.* 1962;5:172–194.

235. Shah CV, Patel MK, Hastreiter AR. Hemodynamics of complete atrioventricular canal and its evolution with age. *Am J Cardiol.* 1969;24:326–334.

236. Rowland TW, Nordstrom LG, Bean MS, Burkhardt H. Chronic upper airway obstruction and pulmonary hypertension in Down's syndrome. *Am J Dis Child.* 1981;135:1050–1052.

237. Spicer RL. Cardiovascular disease in Down syndrome. *Pediatr Clin North Am.* 1984;31:1331–1343.

238. Pueschel SM, Pueschel JK. *Biomedical concerns in persons with Down Syndrome.* Brookes Publishing Company. Baltimore; 1992.

239. Suzuki K, Yamaki S, Mimori S, et al. Pulmonary vascular disease in Down's syndrome with complete atrioventricular septal defect. *Am J Cardiol.* 2000;86:434–437.

240. Holmes LB. Genetic counseling for the older pregnant woman: new data and questions. *N Engl J Med.* 1978;298:1419–1421.

241. Emanuel R, Somerville J, Inns A, Withers R. Evidence of congenital heart disease in the offspring of parents with atrioventricular defects. *Br Heart J.* 1983;49:144–147.

242. Digilio MC, Marino B, Giannotti A, Dallapiccola B. Familial atrioventricular septal defect: possible genetic mechanism. *Br Heart J.* 1994;72:301.

243. Kumar A, Williams CA, Victorica BE. Familial atrioventricular septal defect: possible genetic mechanisms. *Br Heart J.* 1994;71:79–81.

244. Huggon IC, Cook AC, Smeeton NC, Magee AG, Sharland GK. Atrioventricular septal defects diagnosed in fetal life: associated cardiac and extra-cardiac abnormalities and outcome. *J Am Coll Cardiol.* 2000;36:593–601.

245. Tandon R, Moller JH, Edwards JE. Unusual longevity in persistent common atrioventricular canal. *Circulation.* 1974;50:619–626.

246. Zion MM, Rosenman D, Balkin J, Glaser J. Complete atrioventricular canal with survival to the eighth decade. *Chest.* 1984;85:437–438.

247. Hwang B, Hsieh KS, Meng CC. Importance of spontaneous closure of the ventricular part in atrioventricular septal defect. *Jpn Heart J.* 1992;33:205–211.

248. Pahl E, Park SC, Anderson RH. Spontaneous closure of the ventricular component of an atrioventricular septal defect. *Am J Cardiol.* 1987;60:1203–1205.

249. Baird PA, Sadovnick AD. Life expectancy in Down syndrome. *J Pediatr.* 1987;110:849–854.

250. Marino B, Vairo U, Corno A, et al. Atrioventricular canal in Down syndrome. Prevalence of associated cardiac malformations compared with patients without Down syndrome. *Am J Dis Child.* 1990;144:1120–1122.

251. Potter H. Review and hypothesis: Alzheimer disease and Down syndrome–chromosome 21 nondisjunction may underlie both disorders. *Am J Hum Genet.* 1991;48:1192–1200.

252. Van Camp G, Stinissen P, Van Hul W, et al. Selection of human chromosome 21-specific DNA probes for genetic analysis in Alzheimer's dementia and Down syndrome. *Hum Genet.* 1989;83:58–60.

253. Mito T, Pereyra PM, Becker LE. Neuropathology in patients with congenital heart disease and Down syndrome. *Pediatr Pathol.* 1991;11:867–877.

254. Friedman DL, Kastner T, Pond WS, O'Brien DR. Thyroid dysfunction in individuals with Down syndrome. *Arch Intern Med.* 1989;149:1990–1993.

255. Tandon R, Edwards JE. Cardiac malformations associated with Down's syndrome. *Circulation.* 1973;47:1349–1355.

256. Down JLH. Observations on an ethnic classification of idiots. *Clinical Lectures and Reports of the London Hospital.* 1866;3:259–262.

257. Garrod AE. On the association of cardiac malformations with other congenital defects. *Saint Bartholomew's Hospital reports.* 1894;30:53.

258. Abbott ME. New accessions in cardiac anomalies. Pulmonary atresia of inflammatory origin; persistent ostium primum with Mongolian idiocy. *Bulletin of the International Association of Medical Museums.* 1924;10:111–116.

259. Emanuel I, Huang SW, Yeh EK. Physical features of Chinese children with Down's syndrome. *Am J Dis Child.* 1968;115:461–468.

260. Brandenburg RO, Burchell HB, Toscano-Barbosa E. Electrocardiographic studies of cases with intracardiac malformations of the atrioventricular canal. *Proc Staff Meet Mayo Clin.* 1956;31: 513–523.

261. Jacobsen JR, Gillette PC, Corbett BN, Rabinovitch M, Mcnamara DG. Intracardiac electrography in endocardial cushion defects. *Circulation.* 1976;54:599–603.

262. Waldo AL, Kaiser GA, Bowman Jr. FO, Malm JR. Etiology of prolongation of the P-R interval in patients with an endocardial cushion defect. Further observations on internodal conduction and the polarity of the retrograde P wave. *Circulation.* 1973;48: 19–26.

263. Feldt RH, Dushane JW, Titus JL. The atrioventricular conduction system in persistent common atrioventricular canal defect: correlations with electrocardiogram. *Circulation.* 1970;42:437–444.

264. Perloff JK, Roberts NK, Cabeen Jr. WR. Left axis deviation: a reassessment. *Circulation.* 1979;60:12–21.

265. Lev M. The architecture of the conduction system in congenital heart disease. I. Common atrioventricular orifice. *AMA Arch Pathol.* 1958;65:174–191.

266. Horns JW, O'Loughlin BJ. Multiple manubrial ossification centers in Mongolism. *Am J Roentgenol Radium Ther Nucl Med.* 1965;93: 395–398.

267. Delisle MF, Sandor GG, Tessier F, Farquharson DF. Outcome of fetuses diagnosed with atrioventricular septal defect. *Obstet Gynecol.* 1999;94:763–767.

268. Allan LD. Atrioventricular septal defect in the fetus. *Am J Obstet Gynecol.* 1999;181:1250–1253.

269. Falcao S, Daliento L, Ho SY, Rigby ML, Anderson RH. Cross sectional echocardiographic assessment of the extent of the atrial septum relative to the atrioventricular junction in atrioventricular septal defect. *Heart.* 1999;81:199–205.

270. Greene AC, Kotler MN, Mintz GS. Isolated cleft mitral valve: rare cause of mitral regurgitation. *Journal of Cardiovascular Ultrasonography.* 1982;1:13–18.

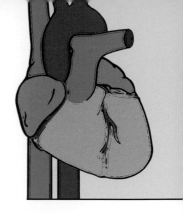

Chapter 16

Pulmonary Stenosis with Interatrial Communication

In 1769, Giovanni Battista Morgagni[1] described pulmonary stenosis with a patent foramen ovale, and in 1848, Thomas Peacock[2] published "Contraction of the Orifice of the Pulmonary Artery and Communication Between the Cavities of the Auricles by a Foramen Ovale."

Pulmonary stenosis with reversed interatrial shunt has been called the triologie de Fallot.[3] Right ventricular outflow obstruction resides in a stenotic mobile dome-shaped pulmonary valve (Figure 16-1) and is occasionally represented by stenosis of the pulmonary artery and its branches (Figure 16-2).[4-7] Infundibular obstruction takes the form of secondary hypertrophic subpulmonary stenosis (Figure 16-3).[8-11] The interatrial communication is by a patent foramen ovale or an ostium secundum atrial septal defect,[4,6,8,12-15] less commonly by an ostium primum[16] or sinus venosus atrial defect,[14] or much less commonly by anomalous pulmonary venous connection.[17] This chapter deals with pulmonary valve stenosis and a patent foramen ovale or a nonrestrictive ostium secundum atrial septal defect.[4]

Severe pulmonary valve stenosis with a right-to-left shunt through a patent foramen ovale is more common than pulmonary valve stenosis with a nonrestrictive atrial septal defect, irrespective of the direction of the shunt.[4] A *restrictive* interatrial communication is almost always a patent foramen ovale, the shunt is right-to-left, and pulmonary stenosis is necessarily severe.[4,18] A *nonrestrictive* interatrial communication is almost always an ostium secundum atrial septal defect, the shunt is left-to-right, and pulmonary stenosis is necessarily mild to moderate.[4-6,12]

The *physiologic consequences* of pulmonary stenosis with an interatrial communication depend on the degree of obstruction to right ventricular outflow and the size of the interatrial communication.[4,18] Patients with pulmonary stenosis and a *right-to-left* interatrial shunt (Figure 16-4) almost always have a severely stenotic pulmonary valve and a patent foramen ovale (see previous).[4] Patients with pulmonary stenosis and a *left-to-right* interatrial shunt almost always have a mild to moderate pulmonary valve stenosis and a nonrestrictive ostium secundum atrial septal defect (see previous).[4]

Severe pulmonary stenosis with right ventricular hypertrophy results in an increase in force of right atrial contraction (Figures 16-5 and 16-6) that generates a presystolic right-to-left interatrial shunt. High right atrial pressure stretches the margins of the foramen ovale and increases its patency. When right atrial blood escapes through the interatrial communication, pulmonary flow tends to fall reciprocally.

A nonrestrictive atrial septal defect with a large left-to-right shunt and mild to moderate pulmonary valve stenosis clinically resembles an isolated atrial septal defect (see Chapter 15). The small gradients generated by hyperkinetic right ventricular ejection across a normal pulmonary valve can generate a small gradient that should not be mistaken for mild pulmonary stenosis.

HISTORY

Familial pulmonary valve stenosis with atrial septal defect has been reported in a mother and her two children.[19] *Severe pulmonary stenosis with a right-to-left shunt across a patent foramen ovale* is clinically analogous to *isolated* severe pulmonary valve stenosis, except for cyanosis that can be present at birth[13,18] or can develop in childhood, puberty, or young adulthood.[6,8,13,20] Infants usually come to attention because of a murmur; although in neonates with pinpoint pulmonary valve stenosis (see Figure 16-1), the murmur is disarmingly soft. Symptoms can be appreciable even when cyanosis is mild[13,21] because right ventricular pressure can exceed systemic before the right-to-left interatrial shunt is established. However, among the author's patients are a teenager who became cyanotic only when he engaged in sports,[8] a woman with severe pulmonary stenosis and reversed interatrial shunt who was in good health until age 40 years,[14] and a woman with a gradient of 120 mm Hg who underwent surgical repair at age 58 years (see Figure 16-5).

Giddiness, light-headedness, and syncope are provoked by exertion. Large jugular venous A waves (see Figure 16-5) are sometimes subjectively sensed, especially after effort or excitement. Chest pain that resembles angina pectoris is attributed to ischemia in the high-pressure hypertrophied right ventricle. Death is usually from right ventricular failure and less commonly from hypoxia, cerebral abscess, or infective endocarditis.[5,6]

Mild to moderate pulmonary stenosis with a nonrestrictive atrial septal defect clinically resembles an isolated nonrestrictive ostium secundum atrial septal defect (see Chapter 15), except for the conspicuous murmur of pulmonary stenosis.[18] Relatively asymptomatic survival into the sixth and seventh decades is not uncommon. A 59-year-old man had a nonrestrictive sinus venosus defect and calcific pulmonary stenosis.[14]

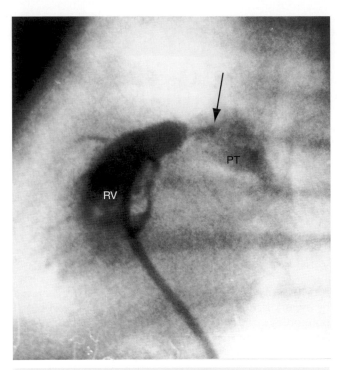

FIGURE 16-1 Lateral right ventricular angiocardiogram (RV) from a 2-day-old male with pinpoint pulmonary valve stenosis, reversed shunt through a patent foramen ovale, and tricuspid regurgitation. The arrow identifies a tiny jet into a dilated pulmonary trunk (PT).

PHYSICAL APPEARANCE

Retarded growth and development are consequences of right ventricular failure that begins in infancy or early childhood. Cyanosis associated with pulmonary stenosis and a patent foramen ovale can be obvious or evident only during exercise.[8,22,23] Mild or intermittent right-to-left shunts are sometimes manifested by highly colored cheeks or by distinctive erythema of the fingertips and toes (see Figure 16-4).[8,20,21] The central cyanosis of a right-to-left shunt must be distinguished from the peripheral cyanosis of diminished skin blood flow caused by the low cardiac output of severe pulmonary stenosis. Peripheral cyanosis is accompanied by cold hands and feet and tends to be more pronounced in the lower extremities. When skin blood flow is improved by warmth, peripheral cyanosis diminishes or may vanish, and central cyanosis becomes more evident.

Children with a nonrestrictive atrial septal defect and mild to moderate pulmonary stenosis may have a delicate gracile body habitus, with weight more affected than height (see Figure 15-14). Noonan's syndrome (see Figure 11-8C) is a distinctive appearance associated with dysplastic pulmonary valve stenosis that may coexist with an atrial septal defect.

ARTERIAL PULSE

In severe pulmonary stenosis with a right-to-left interatrial shunt, the systemic arterial pulse is small unless the reversed shunt is sufficient to maintain adequate left ventricular stroke volume. With the advent of right ventricular failure, the arterial pulse decreases despite right atrial blood shunted into the left side of the heart.

JUGULAR VENOUS PULSE

When pulmonary stenosis coexists with a nonrestrictive atrial septal defect, the hypertrophied right ventricle is less distensible, the right atrium contracts with greater force, and the A wave is prominent. The contour and height of the jugular pulse are determined by the presence and degree of pulmonary stenosis, not by the atrial

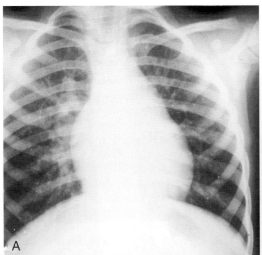
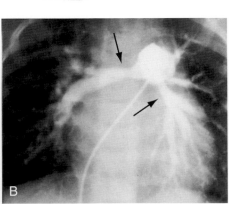

FIGURE 16-2 X-rays from a 5-year-old boy with stenosis of the pulmonary arterial branches (gradient, 50 mm Hg) and a 2.2 to 1 left-to-right shunt through an ostium secundum atrial septal defect. **A,** Posteroanterior projection shows vascular lung fields, moderate dilation of the pulmonary trunk, an inconspicuous ascending aorta, and a prominent right atrial convexity. **B,** Angiocardiogram with contrast material injected into the pulmonary trunk delineates stenoses of the right and left pulmonary arteries (arrows) with distal dilation.

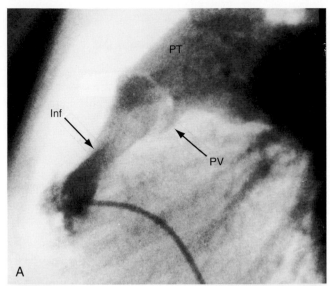

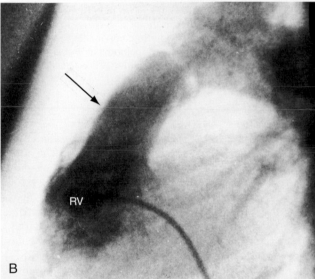

FIGURE 16-3 **A,** Lateral right ventricular angiocardiogram in a 5-year-old girl with severe mobile pulmonary valve stenosis (PV) and secondary dynamic systolic narrowing of the infundibulum (Inf). There was a 1.4 to 1 left-to-right shunt through an atrial septal defect despite suprasystemic right ventricular systolic pressure. The pulmonary trunk (PT) was dilated. **B,** Infundibular narrowing disappeared during diastole (arrow). (RV = right ventricle.)

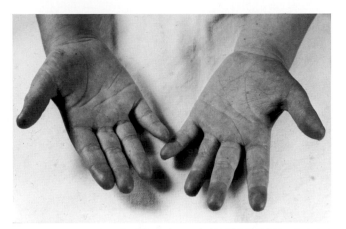

FIGURE 16-4 Red fingertips without cyanosis or clubbing in a 6-year-old boy with severe mobile pulmonary valve stenosis (gradient, 108 mm Hg), a small intermittent right-to-left shunt across a patent foramen ovale, and normal systemic arterial oxygen saturation.

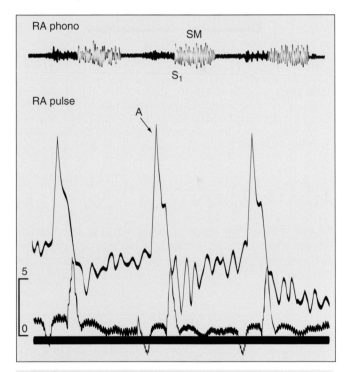

FIGURE 16-5 Tracings from a cyanotic woman who underwent surgical repair at age 58 years for severe mobile pulmonary valve stenosis (gradient, 120 mm Hg) with a reversed shunt through a patent foramen ovale. Large A waves (arrow) appear in the right atrium (RA). The right atrial intracardiac phonocardiogram (RA PHONO) recorded the holosystolic murmur (SM) of tricuspid regurgitation. A soft presystolic murmur is represented by vibrations just before the first heart sound (S_1).

defect. When pulmonary stenosis is severe enough to reverse the shunt, the jugular venous A wave is large, even giant (see Figures 16-5 and 16-6A). With the advent of right ventricular failure, the mean jugular venous pressure rises, and with it the V wave, especially if tricuspid regurgitation coexists.

PRECORDIAL MOVEMENT AND PALPATION

Pulmonary stenosis with a right-to-left interatrial shunt is associated with precordial palpation similar to severe *isolated* pulmonary valve stenosis (see Chapter 11). A nonrestrictive atrial septal defect with mild to moderate pulmonary stenosis is associated with precordial signs similar to an isolated atrial septal defect of equivalent size, except for a systolic thrill of coexisting pulmonary valve stenosis.[23]

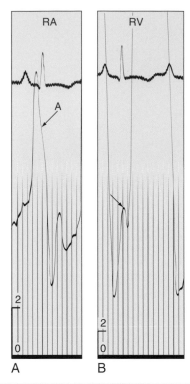

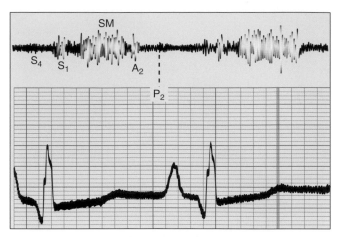

FIGURE 16-7 Phonocardiogram from the second left intercostal space of a 5-month-old cyanotic female with severe mobile pulmonary valve stenosis, a right-to-left shunt across a patent foramen ovale, and suprasystemic right ventricular systolic pressure. The fourth heart sound (S_4) in the first cycle became a short presystolic murmur in the next cycle. A long systolic murmur (SM) goes up to the aortic component of the second heart sound (A_2). The pulmonary component (P_2) is late and diminutive (arrow). Tall peaked right atrial P waves appear in lead 2 of the electrocardiogram.

FIGURE 16-6 Right atrial (RA) and right ventricular (RV) pressure pulses from a 15-month-old cyanotic male with severe mobile pulmonary valve stenosis (gradient, 105 mm Hg) and a right-to-left shunt across a patent foramen ovale. A, Large A waves (arrow) appear in the right atrial pressure pulse. B, The large A wave was transmitted into the right ventricle (RV) as presystolic distention (arrow).

AUSCULTATION

Severe pulmonary valve stenosis with a right-to-left interatrial shunt is accompanied by auscultatory signs analogous to isolated severe pulmonary stenosis (see Chapter 11). The systolic murmur is maximal in the second left intercostal space (Figure 16-7); radiates upward and to the left; extends up to or beyond the aortic component of the second heart sound, which it obscures (Figures 16-7 and 16-8A and D);[24] and has a late systolic peak with a kite-shaped configuration.[24,25] In neonates with critical pulmonary valve stenosis and right ventricular failure, the murmur is short and soft (see previous), and the pulmonary component of the second heart sound is delayed, soft, or absent (see Figures 16-7 and 16-8D). The most prominent auscultatory sign is then a holosystolic murmur of tricuspid regurgitation (see Figure 16-5).

Presystolic distention of the right ventricle (see Figure 16-6B) is accompanied by a fourth heart sound

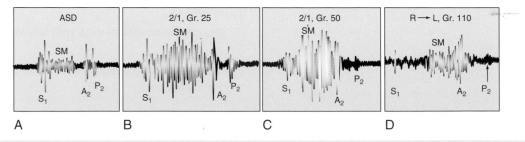

FIGURE 16-8 Phonocardiograms from the second left intercostal space of four patients whose malformations include an isolated atrial septal defect (ASD) and atrial septal defects with mild, moderate, or severe pulmonary valve stenosis. A, Isolated atrial septal defect (ASD) with 2.5 to 1 left-to-right shunt. The short soft systolic murmur (SM) ends well before both components of the split second heart sound. B, Atrial septal defect with a 2 to 1 left-to-right shunt and a 25–mm Hg gradient across a stenotic pulmonary valve. The systolic murmur is relatively loud and long and goes up to but does not obscure the aortic component of the second heart sound. The splitting is wider because pulmonary closure is more delayed. C, Atrial septal defect with a 2 to 1 left-to-right shunt and 50–mm Hg gradient across a stenotic pulmonary valve. The loud long systolic murmur extends beyond the aortic component of the second heart sound. The pulmonary component is soft and even later. D, Severe pulmonary valve stenosis (gradient, 110 mm Hg) with a right-to-left shunt through a patent foramen ovale. A kite-shaped systolic murmur envelopes the aortic component of the second sound. The pulmonary component is delayed and diminutive. (A_2 = aortic component; P_2 = pulmonary component.)

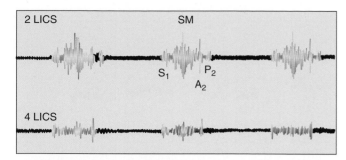

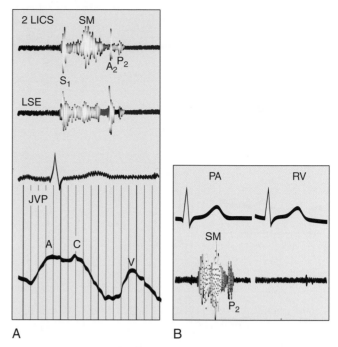

A   B

FIGURE 16-9 Phonocardiogram from a 23-year-old man with a 2.4 to 1 left-to-right shunt through an ostium secundum atrial septal defect and a 45–mm Hg gradient across a mobile stenotic pulmonary valve. The first heart sound (S_1) is normal. A prominent crescendo-decrescendo systolic murmur (SM) is maximal in the second left intercostal space (2 LICS) and goes up to but does not envelope the aortic component of the second heart sound (A_2). The pulmonary component (P_2) is delayed and soft. (4 LICS = fourth left intercostal space.)

FIGURE 16-10 Phonocardiograms from a 6-year-old girl with a 2.3 to 1 left-to-right shunt through an ostium secundum atrial septal defect and a 25–mm Hg gradient across a mobile stenotic pulmonary valve. **A,** The prominent crescendo-decrescendo systolic murmur (SM) in the second left intercostal space (2 LICS) ends before the aortic component of the second heart sound (A_2). The pulmonary component (P_2) is moderately delayed and relatively soft. The systolic murmur is shorter and softer at the lower left sternal edge (LSE) where both components of the split second heart sound are recorded. The jugular venous pulse (JVP) exhibits a small dominant A wave and a blunted X descent (lower tracing). **B,** Intracardiac phonocardiogram from within the main pulmonary artery (PA) recorded a prominent crescendo-decrescendo systolic murmur (SM) that ends before pulmonary valve closure (P_2). The murmur vanished when the microphone was withdrawn into the right ventricle (RV).

that is occasionally long enough to qualify as a murmur (see Figures 16-5 and 16-7). A short presystolic murmur is also generated when powerful right atrial contraction forces blood across a restrictive patent foramen ovale. A large right atrial A wave that is transmitted into the right ventricle (see Figure 16-6) can exceed the diastolic pressure in the main pulmonary artery, open the pulmonary valve, and generate presystolic flow and a presystolic murmur.

When a nonrestrictive atrial septal defect is associated with mild to moderate pulmonary stenosis, the auscultatory signs resemble an isolated nonrestrictive ostium secundum atrial septal defect with three exceptions: 1, an ejection sound is generated by the mobile stenotic pulmonary valve; 2, the pulmonary systolic murmur is loud and long (Figures 16-9 and 16-10); and 3, the second heart sound is more widely split because of a greater delay in the pulmonary component (see Figures 16-8B and C, 16-9, and 16-10). The more severe the pulmonary stenosis, the later and softer the pulmonary component of the second heart sound (see Figures 16-7 and 16-8).

Stenosis of the pulmonary artery and its branches with an ostium secundum atrial septal defect (Figure 16-11) is accompanied by conspicuously wide thoracic distribution of systolic murmurs because the murmurs of pulmonary artery stenosis are reinforced by hyperkinetic pulmonary blood flow of the atrial septal defect. Persistent splitting of the second heart sound is the result of the atrial septal defect (see Figure 16-11).

ELECTROCARDIOGRAM

In *pulmonary valve stenosis with a right-to-left interatrial shunt*, the electrocardiogram is similar to that of severe isolated pulmonary stenosis (Figures 16-12 and 16-13; see Chapter 11).[26] Peaked right atrial P waves appear in lead 2 and in right precordial leads (see Figures 16-7, 16-12, and 16-13) and occasionally are exceptionally tall (see Figures 16-7 and 16-12).[8,22] P wave duration in lead 2 is prolonged when a large right atrium writes the

terminal inscription of the P wave.[27] Right axis deviation (see Figure 16-12) can be extreme (see Figure 16-13). The terminal force of the QRS can be prolonged and slurred (see Figure 16-13). Right ventricular hypertrophy caused by suprasystemic right ventricular systolic pressure is manifested by R waves of great amplitude in right and mid precordial leads with upward convexity of ST segments and deeply inverted T waves, together with deep left precordial S waves (see Figures 16-12 and 16-13).[26] The striking ST segment and T wave patterns sometimes extend to lead V_4. Small q waves appear in lead V_1 (see Figure 16-13) when the precordial electrode topographically overlies a large right atrium (see Chapter 13).

In *a nonrestrictive atrial septal defect with a left-to-right shunt and mild to moderate pulmonary stenosis*, the electrocardiogram is a combination of isolated ostium secundum atrial septal defect (see Chapter 15) and the right ventricular hypertrophy of pulmonary stenosis (Figures 16-14 and 16-15). P waves can be peaked and

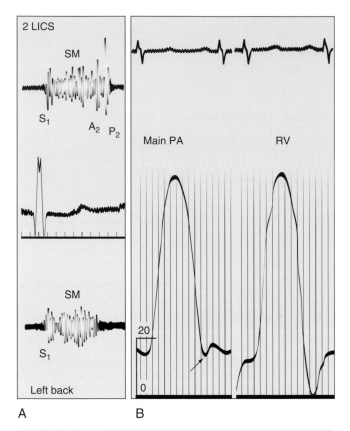

FIGURE 16-11 Tracings from a 5-year-old boy with bilateral *pulmonary artery stenosis* (gradient, 50 mm Hg), an ostium secundum atrial septal defect, and a 2.2 to 1 left-to-right shunt. **A,** The phonocardiograms show systolic murmurs (SM) of approximately equal intensity in the second left intercostal space (2 LICS) and in the left back. Persistent splitting of the second heart sound (A_2/P_2) was the result of the atrial septal defect. **B,** Pressure pulse in the main pulmonary artery (PA) shows the characteristic contour of bilateral stenosis of the pulmonary arterial branches, with a steep rise and a rapid fall to a low dicrotic notch (arrow). The right ventricular pulse (RV) is for comparison.

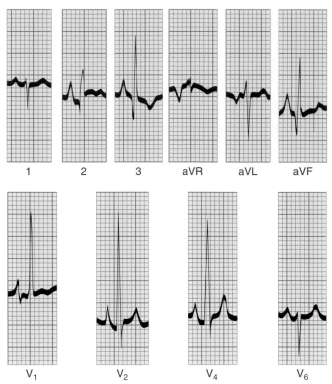

FIGURE 16-12 Electrocardiogram from the 5-month-old cyanotic female referred to in Figure 16-7 with severe pulmonary valve stenosis and a right-to-left shunt across a patent foramen ovale. Tall peaked right atrial P waves appropriate for the 20–mm Hg A wave in the right atrium appear in leads 2, 3, aVF, and V_{1-4}. Right axis deviation and right ventricular hypertrophy are manifested by tall monophasic R waves in leads V_{1-4} and a deep S wave in lead V_6, findings appropriate for suprasystemic right ventricular systolic pressure.

moderately tall (see Figure 16-14). The QRS axis is vertical or rightward (see Figures 16-14 and 16-15). Terminal force prolongation widens the R wave in lead aVR and widens the S waves in leads 1, aVL, and V_6 (see Figures 16-14 and 16-15). The rsR prime in lead V_1 is characterized by a relatively small *s* wave and a relatively tall *R* prime compared with an atrial septal defect without pulmonary stenosis (see Figures 16-14 and 16-15).

X-RAY

Nonrestrictive atrial septal defects with mild to moderate pulmonary stenosis have x-rays indistinguishable from isolated ostium secundum defects (Figure 16-16).[28] *Severe pulmonary stenosis with a right-to-left interatrial shunt through a patent foramen ovale* is associated with an x-ray that resembles that of isolated severe pulmonary valve stenosis (Figure 16-17; see Chapter 11). Lung fields are oligemic because right atrial blood is shunted away

from the lungs across the atrial septum. The reduced right ventricular output and pulmonary blood flow become even more apparent with the advent of right ventricular failure. The pulmonary trunk is dilated (Figures 16-1, 16-3, 16-17, and 16-18) for reasons analogous to dilation in isolated mobile pulmonary valve stenosis (see Chapter 11).[5,8] Heart size is increased because of enlargement of the right atrium and right ventricle (see Figures 16-17 and 16-18).[8,13] The right ventricular apex is not boot-shaped as in Fallot's tetralogy because the size of the left ventricle is not reduced (see Figure 16-17; see Chapter 18).

ECHOCARDIOGRAM

Mobile pulmonary valve stenosis with a right-to-left shunt through a patent foramen ovale is associated with an echocardiogram similar to isolated severe pulmonary valve stenosis (see Chapter 11). Color flow imaging records a high-velocity jet directed toward the left pulmonary artery (Figure 16-19A and Videos 16-1A through 16-1C), and continuous-wave Doppler scan establishes the peak velocity and the gradient (Figure 16-19B). Two-dimensional imaging identifies the patent foramen ovale with its valve

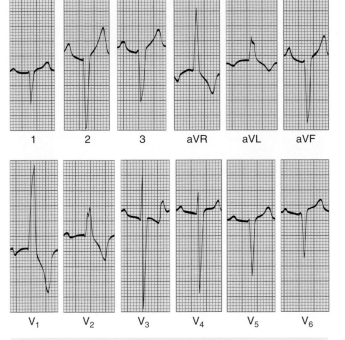

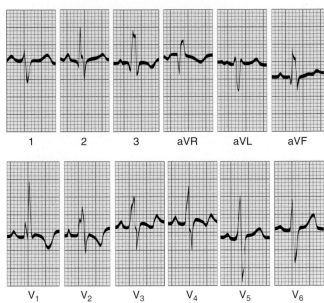

FIGURE 16-13 Electrocardiogram from a 20-year-old man with severe mobile pulmonary valve stenosis (gradient, 110 mm Hg) and a right-to-left shunt through a patent foramen ovale. A tall right atrial P wave appears in lead 2. Small q waves in right precordial leads are evidence of right atrial enlargement. The PR interval is prolonged. Right ventricular hypertrophy is reflected in striking right axis deviation, tall monophasic R wave, and deeply inverted T wave in V_1 and deep S waves in mid to left precordial leads.

FIGURE 16-14 Electrocardiogram from an 18-year-old man with a 2 to 1 left-to-right shunt through an ostium secundum atrial septal defect and a 25–mm Hg gradient across a mobile stenotic pulmonary valve. The P waves in lead 2 and in leads V_{2-4} are peaked but not tall. Right ventricular hypertrophy is manifested by right axis deviation, a tall R prime in lead V_1, and deep S waves in leads V_{5-6}. Prolongation of the terminal portion of the QRS axis in lead aVR is appropriate for the atrial septal defect.

(see Chapter 15), and color flow imaging confirms the right-to-left shunt.

A nonrestrictive ostium secundum atrial septal defect with mild to moderate pulmonary valve stenosis is associated with an echocardiogram similar to that of an isolated atrial septal defect of the same location and size (see Chapter 15), except for coexisting pulmonary stenosis. Real-time imaging identifies the mobile stenotic pulmonary valve, and Doppler interrogation establishes the gradient (Figure 16-20).

SUMMARY

Pulmonary valve stenosis with a right-to-left shunt through a patent foramen ovale is accompanied by a conspicuous systolic murmur, except for the disarmingly soft murmur of pinpoint pulmonary valve stenosis and right ventricular failure. Mild or intermittent cyanosis or digital erythema precedes persistent cyanosis. Symptoms can be appreciable even when cyanosis is mild. Giddiness, lightheadedness, and syncope are typically related to effort. Physical underdevelopment coincides with the catabolic effects of right ventricular failure. Large A waves in the jugular venous pulse are in contrast to the small systemic arterial pulse. The right ventricular impulse is strong

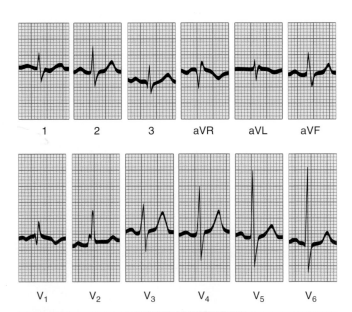

FIGURE 16-15 Electrocardiogram from the 23-year-old man referred to in Figure 16-9 with a 2.4 to 1 left-to-right shunt through an ostium secundum atrial septal defect and a 45–mm Hg gradient across a mobile stenotic pulmonary valve. The normal P waves, the vertical QRS axis, the rsR prime in lead V_1, and the slight prolongation of the terminal force in leads V_1 and aVR are appropriate for the atrial septal defect.

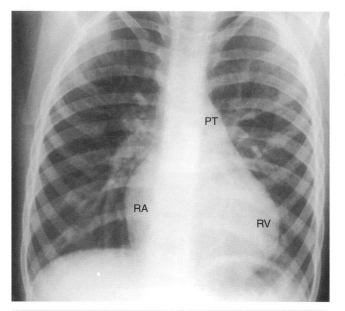

FIGURE 16-16 X-ray from a 10-year-old girl with a 2.1 to 1 left-to-right shunt through an ostium secundum atrial septal defect and a 25–mm Hg gradient across a mobile stenotic pulmonary valve. The x-ray closely resembles that of an isolated ostium secundum atrial septal defect with increased pulmonary blood flow, a dilated pulmonary trunk (PT), an inconspicuous ascending aorta, a prominent right atrium (RA), and an enlarged right ventricle (RV).

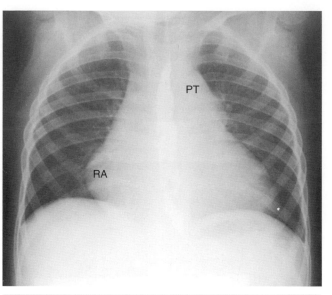

FIGURE 16-18 X-ray from a 30-month-old cyanotic male with severe mobile pulmonary valve stenosis, a right ventricular systolic pressure of 130 mm Hg, and a right-to-left shunt through a patent foramen ovale. The pulmonary trunk (PT) is dilated. Appreciable right atrial enlargement (RA) was the result of severe tricuspid regurgitation.

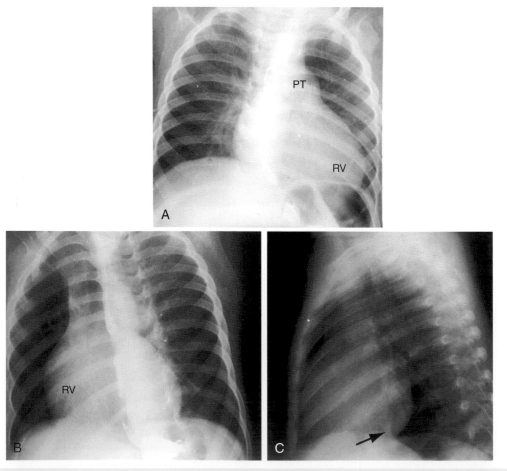

FIGURE 16-17 X-rays from the 15-month-old cyanotic male referred to in Figure 16-6 with severe mobile pulmonary valve stenosis, suprasystemic right ventricular systolic pressure, and a right-to left shunt through a patent foramen ovale. A, The pulmonary trunk (PT) is dilated. An enlarged right ventricle (RV) occupies the apex. B, The left anterior oblique shows a dilated right ventricle (RV) displacing the left ventricle posteriorly. C, In this lateral projection, the normal location of the inferior vena cava (arrow) at the junction of the left ventricle and diaphragm indicates that the left ventricle in not enlarged.

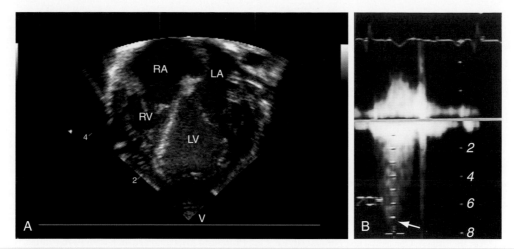

FIGURE 16-19 A, A 28-year-old woman with severe mobile pulmonary valve stenosis and a right-to-left shunt through a patent foramen ovale. The high-velocity jet across the pulmonary valve (PV) traverses the pulmonary trunk (PT) and enters the left pulmonary artery (LPA). **B,** Continuous wave Doppler scan across the pulmonary valve records a velocity of 7.0 msec, which indicates an astonishing peak instantaneous gradient of 190 mm Hg (Videos 16-1A through 16-1C). (Ao = aorta.)

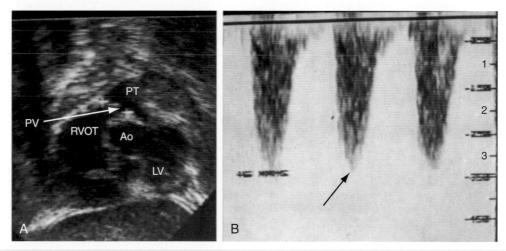

FIGURE 16-20 Echocardiogram with Doppler interrogation from a 7-year-old girl with mobile pulmonary valve stenosis and a left-to-right shunt through an ostium secundum atrial septal defect. **A,** Subcostal view shows the stenotic pulmonary valve (PV) above a well-formed right ventricular outflow tract (RVOT). The pulmonary trunk (PT) is dilated. **B,** Continuous-wave Doppler scan across the stenotic pulmonary valve records a peak velocity (arrow) of 3.4 msec, which indicates a peak instantaneous gradient of 46 mm Hg. (Ao = aorta; LV = left ventricle.)

and sustained and is accompanied by presystolic distention and a systolic thrill in the second left intercostal space. A pulmonary ejection sound precedes the pulmonary stenotic murmur, which is loud and long and extends up to or beyond the aortic component of the second heart sound. The pulmonary component is delayed, soft, or inaudible. Right atrial P waves can be strikingly tall, and right axis deviation can be extreme. Right precordial leads show R waves of great amplitude followed by upward convexity of the ST segments and deep inversion of the T waves, and left precordial leads exhibit deep S waves and upright T waves. The lungs are oligemic, the pulmonary trunk is dilated, the ascending aorta is inconspicuous, and the cardiac silhouette reflects enlargement of the right atrium and right ventricle. Real-time

echocardiography identifies the mobile stenotic pulmonary valve, Doppler interegation determines the gradient, and color flow imaging detects the right-to-left shunt across a patent foramen ovale.

Nonrestrictive atrial septal defect with left-to-right shunt and mild to moderate pulmonary stenosis clinically resembles an isolated ostium secundum atrial septal defect, although the malformation announces itself early because of the prominent pulmonary stenotic murmur. The jugular venous pulse shows a dominant A wave rather than equal A and V crests. The right ventricular impulse is dynamic, and a pulmonary stenotic thrill is consistent. Auscultatory signs are a combination of isolated ostium secundum atrial septal defect and mobile pulmonary valve stenosis. A pulmonary ejection sound introduces a relatively long loud pulmonary stenotic murmur, and fixed splitting of the second heart sound is associated with a more delayed and softer pulmonary component. The electrocardiogram shows right ventricular hypertrophy inappropriate for an isolated atrial septal defect. The x-ray and echocardiogram resemble isolated ostium secundum atrial septal defect except for the pulmonic stenotic Doppler gradient.

REFERENCES

1. Morgagni J. *Seats and causes of diseases.* London: Millar & Cadell in the Strand and Johnson & Payne in Pater-Noster Row; 1769.
2. Peacock T. Contraction of the orifice of the pulmonary artery and communication between the cavities of the auricles by the foramen ovale. *Transactions of the Pathological Society of London.* 1848;1:200.
3. Joly F, Carlotti J, Sicot JR, Piton A. Congenital heart disease. II. Fallot's trilogies. *Arch Mal Coeur Vaiss.* 1950;43:687–704.
4. Roberts WC, Shemin RJ, Kent KM. Frequency and direction of interatrial shunting in valvular pulmonic stenosis with intact ventricular septum and without left ventricular inflow or outflow obstruction. An analysis of 127 patients treated by valvulotomy. *Am Heart J.* 1980;99:142–148.
5. Selzer A, Carnes WH. The types of pulmonary stenosis and their clinical recognition. *Mod Concepts Cardiovasc Dis.* 1949;18:45.
6. Selzer A, Carnes WH, et al. The syndrome of pulmonary stenosis with patent foramen ovale. *Am J Med.* 1949;6:3–23.
7. Shafter HA, Bliss HA. Pulmonary artery stenosis. *Am J Med.* 1959; 26:517–526.
8. Campbell M. Simple pulmonary stenosis; pulmonary valvular stenosis with a closed ventricular septum. *Br Heart J.* 1954;16:273–300.
9. Johnson AM. Hypertrophic infundibular stenosis complicating simple pulmonary valve stenosis. *Br Heart J.* 1959;21:429–439.
10. Little JB, Lavender JP, Desanctis RW. The narrow infundibulum in pulmonary valvular stenosis: its preoperative diagnosis by angiocardiography. *Circulation.* 1963;28:182–189.
11. White PD, Hurst JW, Fennell RH. Survival to the age of seventy-five years with congenital pulmonary stenosis and patent foramen ovale. *Circulation.* 1950;2:558–564.
12. Arnett EN, Aisner SC, Lewis KB, Tecklenberg P, Brawley RK, Roberts WC. Pulmonic valve stenosis, atrial septal defect and left-to-right interatrial shunting with intact ventricular septum. A distinct hemodynamic-morphologic syndrome. *Chest.* 1980;78: 759–762.
13. Engle MA, Taussig HB. Valvular pulmonic stenosis with intact ventricular septum and patent foramen ovale; report of illustrative cases and analysis of clinical syndrome. *Circulation.* 1950;2: 481–493.
14. Hardy WE, Gnoj J, Ayres SM, Giannelli Jr S, Christianson LC. Pulmonic stenosis and associated atrial septal defects in older patients. Report of three cases, including one with calcific pulmonic stenosis. *Am J Cardiol.* 1969;24:130–134.
15. Ordway NK, Levy 2nd L, Hyman AL, Bagnetto RL. Pulmonary stenosis with patent foramen ovale. *Am Heart J.* 1950;40:271–284.
16. Rudolph AM, Nadas AS, Goodale WT. Intracardiac left-to-right shunt with pulmonic stenosis. *Am Heart J.* 1954;48:808–816.
17. Neptune WB, Bailey CP, Goldberg H. The surgical correction of atrial septal defects associated with transposition of the pulmonary veins. *J Thorac Surg.* 1953;25:623–634.
18. De Castro CM, Nelson WP, Jones RC, Hall RJ, Hopeman AR, Jahnke EJ. Pulmonary stenosis: cyanosis, interatrial communication and inadequate right ventricular distensibility following pulmonary valvotomy. *Am J Cardiol.* 1970;26:540–543.
19. Ciuffo AA, Cunningham E, Traill TA. Familial pulmonary valve stenosis, atrial septal defect, and unique electrocardiogram abnormalities. *J Med Genet.* 1985;22:311–313.
20. Abrahams DG, Wood P. Pulmonary stenosis with normal aortic root. *Br Heart J.* 1951;13:519–548.
21. Silverman BK, Nadas AS, Wittenborg MH, Goodale WT, Gross RE. Pulmonary stenosis with intact ventricular septum; correlation of clinical and physiologic data, with review of operative results. *Am J Med.* 1956;20:53–64.
22. Allanby K, Campbell M. Congenital pulmonary stenosis with closed ventricular septum. *Guys Hosp Rep.* 1949;98:18.
23. Evans JR, Rowe RD, Keith JD. The clinical diagnosis of atrial septal defect in children. *Am J Med.* 1961;30:345–356.
24. Vogelpoel L, Schrire V. Auscultatory and phonocardiographic assessment of pulmonary stenosis with intact ventricular septum. *Circulation.* 1960;22:55.
25. Gamboa R, Hugenholtz PG, Nadas AS. Accuracy of the phonocardiogram in assessing severity of aortic and pulmonic stenosis. *Circulation.* 1964;30:35–46.
26. Burch GE, Depasquale NP. The electrocardiogram, vectorcardiogram and ventricular gradient in combined pulmonary stenosis and interatrial communication. *Am J Cardiol.* 1961;7:646–656.
27. Macruz R, Perloff JK, Case RB. A method for the electrocardiographic recognition of atrial enlargement. *Circulation.* 1958;17: 882–889.
28. Magidson O, Cosby RS, Dimitroff SP, Levinso DC, Griffith GC. Pulmonary stenosis with left to right shunt. *Am J Med.* 1954;17: 311–321.

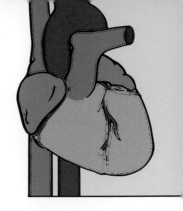

Chapter 17

Ventricular Septal Defect

In 1879, Henri Roger wrote, "A developmental defect of the heart occurs from which cyanosis does not ensue in spite of the fact that a communication exists between the cavities of the two ventricles and in spite of the fact that admixture of venous blood and arterial blood occurs. This congenital defect, which is even compatible with a long life, is a simple one. It comprises a defect in the interventricular septum."[1]

Roger went on to say that at necropsy, "The ventricular walls show no alteration, but in the upper portion of the interventricular septum beneath the mitral valve is an orifice which establishes a communication between the two ventricles."[1] And still further, "Among the congenital defects of the heart compatible with life and perhaps a long one, one of the most frequent which I have encountered . . . is the communication between the two ventricles because of failure of occlusion of the interventricular septum."[1]

Ventricular septal defects remain the most common congenital malformation of the heart, occurring in 50% of children with congenital heart disease.[2] Detection has increased dramatically with advances in imaging and with the facility of echocardiographic diagnosis in neonates, with spontaneous closure and detection of small defects in the muscular trabecular septum taken into account.[3,4] A comprehensive review estimated the median incidence rate of ventricular septal defects to be 2,829 per million live births[5]; the defects are found to be the most common gross morphologic congenital malformation of the heart and circulation in adults, except for the bicuspid aortic valve.[3,6–8]

Although Roger believed that "this congenital defect . . . is a simple one,"[1] there is still no uniform consensus on how best to characterize and classify the diverse types of defects to which the ventricular septum is subject. The ventricular septum is a complex nonplanar partition whose components are best defined according to anatomic landmarks on the right side of the septal surface (Figure 17-1).[9–12] Defects are classified according to their relationship to the membranous, inlet, trabecular, and infundibular septum.[2,12] The *membranous septum* is divided by the tricuspid annulus into ventriculoatrial and interventricular components that abut the three major segments of the muscular septum: namely, the *inlet septum*, which is lightly trabeculated; the *trabecular septum*, which is, as the name implies, heavily trabeculated; and the *infundibular septum*, which is nontrabeculated. The inlet septum is limited by the tensor attachments

of the tricuspid valve and is so named according to its location. The trabecular septum lies between the inlet septum and the infundibular septum (see Figure 17-1). *Atrioventricular conduction tissue* penetrates the ventriculoatrial portion of the membranous septum. The His bundle and bundle branches run beneath the deficient interventricular component of the membranous septum close to the free edge of the ventricular septal defect.[10,13]

Approximately 80% of ventricular septal defects are *perimembranous*. The prefix *peri* underscores extension into adjacent portions of the inlet, trabecular, and infundubular septum. Large perimembranous defects encroach upon all three portions of the muscular septum (Figure 17-2A). *Muscular ventricular septal defects* are prevalent in neonates, with estimates as high as 53 of every 1000 live births. Approximately 90% of the defects close spontaneously within the first 10 months of life.

The most common types of *muscular* defects lie within the trabecular septum.[10,14,15] These malformations are more apparent on the *left* septal surface and vary from small to large, from single to multiple (Figure 17-3), to a honeycombed or Swiss cheese–like structure with sieve-like fenestrations, to tortuous sinusoidal tracks threaded among septal trabeculae without through-and-through perforations.[10,15] Sieve-like fenestrations or multiple small muscular defects have the net functional effect of a single large defect.

Isolated defects in the *inlet septum* represent approximately 8% of ventricular septal defects at surgery.[16] An inlet ventricular septal defect that is bordered entirely by myocardium differs from an inlet defect that involves the basal portion of the septum near the crux where it is partially bordered by bridging atrioventricular valve tissue (see Chapter 15).[10–12]

The *infundibular septum* is represented by a small portion of muscle interposed between the outflow components of the left and right ventricles.[17] A sleeve of subpulmonary infundibulum supports the leaflets of the pulmonary valve and separates the right ventricular outflow tract from the surface of the heart rather than from the left ventricular outflow track. Ventricular septal defects in the infundibular septum are also called supracristal, subpulmonary, subarterial, or doubly committed and account for approximately 5% to 7% of ventricular septal defects in North America and Western Europe, but for approximately 30% in Asian patients.[14,16,17] Infundibular septal defects can be entirely muscular or can be partially rimmed by semilunar valve tissue (subarterial). Defects

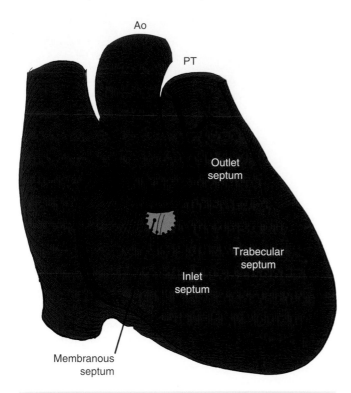

FIGURE 17-1 The four major components of the ventricular septum from the right ventricular aspect. The membranous septum borders on the outlet septum, the trabecular septum, and the inlet septum. (Ao = aorta; PT = pulmonary trunk.) *(Modified from Anderson RH, Becker AE, Lucchese FE, Meier MA, Rigby ML, Soto B. Morphology of congenital heart disease. Baltimore: University Park Press; 1983.)*

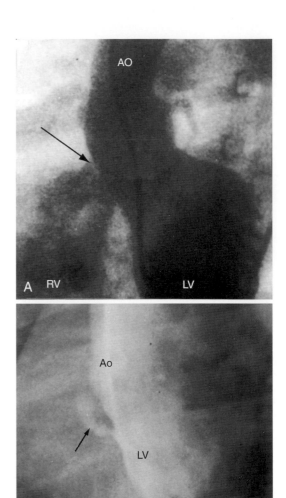

FIGURE 17-2 **A,** Left anterior oblique left ventriculogram from a 4-year-old boy with a moderately restrictive perimembranous ventricular septal defect (arrow). (RV = right ventricle; LV = left ventricle; AO = aorta.) **B,** Left anterior oblique left ventriculogram from a 21-year-old man with a tiny perimembranous ventricular septal defect (arrow).

are considered *doubly committed subarterial* when little or no muscle is interposed between the outflow components of the left and right ventricles and when there is absence of the septal component of the subpulmonary infundibulum, so the aortic and pulmonary leaflets are in fibrous continuity.[10,12,14,16,17] Doubly committed subarterial defects lie immediately beneath the valves of both arterial trunks, so the left and right coronary cusps of the aortic valve tend to prolapse into the outflow tract of the right ventricle (see section on Ventricular Septal Defect with Aortic Regurgitation). Much less commonly, a pulmonary cusp prolapses through the defect.[18]

Atrioventricular septal malalignment necessarily involves an inlet ventricular septal defect and is usually accompanied by straddling of the tensor apparatus of an atrioventricular valve that inserts (straddles) onto both sides of the ventricular septum.[19] So-called *Eisenmenger's malalignment* is represented by a perimembranous ventricular septal defect with anterior deviation of the infundibular septum.[20] Not relevant to this chapter is *malalignment between infundibular and trabecular septum* that is associated with Fallot's tetralogy (see Chapter 18) or much less commonly with coarctation of the aorta (see Chapter 8).

Henri Roger did not anticipate spontaneous closure. "The pathologic state of the heart existing before birth and consisting of an arrest of development is not susceptible to favorable changes, either by spontaneous evolution or by

medical or surgical intervention."[1] However, in 1918, two reports speculated that ventricular septal defects might undergo spontaneous closure.[21,22] One report was entitled "The Possibility of a Loud Congenital Heart Murmur Disappearing When a Child Grows Up."[21] The other report carried the title "Can the Clinical Manifestations of Congenital Heart Disease Disappear with the General Growth and Development of the Patient?"[22] However, four decades elapsed before spontaneous closure was firmly documented.[23–29] In 1960, Paul Wood wrote, "In any large series of geriatric necropsies . . . atrial septal defect is always well represented, but where's the maladie de Roger? Assuming it does not provide immortality, it must either close spontaneously in middle life or have long since run its mortal course."[30]

A defect may remain anatomically open but functionally closed (i.e., with absent or negligible shunt; Figures 17-2B and 17-4). The tendency for ventricular

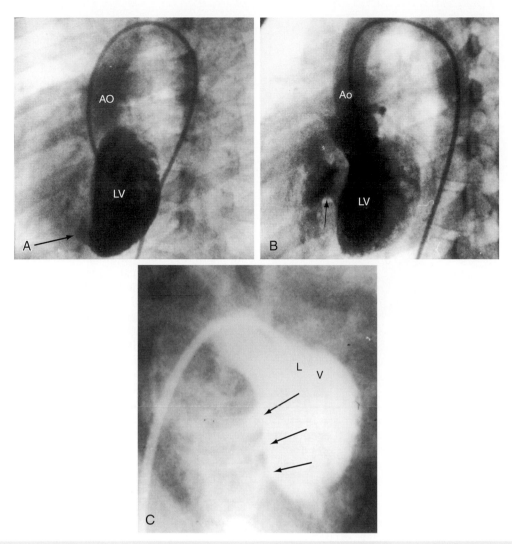

FIGURE 17-3 A, Left anterior oblique left ventriculogram from a 5-year-old girl with a restrictive ventricular septal defect low in the muscular/trabecular septum (arrow). (AO = aorta; LV = left ventricle.) **B,** Left anterior oblique left ventriculogram from a 6-year-old girl with a nonrestrictive ventricular septal defect in the mid portion of the muscular/trabecular septum (arrow). **C,** Lateral left ventriculogram from a 3-week-old male with three moderately restrictive defects (arrows) in the muscular/trabecular septum.

septal defects, especially perimembranous and trabecular muscular defects, to decrease in size finds an ultimate expression in *complete* closure[24,31–33] that has been called the therapeutics of nature—the invisible sutures of spontaneous closure.[34] The incidence rate of spontaneous closure varies considerably depending on the population under study, the method of diagnostic investigation, the type of defect, and whether or not the defect is solitary[35] and has been estimated at 50% to 75% for restrictive perimembranous and trabecular muscular defects observed from birth.[29,36,37] The incidence rate for trabecular muscular defects[35] is reportedly equal to or somewhat higher than that for perimembranous defects. Moderately restrictive and nonrestrictive defects also close spontaneously, but the probability is comparatively low, with an incidence rate estimated at 5% to 10%.[23–25,35,38,39] Most defects that are destined to close do so within the first year of life,[35] with approximately 60% closing before 3 years of age and 90% closing before age 8 years.[36,37] However, spontaneous closure also occurs

in older children and young adults[40] and has been documented at age 23 years,[26] between 26 years and 33 years of age,[41] and at age 46 years. *Multiple* muscular trabecular ventricular septal defects have a strong tendency to close, a conclusion in accord with the observation that multiple defects are three times more prevalent in neonates than after 1 year of age.[42] In preterm infants, ventricular septal defects are about twice as frequent as in full-term infants, but the rate of spontaneous closure is the same,[35] which calls into question the notion that defects reflect incomplete ventricular septation. Spontaneously closed defects in the muscular trabecular septum are funnel-shaped with a sealed orifice on the right ventricular aspect and residual patency on the left ventricular aspect, with endocardial proliferation in the lumen of the funnel and hypertrophy around the exit. Muscular defects represented by "Swiss cheese" fenestrations do not close spontaneously. Defects in the inlet septum seldom decrease in size[43] but are occasionally occluded by bridging atrioventricular valve tissue (see Figure 15-87B). Infundibular defects can be closed by

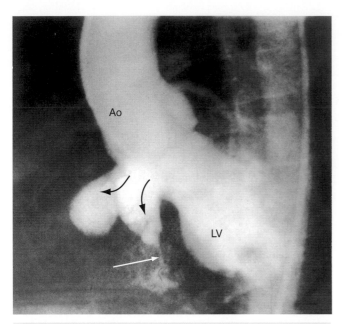

FIGURE 17-4 Lateral left ventriculogram from a 9-year-old girl with a perimembranous ventricular septal defect, a septal aneurysm (black curved arrows), and a persistent small shunt (white arrow). (Ao = aorta; LV = left ventricle.)

prolapse of the right aortic cusp.[2] Perimembranous ventricular septal defects close by adherence of the septal tricuspid leaflet to the margins of the defect, less commonly by prolapse of an aortic cusp,[24,31,44] and rarely by intrusion of a sinus of Valsalva aneurysm. Adherence of tricuspid leaflet tissue is seldom accompanied by tricuspid regurgitation, but there is a tendency for aneurysm formation when perimembranous defects are closed by the tricuspid valve (see Figures 17-4 and 17-31B).[2,32,45–49] Ventricular septal aneurysms were described by Laennec in 1826 and are, as a rule, relatively small (see Figure 17-4). Exceptionally, however, septal aneurysms expand to considerable size, and a giant aneurysm of the membranous septum revealed itself as a mediastinal mass.[50] A *blind septal aneurysm* occasionally represents a *sui generis* congenital malformation of the interventricular portion of the membranous septum rather than a sequel to spontaneous closure of a perimembranous defect.[51] Familial congenital septal aneurysms have been reported, although rarely.[52] With notable exceptions, aneurysms are well tolerated and have been discovered incidentally at necropsy in patients beyond the eighth decade. Complications of septal aneurysms include infective endocarditis, conduction disturbances, intraaneurysmal thrombosis with systemic embolism, aortic or tricuspid regurgitation, and obstruction to right ventricular outflow (see Figure 18-11).[51] Blind congenital aneurysms may spontaneously perforate, establishing a left-to-right shunt into either the right ventricle or right atrium.[51]

The *hemodynamic classification* of ventricular septal defects is relatively straightforward because *physiologic consequences* depend essentially on the size of the defect and the pulmonary vascular resistance.[53] These two variables change with time, and the physiologic and clinical manifestations change accordingly. A defect in the

ventricular septum, even if spontaneously closed, has been postulated to constitute an abnormality that might adversely affect left ventricular systolic function.[54] This postulation is relevant to impaired function or left ventricular failure in an occasional patient with a restrictive defect and a negligible shunt.[54]

When the resistance that limits—*restricts*—the left-to-right shunt resides at the site of the ventricular septal defect, the term *restrictive* is applied, which indicates that left ventricular systolic pressure is higher than right ventricular systolic pressure. Restrictive defects include those with normal right ventricular systolic pressure and those with elevated but less than systemic right ventricular systolic pressure. When the left-to-right shunt is not restricted at the site of the defect, the term *nonrestrictive* is applied. Right and left ventricular systolic pressure, and therefore pulmonary arterial and aortic systolic pressure, are identical, so the magnitude of the left-to-right shunt is governed by pulmonary vascular resistance.

Ventricular septal defects fall into four *anatomic/physiologic categories* (Figure 17-5): (1) *restrictive defects* with normal right ventricular and pulmonary artery systolic pressure and normal pulmonary vascular resistance; (2) *moderately restrictive defects* with elevated right ventricular and pulmonary artery systolic pressures and low but variable pulmonary vascular resistance; (3) *nonrestrictive defects* with identical right ventricular and left ventricular systolic pressure and elevated but subsystemic pulmonary vascular resistance that is variable; and (4) *nonrestrictive defects* with identical right and left ventricular systolic pressures, suprasystemic pulmonary vascular resistance, and a right-to-left shunt—*Eisenmenger's syndrome*.

Henri Roger's account of the physiology of a restrictive ventricular septal defect with normal pulmonary vascular resistance still applies[1]:

> *The mixture of arterial and venous blood which must take place is scarcely contestable when we recall the differences of pressure which exist, according to the experiments of Marey, between the two ventricles. The force of contraction of the left is equal to 128 millimeters of mercury, that of the right only 25 millimeters of mercury.*

Restrictive ventricular septal defects—maladie de Roger—cause little or no functional derangement because the shunt is small and the pressure and resistance in the pulmonary circulation are normal (see Figure 17-5A). A restrictive defect represents a site of obligatory resistance between the left and right ventricles, thus limiting (restricting) the magnitude of the left-to-right shunt (see previous) and precluding delivery of left ventricular systolic pressure into the right ventricle and pulmonary trunk. Shunt flow is systolic. Minor diastolic flow is generated by the normal differences in left and right ventricular distensibility and end diastolic pressure.

A *moderately restrictive* ventricular septal defect is characterized by right ventricular systolic pressure that is above normal but less than systemic and by low but variable pulmonary vascular resistance that rarely progresses. The left ventricle adapts to a moderate increase in volume, and the right ventricle adapts to a moderate

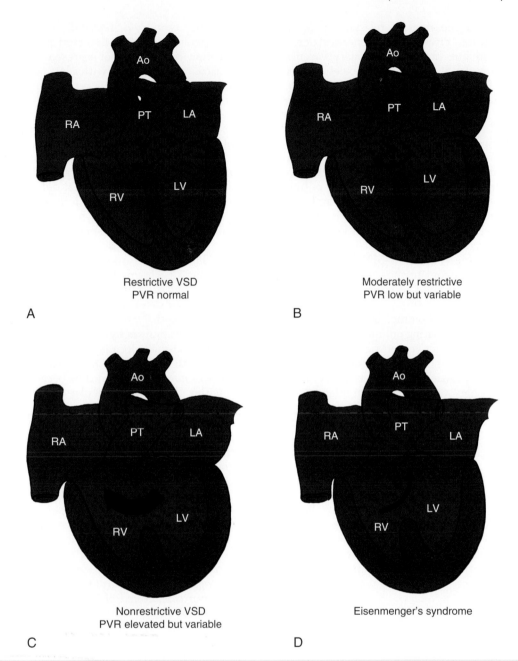

A — Restrictive VSD
PVR normal

B — Moderately restrictive
PVR low but variable

C — Nonrestrictive VSD
PVR elevated but variable

D — Eisenmenger's syndrome

FIGURE 17-5 Schematic illustrations of restrictive, moderately restrictive, and nonrestrictive ventricular septal defects (VSD). **A,** Restrictive VSD with normal pulmonary vascular resistance (PVR) and a small left-to-right shunt (arrow). **B,** Moderately restrictive VSD with low but variable pulmonary vascular resistance and a moderate left-to-right shunt. **C,** Nonrestrictive VSD with a large left-to-right shunt. **D,** Nonrestrictive VSD with suprasystemic pulmonary vascular resistance and reversed shunt (Eisenmenger's syndrome). (Ao = aorta; RA = right atrium; RV = right ventricle; LV = left ventricle; LA = left atrium; PT = pulmonary trunk.)

increase in pressure. Instant-to-instant right-to-left shunting occurs because left ventricular systolic pressure falls more rapidly than right ventricular systolic pressure. However, left ventricular systolic pressure *rises* more rapidly than right ventricular systolic pressure, so the small right-to-left shunts are quantitatively returned to the right ventricle with the next cardiac cycle. An increase in end-diastolic pressure in the volume-loaded left ventricle results in diastolic shunting.[55] Moderately restrictive defects in the trabecular muscular septum

decrease in size during ventricular contraction and, in so doing, decrease the systolic shunt.[56] With isotonic exercise, systemic vascular resistance falls while pulmonary vascular resistance changes little if at all,[57] so a normal increment in systemic flow is achieved without a corresponding increase in left-to-right shunt.[57]

With a *nonrestrictive ventricular septal defect*, the right and left ventricles behave physiologically as a common chamber. Peak systemic systolic pressures are identical, so the volume and direction of flow through the defect depend on the relative resistances in the pulmonary and systemic circulations. A nonrestrictive defect with elevated but variable pulmonary vascular resistance (see Figure 17-5C) imposes an excessive volume load on the left ventricle and systemic afterload on the right ventricle. A persistently large left-to-right shunt culminates in depressed systolic function of the volume overloaded left ventricle.[58] A rise in pulmonary vascular resistance results in a reciprocal fall in left-to-right shunt and a comparable reduction in volume overload of the left ventricle, but systolic pressure in the two ventricles necessarily remains identical. When pulmonary vascular resistance is suprasystemic, the architecture of the pulmonary vascular bed resembles primary pulmonary hypertension (see Chapter 14) and the left-to-right shunt is replaced by a right-to-left shunt, Eisenmenger's syndrome (Figure 17-5D).[37,59-65] Right ventricle function is analogous to the function of a fetal right ventricle that is equipped to cope with systemic vascular resistance.[66]

The vasoreactive immature pulmonary resistance vessels play a pivotal role in regulating pulmonary blood flow in neonates with a nonrestrictive ventricular septal defect. The physiologic fall in neonatal pulmonary vascular resistance is delayed because of the interplay between shunt size and pulmonary vasoreactivity. In infants with a *moderately restrictive ventricular septal defect*, two additional mechanisms serve to regulate the volume and direction of the shunt and the level of pulmonary arterial pressure. The most favorable mechanism is a decrease in size of the defect. A much less common mechanism is acquired obstruction to right ventricular outflow that reduces left ventricular volume overload and protects the pulmonary vascular bed (see Chapter 18).[67] When and to what extent these regulatory mechanisms exert their influence determines the hemodynamic and clinical course in patients with moderately restrictive and nonrestrictive ventricular septal defects.[37,62,68,69]

History

Ventricular septal defects are found in a wide range of mammals and in birds with four-chambered hearts.[4] The incidence in humans is unrelated to gender, race, maternal age, or birth order.[4,70] Ventricular septal defects have been reported in 3.3% of first-degree relatives of index patients.[71] One third of first-degree relatives of patients with congenital heart disease have ventricular septal defects.[4] Between 30% and 60% of siblings of index patients have ventricular septal defects,[72] and siblings of patients with ventricular septal defects have three times the incidence of ventricular septal defects compared to the general population.[4] Ventricular septal defects have been reported in identical twins,[73,74] but with a high frequency of discordance.[4] A parent with a spontaneously closed ventricular septal defect can have offspring with a ventricular septal defect. Birth weights are low in about 18% of full-term infants with ventricular septal defects.[75] Dysmaturity is in addition to and apart from occurrence of ventricular septal defects in preterm infants. Heterotrisomy is a significant factor in ventricular septal defects with Down syndrome.[76]

Restrictive ventricular septal defects come to light because a systolic murmur is detected at the first well-baby examination. A murmur that is present at birth is a feature of ventricular septal defect with a left ventricular-to-right atrial communication in which the shunt exists *in utero* and is therefore present at birth (see subsequent).[77] *Very small defects* with trivial early systolic shunts escape detection because the early systolic murmurs are soft and are either undetected or mistaken for a normal or innocent murmur (see section Auscultation). Spontaneous closure accounts for the striking age-related disparity in the incidence of ventricular septal defects from birth to maturity.[31,35,62] The patient is left with no shunt and a functionally normal heart that harbors a morphologic abnormality (see previous), especially if spontaneous closure is followed by a septal aneurysm (see Figure 17-4).[32] The defect is necessarily missed if the physical examination is performed after spontaneous closure.

Infective endocarditis is a tangible risk in restrictive ventricular septal defects, but rarely occurs before eruption of the second teeth.[62,67,78-80] Roger aptly stated, "Prevention of complications is by means of hygiene."[1] Infective endocarditis is usually located on the septal tricuspid leaflet at site of the jet impact. Muscular defects have a low incidence of infective endocarditis because the jet is dissipated within the right ventricular cavity without striking the septal tricuspid leaflet.[15] Occasionally, the site of infective endocarditis is on an aneurysm of the ventricular septum,[81] and rarely, vegetations at the base of the septal tricuspid leaflet cause perforation and a left ventricular-to-right atrial shunt, an acquired Gerbode defect.[82]

Longevity is likely to be normal, as Roger stated:

Several subjects whom I have been able to observe, I have attended for periods of five, twelve and fifteen years; these children have grown like others, not one has died prematurely. I have occasionally visited as physician a woman whose children I attended from early ages. She had always been in excellent health and had never complained of cardiac difficulties. On auscultation I was greatly surprised to hear a murmur. I asked her if physicians had ever found anything wrong with her heart, and she told me that Guersant the Elder (the famous pediatrician who was my first master in infantile pathology) had recognized in her a few days after birth a cardiac malformation. This woman has now passed her fiftieth year; her health continues to be perfect and she is the mother of four children. In spite of the existence of an uncomplicated defect in the interventricular septum, patients may attain or even surpass the average span of human life.[1]

Moderately restrictive ventricular septal defects with low but variable pulmonary vascular resistance (Figure 17-5B) escape detection in the newborn nursery because the delayed fall in neonatal pulmonary vascular resistance delays the onset of the shunt and the onset of the murmur. Congestive heart failure within the first few months of life is in response to a large left-to-right shunt that is established after the fall in pulmonary vascular resistance. Parents report that their infant fatigues and coughs while feeding,

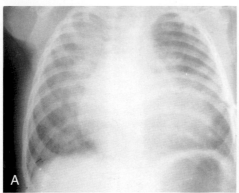
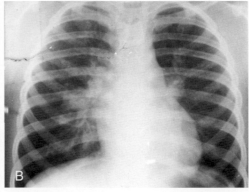

FIGURE 17-6 X-rays at age 3 months (**A**) and 6 years (**B**) from the same patient with a moderately restrictive perimembranous ventricular septal defect that closed spontaneously. **A,** X-ray at 3 months with congestive heart failure, a 3.5 to 1 left-to-right shunt, and a pulmonary artery pressure of 68/22 mm Hg. Pulmonary venous congestion and cardiac enlargement are striking. **B,** At age 6 years, pulmonary vascularity was normal. There was mild residual enlargement of the pulmonary trunk and its proximal branches and a moderately convex left ventricle that extended below the left hemidiaphagm.

sweats excessively, is restless when recumbent, and sleeps poorly. Parents may detect a thrill when they touch their infant's chest and may detect a hyperactive precordium when holding the infant next to their chest. Symptomatic improvement is related to a spontaneous decrease in size of the defect, a favorable trend that may culminate in spontaneous closure (Figure 17-6; see previous).

Patients with moderately restrictive defects and moderate left-to-right shunts tolerate isotonic exercise because the exercise-induced increment in systemic blood flow is achieved without a corresponding increase in shunt flow (see previous).[57] However, persistence of a significant shunt incurs the risk of infective endocarditis, and protracted volume overload of the left ventricle incurs the risk of congestive heart failure.[67] Only an

occasional patient achieves adulthood (Figure 17-7), with one reaching age 65 years (Figure 17-8B) and another reaching age 79 years.[83]

Nonrestrictive ventricular septal defects with elevated but variable pulmonary vascular resistance (see Figure 17-5C) present in infancy with congestive heart failure and with little prospect that the defect will decrease in size. Poor growth and development, labored breathing, frequent lower respiratory infections, difficulty feeding, and excessive diaphoresis are typical.[37,67,84] Dyspnea and irritability are especially pronounced when the infant is supine and improve when the baby is held upright or is placed in an infant seat. Feeding patterns are also typical. A hungry infant awakens from a fretful sleep and feeds vigorously only to stop short of satisfaction

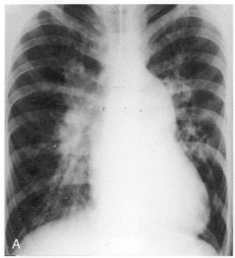
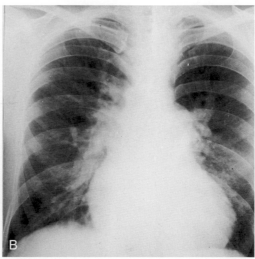

FIGURE 17-7 **A,** X-ray from a 17-year-old boy with a moderately restrictive perimembranous ventricular septal defect, a 2.6 to 1 left-to-right shunt, and a pulmonary artery pressure of 75/23 mm Hg. Pulmonary arterial vascularity is increased, the pulmonary trunk and its proximal branches are markedly dilated, and a moderately enlarged convex left ventricle occupies the apex. **B,** X-ray from a 39-year-old man with a nonrestrictive perimembranous ventricular septal defect and a bidirectional shunt (arterial oxygen saturation, 88%). Pulmonary arterial vascularity is increased, the pulmonary trunk and its proximal branches are markedly dilated, an enlarged convex left ventricle occupies the apex, and a prominent right atrium forms the right lower cardiac border.

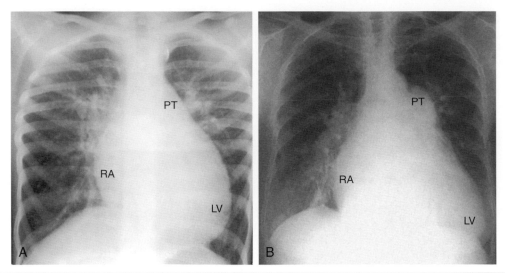

FIGURE 17-8 X-rays from two patients 60 years apart in age, both of whom had perimembranous ventricular septal defects. **A,** The 5-year-old boy had a moderately restrictive ventricular septal defect, a left-to-right shunt of 2.6 to 1, and a pulmonary artery pressure of 43/13 mm Hg. Pulmonary arterial vascularity is increased, the pulmonary trunk (PT) is moderately dilated, an enlarged left ventricle (LV) occupies the apex, and a prominent right atrium occupies the right lower cardiac border. **B,** The 65-year-old woman had a moderately restrictive perimembranous ventricular septal defect, a 2.7 to 1 left-to-right shunt, and pulmonary artery pressure of 55/32 mm Hg. Pulmonary arterial vascularity is increased, the pulmonary trunk (PT) is markedly dilated, an enlarged left ventricle (LV) occupies the apex, and a prominent right atrium (RA) occupies the lower right cardiac border.

because of dyspnea, falls asleep again, exhausted by the effort, and awakens with renewed hunger and repeats the frustrating cycle. Regulation of the large left-to-right shunt with amelioration of symptoms is almost always the result of a rise in pulmonary vascular resistance.[25,38,62,68] A minority of these patients undergo relatively little fall in neonatal pulmonary vascular resistance, so the shunts are small and the early clinical course is deceptively benign. When pulmonary resistance exceeds systemic, the shunt is reversed, the patient is cyanotic,[37,60,64] and the condition that Maude Abbott called *Eisenmenger's complex* exists.[85] Victor Eisenmenger published his account in 1897 in a paper entitled "Congenital Defects of the Ventricular Septum."[86,87] Paul Wood, in his landmark publication of 1958, introduced the term *Eisenmenger's syndrome* (Figure 17-9),

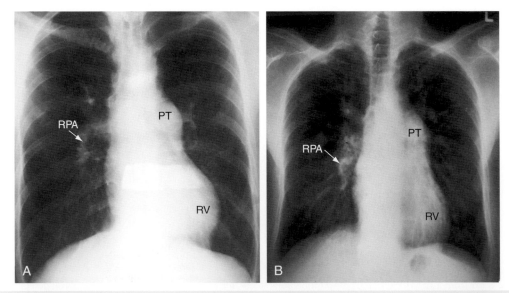

FIGURE 17-9 X-rays from two patients 42 years apart in age, both of whom had a nonrestrictive perimembranous ventricular septal defect and suprasystemic pulmonary vascular resistance (Eisenmenger's syndrome). **A,** X-ray from the 25-year-old man shows clear lung fields, a markedly dilated pulmonary trunk (PT), an enlarged right pulmonary artery (RPA), and a nondilated convex right ventricle (RV) at the apex. **B,** X-ray from the 67-year-old man who died at age 69 years of Legionnaires disease. The lung fields are clear, the pulmonary trunk and the right pulmonary artery are markedly dilated, and a nondilated convex right ventricle (RV) occupies the apex.

which he defined as *pulmonary hypertension with reversed shunt.*[64] Wood quoted Eisenmenger:

The patient was a powerfully built man of 32 who gave a history of cyanosis and moderate breathlessness since infancy. He managed well enough ... until January, 1894 when dyspnea increased and edema set in. Seven months later, he was admitted to hospital in a state of heart failure. ... He improved with rest and digitalis, but collapsed and died more or less suddenly ... following a large hemoptysis. At necropsy, a 2 to 2.5 cm defect was found in the perimembranous septum.

Cyanotic congenital heart disease, represented here by Eisenmenger's syndrome, is a multisystem systemic disorder that involves red cell mass, hemostasis, the central nervous system, bilirubin kinetics, the systemic vascular bed, the coronary circulation, the myocardium, uric acid clearance, the kidneys, respiration, the digits, the long bones, and gynecologic endocrinology.[88,89] Morbidity and mortality take into account contemporary medical management of the multisystem disorders.[88–90] Longevity is about one to two decades longer than in early reports.[63,89,91] Right ventricular failure is uncommon[66] unless acquired systemic hypertension imposes disproportionate afterload.

Erythrocytosis is an adaptive response to the decrease in tissue oxygenation—arterial hypoxemia—that stimulates renal release of erythropoietin, which in turn stimulates an increase in the number of red blood cells. Equilibrium conditions are established at elevated hematocrit levels. Erythrocytosis is a desirable adaptive response designed to offset the hypoxemic deficit in tissue oxygenation and does not incur a risk of stroke from cerebral arterial thrombosis irrespective of hematocrit level, iron stores, or cerebral symptoms of hyperviscosity.[88] However, in cyanotic children younger than age 4 years, iron-deficient erythrocytosis incurs the risk of thrombosis of intracranial venous sinuses.[88] The right-to-left shunts of cyanotic congenital heart disease are pathways for paradoxical emboli that cause transient ischemic attacks and strokes.

Hemostatic abnormalities have been recognized for more than 50 years in patients with cyanotic congenital heart disease.[88] Platelet counts are in the low range of normal, and many clotting factor disorders have been identified, most recently acquired abnormalities of the von Willebrand's factor.[92] A mucocutaneous bleeding tendency is characterized by easy bruising, gingival bleeding, epistaxis, menorrhagia, and increased risk of traumatic bleeding. Pulmonary hemorrhage can be external (hemoptysis) or intrapulmonary, is the most serious type of bleeding, and varies from mild and occasional to copious, recurrent, massive, and fatal.[64,88,93] Massive intrapulmonary hemorrhage is a common cause of sudden death in Eisenmenger's syndrome.[89] Victor Eisenmenger's patient "died more or less suddenly ... following a large hemoptysis."[64]

Bilirubin is formed from the breakdown of heme, a process that is excessive in cyanotic congenital heart disease and that coincides with a substantial increase in the amount of unconjugated bilirubin in the bile.[88] Calcium bilirubinate gallstones develop because unconjugated bilirubin is virtually water insoluble at physiologic pH.[88]

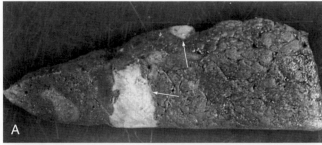

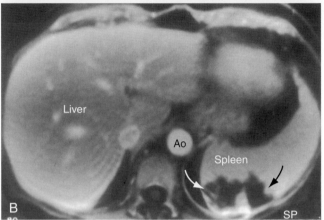

FIGURE 17-10 A, Two splenic infarcts (white arrows) caused by paradoxical emboli in a 42-year-old woman with a nonrestrictive perimembranous ventricular septal defect and Eisenmenger's syndrome. **B,** An an abdominal computed tomographic scan that shows splenic infarcts (curved arrows) caused by paradoxical emboli in a 19-year-old man with a nonrestrictive perimembranous ventricular septal defect and Eisenmenger's syndrome.

Systemic vascular dilation is the result of endothelial-derived nitric oxide and prostaglandins that are released in response to the increase in shear stress inherent in the erythrocytotic perfusate. Increased arteriolar dilation and tissue vascularity contribute to the bleeding tendency (Figure 17-10).[88] Syncope can be caused by the heat-induced vasodilation of hot humid weather or by a hot shower or bath, especially when standing.

The *extramural coronary arteries* are dilated, elongated, and tortuous, even aneurysmal (coronary ectasia).[88] Vasodilator nitric oxide and prostaglandins are released from coronary artery endothelium by the increased shear stress of erythrocytosis. Dilation of the coronary arteries is accompanied by an increase in extramural coronary artery blood flow that does not encroach on coronary vascular reserve because of remodeling of the myocardial microvascular circulation.[94]

Hyperuricemia results from decreased renal clearance and increased production of urate. Elevated plasma uric acid levels are common in cyanotic adults and are secondary to enhanced urate reabsorption that results from renal hypoperfusion reinforced by a high filtration fraction.[88] Acute gouty arthritis is uncommon but not rare.

Renal involvement is represented by abnormalities of both structure and function.[88,89] Decreased clearance of urate is a *functional abnormality*, but the resulting hyperuricemia in turn exerts little or no deleterious effect on renal function.[88,89] Proteinuria is a functional abnormality caused by increased glomerular hydraulic pressure in response to the high viscosity of erythrocytotic blood entering the afferent glomerular arteriole in concert with obligatory ultrafiltration from afferent to afferent arterioles.

Two distinct *structural (morphologic) glomerular abnormalities* are found in cyanotic adults.[89,95] The vascular abnormality is characterized by dilation of hilar arterioles and glomerular capillaries because of intraglomerular release of nitric oxide.[95] The nonvascular abnormality is characterized by an increase in glomerular cellularity in response to platelet-derived growth factor and transforming growth factor beta in the cytoplasm of systemic venous megakaryocytes that are shunted into the systemic arterial circulation and lodge in glomerular tufts.[95]

Cardiorespiratory responses to isotonic exercise in cyanotic congenital heart disease significantly influence the dynamics of oxygen uptake and ventilation.[88,96] Prolonged onset and recovery of oxygen uptake kinetics incur large oxygen deficits that result in hypoxemia even with low levels of exercise, which suggests that patients with right-to-left shunts rely heavily on anaerobic metabolism. Hyperventilation, which is subjectively perceived as dyspnea, is present at rest and increases excessively during exercise because augmentation of the right-to-left shunt induced by exercise is accompanied by an increase in systemic arterial carbon dioxide and a decrease in pH that stimulate the respiratory center and carotid bodies.[88,96]

Clubbing of the digits and *hypertrophic osteoarthropathy* share a common pathogenesis.[88] Systemic venous megakaryocytes are shunted into the systemic arterial circulation (see previous) and impact in the digits and subperiostium. Platelet-derived growth factor and transforming growth factor beta are released from megakaryocytic cytoplasm and promote cell proliferation, protein synthesis, connective tissue formation, and deposition of extracellular matrix that are responsible for clubbing and hypertrophic osteoarthropathy.[88]

Pregnancy poses an excessive risk for women with Eisenmenger's syndrome.[87] The maternal mortality rate exceeds 50%, and there is an independent excessive risk of fetal wastage because of uterine hypoxemia associated with cyanosis.[62,89,97,98]

Sudden death often results from massive intrapulmonary hemorrhage,[89] less commonly from rupture (dissection) of a dilated hypertensive pulmonary trunk,[65,99] and rarely from ventricular tachycardia. A cerebral abscess in early life can result in a *seizure disorder* in adulthood, or the abscess can originate in adulthood.[64,88]

Physical Appearance

The abnormalities in physical appearance are the result of cyanosis caused by the reversed shunt in Eisenmenger's syndrome, the catabolic effects of congestive heart failure in infants (poor growth and development, frailty, and cachexia),[62] and Harrison's grooves caused by the thoracic retractions of chronic dyspnea (Figure 17-11). Growth and development are also influenced by intrauterine and genetic factors and by low birth weight.[75] Infants and young patients with nonrestrictive ventricular septal defects and balanced shunts may become cyanotic only after crying or exercise.[100] Doubly committed subarterial ventricular septal defects are more common among

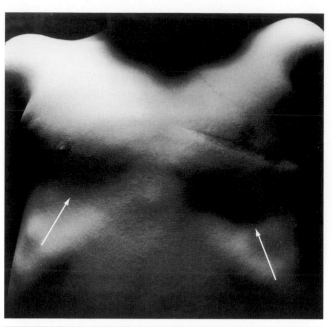

FIGURE 17-11 Photograph of the chest of an 8-year-old boy with a moderately restrictive perimembranous ventricular septal defect and a 2.7 to 1 left-to-right shunt. Lighting was adjusted to highlight the prominent Harrison's grooves (white arrows) caused by chronic dyspnea. The left thoracotomy scar was from repair of coarctation of the aorta.

Asians (see previous).[17] The physical appearance of trisomy 18 Down syndrome (see Figures 19-5 and 20-11) coincides with the presence of an inlet ventricular septal defect (see Figures 15-90 and 15-91).[101–104] In addition, a relationship exists between ventricular septal defect and physical appearance in trisomy 13; trisomy 8 and 9 mosaic; rare aberrations, such as 5p *(cri du chat)* and 13a- and 18q-[105]; Holt-Oram syndrome[29]; Cornelia de Lange's syndrome[72]; Klippel-Feil syndrome[54]; cardiofacial syndrome[106]; and fetal alcohol syndrome.[107]

Arterial Pulse

Moderately restrictive defects with relatively low pulmonary vascular resistance are associated with a brisk arterial pulse because of vigorous ejection from a normal volume-loaded left ventricle. A diminished arterial pulse with pulsus alternans accompanies nonrestrictive defects with large left-to-right shunts and congestive heart failure. The arterial pulse in Eisenmenger's syndrome is normal because systemic stroke volume is maintained (Figure 17-12).[64]

Jugular Venous Pulse

Moderately restrictive and nonrestrictive ventricular septal defects with congestive heart failure are accompanied by an elevated mean jugular venous pressure and an increase in A and V waves. However, the jugular venous pulse in Eisenmenger's syndrome is normal or nearly so, with a small dominant A wave (Figure 17-13). Large A waves are exceptional because right ventricular systolic pressure does not exceed systemic. Systemic afterload exists from birth, so the right ventricle requires little extra help from its atrium.

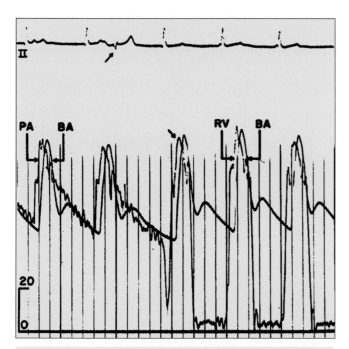

FIGURE 17-12 Pressure pulses from an 18-year-old man with a nonrestrictive perimembranous ventricular septal defect and Eisenmenger's syndrome. The brachial artery pulse (BA) was identical with the pulmonary artery pulse (PA). The diastolic portions of the brachial and pulmonary artery pulses were the same because pulmonary vascular resistance was the same as systemic vascular resistance. As the catheter was withdrawn into the right ventricle (RV), the peak systolic pressure remained the same as the brachial arterial systolic pressure (BA).

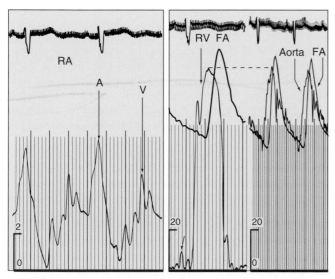

FIGURE 17-13 Tracings from an 11-year-old boy with a nonrestrictive perimembranous ventricular septal defect and Eisenmenger's syndrome. A small dominant wave is present in the right atrial (RA) pressure pulse. The second panel shows identical *diastolic* pressure in the aorta and femoral artery (FA). The femoral artery *systolic* pressure is slightly higher than the right ventricular and aortic systolic pressure because of peripheral amplification.

Precordial Movement and Palpation

Roger stated that when a ventricular septal defect is restrictive, "it coincides with no other sign of organic disease with the exception of the harsh thrill which accompanies it."[1] The thrill is maximal in the third or fourth left intercostal space at the left sternal border. A subarterial ventricular septal defect directs its shunt into the pulmonary trunk, so the accompanying thrill is maximal in the second or first and second left intercostal space with radiation upward, to the left, and into the neck.[108]

In a *moderately restrictive* ventricular septal defect with a large left-to-right shunt, the volume-overloaded left ventricle is dynamic, the dilated pulmonary trunk is palpable in the second left intercostal space, and the moderately afterloaded right ventricle is less impressive.

A *nonrestrictive* ventricular septal defect with low pulmonary vascular resistance and obligatory systemic pressure in the right ventricle and the pulmonary trunk is associated with a dynamic volume-overloaded *left* ventricle, a pressure-overloaded systemic *right* ventricle, a palpable dilated hypertensive pulmonary trunk, and a palpable pulmonary closure sound. In Eisenmenger's syndrome, the hypertensive right ventricular impulse displaces the left ventricle from the apex.

Auscultation

A *very restrictive* defect in the perimembranous or trabecular septum (see Figure 17-2B) is accompanied by a soft, localized, high-frequency, decrescendo, early systolic murmur (Figure 17-14) that is easily missed in restless infants. Early systolic timing indicates that the shunt is early systole because small perimembranous or muscular defects decrease in size or obliterate in late systole.[109] The early systolic murmur lengthens *during a premature ventricular beat* because reduced left ventricular contractility fails to close the defect in late systole.[78] Conversely, vigorous left ventricular contraction *during a postpremature* beat closes the defect early and shortens the murmur still further. During the evolution of spontaneous closure, a holosystolic murmur becomes early systolic before disappearing altogether (see Figure 17-18).[23]

Moderately restrictive ventricular septal defects with pulmonary vascular resistance that is below systemic are accompanied by a loud harsh holosystolic murmur (see Figure 17-16) that is sometimes accentuated in midsystolic because of superimposition of a pulmonary flow murmur. The murmur of a *restrictive perimembranous ventricular septal defect* is also holosystolic, high-frequency, grade 4/6 or louder, and maximal in the third and fourth intercostal spaces at the left sternal border (Figures 17-15 and 17-16). These precordial sites are topographically appropriate for the intracardiac location of the murmur (see Figure 17-15).[110]

The typical holosystolic murmur (see Figures 17-15 and 17-16) corresponds to the holosystolic pressure difference across the defect. Roger recognized this mechanism when he described the murmur as "extending right through systole covering both heart sounds..." and "accompanied by no other physical signs save only the purring thrill."[1,30] When tricuspid chordae tendineae traverse the

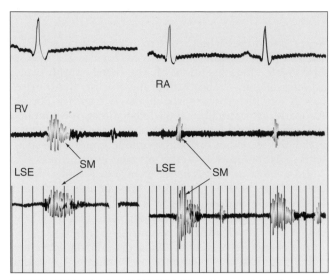

FIGURE 17-14 Phonocardiograms from a 4-year-old girl with a tiny perimembranous ventricular septal defect and a trivial left-to-right shunt. A soft pure high-frequency early systolic murmur (SM) was recorded within the cavity of the right ventricle (RV), and an identical precordial murmur was recorded externally at the lower left sternal edge (LSE). When the intracardiac microphone was withdrawn from right ventricle into right atrium (RA), the murmur vanished, establishing its origin within the right ventricular cavity.

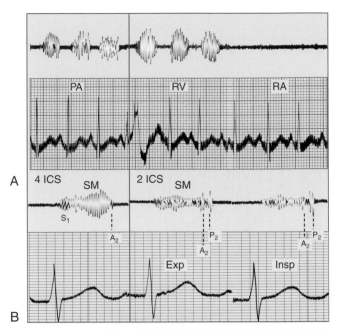

FIGURE 17-15 Phonocardiograms from a 4-year-old girl with a restrictive perimembranous ventricular septal defect, a 1.4 to 1 left-to-right shunt, and normal pulmonary artery pressure. **A,** The intracardiac microphone recorded a prominent midsystolic systolic murmur (SM) in the main pulmonary artery (PA). When the microphone was withdrawn into the outflow tract of the right ventricle (RV), the holosystolic murmur of a ventricular septal defect was recorded. The holosystolic murmur vanished when the microhpone was withdrawn into the right atrium (RA). **B,** Thoracic wall phonocardiogram at the fourth left intercostal space (4 ICS) recorded a holosystolic murmur identical with the holosystolic murmur in the right ventricular outflow tract. The second heart sound in the second left intercostal space (2 ICS) exhibited persistent but not fixed splitting. (S_1 = first heart sound; A_2 = aortic component; P_2 = pulmonary component.)

defect, the murmur is musical, assuming the pitch of an Aeolian harp. Muscular trabecular ventricular septal defect murmurs are maximal at the same precordial sites as murmurs of perimembranous defects.

The shunt in a *subarterial ventricular septal defect* is directly into the pulmonary trunk, so the accompanying murmur and thrill are maximal in the second or first and second left intercostal space (Figure 17-17) with radiation upward toward the left clavicle into the suprasternal notch and into the left side of the neck (see Figure 17-17).[108]

A decrease in size or spontaneous closure of a perimembranous ventricular septal defect is sometimes accompanied by a *septal aneurysm*[111] that may harbor a small residual left-to-right shunt (see Figure 17-4). Otherwise, the aneurysm resembles a blind congenital membranous septal aneurysm (see previous).[44] Septal aneurysms are usually occult, but occasionally there are auscultatory clues. The aneurysm may contain one or more small perforations (see Figure 17-4) that generate a late systolic murmur, or a holosystolic murmur with late systolic accentuation, because stretching of the aneurysmal pouch accentuates late systolic patency of small perforations.[112–114] Murmurs have also been attributed to the entry of blood into a *sealed blind aneurysmal pouch* during ventricular systole. Systolic tensing of the aneurysm sometimes produces a midsystolic click that introduces a late systolic murmur.[113] The aneurysm occasionally protrudes into the right ventricular outflow tract outflow tract (see Figure 17-4), causing a midsystolic murmur in the second left intercostal space. A septal aneurysm may cause tricuspid regurgitation[115] with the murmur identified during active respiration (Carvallo's sign).[116]

The prominent holosystolic murmur of a moderately restrictive ventricular septal defect usually buries both components of the second sound, rendering the pulmonary component audible only during inspiration as it emerges from the murmur (see Figure 17-17). Analysis of the second heart sound benefits from exaggerated splitting (see Figure 17-15B).[117] Attention has been called to wide splitting with subarterial defects (see Figure 17-17).[108]

Moderately restrictive or nonrestrictive ventricular septal defects with large left-to-right shunts are associated with short mid-diastolic murmurs at the apex because of torrential flow across the mitral valve (see Figure 17-16)[118] as originally described by Laubry and Pezzi in 1921.[119] These murmurs are often preceded by a third heart sound, especially in the presence of left ventricular failure. Intracardiac phonocardiograms confirm the presence of mid-diastolic murmurs within the inflow tract of the left ventricle just beyond the mitral valve.[110]

Nonrestrictive ventricular septal defects with a progressive increase in pulmonary vascular resistance illustrate the effects of pulmonary vascular disease on the length and loudness of the accompanying systolic murmur.[120] As pulmonary resistance approaches systemic, the holosystolic murmur shortens and softens (Figures 17-18C, 17-18D, and 17-19), and its shape becomes decrescendo

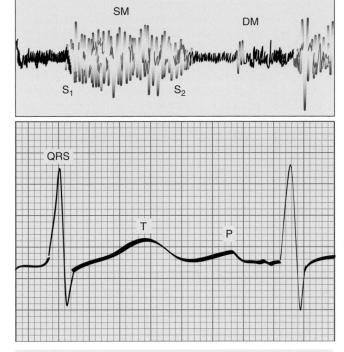

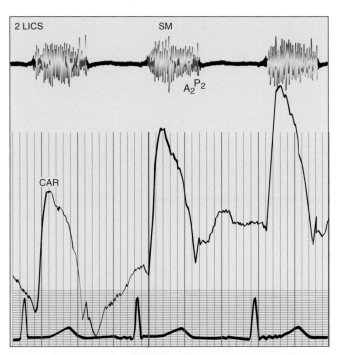

FIGURE 17-16 Phonocardiogram recorded over the left ventricular impulse of a 2-year-old girl with a moderately restrictive perimembranous ventricular septal defect and a 2.5 to 1 left-to-right shunt. A holosystolic murmur (SM) is followed by a mid-diastolic–presystolic murmur (DM) caused by increased flow across the mitral valve. (S_1 = first heart sound; S_2 = second heart sound.)

FIGURE 17-17 Phonocardiogram from a 5-year-old boy with a moderately restrictive subarterial ventricular septal defect, a 2 to 1 left-to-right shunt, and a pulmonary artery pressure of 80/36 mm Hg. The holosystolic systolic murmur (SM) was maximal in the second left intercostal costal space (2 LICS) because blood was shunted from the left ventricle through the subarterial ventricular septal defect directly into the pulmonary trunk. There is relatively wide splitting of the second heart sound from delayed closure of the pulmonary valve. The aortic component of the second sound is buried by the holosystic murmur. (A_2/P_2 = aortic and pulmonary components of the second heart sound; CAR = carotid pulse.)

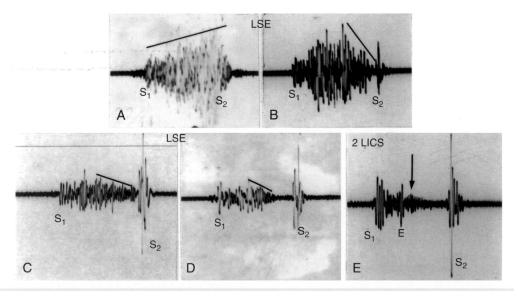

FIGURE 17-18 Phonocardiograms from five patients with perimembranous ventricular septal defects and pulmonary vascular resistance ranging from normal (**A**) to suprasystemic (**E**). The tracings show modifications of the murmur from a restrictive nonpulmonary hypertensive left-to-right shunt (**A**) to a pulmonary hypertensive right-to-left shunt (**E**). In Eisenmenger's syndrome (**E**), a pulmonary ejection sound (**E**) introduces a short midsystolic murmur (arrow) caused by flow into a dilated hypertensive pulmonary trunk. (LSE = left sternal edge; PA = pulmonary artery; 2 LICS = second left intercostal space.)

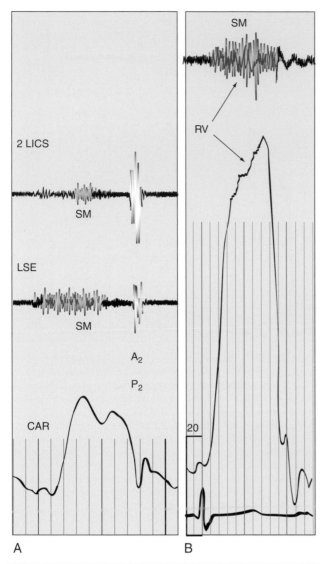

FIGURE 17-19 Tracings from a 6-year-old boy with a non-restrictive perimembranous ventricular septal defect, elevated pulmonary vascular resistance, and a 1.8 to 1 left-to-right shunt. **A,** The murmur (SM) at the left sternal edge (LSE) was early systolic, ending before both components of the second heart sound (A_2/P_2) even though the same murmur recorded by an intracardiac microphone within the cavity of the right ventricle was holosystolic **(B).** (RV = right ventricle; 2 LICS = second left intercostal space; A_2 = aortic component; P_2 = pulmonary component; CAR = carotid pulse.)

(see Figures 17-18 and 17-19). The murmur is early systolic (see Figure 17-18D) before disappearing altogether as the shunt is reversed (see Figure 17-18E).[64,120]

Auscultatory analysis of the *second heart sound* benefits from an increase in intensity of the pulmonary component and from a rise in pulmonary vascular resistance that softens the murmur in latter systole.[120] As pulmonary resistance increases, the degree of splitting decreases (see Figure 17-19),[120] so the second sound is single in Eisenmenger's syndrome (see Figure 17-18E).[64,120,121] The two components fuse because the respective descending limbs of the left and

right ventricular pressure pulses cross the aortic and pulmonary arterial pressure pulses simultaneously. Because the aortic and pulmonary arterial dicrotic notches are synchronous, the two components of the second sound are synchronous.

When suprasystemic pulmonary vascular resistance abolishes the left-to-right shunt, the auscultatory signs are those of pure pulmonary hypertension (see Figure 17-18E and Chapter 14).[120] Flow into the dilated hypertensive pulmonary trunk causes a pulmonary ejection sound that introduces a short, soft, midsystolic murmur.[120] A high-frequency Graham Steell murmur issues from a loud pulmonary component of the second heart sound and is the only diastolic murmur when the shunt is reversed. The mid-diastolic murmur across the mitral valve disappears as pulmonary blood flow decreases. Rarely, the murmur of pulmonary regurgitation is caused by prolapse of a pulmonary cusp through a subarterial ventricular septal defect.[18]

Electrocardiogram

The electrocardiogram is an important indication of the physiologic derangements of ventricular septal defects, but not of their anatomic location. The scalar tracing is influenced by the size of the defect, the size of the left-to-right shunt, and the pulmonary vascular resistance (see Figure 17-5; i.e., by the presence and degree of volume overload of the left ventricle and the presence and degree of pressure overload of the right ventricle).

A *restrictive* ventricular septal defect with normal pulmonary artery pressure is associated with a normal electrocardiogram and an occasional rsr prime pattern in lead V_1.[122,123] When a restrictive perimembranous defect is accompanied by a septal aneurysm, there is an increase in the incidence of rhythm and conduction disturbances, especially atrial fibrillation, paroxysmal atrial tachycardia, junctional rhythm, atrial flutter, and complete heart block.[51]

Moderately restrictive ventricular septal defects with a large left-to-right shunt are associated with broad notched left atrial P waves in lead 1 and 2 and with a broad deep P terminal force in lead V_1 (Figure 17-20).[122] The QRS axis is normal (see Figure 17-20), although left axis deviation occurs in about 5% of restrictive or moderately restrictive perimembranous defects (Figure 17-21).[124–126] Inlet defects are associated with left axis deviation when they are a component of an atrioventricular septal defect (see Chapter 15).[127] In the presence of ventricular septal aneurysms, the incidence rate of left axis deviation increases; it has been found in as many as 40% of patients with multiple ventricular septal defects. Volume overload of the left ventricle is reflected in tall R waves and tall peaked T waves in leads 2, 3, and aVF and in prominent Q waves, tall R waves, and tall peaked T waves in leads V_{5-6} (see Figure 17-20).[123,128]

A *nonrestrictive* ventricular septal defect with a large left-to-right shunt exhibits right atrial or combined right and left atrial P wave abnormalities, especially in lead 2

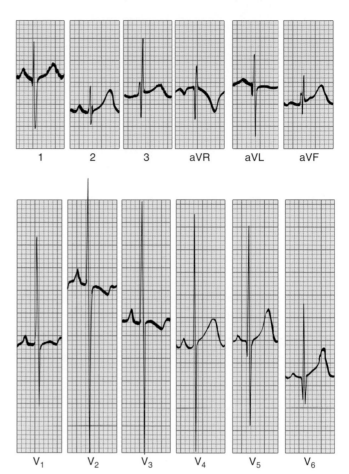

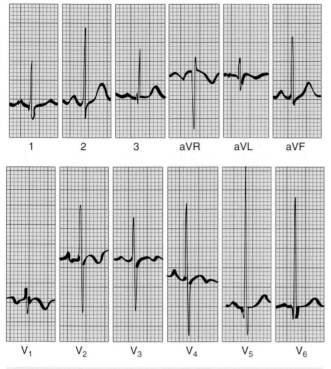

FIGURE 17-20 Electrocardiogram from a 14-month-old female with a moderately restrictive perimembranous ventricular septal defect, a 2.5 to 1 left-to-right shunt, and a pulmonary artery pressure of 38/16 mm Hg. A bifid left atrial P wave abnormality is present in lead 1, and the P wave in lead V_1 has a deep broad terminal left artial component. The QRS axis is normal. Deep Q waves, tall R waves, and upright T waves in leads V_{5-6} are signs of left ventricular volume overload.

FIGURE 17-22 Electrocardiogram from a 3-month-old female with a nonrestrictive perimembranous ventricular septal defect and a 3.5 to 1 left-to-right shunt. Peaked right atrial P waves appear in leads 1, 2, and V_{1-4}. Right ventricular hypertrophy is manifested by prominent R waves in right precordial leads and prominent S waves in left precordial leads. Left ventricular volume overload is reflected in the deep Q waves, well-developed R waves, and tall peaked T waves in leads V_{5-6}. Combined ventricular hypertrophy is represented by the large RS complexes in leads V_{2-5}.

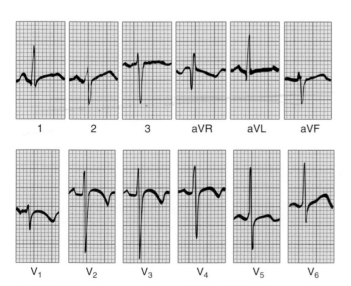

FIGURE 17-21 Electrocardiogram from a 3-year-old girl with a moderately restrictive perimembranous ventricular septal defect, a 2 to 1 left-to-right shunt, and a pulmonary artery pressure of 32/15 mm Hg. There is left axis deviation with counterclockwise depolarization.

and in leads V_{1-2} (Figure 17-22). The QRS axis shifts moderately to the right (Figures 17-22 and 17-23). Biventricular hypertrophy is reflected in the increased R wave amplitude in lead V_1, the deep Q waves, tall R waves, and tall peaked T waves in leads V_{5-6} and in large equidiphasic RS complexes (the Katz-Wachtel pattern) in midprecordial leads (see Figures 17-22 and 17-23).[122,129] Infants with a nonrestrictive ventricular septal defect and large left-to-right shunts occasionally exhibit marked right axis deviation and pure or relatively pure right ventricular hypertrophy, except for large equidiphasic complexes in one or more midprecordial leads (Figure 17-24).

In Eisenmenger's syndrome, P waves are often normal (Figure 17-25) in younger patients and moderately peaked in older patients. Right axis deviation is moderate. Lead V_1 exhibits a tall monophasic R wave (see Figure 17-25)

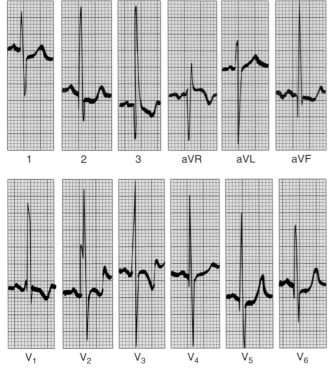

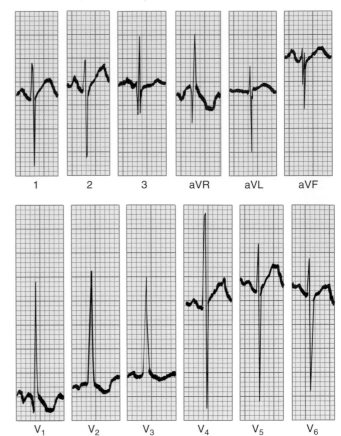

FIGURE 17-23 Electrocardiogram from a 6-year-old girl with a nonrestrictive perimembranous ventricular septal defect and a 3 to 1 left-to-right shunt. The QRS axis is plus 90 degrees. Volume overload of the left ventricle is indicated by deep Q waves, prominent R waves, and tall peaked T waves in leads V_{5-6}, and by deep Q waves and tall R waves in leads 2, 3, and aVF. Right ventricular hypertrophy is indicated by tall right precordial R waves and deep left precordial S waves. Biventricular hypertrophy is manifested by large RS complexes in mid precordial leads.

FIGURE 17-24 Electrocardiogram from a 3-month-old female with a nonrestrictive muscular ventricular septal defect and a 3.4 to 1 left-to-right shunt. A right atrial abnormality is indicated by the peaked P wave in lead 2, and right atrial enlargement is indicated by the q wave in lead V_1. The QRS shows pure right ventricular hypertrophy with marked right axis deviation, a tall R wave in lead aVR, a 23-mm R wave in lead V_1, and deep left precordial S waves. A left ventricular contribution is confined to the large equidiphasic RS complex in V_4.

that is occasionally notched on its upstroke and followed by a small s wave. Prominent S waves appear in left precordial leads, but combined ventricular hypertrophy is lacking (see Figure 17-25).

X-Ray

Vaquez and Bordet[130] described the radiologic signs of ventricular septal defect in 1913. *Small defects* that were moderately restrictive at birth show residual signs of an initially larger left-to-right shunt, especially an increase in size of the left ventricle and dilation of the pulmonary trunk (Figures 17-6B and 17-26).

Moderately restrictive ventricular septal defects with low but variable pulmonary vascular resistance (see Figure 17-5B) exhibit radiologic signs appropriate for the magnitude of the left-to-right shunt and the presence and degree of pulmonary hypertension. When pulmonary vascular resistance is relatively low, increased pulmonary arterial vascularity and pulmonary venous congestion coexist (Figures 17-6A and 17-27). Large shunts in infants are accompanied by hyperinflated lungs with flat hemidiaphragms.[131] Right atrial dilation accompanies congestive

heart failure (see Figures 17-6A and 17-27). Enlargement of the left atrium is best recognized in the lateral projection (see Figure 17-27B) and can be more impressive than enlargement of the left ventricle. An increase in size of the pulmonary trunk and its branches reflects the magnitude and chronicity of pulmonary arterial blood flow and the level of pulmonary arterial pressure (see Figures 17-7 and 17-8).[132] The size of the ascending aorta is not increased because the left-to-right shunt is intracardiac and therefore does not traverse the aortic root (see Figure 17-8). In the lateral projection, the *lower* sternum is apt to protrude anteriorly whereas the *upper* sternum is relatively straight.

Nonrestrictive ventricular septal defects with elevated but variable pulmonary vascular resistance present in infancy with congestive heart failure, pulmonary venous congestion, and enlargement of all four chambers. The x-rays resemble those of moderately restrictive defects with large left-to-right shunts (see Figures 17-6A and 17-7). In the exceptional adult, the

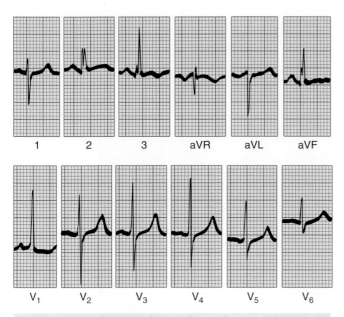

FIGURE 17-25 Electrocardiogram from a 19-year-old man with a nonrestrictive perimembranous ventricular septal defect and Eisenmenger's syndrome. The shunt was balanced at age 5 years and reversed at age 9 years. The P waves are normal. Right axis deviation is mild. Right ventricular hypertrophy is manifested by the tall monophasic R wave in lead V₁.

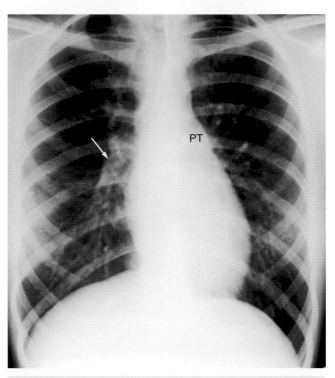

FIGURE 17-26 X-ray from a 15-year-old girl with a restrictive perimembranous ventricular septal defect, a left-to-right shunt of 1.4 to 1, and normal pulmonary artery pressure. The pulmonary trunk (PT) and its right branch (arrow) are moderately prominent because the ventricular septal defect was previously larger. The film is otherwise normal.

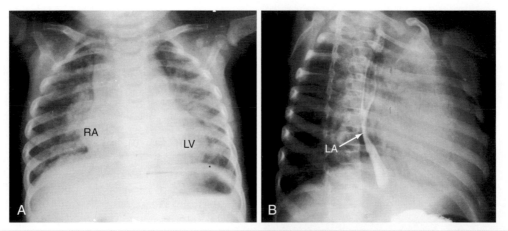

FIGURE 17-27 X-rays from a 7-month-old female with a moderately restrictive perimembranous ventricular septal defect, a 3 to 1 left-to-right shunt, and a pulmonary artery pressure of 45/18 mm Hg. **A,** There is increased pulmonary blood flow, a marked increase in pulmonary venous vascularity, a dilated left ventricle at the apex, and a prominent right atrium at the right lower cardiac border. **B,** The right anterior oblique shows retrodisplacement of the barium esophagram by an enlarged left atrium (LA).

pulmonary trunk and its branches are aneurysmal (Figure 17-28). As pulmonary vascular resistance rises, the left-to-right shunt falls reciprocally, congestive heart failure is ameliorated, and the heart size decreases, but enlargement of the pulmonary trunk and its branches persists (see Figure 17-6B) When the shunt is reversed by suprasystemic pulmonary vascular resistance, *Eisenmenger's*

syndrome (see Figure 17-5D), the lung fields are oligemic; right atrial, left atrial, and left ventricular sizes are normal; and the hypertrophied but nondilated right ventricle occupies the apex (see Figure 17-9). Except for enlargement of the pulmonary trunk and its branches and a convex apical right ventricle, the cardiac silhouette is deceptively unimpressive (see Figure 17-9).

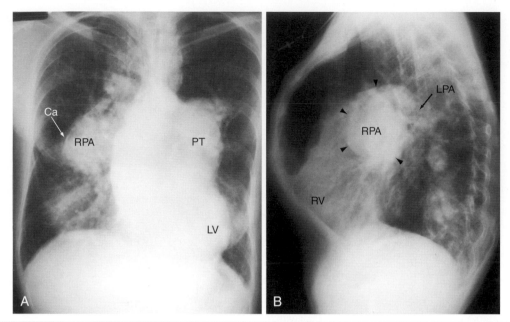

FIGURE 17-28 Remarkable x-rays from a 39-year-old woman with a nonrestrictive perimembranous ventricular septal defect and a 2.3 to 1 left-to-right shunt. **A,** Rightward scoliosis is apparent. There is aneurysmal dilation of the pulmonary trunk (PT) and the right pulmonary artery (RPA), which contains a thin rim of calcium (Ca). Pulmonary arterial vascularity is increased, and a dilated left ventricle (LV) occupies the apex. **B,** Lateral view shows the aneurysmal right pulmonary artery end-on, a dilated left pulmonary artery (LPA), an enlarged right ventricle (RV), and striking pectus corinatum.

Echocardiogram

Tranthoracic and tranesophageal echocardiography with color flow imaging and Doppler interrogation establish the presence, location, and physiologic consequences of ventricular septal defects (Figure 17-29 and Video 17-1).[133–135] Shunt flow can be examined in the fetus with color Doppler M-mode scan.[136] Three-dimensional echocardiography improves assessment[137,138] and has proven accurate in quantifying shunts.[2] Small multiple defects in the muscular septum,[139] spontaneous closure of perimembranous or muscular defects, and septal aneurysms[140] can be identified, and Swiss cheese defects in the trabecular muscular septum can be recognized with color flow imaging. Right ventricular systolic pressure and pulmonary artery systolic and diastolic pressure can be estimated (Figure 17-30).

The complex shunt flow across a ventricular septal defect was first characterized with angiocardiography[141] but is now characterized with echocardiography.[139] Isovolumetric contraction is accompanied by left-to-right shunting, with flow patterns during ventricular ejection depending in part on the size of the ventricular septal defect (see Figure 17-30). In nonrestrictive defects, the direction of shunt flow is determined by the relative resistances in the pulmonary and systemic vascular beds. Isovolumetric relaxation coincides with right-to-left flow. Two patterns have been identified during ventricular diastole: transient right-to-left flow at the time of mitral valve opening followed by left-to-right flow from mid-diastole to the time of mitral valve closure.

Echocardiography with color flow imaging identifies the ventricular septal defect in the perimembranous septum (Figure 17-31 and Video 17-2), in the muscular septum (Figures 17-32 and 17-33 and Videos 17-3 and 17-4), in the infundibular septum, or in the inlet septum (Figure 17-34). Two-dimensional imaging identifies a septal aneurysm (Figures 17-31B and 17-35A and Video 17-5A), and color flow imaging determines whether or not the aneurysm harbors a residual shunt (Figure 17-35B and Video 17-5B). Aneurysm formation warrants color flow interrogation of the tricuspid valve for the presence of regurgitation.[115] Inlet ventricular septal defects can be accompanied by atrioventricular valve straddling (see

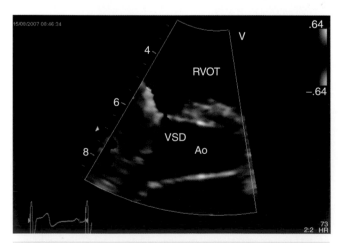

FIGURE 17-29 Short-axis color flow image from a 23-year-old woman with a restrictive perimembranous ventricular septal defect (VSD) (Video 17-1). (RVOT = right ventricular outflow tract; Ao = aorta.)

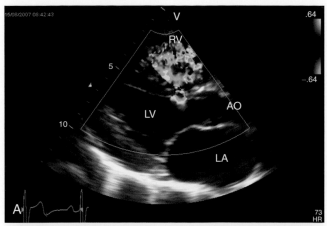

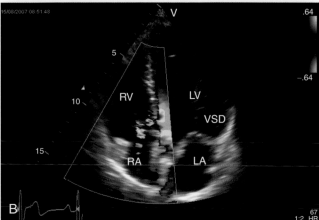

FIGURE 17-30 **A,** Short-axis color flow image from a 40-year-old woman with a restrictive perimembranous ventricular septal defect. A high-velocity jet is directed into the outflow tract of the right ventricle (RV). (LV/LA=left ventricle/left atrium; AO=aorta.) **B,** Apical four-chamber view shows the high-velocity jet traversing the perimembranous ventricular septal defect.

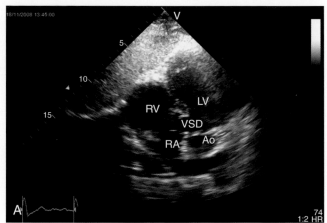

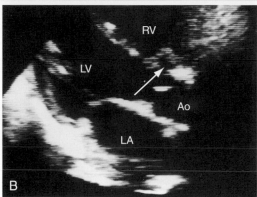

FIGURE 17-31 **A,** Subcostal four-chamber view shows a moderately restrictive perimembranous ventricular septal defect (VSD) and defines the relationship of the defect to the aorta (Ao) and tricuspid valve (TV) (Video 17-2). (RV/LV=right ventricle/left ventricle; RA/LA = right atrium/left atrium.) **B,** Echocardiogram from a 3-year-old girl with a restrictive perimembranous ventricular septal defect that closed spontaneously. Parasternal long-axis view shows a septal aneurysm (arrow) projecting into the outflow tract of the right ventricle (RV).

Figure 17-34). A subarterial defect is associated with flow directed toward the pulmonary trunk (Figure 17-36), with continuity of aortic and pulmonary valves in the roof of the defect[43,133] and with aortic regurgitation from prolapse of the right or noncoronary cusp (see Figure 17-45 and Videos 17-6A and 17-6B).

Summary

Perimembranous and trabecular muscular ventricular septal defects that are trivial at birth go unrecognized unless the soft high-frequency early systolic murmur is identified before the defect spontaneously closes. *A restrictive but not trivial* defect comes to light because of a left parasternal holosystolic murmur. Restrictive defects in the perimembranous or muscular septum usually close spontaneously. During the time course of spontaneous closure, the holosystolic murmur becomes early systolic before disappearing. Restrictive perimembranous defects are substrates for infective endocarditis.

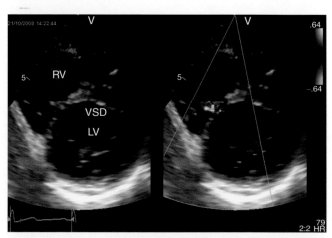

FIGURE 17-32 Echocardiogram in the short axis from a 1-year-old boy with a moderately restrictive ventricular septal defect (VSD) in the trabecular muscular septum (Video 17-3). (LV = left ventricle; RV = right ventricle.)

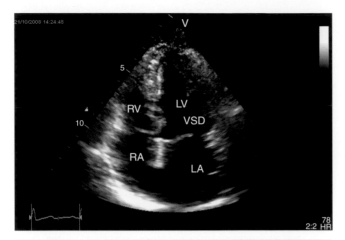

FIGURE 17-33 Apical echocardiogram from a 3-month-old male with a restrictive ventricular septal defect (VSD) in the midportion of the trabecular muscular septum (Video 17-4). (RV/LV = right ventricle/left ventricle.)

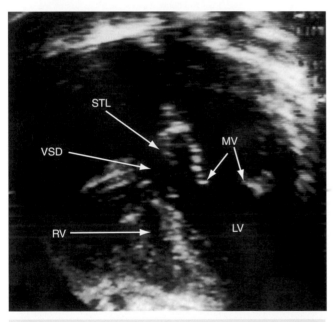

FIGURE 17-34 Subcostal echocardiogram from a 4-year-old girl with an inlet ventricular septal defect (VSD) and straddling of the septal tricuspid leaflet (STL). The right ventricle (RV) was significantly reduced in size. (LV = left ventricle; MV = mitral valve.)

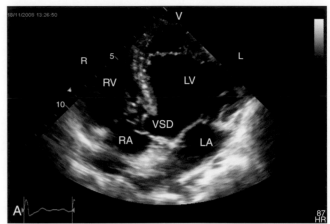

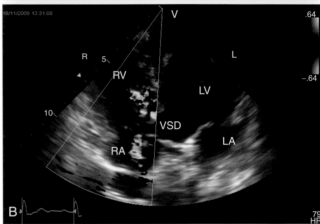

FIGURE 17-35 A, Echocardiograms from a 4-year-old boy with aneurysm formation after spontaneous closure of a moderately restrictive perimembranous ventricular septal defect. (LV/RV = left ventricle/right ventricle.) B, Color flow image from the same patient showing the sealed aneurysm that filled during ventricular systole (Videos 17-5A and 17-5B).

Moderately restrictive ventricular septal defects with low but variable pulmonary vascular resistance present with congestive heart failure in infancy. Holosystolic murmurs are absent at birth but are obvious at the first well-baby examination. Infants with large shunts and congestive heart failure thrive poorly. The physical examination reveals retarded growth and development, a hyperdynamic left ventricular impulse, a variable right ventricular impulse, a left parasternal systolic thrill with a prominent holosystolic murmur, and an apical mid-diastolic flow murmur across the mitral valve. The electrocardiogram shows left atrial P wave abnormalities and

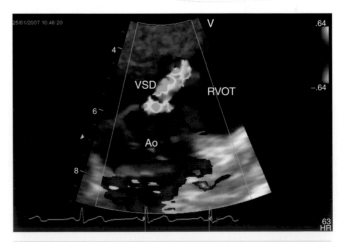

FIGURE 17-36 Short-axis color flow image from a 10-year-old girl with a subarterial ventricular septal defect (VSD). The systolic jet is directed into the pulmonary trunk (PT). There was no aortic regurgitation. (Ao = aorta; RV = right ventricle.)

volume overload of the left ventricle with variable degrees of right ventricular hypertrophy. X-rays reveal vascular lung fields that are a combination of increased pulmonary arterial blood flow and pulmonary venous congestion. All four cardiac chambers and the pulmonary trunk are dilated. Echocardiography with color flow imaging and Doppler interrogation establishes the presence and location of the ventricular septal defects and determines the physiologic consequences. Perimembranous and trabecular muscular defects tend to decrease in size and close spontaneously, except Swiss cheese defects. Reduction in size of the defect curtails excessive pulmonary arterial blood flow, curtails left ventricular volume overload, and ameliorates congestive heart failure.

Nonrestrictive ventricular septal defects with elevated but variable pulmonary vascular resistance presents in infancy with congestive heart failure and its catabolic effects. If pulmonary vascular resistance remains sufficiently high to limit the shunt, the infant deceptively escapes heart failure with its ill effects but goes on to confront a progressive rise in pulmonary vascular resistance. When the shunt is large, the physical examination reveals a dynamic precordium from volume overload of the left ventricle and dilation of the hypertensive right ventricle. A systolic thrill and a holosystolic murmur are accompanied by a loud pulmonary closure sound and an apical mid-diastolic flow murmur across the mitral valve. The electrocardiogram shows biatrial P waves and biventricular hypertrophy. The x-ray discloses shunt vascularity and pulmonary venous congestion with dilation of the pulmonary trunk and all four cardiac chambers. A rise in pulmonary vascular resistance decreases pulmonary blood flow and ameliorates congestive heart failure. When pulmonary resistance is suprasystemic, the shunt is reversed and Eisenmenger's syndrome exists. The physical examination then reveals symmetric cyanosis, a normal jugular venous pulse with a small dominant A wave, a relatively modest right ventricular impulse, a palpable pulmonary trunk, and a palpable pulmonary component of the second heart sound. Auscultation discloses signs of pure pulmonary hypertension: a pulmonary ejection sound, a short pulmonary midsystolic murmur, a loud single second heart sound, and a Graham Steell murmur. The electrocardiogram shows right atrial P waves and relatively pure right ventricular hypertrophy. The x-ray reveals oligemic lung fields and an unimpressive cardiac silhouette except for a dilated pulmonary trunk and a convex right ventricle at the apex.

VENTRICULAR SEPTAL DEFECT WITH AORTIC REGURGITATION

In 1921, Laubry and Pezzi[119] published a postmortem account of ventricular septal defect with an incompetent aortic valve. Eleven years later, Laubry, Routier, and Soulie[142] described two patients with a ventricular septal defect, a loud aortic diastolic murmur, a wide pulse pressure, and at necropsy, prolapsed aortic cusps. The prevalence of aortic regurgitation with ventricular septal defect depends largely on the relative prevalence of

perimembranous versus doubly committed subarterial defects.[17,143,144] *Perimembranous* defects are more common in whites, with an incidence rate of aortic regurgitation of approximately 5% to 8%.[143,144] *Subarterial* defects are more common in Asians, with an incidence rate of aortic regurgitation of approximately 30%.[17,144]

Perimembranous defects are located immediately beneath the commissure between the right coronary cusp and the noncoronary cusp.[143] Aortic regurgitation is associated with sagging or herniation of the right coronary cusp or the right coronary cusp and the noncoronary cusp (Figures 17-37 and 17-38).[32,144] Herniation sometimes protrudes into the right ventricular outflow tract and causes obstruction[145] or protrudes through the ventricular septal defect and reduces the left-to-right shunt.[143]

The inherent morphologic basis for aortic regurgitation has been assigned to the right coronary/noncoronary commissure where a structural abnormality is aggravated if not caused by the high-velocity jet accompanying the ventricular septal defect shunt.[145,146] This is in accord with observations that aortic regurgitation develops years *after* birth[147] and that when the high-velocity jet is absent as in Eisenmenger's syndrome, aortic regurgitation is virtually unknown.[143]

The typical sequence begins with the basic structural abnormality responsible for faulty aortic leaflet apposition, followed by sagging of the noncoronary cusp and right coronary cusp (see Figures 17-37 and 17-38).[145,146] Once the cusps fall below the normal closure line, the aortic valve becomes incompetent, the impact of the regurgitant jet provokes leaflet elongation and thickening, and aortic regurgitation begets aortic regurgitation.[146]

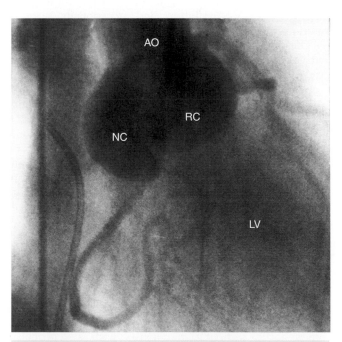

FIGURE 17-37 Right anterior oblique aortogram from a 19-year-old man with a restrictive perimembranous ventricular septal defect. Mild to moderate aortic regurgitation opacified the left ventricle (LV). There is sagging of the noncoronary cusp (NC) and right coronary cusp (RC). (AO = aorta.)

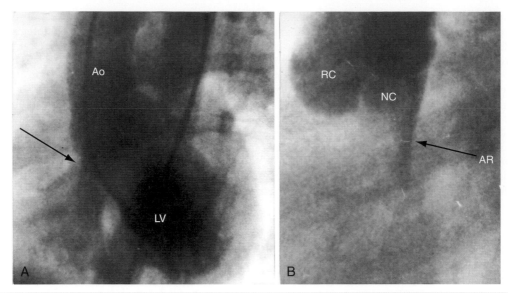

FIGURE 17-38 Angiograms from a 5-year-old boy with a moderately restrictive perimembranous ventricular septal defect and mild aortic regurgitation. **A,** Left anterior oblique left ventriculogram (LV) discloses the shunt (arrow). (AO = aorta.) **B,** Lateral aortogram shows sagging of the right coronary cusp (RC) and noncoronary cusp (NC) with mild aortic regurgitation (AR).

Ventricular septal defects in the infundibular septum lie immediately beneath the aortic and pulmonary valves that constitute a contiguous roof over the defect, which is therefore doubly committed and subarterial.[17] The aortic and pulmonary valves are in fibrous continuity because the infundibular septum, including the septal portion of the subpulmonary infundibulum, is deficient.[17] The aortic valve lacks support, so the right and noncoronary sinuses move into the right ventricular outflow tract, causing aortic regurgitation and occasionally a subpulmonary gradient.[12,143,145]

The *physiologic consequences* of aortic regurgitation with a ventricular septal defect are borne by the left ventricle, which receives the sum of the regurgitant volume from the aorta and the shunt volume from the ventricular septal defect. Aortic regurgitation begins insidiously and progresses gradually unless infective endocarditis supervenes (see section The History). The left-to-right shunt is larger for a given degree of incompetence when regurgitation is associated with a *subarterial* defect, which does not decrease in size unless partially occluded by the prolapsed right coronary cusp. Conversely, a *perimembranous* ventricular defect tends to get smaller as the degree of aortic regurgitation increases, so aortic regurgitant volume rather than shunt volume becomes the major contributor to left ventricular volume overload.[143] The shunt can then be trivial or even absent in the presence of severe aortic regurgitation (Figure 17-39).[143]

History

When aortic regurgitation coexists with a ventricular septal defect, the male:female ratio is as high as 2:1, in contrast to the equal gender distribution when a ventricular septal defect occurs in isolation (see previous).[143,144] Echocardiography and aortography in perimembranous and subarterial ventricular septal defects detect herniation

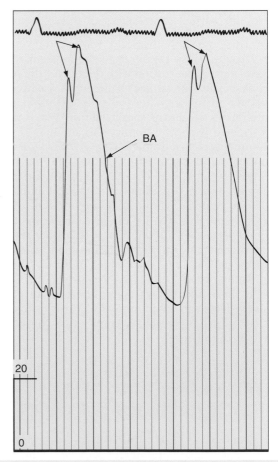

FIGURE 17-39 Brachial arterial pulse (BA) from a 21-year-old man with a restrictive perimembranous ventricular septal defect and severe aortic regurgitation. The brachial pulse shows a brisk rise, bisferiens (twin) peaks, and a wide pulse pressure (115/55 mm Hg). The left-to-right shunt was 1.5 to 1. The pulmonary artery pressure was normal.

of the right and noncoronary cusps before the onset of regurgitation,[17] which seldom begins before age 2 years or after age 10 years and peaks between 5 and 9 years of age.[143,147]

The diagnosis can sometimes be suspected based on the history. The typical murmur of ventricular septal defect is known for years, more likely in a male. Between age 5 years and 9 years, an additional murmur is discovered. The patient gradually becomes aware of neck pulsations, chest pain, diaphoresis, and vigorous precordial movement, especially at night when lying in the left lateral recumbent position. Infective endocarditis, to which the incompetent aortic valve is highly susceptible, dramatically accelerates regurgitant flow,[144] and the occasional coexistence of a bicuspid aortic valve increases susceptibility to infection.[148]

Arterial Pulse

In *gradually progressive chronic severe aortic regurgitation*, the arterial pulse is the classic bounding Corrigan water hammer with a wide pulse pressure, a brisk rate of rise, bisferiens peaks (see Figure 17-39), pistol shot sounds over the femoral arteries, and capillary pulsations in the nail beds (see Chapter 7).[143] Taussig said of one patient, "The head shook with each cardiac impulse and the pulsations of the dorsalis pedis were readily felt through the bed clothes."[149]

In *acute severe aortic regurgitation*, the arterial pulse differs considerably from the previous description.[150] The left ventricle cannot adapt to the sudden increase in volume, so contractility is depressed, the velocity of ejection declines, stroke volume and peak systolic pressure cannot increase, and end diastolic pressure rises steeply. Accordingly, the pulse pressure is not increased, and the rate of rise is not brisk.

Precordial Movement and Palpation

The greater the degree of aortic regurgitation, the more dynamic the left ventricular impulse; a right ventricular impulse is conspicuous by its absence.

Auscultation

The murmurs of ventricular septal defect with aortic regurgitation are *not continuous* (see Figure 17-41B) but are contiguous *holosystolic and early diastolic* (Figures 17-40 and 17-41A).[116,143] The systolic portion of the murmur is typical of ventricular septal defect (see Figures 17-40 and 17-41A),[110] and the diastolic portion is typical of chronic aortic regurgitation (see Figures 17-40 and 17-41A).[150] These contiguous murmurs do not peak around the second heart sound and therefore differ from the continuous murmur of a patent ductus arteriosus that envelops the second heart sound and peaks around it (see Figure 17-41B and Chapter 20).

The systolic and diastolic portions of the continuous murmur of patent ductus are both maximal in the first or second left intercostal space, the *systolic* portion of the murmur of ventricular septal defect is loudest in the third or fourth intercostal space, and the *diastolic* aortic regurgitation portion is best heard at the mid to lower left

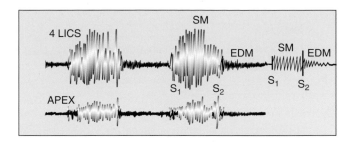

A

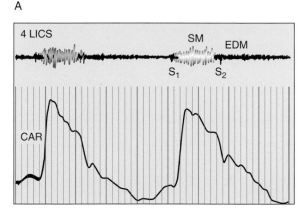

B

FIGURE 17-40   **A,** Tracings from an 8-year-old boy with a moderately restrictive perimembranous ventricular septal defect, a 2 to 1 left-to-right shunt, and mild aortic regurgitation. A prominent holosystolic murmur (SM) is followed by a soft, high-frequency early diastolic murmur of aortic regurgitation (EDM). The holosystolic and early diastolic murmurs are schematically illustrated on the right of the same strip (also see Figure 17-41A). At the apex, the holosystolic murmur remained prominent, but the aortic regurgitation murmur was absent. **B,** Tracings from a 17-year-old boy with a restrictive perimembranous ventricular septal defect, a 1.3 to 1 shunt, and moderate aortic regurgitation (brachial arterial pressure, 135/50 mm Hg). In the fourth left intercostal space (4 LICS), there was the high-frequency holosystolic murmur of a restrictive ventricular septal defect and a soft early diastolic murmur (EDM) of aortic regurgitation. (CAR = carotid pulse.)

sternal border (see Figure 17-40). Uncertainty arises in the *third* left intercostal space where the systolic and diastolic murmurs are both prominent and sometimes create the mistaken impression of a continuous murmur. Distinctive eddy sounds punctuate the ductus murmur.[116]

The distinction between the murmur of aortic regurgitation and a Graham Steell murmur is difficult if not impossible on purely auscultatory grounds.[116] However, aortic regurgitation rarely occurs with the Eisenmenger's syndrome (see previous), so a high-frequency early diastolic murmur in that contest is likely to be Graham Steell.[120] Conversely, in the presence of a restrictive ventricular septal defect, an early diastolic murmur is likely to be aortic regurgitation, especially if the patient is male and certainly if the systemic arterial pulse is water hammer. When the shunt is small and aortic regurgitation is severe, an apical mid-diastolic murmur is an Austin Flint rumble and not increased shunt flow across the mitral valve.[143]

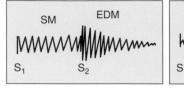
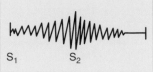

A   B

FIGURE 17-41 Schematic illustrations of (A) the holosystolic murmur (SM) followed by an early diastolic murmur (EDM) in contrast to (B) the continuous murmur of a patent ductus that envelops the second heart sound and peaks around it.

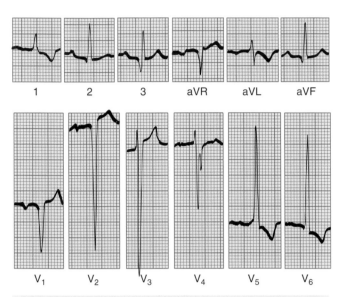

FIGURE 17-42 Electrocardiogram from a 21-year-old man with a restrictive perimembranous ventricular septal defect and severe aortic regurgitation. The tracing resembles isolated severe aortic regurgitation with PR interval prolongation, deep S waves in right precordial leads, and tall R waves with deeply inverted T waves and coved ST segments in left precordial leads, typical of left ventricular volume overload.

Electrocardiogram

The scalar tracing is useful in calling attention to the left ventricular hypertrophy of aortic regurgitation unexplained by a restrictive ventricular septal defect (Figure 17-42) (i.e., the electrocardiogram resembles aortic regurgitation rather than ventricular septal defect). Deep Q waves, tall R waves, deeply inverted T waves, and coved ST segments appear in left precordial leads (Figure 17-42). When a subarterial ventricular septal defect coexists with moderate aortic regurgitation and a moderate left-to-right shunt, these distinctions are less clear.

X-Ray

A key point in the x-ray is the contrast between appreciable enlargement of the left ventricle in the context of no more than a modest left-to-right shunt (Figure 17-43).[143] The x-ray resembles severe aortic regurgitation rather

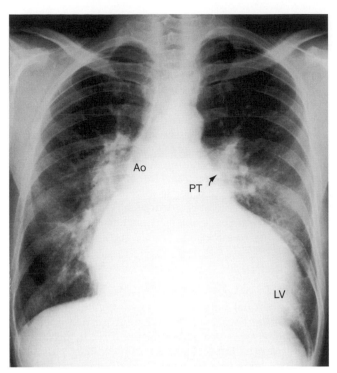

FIGURE 17-43 X-ray from a 21-year-old man with a restrictive perimembranous ventricular septal defect, a left-to-right shunt of 1.4 to 1, and severe aortic regurgitation. The electrocardiogram is shown in Figure 17-42. The pulmonary trunk (PT) only mildly convex, but the relatively prominent pulmonary vascularity implies that the shunt had previously been larger and the ventricular septal defect had decreased in size. The large left ventricle (LV) and the dilated ascending aorta (Ao) are the result of the aortic regurgitation, not the left-to-right shunt of the ventricular septal defect.

than ventricular septal defect (see Figure 17-43). The ascending aorta is prominent and pulsates vigorously on fluoroscopy. When the ventricular septal defect is subarterial, the aortic root is inconspicuous despite appreciable regurgitant flow because the ventricular septal defect remains large enough to divert a sizable fraction of left ventricular stroke volume into the pulmonary circulation (Figure 17-44). Whether the ventricular septal defect is perimembranous or subarterial, the onset of aortic regurgitation is insidious, so the x-ray initially reflects the left-to-right shunt. As time goes on, the balance shifts as described previously.

Echocardiogram

Transthoracic and transesophageal echocardiography with Doppler interrogation and color flow imaging identify the ventricular septal defect as perimembranous or subarterial, identify prolapse of the right and noncoronary cusps, and establish the presence and degree of aortic regurgitation (Figure 17-45 and Videos 17-6A and 17-6B).[2,17,151] Prolapse of the right coronary artery can be distinguished from an aneurysm of the membranous septum. Color flow imaging identifies flow across a perimembranous ventricular septal defect (Figure 17-46A) and

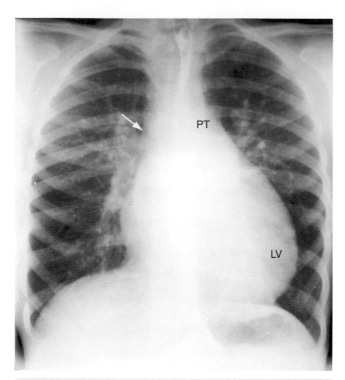

FIGURE 17-44 X-ray from a 14-year-old boy with moderately severe aortic regurgitation and a 2 to 1 left-to-right shunt through a subarterial ventricular septal defect. The left ventricle (LV) is considerably enlarged because of a combination of volume overload from moderately severe aortic regurgitation and a 2 to 1 left-to-right shunt. Pulmonary vascularity is increased, the pulmonary trunk (PT) is only slightly convex, and the aortic root (arrow) is inconspicuous.

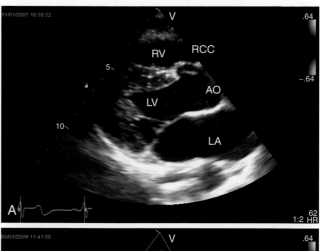

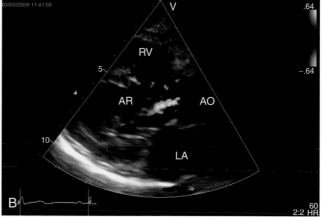

FIGURE 17-45 Echocardiograms from a 4-year-old boy with a moderately restrictive perimembranous ventricular septal defect and mild aortic regurgitation. **A,** The parasternal long-axis view shows prolapse of the right coronary cusp (RCC) into the ventricular septal defect. (AO = aorta; RV/LV = right ventricle/left ventricle; LA = left atrium.) **B,** Color flow image in the short axis showing aortic regurgitation (AR) (Videos 17-6A and 17-6B).

establishes the presence and degree of aortic regurgitation (see Figures 17-45B and 17-46B). A subarterial ventricular septal defect is recognized by its proximity to the pulmonary and aortic valves, whose sinuses are contiguous without interposition of an infundibular septum. The systolic jet through the subarterial ventricular septal defect is directed into the pulmonary trunk (see Figure 17-36). Echocardiography with color flow imaging identifies prolapse of the right coronary cusp or noncoronary aortic cusp before the onset of aortic regurgitation.[17] Doppler interrogation determines the presence and degree of right ventricular outflow obstruction caused by prolapse of an elongated right coronary cusp through the ventricular septal defect.

Summary

Patients with ventricular septal defect and aortic regurgitation are likely to be male. The murmur of ventricular septal defect dates from infancy. Between 5 and 9 years of age, the aortic regurgitation murmur makes its appearance and is followed by insidious progression of regurgitant flow with gradual development of a bounding arterial pulse and a dynamic left ventricular impulse. The systolic or diastolic murmurs of ventricular septal defect and aortic regurgitation are contiguous holosystolic or early diastolic, do not peak around the second heart sound, and are devoid of eddy sounds. The electrocardiogram and x-ray disclose

left ventricular hypertrophy and left ventricular enlargement out of proportion to the size of the left- to-right shunt. Echocardiography with color flow imaging and Doppler interrogation identify the ventricular septal defect in the perimembranous or infundibular septum and establish the presence and degree of aortic regurgitation.

LEFT VENTRICULAR TO RIGHT ATRIAL COMMUNICATION

In 1838, Thurnman[152] described a left ventricular–to–right atrial communication in which a cleft tricuspid septal leaflet adhered to a ventricular septal defect. Two decades later, Hillier[153] reported on "Congenital Malformation of the Heart; Perforation of the Septum Ventriculorum, Establishing a Communication between the Left Ventricle and the Right Atrium." Similar if not identical reports appeared from Merkel in 1869 and from Preicz in 1890.[154] The 1958 publication by

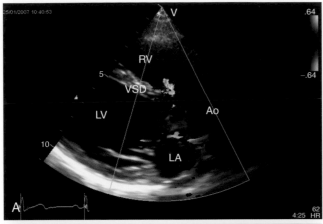

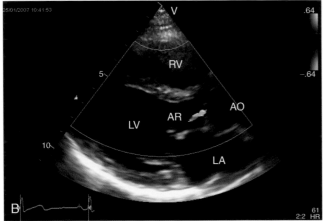

FIGURE 17-46 Color flow images in the parasternal long axis from an 8-year-old girl with a restrictive perimembranous ventricular septal defect and aortic regurgitation. **A,** There is a high-velocity jet across the ventricular septal defect (VSD). (Ao=aorta; LV=left ventricle; RV = right ventricle; LA=left atrium.) **B,** Diastolic frame shows the high-velocity jet of moderate aortic regurgitation (AR).

FIGURE 17-47 Schematic illustrations of the two varieties of left ventricular–to–right atrial communications originally proposed by Perry, Burchell, and Edwards[156] in 1949. The variety depicted in (A), the large sketch, consists of a defect in the *intraventricular* portion of the membranous septum with tethering of the septal tricuspid leaflet to the crest of the ventricular septal defect. (RA/LA=right atrium/left atrium; RV/LV=right ventricle/left ventricle.) Circular insert (E) depicts the variety in which a defect in the *atrioventricular* portion of the membranous septum creates a direct communication from left ventricle into right atrium (arrow). Inserts B, C, and D are variations of a *subanular* defect in the membranous septum. *(With permission from Perry EL, Burchell HB, Edwards JE. Congenital communication between left ventricle and right atrium. Proc Staff Meet Mayo Clin 1949;24:198.)*

Gerbode and associates[155] stimulated renewed interest in the malformation that is sometimes called the Gerbode defect.

A perimembranous ventricular septal defect is an obligatory component of the two types of left ventricular–to–right atrial communications illustrated in Figure 17-47.[77,155–158] The first and more common type is characterized by a defect in the *intraventricular portion* of the membranous septum that opens into the right ventricle and then communicates with the right atrium through an anatomic deficiency in the septal tricuspid leaflet, which is tethered to the crest of the ventricular septum (see Figure 17-47A). The deficiency in the septal tricuspid leaflet takes the form of perforations, clefts, and widening or absence of the commissure between the anterior and septal tricuspid leaflets.[157] A septal aneurysm is almost always present.[159,160] The ventriculoatrial communication originally described by Thurnman was this first type.[152] In the second and much less common type, the defect is in the *atrioventricular* portion of the membranous septum, so left

ventricular blood enters the right atrium directly (see Figure 17-47E). This type of communication differs structurally from the atrioventricular septal defect discussed in Chapter 15.

The *physiologic consequences* of left ventricular to right atrial communications depend on the size of the defect and on the pulmonary vascular resistance, as is the case with other types of ventricular septal defects. Shunt flow begins *in utero* because of the obligatory difference in systolic pressure between the left ventricle and right atrium.[77] The right atrium accepts the shunt with little or no elevation of pressure because right atrial distensibility and volume increase appropriately and because the ventricular septal defect is usually restrictive,[77,155] a feature that also accounts for normal or near-normal pulmonary artery pressure. Left ventricular blood that is received by the right atrium during ventricular systole (Figure 17-48) enters the right ventricle during the next diastole, establishing right ventricular volume overload. The shunt volume then finds its way through the pulmonary circulation, so volume overload of the left side of the heart coexists.

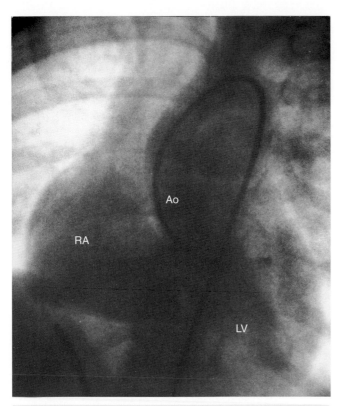

FIGURE 17-48 Angiocardiogram from a 4-year-old girl with a perimembranous ventricular septal defect and a left ventricular (LV) to right atrial (RA) shunt. (Ao = ascending aorta.)

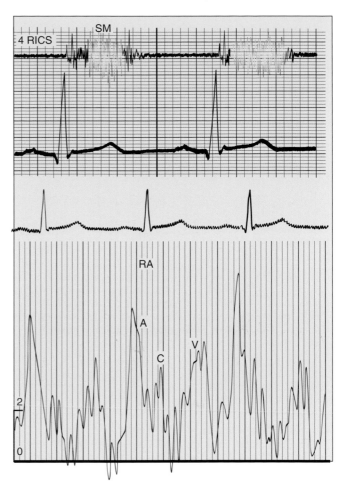

FIGURE 17-49 Tracings from a 17-year-old boy with a left ventricular–to–right atrial communication and a 2 to 1 left-to-right shunt. A prominent holosystolic murmur (SM) was present in the fourth *right* intercostal space (4 RICS). The right atrial (RA) pressure pulse did not show a large V wave even though the right atrium received shunt from the left ventricle.

History

Gender distribution is equal or with slight female preponderance.[77,161] One patient with a left ventricular–to–right atrial communication had a sibling with an isolated perimembranous ventricular septal defect.[160] The clinical course is, for all practical purposes, indistinguishable from that described previously for restrictive or moderately restrictive perimembranous ventricular septal defects. However, an important difference is the *chronology* of the murmur because onset of the shunt and therefore the onset of the murmur do not depend on the neonatal fall in pulmonary vascular resistance. The shunt is present *in utero* (see previous) because of the obligatory differences in systolic pressure between left ventricle and right atrium, so the murmur generated by the shunt is necessarily present at birth.[77] The lesion is susceptible to infective endocarditis as with other perimembranous ventricular septal defects.[162] Occasionally, infective endocarditis is responsible for creating an acquired Gerbode defect (see previous).[82]

Jugular Venous Pulse

Because right atrial volume and distensibility increase in proportion to the shunt,[77,155] large V waves are seldom present and the mean jugular venous pressure is seldom elevated (Figure 17-49), even though the left ventricle ejects into the right atrium (see previous).[155]

Precordial Movement and Palpation

The left-to-right shunt received by the right atrium then enters the right ventricle, which is therefore volume overloaded. The right ventricular impulse is disproportionately prominent compared with ventricular septal defects of comparable size in other locations and is analogous to the volume-overloaded right ventricular impulse of an ostium secundum atrial septal defect (see Chapter 15). However, the apex is occupied by a volume-overloaded *left* ventricle.

Auscultation

The quality, configuration, and intensity of the systolic murmur generated by a left ventricular–to–right atrial communication are indistinguishable from murmurs of other ventricular septal defects of comparable size.[155] The *topographic location* of the murmur is its only distinguishing feature. Because the shunt is received by a right atrium that underlies the *right* lower sternal border (see Figure 17-49), the systolic murmur is recorded within the right atrial cavity (Figure 17-50)[163] and is located in a relatively rightward

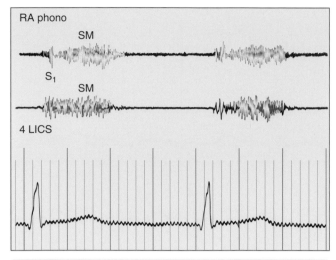

FIGURE 17-50 Tracings from the 17-year-old boy referred to in Figure 17-49. Intracardiac phonocardiogram within the right atrial cavity (RA pHONO) recorded a holosystolic murmur (SM), and the thoracic wall phonocardiogram in the fourth left intercostal space (4 LICS) recorded an identical murmur.

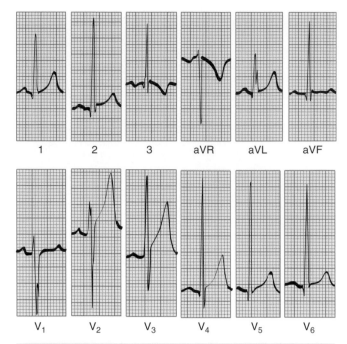

FIGURE 17-51 Electrocardiogram from the 17-year-old boy referred to in Figure 17-49. The tracing resembles an isolated ventricular septal defect. Volume overload of the left ventricle is represented by prominent Q waves, tall R waves, and peaked T waves in leads V_{5-6}. Slight peaking of the P wave in lead V_2 is the only suggestion of a right atrial abnormality.

thoracic position (see Figure 17-49).[164] Equal volumes of blood traverse the tricuspid and mitral valves, so middiastolic murmurs are generated across both atrioventeicular valves, depending on shunt volume.

The intensity, splitting, and respiratory movement of the second heart sound are the same as in comparable isolated perimembranous ventricular septal defects. The split widens normally during inspiration because systemic venous return to the right side of the heart increases without a reciprocal decline in left-to-right shunt. The systolic shunt that is responsible for volume overload of the right ventricle also traverses the left ventricle, so both ventricles handle equal volumes that are ejected against different resistances. Low pulmonary vascular resistance and increased pulmonary capacitance delay the pulmonary component of the second sound. The split is persistent but moves normally with respiration because an intact atrial septum prevents a reciprocal decline in left-to-right shunt that accompanies an ostium secundum atrial septal defect (see Chapter 15). Normal intensity of the pulmonary component is a useful sign because it indicates that right ventricular enlargement is not the result of pulmonary hypertension but instead of volume overload.

Electrocardiogram

There is an age-related increase in the incidence of supraventricular tachycardia, atrial flutter, and atrial fibrillation.[77,165] Tall peaked right atrial P waves date from infancy because the right atrium is the early recipient of the left-to-right shunt. PR interval prolongation reflects right atrial enlargement, and biatrial P wave abnormalities are common because both atria handle an equivalent increase in volume (Figure 17-51).[77,166]

An rSr prime in lead V_1 and a terminal r wave in aVR and V_3R are electrocardiographic signs of right ventricular

volume overload. Prominent left precordial Q waves, tall R waves, and upright T waves are signs of coexisting left ventricular volume overload (see Figure 17-51). A useful electrocardiographic sign is the combination of tall peaked *right* atrial P waves with *left* ventricular hypertrophy.[77,155]

X-Ray

The most distinctive feature in the x-ray is disproportionate right atrial enlargement (Figure 17-52).[155,161,165] The cardiac silhouette occasionally has a ball-like shape with the right side of the ball formed by the large right atrium and the left side of the ball formed by dilation of the right ventricular infundibulum and the left ventricle (see Figure 17-52A).[77,165]

Echocardiogram

Echocardiography identifies the perimemranous ventricular septal defect, and color flow imaging identifies the flow pattern from left ventricle into right atrium.[133,135] The relationship of the ventricular septal defect to the tricuspid valve can be established, and a ventricular septal aneurysm can be identified.

Summary

Clinical features of a left ventricular–to–right atrial communication resemble those of an isolated perimembranous ventricular septal defect of comparable size, but with a number of important differences. The systolic

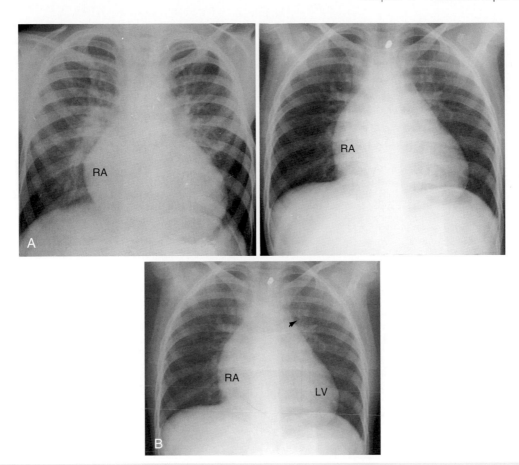

FIGURE 17-52 A, X-ray from a 4-year-old girl with a left ventricular–to–right atrial communication and a 2 to 1 left-to-right shunt. Pulmonary vascularity is increased. The right atrium (RA) is disproportionately enlarged compared to an inconspicuous pulmonary trunk. A dilated left ventricle occupies the apex and extends below the left hemidiaphragm. **B,** X-ray from a 10-year-old boy with a left ventricular–to–right atrial communication and a 2 to 1 left-to-right shunt. Pulmonary arterial vascularity is increased. The right atrium (RA) is disproportionately enlarged compared to the inconspicuous pulmonary trunk (arrow). A dilated left ventricle (LV) occupies the apex and extends below the left hemidiaphragm.

murmur is present *in utero* and therefore at birth, and the murmur occupies a relatively rightward thoracic position because it originates within the right atrium. Precordial palpation identifies both right and left ventricular impulses. The electrocardiogram shows tall peaked right atrial P waves without right ventricular hypertrophy, but instead with evidence of left ventricular volume overload. Atrial arrhythmias are relatively common. The x-ray reveals right atrium enlargement that is disproportionate to the relatively small size of the pulmonary trunk. Echocardiography identifies the perimembranous ventricular septal defect, and color flow imaging establishes shunt flow from left ventricle into right atrium. The relationship of the ventricular septal defect to the tricuspid valve can be established, and a ventricular septal aneuyrsm can be identified.

REFERENCES

 1. Roger H. Clinical researches on the congenital communication of the two sides of the heart by failure of occlusion of the interventricular septum. Bull, de l'Acad. de Méd. 8:1074,1879. In: Willius EA, Keys TE, eds. *Classics of Cardiology*. Malabar: Floida Robert E. Krieger Publishing Company; 1983.

 2. Minette MS, Sahn DJ. Ventricular septal defects. *Circulation*. 2006;114:2190–2197.

 3. Martin GR, Perry LW, Ferencz C. Increased prevalence of ventricular septal defect: epidemic or improved diagnosis. *Pediatrics*. 1989;83:200–203.

 4. Newman TB. Etiology of ventricular septal defects: an epidemiologic approach. *Pediatrics*. 1985;76:741–749.

 5. Hoffman JI, Kaplan S. The incidence of congenital heart disease. *J Am Coll Cardiol*. 2002;39:1890–1900.

 6. Ferencz C, Rubin JD, Mccarter RJ, et al. Congenital heart disease: prevalence at livebirth. The Baltimore-Washington Infant Study. *Am J Epidemiol*. 1985;121:31–36.

 7. Fyler DC. Report of the New England Regional Infant Cardiac Program. *Pediatrics*. 1980;65:375–461.

 8. Hoffman JI, Christianson R. Congenital heart disease in a cohort of 19,502 births with long-term follow-up. *Am J Cardiol*. 1978;42: 641–647.

 9. Mcdaniel NL. Ventricular and atrial septal defects. *Pediatr Rev*. 2001;22:265–270.

10. Anderson RH, Wilcox BR. The surgical anatomy of ventricular septal defect. *J Card Surg*. 1992;7:17–35.

11. Baker EJ, Leung MP, Anderson RH, Fischer DR, Zuberbuhler JR. The cross sectional anatomy of ventricular septal defects: a reappraisal. *Br Heart J*. 1988;59:339–351.

12. Soto B, Becker AE, Moulaert AJ, Lie JT, Anderson RH. Classification of ventricular septal defects. *Br Heart J*. 1980;43:332–343.

13. Titus JL, Daugherty GW, Edwards JE. Anatomy of the atrioventricular conduction system in ventricular septal defect. *Circulation*. 1963;28:72–81.

14. Becu LM, Burchell HB, Dushane JW, Edwards JE, Fontana RS, Kirklin JW. Anatomic and pathologic studies in ventricular septal defect. *Circulation.* 1956;14:349–364.

15. Saab NG, Burchell HB, Dushane JW, Titus JL. Muscular ventricular septal defects. *Am J Cardiol.* 1966;18:713–723.

16. Lincoln C, Jamieson S, Joseph M, Shinebourne E, Anderson RH. Transatrial repair of ventricular septal defects with reference to their anatomic classification. *J Thorac Cardiovasc Surg.* 1977;74:183–190.

17. Griffin ML, Sullivan ID, Anderson RH, Macartney FJ. Doubly committed subarterial ventricular septal defect: new morphological criteria with echocardiographic and angiocardiographic correlation. *Br Heart J.* 1988;59:474–479.

18. Gould L, Lyon AF. Prolapse of the pulmonic valve through a ventricular septal defect. *Am J Cardiol.* 1966;18:127–131.

19. Wenink AC, Gittenberger-De Groot AC. Straddling mitral and tricuspid valves: morphologic differences and developmental backgrounds. *Am J Cardiol.* 1982;49:1959–1971.

20. Zielinsky P, Rossi M, Haertel JC, Vitola D, Lucchese FA, Rodrigues R. Subaortic fibrous ridge and ventricular septal defect: role of septal malalignment. *Circulation.* 1987;75:1124–1129.

21. French H. Possibility of loud congenital heart murmur disappearing when child grows up. *Guys Hospital Reports.* 1918;32:87.

22. Weber FP. Can the clinical manifestation of congenital heart disease disappear with the general growth and development of the patient? *British Journal of Children's Diseases.* 1918;15:113.

23. Evans JR, Rowe RD, Keith JD. Spontaneous closure of ventricular septal defects. *Circulation.* 1960;22:1044–1054.

24. Glancy DL, Roberts WC. Complete spontaneous closure of ventricular septal defect: necropsy study of five subjects. *Am J Med.* 1967;43:846–853.

25. Moore D, Vlad P, Lambert EC. Spontaneous closure of ventricular septal defect following cardiac failure in infancy. *J Pediatr.* 1965;66:712–721.

26. Schott GD. Documentation of spontaneous functional closure of a ventricular septal defect during adult life. *Br Heart J.* 1973;35:1214–1216.

27. Simmons RL, Moller JH, Edwards JE. Anatomic evidence for spontaneous closure of ventricular septal defect. *Circulation.* 1966;34:38–45.

28. Wade G, Wright JP. Spontaneous closure of ventricular septal defects. *Lancet.* 1963;1:737–740.

29. Krovetz LJ. Spontaneous closure of ventricular septal defect. *Am J Cardiol.* 1998;81:100–101.

30. Wood PH. *Diseases of the heart and circulation.* Philadelphia: Lippincott; 1956.

31. Anderson RH, Lenox CC, Zuberbuhler JR. Mechanisms of closure of perimembranous ventricular septal defect. *Am J Cardiol.* 1983;52:341–345.

32. Eroglu AG, Oztunc F, Saltik L, Bakari S, Dedeoglu S, Ahunbay G. Evolution of ventricular septal defect with special reference to spontaneous closure rate, subaortic ridge and aortic valve prolapse. *Pediatr Cardiol.* 2003;24:31–35.

33. Garne E. Atrial and ventricular septal defects - epidemiology and spontaneous closure. *J Matern Fetal Neonatal Med.* 2006;19:271–276.

34. Perloff JK. Therapeutics of nature–the invisible sutures of "spontaneous closure". *Am Heart J.* 1971;82:581–585.

35. Moe DG, Guntheroth WG. Spontaneous closure of uncomplicated ventricular septal defect. *Am J Cardiol.* 1987;60:674–678.

36. Alpert BS, Mellits ED, Rowe RD. Spontaneous closure of small ventricular septal defects: probability rates in the first five years of life. *Am J Dis Child.* 1973;125:194–196.

37. Collins G, Calder L, Rose V, Kidd L, Keith J. Ventricular septal defect: clinical and hemodynamic changes in the first five years of life. *Am Heart J.* 1972;84:695–705.

38. Diehl AM, Kittle CF, Crockett JE. Spontaneous complete closure of a high-flow, high-pressure ventricular septal defect. *J Lancet.* 1961;81:572–576.

39. Nadas AS, Scott LP, Hauck AJ, Rudolph AM. Spontaneous functional closing of ventricular septal defects. *N Engl J Med* 1961;201:303–310.

40. Suzuki H, Lucas Jr RV. Spontaneous closure of ventricular septal defects. Anatomic evidence in three patients. *Arch Pathol.* 1967;84:31–36.

41. Wise Jr JR, Wilson WS. Angiographic documentation of spontaneous closure of ventricular septal defect in an adult. *Chest.* 1979;75:90–93.

42. Fellows KE, Westerman GR, Keane JF. Angiocardiography of multiple ventricular septal defects in infancy. *Circulation.* 1982;66:1094–1099.

43. Shirali GS, Smith EO, Geva T. Quantitation of echocardiographic predictors of outcome in infants with isolated ventricular septal defect. *Am Heart J.* 1995;130:1228–1235.

44. Chesler E, Korns ME, Edwards JE. Anomalies of the tricuspid valve, including pouches, resembling aneurysms of the membranous ventricular septum. *Am J Cardiol.* 1968;21:661–668.

45. Beerman LB, Park SC, Fischer DR, et al. Ventricular septal defect associated with aneurysm of the membranous septum. *J Am Coll Cardiol.* 1985;5:118–123.

46. Hamby RI, Raia F, Apiado O. Aneurysm of the pars membranacea. Report of three adult cases and a review of the literature. *Am Heart J.* 1970;79:688–699.

47. Misra KP, Hildner FJ, Cohen LS, Narula OS, Samet P. Aneurysm of the membranous ventricular septum. A mechanism for spontaneous closure of ventricular septal defect. *N Engl J Med.* 1970;283:58–61.

48. Ramaciotti C, Keren A, Silverman NH. Importance of (perimembranous) ventricular septal aneurysm in the natural history of isolated perimembranous ventricular septal defect. *Am J Cardiol.* 1986;57:268–272.

49. Varghese PJ, Izukawa T, Celermajer J, Simon A, Rowe RD. Aneurysm of the membranous ventricular septum: A method of spontaneous closure of small ventricular septal defect. *Am J Cardiol.* 1969;24:531–536.

50. Sethia B, Cotter L. Giant aneurysm of membranous septum. Unusual cause of mediastinal mass. *Br Heart J.* 1981;46:107–109.

51. Thery C, Lekieffre J, Dupuis C. Atrioventricular block secondary to a congenital aneurysm of the membranous septum. Histological examination of conduction system. *Br Heart J.* 1975;37:1097–1100.

52. Chen MR, Rigby ML, Redington AN. Familial aneurysms of the interventricular septum. *Br Heart J.* 1991;65:104–106.

53. Rudolph AM. The changes in the circulation after birth. Their importance in congenital heart disease. *Circulation.* 1970;41:343–359.

54. Nora JJ, Cohen M, Maxwell GM. Klippel-Feil syndrome with congenital heart disease. *Am J Dis Child.* 1961;102:110.

55. Graham Jr TP, Atwood GF, Boucek Jr RJ, Cordell D, Boerth RC. Right ventricular volume characteristics in ventricular septal defect. *Circulation.* 1976;54:800–804.

56. Herbert WH. Hydrogen-detected ventricular septal defects. *Br Heart J.* 1969;31:766–769.

57. Bendien C, Bossina KK, Buurma AE, et al. Hemodynamic effects of dynamic exercise in children and adolescents with moderate-to-small ventricular septal defects. *Circulation.* 1984;70:929–934.

58. Jarmakani JM, Graham Jr TP, Canent Jr RV. Left ventricular contractile state in children with successfully corrected ventricular septal defect. *Circulation.* 1972;45:I102–110.

59. Friedli B, Kidd BS, Mustard WT, Keith JD. Ventricular septal defect with increased pulmonary vascular resistance. Late results of surgical closure. *Am J Cardiol.* 1974;33:403–409.

60. Haworth SG. Pulmonary vascular disease in ventricular septal defect: structural and functional correlations in lung biopsies from 85 patients, with outcome of intracardiac repair. *J Pathol.* 1987;152:157–168.

61. Wagenvoort CA, Neufeld HN, Dushane JW, Edwards JE. The pulmonary arterial tree in ventricular septal defect. A quantitative study of anatomic features in fetuses, infants. and children. *Circulation.* 1961;23:740–748.

62. Walker WJ, Garcia-Gonzalez E, Hall RJ, et al. Interventricular septal defect: Analysis of 415 catheterized cases, ninety with serial hemodynamic studies. *Circulation.* 1965;31:54–65.

63. Warnes CA, Boger JE, Roberts WC. Eisenmenger ventricular septal defect with prolonged survival. *Am J Cardiol.* 1984;54:460–462.

64. Wood P. The Eisenmenger syndrome, or pulmonary hypertension with reversed central shunt. *Br Med J*. 1958;2:701–709, 755–762.

65. Shuhaiber JH. Eisenmenger's syndrome and pulmonary-artery dissection. *N Engl J Med*. 2007;357:718; author reply 718–719.

66. Hopkins WE, Waggoner AD. Severe pulmonary hypertension without right ventricular failure: the unique hearts of patients with Eisenmenger syndrome. *Am J Cardiol*. 2002;89:34–38.

67. Van Hare GF, Soffer LJ, Sivakoff MC, Liebman J. Twenty-five-year experience with ventricular septal defect in infants and children. *Am Heart J*. 1987;114:606–614.

68. Bliss HA, Moffat JE. Hemodymaic events during the development of cyanosis and heart failure in a patient with large ventricular septal defect. *Circulation*. 1964;30:101–105.

69. Lucas Jr. RV, Adams Jr P, Anderson RC, Meyne NG, Lillehei CW, Varco RL. The natural history of isolated ventricular septal defect. A serial physiologic study. *Circulation*. 1961;24: 1372–1387.

70. Weidman WH, Blount Jr. SG, Dushane JW, Gersony WM, Hayes CJ, Nadas AS. Clinical course in ventricular septal defect. *Circulation*. 1977;56:I56–69.

71. Czeizel A, Meszaros M. Two family studies of children with ventricular septal defect. *Eur J Pediatr*. 1981;136:81–85.

72. Nora JJ, Nora AH. The genetic contribution to congenital heart disease. In: Nora JJ, Takao A, eds. *Congenital Heart Disease Mount Kisco*. New York: Futura Publishing Company; 1984.

73. Blair E, Herman R, Cowley RA. Interventricular septal defect in identical twins. *J Thorac Cardiovasc Surg*. 1965;50:197–201.

74. Rubenstein HJ, Weaver KH. Monozygotic twins concordant for ventricular septal defects. Case report and review of the literature of congenital heart disease in monozygotic twins. *Am J Cardiol*. 1965;15:386–390.

75. Levy RJ, Rosenthal A, Miettinen OS, Nadas AS. Determinants of growth in patients with ventricular septal defect. *Circulation*. 1978;57:793–797.

76. Baptista MJ, Fairbrother UL, Howard CM, et al. Heterotrisomy, a significant contributing factor to ventricular septal defect associated with Down syndrome? *Hum Genet*. 2000;107: 476–482.

77. Riemenschneider TA, Moss AJ. Left ventricular-right atrial communication. *Am J Cardiol*. 1967;19:710–718.

78. Mudd JG, Aykent Y, Willman VL, Hanlon CR, Fagan LF. The natural and postoperative history of 252 patients with proved ventricular septal defects. *Am J Med*. 1965;39:946–951.

79. Shah P, Singh WS, Rose V, Keith JD. Incidence of bacterial endocarditis in ventricular septal defects. *Circulation*. 1966;34: 127–131.

80. Zakrzewski T, Keith J. Bacterial endocarditis in infants and children. *J Pediatr*. 1965;67:1179.

81. Walpot J, Peerenboom P, Van-Wylick A, Klazen C. Aneurysm of the membranous septum with ventricular septal defect and infective endocarditis. *Eur J Echocardiogr*. 2004;5:391–393.

82. Matt P, Winkler B, Gutmann M, Eckstein F. Acquired Gerbode defect after endocarditis. *Eur J Cardiothorac Surg*. 2009;36: 402.

83. Fontana RS, Edwards JE. *Congenital Cardiac Disease*. Philadelphia: W.B. Saunders Company; 1962.

84. Alter BP, Czapek EE, Rowe RD. Sweating in congenital heart disease. *Pediatrics*. 1968;41:123–129.

85. Abbott ME. *Congenital Heart Disease*. New York: Thomas Nelson & Sons; 1932.

86. Eisenmenger V. Die angeborenen Defecte der Kammerscheidewand des Herzens. *Z Klin Med*. 1897;32(suppl 1).

87. Kumar RK, Sandoval J. Advanced pulmonary vascular disease: the Eisenmenger syndrome. *Cardiol Young*. 2009;19:622–626.

88. Perloff JK, Rosove MH, Sietsema KE, Territo MC. Cyanotic congenital heart disease: A multisystem systemic disorder. In: Perloff JK, Child JS, Aboulhosn J, eds. *Congenital Heart Disease in Adults*. 3rd ed. Philadelphia: W.B. Saunders; 2009.

89. Niwa K, Perloff JK, Kaplan S, Child JS, Miner PD. Eisenmenger syndrome in adults: ventricular septal defect, truncus arteriosus, univentricular heart. *J Am Coll Cardiol*. 1999;34:223–232.

90. Territo MC, Rosove MH. Cyanotic congenital heart disease: hematologic management. *J Am Coll Cardiol*. 1991;18:320–322.

91. Rosove MH, Perloff JK, Hocking WG, Child JS, Canobbio MM, Skorton DJ. Chronic hypoxaemia and decompensated erythrocytosis in cyanotic congenital heart disease. *Lancet*. 1986;2:313–315.

92. Terito M, Perloff J, Rosove M, Moake J, Runge A. Acquired von Willebrand factor abnormalities in adults with congenital heart disease. *Clin Appl Thromb Hemost*. 1998;4:257.

93. Clarkson PM, Frye RL, Dushane JW, Burchell HB, Wood EH, Weidman WH. Prognosis for patients with ventricular septal defect and severe pulmonary vascular obstructive disease. *Circulation*. 1968;38:129–135.

94. Brunken RC, Perloff JK, Czernin J, et al. Coronary blood flow and myocardial perfusion reserve in adults with cyanotic congenital heart disease. *Am J Physiol*. 2005;H1798–H1806.

95. Tutar HE, Atalay S, Turkay S, Imamoglu A. QRS axis in isolated perimembranous ventricular septal defect and influences of morphological factors on QRS axis. *J Electrocardiol*. 2001;34: 197–203.

96. Sietsema KE, Cooper DM, Perloff JK, et al. Dynamics of oxygen uptake during exercise in adults with cyanotic congenital heart disease. *Circulation*. 1986;73:1137–1144.

97. Perloff JK. Pregnancy in congenital heart disease: The mother and the fetus. In: Perloff JK, Child JS, Aboulhosn J, eds. *Congenital Heart Disease in Adults*. 3rd ed. Philadelphia: WB Saunders; 2009.

98. Pitts JA, Crosby WM, Basta LL. Eisenmenger's syndrome in pregnancy: does heparin prophylaxis improve the maternal mortality rate? *Am Heart J*. 1977;93:321–326.

99. Niwa K, Perloff JK, Bhuta SM, et al. Structural abnormalities of great arterial walls in congenital heart disease: light and electron microscopic analyses. *Circulation*. 2001;103:393–400.

100. Albers HJ, Carroll SE, Coles JC. Spontaneous closure of a membranous ventricular septal defect. Necrospy finding with clinical application. *Br Med J*. 1962;2:1162–1163.

101. Balderston SM, Shaffer EM, Washington RL, Sondheimer HM. Congenital polyvalvular disease in trisomy 18: echocardiographic diagnosis. *Pediatr Cardiol*. 1990;11:138–142.

102. Matsuoka R, Misugi K, Goto A, Gilbert EF, Ando M. Congenital heart anomalies in the trisomy 18 syndrome, with reference to congenital polyvalvular disease. *Am J Med Genet*. 1983;14: 657–668.

103. Moene RJ, Sobotka-Plojhar M, Oppenheimer-Dekker A, Lindhout D. Ventricular septal defect with overriding aorta in trisomy-18. *Eur J Pediatr*. 1988;147:556–557.

104. Van Praagh S, Truman T, Firpo A, et al. Cardiac malformations in trisomy-18: a study of 41 postmortem cases. *J Am Coll Cardiol*. 1989;13:1586–1597.

105. Lin AE, Perloff JK. Upper limb malformations associated with congenital heart disease. *Am J Cardiol*. 1985;55:1576–1583.

106. Cayler GG. Cardiofacial syndrome. Congenital heart disease and facial weakness, a hitherto unrecognized association. *Arch Dis Child*. 1969;44:69–75.

107. Steeg CN, Woolf P. Cardiovascular malformations in the fetal alcohol syndrome. *Am Heart J*. 1979;98:635–637.

108. Farru O, Duffau G, Rodriguez R. Auscultatory and phonocardiographic characteristics of supracristal ventricular septal defect. *Br Heart J*. 1971;33:238–245.

109. Moncada R, Bicoff JP, Arcilla RA, Agustsson MH, Lendrum BL, Gasul BM. Retrograde left ventricular angiocardiography in ventricular septal defect. *Am J Cardiol*. 1963;11:436–446.

110. Feruglio GA, Gunton RW. Intracardiac phonocardiography in ventricular septal defect. *Circulation*. 1960;21:49–58.

111. Carr M, Kearney DL, Eidem BW. Congenital aneurysm of the muscular interventricular septum. *J Am Soc Echocardiogr*. 2008; 21:1282.e1281–1282.e1286.

112. Linhart JW, Razi B. Late systolic murmur: a clue to the diagnosis of aneurysm of the membranous ventricular septum. *Chest*. 1971;60: 283–286.

113. Pickering D, Keith JD. Systolic clicks with ventricular septal defects. A sign of aneurysm of ventricular septum? *Br Heart J*. 1971;33:538–539.

114. Pieroni DR, Bell BB, Krovetz LJ, Varghese PJ, Rowe RD. Auscultatory recognition of aneurysm of the membranous ventricular septum associated with small ventricular septal defect. *Circulation*. 1971;44:733–739.

115. Winslow TM, Redberg RF, Foster E, Schiller NB. Transesophageal echocardiographic detection of abnormalities of the tricuspid valve in adults associated with spontaneous closure of perimembranous ventricular septal defect. *Am J Cardiol.* 1992;70:967–969.

116. Perloff JK. *Physical Examination of the Heart and Circulation.* 4th ed. Shelton, Connecticut: People's Medical Publishing House; 2009.

117. Harris C, Wise Jr. J, Oakley CM. "Fixed" splitting of the second heart sound in ventricular septal defect. *Br Heart J.* 1971;33:428–431.

118. Nadas AS, Ellison RC. Phonocardiographic analysis of diastolic flow murmurs in secundum atrial septal defect and ventricular septal defect. *Br Heart J.* 1967;29:684–688.

119. Laubry C, Pezzi C. *Traits des Maladies Congenitales du Coeur.* Paris: J. B. Bailliere et Fits; 1921.

120. Perloff JK. Auscultatory and phonocardiographic manifestations of pulmonary hypertension. *Prog Cardiovasc Dis.* 1967;9:303–340.

121. Sutton G, Harris A, Leatham A. Second heart sound in pulmonary hypertension. *Br Heart J.* 1968;30:743–756.

122. Toscano-Barboza E, Dushane JW. Ventricular septal defect: correlation of electrocardiographic and hemodynamic findings in 60 proved cases. *Am J Cardiol.* 1959;3:721–732.

123. Vince DJ, Keith JD. The electrocardiogram in ventricular septal defect. *Circulation.* 1961;23:225–240.

124. Backman H. Influence of structural and functional features of ventricular septal defect on frontal plane QRS axis of the electrocardiogram. *Br Heart J.* 1972;34:274–283.

125. Farru-Albohaire O, Arcil G, Hernandez I. An association between left axis deviation and an aneurysmal defect in children with a perimembranous ventricular septal defect. *Br Heart J.* 1990;64:146–150.

126. Shaw NJ, Godman MJ, Hayes A, Sutherland GR. Superior QRS axis in ventricular septal defect. *Br Heart J.* 1989;62:281–283.

127. Neufeld HN, Titus JL, Dushane JW, Burchell HB, Edwards JE. Isolated ventricular septal defect of the persistent common atrioventricular canal type. *Circulation.* 1961;23:685–696.

128. Witham AC, Mcdaniel JS. Electrocardiogram, vectorcardiogram, and hemodynamics in ventricular septal defect. *Am Heart J.* 1970;79:335–346.

129. Katz LN, Wachtel H. Diphasic QRS type of electrocardiogram in congenital heart disease. *Am Heart J.* 1937;13:202.

130. Vaquez H, Bordet E. *Le Coeur et l'Aorte, Etudes Radiographiques.* Paris: J. B. Bailliere et Fils; 1913.

131. Davies H, Williams J, Wood P. Lung stiffness in states of abnormal pulmonary blood flow and pressure. *Br Heart J.* 1962;24:129–138.

132. Jarmakani JM, Graham Jr TP, Benson Jr DW, Canent Jr RV, Greenfield Jr JC. In vivo pressure-radius relationships of the pulmonary artery in children with congenital heart disease. *Circulation.* 1971;43:585–592.

133. Helmcke F, De Souza A, Nanda NC, et al. Two-dimensional and color Doppler assessment of ventricular septal defect of congenital origin. *Am J Cardiol.* 1989;63:1112–1116.

134. Sutherland GR, Godman MJ, Smallhorn JF, Guiterras P, Anderson RH, Hunter S. Ventricular septal defects. Two dimensional echocardiographic and morphological correlations. *Br Heart J.* 1982;47:316–328.

135. Child J. Transthoracic and transesophageal echocardiographic imaging: Anatomic and homodynamic assessment. In: Perloff J, Child J, eds. *Congenital Heart Disease in Adults.* 2nd ed. Phialdelphia: WB Saunders Co; 1998.

136. Lethor JP, Marcon F, De Moor M, King ME. Physiology of ventricular septal defect shunt flow in the fetus examined by color Doppler M-mode. *Circulation.* 2000;101:E93.

137. Ishii M, Hashino K, Eto G, et al. Quantitative assessment of severity of ventricular septal defect by three-dimensional reconstruction of color Doppler-imaged vena contracta and flow convergence region. *Circulation.* 2001;103:664–669.

138. Dall'agata A, Cromme-Dijkhuis AH, Meijboom FJ, et al. Three-dimensional echocardiography enhances the assessment of

ventricular septal defect. *Am J Cardiol.* 1999;83:1576–1579 A1578.

139. Sutherland GR, Fraser AG. Colour flow mapping in cardiology: indications and limitations. *Br Med Bull.* 1989;45:1076–1091.

140. Dipchand AI, Boutin C. Left ventricular septal aneurysm. *Circulation.* 1998;98:1697.

141. Levin AR, Spach MS, Canent Jr RV, et al. Intracardiac pressure-flow dynamics in isolated ventricular septal defects. *Circulation.* 1967;35:430–441.

142. Laubry C, Routier D, Soulie P. Les souffles de la maladie de Roger. *Revue de Medécine.* 1933;50:439.

143. Nadas AS, Thilenius OG, Lafarge CG, Hauck AJ. Ventricular septal defect with aortic regurgitation: Medical and pathologic aspects. *Circulation.* 1964;29:862–873.

144. Rhodes LA, Keane JF, Keane JP, et al. Long follow-up (to 43 years) of ventricular septal defect with audible aortic regurgitation. *Am J Cardiol.* 1990;66:340–345.

145. Van Praagh R, Mcnamara JJ. Anatomic types of ventricular septal defect with aortic insufficiency. Diagnostic and surgical considerations. *Am Heart J.* 1968;75:604–619.

146. Tatsuno K, Konno S, Ando M, Sakakibara S. Pathogenetic mechanisms of prolapsing aortic valve and aortic regurgitation associated with ventricular septal defect. Anatomical, angiographic, and surgical considerations. *Circulation.* 1973;48:1028–1037.

147. Halloran KH, Talner NS, Browne MJ. A study of ventricular septal sefect associated with aortic insufficiency. *Am Heart J.* 1965;69:320–326.

148. Hor KN, Border WL, Cripe LH, Benson DW, Hinton RB. The presence of bicuspid aortic valve does not predict ventricular septal defect type. *Am J Med Genet Part A.* 2008;146A:3202–3205.

149. Taussig HB, Semans JH. Severe aortic insufficiency in association with a congenital malformation of the heart of the Eisenmenger type. *Bull Johns Hopkins Hosp.* 1940;66:157.

150. Morganroth J, Perloff JK, Zeldis SM, Dunkman WB. Acute severe aortic regurgitation. Pathophysiology, clinical recognition, and management. *Ann Intern Med.* 1977;87:223–232.

151. Nishimura RA, Miller Jr FA, Callahan MJ, Benassi RC, Seward JB, Tajik AJ. Doppler echocardiography: theory, instrumentation, technique, and application. *Mayo Clinic Proceedings.* 1985;60:321–343.

152. Thurman J. On aneurysms of the heart. *Trans Med Soc Lond.* 1838;21:187.

153. Hillier T. Congenital malformation of the heart; perforation of the septum ventriculorum, establishing a communication between the left ventricle and the right atrium. *Trans Pathol Soc Lond.* 1859;10:110.

154. Preicz H. Beitrage zur Lehre von den angeborenen Herzanomalien. *Beitr Pathol Anat.* 1890;7:234.

155. Gerbode F, Hultgren H, Melrose D, Osborn J. Syndrome of left ventricular-right atrial shunt; successful surgical repair of defect in five cases, with observation of bradycardia on closure. *Ann Surg.* 1958;148:433–446.

156. Perry EL, Burchell HB, Edwards JE. Congenital communication between the left ventricle and the right atrium; co-existing ventricular septal defect and double tricuspid orifice. *Mayo Clinic Proceedings.* 1949;24:198–206.

157. Rosenquist GC, Sweeney LJ. Normal variations in tricuspid valve attachments to the membranous ventricular septum: a clue to the etiology of left ventricle-to-right atrial communication. *Am Heart J.* 1975;89:186–188.

158. Stahlman M, Kaplan S, Helmsworth JA, Clark LC, Scott Jr HW. Syndrome of left ventricular-right atrial shunt resulting from high interventricular septal defect associated with defective septal leaflet of the tricuspid valve. *Circulation.* 1955;12:813–818.

159. Burrows PE, Fellows KE, Keane JF. Cineangiography of the perimembranous ventricular septal defect with left ventricular-right atrial shunt. *J Am Coll Cardiol.* 1983;1:1129–1134.

160. Grenadier E, Shem-Tov A, Motro M, Palant A. Echocardiographic diagnosis of left ventricular-right atrial communication. *Am Heart J.* 1983;106:407–409.

161. Edwards J, Carey LS, Neufeld HN, Lester RG. *Congenital Heart Disease*. Philadelphia: WB. Saunders Company; 1965.
162. Yacoub MH, Mansur A, Towers M, Westbury H. Bacterial endocarditis complicating left ventricle to right atrium communication. *Br J Dis Chest*. 1972;66:78–82.
163. Bouchard F, Wolff F, Kalmanson D. Left ventricle-right atrium communication: diagnosis by catheterization and intracardiac phonocardiography. *Arch Mal Coeur Vaiss*. 1961;54:1310–1325.
164. Sakakibara S, Konno S. Left ventricular-right atrial communication. *Ann Surg*. 1963;158:93–99.
165. Levy M, Lillehei CW. Left ventricular-right atrial canal. Ten cases treated surgically. *Am J Cardiol*. 1962;10:623–633.
166. Macruz R, Perloff JK, Case RB. A method for the electrocardiographic recognition of atrial enlargement. *Circulation*. 1958;17:882–889.

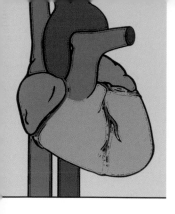

Chapter 18

Ventricular Septal Defect with Pulmonary Stenosis

Ventricular septal defects with obstruction to right ventricular outflow encompass a wide range of anatomic malformations and their physiologic and clinical expressions. *Nonrestrictive* ventricular septal defects occur with pulmonary stenosis that varies from *mild* to *severe* to *complete* (pulmonary atresia). *Restrictive* ventricular septal defects occur with pulmonary stenosis that varies from *mild* to *severe*. This chapter focuses on *Fallot's tetralogy*, which is the most familiar and prevalent combination of these two defects.

Etienne-Louis Arthur Fallot's classic publication, *L'Anatomie Pathologique de La Maladie Bleue* (Figure 18-1A), appeared in 1888 in an obscure journal published in Marseille where Fallot lived throughout his life.[1] The malformation reported by Fallot was originally described 1671 by Niels Stensen,[2] better known by his Latinized name, Nicholas Steno, who was equally distinguished as anatomist, geologist, and theologian.[3,4] Steno wrote, "When I opened the right ventricle ... the probe that was passed forward and upward along the interventricular septum entered directly into the aorta just as readily as the probe passed from left ventricle into aorta. The same aortic canal ... was common to both ventricles. Thus, the aorta receives blood from both ventricles at the same time ... as it partly straddles the right ventricle"[4] (Figure 18-1B). In 1872, 16 years before Fallot's publication, Sir Thomas Watson[5] wrote, "The septum between the ventricles was imperfect in its upper part; and the aorta belonged as much to one ventricle as to the other. The pulmonary artery would not admit a goose-quill; the walls of the right ventricle were as thick as those of the left." The anatomic and clinical features of Fallot's tetralogy were also described by Eduard Sandifort (1777),[4,6] William Hunter (1784),[7] James Hope (1839),[8] and Thomas Peacock (1866).[9] Fallot made an anatomic diagnosis at the bedside, was proven right at postmortem, and coined the term *tetralogy*.[10] He said, "This malformation consists of a true anatomo-pathologic type represented by the following tetralogy: 1) stenosis of the pulmonary artery; 2) interventricular communication; 3) deviation of the origin of the aorta to the right; 4) hypertrophy, almost always concentric, of the right ventricle."[10] Fallot requested that no eulogy be published after his death, but the tetralogy that bears his name remains one of the most familiar eponyms in cardiovascular medicine. The incidence rate is estimated at 1 in 3600 live births.[11,12]

The four salient anatomic components of Fallot's tetralogy result from a specific morphogenetic abnormality: *malalignment of the infundibular septum.*[13] In the normal heart, division of the fetal conotruncus culminates in alignment of the infundibular septum with the muscular trabecular septum. In Fallot's tetralogy, the infundibular septum deviates anteriorly and cephalad and is therefore not aligned with the trabecular septum, creating a ventricular septal defect at the site of malalignment. The deviation of the infundibular septum encroaches on the right ventricular outflow tract and causes infundibular stenosis and a biventricular (overriding) aorta (Figure 18-2).[13] The degree of override and the size of the biventricular aorta are determined chiefly by the degree of malalignment, but aortic size is also influenced by an inherent medial abnormality.[14] The nonrestrictive malaligned ventricular septal defect accounts for systemic systolic pressure in the right ventricle and concentric right ventricular hypertrophy.

Malaligned ventricular septal defects are located in the perimembranous septum with extension into the infundibular septum.[13] Atrioventricular conduction is normal. The crest of the muscular trabecular septum forms the floor of the defect, which is roofed by the valve of the overriding aorta, setting the stage for aortic regurgitation. *Subarterial* ventricular septal defects, which are more frequent among Asians, are understandably accompanied by aortic regurgitation because a supporting infundibulum is absent.[15] Rarely, the ventricular septal defect is part of an atrioventricular septal defect (see Chapter 15).[16–18] Muscular ventricular septal defects sometimes coexist but usually close spontaneously in the first year of life. Occasionally, a nonrestrictive malaligned defect is reduced in size by intrusion of accessory or excessive tricuspid valve tissue (see Figure 18-18) that is fixed to the edges of the defect by short chordae tendineae or tethered by long chordae, which permit wide excursions through the defect.[19]

Malalignment of the infundibular septum is the essential but not the only cause of obstruction to right ventricular outflow,[13] which also results from hypertrophy of the septoparietal trabeculations, the trabecula septomarginalis, and the infundibular septum (Figure 18-3A). Anterior and cephalad malalignment of the infundibular septum can narrow the entire right ventricular outflow tract (see Figure 18-3).[13,20] The pulmonary valve is frequently stenotic and bicuspid (see Figure 18-3B),[21] and less frequently unicommissural unicuspid.[22] Occasionally, the main site of obstruction is a hypoplastic pulmonary annulus or the ostium of the infundibulum

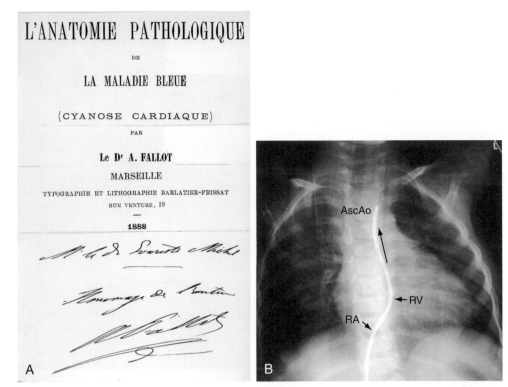

FIGURE 18-1 **A,** Cover of Arthur Fallot's 1888 publication inscribed to Messieur le Docteur S. Michel, *"Homage from the author,"* and signed *"A Fallot."* **B,** Catheter following the path of Nicholas Steno's probe, *"When I opened the right ventricle, . . . the probe that was passed forward and upward along the interventricular septum entered directly into aorta. . ."* (RA = right atrium; RV = right ventricle; Asc Ao = ascending aorta.)

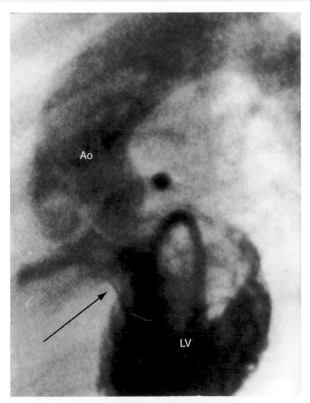

FIGURE 18-2 Left anterior oblique left ventriculogram from an 8-month-old female with cyanotic Fallot's tetralogy. The enlarged aorta (Ao) significantly overrides the ventricular septum (arrow). (LV = left ventricle.)

(Figure 18-4).[23] The pulmonary trunk, its bifurcation, and its right and left branches may be segmentally or diffusely hypoplastic (Figure 18-5B).[23] Rarely, the pulmonary arteries cross as they proceed to their respective lungs.[24] Even more rarely, the tetralogy is associated with the scimitar syndrome.[25]

Pulmonary atresia with Fallot's tetralogy is the ultimate expression of severity.[26] The right ventricle terminates blindly against an atretic pulmonary valve or against imperforate muscle (Figures 18-6A and 18-7B). The pulmonary trunk is either a vestigial cord or a hypoplastic funnel-shaped channel that widens as it approaches the bifurcation. The proximal pulmonary arteries are hypoplastic (Figure 18-7D) and may be discontinuous.[26] The entire right ventricular output enters the systemic circulation via the nonrestrictive malaligned ventricular septal defect (see Figures 18-6A and 18-7B). The biventricular aorta is dilated (see Figures 18-6A and 18-7A, B) and often continues as a right aortic arch (Figure 18-8A). The lungs are perfused by systemic-to-pulmonary arterial collaterals (see Figures 18-6B and 18-7C, D), on which survival depends (see subsequent).[27,28] Exceptionally, the pulmonary circulation is supplied primarily, if not exclusively, by a long, narrow sigmoid-shaped ductus arteriosus (see Figure 18-38B) that is structurally a muscular systemic artery similar to a systemic arterial collateral. This ductal structure is appropriate for intrauterine flow, which is directed *from* the aorta *into* the pulmonary artery.

One of the most characteristic features of Fallot's tetralogy with pulmonary atresia is a pulmonary circulation

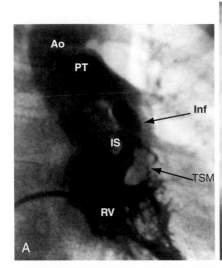

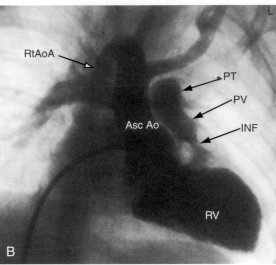

FIGURE 18-3 **A,** Right ventriculogram from a 5-year-old boy with Fallot's tetralogy. The infundibular septum (Inf) and the trabecula septomarginalis (TSM) are hypertrophied. The aorta (Ao) visualizes from the right ventricle (RV) and is larger than the pulmonary trunk (PT). **B,** Right ventriculogram from a 15-month-old male with Fallot's tetralogy. There is hourglass narrowing of the hypertrophied infundibulum (INF), a dome-shaped stenotic pulmonary valve (PV), and a well-formed annulus and pulmonary trunk (PT). The dilated ascending aorta (Asc Ao) visualizes from the right ventricle (RV) and continues as a right aortic arch (RtAoA).

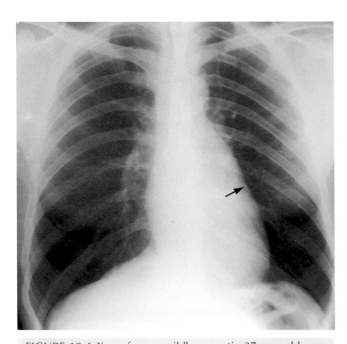

FIGURE 18-4 X-ray from a mildly cyanotic 37-year-old man with Fallot's tetralogy. Arrow points to a localized indentation at the site of stenosis of the ostium of the infundibulum, above which the infundibular chamber is mildly convex. The x-ray is otherwise normal.

supplied entirely by collateral arteries that serve both a nutritive function and a respiratory function (gas exchange). The three types of arterial blood supply to the lungs include systemic arterial collaterals; the distinctive ductus arteriosus, which is a muscular systemic artery (see previous); and small diffuse pleural arterial plexuses.[27]*Systemic arterial collaterals* are classified according to their origins as: (1) *bronchial*, which originate where their name indicates and anastomose to pulmonary arteries within the lung (see Figure 18-6B)[28,29]; (2) *direct systemic arterial collaterals*, which originate from the descending aorta, enter the hilum, and then assume the structure and distribution of intrapulmonary arteries (see Figure 18-7C, D)[28]; and (3) *indirect systemic arterial collaterals*, which originate from the internal mammary, innominate, and subclavian arteries and anastomose to proximal pulmonary arteries outside the lung (see Figure 18-8B).[28] Bronchial arterial collaterals are characterized by *intrapulmonary* anastomoses, direct arterial collaterals by *hilar* anatomoses, and indirect arterial collaterals by *extrapulmonary* anatomoses.[28] Thus, systemic arterial collaterals anatomose with pulmonary arteries in three locations: (1) intrapulmonary; (2) extrapulmonary; and (3) hilar.[28] All three major types of collaterals are present when Fallot's tetralogy occurs with *pulmonary atresia*, but only bronchial collaterals are present when the tetralogy occurs with *pulmonary stenosis*, irrespective of severity.[28] About 10% of arterial collaterals originate from coronary arteries.[30–32] The pulmonary circulation is effective in gas exchange regardless of the type of systemic arterial collateral.

Direct aortic to pulmonary collaterals originate from intersegmental branches of the dorsal aorta during the third and fourth weeks of gestation.[28,29]*Bronchial arterial collaterals* develop in the ninth gestational week after the paired intersegmental arteries have been resorbed[28,29] and do not coexist with direct aortic collaterals.[28]*Indirect collaterals* arise later in gestation and therefore coexist with bronchial collaterals but not with direct aortic collaterals.[28] A particular collateral artery supplies a particular segment of lung, but duplicate blood supplies occasionally occur. A single type of collateral usually predominates in a given patient.[28] Lung growth and survival depend on the size and patency of

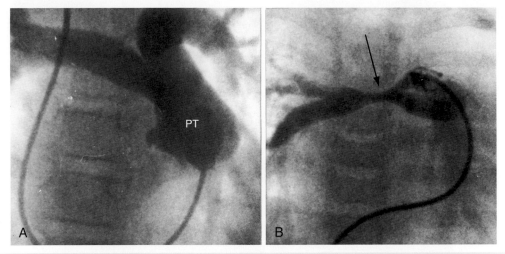

FIGURE 18-5 A, Pulmonary arteriogram from a 12-year-old boy with Fallot's tetralogy and a normally formed pulmonary trunk (PT) and proximal branches. **B,** Pulmonary arteriogram from a 9-month-old female with Fallot's tetralogy and tubular hypoplasia of the right pulmonary artery (arrow). Similar obstruction was present in the left pulmonary artery.

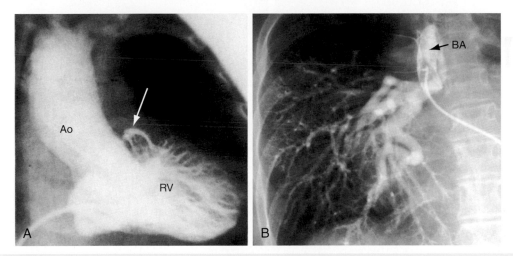

FIGURE 18-6 A, Right ventriculogram from a 5-year-old boy with Fallot's tetralogy and pulmonary atresia. Arrow points to the blind infundibulum. The aortic root (Ao) is conspicuously dilated and continues as a right aortic arch. **B,** Selective opacification of a large right bronchial arterial collateral (BA) that connects to intrapulmonary arteries. (RV = right ventricle.)

the collateral arteries. Diminished pulmonary blood flow adversely effects the growth of peripheral pulmonary arteries.[28]

Systemic arterial collaterals have a strong tendency to harbor *intimal cushions* (proliferations) that serve as sites of potential segmental stenosis (see Figure 18-8B).[28] In the absence of these obstructing cushions, large collateral arteries transmit systemic arterial pressure into the pulmonary vascular bed, resulting in morphologic changes analogous to pulmonary vascular disease (see Chapter 14).[28,33] Although stenotic sites protect the intrapulmonary resistance vessels from systemic pressure, regional pulmonary blood flow is compromised.

In 1947, Taussig observed that the ductus arteriosus was not structurally normal in Fallot's tetralogy with pulmonary atresia.[34,35] The *normal* fetal ductus functions as a conduit for right ventricular flow into pulmonary trunk, a function that cannot be served when pulmonary atresia

diverts the entire right ventricular output into the aorta via the nonrestrictive malaligned ventricular septal defect. Not surprisingly, the ductus is malformed or absent when pulmonary atresia exists from early fetal life. Absence of a ductus indicates that normal intrauterine ductal function was usurped, rendering the ductus superfluous. If a ductus is present, it is represented by a long narrow branch of the aorta that carries systemic arterial blood *from* the aorta *into* the pulmonary trunk.[27] This ductus is narrow because it delivers blood only to the lungs, which represents no more than 5% to 10% of the combined ventricular output. The ductus is long because it first runs distally, diverging from the aortic arch, and then turns back to join the proximal left pulmonary artery.

Aortic regurgitation in Fallot's tetralogy occurs because the malaligned ventricular septal defect is partially roofed by the aortic valve.[13,36] Herniation of aortic cusps

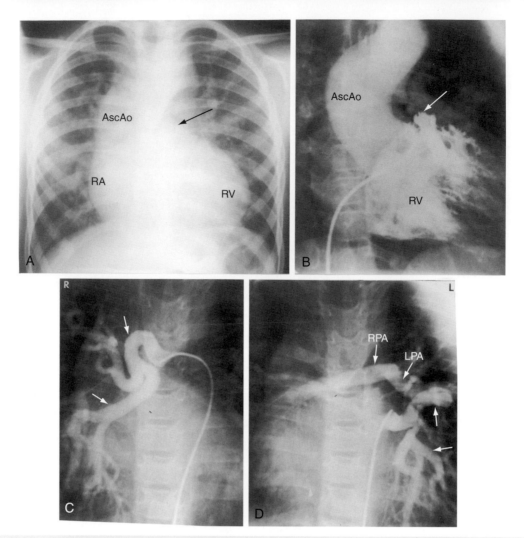

FIGURE 18-7 **A,** X-ray from a 3-year-old boy with Fallot's tetralogy and pulmonary artresia. The ascending aorta (AscAo) is conspic-uously dilated, the main pulmonary artery segment (arrow) is not border-forming, the right lower cardiac border is occupied by a convex right arium (RA), and the apex is occupied by a convex right ventricle (RV). **B,** Right ventriculogram showing the blind outflow tract of pulmonary atresia (arrow) and a conspicoulsy dilated ascending aorta (AscAo). **C,** Selective visualization of a direct right arterial collateral (arrows) that arises from the descending thoracic aorta and had a hilar anastomosis. **D,** The right pulmonary artery (RPA) and left pulmonary artery (LPA) are hypoplastic but continuous. A direct systemic arterial collateral (two unmarked arrows) arose from the descending aorta and had a hilar anastomosis. A vestigial pulmonary trunk was not visualized.

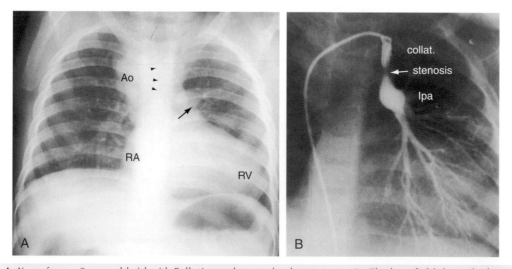

FIGURE 18-8 **A,** X-ray from a 2-year-old girl with Fallot's tetralogy and pulmonary atresia. The lung fields have the lacy appearance of systemic arterial collateral circulation. The ascending aorta (Ao) continues as a prominent right aortic arch and displaces the trachea to the left (three unmarked arrowheads). An enlarged boot-shaped right ventricle (RV) occupies the apex, and a convex right atrium (RA) occupies the lower right cardiac border. **B,** Selective opacification of an indirect systemic arterial collateral (SAC) that originated from the left subclavian artery. There was a zone of stenosis in the collateral before the left pulmonary artery (lpa) visualized.

is more frequent with an isolated subarterial ventricular septal defects than with Fallot's tetralogy, a difference ascribed to dissimilar flow patterns and their impact on the aortic valve. In cyanotic Fallot's tetralogy, the aortic valve is not subjected to turbulent flow because the left ventricle ejects directly into the aorta without generating a left-to-right jet. Nevertheless, there is an age-related increase in aortic regurgitation,[37] in part as a result of progressive aortic root dilation associated with an inherent medial abnormality.[14,38,39] Aortic regurgitation causes volume overload of *both* ventricles because the aorta is biventricular.[37] The incompetent aortic valve is susceptible to infective endocarditis, which can suddenly and catastrophically augment the degree of biventricular regurgitation (see section The History).[37] *A right aortic arch* is a feature of Fallot's tetralogy.[40] Its incidence rate increases as the severity of right ventricular outflow obstruction increases (see Figure 18-3) and reaches approximately 25% with pulmonary atresia (see Figures 18-6A and 18-8A).

Anomalous origin and distribution of *coronary arteries* are common (see Chapter 32)[30,41,42] and may be of no *functional* importance but are of considerable *surgical* importance. The incidence of coronary artery anomalies is influenced by aortopulmonary rotation[43] and is higher when the aortic root is anterior to or side-by-side the pulmonary trunk. The most common anomalies are origin of a conus artery or the left anterior descending artery from the right coronary artery or from the right sinus of Valsalva (Figure 18-9).[41] Origin of a single coronary artery from the right sinus of Valsalva is less common. Relatively frequent are fistulous communications between coronary arteries and the pulmonary artery[30,44] or the right atrium and between coronary arteries and bronchial arteries.[32] Rarely, the left anterior descending coronary artery originates from the pulmonary artery,[45] or the left coronary artery is intramural.[46]

Etienne-Louis Fallot recognized that "... at times, there is an additional entirely accessory defect, namely, patency of the foramen ovale."[10] An atrial septal defect occasionally coexists with Fallot's tetralogy, but the term *pentalogy* is longer used. Rarely, the tetralogy is associated with total anomalous pulmonary venous connection and an atrial septal defect.[47]

The combination of right ventricular outflow obstruction and ventricular septal defect is not confined to Fallot's tetralogy. *Pulmonary valve stenosis* occasionally occurs with an isolated *perimembranous* ventricular septal defect (Figure 18-10). The degree of stenosis varies from trivial to severe, the size of the ventricular septal defect varies from small to nonrestrictive, and right ventricular systolic pressure varies from normal to suprasystemic. Other examples of the combination include pulmonary valve stenosis with a *muscular* ventricular septal defect,[48] obstruction to right ventricular outflow caused by protrusion of a large *ventricular septal aneurysm* into the right ventricular outflow tract (Figure 18-11), and double-chambered right ventricle with a *perimembranous*[49–51] or a *malaligned* ventricular septal defect (Figure 18-12).[20,52] Sir Arthur Keith in his 1909 Hunterian lecture focused on obstructing right ventricular muscular bundles, which consist

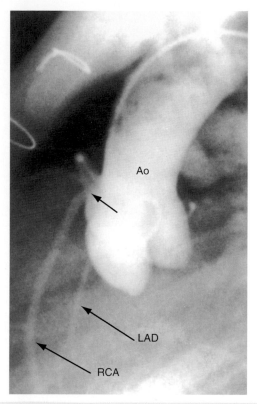

FIGURE 18-9 Aortogram from a 6-year-old boy with Fallot's tetralogy. A single ostium (arrow) gave rise to the left anterior descending coronary artery (LAD) and to the right coronary artery (RCA). A branch of the left anterior descending artery crossed the right ventricular outflow tract. The circumflex coronary (not shown) originated from the right coronary artery. (Ao = aorta.)

of an hypertrophied moderator band, an hypertrophied trabecula, or a fibromuscular diaphragm,[53] with obstruction ranging from nil to severe to complete.[50,54] A ventricular septal defect that communicates with the proximal high-pressure compartment results in a right-to-left shunt.[50]

Taussig[55] described two infants with a loud holosystolic murmur at the lower left sternal border and increased pulmonary blood flow, prompting the diagnosis of ventricular septal defect. Several years later, both patients were cyanotic with pulmonary stenotic murmurs and decreased pulmonary blood flow, appropriate for the diagnosis to Fallot's tetralogy. Gasul formalized the notion that progressive infundibular obstruction sometimes occurs with ventricular septal defect (Figure 18-13), and confirmatory reports soon appeared.[56–58] The acquired obstruction usually results from hypertrophy of right ventricular muscle bundles, and only rarely from a malaligned infundibular septum.[57]

The *physiologic consequences* of Fallot's tetralogy depend essentially on two variables: the degree of obstruction to right ventricular outflow and, to a lesser extent, systemic vascular resistance. The magnitude and direction of the shunt are determined by the resistance at the site of pulmonary stenosis relative to systemic vascular resistance. When pulmonary stenosis offers lesser resistance, the shunt is left-to-right. When the resistances are equal, the shunt is balanced. When right ventricular

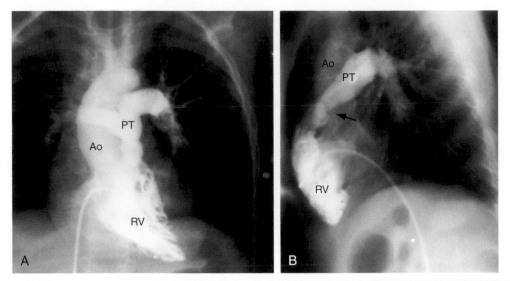

FIGURE 18-10 Right ventriculograms from a 23-month-old male with pulmonary valve stenosis, a nonrestrictive perimembranous ventricular septal defect, and a balanced shunt. **A,** The plane of the ventricular septum is relatively vertical because a well-developed left ventricle occupied the apex. The pulmonary trunk (PT) and a normal-sized aorta (Ao) fill simultaneously. **B,** In the lateral projection, pulmonary stenosis originates in a slightly thickened valve. The pulmonary trunk is mildly dilated. The infundibulum is normal. (RV = right ventricle.)

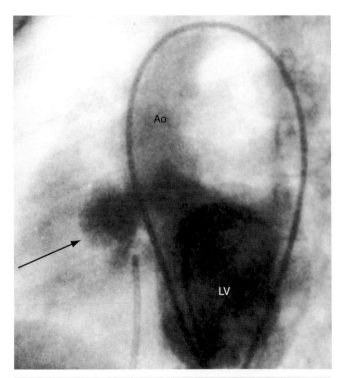

FIGURE 18-11 Lateral left ventriculogram from an 8-year-old boy with a large ventricular septal aneurysm (arrow) that obstructed the right ventricular outflow tract. A restrictive perimembranous ventricular septal defect had spontaneously closed. Systolic pressure proximal to the obstructing aneurysm was 70 mm Hg and distal to the aneurysm was 30 mm Hg. (Ao = aorta; LV = left ventricle.)

outflow resistance exceeds systemic resistance, the shunt is right-to-left. The amount of aortic override is not the issue, although the degree of override tends to coincide with the degree of right ventricular outflow obstruction, which is the issue. When right ventricular

blood preferentially flows into the aorta, pulmonary blood flow falls reciprocally, so the left side of the heart is underfilled.[59,60] The ultimate expression of right ventricular outflow obstruction is *pulmonary atresia*, which commits the entire right ventricular output to the aorta. Pulmonary blood flow then depends on systemic arterial collaterals (see previous), which provide the lungs with normal or increased flow, so cyanosis can be mild or even absent.[61] Unobstructed flow through arterial collaterals sets the stage for pulmonary vascular disease. Stenoses at *intimal cushions* in arterial collaterals (see previous) protect the pulmonary vascular bed, but at the price of reduced pulmonary blood flow.

Irrespective of the degree of right ventricular outflow obstruction, right ventricular systolic pressure cannot exceed systemic because the ventricular septal defect is nonrestrictive. Accordingly, a systemic ceiling is placed on the pressure overload that pulmonary stenosis can impose on the right ventricle. When pulmonary stenosis is severe, right ventricular pressure overload is determined by systemic vascular resistance. Increased resistance associated with systemic hypertension or, less commonly, with acquired calcific aortic stenosis (see Figure 18-33B) improves pulmonary blood flow but increases right ventricular afterload. Aortic regurgitation imposes volume load on the already pressure-overloaded right ventricle.

In addition to concentric hypertrophy of the right ventricle, certain morphologic changes are *secondary* to the physiologic derangements of Fallot's tetralogy. Tricuspid leaflets develop fibrous thickening because right ventricular systolic pressure is systemic, but the thickened leaflets are seldom incompetent. The right ventricle ejects against systemic resistance without an increase in filling pressure, so right atrial pressure remains normal, and overall systolic function of the hypertrophied right ventricle remains normal (Figure 18-14B, C; see subsequent).[60] The *underfilled left ventricle* tends to be

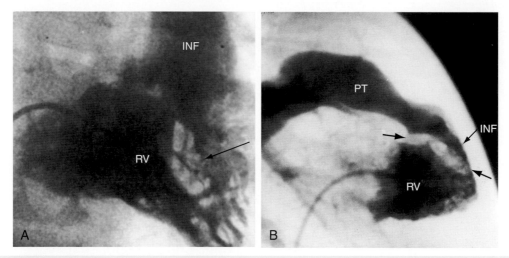

FIGURE 18-12 A, Right ventriculogram from an acyanotic 8-year-old boy with a *double-chambered right ventricle* caused by an hypertrophied trabecula septomarginalis (arrow). A restrictive perimembranous ventricular septal defect coexisted. Systolic pressure in the inflow tract of the right ventricle was 50 mm Hg higher than systolic pressure in the pulmonary trunk and infundibulum (INF). **B,** Lateral right ventriculogram showing the prominent muscular partition (arrows) that separated the high-pressure inflow portion of the right ventricle (RV) from the low-pressure infundibular portion, creating a *two-chambered right ventricle.*

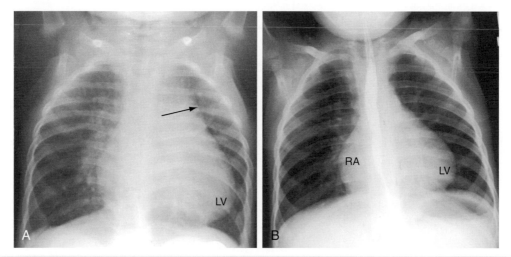

FIGURE 18-13 A, X-ray from an acyanotic 7-month-old female with a large left-to-right shunt through a moderately restrictive perimembranous ventricular septal defect. Pulmonary arterial vascularity is increased, an enlarged convex left ventricle (LV) occupies the apex, the right atrium occupies the right lower cardiac border, and the left thoracic inlet is obscured by thymus (arrow). **B,** X-ray at 2 years of age after progressive acquired obstruction to right ventricular outflow had reversed the shunt. Pulmonary arterial vascularity is reduced and the left ventricle (LV) is no longer dilated, but the right atrium (RA) remains prominent.

reduced in size with reduced stroke volume.[59,60] Low pressure and low flow in the pulmonary circulation alter the small muscular arteries and arterioles and cause thinning of the media with interruption of elastic tissue and widespread thromboses.[62–64]

When *severe* pulmonary stenosis occurs with a *restrictive* ventricular septal defect, right ventricular systolic pressure exceeds systemic and the hypertrophied right ventricle dilates and fails. A physiologically analogous state exists when accessory tricuspid leaflet tissue partially occludes the malaligned ventricular septal defect (see Figure 18-18).[19]

History

Gender distribution in Fallot's tetralogy is approximately equal. The malformation recurs in families and has been reported in siblings,[65–67] including triplets,[68] and in parents and offspring.[67,69] Two brothers with DiGeorge syndrome had Fallot's tetralogy. Birth weight tends to be lower than normal, and growth and development are generally retarded. Hereditary cardiovascular defects in Keeshond dogs include typical Fallot's tetralogy and isolated ventricular septal defect with pulmonary stenosis.[70] Familial tetralogy has been associated with mutation of

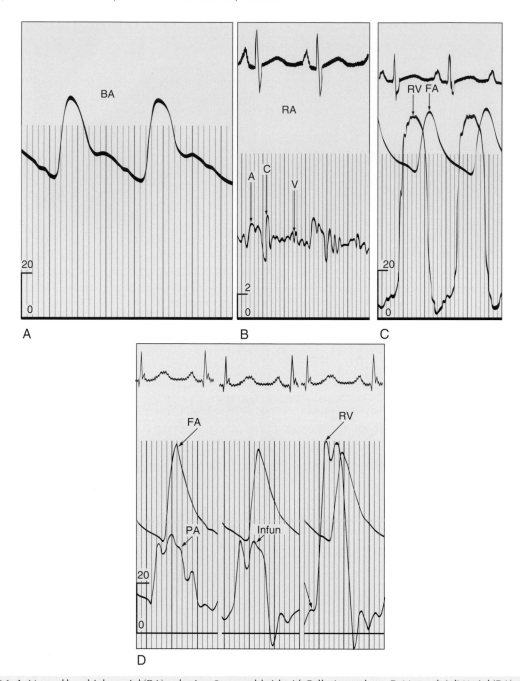

FIGURE 18-14 A, Normal brachial arterial (BA) pulse in a 9-year-old girl with Fallot's tetralogy. **B,** Normal right atrial (RA) pressure pulse from a 5-year-old boy with Fallot's tetralogy. **C,** Right ventricular (RV) systolic pressure is virtually identical with femoral arterial (FA) systolic pressure. Right ventricular end-diastolic pressure is normal. **D,** Catheter withdrawal tracings from a 3-year-old mildly cyanotic girl with Fallot's tetralogy. Identical systolic pressures of 40 mm Hg in the pulmonary artery (PA) and infundibulum (Infun) abruptly increase to systemic level in the right ventricle (RV) where the end-diastolic pressure was normal (lower right arrow).

the jagged 1 gene,[71] with NKX2.5 mutations,[72] and with chromosome 22q11.2 deletion.[73]

The tetralogy usually comes to light in neonates and infants. When the shunt is left-to-right, initial suspicion is a prominent systolic murmur. When the shunt is balanced, the murmur persists in addition to mild, intermittent, or stress-induced cyanosis. When the shunt is reversed, the prominence of the systolic murmur is inversely proportional to the degree of cyanosis (see section Auscultation).

The clinical course in early infancy is often benign. Mild to moderate neonatal cyanosis tends to increase, but cyanosis may be delayed for months and is coupled with increased oxygen requirements of the growing infant rather than with progressive obstruction to right ventricular outflow.[74] Patients seldom remain acyanotic after the first few years of life, and by 5 to 8 years of age, most children are conspicuously cyanotic, with cyanosis closely coupled to the severity of pulmonary stenosis. Infants with Fallot's tetralogy and pulmonary atresia are mildly cyanotic or acyanotic when collateral flow is abundant.[61]

In an analysis of survival patterns based on 566 necropsy cases of Fallot's tetralogy, two thirds of patients reached their first birthday, approximately half reached age 3 years, and approximately a quarter completed the first decade of life.[75,76] The attrition rate was then 6.4% per year with 11% alive at age 20 years, 6% at age 30 years, and 3% at age 40 years.[75,76] Nevertheless, Fallot's tetralogy remains the most common cyanotic congenital heart disease after 4 years of age and constitutes a large proportion of adults with cyanotic congenital heart disease. Fallot recognized this tendency when he wrote, "We have seen from our observations that cyanosis, especially in the adult, is the result of a small number of cardiac malformations well determined. One of these cardiac malformations is much more frequent than others...," namely, the tetralogy to which he referred.[10] Fallot's oldest patient was 36 years of age.[10] Survivals between the fifth and seventh decades are uncommon but not rare.[12,77–79] A 64-year-old woman with the tetralogy was diagnosed in 1895 by G.A. Gibson, best known for his description of the continuous murmur of patent ductus arteriosus. In 1929, White and Sprague[80] published an account of the American composer Henry F. Gilbert who lived a productive life to age 60 years. Another patient played cricket and football as a schoolboy and survived to age 62 years. Patients without repair have lived to age 75 years,[81] 78 years,[82] 84 years,[83] and 86 years.[84] In Fallot's tetralogy with *pulmonary atresia*, life expectancy without surgery is as low as 50% in 1 year and 8% in 10 years,[75] but adequate collateral blood flow occasionally permits survival into adolescence and adulthood.[18,37,78,85,86] One such patient lived to age 54 years,[78] and another lived to age 55 years, despite acquired calcific aortic stenosis and regurgitation (see Figure 18-33B.)

Pregnancy is poorly tolerated in females who reach childbearing age.[87] The gestational fall in systemic vascular resistance increases the right-to-left shunt, and labile systemic vascular resistance during labor and delivery results in abrupt oscillations in hypoxemia. Fetal wastage is high,[23] and live born infants are dysmature.

The neonatal right ventricle is well equipped to eject against systemic vascular resistance because the nonrestrictive ventricular septal defect permits decompression into the aorta.[60] The right ventricle has been analyzed in terms of its inlet, apical trabecular, and outlet portions.[88] The apical trabecular portion took up the greatest portion of the overload, the outlet portion had decreased ejecting force, and the inlet portion was not significantly affected.[88] Right ventricular failure is uncommon.[89] However, biventricular failure in the first few weeks of life accompanies pulmonary atresia with excessive flow through large systemic arterial collaterals.[61] Accessory tricuspid leaflet tissue that partially occludes the ventricular septal defect results in suprasystemic right ventricular systolic pressure and the right ventricular failure.[19,89] Absence of the pulmonary valve (see subsequent section) results in volume overload of the pressure-overloaded right ventricle.[90] Systemic hypertension increases left *and* right ventricular afterload and can induce right ventricular or biventricular failure.[89,91] Acquired calcific stenosis of the biventricular aortic valve imposes increased afterload on both the right and the left ventricles (see Figure 18-33B). Regurgitation of a biventricular aortic valve sets the stage for right ventricular failure by imposing volume overload on the already pressure-overloaded right ventricle.[37] Infective endocarditis on an incompetent aortic valve can result in catastrophic acute severe biventricular aortic regurgitation.

Isotonic exercise is accompanied by a fall in systemic vascular resistance in the face of fixed obstruction to right ventricular outflow, increasing venoarterial mixing and significantly influencing the dynamics of O_2 uptake and ventilation.[92,93] Exercise-induced hypoxemia and increased carbon dioxide content stimulate the respiratory center and the carotid body, provoking hyperventilation that is subjectively perceived as dyspnea.[92,93]

Hypoxic spells, variously called paroxysmal hyperpnea, syncopal attacks, hypoxic or hypercyanotic spells, are dramatic and alarming features of Fallot's tetralogy.[94–96] A typical spell begins with a progressive increase in the rate and depth of breathing and culminates in paroxysmal hyperpnea, deepening cyanosis, limpness, syncope, and occasionally convulsions, cerebrovascular accidents, and death.[95,96] Electroencephalographic abnormalities during an hypoxic spell are similar to those of hypoxic episodes of other causes.[97] Peak incidence is between the second and sixth month of life, with an occasional spell as early as the first month but comparatively few spells after age 2 years, and only rarely in adults.[98] Spells in infants are typically initiated by the stress of feeding, crying, or a bowel movement, particularly after awakening from a long deep sleep.[94,95] However, attacks sometimes occur without an apparent precipitating cause, especially in deeply cyanotic infants, although spells are not necessarily related to the degree of cyanosis.[95] Spells were originally attributed to infundibular contraction caused by sympathetic stimulation, which was believed to divert right ventricular blood into the aorta,[96] but occurrence in patients with pulmonary *atresia* argued against this theory. It is now believed that vulnerable respiratory control mechanisms, which are especially sensitive after prolonged deep sleep, react to the sudden increase in cardiac output provoked by feeding, crying, or straining, by initiating the following vicious cycle.[94,95] As heart rate and cardiac output increase, venous return increases in the face of fixed obstruction to right ventricular outflow, so the right-to-left shunt increases. Infundibular contraction reinforces this pattern but does not initiate it. The increased right-to-left shunt causes a fall in systemic arterial pO_2 and pH and a rise in pCO_2, a blood gas composition to which a sleep-sensitive respiratory center and carotid body overreact, provoking hyperpnoea, which in turn further increases the cardiac output and perpetuates the cycle. *Supraventricular tachycardia* and *rapid atrial pacing* initiate spells by inducing infundibular narrowing, which increases the right-to-left shunt.[99] Five mechanisms are therefore involved in the pathogenesis of Fallot spells: (1) an acceleration in heart rate; (2) an increase in cardiac output and venous return; (3) an increase in right-to-left shunt; (4) vulnerable respiratory control centers; and (5) infundibular contraction. Manual

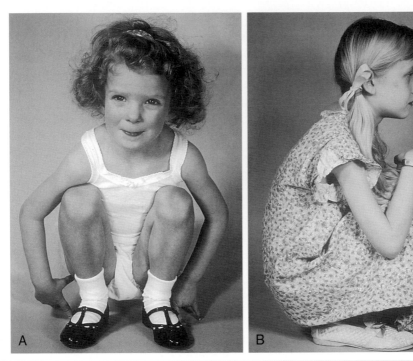

FIGURE 18-15 Typical squatting postures assumed effortlessly in two children with Fallot's tetralogy.

compression of the abdominal aorta can abort a spell by decreasing cardiac output and venous return.[100] *Squatting* for relief of dyspnea is a time-honored hallmark of Fallot'stetralogy (Figure 18-15).[101,102] In 1784, William Hunter[7] made the following observations on the effects of posture: "Any hurry upon his spirits or brisk motion of his body would generally occasion a fit. And for some of the last years of his life he found out by his own observations that when the fit was coming upon him, he would escape it altogether, or at least take considerably from its violence or duration by instantly lying down upon the carpet on his left side, and remaining immovable in that position for about 10 minutes. I saw the experiments made with success."

Taussig described the preference for certain postures other than squatting, namely, the knee-chest position, lying down, or sitting with legs drawn underneath (Figure 18-16).[103] Parents may hold their breathless

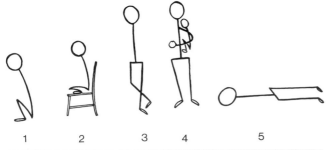

FIGURE 18-16 Line drawings illustrating various postures assumed for relief of dyspnea in Fallot's tetralogy: *1,* squatting; *2,* sitting with legs drawn underneath (squatting equivalent); *3,* legs crossed while standing; *4,* infant held with legs flexed on abdomen, and *5,* lying down. (*Modified from Lurie PR. Postural effects in tetralogy of Fallot. Am J Med 15;297:1953.*)

infant upright with its legs flexed against its abdomen (see Figure 18-16, panel 4). Young adults cross their legs during quiet standing or sitting, a relatively ineffective variation. Habitual squatters assume the position effortlessly (see Figure 18-15). The mechanisms by which squatting exerts its beneficial effects are as follows.[101,102,104,105] (1) Quiet standing after exercise-induced peripheral vasodilation predisposes to orthostatic hypotension and faintness, a tendency that is exaggerated in hypoxemic patients. Squatting counteracts orthostatic hypotension and diminishes or prevents postexertion orthostatic faintness.[102,104] (2) Squatting increases systemic vascular resistance, diverts right ventricular blood into the pulmonary circulation, and increases the amount of oxygenated blood entering the left side of the heart.[102,104,106] The left ventricle delivers the larger volume of oxygenated blood into the systemic circulation, so systemic arterial pO_2 and pH increase and pCO_2 decreases, blunting the stimulus to the respiratory center and carotid body and relieving hyperventilatory dyspnea.[104] The effect of squatting on *systemic venous return* is an even more effective means by which hyperventilatory dyspnea is relieved.[104] (3) Isotonic leg exercise reduces the oxygen saturation of venous effluent returning to the heart from the lower extremities. Squatting mechanically curtails lower extremity venous return, decreases the volume of unsaturated venous blood delivered to the heart, and increases the oxygen saturation of right ventricular blood. (4) Right ventricular blood shunted into systemic circulation has a higher oxygen content and pH and a lower pCO_2 content.[104] (5) The higher pO_2 and pH and the lower pCO_2 reduce the stimulus to the respiratory center and carotid body and reduce the hyperventilatory dyspnea.

Recurrent hypoxic spells sometimes lead to brain damage and mental retardation. Cerebral venous sinus thromboses and small occult thromboses may become manifest after prolonged hypoxic spells. Hypernasal resonance or nasal speech (velopharyngeal insufficiency) may develop after repeated or prolonged spells because nasal resonance is compromised by improper approximation of the velum (soft palate) and the pharyngeal walls, a disturbance that has been ascribed in part to central nervous system damage caused by hypoxic spells.[107]

Brain abscess and cerebral embolism add to the list of central nervous system complications.[108-110] Iron-deficient erythrocytosis in patients less than 4 years of age increases the risk of cerebral venous sinus thrombosis.[110] Wheezing and stridor have been attributed to tracheal compression by an enlarged aorta.[14,111] A stenotic pulmonary valve[112] and an incompetent aortic valve[113] are substrates for infective endocarditis.

The *physiologic consequences and clinical course* of a nonrestrictive ventricular septal defect are favorably influenced by mild to moderate *acquired* obstruction to right ventricular outflow (see previous[57] and Chapter 17). The clinical picture initially resembles an isolated nonrestrictive ventricular septal defect with large left-to-right shunt (see Figure 18-13A.) With the development of right ventricular outflow obstruction, excessive pulmonary blood flow and volume overload of the left ventricle are curtailed,[56,58,74] symptoms related to the left-to-right shunt diminish, and physical development improves. Obstruction to right ventricular outflow may progress sufficiently to reverse the shunt, resulting in late onset cyanosis (see Figure 18-13B).

When a *restrictive* ventricular septal defect is accompanied by *severe* pulmonary valve stenosis, the clinical picture resembles isolated pulmonary stenosis with intact ventricular septum (see Chapter 11). A *restrictive* ventricular septal defect with *mild* pulmonary stenosis is associated with a conspicuous murmur and few or no symptoms but with the risk of infective endocarditis.

Physical Appearance

Patients with cyanotic Fallot's tetralogy are as a rule physically underdeveloped,[114] and infants with excessive collateral arterial blood flow accompanying pulmonary atresia have development of congestive heart failure and the catabolic effects of poor physical development.

Cyanosis varies from absent to severe and is symmetrically distributed. John Hunter described such a patient: "I was consulted about a young gentleman's health. From his infancy, every considerable exertion produced a seeming tendency to suffocation and a change from the scarlet tinge to the modena or purple."[115] Cyanosis may become manifest only after crying, feeding, or exercise when the accompanying stress increases venous return to the obstructed right ventricle and augments the right-to-left shunt. When there is a history of squatting or an analogous posture, it is useful to have the patient or parent illustrate the posture, so it can be witnessed by the examiner (see Figures 18-15 and 18-16).

Fallot's tetralogy is associated with a number of distinctive phenotypes[116]: CATCH 22 monosomy 22q11.2,[117,118] Down trisomy 21,[16,17] velocardiofacial (Shprintzen-Goldberg) syndrome,[119] Goldenhar's syndrome[120] (oculo-auriculo-vertebral dysplasia), absent thumb and first metacarpal,[121] absence of a pectoralis major muscle (congenital pectoral dysplasia or Poland's syndrome; Figure 18-17),[1] syndactyly, brachydactyly with hypoplasia of the ipsilateral hand,[122] underdevelopment of the left arm secondary to an isolated left subclavian artery, and hypoplsia of a hand.[123]

Arterial Pulse

The arterial pulse is normal, irrespective of the severity of pulmonary stenosis (see Figure 18-14C, D). When the shunt is balanced, the left ventricle maintains a normal stroke volume, and when there is severe pulmonary stenosis or atresia, a reduced left ventricular stroke volume is supplemented by right ventricular blood ejected directly into the aorta.[60] A *brisk* arterial pulse with wide pulse pressure is reserved for large systemic arterial collateral flow[61] or aortic regurgitation.

An accurate estimate of the right ventricular outflow gradient requires little more than the bedside determination of blood pressure. Right ventricular systolic pressure is systemic (see Figure 18-14C, D) so the stenotic gradient is the difference between the cuff brachial arterial systolic pressure and an estimated pulmonary arterial

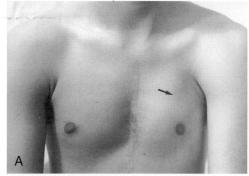
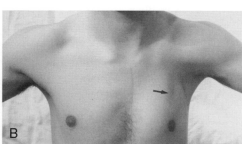

FIGURE 18-17 Photographs of a 16-year-old boy with Fallot's tetralogy and Poland's syndrome. **A,** The left chest is mildly flattened (arrow). **B,** Raising the arms exaggerated the appearance of agenesis of the left pectoralis major muscle (arrow) and displaced the nipple to the left. Compare with the right chest, which is normal.

systolic pressure of 15 to 25 mm Hg, depending on age and the severity of pulmonary stenosis. The estimate is further refined by taking into account that pulmonary arterial pressure is lowest when cyanosis is severe and normal when cyanosis is mild.

Jugular Venous Pulse

The neonatal right ventricle has an inherent capacity to eject against systemic resistance without extra help from its atrium. In Fallot's tetralogy, resistance to right ventricular discharge is at, but not above, systemic because the nonrestrictive ventricular septal defect permits decompression into the aorta (see Figure 18-14C, D.) The right ventricle maintains its neonatal capacity to eject at systemic resistance without increasing its filling pressure. Accordingly, the right atrium is not required to increase its contractile force, so the jugular venous pulse is normal in height and wave form (see Figure 18-14B).[60] If accessory tricuspid leaflet tissue partially occludes the ventricular septal defect, right ventricular systolic pressure exceeds systemic (Figure 18-18) and the jugular A wave becomes prominent. With systemic hypertension, the right ventricle contracts from an increased end-diastolic fiber length induced by forceful right atrial contraction, which is reflected in the jugular venous pulse as an increase in the A wave. Acquired stenosis of the biventricular aortic valve has a similar effect on the right ventricle and right atrium. A minor feature of the jugular venous pulse is related to a persistent left superior vena cava.[124] The left jugular pulse is then more prominent than the right.[124,125]

Precordial Movement and Palpation

In 1839, James Hope[8] described an *"increase of pulsation at the inferior part of the sternum"* as a sign of right ventricular hypertrophy. The right ventricle in Fallot's tetralogy ejects at systemic pressure with little or no increase in its force of contraction. Accordingly, the accompanying precordial impulse is gentle, analogous to the impulse of a normal neonatal right ventricle. The right ventricular impulse is relegated to the fourth and fifth left intercostal spaces and subzyphoid area because the stenosis is infundibular (see Figure 18-14D.) A *left* ventricular impulse is conspicuous by its absence because the left ventricle is underfilled. Abundant flow through large systemic arterial collaterals augments left ventricular filling, but even then, a left ventricular impulse is seldom palpated. *Subinfundibular* stenosis or double-chambered right ventricle (see Figure 18-12) relegates the right ventricular impulse to the *fifth* left intercostal space and subxyphoid area.

A dilated *right aortic arch* (see Figure 18-6) reveals itself by an impulse at the right sternoclavicular junction. The aortic component of the second heart sound is often palpable in the second left intercostal space because a hypoplastic or atretic anterior pulmonary trunk is all that guards the enlarged aortic root. Systolic thrills do not originate at sites of severe stenosis because right ventricular blood flow is diverted from the pulmonary trunk into the aorta. In acyanotic Fallot's tetralogy, the lesser degree

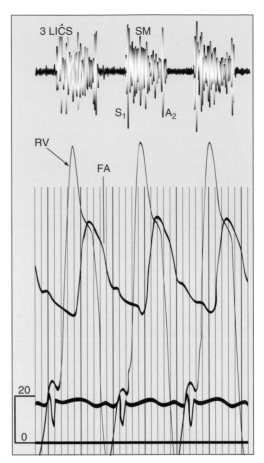

FIGURE 18-18 Tracings from a 3-year-old girl with Fallot's tetralogy. Right ventricular (RV) systolic pressure exceeded femoral artery systolic pressure (FA) because accessory tricuspid leaflet tissue partially occluded the ventricular septal defect. As a result, the pulmonary stenotic murmur (SM) was long and loud and went up to the aortic component of the second heart sound (A₂). Right ventricular end-diastolic pressure was 28 mm Hg (see calibration below). (S₁ = first heart sound.)

of obstruction permits sufficient flow across the stenotic site to generate a thrill.

Auscultation

The physiology of Fallot's tetralogy is nicely reflected in the accompanying auscultatory signs. Ejection sounds originate in a dilated *aorta* (see Figures 18-6A and 18-7A) and are therefore important auscultatory signs of severe pulmonary stenosis or atresia (Figures 18-19 through 18-23).[74,86,112] The aortic ejection sound is maximal at the upper *right* sternal border, but when loud, it is heard along the left sternal border and toward the apex. The ejection sound may selectively decrease with inspiration (see Figure 18-19), even though it originates in the aortic root rather than in the pulmonary valve (see Chapter 11). *Pulmonary* ejection sounds are absent because the stenotic bicuspid pulmonary valve is not sufficiently mobile (see Figure 18-3).

Nearly 50 years before Fallot's report, James Hope[0] wrote: "A loud superficial murmur with the first heart

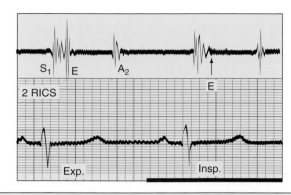

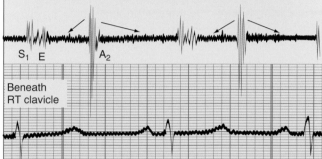

FIGURE 18-19 Phonocardiograms from an 11-year-old girl with Fallot's tetralogy and pulmonary atresia. Tracing from the second right intercostal space (2 RICS) shows an aortic ejection sound (E) that was prominent during expiration (Exp) but absent during inspiration (Insp). Phonocardiogram from beneath the right clavicle shows a soft continuous murmur (paired arrows). (S_1 = first heart sound; A_2 = aortic component of the second sound.)

sound in the third left intercostal space may proceed from a contraction of the pulmonary orifice or from an opening out of the right ventricle into the left ventricle, or from both these lesions conjoined. When these lesions coincide with cyanosis, the double lesion is almost positive and an increase of pulsation at the inferior part of the sternum, indicative of right ventricular hypertrophy is a corroborative circumstance." The murmur that Hope described referred to cyanotic Fallot's tetralogy and originated at the site of stenosis rather than across the ventricular septal defect (Figure 18-24).[126] The murmur is maximal in the third left intercostal space because the stenosis is infundibular. *Subinfundibular* stenosis results in a lower location of the murmur.[51] The duration and configuration of the systolic murmur are determined by the balance between resistance at the site of stenosis and resistance in the systemic vascular bed. Changes in this balance are reflected in changes in the length and loudness of the systolic murmur. These auscultatory signs are closely coupled with the severity of pulmonary stenosis (see Figure 18-20).[112] A holosystolic murmur extending up to the aortic component of the second heart sound reflects a *left-to-right* shunt across the ventricular septal defect (see Figure 18-20B). As pulmonary stenosis increases, the shunt murmur becomes decrescendo, diminishing and ending before the aortic component of the second sound (see Figure 18-20C). When the shunt is balanced, the ventricular septal defect is silent and

the previously obscured pulmonary stenotic murmur emerges (see Figure 18-20D). A further increase in the degree of pulmonary stenosis diverts right ventricular blood into the aorta and away from the pulmonary trunk, so the pulmonary stenotic murmur becomes shorter and softer (Figure 18-20E). Severe pulmonary stenosis is reflected in an even shorter and softer systolic murmur and by an ejection sound that is generated in the dilated aortic root (see Figure 18-20F). Pulmonary atresia abolishes right ventricular-to-pulmonary arterial flow and abolishes the pulmonary stenotic murmur. An aortic ejection sound may be followed by no murmur at all (see Figure 18-20G) or a trivial midsystolic murmur into the dilated aorta.

During hypoxic spells, pulmonary arterial blood flow sharply declines, the pulmonary stenotic murmur shortens and softens, and with loss of consciousness, the murmur disappears.[96,112] Vasoactive drugs induce analogous changes by altering systemic vascular resistance.[112,127] Pressor agents increase systemic vascular resistance and increase the resistance to right ventricular discharge into the aorta.[91] The right-to-left shunt decreases, right ventricular blood is diverted into the pulmonary artery, and the pulmonary stenotic murmur becomes louder and longer. Amyl nitrite has the opposite effect, inducing a decrease in systemic vascular resistance, a decrease in resistance to right ventricular discharge into the aorta, and a decrease in flow into the pulmonary trunk, with softening and shortening of the stenotic murmur (Figure 18-25).

Continuous murmurs are auscultatory signs of pulmonary *atresia* and occur in more than 80% of such patients (see Figures 18-19 and 18-21 through 18-23). Continuous murmurs originate in direct and indirect systemic arterial collaterals (see previous) and therefore do not occur in Fallot's tetralogy with pulmonary stenosis in which collaterals are confined to bronchial arteries (see Figure 18-6B).[28] The intensity of continuous murmurs ranges from grade 3/6 to soft and easily overlooked, especially at nonprecordial sites. Continuous murmurs are heard beneath the clavicles, in the back, to the right and left of the sternum, and in the right and left axillae (see Figures 18-21 through 18-23). Thoracic locations vary from patient to patient, and from time to time, in the same patient.[86,128] Continuous murmurs may peak before and after the second heart sound (see Figures 18-21 and 18-23) or may be more prominent in systolic, as with other arterial continuous murmurs (see Figure 18-22), creating the mistaken impression of a long intracardiac systolic murmur, especially if the murmur is located at the left sternal edge.

The murmur of tricuspid regurgitation is reserved for the occasional adult with right ventricular failure caused by systemic hypertension or acquired aortic stenosis or in the occasional patient with suprasystemic right ventricular pressure from partial occlusion of the ventricular septal defect by tricuspid leaflet tissue.

Diastolic murmurs are caused by aortic regurgitation, or much less frequently, by absent pulmonary valve (see subsequent section).[112] The aortic regurgitant murmur is typically high-frequency decrescendo, beginning with the prominent single aortic component of the second heart

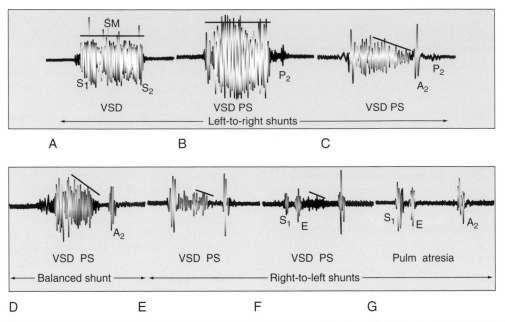

FIGURE 18-20 Series of phonocardiograms showing auscultatory modifications incurred when varying degrees of pulmonary stenosis (PS) are imposed on a nonrestrictive ventricular septal defect (VSD). **A,** Holosystolic murmur of isolated ventricular septal defect. **B,** Holosystolic murmur of ventricular septal defect with mild pulmonary stenosis. The pulmonary component of the second heart sound (P₂) was delayed but readily heard. **C,** The ventricular septal defect murmur decreases in latter systole as moderately severe pulmonary stenosis decreases left-to-right shunt. The pulmonary component of the second heart sound is soft and further delayed. **D,** The ventricular septal defect murmur is replaced by a relatively long pulmonary stenotic murmur because right ventricular outflow resistance equals systemic vascular resistance. The shunt is balanced, and the ventricular septal defect is silent. The second sound is the single aortic component (A₂) because the pulmonary component is inaudible. **E,** The pulmonary stenotic murmur shortens and softens when right ventricular outflow resistance exceeds systemic vascular resistance because right ventricular blood is diverted into the aorta. The single second sound is the aortic component. **F,** The systolic murmur is shorter and softer because severe pulmonary stenosis diverts still more right ventricular blood into the aorta away and from the pulmonary artery. An ejection (E) originates in the dilated ascending aorta. The single second sound is the aortic component. **G,** The pulmonary stenotic murmur vanishes because of pulmonary atresia. An ejection sound (E) originates in the dilated ascending aorta. The single second sound is the aortic component (A₂).

sound (see Figure 18-22A). Continuous murmurs from collateral circulation obscure the murmur of aortic regurgitation. A brisk arterial pulse may result from abundant collateral flow rather than aortic regurgitant flow. However, conspicuous cyanosis with a brisk arterial pulse favors aortic regurgitation because arterial collaterals large enough to cause bounding pulses are also large enough to increase pulmonary arterial blood flow and minimize the cyanosis. Large collateral arteries that deliver abundant pulmonary blood flow occasionally cause a mitral mid-diastolic murmur (see Figure 18-22A). Rarely, a bicuspid pulmonary valve is incompetent, generating a delayed medium-frequency diastolic murmur of low-pressure pulmonary regurgitation (see Figure 18-22B).

The pulmonary component of the second heart sound is *soft or absent* because right ventricular blood preferentially enters the aorta, so pulmonary blood flow and artery pressure are abnormally low. A *delay* in the pulmonary component is the result of the relatively long interval required for high right ventricular systolic pressure to fall below the low pulmonary arterial diastolic incisura and to delayed relaxation of the infundibulum that contributes to late pulmonary valve closure by supporting the column of blood in the pulmonary trunk after the right ventricle has begun to relax.[112,129]

With mild or absent cyanosis, a soft delayed pulmonary component can be detected (see Figures 18-20C and 18-24).[129,130] When cyanosis is marked, the pulmonary component is typically inaudible, and with pulmonary atresia, there can be no pulmonary component because there is no functional pulmonary valve. Amyl nitrite inhalation reduces pulmonary arterial flow still further, so an audible pulmonary second sound disappears (see Figure 18-25).[127,131] Inaudibility also results from thickened bicuspid pulmonary leaflets that preclude brisk closing excursions. In 1866, Thomas Peacock[9] wrote: "The aorta is unusually large and from the powerful reaction on the valves during diastole of the heart, a loud ringing second sound is heard on listening at the upper part of the sternum." Peacock's loud ringing second sound was the loud aortic component (Figures 18-23 and 18-26).

Fourth heart sounds are exceptional because the force of right atrial contraction is not increased. Third heart sounds rarely occur on either side of the heart because right ventricular failure is uncommon and left ventricular filling is reduced. With systemic hypertension, right ventricular or biventricular failure may be accompanied by third and fourth heart sounds. With pulmonary atresia and large systemic to pulmonary arterial collaterals, increased blood flow across the mitral valve sometimes

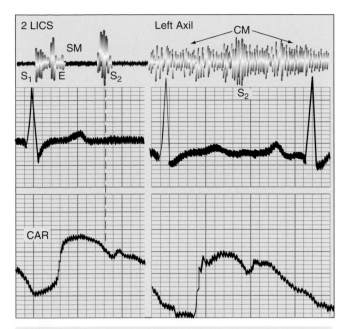

FIGURE 18-21 Phonocardiograms from an 11-year-old girl with Fallot's tetralogy and pulmonary atresia. In the second left intercostal space (2 LICS), an aortic ejection sound (E) follows the first heart sound (S₁) by a delay appropriate for the isometric contraction time incurred by systemic vascular resistance. The ejection sound introduces a soft short systolic murmur that originated in the dilated ascending aorta. The aortic component second sound (A₂) is loud because the aorta was dilated and guarded anteriorly by a hypoplastic pulmonary trunk. In the left axilla (Left Axil.), a continuous murmur (CM) peaked before and after the second heart sound.

generates a left ventricular third sound and a short mid-diastolic murmur (see Figure 18-22).

Auscultatory signs in *severe* pulmonary valve stenosis with a *restrictive* perimembranous ventricular septal defect are similar to if not identical to the auscultatory signs of severe *isolated* pulmonary stenosis. Suprasystemic right ventricular systolic pressure abolishes the left-to-right shunt through the ventricular septal defect, so a long pulmonary stenotic murmur exists alone.[132] A loud long pulmonary stenotic murmur is also heard when accessory tricuspid leaflet tissue partially occludes the ventricular septal defect (see Figure 18-18).[132]

Mild pulmonary valve stenosis with a *restrictive* ventricular septal defect results in auscultatory signs dominated by the holosystolic murmur of the ventricular septal defect. Suspicion of coexisting pulmonary valve stenosis depends on the presence of a pulmonary ejection sound and a right ventricular impulse.

Electrocardiogram

The electrocardiogram tends to be a reliable reflection of the physiology of Fallot's tetralogy.[133,134] Because the force of right atrial contraction is not increased and the right atrium is not enlarged, P waves are often normal in young patients and are seldom increased in amplitude but may be peaked (Figures 18-27 and 18-28). P wave duration tends to be short (see Figure 18-27) because the underfilled and relatively small left atrium writes the terminal force.[135–137] The PR interval is normal because the conduction system is normal.

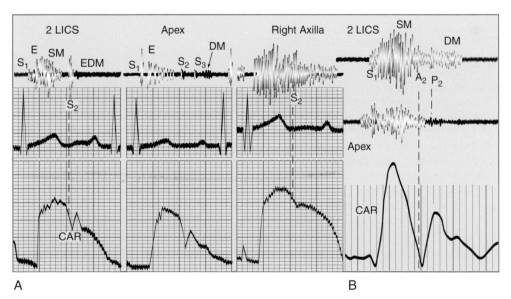

FIGURE 18-22 A, Phonocardiograms from a 15-year-old boy with Fallot's tetralogy and pulmonary atresia. In the second left intercostal space (2 LICS), an aortic ejection sound (E) merges with a prominent short midsystolic murmur (SM). The single second sound (S₂) is the aortic component that introduces an early diastolic murmur (EDM) of aortic regurgitation. The aortic ejection sound is more obvious at the apex where the systolic murmur is softer. A third heart sound (S₃) is followed by a soft short mid-diastolic murmur (DM) across the mitral valve. A continuous murmur in the right axilla is louder in systole. **B,** Tracings from a mildly cyanotic 12-year-old boy with Fallot's tetralogy and a stenotic and incompetent bicuspid pulmonary valve. A long loud midsystolic murmur of pulmonary stenosis envelopes the aortic component of the second heart sound (A₂). A medium-pitched low-pressure mid-diastolic murmur (DM) begins with the delayed pulmonary component of the second sound (P₂). (CAR = carotid pulse.)

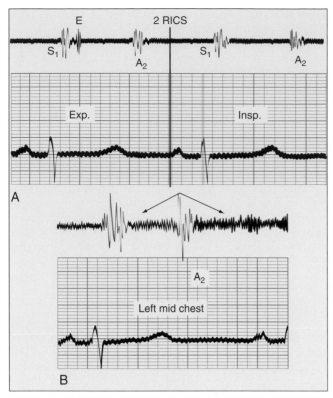

FIGURE 18-23 Phonocardiograms from a 4-year-old child with Fallot's tetralogy and pulmonary atresia. **A,** In the second right intercostal space (2 RICS), an aortic ejection sound (E) is prominent during expiration (Exp.) and absent during inspiration (Insp.) **B,** In the left midchest, a soft continuous murmur is of equal intensity in systole and diastole (paired arrows). (S_1 = first heart sound; A_2 = aortic component of the second heart sound.)

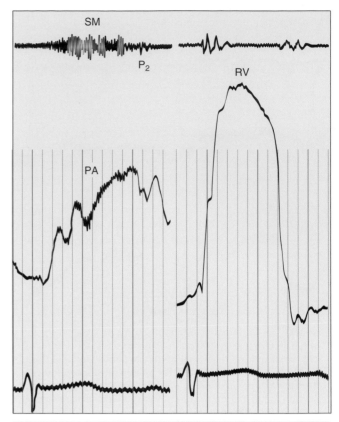

FIGURE 18-24 Intracardiac phonocardiogram, pulmonary arterial (PA) pressure pulse, and right ventricular (RV) pressure pulse in a 10-year-old girl with severe Fallot's tetralogy. A soft systolic stenotic murmur (SM) was recorded in the main pulmonary artery (PA) but not in the right ventricle (RV). The faint pulmonary component of the second heart sound (P_2) was recorded with the intracardiac microphone but was neither heard nor recorded on the chest wall.

The QRS axis is the same as that of a healthy newborn (see Figure 18-27).[134,138] However, the axis and direction of ventricular depolarization do not change as the neonate matures because the functional demands on the right ventricle do not change (see Figures 18-27 and 18-28).[134,138] The QRS complex is neither notched or slurred, and the duration is normal,[133,134] but peripheral conduction delay occurs in an occasional adult.[139] Left axis deviation with counterclockwise depolarization is reserved for Fallot's tetralogy with an atrioventricular septal defect (see Chapter 15).[140]

Right ventricular hypertrophy is characterized by a tall monophasic R wave confined to lead V_1, with an abrupt change to an rS pattern in V_2 (Figures 18-27, 18-28, and 18-29).[133,134,136,138] The presence and depth of Q waves and the amplitude of R waves in leads V_{5-6} are sensitive signs of the magnitude of pulmonary blood flow and of left ventricular filling. Reduced pulmonary flow with an underfilled left ventricle is accompanied by rS patterns in leads V_{2-6} (see Figure 18-27). A balanced shunt is accompanied by small q waves and well-developed R waves in lead V_{5-6} (see Figure 18-28). A left-to-right shunt is accompanied by deeper left precordial Q waves and relatively tall R waves (see Figure 18-29).

Right precordial T waves are upright or inverted with almost equal frequency (see Figures 18-27 through 18-29). The deeply inverted right precordial T waves that

characterize severe pulmonary stenosis with an intact ventricular septum seldom occur because right ventricular systolic pressure seldom exceeds systemic.

With pulmonary atresia and an abundant collateral arterial circulation, P waves are broad and bifid because of increased flow into the left atrium. Q waves with well-developed R waves appear in leads V_{5-6} because of increased flow into the left ventricle. ST segment and T wave abnormalities may be found in midprecordial leads (Figure 18-30).

Acquired obstruction to right ventricular outflow with a nonrestrictive ventricular septal defect results in an electrocardiogram that initially resembles isolated ventricular septal defect of equivalent size. Right ventricular systolic pressure remains unchanged, but pulmonary blood flow and left ventricular volume necessarily decrease. As outflow obstruction increases, left precordial qR complexes are less prominent and tall right precordial R waves persist.[74]

In *double-chambered right ventricle*, the increase in right ventricular pressure and mass are confined to the hypertensive proximal compartment, so precordial leads display a normal QRS progression from V_{1-6} (Figure 18-31).[49,141] An upright T wave in lead V_3R

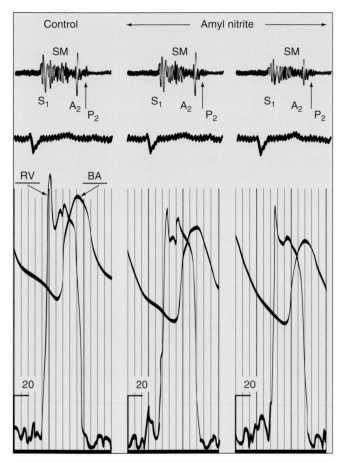

FIGURE 18-25 Tracings from a mildly cyanotic 3-year-old girl with Fallot's tetralogy and a balanced shunt. Amyl nitrite inhalation induced a fall in systemic vascular resistance and a parallel fall in right ventricular (RV) and brachial arterial (BA) pressure. Blood from the right ventricle preferentially entered the aorta, pulmonary blood flow reciprocally decreased, the pulmonary stenotic murmur (SM) shortened and softened, and the faint pulmonary component of the second sound (P$_2$) disappeared altogether.

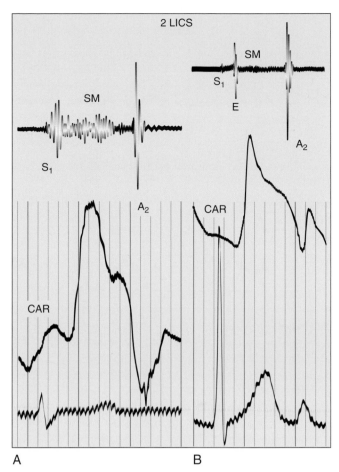

FIGURE 18-26 A, Tracings from a moderately cyanotic 2-year-old female with Fallot's tetralogy. A grade 3/6 pulmonary stenotic murmur (SM) ends before the aortic component of the second sound (A$_2$), which was loud because a dilated aorta was guarded by a small anterior pulmonary trunk. **B,** Tracings from an 18-month-old female with Fallot's tetralogy and pulmonary atresia. A prominent aortic ejection sound (E) introduces a soft short systolic murmur (SM) that originated in the dilated aortic root. The interval between the first heart sound and ejection sound is appropriate for the isovolumetric contraction time incurred by systemic vascular resistance. The aortic component of the second sound (A$_2$) was loud because a dilated aorta was guarded by a hypoplastic anterior pulmonary trunk. (2 LICS = second left intercostal space; CAR = carotid pulse.)

may be the only electrocardiographic sign of right ventricular hypertrophy.[49]

The electrocardiogram of a *restrictive* ventricular septal defect with *severe* pulmonary valve stenosis is indistinguishable from isolated pulmonary stenosis with intact ventricular septum.[132] *Restrictive* ventricular septal defects with *mild* pulmonary stenosis are associated with modest signs of right ventricular hypertrophy manifested by a relatively vertical QRS axis, an rSr′ pattern in lead V$_1$, and persistent upright right precordial T waves.

X-Ray

In cyanotic Fallot's tetralogy, pulmonary vascularity is reduced and the middle and outer thirds of the lung fields display a paucity of vascular markings because of a reduction in size of intrapulmonary arteries and veins (Figure 18-32).[142] The right lung is occasionally less vascular than the left.[143] In pulmonary atresia, there is a lacy reticular pattern without the normal diminution in vessel caliber toward the periphery because systemic arterial collaterals anastomose with *segmental* or *lobar intrapulmonary* arteries (Figure 18-33A).[133,144] When systemic arterial collaterals or bronchial collaterals anastomose with *hilar* or *extrapulmonary* arteries, intrapulmonary branching is normal (see Figures 18-6A, 18-7C, D, and 18-8B). The patterns of collateral arterial circulation are not uniform, with some areas oligemic and others normal or hypervascular (Figure 18-34). Systemic collateral arteries rarely cause rib notching because they do not run in intercostal grooves.[145]

The *concave* main pulmonary artery segment of pulmonary atresia stands out in bold contrast to the dilated right aortic arch (see Figures 18-32 and 18-33A).[86] The size of the ascending aorta tends to vary inversely with

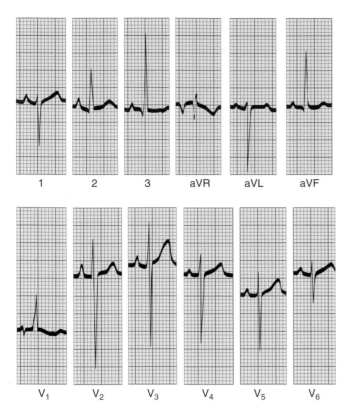

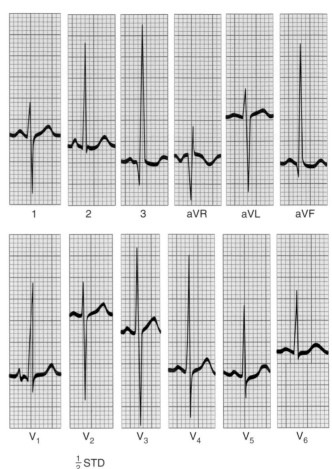

FIGURE 18-27 Electrocardiogram from a 2-year-old girl with cyanotic Fallot's tetralogy. P waves in leads 1, 2, 3, and V_{2-3} are peaked but not tall. There is moderate right axis deviation with clockwise depolarization. Right ventricular hypertrophy is represented by a notched monophasic R wave in lead V_1. Right precordial T waves were normal because right ventricular systemic pressure did not exceed systemic. There is the typical abrupt change from an R wave in lead V_1 to an rS in lead V_2. Q waves are absent in left precordial leads because the left ventricle was underfilled.

$\frac{1}{2}$ STD

FIGURE 18-28 Electrocardiogram from a mildly cyanotic 3-year-old girl with Fallot's tetralogy. P waves are normal. There is moderate right axis deviation with clockwise depolarization. Right ventricular hypertrophy is represented by a tall monophasic R wave in lead V_1 with a typical abrupt change to an rS complex in lead V_2. Right precordial T waves remain upright because right ventricular systolic pressure did not exceed systemic. Prominent R waves in left precordial leads reflect an adequately filled well-developed left ventricle. The large equidiphasic in RS complex in lead V_3 suggests biventricular hypertrophy. Leads V_{2-3} are half standardized.

the size of the pulmonary trunk (see Figure 18-3), culminating in the conspicuously dilated ascending aorta of pulmonary atresia (see Figure 18-33). However, dilation of the ascending aorta is also determined by inherent medial abnormalities.[14,38,39,146] There is a *right aortic arch* in 20% to 30% of patients with Fallot's tetralogy, with the highest incidence rate in pulmonary atresia (see Figures 18-6A and 18-33A).[40,86] A right arch is typically accompanied by a right descending aorta, which runs as a fine line parallel to the vertebral column (Figures 18-33 and 18-36). A right aortic arch indents the *right side* of the trachea (see Figure 18-8A), and a left aortic arch indents the *left side* of the trachea (see Figure 18-33B). Occasionally, there is a double aortic arch.[147] A dilated anomalous left subclavian artery may pass behind the esophagus and cause localized posterior indentation (Figure 18-35).[148] A left superior vena cava casts its shadow at the left thoracic inlet.[149]

The *size* of the heart in cyanotic Fallot's tetralogy is normal (see Figure 18-32).[103] The right atrium and right ventricle cope with systemic resistance without dilating, and the left atrium and left ventricle are underfilled and are therefore small. In pulmonary atresia, cardiac size

tends to be larger in response to flow through systemic arterial collaterals (see Figures 18-33 and 18-34).[86]

The *configuration* of the heart has long been a subject of interest in Fallot's tetralogy because of the distinctive boot-shaped or *coeur en sabot* appearance (see Figure 18-32).[103,150] The configuration has also been likened to a golf club wood or driver, especially when a right aortic arch and a concave pulmonary artery segment accentuate the configuration of the left cardiac border (see Figures 18-6A and 18-8A). The boot shape results from the combination of a small underfilled left ventricle that lies above a horizontal ventricular septum, inferior to which is a concentrically hypertrophied but nondilated right ventricle (see Figure 18-32).[150] The *coeur en sabot* is uncommon in neonates because intrauterine left ventricular volume is normal. In pulmonary atresia, the boot shape may be present at birth because of a reduction in

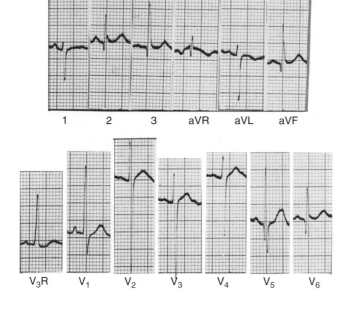

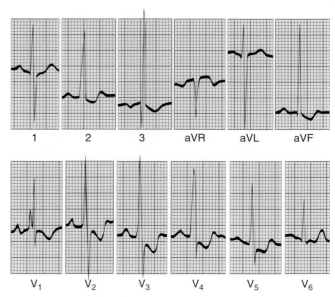

FIGURE 18-29 Electrocardiogram from a 2-year-old girl with acyanotic Fallot's tetralogy and a left-to-right shunt of 1.4/1. P wave in leads 1 and V_1 are slightly peaked. There is moderate right axis deviation with clockwise depolarization. Right ventricular hypertrophy is represented by tall monophasic R waves in leads V_3R and V_1 with the typical abrupt change to rS complexes in lead V_2. T waves are upright in right precordial leads because right ventricular systolic pressure did not exceed systemic. The well-developed R waves and prominent Q waves in leads V_{5-6} indicate adequate filling of a well-developed left ventricle.

FIGURE 18-30 Electrocardiogram from a 15-year-old boy with Fallot's tetralogy and pulmonary atresia. P waves are slightly peaked in leads V_{1-2}. Right axis deviation is moderate. Right ventricular hypertrophy is represented by a tall notched R wave in lead V_1 with atypical extension of the tall R wave to midprecordial leads, together with inverted T waves and ST segment depressions. Prominent R waves in left precordial leads and the q wave in lead V_6 indicate an adequately filled well-developed left ventricle from abundant aortopulmonary collaterals.

pulmonary blood flow and left ventricular volume caused by atresia of the fetal ductus arteriosus (see Figure 18-33A). In *acyanotic* Fallot's tetralogy or with pulmonary atresia and *large systemic arterial collaterals*, a well-formed convex apex is the result of normal if not increased left ventricular filling (see Figure 18-34). When right ventricular outflow obstruction is caused by stenosis of the *ostium of the infundibulum*, a localized indentation marks the site of obstruction, above which the infundibular chamber is slightly convex (see Figures 18-4 and 18-36).

A nonrestrictive ventricular septal defect with *acquired* obstruction to right ventricular outflow exhibits an initial increase in pulmonary vascularity, with enlargement of the left ventricle, left atrium, and pulmonary trunk (see Figure 18-13A). Progressive obstruction results in a decline in pulmonary arterial blood flow and in normalization of the size of the left atrium and left ventricle (see Figure 18-13B).[74] When a nonrestrictive *perimembranous* ventricular septal defect occurs with *pulmonary valve stenosis*, the radiologic picture is determined by the degree of pulmonary stenosis. The size of the ascending is normal, the pulmonary trunk is dilated, and the ventricular septum is vertical rather than horizontal (see Figure 18-10). When a malaligned ventricular septal defect is partially occluded by tricuspid leaflet tissue, the right ventricle may fail and dilate. When

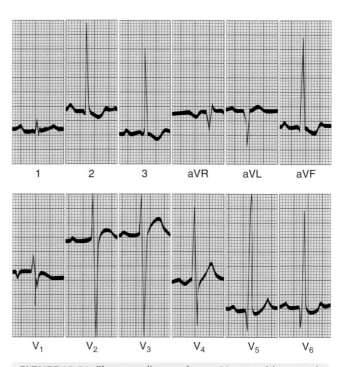

FIGURE 18-31 Electrocardiogram from a 23-year-old man with a nonrestrictive perimembranous ventricular septal defect and a *double-chambered* right ventricle. Right ventricular hypertrophy is conspicuously absent in both limb leads and precordial leads because only the most proximal portion of the right ventricle was hypertensive. The left ventricular volume overload pattern in leads V_{5-6} was the result of a surgical shunt.

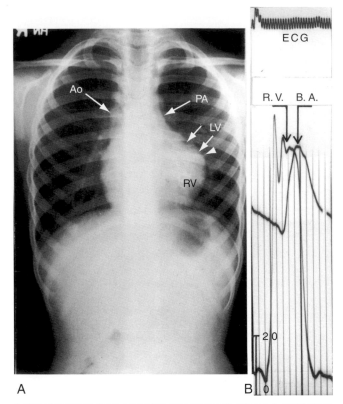

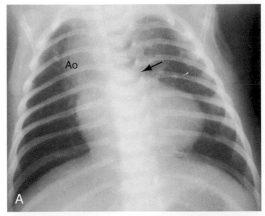

A

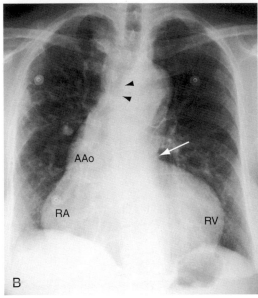

B

FIGURE 18-32 A, X-ray from a 4-year-old girl with classic cyanotic Fallot's tetralogy. The heart is typically boot-shaped because a small underfilled left ventricle (LV) lies superior to a relatively horizontal ventricular septum and an elevated interventricular sulcus (unmarked arrowhead) inferior to which lies the concentrically hypertrophied apical right ventricle (RV). The ascending aorta (Ao) is prominent, the main pulmonary artery segment (PA) is concave, and the lungs are oligemic. **B,** Systolic pressures are identical in the right ventricular (RV) and brachial artery (BA) because the ventricular septal defect was nonrestrictive.

FIGURE 18-33 X-rays from two patients 55 years apart in age. **A,** A 20-day-old male infant with Fallot's tetralogy and pulmonary atresia. The boot-shaped apex is emphasized by the concave main pulmonary artery segment (arrow) and the right aortic arch (Ao). The lung fields show the lacy appearance of systemic arterial collaterals. **B,** X-ray from a 55-year-old woman with Fallot's tetralogy, pulmonary atresia, and acquired calcific stenosis and aortic regurgitation. Death was from biventricular failure. The lung fields show the lacy appearance of systemic arterial collaterals. The dilated ascending aorta (AAo) continues as a left aortic arch that deviates the trachea to the right (arrowheads) and descends along the left side of the vertebral column. The main pulmonary artery segment is concave (arrow). An enlarged right atrium (RA) occupies the lower right cardiac border. The apex-forming right ventricle (RV) is convex and not boot-shaped because the left ventricle was well-developed.

a restrictive perimembranous ventricular septal defect occurs with mild pulmonary valve stenosis, the x-ray resembles isolated pulmonary valve stenosis.

Echocardiogram

Echocardiography with color flow imaging and Doppler interrogation provides morphologic and physiologic assessment of Fallot's tetralogy and its variations.[151,152] Thymic aplasia or hypoplasia identifies patients with DiGeorge syndrome.[153] Continuous wave Doppler scan establishes the outflow gradient and the combination of valvular and infundibular pulmonary stenosis (Figure 18-37). The malaligned ventricular septal defect is recognized by anterior and cephalad deviation of the infundibular septum and a biventricular aorta (Figures 18-38 and 18-39). The pulmonary trunk and its proximal branches can be visualized (see Figure 18-39). A right aortic arch is imaged from suprasternal notch and subclavicular windows and the presence and degree of aortic regurgitation can be established with color flow. Echocardiography identifies tricuspid leaflet

tissue partially occluding the malaligned ventricular septal defect, and color flow imaging with continuous-wave Doppler interrogation establishes the degree of restriction across the partially obstructed defect. Pulmonary atresia is diagnosed when pulmonary valve echoes are absent and when color flow imaging and continuous wave Doppler scan detect no flow across the right ventricular outflow tract (see Figure 18-38A). The distinctive narrow serpentine elongated arterialized ductus arteriosus can be identified (see Figure 18-38B).

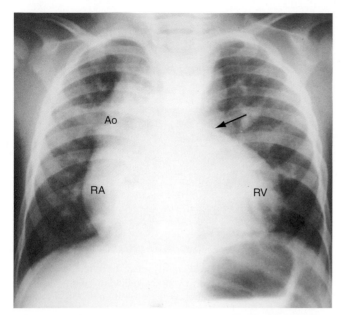

FIGURE 18-34 X-ray from the 3-year-old boy with Fallot's tetralogy and pulmonary atresia (angiograms in Figure 18-7). Pulmonary vascularity is not homogeneous because systemic arterial collateral flow is not uniform (see Figure 18-7). The ascending aorta (Ao) is dilated, and the main pulmonary artery segment is concave (arrow). A prominent right atrium (RA) occupies the lower right cardiac border. The apex-forming right ventricle (RV) is not boot-shaped because the left ventricle was well-developed from adequate filling from systemic arterial collaterals.

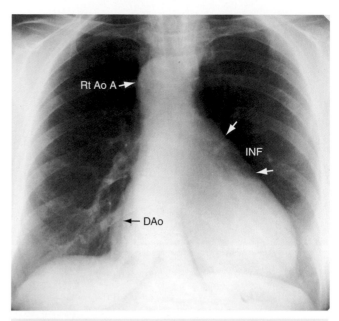

FIGURE 18-36 X-ray from a 62-year-old woman with localized stenosis of the ostium of the infundibulum (INF) and a restrictive perimembranous ventricular septal defect. Paired arrows bracket the slightly convex infundibulum. A right aortic arch (Rt AoA) continued as a right descending aorta (DAo).

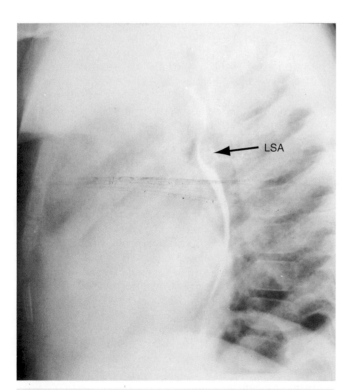

FIGURE 18-35 Lateral x-ray from a 5-year-old girl with Fallot's tetralogy, pulmonary atresia, a right aortic arch, and an aberrant retroesophageal left subclavian artery (LSA).

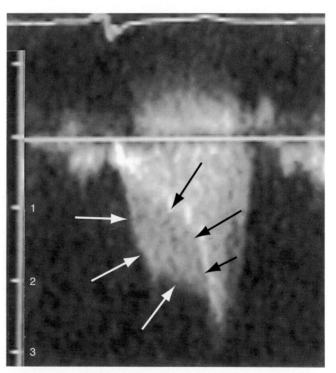

FIGURE 18-37 Continuous wave Doppler scan from an 18-month-old female with Fallot's tetralogy, a stenotic bicuspid pulmonary valve, and a stenotic infundibulum. The Doppler signal across the pulmonary valve (white arrows) contains the profile of coexisting infundibular stenosis (black arrows).

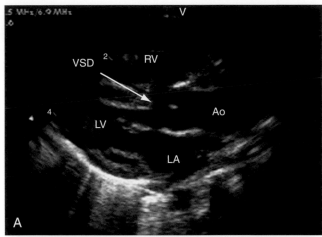

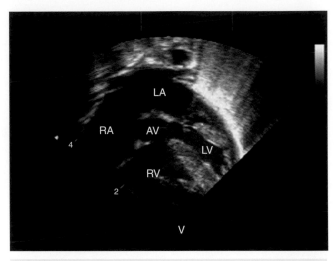

FIGURE 18-39 Echocardiogram (subcostal view) from an 18-month-old female with cyanotic Fallot's tetralogy, a malaligned infundibular septum. A large ventricular septal defect lies beneath the biventricular aorta. (RV = right ventricle; LV = left ventricle.)

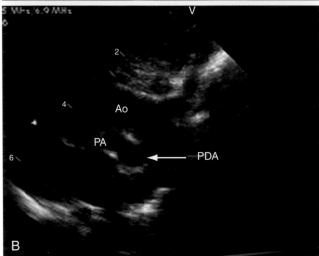

FIGURE 18-38 **A,** Echocardiogram (parasternal long axis) from a 22-year-old man with Fallot's tetralogy and pulmonary atresia. A nonrestrictive malaligned ventricular septal defect (VSD) lies beneath a dilated biventricular aorta (Ao). (LA = left atrium; RV = right ventricle; LV = left ventricle.) **B,** Echocardiogram (arch view) from a neonate with Fallot's tetralogy and pulmonary atresia. The arterialized ductus is typically narrow, serpentine, and elongated. (Ao = aorta; PDA = patent ductus arteriosus.)

Obstructing or nonobstructing subinfundibular muscle bundles of a double-chambered right ventricle can be identified, the degree of obstruction can be established with color flow and Doppler interrogation (Figure 18-40 and Videos 18-1A and 18-1B), and a coexisting perimembranous ventricular septal defect can be detected.[154]

FALLOT'S TETRALOGY WITH ABSENT PULMONARY VALVE

In 1847, Chevers[155] described the combination of absent pulmonary valve, ventricular septal defect, annular stenosis, and dilation of the pulmonary trunk and its branches. The malformation was confirmed in 1908 by Royer and

Wilson[156] and reconfirmed in 1927 by Kurtz, Sprague, and White.[157] The incidence rate of absent pulmonary valve with Fallot's tetralogy ranges from 2.4% to 6.3%.[158] Pulmonary valve tissue is lacking completely or consists of rudimentary remnants of avascular myxomatous connective tissue. Rarely, absence of the pulmonary valve occurs with absence of a pulmonary artery (see subsequent section)[159,160] and with systemic to pulmonary artery collaterals.[161] Obstruction to right ventricular outflow resides at the narrow pulmonary annulus, not at the malaligned infundibular septum.[159] The pulmonary trunk, especially its proximal branches, dilates massively (Figure 18-41) together with the infundibulum (see Figure 18-41C).[90,159,162]

The malformation can be recognized in the fetus.[163] Regurgitant volume *in utero* is returned to the pulmonary trunk during each right ventricular systole, distending the pulmonary trunk and its branches, more so when egress is curtailed by agenesis of the ductus arteriosus,[163] even though decompression is achieved via the nonrestrictive ventricular septal defect.[163] *Diastolic collapse* of the central pulmonary arteries occurs after each systole, and diastolic flow is accelerated by elastic recoil of the proximal pulmonary arteries.[163] Medial abnormalities in the walls of the dilated proximal pulmonary arteries have been attributed to abnormal flow patterns *in utero*, but inherent medial abnormalities contribute materially to the massive dilation (Figures 18-41 and 18-42).[14,164] Morphometric studies reveal a bizarre pattern of abnormal hilar branching in addition to abnormalities of the proximal pulmonary artery.[165] Tufts of pulmonary arteries are entwined among compressed intrapulmonary bronchi. Compression of small bronchi by abnormal branching patterns of intrapulmonary arteries together with compression of the trachea and bronchi by dilated *proximal* pulmonary arteries are major complications of the malformation.[159,166] An important feature of the

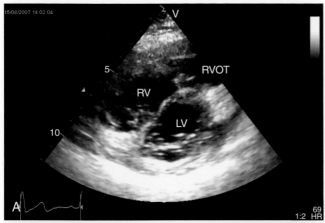

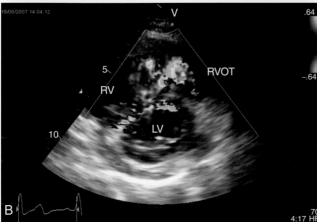

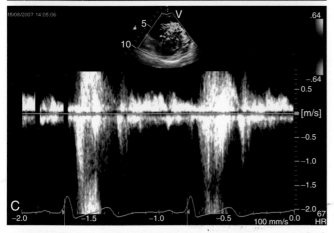

FIGURE 18-40 A, Echocardiogram (short axis) from a 2-year-old girl with double-chambered right ventricle. **B,** Color flow image showing the site of subinfundibular obstruction. **C,** Continuous wave Doppler across the obstruction.

experimental fetal rat model of congenitally absent pulmonary valve is the degree of bronchial deformity that suggests an inherent bronchial abnormality as an essential part of the syndrome.[167]

The *physiologic consequences* of Fallot's tetralogy with absent pulmonary valve are borne by the right ventricle, which is subjected to the massive volume overload of severe pulmonary regurgitation in addition to the resistance to discharge incurred by annular obstruction.[160]

The doubly beset right ventricle dilates and fails, its filling pressure rises and equilibrates with pulmonary arterial diastolic pressure, and right atrial pressure rises in parallel. Right ventricular failure and tracheobronchial compression are responsible for the high morbidity and mortality rates.[168]

History

The malformation causes respiratory distress (tracheobronchial obstruction) and right ventricular failure soon after birth, but an occasional patient experiences infancy with surprisingly few symptoms.[159] The symptoms occasionally improve during the course of tracheobronchial maturation, although emphysema, atelectasis, and pulmonary infection are common.[159] Early cyanosis is the result of respiratory distress, and a right-to-left shunt diminishes with age because a fall in pulmonary vascular resistance decreases pulmonary regurgitant flow, decreases volume overload of the pressure-overloaded right ventricle, and decreases the right-to-left shunt.

Arterial Pulse, Jugular Venous Pulse, and Precordial Palpation

Right ventricular failure curtails aortic flow and reduces the systemic arterial pulse. The jugular venous pulse is elevated in parallel with the elevated right ventricular filling pressure. The A wave remains dominant until tricuspid regurgitation obliterates the X descent and increases the crest of the V wave. The right ventricular impulse is especially dynamic because of the combined effects of volume and pressure overload. A dilated infundibulum (see Figure 18-41C) is readily palpated in the third left intercostal space, and a dilated pulsatile pulmonary trunk is palpated in the *second left* intercostal space (see Figure 18-41A). A systolic thrill is common because augmented right ventricular stroke volume is ejected rapidly across a hypoplastic pulmonary annulus. A diastolic thrill of pulmonary regurgitation is common because diastolic flow is accelerated by recoil of the dilated proximal pulmonary arteries.

Auscultation

The wheezing and stertorous breathing of tracheobronchial compression compromise auscultation. A pulmonary ejection sound is absent because the pulmonary valve is absent. The pulmonary component of the second heart sound is necessarily absent because the pulmonary valve mechanism is absent.[90] The aortic component of the second sound is muted by anterior interposition of the dilated pulmonary trunk. A midsystolic murmur is maximal in the second left intercostal space and is loud, harsh, and long because a large right ventricular stroke volume is ejected across a narrow annulus into a dilated pulmonary trunk (see Figure 18-42).[169] The pulmonary regurgitant murmur is analogous to the diastolic murmur of isolated severe congenital pulmonary valve regurgitation (see Chapter 12).[112,169] A distinct gap exists between the aortic component of the second heart sound

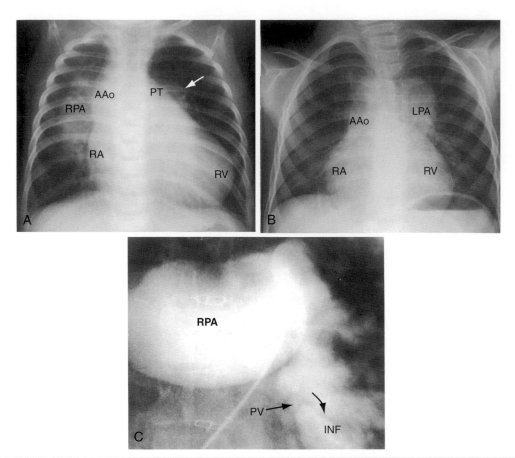

FIGURE 18-41 **A,** X-ray from a 6-month-old male with Fallot's tetralogy and absent pulmonary valve. The *right* pulmonary artery (RPA) is aneurysmal. A dilated left pulmonary artery (arrow) is partially obscured by the large pulmonary trunk (PT). The ascending aorta (AAo) is dilated. A large right atrium (RA) occupies the right lower cardiac border, and an enlarged right ventricle (RV) occupies the apex. **B,** X-ray from an 8-month-old male with Fallot's tetralogy and absent pulmonary valve. The *left* pulmonary artery (LPA) is aneurysmal. The ascending aorta (AAo) is dilated. An enlarged right atrium occupies the right lower cardiac border. An enlarged right ventricle (RV) occupies the apex and extends below the left hemidiaphragm. **C,** Pulmonary arteriogram from a 26-year-old man with Fallot's tetralogy and absent pulmonary valve. The right pulmonary artery (RPA) is aneurysmal. The site of the absent pulmonary valve (PV) is identified by the straight arrow. The curved arrow identifies regurgitant flow into the dilated infundibulum (INF).

and the onset of the diastolic murmur, which coincides with the delayed timing of the absent pulmonary closure sound. The diastolic murmur is usually grade 3/6 and is impure and often harsh, ending well before the subsequent first heart sound (see Figure 18-42). The crescendo portion of the diastolic murmur may be comparatively long because a delayed fall in pressure is associated with impaired infundibular relaxation and increased diastolic stiffness.[169] The combination of a long, loud, harsh systolic murmur followed by a shorter harsh diastolic murmur creates the auscultatory impression of *sawing wood*.

Electrocardiogram

The P wave is usually peaked and tall (Figure 18-43). The QRS axis is rightward. However, the chief electrocardiographic distinction between Fallot's tetralogy with absent pulmonary valve and classic cyanotic Fallot's tetralogy is the precordial lead pattern of right ventricular hypertrophy. When the pulmonary valve is absent, the tall

monophasic R wave in lead V_1 extends to adjacent precordial leads (see Figure 18-43), in contrast to Fallot's tetralogy in which the tall right precordial R wave is confined to lead V_1 (see Figure 18-27).

X-Ray

Radiologic features of Fallot's tetralogy with absent pulmonary valve are striking.[90] The pulmonary trunk and proximal branches dilate massively (see Figures 18-41 and 18-42). Infundibular dilation (see Figure 18-41C) projects leftward as a hump-shaped shadow.[90] A conspicuously dilated right ventricle occupies the apex, and an enlarged right atrium forms the right lower cardiac silhouette (see Figure 18-41A, B). Pulmonary vascularity is normal rather than decreased, although assessment is compromised by emphysema, hyperinflation, and atelectasis. Rarely, the right or left pulmonary artery arises directly from the aorta; lung vascularity is greater on the ipsilateral side.[158]

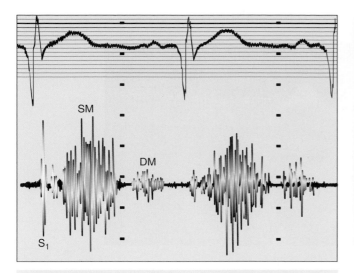

FIGURE 18-42 Phonocardiogram (third left intercostal space) from a 2-month-old female with Fallot's tetralogy and absent pulmonary valve. A long loud midsystolic murmur (SM) is followed by a murmur-free interval before the onset of a middiastolic murmur (DM). The pulmonary component of the second heart sound is absent because the pulmonary valve is absent. The aortic component of the second heart sound is obscured by the long systolic murmur.

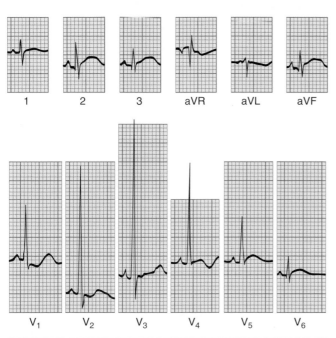

FIGURE 18-43 Electrocardiogram from a female neonate with Fallot's tetralogy and absent pulmonary valve. P waves are peaked and tall in leads 2 and aVF and in the midprecordium. The QRS axis is plus 90 degrees. Tall monophasic R waves of right ventricular hypertrophy in lead V_1 extend into contiguous mid precordial leads.

Echocardiogram

Echocardiography with color flow imaging and Doppler interrogation establishes the diagnosis and hemodynamics consequences of Fallot's tetralogy with absent pulmonary valve.[163] The malaligned ventricular septal

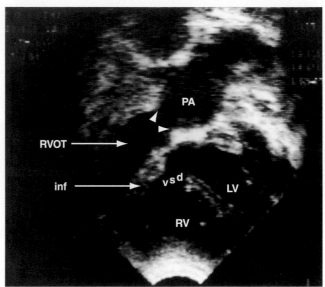

FIGURE 18-44 Echocardiogram (subcostal view) from a 23-month-old male with Fallot's tetralogy and absent pulmonary valve. The main pulmonary artery (PA) and right ventricular outflow tract (RVOT) are dilated. Echogenic ridges project into the lumen at the expected site of the pulmonary valve (paired arrowheads). The infundibular septum (inf) is malaligned, and the ventricular septal defect (vsd) is nonrestrictive. (RV = right ventricle; LV = left ventricle.)

defect is nonrestrictive (Figures 18-44 and 18-45). An echodense ridge projects into the lumen at the expected site of the absent pulmonary valve (see Figures 18-44 and 18-45A). The infundibulum, pulmonary trunk, and proximal branches are dilated, but the annulus is obstructed (see Figures 18-44 and 18-45A). Color flow imaging and Doppler interrogation characterize the pulmonary regurgitation and the flow patterns across the absent pulmonary valve and the narrow pulmonary annulus (Figure 18-45B).

Fallot's Tetralogy with Absence of a Pulmonary Artery

Congenital absence of a pulmonary artery almost always involves the *left* pulmonary artery[143,170] and only rarely occurs in isolation (Figures 18-46 and 18-47).[139] Congenital *absence* of a pulmonary artery differs from *anomalous origin* of a pulmonary artery from the ascending aorta, a malformation that also occurs with the tetralogy.[171] When the left pulmonary artery is absent, the murmur of pulmonary stenosis radiates into the *right* pulmonary artery and *right* upper chest.[170] The x-ray is diagnostically useful because the left hemithorax is small, the left hemidiaphragm is elevated, the left lung is hypovascular (see Figure 18-46A),[143,170] and the aortic arch is on the *right* (see Figure 18-46).[172,173] When the left pulmonary artery originates from the ascending aorta, the *ipsilateral* lung is relatively *hypervascular*. When the *right* pulmonary artery is absent, the blood supply to the ipsilateral lung is usually derived from the coronary arteries.[174]

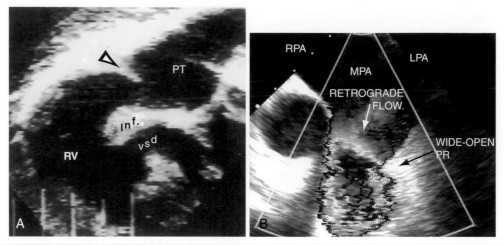

FIGURE 18-45 A, Echocardiogram (subcostal view) from a 4-year-old boy with Fallot's tetralogy and absent pulmonary valve. The large arrowhead points to an echogenic ridge at the site of the absent pulmonary valve. The pulmonary trunk (PT) is dilated. (inf. = infundibulum; vsd = ventricular septal defect.) **B,** Echocardiogram from a 26-year-old man with Fallot's tetralogy and absent pulmonary valve. Color flow image shows retrograde flow and wide-open pulmonary regurgitation (PR). (MPA = main pulmonary artery; RPA/LPA = right/left pulmonary artery.)

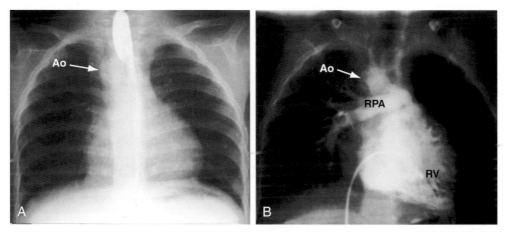

FIGURE 18-46 A, X-ray from an infant with Fallot's tetralogy and absent left pulmonary artery. The left hemithorax is smaller than the right hemithorax (posterior ribs are closer). Lung vascularity is not reduced. The aortic arch (Ao) and descending aorta are right-sided. **B,** The right ventriculogram from the same patient opacifies the right pulmonary artery (RPA). The left pulmonary artery is absent. The right aortic arch (Ao) visualized simultaneously. (RV = right ventricle.)

Summary

In *classic Fallot's tetralogy*, cyanosis is usually detected a few weeks after birth, and most patients are overtly cyanotic within 6 months. In Fallot's tetralogy with *pulmonary atresia*, cyanosis is mild or absent when pulmonary blood flow is appreciably increased by large systemic-to-pulmonary artery collaterals. Physical underdevelopment is common. Distinctive attacks of hyperpnea, deepening cyanosis, and syncope occur, especially in the first 6 months of life, and are provoked by feeding, straining, or crying. Squatting is the characteristic posture assumed for symptomatic relief. With few exceptions, right ventricular failure is conspicuous by its absence. The arterial pulse and the jugular venous pulse are

normal. Precordial palpation detects a gentle right ventricular impulse confined to the lower left sternal border and subxyphoid area. A right sternoclavicular impulse indicates a right aortic arch with a dilated ascending aorta. The length and loudness of the pulmonary stenotic murmur vary inversely with the severity of right ventricular outflow obstruction. An aortic ejection sound can be anticipated when the aortic root is dilated and is consistently present in the dilated ascending aorta of pulmonary atresia. Pulmonary ejection sounds are absent because the bicuspid pulmonary valve is not sufficiently mobile. A single second heart sound represents the aortic component. A soft delayed pulmonary component is reserved for the occasional patient with adequate flow into a

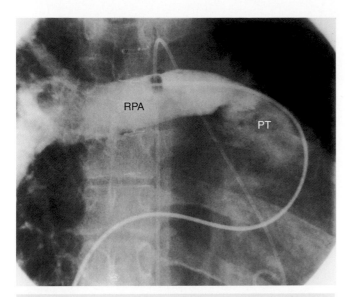

FIGURE 18-47 Selective pulmonary arteriogram from a 28-year-old man with Fallot's tetralogy and absent left pulmonary artery. The pulmonary trunk (PT) continues as the right pulmonary artery (RPA). The aortic arch (not shown) was atypically left-sided.

well-formed pulmonary trunk. Continuous murmurs originate in aortopulmonary collaterals that accompany Fallot's tetralogy with pulmonary atresia. P waves are normal or peaked but not tall. The QRS axis retains its normal neonatal direction. Right ventricular hypertrophy is characterized by a tall monophasic R wave confined to lead V_1 with abrupt transition to an rS complex in lead V_2. Q waves and well-developed R waves in left precordial leads reflect adequate pulmonary arterial blood flow and adequate left ventricular filling. The x-ray shows reduced pulmonary vascularity except for aortopulmonary collateral blood flow with pulmonary atresia. The ascending aorta is enlarged and often right-sided. The main pulmonary artery segment is concave. Cardiac size is normal, but the contour is characteristically boot-shaped. The echocardiogram reveals a biventricular aorta, a malaligned ventricular septal defect, and a narrow right ventricular outflow tract.

Fallot's tetralogy with absent pulmonary valve announces itself shortly after birth with symptoms of tracheobronchial compression and right ventricular failure. Neonatal cyanosis lessens with age. The jugular venous pulse is elevated because right ventricular filling pressure is elevated. A systolic impulse is palpated over the volume-overloaded right ventricle, over the dilated infundibulum, and over an aneurysmal pulmonary trunk. There is a systolic thrill in the second left intercostal space. The mid-diastolic murmur of pulmonary regurgitation begins at an interval after the aortic component of the second heart sound at the expected timing of the absent pulmonary component or after the end of the long harsh systolic murmur. The systolic/diastolic murmurs are not continuous, but to and fro. The x-ray discloses massive, often aneurysmal dilation of the pulmonary trunk and its

proximal branches. The right atrium and especially the right ventricle are appreciably enlarged. The electrocardiogram is characterized by P waves that are peaked and tall, a rightward QRS axis, and tall monophasic R waves of right ventricular hypertrophy that extend beyond lead V_1. Echocardiography identifies a dense band of echoes at the expected site of the absent pulmonary valve and identifies the malaligned ventricular septal defect and the biventricular aorta. Color flow imaging establishes severe pulmonary regurgitation, and Doppler interrogation records the systolic/diastolic flow patterns across the right ventricular outflow tract.

Fallot's tetralogy with absent left pulmonary artery is characterized by a relatively small left hemithorax, an elevated left hemidiaphragm, and an ipsilateral decrease in pulmonary vascularity. The murmur of pulmonary stenosis radiates preferentially into the right pulmonary artery and the right upper chest.

REFERENCES

1. Acierno LJ. Etienne-Louis Fallot: is it his tetralogy? *Clin Cardiol.* 1999;22:321–322.
2. Steno N. Anatomicus regij hafniensis embryo monstro affinis paisiis dissectus. *Acta Med et Philosophia, Hafminsia.* 1671;1:200.
3. Maas V. Nicolai Steno. *Opera Philosophica.* 1910;2:49.
4. Willius FA. An unusually early description of the so-called tetralogy of Fallot. *Mayo Clin Proc.* 1948;23:316–320.
5. Watson T. *Lectures on the principles and practice of physic.* Philadelphia: Henry C- Lea; 1872.
6. Sandifort E. *Observationes Anatomico-pathological.* Lugduni Batavorum: Eyk and D. Vygh; 1777.
7. Hunter W. Three cases of malformation of the heart. *Medical Observations and Inquiries by a Society of Physicians in London.* 1784;6:291.
8. Hope J. *Diseases of the heart.* 3rd ed. London: John Churchill & Sons; 1839.
9. Peacock T. *On malformations of the human heart.* London: J. Churchill & Sons; 1866.
10. Fallot A. Contribution à. l'anatomie pathologique de la maladie bleue (cyanose cardiaque). *Mars Med.* 1888;25:77–93.
11. Apitz C, Webb GD, Redington AN. Tetralogy of Fallot. *Lancet.* 2009;374:1462–1471.
12. Shinebourne EA, Babu-Narayan SV, Carvalho JS. Tetralogy of Fallot: from fetus to adult. *Heart.* 2006;92:1353–1359.
13. Soto B, Pacifico AD, Ceballos R, Bargeron Jr LM. Tetralogy of Fallot: an angiographic-pathologic correlative study. *Circulation.* 1981;64:558–566.
14. Niwa K, Perloff JK, Bhuta SM, et al. Structural abnormalities of great arterial walls in congenital heart disease: light and electron microscopic analyses. *Circulation.* 2001;103:393–400.
15. Ando M, Takahashi Y, Kikuchi T, Tatsuno K. Tetralogy of Fallot with subarterial ventricular septal defect. *Ann Thorac Surg.* 2003;76:1059–1064; discussion 1064–1055.
16. Tandon R, Moller JH, Edwards JE. Tetralogy of Fallot associated with persistent common atrioventricular canal (endocardial cushion defect). *Br Heart J.* 1974;36:197–206.
17. Uretzky G, Puga FJ, Danielson GK, et al. Complete atrioventricular canal associated with tetralogy of Fallot. Morphologic and surgical considerations. *J Thorac Cardiovasc Surg.* 1984;87:756–766.
18. Okamura T, Nagase Y, Matsumoto Y, Park I-S, Mitsui F, Shibairi M. Complete atrioventricular canal and tetralogy of Fallot with pulmonary atresia. *Ann Thorac Surg.* 2004;78:e69–71.
19. Faggian G, Frescura C, Thiene G, Bortolotti U, Mazzucco A, Anderson RH. Accessory tricuspid valve tissue causing obstruction of the ventricular septal defect in tetralogy of Fallot. *Br Heart J.* 1983;49:324–327.
20. Daliento L, Grisolia EF, Frescura C, Thiene G. Anomalous muscle bundle of the sub-pulmonary outflow in tetralogy of Fallot. *Int J Cardiol.* 1984;6:547–550.

21. Nair V, Thangaroopan M, Cunningham KS, et al. A bicuspid pulmonary valve associated with tetralogy of fallot. *J Card Surg.* 2006; 21:185–187.

22. Altrichter PM, Olson LJ, Edwards WD, Puga FJ, Danielson GK. Surgical pathology of the pulmonary valve: a study of 116 cases spanning 15 years. *Mayo Clin Proc.* 1989;64:1352–1360.

23. Sharma SN, Sharma S, Shrivastava S, Rajani M, Tandon R. Pulmonary arterial anatomy in tetralogy of Fallot. *Int J Cardiol.* 1989;25: 33–37.

24. Chaturvedi R, Mikailian H, Freedom RM. Crossed pulmonary arteries in tetralogy of Fallot. *Cardiol Young.* 2005;15:537.

25. Azhari N, Al-Fadley F, Bulbul ZR. Tetralogy of Fallot associated with scimitar syndrome. *Cardiol Young.* 2000;10:70–72.

26. Edwards JE, Mcgoon DC. Absence of anatomic origin from heart of pulmonary arterial supply. *Circulation.* 1973;47:393–398.

27. Liao PK, Edwards WD, Julsrud PR, Puga FJ, Danielson GK, Feldt RH. Pulmonary blood supply in patients with pulmonary atresia and ventricular septal defect. *J Am Coll Cardiol.* 1985;6: 1343–1350.

28. Rabinovitch M, Herrera-Deleon V, Castaneda AR, Reid L. Growth and development of the pulmonary vascular bed in patients with tetralogy of Fallot with or without pulmonary atresia. *Circulation.* 1981;64:1234–1249.

29. Deruiter MC, Gittenberger-De Groot AC, Poelmann RE, Vaniperen L, Mentink MM. Development of the pharyngeal arch system related to the pulmonary and bronchial vessels in the avian embryo. With a concept on systemic-pulmonary collateral artery formation. *Circulation.* 1993;87:1306–1319.

30. Wu L, Liu F. Anomalous origin of the pulmonary arteries from the left coronary artery in tetralogy of Fallot with pulmonary atresia. *Cardiol Young.* 2009;19:620–621.

31. Amin Z, Mcelhinney DB, Reddy VM, Moore P, Hanley FL, Teitel DF. Coronary to pulmonary artery collaterals in patients with pulmonary atresia and ventricular septal defect. *Ann Thorac Surg.* 2000;70:119–123.

32. Pahl E, Fong L, Anderson RH, Park SC, Zuberbuhler JR. Fistulous communications between a solitary coronary artery and the pulmonary arteries as the primary source of pulmonary blood supply in tetralogy of Fallot with pulmonary valve atresia. *Am J Cardiol.* 1989;63:140–143.

33. Andriko JA, Robinowitz M, Moore J, Virmani R. Necrotizing arteritis in uncorrected tetralogy of Fallot with pulmonary artery. *Pediatr Cardiol.* 1992;13:233–236.

34. Berry TE, Muster AJ, Paul MH. Transient neonatal tricuspid regurgitation: possible relation with premature closure of the ductus arteriosus. *J Am Coll Cardiol.* 1983;2:1178–1182.

35. Taussig HB. Clinical and pathological findings in cases of truncus arteriosus in infancy. *Am J Med.* 1947;2:26–34.

36. Glancy DL, Morrow AG, Roberts W. Malformations of the aortic valve in patients with the tetralogy of Fallot. *Am Heart J.* 1968;76: 755–759.

37. Marelli AJ, Perloff JK, Child JS, Laks H. Pulmonary atresia with ventricular septal defect in adults. *Circulation.* 1994;89: 243–251.

38. Chowdhury UK, Mishra AK, Ray R, Kalaivani M, Reddy SM, Venugopal P. Histopathologic changes in ascending aorta and risk factors related to histopathologic conditions and aortic dilatation in patients with tetralogy of Fallot. *J Thorac Cardiovasc Surg.* 2008;135:69–77.

39. Niwa K, Siu SC, Webb GD, Gatzoulis MA. Progressive aortic root dilatation in adults late after repair of tetralogy of Fallot. *Circulation.* 2002;106:1374–1378.

40. Hastreiter AR, D'cruz IA, Cantez T, Namin EP, Licata R. Right-sided aorta. I. Occurrence of right aortic arch in various types of congenital heart disease. II. Right aortic arch, right descending aorta, and associated anomalies. *Br Heart J.* 1966;28: 722–739.

41. Fellows KE, Freed MD, Keane JF, Praagh R, Bernhard WF, Castaneda AC. Results of routine preoperative coronary angiography in tetralogy of Fallot. *Circulation.* 1975;51:561–566.

42. Gupta D, Saxena A, Kothari SS, et al. Detection of coronary artery anomalies in tetralogy of Fallot using a specific angiographic protocol. *Am J Cardiol.* 2001;87:241–244, A310.

43. Chiu IS, Wu CS, Wang JK, et al. Influence of aortopulmonary rotation on the anomalous coronary artery pattern in tetralogy of fallot. *Am J Cardiol.* 2000;85:780–784, A789.

44. Talwar S, Sharma P, Gulati GS, Kothari SS, Choudhary SK. Tetralogy of fallot with coronary artery to pulmonary artery fistula and unusual coronary pattern: missed diagnosis. *J Card Surg.* 2009; 24:752–755.

45. Yamaguchi M, Tsukube T, Hosokawa Y, Ohashi H, Oshima Y. Pulmonary origin of left anterior descending coronary artery in tetralogy of Fallot. *Ann Thorac Surg.* 1991;52:310–312.

46. Gandhi SK, Pigula FA, Siewers RD. Intramural left coronary artery associated with right ventricular outflow tract obstruction. *J Thorac Cardiovasc Surg.* 2003;125:729–730.

47. Talwar S, Choudhary SK, Shivaprasad MB, et al. Tetralogy of Fallot with total anomalous pulmonary venous drainage. *Ann Thorac Surg.* 2008;86:1937–1940.

48. Sautter RD, Emanuel DA, Doege KH. Association of pulmonary valvular stenosis and muscular ventricular septal defect. Report of a case in a patient aged 75 years. *Am J Cardiol.* 1965;16: 743–745.

49. Goitein KJ, Neches WH, Park SC, Mathews RA, Lenox CC, Zuberbuhler JR. Electrocardiogram in double chamber right ventricle. *Am J Cardiol.* 1980;45:604–608.

50. Hartmann Jr AF, Tsifutis AA, Arvidssonh D, Goldring D. The two-chambered right ventricle. Report of nine cases. *Circulation.* 1962;26:279–287.

51. Perloff JK, Ronan Jr JA, De Leon Jr AC. Ventricular septal defect with the "two-chambered right ventricle" *Am J Cardiol.* 1965;16: 894–900.

52. Wang JK, Wu MH, Chang CI, et al. Malalignment-type ventricular septal defect in double-chambered right ventricle. *Am J Cardiol.* 1996;77:839–842.

53. Bashour TT, Kabbani S, Sandouk A, Cheng TO. Double-chambered right ventricle due to fibromuscular diaphragm. *Am Heart J.* 1984; 107:792–794.

54. Hindle Jr WV, Engle MA, Hagstrom JW. Anomalous right ventricular muscles: a clinicopathologic study. *Am J Cardiol.* 1968;21: 487–495.

55. Taussig HB. Left to right shunts in infancy. In: Lam CR, ed. *Henry Ford Hospital International Symposium on Cardiovascular Surgery.* Philadelphia: W. B. Saunders Company; 1955.

56. Maron BJ, Ferrans VJ, White Jr RI. Unusual evolution of acquired infundibular stenosis in patients with ventricular septal defect. Clinical and morphologic observations. *Circulation.* 1973;48:1092–1103.

57. Pongiglione G, Freedom RM, Cook D, Rowe RD. Mechanism of acquired right ventricular outflow tract obstruction in patients with ventricular septal defect: an angiocardiographic study. *Am J Cardiol.* 1982;50:776–780.

58. Shepherd RL, Glancy DL, Jaffe RB, Perloff JK, Epstein SE. Acquired subvalvular right ventricular outflow obstruction in patients with ventricular septal defect. *Am J Med.* 1972;53:446–455.

59. Fukuda J, Izumi T, Matsukawa T, Eguchi S. Development of left ventricular muscle in tetralogy of Fallot. *Jpn Circ J.* 1984;48: 465–473.

60. Jarmakani JM, Graham Jr TP, Canent Jr RV, Jewett PH. Left heart function in children with tetralogy of Fallot before and after palliative or corrective surgery. *Circulation.* 1972;46:478–490.

61. Danilowicz D, Ross Jr J. Pulmonary atresia with cyanosis. Report of two cases with ventricular septal defect and increased pulmonary blood flow. *Br Heart J.* 1971;33:138–141.

62. Best PV, Heath D. Pulmonary thrombosis in cyanotic congenital heart disease without pulmonary hypertension. *J Pathol Bacteriol.* 1958;75:281–291.

63. Ferencz C. The pulmonary vascular bed in tetralogy of Fallot. I. Changes associated with pulmonic stenosis. *Bull Johns Hopkins Hosp.* 1960;106:81–99.

64. Rich AR. A hitherto unrecognized tendency to the development of widespread pulmonary vascular obstruction in patients with congenital pulmonary stenosis (tetralogy of Fallot). *Bull Johns Hopkins Hosp.* 1948;82:389–401.

65. Der Kalouetian VM, Ratl H, Malouf J, et al. Tetralogy of Fallot with pulmonary atresia in siblings. *Am J Med Genet.* 1985;21: 119–122.

66. Pankau R, Siekmeyer W, Stoffregen R. Tetralogy of Fallot in three sibs. *Am J Med Genet.* 1990;37:532–533.

67. Zellers TM, Driscoll DJ, Michels VV. Prevalence of significant congenital heart defects in children of parents with Fallot's tetralogy. *Am J Cardiol.* 1990;65:523–526.

68. Cassidy SC, Allen HD. Tetralogy of Fallot in triplet siblings. *Am J Cardiol.* 1991;67:1442–1444.

69. Dichiara JA, Pieroni DR, Gingell RL, Bannerman RM, Vlad P. Familial pulmonary atresia. Its occurrence with a ventricular septal defect. *Am J Dis Child.* 1980;134:506–508.

70. Patterson DF, Pyle RL, Van Mierop L, Melbin J, Olson M. Hereditary defects of the conotruncal septum in Keeshond dogs: pathologic and genetic studies. *Am J Cardiol.* 1974;34:187–205.

71. Eldadah ZA, Hamosh A, Biery NJ, et al. Familial Tetralogy of Fallot caused by mutation in the jagged1 gene. *Hum Mol Genet.* 2001;10:163–169.

72. Goldmuntz E, Geiger E, Benson DW. NKX2.5 mutations in patients with tetralogy of fallot. *Circulation.* 2001;104: 2565–2568.

73. Momma K. Coarctation with tetralogy and pulmonary astresia. *Cardiol Young.* 2001;11:478.

74. Lendrum B, Agustsson M, Arcilla R, Gasul B. Natural history of patients with" acyanotic" tetralogy of Fallot [abstract]. *Circulation.* 1961;24:979.

75. Bertranou EG, Blackstone EH, Hazelrig JB, Turner ME, Kirklin JW. Life expectancy without surgery in tetralogy of Fallot. *Am J Cardiol.* 1978;42:458–466.

76. Rygg IH, Olesen K, Boesen I. The life history of tetralogy of Fallot. *Dan Med Bull.* 1971;18(suppl 2):25–30.

77. Bain GO. Tetralogy of fallot: survival to seventieth year; report of a case. *AMA Arch Pathol.* 1954;58:176–179.

78. Smitherman TC, Nimetz AA, Friedlich AL. Pulmonary atresia with ventricular septal defect: report of the oldest known surviving case. *Chest.* 1975;67:603–606.

79. Huang M-H, Hu H, Plata ET, Yahia AM, Goldfarb AL, Izzo Jr JL. Exceptional survival of a patient with large ventricular septal defect, bidirectional shunt, and severe pulmonary valve stenosis. *J Am Soc Echocardiogr.* 2002;15:665–667.

80. White PD, Sprague HB. The Tetralogy of fallot. report of a case in a noted musician, who lived to his sixtieth year. *J Am Med Assoc.* 1929;92:787–791.

81. Stanescu CM, Branidou K. A case of 75-year-old survivor of unrepaired tetralogy of Fallot and quadricuspid aortic valve. *Eur J Echocardiogr.* 2008;9:167–170.

82. Chandrasekaran B, Wilde P, Mccrea WA. Tetralogy of fallot in a 78-year-old man. *N Engl J Med.* 2007;357:1160–1161.

83. Gerlis LM, Ho SY, Sheppard MN. Longevity in the setting of tetralogy of Fallot: survival to the 84th year. *Cardiol Young.* 2004;14:664–666.

84. Alonso A, Downey BC, Kuvin JT. Uncorrected tetralogy of Fallot in an 86-year-old patient. *Am J Geriat Cardiol.* 2007;16:38–41.

85. Garcia R, Cargill JW, Drake EH. Pseudotruncus arteriosus. Report of the oldest surviving patient. *Am Heart J.* 1969;78:537–540.

86. Lafargue RT, Vogel JH, Pryor R, Blount Jr SG. Pseudotruncus arteriosus. A review of 21 cases with observations on oldest reported case. *Am J Cardiol.* 1967;19:239–246.

87. Perloff JK. Pregnancy in congenital heart disease. In: Perloff JK, Child JS, Aboulhosn J, eds. *Congenital heart disease in adults.* 3rd ed. Philadelphia: WB Saunders; 2009.

88. Bodhey NK, Beerbaum P, Sarikouch S, et al. Functional analysis of the components of the right ventricle in the setting of tetralogy of Fallot. *Circulation.* 2008;1:141–147.

89. Chesler E, Joffe HS, Beck W, Schrire V. Tetralogy of Fallot and heart failure. *Am Heart J.* 1971;81:321–326.

90. Ruttenberg HD, Carey LS, Adams P, Adams Jr P, Edwards JE. Absence of the pulmonary valve in the tetralogy of Fallot. *Am J Roentgenol Radium Ther Nucl Med.* 1964;91:500–510.

91. Benge W, White CW. Systemic hypertension complicating tetralogy of Fallot: effects of antihypertensive therapy. *Am J Cardiol.* 1978;42:294–298.

92. Sietsema KE, Cooper DM, Perloff JK, et al. Dynamics of oxygen uptake during exercise in adults with cyanotic congenital heart disease. *Circulation.* 1986;73:1137–1144.

93. Sietsema KE, Cooper DM, Perloff JK, et al. Control of ventilation during exercise in patients with central venous-to-systemic arterial shunts. *J Appl Physiol.* 1988;64:234–242.

94. Guntheroth WG, Morgan BC, Mullins GL. Physiologic studies of paroxysmal hyperpnea in cyanotic congenital heart disease. *Circulation.* 1965;31:70–76.

95. Morgan BC, Guntheroth WG, Bloom RS, Fyler DC. A clinical profile of paroxysmal hyperpnea in cyanotic congenital heart disease. *Circulation.* 1965;31:66–69.

96. Wood P. Attacks of deeper cyanosis and loss of consciousness (syncope) in Fallot's tetralogy. *Br Heart J.* 1958;20:282–286.

97. Daniels SR, Bates SR, Kaplan S. EEG monitoring during paroxysmal hyperpnea of tetralogy of Fallot: an epileptic or hypoxic phenomenon? *J Child Neurol.* 1987;2:98–100.

98. Weng Y-M, Chang Y-C, Chiu T-F, Weng C-S. Tet spell in an adult. *Am J Emerg Med.* 2009;27:130.e133–e135.

99. King SB, Franch RH. Production of increased right-to-left shunting by rapid heart rates in patients with tetralogy of Fallot. *Circulation.* 1971;44:265–271.

100. Van Roekens CN, Zuckerberg AL. Emergency management of hypercyanotic crises in tetralogy of Fallot. *Ann Emerg Med.* 1995;25:256–258.

101. Brotmacher L. Haemodynamic effects of squatting during recovery from exertion. *Br Heart J.* 1957;19:567–573.

102. O'donnell TV, Mc IM. The circulatory effects of squatting. *Am Heart J.* 1962;64:347–356.

103. Taussig HB. *Congenital malformations of the heart.* New York: The Commonwealth Fund; 1947.

104. Guntheroth WG, Mortan BC, Mullins GL, Baum D. Venous return with knee-chest position and squatting in tetralogy of Fallot. *Am Heart J.* 1968;75:313–318.

105. Lurie PR. Postural effects in tetralogy of Fallot. *Am J Med.* 1953; 15:297–306.

106. Sharpey-Schafer EP. Effects of squatting on the normal and failing circulation. *Br Med J.* 1956;1:1072–1074.

107. Laskin RL, Salazer R, Witzel MA, Rose V. Velopharyngeal insufficiency in tetralogy of Fallot: a report of four cases. *Pediatr Cardiol.* 1983;4:41–44.

108. Berthrong M, Sabiston Jr DC. Cerebral lesions in congenital heart disease, a review of autopsies on 162 cases. *Bull Johns Hopkins Hosp.* 1951;89:384–406.

109. Martelle RR, Linde LM. Cerebrovascular accidents with tetralogy of Fallot. *Am J Dis Child.* 1961;101:206–209.

110. Perloff JK, Marelli A. Neurological and psychosocial disorders in adults with congenital heart disease. *Heart Dis Stroke.* 1992;1: 218–224.

111. Capitanio MA, Wolfson BJ, Faerber EN, Williams JL, Balsara RK. Obstruction of the airway by the aorta: an observation in infants with congenital heart disease. *AJR Am J Roentgenol.* 1983;140: 675–679.

112. Vogelpoel L, Schrire V. Auscultatory and phonocardiographic assessment of Fallot's tetralogy. *Circulation.* 1960;22:73.

113. Emanuel R, Somerville J, Prusty S, Ross DN. Aortic regurgitation from infective endocarditis in Fallot's tetralogy and pulmonary atresia. *Br Heart J.* 1975;37:365–370.

114. Baum D, Stern MP. Adipose hypocellularity in cyanotic congenital heart disease. *Circulation.* 1977;55:916–920.

115. Qvist G. *John Hunter 1728–1793.* London: William Heinemann Medical Books Limited; 1981.

116. Kinouchi A, Mori K, Ando M, Takao A. Facial appearance of patients with conotruncal anomalies. *Pediatr Jap.* 1976;17: 84–87.

117. Hofbeck M, Rauch A, Buheitel G, et al. Monosomy 22q11 in patients with pulmonary atresia, ventricular septal defect, and major aortopulmonary collateral arteries. *Heart.* 1998;79: 180–185.

118. Momma K, Kondo C, Ando M, Matsuoka R, Takao A. Tetralogy of Fallot associated with chromosome 22q11 deletion. *Am J Cardiol.* 1995;76:618–621.

119. Pauliks LB, Chan K-C, Lorts A, Elias ER, Cayre RO, Valdes-Cruz LM. Shprintzen-Goldberg syndrome with tetralogy of fallot and subvalvar aortic stenosis. *J Ultrasound Med.* 2005;24: 703–706.

120. Greenwood RD, Rosenthal A, Sommer A, Wolff G, Craenen J. Cardiovascular malformations in oculoauriculovertebral dysplasia (Goldenhar syndrome). *J Pediatr*. 1974;85:816–818.

121. Sajeev CG, Fassaludeen M, Venugopal K. Tetralogy of Fallot with absent thumb and first metacarpal. *Int J Cardiol*. 2005;102: 349–350.

122. Mace JW, Kaplan JM, Schanberger JE, Gotlin RW. Poland's syndrome. Report of seven cases and review of the literature. *Clin Pediatr (Phila)*. 1972;11:98–102.

123. Carnero Alcazar M, Marianeschi S, Ruiz Alonso E, Garcia Torres E, Comas JV. Left arm underdevelopment secondary to an isolated left subclavian artery in tetralogy of Fallot. *Ann Thorac Surg*. 2010;89:637–639.

124. Horwitz S, Esquivel J, Attie F, Lupi E, Espino-Vela J. Clinical diagnosis of persistent left superior vena cava by observation of jugular pulses. *Am Heart J*. 1973;86:759–763.

125. Colman AL. Diagnosis of left superior vena cava by clinical inspection, a new physical sign. *Am Heart J*. 1967;73:115–120.

126. Feruglio GA, Gunton RW. Intracardiac phonocardiography in ventricular septal defect. *Circulation*. 1960;21:49–58.

127. Vogelpoel L, Schrire V, Nellen M, Swanepoel A. The use of amyl nitrite in the differentiation of Fallot's tetralogy and pulmonary stenosis with intact ventricular septum. *Am Heart J*. 1959;57: 803–819.

128. Campeau L, Gilbert G, Aerichide N. Absence of the pulmonary valve. Report of two cases associated with other congenital lesions. *Am J Cardiol*. 1961;8:113–124.

129. Bousvaros GA. Pulmonary second sound in the tetralogy of Fallot. *Am Heart J*. 1961;61:570–571.

130. Tofler OB. The pulmonary component of the second heart sound in Fallot's tetralogy. *Br Heart J*. 1963;25:509–513.

131. Perloff JK, Calvin J, Deleon AC, Bowen P. Systemic hemodynamic effects of amyl nitrite in normal man. *Am Heart J*. 1963; 66:460–469.

132. Padmanabhan J, Varghese PJ, Lloyd S, Haller Jr JA. Tetralogy of Fallot with suprasystemic pressure in the right ventricle. A case report and review of the literature. *Am Heart J*. 1971;82:805–811.

133. Bender SR, Dreifus LS, Downing D. Anatomic and electrocardiographic correlation of Fallot's tetralogy: a study of 100 proved cases. *Am J Cardiol*. 1961;7:475–480.

134. Depasquale NP, Burch GE. The electrocardiogram, vectorcardiogram, and ventricular gradient in the tetralogy of Fallot. *Circulation*. 1961;24:94–109.

135. Macruz R, Perloff JK, Case RB. A method for the electrocardiographic recognition of atrial enlargement. *Circulation*. 1958;17: 882–889.

136. Coelho E, De P, et al. Tetralogy of Fallot. Angiocardiographic, electrocardiographic, vectorcardiographic and hemodynamic studies of the Fallot-type complex. *Am J Cardiol*. 1961;7: 538–564.

137. Lev M. The architecture of the conduction system in congenital heart disease. II. Tetralogy of Fallot. *AMA Arch Pathol*. 1959; 67:572–587.

138. Pileggi F, Bocanegra J, Tranchesi J, et al. The electrocardiogram in tetralogy of Fallot: a study of 142 cases. *Am Heart J*. 1960;59: 667–680.

139. Abraham KA, Cherian G, Rao VD, Sukumar IP, Krishnaswami S, John S. Tetralogy of Fallot in adults. A report on 147 patients. *Am J Med*. 1979;66:811–816.

140. Feldt RH, Dushane JW, Titus JL. The anatomy of the atrioventricular conduction system in ventricular septal defect and tetralogy of fallot: correlations with the electrocardiogram and vectorcardiogram. *Circulation*. 1966;34:774–782.

141. Gale GE, Heimann KW, Barlow JB. Double-chambered right ventricle. A report of five cases. *Br Heart J*. 1969;31:291–298.

142. Hislop A, Reid L. Structural changes in the pulmonary arteries and veins in tetralogy of Fallot. *Br Heart J*. 1973;35:1178–1183.

143. Wilson WJ, Amplatz K. Unequal vascularity in tetralogy of Fallot. *Am J Roentgenol Radium Ther Nucl Med*. 1967;100:318–321.

144. Campbell M, Gardner F. Radiological features of enlarged bronchial arteries. *Br Heart J*. 1950;12:183–200.

145. Wong HO, Ang AH. Unilateral rib notching in Fallot's tetralogy due to systemic-pulmonary collateral vessels. *Br Heart J*. 1973; 35:226–228.

146. Tan JL, Davlouros PA, Mccarthy KP, Gatzoulis MA, Ho SY. Intrinsic histological abnormalities of aortic root and ascending aorta in tetralogy of Fallot: evidence of causative mechanism for aortic dilatation and aortopathy. *Circulation*. 2005;112: 961–968.

147. Emmel M, Schmidt B, Schickendantz S. Double aortic arch in a patient with Fallot's tetralogy. *Cardiol Young*. 2005;15:52–53.

148. Velasquez G, Nath PH, Castaneda-Zuniga WR, Amplatz K, Formanek A. Aberrant left subclavian artery in tetralogy of Fallot. *Am J Cardiol*. 1980;45:811–818.

149. Fraser RS, Dvorkin J, Rossall RE, Eidem R. Left superior vena cava: a review of associated congenital heart lesions, catheterization data and roentgenologic findings. *Am J Med*. 1961;31: 711–716.

150. Haider EA. The boot-shaped heart sign. *Radiology*. 2008;246: 328–329.

151. Dadlani GH, John JB, Cohen MS. Echocardiography in tetralogy of Fallot. *Cardiol Young*. 2008;18(suppl 3):22–28.

152. Moon-Grady AJ, Tacy TA, Brook MM, Hanley FL, Silverman NH. Value of clinical and echocardiographic features in predicting outcome in the fetus, infant, and child with tetralogy of Fallot with absent pulmonary valve complex. *Am J Cardiol*. 2002;89: 1280–1285.

153. Moran AM, Colan SD, Mayer Jr JE, Van Der Velde ME. Echocardiographic identification of thymic hypoplasia in tetralogy of fallot/tetralogy pulmonary atresia. *Am J Cardiol*. 1999;84: 1268–1271, A1269.

154. Von Doenhoff LJ, Nanda NC. Obstruction within the right ventricular body: two-dimensional echocardiographic features. *Am J Cardiol*. 1983;51:1498–1501.

155. Chevers N. Rétrécissement congenital de l'orifice pulmonaire. *Arch Gen Med Fourth Series*. 1847;15:488.

156. Royer BE, Wilson JD. Incomplete heterotaxy with unusual heart malformations. *Arch Pediatr*. 1908;25:881–896.

157. Kurtz CM, Sprague HB, White PD. Congenital heart disease. Interventricular septal defects with associated anomalies in a series of three cases examined postmortem, and a living patient fifty-eight years old with cyanosis and clubbing of the fingers. *Am Heart J*. 1927;3:77–90.

158. Calder AL, Brandt PW, Barratt-Boyes BG, Neutze JM. Variant of tetralogy of fallot with absent pulmonary valve leaflets and origin of one pulmonary artery from the ascending aorta. *Am J Cardiol*. 1980;46:106–116.

159. Buendia A, Attie F, Ovseyevitz J, et al. Congenital absence of pulmonary valve leaflets. *Br Heart J*. 1983;50:31–41.

160. Jekel L, Benatar A, Bennink GB, Woolley SR, Van De Wal HJ. Tetralogy of Fallot with absent pulmonary valve. A continuing challenge. *Scand Cardiovasc J*. 1998;32:213–217.

161. Siwik ES, Preminger TJ, Patel CR. Association of systemic to pulmonary collateral arteries with tetralogy of Fallot and absent pulmonary valve syndrome. *Am J Cardiol*. 1996;77:547–549.

162. Kirshbom PM, Kogon BE. Tetralogy of Fallot with absent pulmonary valve syndrome. *Semin Thorac Cardiovasc Surg Pediatr Card Surg Annu*. 2004;7:65–71.

163. Fouron JC, Sahn DJ, Bender R, et al. Prenatal diagnosis and circulatory characteristics in tetralogy of Fallot with absent pulmonary valve. *Am J Cardiol*. 1989;64:547–549.

164. Bedard E, Mccarthy KP, Dimopoulos K, Giannakoulas G, Gatzoulis MA, Ho SY. Structural abnormalities of the pulmonary trunk in tetralogy of Fallot and potential clinical implications: a morphological study. *J Am Coll Cardiol*. 2009;54: 1883–1890.

165. Milanesi O, Talenti E, Pellegrino PA, Thiene G. Abnormal pulmonary artery branching in tetralogy of Fallot with "absent" pulmonary valve. *Int J Cardiol*. 1984;6:375–380.

166. Hiraishi S, Bargeron LM, Isabel-Jones JB, Emmanouilides GC, Friedman WF, Jarmakani JM. Ventricular and pulmonary artery volumes in patients with absent pulmonary valve. Factors affecting the natural course. *Circulation*. 1983;67:183–190.

167. Momma K, Ando M, Takao A. Fetal cardiac morphology of tetralogy of Fallot with absent pulmonary valve in the rat. *Circulation*. 1990;82:1343–1351.

168. Donofrio MT, Jacobs ML, Rychik J. Tetralogy of Fallot with absent pulmonary valve: echocardiographic morphometric features of the

right-sided structures and their relationship to presentation and outcome. *J Am Soc Echocardiogr.* 1997;10:556–561.

169. Fontana ME, Wooley CF. The murmur of pulmonic regurgitation in tetralogy of Fallot with absent pulmonic valve. *Circulation.* 1978;57:986–990.

170. Nadas AS, Rosenbaum HD, Wittenborg MH, Rudolph AM. Tetralogy of Fallot with unilateral pulmonary atresia. A clinically diagnosable and surgically significant variant. *Circulation.* 1953;8:328–336.

171. Morgan JR. Left pulmonary artery from ascending aorta in tetralogy of Fallot. *Circulation.* 1972;45:653–657.

172. Barrett OJ, Walker W. Tetralogy of Fallot with absent left pulmonary artery: report of a case with anomalous development of the right hilar vasculature and non-functioning right lung. *Am Heart J.* 1958;55:357.

173. Pool PE, Vogel JH, Blount Jr SG. Congenital unilateral absence of a pulmonary artery. The importance of flow in pulmonary hypertension. *Am J Cardiol.* 1962;10:706–732.

174. Gupta K, Livesay JJ, Lufschanowski R. Absent right pulmonary artery with coronary collaterals supplying the affected lung. *Circulation.* 2001;104:E12–E13.

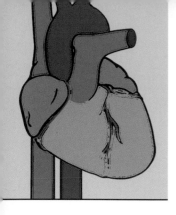

Chapter 19

Double Outlet Ventricle

The earliest report that alluded to *double outlet right ventricle* was published in French in 1703.[1] Ninety years elapsed before an English-language publication appeared.[2] In 1793, John Abernathy,[2] an assistant surgeon at St Bartholomew's Hospital in London, described "partial transposition" of the great arteries, and in 1898, Karl von Vierordt[3] called double outlet right ventricle *partial transposition* to signify that the aorta was transposed but the pulmonary trunk was normally aligned. It was not until 1957 that Witham[4] introduced *double outlet right ventricle* as a diagnostic term for a partial transposition complex. Witham's term is now preferred to the synonymous *right ventricular origin of both great arteries*. Double outlet *left ventricle* is the rarest of the ventriculoarterial malalignments (see subsequent section).[5,6]

The question of how best to define double outlet right ventricle has been much debated, and the debate continues without a consensus.[7,8] It has been argued that the malformation is virtually unclassifiable because of its excessively complex and diverse anatomy. Should double outlet right ventricle be defined as a connection between the great arterial trunks and the right ventricular mass, or as a malformation in which the leaflets of both great arterial valves are supported by right ventricular infundibular musculature?[7] How much overriding of one or the other arterial valves is acceptable? In this chapter, double outlet right ventricle is defined pragmatically as a malformation in which the greater part of the circumference of both arterial valves is supported within a morphologic right ventricle in hearts with two distinct ventricular chambers and concordant atrioventricular connections (Table 19-1).[7] The aorta and main pulmonary artery are separated by an outlet septum housed exclusively in the right ventricle. A conus resides beneath each of the two great arterial valves (double conuses), although either conus may be attenuated. The position of the outlet septum establishes two types of infundibular relationships: namely, anterior/posterior and side-by-side. In the more common anterior/posterior relationship, the aorta arises from the posterior infundibulum, and the ventricular septal defect is subaortic. In the less common side-by-side relationship, the pulmonary trunk arises from the medial infundibulum, and the ventricular septal defect is subpulmonary.

CONNECTIONS OF THE GREAT ARTERIES TO THE VENTRICLES

The aorta is either to the right of and anterior to the pulmonary trunk or side-by-side with the aorta to the right.[9] Each great artery arises above a conus that prevents fibrous continuity with atrioventricular valve tissue, but conal attenuation occasionally permits fibrous continuity.[9–11] When each great artery is equipped with a separate conus, and both great arteries arise exclusively from the right ventricle, the term *double outlet right ventricle* is not disputed. However, the appropriate terminology for hearts with a biventricular great arterial valve is unresolved.

Double outlet right ventricle with a *subaortic* ventricular septal defect, pulmonary stenosis, and an aortic override greater than 50% resembles Fallot's tetralogy (Box 19-1; see Chapter 18). Double outlet right ventricle with a *subpulmonary* ventricular septal defect and a posterior non–border-forming biventricular pulmonary trunk resembles complete transposition of the great arteries (see Box 19-1; see Chapter 27). Double outlet right ventricle, Fallot's tetralogy, and complete transposition have been proposed to represent a spectrum of anomalies resulting from embryonic arrest of the normal rotation of the junction of the outflow tract and the great arteries. In 1949, Taussig and Bing[12] published a case of *complete transposition of the aorta* and *levoposition of the pulmonary artery*, which arose chiefly from the right ventricle (see subsequent section).

RELATIONSHIP OF THE VENTRICULAR SEPTAL DEFECT TO THE GREAT ARTERIES

A ventricular septal defect is usually subaortic or subpulmonary and provides the left ventricle with its only outlet (Figure 19-1). Less often, the defect is committed to both great arteries, or the ventricular septum is intact (see Table 19-1).[9,13,14] Rarely, the defect is in muscular or inlet septum and is therefore not committed to either great artery.[15,16]

Table 19-1 **Double Outlet Right Ventricle: Clinical Classification**

The More Common Types

A. Subaortic ventricular septal defect without pulmonary stenosis:
   a. Low pulmonary vascular resistance
   b. High pulmonary vascular resistance
B. Subpulmonary ventricular septal defect without pulmonary stenosis:
   a. Low pulmonary vascular resistance
   b. High pulmonary vascular resistance

The Less Common Types

A. Doubly committed ventricular septal defect
B. Uncommitted ventricular septal defect
C. Intact ventricular septum

BOX 19-1 **DOUBLE OUTLET RIGHT VENTRICLE: MAJOR CLINICAL PATTERNS**

Subaortic ventricular septal defect, no pulmonary stenosis, low pulmonary vascular resistance: resembles nonrestrictive perimembranous ventricular septal defect.

Subaortic ventricular septal defect, no pulmonary stenosis, high pulmonary vascular resistance: resembles Eisenmenger's syndrome.

Subaortic ventricular septal defect with pulmonary stenosis: resembles Fallot's tetralogy.

Subpulmonary ventricular septal defect with no pulmonary stenosis: resembles complete transposition of the great arteries with nonrestrictive ventricular septal defect.

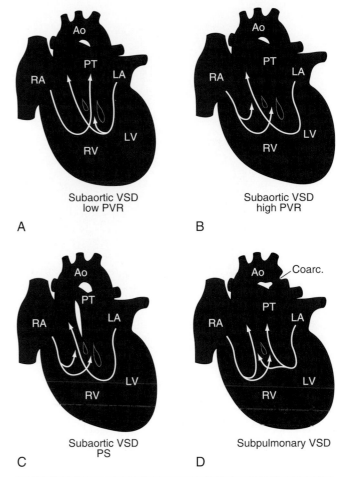

FIGURE 19-1 Illustrations of four major clinical patterns of double outlet right ventricle (see Table 19-1 and Box 19-1). **A,** *Subaortic* ventricular septal defect (VSD), low pulmonary vascular resistance, no pulmonary stenosis. **B,** *Subaortic* ventricular septal defect, high pulmonary vascular resistance. **C,** *Subaortic* ventricular septal defect with pulmonary stenosis. **D,** *Subpulmonary* ventricular septal defect. (Ao = aorta; RA = right atrium; PT = pulmonary trunk; LA = left atrium; LV = left ventricle; RV = right ventricle.)

The location of the ventricular septal defect is the major determinant of intracardiac streaming. When the defect is committed to the aorta, blood flow is preferentially channeled into the aorta (see Figure 19-1A). Streaming is secondarily influenced by pulmonary vascular resistance and pulmonary stenosis. In the Taussig-Bing anomaly (see previous), which constitutes less than 10% of cases of double outlet right ventricle, the aorta arises completely from the right ventricle, a nonrestrictive ventricular septal defect is subpulmonary, and the pulmonary trunk is biventricular, although principally in the right ventricle.[12] Left ventricular blood preferentially enters the pulmonary artery through the subpulmonary ventricular septal defect (Figures 19-1D and 19-2).[10–12,17]

OBSTRUCTION TO VENTRICULAR OUTFLOW

Pulmonary stenosis occurs in 40% to 70% of cases of double outlet right ventricle with *subaortic* ventricular septal defect (see Figure 19-1C)[10,18] and is represented by an underdeveloped subpulmonary conus or by a stenotic bicuspid pulmonary valve.[9] A *subpulmonary* ventricular septal is rarely accompanied by pulmonary stenosis.[19]

When there is pulmonary artesia (Figure 19-3), the right ventricle has a single functional outlet—the aorta—so *double outlet* then refers to ventriculoarterial *alignment*.

A nonrestrictive ventricular septal defect is physiologically advantageous because it provides the left ventricle with an unobstructed exit. An inherently *restrictive* subaortic ventricular septal defect or a spontaneous decrease in size is a form of subaortic stenosis.[20–22] The decrease in size may culminate in complete closure,[13,22] or rarely, the ventricular septum is congenitally intact and the left ventricle is hypoplastic.[13,23] Aortic stenosis can also be caused by an underdeveloped subaortic infundibulum, which occurs in about 50% of cases with a subaortic ventricular septal defect.

Nearly a third of patients with *straddling atrioventricular valves* (biventricular insertion of chordae tendineae) have a double outlet right ventricle (see Figure 19-10 and Video 9-1).[24] The straddle involves the right-sided or left-sided portion of the atrioventricular valve.[24]

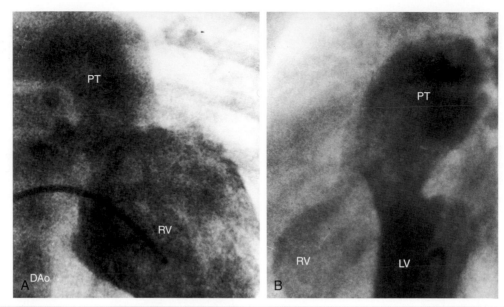

FIGURE 19-2 Angiocardiograms from a 20-month-old male with double outlet right ventricle and a subpulmonary ventricular septal defect. **A,** The right ventriculogram visualized a large pulmonary trunk (PT) arising from a dilated right ventricle. (DAo = descending aorta.) **B,** Left oblique left ventriculogram in the same patient showing selective flow from the left ventricle (LV) into a dilated biventricular pulmonary trunk (PT). The right ventricle (RV) faintly visualizes.

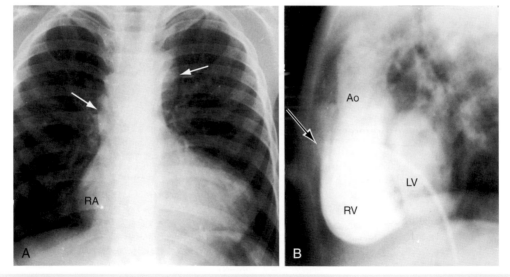

FIGURE 19-3 **A,** X-ray from a 3-year-old boy with double outlet right ventricle, subaortic ventricular septal defect, and pulmonary atresia. Lung fields show the lacy appearance of systemic-to-pulmonary arterial collaterals. The pulmonary trunk is conspicuously absent, and the ascending and transverse aorta (arrows) are correspondingly large. The prominent apex is boot-shaped. The right atrium (RA) is moderately convex. **B,** Lateral right ventriculogram (RV) showing a blind outflow tract (arrow) and a dilated aorta (Ao) that arises anterior to the ventricular septum. (LV = left ventricle.)

Overriding refers to biventricular commitment of the atrioventricular annulus, which is not a feature of double outlet right ventricle.

The *atrioventricular node* is normally located, and the conduction system penetrates the right side of the central fibrous body (see section Electrocardiogram).[25]

The location of the atrioventricular bundle is related to the ventricular septal defect as in isolated ventricular septal defect (see Chapter 17).

The classification of double outlet right ventricle in Table 19-1 is based on anatomic faults that are principally responsible for the physiologic derangements and clinical expressions of a subaortic or subpulmonary ventricular septal defect and from the absence or presence of pulmonary stenosis or pulmonary vascular disease.

The *physiologic consequences* of double outlet right ventricle with a *subaortic* ventricular septal defect and *no pulmonary stenosis* resemble an isolated nonrestrictive perimembranous ventricular septal defect (see Box 19-1; see Chapter 17). Because the defect is committed to the aorta, left ventricular blood preferentially enters the aorta, and low pulmonary vascular resistance permits a substantial portion of left ventricular blood to stream into the pulmonary circulation and permits right ventricular blood to stream almost exclusively into the pulmonary trunk (see Figure 19-1A). Pulmonary blood flow is increased, and aortic oxygen saturation is virtually normal. As pulmonary vascular resistance rises, right ventricular blood is diverted into the aorta and left ventricular blood is diverted away from the pulmonary trunk (see Figure 19-1B). Pulmonary blood flow declines, and aortic oxygen saturation declines in parallel.

When *pulmonary stenosis* occurs with double outlet right ventricle, the ventricular septal defect is almost always *subaortic*. Pulmonary stenosis may initially be absent or mild and then develop and progress. Pulmonary stenosis diverts right ventricular and left ventricular blood away from the pulmonary artery and into the aorta (see Figure 19-1C), so pulmonary blood flow and aortic oxygen saturation fall. The more severe the pulmonary stenosis, the more blood from right and left ventricles enters the aorta; and in the presence of pulmonary atresia, all blood from both ventricles enters the aorta (see Figure 19-3).[26] Double outlet right ventricle with a nonrestrictive subaortic ventricular septal defect and severe pulmonary stenosis or atresia physiologically resembles Fallot's tetralogy (see Box 19-1; see Chapter 18).[10,26]

When the ventricular septal defect is *subpulmonary*, left ventricular blood preferentially enters the pulmonary trunk, and right ventricular blood preferentially enters the aorta (see Figures 19-1D and 19-2), so pulmonary arterial oxygen saturation exceeds aortic oxygen saturation. When pulmonary vascular resistance is low, pulmonary blood flow is increased, systemic arterial oxygen saturation is high, cyanosis is relatively mild, and the left ventricle is volume overloaded as in complete transposition of the great arteries (see Chapter 27). A rise in pulmonary vascular resistance diverts right ventricular blood from the pulmonary artery into the aorta. Pulmonary blood flow declines, systemic arterial oxygen saturation falls, and left ventricular volume overload is curtailed (see Figure 19-1D).

DOUBLE OUTLET RIGHT VENTRICLE WITH SUBAORTIC VENTRICULAR SEPTAL DEFECT

The clinical manifestations closely resemble isolated nonrestrictive perimembranous ventricular septal defect (see Figure 19-1A and B and Box 19-1). Male:female ratio is estimated at 1.7:1.[27] A large kindred included a second cousin with double outlet right ventricle, a first cousin with complete transposition of the great arteries, and two siblings with truncus arteriosus.[28]

History

The murmur of ventricular septal defect dates from birth because flow from the left ventricle through the defect is obligatory and does not await the neonatal fall in pulmonary vascular resistance. However, the intensity of the murmur increases as neonatal pulmonary resistance falls and as increased left ventricular stroke volume is ejected through the ventricular septal defect into both great arteries. Increased pulmonary blood flow results in volume overload of the left ventricle, congestive heart failure, and poor growth and development. Cyanosis is mild or absent because left ventricular blood preferentially enters the aorta and right ventricular blood preferentially enters the pulmonary artery (see Figure 19-1A). A rise in pulmonary vascular resistance curtails pulmonary blood flow and relieves the left ventricular of volume overload. Patients occasionally reach young adulthood (Figure 19-4A); one patient underwent intracardiac repair at age 53 years (Figure 19-4B), and one survived to age 65 years.[29]

Physical Appearance

Transient neonatal cyanosis coincides with transient elevation in neonatal pulmonary vascular resistance. The subsequent fall in pulmonary vascular resistance is accompanied by an increase in pulmonary blood flow, volume overload of the left ventricle, and the catabolic appearance of congestive heart failure. A subsequent rise in pulmonary resistance diverts left ventricular blood from the pulmonary trunk and diverts right ventricular blood into the aorta (see Figure 19-1B)—Eisenmenger's syndrome—with the appearance of cyanosis and clubbing (see Box 19-1). Double outlet right ventricle is occasionally associated with trisomy 18 and the distinctive overlapping fingers (clinodactyly), rocker-bottom feet, and lax skin (Figure 19-5).[30–32]

Arterial Pulse

The arterial pulse is brisk when pulmonary blood flow is increased and the volume-overloaded left ventricle is functionally normal. A rise in pulmonary vascular resistance curtails left ventricular volume overload and normalizes the arterial pulse.

Jugular Venous Pulse

When increased pulmonary blood flow results in biventricular failure, the jugular venous A wave, V wave, and mean pressure are elevated. The height and waveform of the jugular pulse normalize when pulmonary vascular resistance increases. The right ventricle then ejects at systemic resistance with little extra help from the right atrium, as in Eisenmenger's syndrome (see Chapter 17).

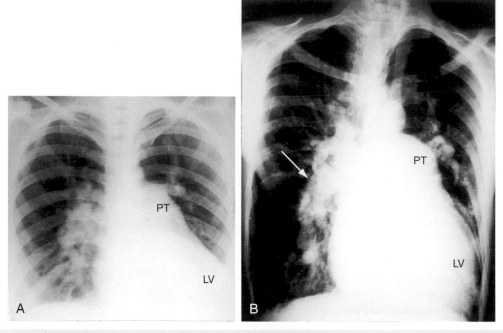

FIGURE 19-4 A, X-ray from an acyanotic 24-year-old woman with double outlet right ventricle, a subaortic ventricular septal defect, and a pulmonary-to-systemic flow ratio of 2 to 1. Pulmonary vascularity is increased, the pulmonary trunk (PT) and its proximal branches are dilated, the ascending aorta is not border-forming, and a large left ventricle (LV) occupies the apex. The x-ray resembles a nonrestrictive perimembranous ventricular septal defect. **B,** X-ray from a 53-year-old man with double outlet right ventricle, a subaortic ventricular septal defect, and a pulmonary to systemic flow ratio of 1.7 to 1. The pulmonary trunk (PT) and its right branch (arrow) are markedly dilated, and an enlarged left ventricle (LV) occupies the apex. Distortion of the clavicles is the result of scoliosis.

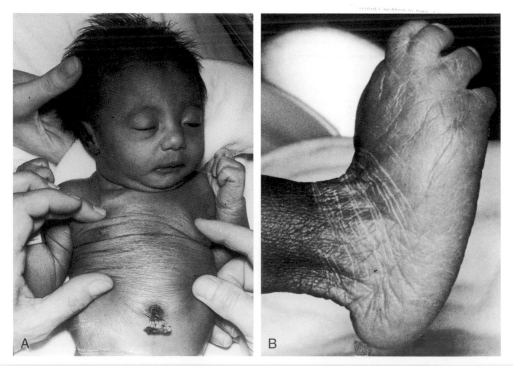

FIGURE 19-5 Photographs of a 6-week-old male with the characteristic clenched fists, overlapping fingers (clinodactyly), lax skin, and rocker-bottom feet of trisomy 18. The infant had double outlet right ventricle with a subaortic ventricular septal defect.

Precordial Movement and Palpation

A hyperactive precordium with Harrison's grooves result from chronic dyspnea. A right ventricular impulse is accompanied by the impulse of a dilated hypertensive pulmonary trunk and a palpable pulmonary valve closure sound. A thrill generated by the ventricular septal defect is maximal in the third and fourth intercostal spaces at the left sternal border (see section Auscultation).

A rise in pulmonary vascular resistance curtails pulmonary blood flow and decreases left ventricular volume overload, so the left ventricular impulse becomes inconspicuous or absent, as in Eisenmenger's syndrome. The right ventricular impulse, the palpable pulmonary trunk, and the palpable pulmonary closure sound persist.

Auscultation

The first heart sound is soft because the PR interval tends to be prolonged (see section Electrocardiogram).[33] *Low pulmonary vascular resistance* results in a holosystolic murmur of ventricular septal defect that is maximal in the third and fourth spaces at the left sternal border. The pulmonary component of the second heart sound is loud because the hypertensive dilated pulmonary trunk is anterior. The aortic component of the second sound is prominent because the aortic valve lies side by side and to the right of the pulmonary trunk rather than posterior. Inspiratory splitting is preserved as long as pulmonary vascular resistance is less than systemic. Increased flow across the mitral valve generates an apical mid-diastolic murmur.

Elevated pulmonary vascular resistance reduces pulmonary blood flow and left ventricular volume overload (see Figure 19-1B). The murmur of ventricular septal defect becomes decrescendo and is softer (Figure 19-6) but does not disappear because flow from left ventricle into aorta is obligatory. Except for the soft decrescendo murmur, the auscultatory signs are analogous to Eisenmenger's syndrome with an isolated nonrestrictive ventricular septal defect: namely, a pulmonary ejection sound, a loud single second heart sound, and a Graham Steell murmur of pulmonary hypertensive pulmonary regurgitation (see Chapter 17).

Electrocardiogram

PR interval prolongation is common (Figure 19-7; see previous) because of the unusually long course of the common atrioventricular bundle.[33] When pulmonary blood flow is increased, peaked right atrial P waves are associated with bifid broad left atrial P waves (Figure 19-8). *Left axis deviation* with counterclockwise depolarization is an important feature of double outlet right ventricle with a subaortic ventricular septal defect, no pulmonary stenosis, and increased pulmonary blood flow (see Figure 19-7).[25,33] The mechanism of left axis deviation is unknown but cannot be related to an abnormality of the conduction system, which is structurally the same when pulmonary vascular resistance is elevated and there is right axis deviation (see Figure 19-8) and when double outlet right ventricle exists with pulmonary stenosis and

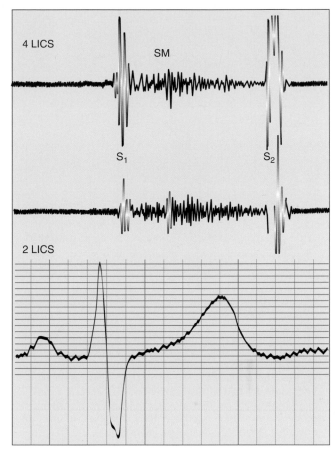

FIGURE 19-6 Phonocardiogram from a 10-year-old boy with double outlet right ventricle, subaortic ventricular septal defect, elevated pulmonary vascular resistance, and a pulmonary-to-systemic flow ratio of 1.2 to 1. A relatively soft decrescendo systolic murmur (SM) was recorded in the fourth left intercostal space (4 LICS). The second heart sound (S_2) is loud and single. Lead 2 of electrocardiogram shows left axis deviation. (2 LICS = second left intercostal space; S_1 = first heart sound.)

right axis deviation.[25] The QRS duration is normal, but right ventricular conduction defects sometimes occur, including right bundle branch block.[33] Right ventricular hypertrophy is obligatory and is manifested by tall R waves in leads V_1 and aVR with deep S waves in left precordial leads (see Figures 19-7 and 19-8). Left ventricular volume overload is indicated by large RS complexes in midprecordial leads and by tall R waves in left precordial leads (see Figure 19-7). Elevated pulmonary vascular resistance is associated with right axis deviation and pure right ventricular hypertrophy (see Figure 19-8).

X-Ray

With double outlet right ventricle, nonrestrictive subaortic ventricular septal defect, and low pulmonary vascular resistance, the x-ray resembles isolated nonrestrictive perimembranous ventricular septal defect with increased pulmonary blood flow (Figures 19-4 and 19-9A).[27] Thymus is present even though there is transposition of the aorta (Figure 19-9B), in contrast to complete

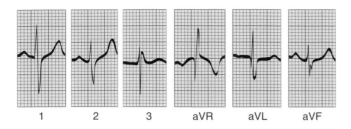

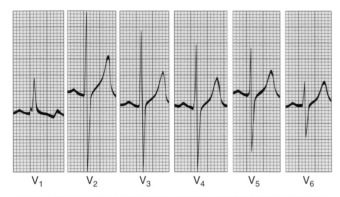

FIGURE 19-7 Electrocardiogram from an acyanotic 24-year-old woman with double outlet right ventricle, subaortic ventricular septal defect, and a pulmonary to systemic flow ratio of 2 to 1. The PR interval is 200 msec. There is left axis deviation with counterclockwise depolarization. The deep S waves in V_{5-6} indicate right ventricular hypertrophy. Biventricular hypertrophy is manifested by large RS complexes in the mid precordial leads (V_{3-6} are half standardized).

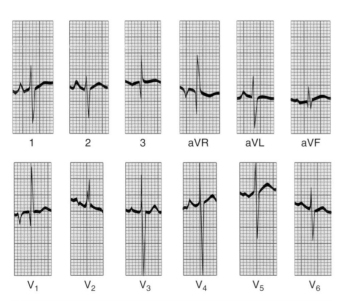

FIGURE 19-8 Electrocardiogram from a 6-week-old male with trisomy 18 (see Figure 19-5) and double outlet right ventricle, subaortic ventricular septal defect, and moderately elevated pulmonary vascular resistance. Peaked right atrial P waves are present in leads 1 and 2, and a broad bifid left atrial P wave is present in lead V_2. Right axis deviation is moderate, and depolarization is clockwise. The q wave in lead V_1 indicates right atrial enlargement. Right ventricular hypertrophy is manifested by tall R waves in leads V_1 and aVR and by deep S waves in left precordial leads.

transposition of *both* great arteries in which thymus is typically absent (see Chapter 27). The pulmonary trunk is prominent because it carries increased volume at systemic pressure and is not posterior to the aorta (see Figure 19-4). Left atrial and left ventricular enlargement reflect the volume overload of increased pulmonary blood flow (see Figure 19-4). With the advent of congestive heart failure, the right atrium and right ventricle dilate conspicuously.

The lung fields are oligemic when left ventricular volume overload is curtailed by *elevated pulmonary vascular resistance*, either before the neonatal fall (see Figure 19-9B) or after the development of pulmonary vascular disease. The right ventricle copes with systemic resistance without enlarging significantly. The x-ray is indistinguishable from a nonrestrictive ventricular septal defect and Eisenmenger's syndrome (see Figure 17-9).

Echocardiogram

Echocardiography with color flow imaging and Doppler interrogation[34] provides diagnostic information on: (1) the right ventricular origin and spatial relationships of the great arteries; (2) the presence and position of the infundibular septum; (3) the size of the ventricular septal defect and its relationship to the aortic and pulmonary valves; (4) mitral/semilunar valve discontinuity (see Figures 19-19 and 19-20)[35]; and (5) straddling of the atrioventricular valve tensor apparatus (Figure 19-10 and Video 19-1). The aortic root and pulmonary trunk are parallel and are separated by a prominent outlet septum. The aorta arises entirely from the right ventricle, and the pulmonary trunk arises predominantly, if not entirely, from the right ventricle (see Figure 19-19). In the short axis, the great arteries appear as double circles, with the aorta to the right of the pulmonary trunk as in complete transposition of the great arteries (see Chapter 27). The pulmonary trunk is identified by its bifurcation, and the aorta is identified by its brachiocephalic branches. Bilateral subarterial conuses separate the aortic and pulmonary valves from the atrioventricular valves. The course of the outlet septum establishes the alignment of the ventricular septal defect with the aortic or the pulmonary valve. If the outlet septum curves leftward toward the ventriculo/infundibular fold, the ventricular septal defect is subaortic. If the outlet septum is straight and parallel to the trabecular septum, the ventricular septal defect is subpulmonary. The echocardiogram can identify a single coronary artery, which is estimated to occur in 11% of cases of double outlet right ventricle.[36] Fetal echocardiography can be used to determine most of the essential anatomic features.[37]

Summary

Double outlet right ventricle with subaortic ventricular septal defect and no pulmonary stenosis comes to light because of *transient neonatal cyanosis*. A fall in pulmonary vascular resistance with increased pulmonary blood flow results in congestive heart failure with poor growth and development. Physical examination reveals hyperactive right and left ventricular impulses, a left parasternal systolic thrill and murmur of ventricular septal defect, a loud

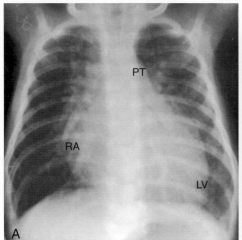
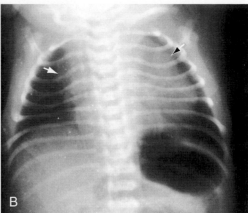

FIGURE 19-9 **A,** X-ray from an acyanotic 8-week-old male with double outlet right ventricle, a subaortic ventricular septal defect, and a pulmonary to systemic flow ratio of 2.4 to 1. The film is overpenetrated, but pulmonary vascularity is increased. The pulmonary trunk (PT) is moderately convex, a dilated left ventricle (LV) occupies the apex, and a prominent right atrium (RA) forms the right lower cardiac border. **B,** X-ray from a 1-day-old male with double outlet right ventricle and a subaortic ventricular septal defect. A large thymus (arrows) and a large gas-filled stomach alter the cardiac silhouette, which is otherwise normal for age.

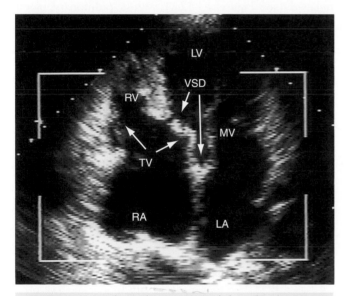

FIGURE 19-10 Echocardiogram (apical four-chamber view) from a 7-year-old boy with double outlet right ventricle and a subaortic ventricular septal defect (VSD). Tensor apparatus of the tricuspid valve (TV) inserts on both sides—straddles—the ventricular septum (Video 19-1). (RV/LV = right and left ventricle; RA/LA = right and left atrium; MV = mitral valve.)

pulmonary component of the second sound with close splitting, and an apical mid-diastolic murmur of augmented flow across the mitral valve. The electrocardiogram is of special diagnostic importance because of left axis deviation with counterclockwise depolarization. The x-ray is indistinguishable from a nonrestrictive perimembranous ventricular septal defect with increased pulmonary blood flow.

Pulmonary vascular disease results in a clinical picture that resembles Eisenmenger's syndrome with a nonrestrictive ventricular septal defect, but double outlet right ventricle should be suspected when pulmonary blood flow remains increased in the presence of cyanosis and when a soft decrescendo systolic murmur persists at the left sternal edge because of obligatory flow from left ventricle through the subaortic ventricular septal defect into the aorta. The echocardiogram with color flow imaging and Doppler interrogation identifies right ventricular origin of both great arteries and establishes the location, size, and great arterial commitments of the ventricular septal defect.

DOUBLE OUTLET RIGHT VENTRICLE WITH SUBAORTIC VENTRICULAR SEPTAL DEFECT AND PULMONARY STENOSIS

More than 50% of patients with double outlet right ventricle and a subaortic ventricular septal defect have pulmonary stenosis (see Box 19-1 and Figure 19-1C). The clinical manifestations closely resemble Fallot's tetralogy (see Chapter 18).

History and Physical Appearance

Pulmonary stenosis, which varies from mild to severe to atresia, can be present at birth or delayed with a progressive increase in severity (Figure 19-11). Cyanotic patients squat as in Fallot's tetralogy. The clinical course and longevity are better than in double outlet right ventricle *without* pulmonary stenosis because pulmonary blood flow is more effectively regulated (see previous).[10,38]

Jugular Venous Pulse and Arterial Pulse

The A wave is normal because the right ventricle ejects at but not above systemic vascular resistance and does not need an increase in right atrial contractile force, analogous

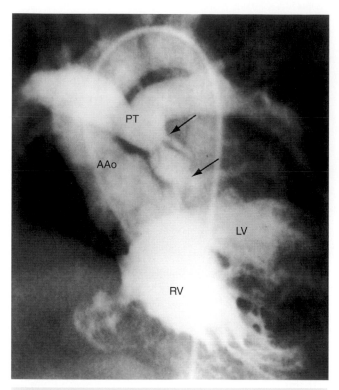

FIGURE 19-11 Angiocardiogram from a 15-month-old male with double outlet right ventricle, a nonrestrictive subaortic ventricular septal defect, and pulmonary stenosis caused by an underdeveloped subpulmonary conus (lower unmarked arrow) and a bicuspid pulmonary valve (upper unmarked arrow). The ascending aorta (AAo) and the pulmonary trunk (PT) arise from the right ventricle (RV). (LV = left ventricle.)

to Fallot's tetralogy (see Chapter 18). The arterial pulse is normal because biventricular ejection into the aorta maintains a normal stroke volume.

Precordial Movement and Palpation

The right ventricular impulse is analogous to the gentle impulse of a normal neonatal heart and is assigned to the fourth and fifth left intercostal spaces and subxyphoid area because the stenosis is subpulmonary (see Figure 19-11). A systolic thrill is maximal in the third left intercostal space for the same reason. A left ventricular impulse is not palpable in cyanotic patients because pulmonary blood flow is reduced, so the left ventricle is underfilled.

Auscultation

Acyanotic patients with mild pulmonary stenosis have a holosystolic murmur of ventricular septal defect at the lower left sternal border and a midsystolic murmur of pulmonary stenosis in the second and third left intercostal spaces (Figure 19-12A, C). The pulmonary component of the second heart sound is appropriately delayed (see Figure 19-12A). When pulmonary blood flow is increased, an apical third heart sound introduces a mid-diastolic murmur across the mitral valve (Figure 19-12B).

Patients with severe pulmonary stenosis or atresia have auscultatory signs indistinguishable from cyanotic Fallot's tetralogy (see Chapter 18). The duration of the pulmonary stenotic murmur varies inversely with the severity of stenosis. Pulmonary atresia is accompanied by an aortic

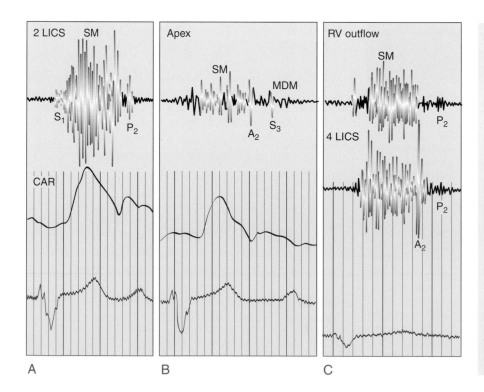

FIGURE 19-12 Phonocardiograms from an 18-year-old man with double outlet right ventricle, subaortic ventricular septal defect, and a 45–mm Hg subpulmonary gradient. **A,** In the second left intercostal space (2 LICS), a loud crescendo-decrescendo systolic murmur (SM) obscures the aortic component of the second heart sound. The pulmonary component (P_2) is delayed and prominent. (CAR = carotid pulse.) **B,** The systolic murmur (SM) radiated to the apex where a prominent third heart sound (S_3) introduced a mid-diastolic murmur (MDM) caused by increased flow across the mitral valve. **C,** Intracardiac phonocardiogram from the right ventricular outflow tract recorded a systolic murmur (SM) similar to the murmur in the second left intercostal space, together with a delayed pulmonary closure sound (P_2). The simultaneous chest wall phonocardiogram in the fourth left intercostal space (4 LICS) recorded a decrescendo holosystolic murmur and the delayed P_2 (A_2 = prominent aortic component of the second sound.)

ejection sound, a soft midsystolic murmur into the dilated aorta, and a loud single second heart sound of aortic valve closure (Figure 19-13). Exceptionally, there is a long decrescendo systolic murmur at the left sternal border because of obligatory flow from left ventricle into aorta through a restrictive ventricular septal defect that constitutes a zone of subaortic stenosis. A left ventricular fourth heart sound can then be heard because the left ventricular hypertrophy of subaortic stenosis is associated with an increased force of left atrial contraction. Audibility of the fourth heart sound is enhanced by prolongation of the PR interval. An early diastolic murmur of aortic regurgitation is occasionally present in double outlet right ventricle with pulmonary stenosis as in Fallot's tetralogy.[17,38]

Electrocardiogram

Because the right ventricle is systemic, peaked right atrial P waves occur even with mild pulmonary stenosis and may be accompanied by left atrial P waves because pulmonary blood flow is increased (Figure 19-14). With severe pulmonary stenosis, the P waves are either normal or peaked and low amplitude (Figure 19-15) but are occasionally peaked and tall (Figure 19-16). The PR interval is likely to be prolonged (see Figures 19-14, 19-15, and 19-16).

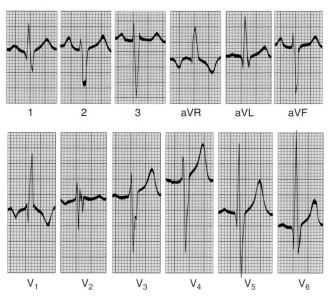

FIGURE 19-14 Electrocardiogram from an 18-year-old man with double outlet right ventricle, subaortic ventricular septal defect, and a 45–mm Hg subpulmonary gradient. The PR interval is 210 msec. The right atrial P wave in lead 2 is tall and peaked. A deep broad left atrial P terminal force appears in lead V_1. Terminal forces are prolonged with slurred S waves in inferior leads and a slurred R wave in lead aVR. There is left axis deviation with counterclockwise depolarization. Right ventricular hypertrophy is manifested by the tall R prime in lead V_1 and by the deep S waves in left precordial leads. Left ventricular volume overload is manifested in leads V_{5-6} by deep Q waves, tall R waves, and tall peaked T waves.

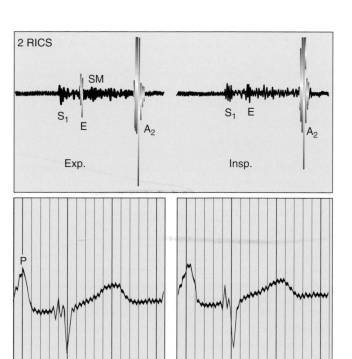

FIGURE 19-13 Phonocardiogram in the second right intercostal space (2 RICS) of a 3-year-old cyanotic boy with double outlet right ventricle, a subaortic ventricular septal defect, and pulmonary atresia. An aortic ejection sound (E) introduces a soft midsystolic murmur (SM) that ends before a loud single second heart sound that was the aortic component (A_2). The ejection sound decreased during inspiration despite aortic origin.

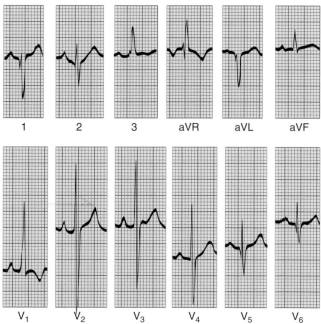

FIGURE 19-15 Electrocardiogram from a 13-year-old cyanotic girl with double outlet right ventricle, subaortic ventricular septal defect, and severe subpulmonary stenosis. Peaked right atrial P waves appear in leads 2 and V_1. The PR interval is 190 msec. Q waves appear in leads 1 and aVL despite right axis deviation. Right ventricular hypertrophy is manifested by tall R waves in leads V_1 and aVR. The qR pattern in leads V_{5-6} indicates that the left ventricle is moderately well-developed.

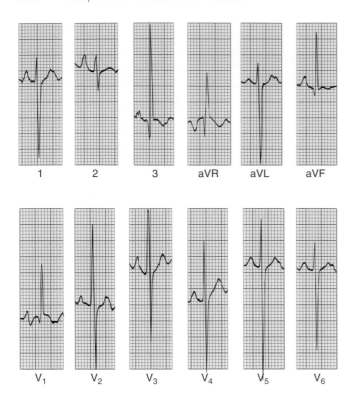

1 2 3 aVR aVL aVF

V₁ V₂ V₃ V₄ V₅ V₆

FIGURE 19-16 Electrocardiogram from a 3-year-old boy with double outlet right ventricle, subaortic ventricular septal defect, and pulmonary atresia. Tall peaked P waves appear in leads 1 and 2 and in midprecordial leads. The PR interval is 190 msec. There is marked right axis deviation. The q wave in lead V₁ reflects right atrial enlargement. Right ventricular hypertrophy is manifested by the tall R wave in lead V₁ and by the deep S waves in left precordial leads.

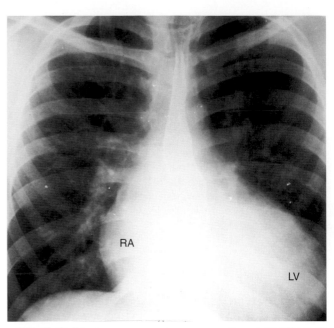

FIGURE 19-17 X-ray from an 18-year-old man with double outlet right ventricle, a subaortic ventricular septal defect, a 40–mm Hg subpulmonary gradient, and a pulmonary to systemic flow ratio of 2.2 to 1. The pulmonary trunk is not dilated, even though pulmonary blood flow is increased. An enlarged left ventricle (LV) occupies the apex, and a prominent right atrium (RA) occupies the right lower cardiac border.

When pulmonary stenosis is *mild*, the electrocardiogram retains the left axis deviation and counterclockwise depolarization that occur in the absence of pulmonary stenosis (see Figure 19-14). As stenosis increases, the QRS axis becomes vertical or rightward. It is here that distinctive albeit subtle features arouse suspicion of double outlet right ventricle with pulmonary stenosis.[33] The distinctive feature is persistence of *counterclockwise* initial forces that generate q waves in leads 1 and aVL even when the axis is vertical or rightward (see Figure 19-15). Q waves in leads 1 and aVL are rare in neonates and young children[39] and are virtually unknown in Fallot's tetralogy (see Chapter 18). The terminal forces are deep and prolonged with a tendency for broad slurred S waves in leads 1, aVL, and V₅₋₆ and a broad R wave in lead aVR (see Figures 19-14 and 19-15).[33] With pulmonary atresia, the electrocardiogram is similar if not indistinguishable from Fallot's tetralogy with pulmonary atresia (see Figure 19-16). A restrictive subaortic ventricular septal defect is functionally subaortic stenosis, which can cause left ventricular hypertrophy.

X-Ray

The pulmonary trunk is not dilated because the stenosis is subpulmonary (Figures 19-10 and 19-17). When the stenosis is mild, pulmonary vascularity is increased and the left ventricle is dilated (see Figure 19-17). When pulmonary stenosis is severe, pulmonary vascularity is reduced, the heart size is normal, and the apex is convex (Figure 19-18A).[27] In the presence of pulmonary atresia, the ascending aorta is enlarged, the main pulmonary artery segment is concave, and the apex is boot-shaped (Figures 19-3A, B and 19-18B).

Echocardiogram

Echocardiography with color flow imaging and Doppler interrogation establishes the subaortic location of the ventricular septal defect and the presence, type, and degree of pulmonary stenosis (Figures 19-19 and 19-20 and Videos 19-2, 19-3A, and 19-3B). Both great arteries are imaged above the right ventricle, and subpulmonary stenosis with a nondilated pulmonary trunk is identified (see Figure 19-19). Continuous wave Doppler scan establishes the pulmonary stenotic gradient (see Figure 19-20B). In the short axis, the great arteries appear as double circles, and a bicuspid stenotic pulmonary valve is occasionally identified at the origin of the pulmonary trunk to the left of the aorta.

Summary

When pulmonary stenosis is mild, cyanosis coexists with increased pulmonary blood flow. When pulmonary stenosis is severe, the electrocardiogram arouses suspicion, especially because of q waves in leads 1 and aVL despite a vertical or rightward QRS axis. The PR interval tends to

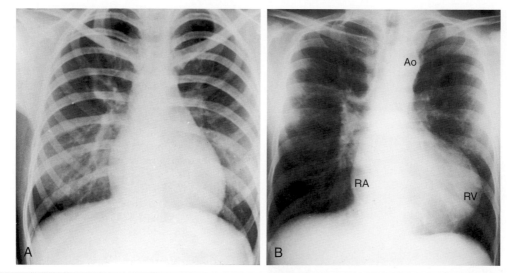

FIGURE 19-18 A, X-ray from a 13-year-old girl with double outlet right ventricle, subaortic ventricular septal defect, and severe sub-pulmonary stenosis. Pulmonary vascularity is normal. The heart size is normal with a slightly rounded apex. **B,** X-ray from a 29-year-old man with double outlet right ventricle, a subaortic ventricular septal defect, and pulmonary atresia (compare with Figure 19-3A). The lung fields have the lacy appearance of systemic-to-pulmonary artery collaterals. The pulmonary trunk is conspicuously absent, but the right and left branches are well-formed. The aortic knuckle (Ao) is prominent and continues as a left descending aorta. The boot-shaped apex is occupied by the right ventricle (RV). The right atrium (RA) is moderately convex.

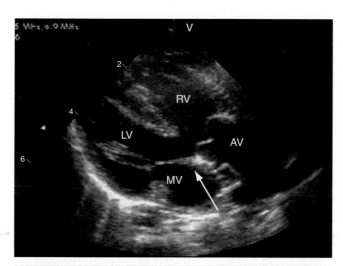

FIGURE 19-19 Echocardiogram (subcostal view) from a 2-month-old male with double outlet right ventricle (RV), a subaortic ventricular septal defect (VSD), valvular and infundibular pulmonary stenosis (PS), and a hypoplastic pulmonary trunk (PT). The large curved arrow indicates the direction of blood flow from left ventricle (LV) through the ventricular septal defect into the aorta (Ao) (Video 19-2).

be prolonged. Terminal forces are slurred in leads 1, aVL, and avR and in leads V_{5-6}. A decrescendo systolic murmur persists at the lower left sternal border because of obligatory flow from left ventricle across the ventricular septal defect into the right ventricular aorta. Echocardiography establishes the diagnosis of double outlet right ventricle with subaortic ventricular septal defect and subpulmonary or pulmonary valve stenosis.

DOUBLE OUTLET RIGHT VENTRICLE WITH SUBPULMONARY VENTRICULAR SEPTAL DEFECT: THE TAUSSIG-BING ANOMALY

Clinical manifestations of the Taussig-Bing anomaly resemble complete transposition of the great arteries with a nonrestrictive ventricular septal defect (see Box 19-1; see Chapter 27). About 50% of these patients have congenital malformations of the aortic arch, including coarctation, isthmic hypoplasia, interruption, and patent ductus arteriosus, in addition to subaortic stenosis.[17,40,41]

History

Cyanosis dates from birth or early infancy because flow from right ventricle into aorta is obligatory (see Figure 19-1D).[12,17,42] As neonatal pulmonary vascular resistance falls, left ventricular blood preferentially enters the pulmonary trunk across the subpulmonary ventricular septal defect (see Figure 19-2). Systemic arterial oxygen saturation is relatively high but at the price of increased pulmonary blood flow, left ventricular volume overload, and congestive heart failure.[10,17] The clinical course is especially poor when coarctation of the aorta elevates systemic systolic pressure, which augments already abundant pulmonary blood flow by diverting still more right ventricular blood into the pulmonary trunk (see Figure 19-1D).[10,41] A rise in pulmonary vascular resistance occasionally regulates pulmonary blood flow and ameliorates congestive heart failure. Cyanosis

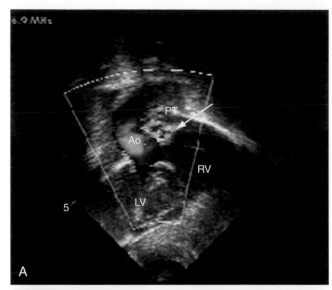

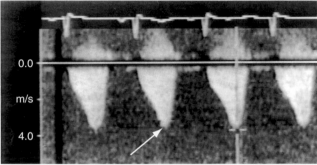

FIGURE 19-20 A, Black and white print of a color flow image from the 2-month-old male with double outlet right ventricle, subaortic ventricular septal defect, and pulmonary stenosis (see Figure 19-19 for two-dimensional echocardiogram). Both great arteries arise from the right ventricle (RV). Blood flow through the ventricular septal defect (VSD) selectively enters the aorta (Ao). The high-velocity jet of pulmonary stenosis (PS) enters the pulmonary trunk (PT). (RV/LV = right and left ventricles.) **B,** Continuous wave Doppler scan records a peak velocity of 4 msec for a peak instantaneous gradient of 64 mm Hg from right ventricle to pulmonary trunk (Videos 19-3A and 19-3B).

increases, but longevity improves; and an occasional patient reaches the second, third, or fourth decade (Figure 19-21).[42]

Physical Appearance

Infants with increased pulmonary blood flow have the catabolic effects of congestive heart failure with poor growth and development. When a moderate elevation in pulmonary vascular resistance curtails pulmonary blood flow, congestive heart failure is relieved and growth and development improve. Suprasystemic pulmonary vascular resistance results in *reversed differential cyanosis*, a distinctive physical appearance that is manifest because ductal flow is right to left (Figure 19-22).[17] The toes are *less* cyanotic and *less* clubbed than the fingers because *oxygenated* blood from the left ventricle flows

through the subpulmonary ventricular septal defect into the pulmonary trunk and through the patent ductus into the descending aorta, whereas *unoxygenated* blood from the right ventricle flows into the aorta and to the upper extremities. Trisomy 18 is another distinctive physical appearance with either a subpulmonary or a subaortic ventricular septal defect (see Figure 19-5).[30–32]

Arterial Pulse

Upper and lower extremity arterial pulses are diagnostically important because of the frequency of coarctation of the aorta.[10,17] However, the femoral pulses are preserved when a nonrestrictive patent ductus is distal to the coarctation (see Figure 19-21).

Jugular Venous Pulse

In the presence of biventricular failure, the right atrial A wave, V wave, and mean pressure are elevated. Increased pulmonary vascular resistance curtails pulmonary blood flow and alleviates congestive heart failure, so the jugular venous pulse normalizes (Figure 19-23, *second panel*).

Precordial Movement and Palpation

An obigatory right ventricular impulse becomes more conspicuous in the presence of biventricular failure. The dilated hypertensive pulmonary trunk (see Figures 19-2 and 19-21) and the loud pulmonary second heart sound can be palpated in the second left intercostal space. Volume overload of the left ventricle is responsible for a left ventricular impulse. A thrill is located as high as the second left intercostal space because the ventricular septal defect is subpulmonary. As pulmonary vascular resistance rises, pulmonary blood flow falls, left ventricular volume overload decreases, the left ventricular impulse may disappear, the right ventricular impulse decreases, and the ventricular septal defect thrill vanishes.

Auscultation

The systolic murmur that originates from a ventricular septal defect can be located as high as the second left intercostal space because the left ventricle ejects directly into the pulmonary trunk through the subpulmonary ventricular septal defect (see Figure 19-1D).[17,42] The pulmonary component of the second heart sound is loud, and splitting is preserved when pulmonary resistance is lower than systemic. An apical mid-diastolic murmur signifies increased pulmonary blood flow with increased flow across the mitral valve. As pulmonary resistance rises, pulmonary blood flow and left ventricular volume overload decline, the murmur through the subpulmonary ventricular septal defect is attenuated (see Figure 19-23), and the mitral flow murmur disappears. A pulmonary ejection sound, a soft short mid-systolic murmur, and a Graham Steell murmur originate in the dilated hypertensive pulmonary trunk. The second heart sound is loud and single because of synchronous closure of aortic and pulmonary valves.

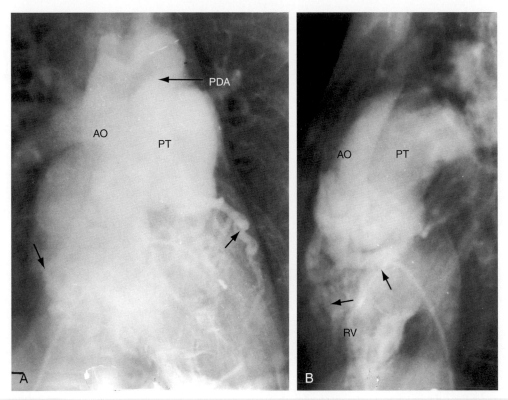

FIGURE 19-21 Right ventriculograms (RV) from a 40-year-old woman with the Taussig-Bing anomaly characterized by double outlet right ventricle, a subpulmonary ventricular septal defect, a biventricular pulmonary trunk, and pulmonary vascular disease **A,** The ascending (AO) and the pulmonary trunk (PT) are side by side with the aorta to the right. A large patent ductus arteriosus (PDA) was distal to an aortic coarctation. **B,** Lateral projection shows the aorta (AO) anterior to the pulmonary trunk (PT). Two unmarked arrows point to dilated ectatic coronary arteries (see Chapter 32). (RV = right ventricle.)

Electrocardiogram

PR interval prolongation is less frequent than with double outlet right ventricle and a subaortic ventricular septal defect (Figure 19-24). Biatrial P wave abnormalities reflect the combination of volume overload of the left atrium and enlargement of the right atrial caused by right ventricular failure. The QRS axis is vertical or rightward with clockwise depolarization (see Figure 19-24), resembling the QRS axis of complete transposition of the great arteries with a nonrestrictive ventricular septal defect (see Chapter 27). Right ventricular hypertrophy is reflected in tall R waves in lead V_1 and aVR and deep S waves in left precordial leads (see Figure 19-24). Volume overload of left ventricle is represented by well-developed R waves in leads V_{5-6} (see Figure 19-24). Elevated pulmonary vascular resistance curtails pulmonary blood flow and reduces volume overload of the left ventricle, but right ventricular pressure overload is unchanged. Accordingly, tall peaked right atrial P waves persist with residual evidence of a left atrial abnormality and with biventricular hypertrophy in mid precordial leads (Figure 19-25).

X-Ray

An increase in pulmonary arterial and pulmonary venous vascularity results from low pulmonary vascular resistance and congestive heart failure (Figure 19-26).

The left atrium and left ventricle are enlarged because of volume overload, and the right atrium and right ventricle are enlarged because of congestive heart failure (Figure 19-26 and 19-27). The dilated pulmonary trunk projects prominently to the left when the great arteries are side-by-side. The x-ray then resembles a nonrestrictive perimembranous ventricular septal defect (Figure 19-28). When the dilated pulmonary trunk is posterior and therefore not border-forming, the x-ray resembles complete transposition of the great arteries (see Figure 19-26),[12,42] except for the presence of a thymus (see Figure 19-27). With the advent of pulmonary vascular disease, pulmonary arterial blood flow decreases, pulmonary venous vascularity disappears, and volume overload of the left ventricle is curtailed, but dilation of the pulmonary trunk persists, so the x-ray resembles a nonrestrictive ventricular septal defect with Eisenmenger's syndrome (Figures 19-28 and 19-29).

Echocardiogram

The following points are relevant in addition to the features described in the section on double outlet right ventricle with *subaortic* ventricular septal defect: (1) the pulmonary trunk overrides a subpulmonary ventricular septal defect (Figure 19-30 and 19-31); (2) pulmonary stenosis is absent; and (3) subaortic stenosis, coarctation of the aorta, and patent ductus arteriosus often coexist.

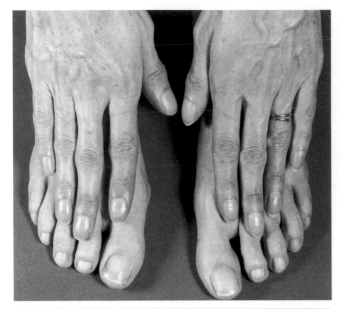

FIGURE 19-22 Hands and feet of the 40-year-old woman with the Taussig-Bing anomaly referred to in Figure 19-21. There is reversed differential cyanosis, with fingers more cyanotic than toes because unoxygenated blood from the right ventricle entered the ascending aorta and the bracheocephalic arteries while oxygenated blood from the left ventricle entered the pulmonary trunk through the subpulmonary ventricular septal defect and preferentially flowed through the patent ductus arteriosus into the descending thoracic aorta. Compare with Figure 20-12, which illustrates the differential cyanosis that characterizes a reversed shunt through an isolated patent ductus arteriosus.

Summary

The Taussig-Bing anomaly, or double outlet right ventricle with subpulmonary ventricular septal defect, resembles complete transposition of the great arteries with a nonrestrictive ventricular septal defect. Both malformations are characterized by cyanosis with increased pulmonary blood flow. However, in the Taussig-Bing anomaly, birth weights are not large, and there is a high incidence of aortic arch malformations, especially coarctation of the aorta and patent ductus arteriosus. Pulmonary vascular disease with a right-to-left shunt through a nonrestrictive patent ductus arteriosus results in distinctive *reversed* differential cyanosis, with fingers more cyanotic than toes. There is a soft early systolic murmur at the left sternal border because of obligatory flow through the subpulmonary ventricular septal defect. The QRS axis is rightward as with complete transposition, rather than the left axis deviation of double outlet right ventricle with subaortic ventricular septal defect. When the dilated pulmonary trunk is posterior and therefore not border-forming, the x-ray resembles complete transposition of the great arteries except for a thymic shadow. The x-ray, the physical signs, and the electrocardiogram otherwise resemble a nonrestrictive ventricular septal defect with Eisenmenger's syndrome, but the early onset of cyanosis with increased pulmonary arterial blood flow should prevent error. The echocardiogram with color

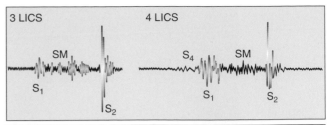

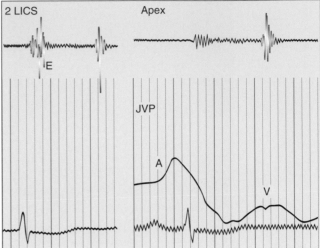

FIGURE 19-23 Phonocardiograms from the 40-year-old woman with the Taussig-Bing anomaly referred to in Figures 19-21 and 19-22. A soft systolic murmur (SM) is maximal in the third left intercostal space (3 LICS) and ends before a loud single second heart sound (S₂). The pulmonary ejection sound (E) originated in a dilated hypertensive pulmonary trunk and was recorded in the second left intercostal space (2 LICS). A soft fourth heart sound (S₄) was present in the fourth left intercostal space (4 LICS). The jugular venous pulse (JVP) shows a small dominant A wave.

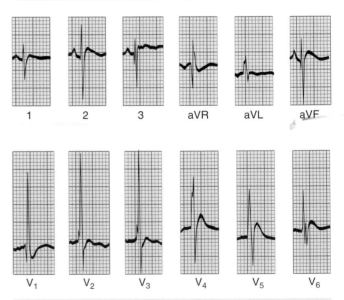

FIGURE 19-24 Electrocardiogram from a 3-month-old male with double outlet right ventricle and a subpulmonary ventricular septal defect. The PR interval is normal. Peaked right atrial P waves appear in leads 2, 3, and aVF. The QRS axis is rightward with clockwise depolarization. Right ventricular hypertrophy is reflected in the tall R waves in leads V₁₋₂ and in lead aVR and by prominent S waves in left precordial leads.

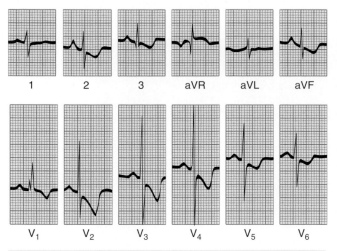

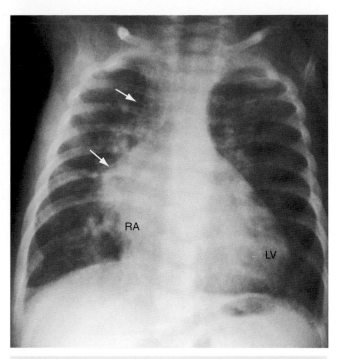

FIGURE 19-25 Electrocardiogram from the 40-year-old woman with the Taussig-Bing anomaly referred to in Figures 19-21 and 19-22. The P wave in lead 2 is tall and peaked (right atrial abnormality) and broad (left atrial abnormality). The PR interval is 180 msec. The QRS axis is plus 90 degrees. Right ventricular hypertrophy is indicated by the rR pattern in lead V_1, the R wave in lead aVR, the deep S waves in left precordial leads, and inverted T waves in right and midprecordial leads. Biventricular hypertrophy from a well-developed left ventricle is implied by the large RS complexes in midprecordial leads.

FIGURE 19-27 X-ray from a 3-month-old female with the Taussig-Bing anomaly and coarctation of the aorta proximal to a ductus arteriosus. Pulmonary vascularity is increased, but the vascular pedicle is narrow because the posterior pulmonary trunk is not border-forming. An enlarged left ventricle (LV) occupies the apex, and an enlarged right atrium (RA) occupies the right lower cardiac border. The film resembles complete transposition of the great arteries except for the thymus (arrows).

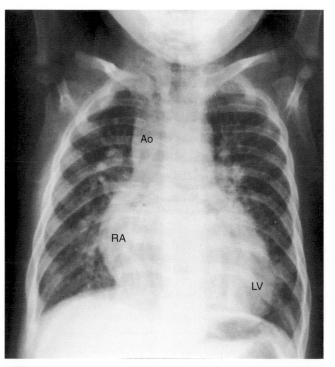

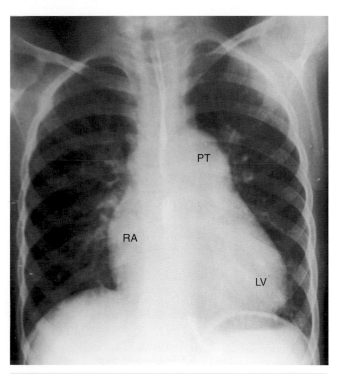

FIGURE 19-26 X-ray from a 4-month-old female with the Taussig-Bing anomaly characterized by double outlet right ventricle, a subpulmonary ventricular septal defect, and a pulmonary-to-systemic flow ratio of 3 to 1. A dilated pulmonary trunk was not border-forming because it was posterior. The rightward and anterior ascending aorta (Ao) is at the right thoracic inlet. Pulmonary vascularity is increased, a convex left ventricle (LV) occupies the apex, and a prominent right atrium (RA) occupies the right lower cardiac border.

FIGURE 19-28 X-ray from a 10-year-old girl with the Taussig-Bing anomaly, pulmonary vascular disease, and reversed shunt through a large patent ductus arteriosus. Pulmonary vascularity is normal, the pulmonary trunk (PT) is dilated, a moderately prominent right atrium (RA) forms the lower right cardiac border, and an enlarged left ventricle (LV) occupies the apex. Death followed a brain abscess.

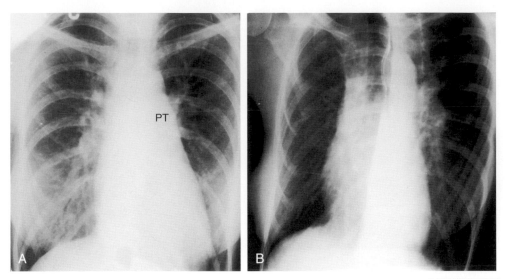

FIGURE 19-29 X-rays from the 40-year-old woman with the Taussig-Bing anomaly referred to in Figures 19-21 and 19-22. **A,** Pulmonary soft tissue densities are enhanced by breast tissue, but pulmonary vascularity is otherwise normal. The cardiac silhouette is normal except for the mildly convex dilated posterior pulmonary trunk (PT). **B,** A left anterior oblique projection confirms the normal size of the right atrium and both ventricles.

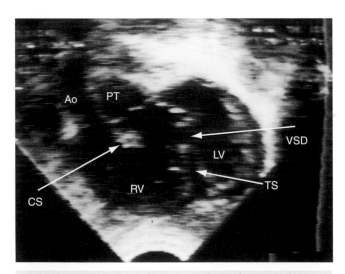

FIGURE 19-30 Echocardiogram (subcostal view) from a 4-month-old female with double outlet right ventricle and a subpulmonary ventricular septal defect (VSD). The ascending aorta (Ao) and pulmonary trunk (PT), which are parallel to each other, are separated by the conal septum (CS) and positioned entirely above the right ventricle (RV). The conal septum is straight and parallel to the trabecular septum (TS), thus committing the ventricular septal defect to the pulmonary trunk. (LV = left ventricle.)

flow imaging and Doppler interrogation establishes the diagnosis of double outlet right ventricle and identifies the subpulmonary location of the ventricular septal defect and coexisting coarctation of the aorta and patent ductus arteriosus.

DOUBLE OUTLET LEFT VENTRICLE

In biventricular hearts, origin of both great arteries from the morphologic *left* ventricle is among the rarest of ventriculoarterial malalignments.[5,43–45] The malformation was described in the early 19th century, rediscovered in 1967, and defined clinically and at necropsy in 1970.[46] Morphogenesis has been assigned to misalignment of the septal anlagen of the embryonic conus and the conal ridges.[9,47] Double outlet left ventricle is the converse of double outlet right ventricle because both great arteries arise entirely or predominantly from the morphologic *left* ventricle (Figure 19-32).[47] The only exit for the right ventricle is a subaortic or subpulmonary ventricular septal defect. Rarely, the ventricular septum is intact.[48]

In hearts with two well-formed noninverted ventricles, this rare malformation is associated with a *subaortic* ventricular septal defect that tends to occur with pulmonary stenosis (see Figure 19-32).[49] Less commonly, the ventricular septal defect is subpulmonary, and the outflow obstruction is *aortic stenosis.*[45]

Double outlet left ventricle with subaortic ventricular septal defect and pulmonary stenosis (see Figure 19-32) resembles cyanotic Fallot's tetralogy, including a right aortic arch, hypoxic spells, and a pulmonary stenotic murmur whose length varies inversely with the severity of obstruction. The electrocardiogram shows right ventricular hypertrophy. The x-ray shows little or no increase in cardiac size and normal or reduced pulmonary vascularity.[45] The echocardiogram with Doppler interrogation identifies two noninverted ventricles with left ventricular origin of both great arteries and establishes the location of the ventricular septal defect and the presence and

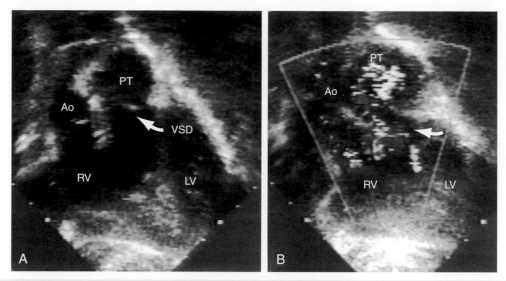

FIGURE 19-31   A, Echocardiogram from a 3-year-old boy with double outlet right ventricle and a nonrestrictive subpulmonary ventricular septal defect. The aorta (Ao) and the dilated pulmonary trunk (PT) arise entirely from the right ventricle (RV). The ventricular septal defect (VSD) is committed to the pulmonary trunk. (LV = left ventricle.) **B,** Black-and-white print of a color flow image showing flow from left ventricle through the ventricular septal defect (curved arrow) into the dilated pulmonary trunk.

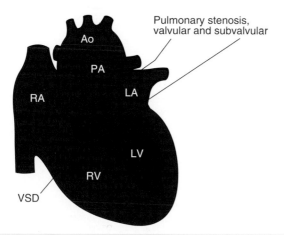

FIGURE 19-32 Drawing of double outlet *left* ventricle with a subaortic ventricular septal defect (VSD) and valvular/subvalvular pulmonary stenosis. The aorta (Ao) and pulmonary artery (PA) both arise from the left ventricle (LV). (RV = right ventricle; RA = right atrium.) *(Modified from Conti V, Adams F, and Mulder DG. Double-outlet left ventricle. Ann Thorac Surg 51:159, 1991.)*

degree of pulmonary stenosis.[20,49] Double outlet *left* ventricle is distinguished from origin of both great arteries from an *inverted morphologic right ventricle* (Figure 19-33).[50]

Double outlet left ventricle with *subaortic ventricular septal defect* and *no pulmonary stenosis* resembles complete transposition of the great arteries with a subaortic ventricular septal defect and a posterior aorta. The two circulations run in parallel, with blood from the left ventricle recirculating within the pulmonary circulation and blood from the right ventricle recirculating within the systemic circulation (see Chapter 27). Cyanosis varies inversely with pulmonary arterial blood flow. When pulmonary vascular resistance is low, cyanosis exists with *increased* pulmonary blood flow as in complete transposition of the great arteries.

Double outlet left ventricle with a nonrestrictive *subpulmonary* ventricular septal defect and no pulmonary stenosis resembles isolated nonrestrictive ventricular septal defect.[45] As neonatal pulmonary vascular resistance falls, left ventricular blood is increasingly diverted into the pulmonary artery. Right ventricular blood preferentially flows into the pulmonary artery because the ventricular septal defect is subpulmonary. Pulmonary blood flow increases, the electrocardiogram shows biventricular hypertrophy, cyanosis is minimal, and congestive heart failure results in poor growth and development.[45] Echocardiography identifies two noninverted ventricles, establishes left ventricular origin of both great arteries, and identifies the subpulmonary ventricular septal defect.[45]

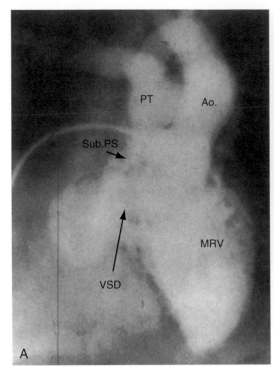

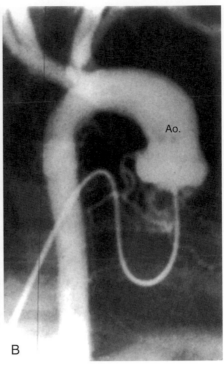

FIGURE 19-33 Angiocardiograms from a 3-year-old boy with congenitally corrected transposition of the great arteries, a ventricular septal defect (VSD), and subpulmonary stenosis (Sub. PS). **A,** The aorta (Ao.) and pulmonary trunk (PT) both arise from the morphologic right ventricle (MRV). The ascending aorta (Ao.) is convex to the left, a feature confirmed in **B.**

REFERENCES

1. Van Praagh S, Davidoff A, Chin A, Shiels F, Reynolds J, Van Praagh R. Double-outlet right ventricle: anatomic types and developmental implications based on a study of 101 autopsied cases. *Coeur.* 1982;13:389–439.
2. Abernathy J. *Surgical and physiological essays. Part II.* London: James Evans; 1793.
3. Vierordt H. Die angeborenen Herzkrankheiten. *Spez Pathol Ther.* 1898;15.
4. Witham AC. Double outlet right ventricle; a partial transposition complex. *Am Heart J.* 1957;53:928–939.
5. Anderson R, Galbraith R, Gibson R, Miller G. Double outlet left ventricle. *Br Heart J.* 1974;36:554–558.
6. Bharati S, Lev M, Stewart R, Mcallister Jr HA, Kirklin JW. The morphologic spectrum of double outlet left ventricle and its surgical significance. *Circulation.* 1978;58:558–565.
7. Anderson RH, Mccarthy K, Cook AC. Continuing medical education. Double outlet right ventricle. *Cardiol Young.* 2001;11:329–344.
8. Anderson RH. Double outlet right ventricle. *Eur J Cardiothorac Surg.* 2002;22:853.
9. Sridaromont S, Feldt RH, Ritter DG, Davis GD, Edwards JE. Double outlet right ventricle: hemodynamic and anatomic correlations. *Am J Cardiol.* 1976;38:85–94.
10. Sondheimer HM, Freedom RM, Olley PM. Double outlet right ventricle: clinical spectrum and prognosis. *Am J Cardiol.* 1977;39:709–714.
11. Van Praagh R. What is the Taussig-Bing malformation? *Circulation.* 1968;38:445–449.
12. Taussig HB, Bing RJ. Complete transposition of the aorta and a levoposition of the pulmonary artery; clinical, physiological, and pathological findings. *Am Heart J.* 1949;37:551–559.
13. Macmahon HE, Lipa M. Double-outlet right ventricle with intact interventricular septum. *Circulation.* 1964;30:745–748.
14. Cheung YF, Yung TC, Leung MP. Left ventriculo-coronary communications in a double-outlet right ventricle with an intact ventricular septum. *Int J Cardiol.* 2000;74:227–229.
15. Beekman RP, Bartelings MM, Hazekamp MG, Gittenberger-De Groot AC, Ottenkamp J. The morphologic nature of noncommitted ventricular septal defects in specimens with double-outlet right ventricle. *J Thorac Cardiovasc Surg.* 2002;124:984–990.
16. Caffarena JM, Gomez-Ullate JM. DORV with non-committed VSD and Taussig-Bing hearts. Controversial anatomic entities. *Eur J Cardio-Thoracic Surg.* 2003;23:136–137.
17. Wedemeyer AL, Lucas Jr RV, Castaneda AR. Taussig-Bing malformation, coarctation of the aorta, and reversed patent ductus arteriosus. Operative correction in an infant. *Circulation.* 1970;42:1021–1027.
18. Bashore TM. Adult congenital heart disease: right ventricular outflow tract lesions. *Circulation.* 2007;115:1933–1947.
19. Michaelsson M, Tuvemo T. Double outlet right ventricle with spontaneously developing pulmonary outflow obstruction. *Br Heart J.* 1974;36:937–940.
20. Lavoie R, Sestier F, Gilbert G, Chameides L, Van Praagh R, Grondin P. Double outlet right ventricle with left ventricular outflow tract obstruction due to small ventricular septal defect. *Am Heart J.* 1971;82:290–299.
21. Mason DT, Morrow AG, Elkins RC, Friedman WF. Origin of both great vessels from the right ventricle associated with severe obstruction to left ventricular outflow. *Am J Cardiol.* 1969;24:118–124.
22. Rao PS, Sissman NJ. Spontaneous closure of physiologically advantageous ventricular septal defects. *Circulation.* 1971;43:83–90.
23. Davachi F, Moller JH, Edwards JE. Origin of both great vessels from right ventricle with intact ventricular septum. *Am Heart J.* 1968;75:790–794.
24. Rice MJ, Seward JB, Edwards WD, et al. Straddling atrioventricular valve: two-dimensional echocardiographic diagnosis, classification and surgical implications. *Am J Cardiol.* 1985;55:505–513.
25. Titus JL, Neufeld H, Edwards JE. The atrioventricular conduction system in hearts with both great vessels originating from the right ventricle. *Am Heart J.* 1964;67:588–592.
26. Rogoff JH, Anthony W. Double-outlet right ventricle with pulmonary valve atresia. Report on a patient surviving to age 25. *Am Heart J.* 1966;72:259–264.
27. Guo DW, Lin ML, Gu ZQ, Cheng TO. Double-outlet right ventricle. A clinical-roentgenologic-pathologic study of 28 consecutive patients. *Chest.* 1984;85:526–532.
28. Rein AJ, Dollberg S, Gale R. Genetics of conotruncal malformations: review of the literature and report of a consanguineous kindred with various conotruncal malformations. *Am J Med Genet.* 1990;36:353–355.

29. Dickinson C, Walker S, Wilmshurst P. Double outlet right ventricle with unprotected pulmonary vasculature presenting in a woman of 65. *Heart.* 1996;76:187.

30. Butler LJ, Snodgrass GJ, Sinclair L, France NE, Russell A. E (16–18) trisomy syndrome: analysis of 13 cases. *Arch Dis Child.* 1965;40: 600–611.

31. Rogers TR, Hagstrom JW, Engle MA. Origin of both great vessels from the right ventricle associated with the trisomy-18 syndrome. *Circulation.* 1965;32:802–807.

32. Rohde RA, Hodgman JE, Cleland RS. Multiple congenital anomalies in the E1-Trisomy (Group 16-18) Syndrome. *Pediatrics.* 1964;33:258–270.

33. Krongrad E, Ritter DG, Weidman WH, Dushane JW. Hemodynamic and anatomic correlation of electrocardiogram in double-outlet right ventricle. *Circulation.* 1972;46:995–1004.

34. Saleeb SF, Juraszek A, Geva T. Anatomic, imaging, and clinical characteristics of double-inlet, double-outlet right ventricle. *Am J Cardiol.* 2010;105:542–549.

35. Child J. Transthoracic and transesophageal echocardiographic imaging: anatomic and hemodynamic assessment. In: Perloff JK, Child JS, Aboulhosn J, eds. *Congenital heart disease in adults.* 3rd ed. Philadelphia: WB Saunders Company; 2009.

36. Ewing S, Silverman NH. Echocardiographic diagnosis of single coronary artery in double-outlet right ventricle. *Am J Cardiol.* 1996; 77:535–539.

37. Gedikbasi A, Oztarhan K, Gul A, Sargin A, Ceylan Y. Diagnosis and prognosis in double-outlet right ventricle. *Am J Perinatol.* 2008;25: 427–434.

38. Khattri HN, Misra KP, Dutta BN. Double outlet right ventricle with long survival. *Br Heart J.* 1968;30:569–570.

39. Robinson BW, Anisman PC, Sandhu S, Sokoloski M, Eshaghpour E. Significance of a Q wave in lead I in the newborn. *Am J Cardiol.* 1999;84:615–617 A619.

40. Khoury GH, Gilbert EF. Taussig-Bing malformation with coarctation of the aorta. *Angiology.* 1970;21:143–150.

41. Parr GV, Waldhausen JA, Bharati S, Lev M, Fripp R, Whitman V. Coarctation in Taussig-Bing malformation of the heart. Surgical significance. *J Thorac Cardiovasc Surg.* 1983;86:280–287.

42. Beuren A. Differential diagnosis of the Taussig-Bing heart from complete transposition of the great vessels with a posteriorly overriding pulmonary artery. *Circulation.* 1960;21:1071–1087.

43. Dadourian BJ, Perloff JK, Drinkwater DC, Child JS, Mulder DG. Double outlet left ventricle—long survival after surgical correction. *Ann Thorac Surg.* 1991;51:159–160.

44. Kerr AR, Barcia A, Bargeron Jr LM, Kirklin JW. Double-outlet left ventricle with ventricular septal defect and pulmonary stenosis: report of surgical repair. *Am Heart J.* 1971;81:688–693.

45. Marino B, Bevilacqua M. Double-outlet left ventricle: two-dimensional echocardiographic diagnosis. *Am Heart J.* 1992;123: 1075–1077.

46. Paul MH, Muster AJ, Sinha SN, Cole RB, Van Praagh R. Double-outlet left ventricle with an intact ventricular septum. Clinical and autopsy diagnosis and developmental implications. *Circulation.* 1970;41:129–139.

47. Manner J, Seidl W, Steding G. Embryological observations on the formal pathogenesis of double-outlet left ventricle with a right-ventricular infundibulum. *Thorac Cardiovasc Surg.* 1997;45: 172–177.

48. Beitzke A, Suppan C. Double outlet left ventricle with intact ventricular septum. *Int J Cardiol.* 1984;5:175–183.

49. Bengur AR, Snider AR, Peters J, Merida-Asmus L. Two-dimensional echocardiographic features of double outlet left ventricle. *J Am Soc Echocardiogr.* 1990;3:320–325.

50. Battistessa S, Soto B. Double outlet right ventricle with discordant atrioventricular connexion: an angiographic analysis of 19 cases. *Int J Cardiol.* 1990;27:253–263 discussion 265–257.

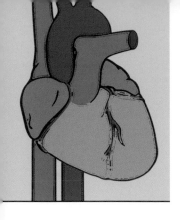

Chapter 20

Patent Ductus Arteriosus
Aortopulmonary Window

In 1593, Giambattista Carcano, Professor of Anatomy in Pavia, an ancient town in northern Italy, described the ductus arteriosus in his book on the great cardiac vessels of the fetus.[1] However, Leo Bottali came to be associated with the arterial duct, the *duktus arteriosus persisten*, even though he misapplied the term to the foramen ovale.[1] It was not until Karl von Rokitansky's handbook of 1844 and his beautifully illustrated monograph of 1852 that patent ductus arteriosus was recognized as a specific congenital malformation.[2] The *first section* of this chapter is concerned with persistent patency of the ductus arteriosus. The *second section* is devoted to aortopulmonary window, often called aortopulmonary or aorticopulmonary septal defect, an anomaly that is embryologically unrelated to patent ductus but that is physiologically and clinically similar.

The incidence rate of isolated persistent patency of the ductus has been estimated at 1:2000 to 1:5000 births, or about 10% to 12% of all varieties of congenital heart disease.[3] The pulmonary orifice of the ductus is located immediately to the left of the bifurcation of the pulmonary trunk near the origin of its left branch (Figures 20-1 and 20-2). The aortic orifice is located immediately distal to the origin of the left subclavian artery (see Figures 20-1 and 20-2). A patent ductus can be long and narrow or short and wide, with all gradations in between (Figures 20-3, 20-4, and 20-5). Closure consistently begins at the pulmonary arterial end, so the ductus assumes the shape of a truncated cone that is larger at its aortic end (see Figures 20-3 and 20-4).[4,5] A widely patent aortic end with a sealed pulmonary end is the substrate for a ductal aneurysm (Figure 20-6).[6-9] Patency confined to the pulmonary end is exceptional.[10] Anatomic variations include bilateral patent ductus,[11,12] left-sided patent ductus with right aortic arch,[13] right-sided patent ductus with right aortic arch,[14] patent ductus or ligamentum arteriosum as a component of a vascular ring (Figure 20-7),[15] and dissection of the aorta with extension into a patent ductus.[16]

Despite its seeming anatomic simplicity, the ductus arteriosus is a complex structure. The *fetal ductus* is a major anatomic component of a contiguous intrauterine great arterial system that consists of pulmonary trunk/ductus/aortic continuity that delivers 85% of right ventricular output into the descending aorta.[17] *Persistent fetal circulation* is a designation applied to an intrauterine right-to-left ductal shunt that persists after birth (see Chapter 14).[18] Persistent patency of the ductus arteriosus is abnormal and therefore undesirable, although certain forms of congenital heart disease depend for survival on neonatal ductal patency. *Ductal dependent circulations* include malformations in which a patent ductus is the only source of pulmonary arterial blood flow (pulmonary atresia with intact ventricular septum), the only source of systemic arterial blood flow (aortic atresia or complete interruption of the aortic arch), or the only source of bidirectional blood flow (simple complete transposition of the great arteries; see relevant chapters).

The ductus arteriosus is derived from the sixth aortic arch. By the fourth month of gestation, ductal tissue has become distinctive, differing histologically from pulmonary arterial and aortic tissue.[19] At 16 weeks of gestation, the ductus consists of a muscular arterial channel with an endothelium separated by an internal elastic lamina and a thin subendothelial layer.[19] The media differs at the aortic and pulmonary ends, so ductal media can be aortic, pulmonary, or mixed.[4] As gestation continues, the intima thickens, and the subendothelial layer is invaded by cells from the media that disrupt the internal elastic lamina. At term, the mature ductus harbors conspicuous intimal cushions that protrude into the lumen. The ductus is then is capable of contraction, *functional closure*, which is followed by *anatomic closure* that uniformally begins at the pulmonary arterial end (see previous).[4] *Anatomic closure* follows a sequence of immunohistochemical and ultrastructural changes, namely[4,19]: (1) separation of endothelium from internal elastic lamina; (2) enfolding and ingrowth of endothelial cells; (3) migration of undifferentiated medial smooth muscle cells into the subendothelium; (4) fragmentation of the internal elastic lamina; (5) sealing of the lumen by endothelial cell apposition; (6) accumulation of lipid droplets; and (7) intimal and subendothelial degenerative changes that spread centrally and peripherally and result in disappearance of endothelial cells at luminal apposition lines.[4] The normal process of *functional closure* begins within 10 to 15 hours after birth and is virtually complete (probe patent) by the second week of extrauterine life. The ductus is an *anatomically closed* ligamentum arteriosum 2 to 3 weeks after birth.[5,17,20] *When a ductus is destined to remain patent*, the intrauterine subendothelial internal elastic lamina lies adjacent to the intimal cushions, endothelial cells adhere to the elastic lamina, and subendothelial edema with enfolding of endothelial cells does not occur.[4,19] A ductus that remains patent in full-term infants after 3 months of extrauterine life harbors the histologic features of persistent patency just described. Spontaneous closure is then unlikely.[19,21,22]

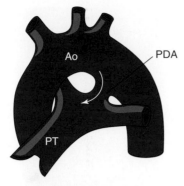

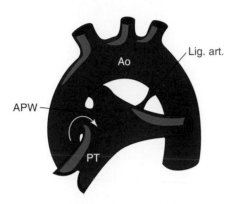

FIGURE 20-1 Illustrations of patent ductus arteriosus (PDA) and aortopulmonary window (APW). The aortic orifice of a *patent ductus arteriosus* inserts immediately distal to the origin of the left subclavian artery. (Ao = aorta.) The pulmonary orifice inserts immediately to the left of the bifurcation of the pulmonary trunk (PT). An *aortopulmonary window* is a communication between adjacent walls of the ascending aorta (Ao) and the pulmonary trunk (PT) proximal to its bifurcation. (Lig. art. = ligamentum arteriosum.)

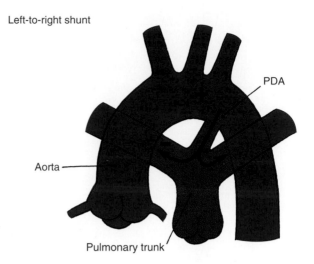

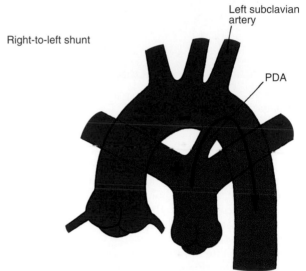

FIGURE 20-2 Illustrations of two major flow patterns in patent ductus arteriosus (PDA). The *upper* drawing illustrates a left-to-right shunt through a patent ductus in which pulmonary vascular resistance is lower than systemic vascular resistance. Shunt flow is from aorta into the pulmonary trunk. The *lower* drawing illustrates a right-to-left shunt through a patent ductus in which pulmonary vascular resistance is suprasystemic. Shunt flow is from pulmonary trunk into the aorta immediately distal to the left subclavian artery.

In utero ductal tone is determined by an interplay between the constricting effect of oxygen (relatively weak because of low fetal pO₂) and the dilating effect of endogenous prostaglandin E₂.[23,24] Prostaglandin synthetase inhibitors administered to mammalian fetuses or to pregnant ewes constrict the fetal ductus and deprive the fetal right ventricle of its only outlet.[24] As term approaches, the ductus becomes less responsive to prostaglandin E₂ and more responsive to oxygen, setting the stage for constriction that begins a few hours after birth in full term infants.[25] Functional closure is closely coupled to the increase in extrauterine ambient oxygen tension that exerts a direct constricting effect on the ductal wall (see previous). Oxygen-induced constriction has been related to inhibition of voltage-gated potassium channels.[26] Flow through the closing ductus is transiently bidirectional. Left-to-right flow[25] then decreases rapidly during the next 12 hours and cannot be detected at 48 hours.[27] Anatomic closure is the culmination of morphologic changes accrued during intrauterine ductal maturation (see previous).[4,19,28] In addition, apoptosis and smooth muscle cell proliferation have been assigned a role in anatomic closure.[29]

In healthy preterm infants, delayed closure of the ductus arteriosus is common.[30–33] Premature neonates with a gestational age of 30 weeks or more usually experience spontaneous ductal closure within a time frame that corresponds to the closure time in full-term infants.[31,32] In full-term infants, spontaneous closure is unlikely after 3 months of age,[21,22] and in premature infants, it is unlikely after 1 year of age (Figure 20-8).[22] Exceptional examples of spontaneous closure have been documented between 5 and 6 years of age, between 7 and 14 years,[34] after 17 years,[35] and at age 19 years.

Persistent patency of the ductus in premature infants sometimes coincides with respiratory distress, but the

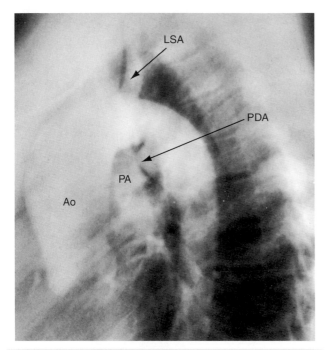

FIGURE 20-3 Lateral aortogram from a 14-year-old girl with a patent ductus arteriosus.

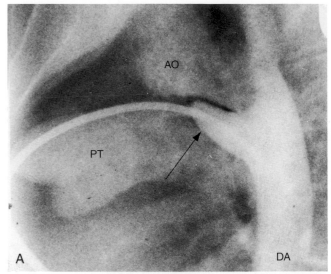

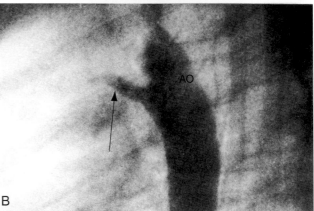

FIGURE 20-4 **A,** Lateral angiogram from a 16-year-old girl. A catheter passed from the pulmonary trunk (PT) through a ductus arteriosus (arrow), which is distinctly larger at its aortic end. (AO = aortic arch; DA = descending aorta.) **B,** Lateral angiogram from an 8-year-old boy with a restrictive tubular ductus arteriosus (arrow) that fills from the aorta (AO) and tapers markedly at its pulmonary end.

distress may not improve with subsequent ductal closure.[31,32,36] Patent ductus in preterm infants is associated with reduced cerebral blood flow from a steal effect caused by the aortic-to-pulmonary shunt, rather than by a limited capacity of the preterm left ventricle to achieve adequate cardiac output.[37,38]

First-trimester *maternal rubella* with rash carries an 80% incidence rate of intrauterine viral infection[39]; deafness and cataracts (Figure 20-9). Congenital heart disease affects two thirds of offspring. Patent ductus arteriosus accounts for a third of the congenital malformations[22] and is characterized by maturational arrest and an immature ductal wall of the type found at 16 weeks of gestation (see previous).[22]

The *physiologic consequences* of persistent patency of the ductus arteriosus depend on five variables: (1) the size of the ductus; (2) pulmonary vascular resistance; (3) the adaptive response of the left ventricle to volume overload; (4) prematurity; and (5) respiratory distress. When the ductus is *restrictive*, pulmonary vascular resistance is normal, right ventricular afterload is normal, and the hemodynamic consequences are negligible. When the ductus is *moderately restrictive* and pulmonary vascular resistance is normal or nearly so, right ventricular afterload is not significantly affected and continuous aortic-to-pulmonary flow imposes only a moderate volume load on the left ventricle. About 95% of isolated patent ductuses are restrictive or moderately restrictive. When the ductus is *nonrestrictive*, systolic pressure in the aorta and pulmonary trunk equalize at systemic level, so the direction of blood flow depends on the relative resistances in the systemic and pulmonary vascular beds.[40] If pulmonary resistance is lower than systemic, a left-to-right shunt is established, imposing volume overload on the left ventricle while right ventricular afterload remains at

systemic level (see Figure 20-2, *upper*). When pulmonary vascular resistance exceeds systemic, the shunt is reversed (see Figure 20-2, *lower*). Volume overload of the left ventricle is then curtailed, pressure overload of the right ventricle remains at systemic level, and the pulmonary vascular bed exhibits histologic changes similar to primary pulmonary hypertension or Eisenmenger's syndrome (see Chapters 14 and 17).[35,41]

HISTORY

A newborn is typically pronounced healthy and discharged as a well baby. As neonatal pulmonary vascular resistance falls, a left-to-right shunt is established, the ductus murmur emerges, and the diagnosis becomes apparent. Less commonly, a neonate comes to attention because of low birth weight, systemic hypoperfusion, or congestive heart failure *without* an incriminating ductus

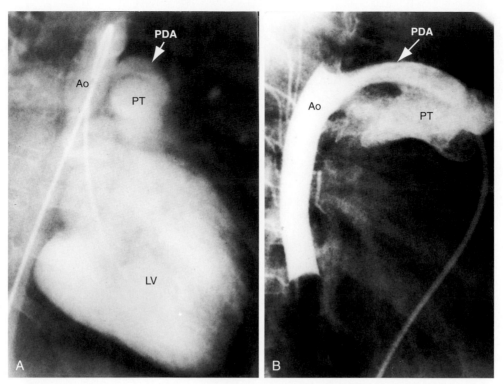

FIGURE 20-5 Angiocardiograms from a 3-year-old boy with a nonrestrictive patent ductus arteriosus (PDA), low pulmonary vascular resistance, and a 3 to 1 left-to-right shunt. **A,** The ascending aorta (Ao) is relatively small. The pulmonary trunk (PT) and left ventricle (LV) are dilated. **B,** The patent ductus arteriosus (PDA) connects a relatively small ascending aorta (Ao) to a dilated pulmonary trunk (PT).

murmur (Figure 20-10).[33,42] Absence of a murmur does not necessarily mean that the ductus has closed.[17] A ductus can be *patent but silent* because of the direction of the jet as it enters the pulmonary artery.[43] No correlation has

been found between the presence of a murmur and the size of the arterial duct.[43] Doppler echocardiography occasionally detects a tiny patent ductus in infants without auscultatory signs of its presence,[44] or auscultation

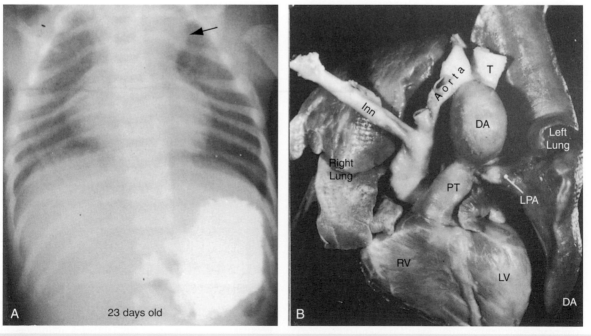

FIGURE 20-6 A, X-ray showing the striking convexity of a large ductal aneurysm (arrow) in a 23-day-old infant. Retention of barium in the stomach was caused by pyloric stenosis. **B,** Necropsy specimen showing the ductal aneurysm (DA), which was sealed at its pulmonary arterial end but patent at its aortic end. (Inn = innominate artery; T = trachea; PT = pulmonary trunk; LPA = left pulmonary artery; RV/LV = right ventricle/left ventricle.)

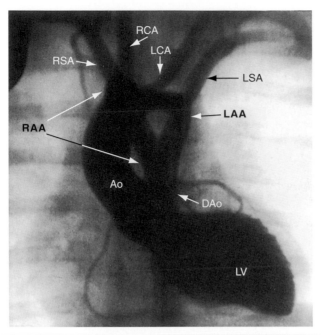

FIGURE 20-7 Angiocardiogram with contrast material injected into the left ventricle (LV) of a 15-year-old boy with a vascular ring. The ascending aorta (Ao) bifurcates into a right aortic arch (RAA) that passes anterior to the trachea and a left aortic arch (LAA) that passes posterior to the esophagus, hence a vascular ring that compressed the trachea and esophagus. The two aortic arches joined to form the descending aorta (DAo). All anatomic components of the vascular ring are visualized except the ligamentum arteriosum, which was surgically divided. (RSA/LSA = right subclavian artery/left subclavian artery; RCA/LCA = right carotid artery/left carotid artery.)

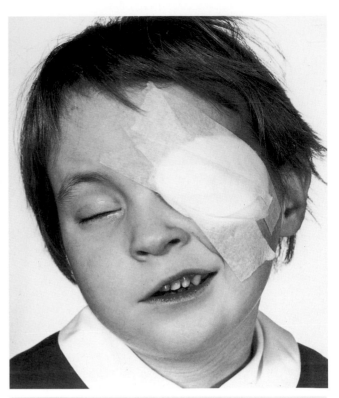

FIGURE 20-9 A 5-year-old girl whose mother had first-trimester rubella. The bandage followed ophthalmic surgery for cataract. The child had a patent ductus arteriosus.

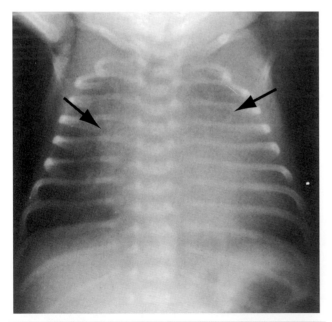

FIGURE 20-8 X-ray from the 21-day-old premature male with a widely patent ductus arteriosus. The phonocardiogram is shown in Figure 20-10. Pulmonary blood flow is increased, the heart is considerably enlarged, and a thymus (arrows) obscures the base. By age 4 months, the ductus had spontaneously closed, the thymus had disappeared, and the x-ray was virtually normal.

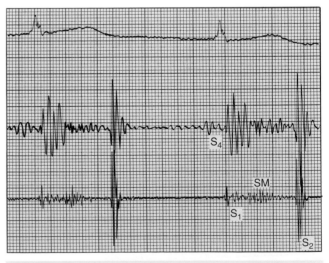

FIGURE 20-10 Phonocardiograms at the second left intercostal space in a 21-day-old premature male with a nonrestrictive patent ductus arteriosus (see x-ray in Figure 20-8). The low-frequency filter (upper tracing) shows a fourth heart sound (S_4). The high-frequency filter (lower tracing) shows a normal first heart sound (S_1) and an unimpressive early to midsystolic ductal murmur (SM) that fades before a loud single second heart sound (S_2).

detects a tiny ductus in adults in whom the diagnosis had been missed (see Figure 20-40). Closure of a patent ductus is occasionally the result of healed infective endocarditis[45,46] or thrombotic occlusion.[47,48]

In 1561, Vesalius described a valve or membrane in a patent ductus arteriosus.[49] A valve-like structure was subsequently found in stillborn human fetuses and in newborn rabbits,[49] and in 1903, a necropsy report called attention to a perforated ductal valve.[50] Taussig[51] confirmed the presence of a membranous valve at the pulmonary end of a ductus and theorized that rupture might account for the sudden appearance of a ductus murmur, an event occasionally witnessed in children or young adults. A continuous murmur intermittently *appeared* and *disappeared* in a patient with a veil-like valve at the pulmonary end of a ductus,[52] and the *abrupt appearance* of a loud continuous murmur was described in a 55-year-old man with a ductal membrane.[53] Rarely, a closed lumen is reopened by spontaneous intramural dissection of a ductal aneurysm or by propagation of aortic dissection into the ductus.[16]

Patent ductus arteriosus predominates in females, with a gender ratio of 2 or 3 to 1.[35] Female prevalence is even greater in older patients.[54] There is a tendency for recurrence of patent ductus in siblings[55–57] and in the offspring of parents with patent ductus.[55] Familial recurrence has been reported in three generations of a single family.[58] Identical twins may both have a patent ductus, or the ductus may be patent in only one twin. Canine patent ductus is more common in females and can be hereditary.[59]

In offspring of gravida with *maternal rubella*, patent ductus arteriosus and pulmonary artery stenosis coexist as congenital malformations (see Chapter 11).[60–62] Maternal rubella resulted in patent ductus arteriosus in one of a twin pair; the other twin had pulmonary artery stenosis. Low birth weight and failure to thrive are features of the rubella syndrome, even if the ductus is restrictive. A seasonal incidence of patent ductus in late winter and early spring coincided with the peak incidence of rubella.[62]

Persistent patency of the ductus arteriosus is about six times more prevalent in high-altitude locations than in sea-level locations.[63] A predilection for increased pulmonary vascular resistance is a feature of high-altitude births with patent ductus.[63] The predilection exists even when the ductus is restrictive.[63]

Congestive heart failure is the most common cause of death directly related to patent ductus.[35] Rarely, death is from dissection or rupture of a ductal aneurysm[64] or from rupture of a hypertensive aneurysmal pulmonary trunk.[65,66] Aneurysm of a *nonpatent* ductus (see Figure 20-6) can be complicated by rupture, by spontaneous intramural dissection, by systemic embolism, by infection, by recurrent laryngeal nerve paralysis, by compression of the pulmonary trunk, or by hemorrhagic erosion into the esophagus or tracheobronchial tree.[8,9]

Infective endarteritis occurs with a restrictive patent ductus because of the high-velocity left-to-right shunt but does not occur with a nonrestrictive ductus and reversed shunt.[35] The infection is located at the narrow pulmonary arterial end of the ductus or at the site of an intimal jet lesion in the pulmonary artery opposite the ductus. Susceptibility has not been determined for a tiny clinically silent ductus detected only with Doppler echocardiography (see Figure 20-40; see previous).[67]

Abnormal patterns of cerebral arterial blood flow in infants, especially preterm neonates with a nonrestrictive patent ductus, predispose to central nervous system ischemia and hemorrhage into the germinal matrix.[38,68,69] Increased pulse pressure and major fluctuations of blood flow velocity caused by opening and closing of a ductus may rupture capillaries of the germinal matrix and cause intraventricular hemorrhage. A sharp decrease in diastolic arterial flow velocity can act as a *steal* from the cerebral circulation.[68]

After the first year of life, most patients with patent ductus arteriosus are asymptomatic. Beginning with the second decade, the risk of infective endarteritis exceeds the risk of congestive heart failure.[35,54,70] In the third decade, more and more patients with a moderately restrictive ductus experience heart failure,[35,54] and those with a restrictive ductus remain asymptomatic. A 20-year-old man with a patent ductus had been a cross-country runner, and an active schoolmistress died at the age of 85 years because of gastrointestinal bleeding. A number of reports have called attention to survival beyond age 60 years (see Figure 20-16)[35,71–75]: an elderly woman presented with biventricular failure in her 81st year,[76] and a patient died at 90 years of age.[77]

A nonrestrictive patent ductus with *Eisenmenger's syndrome* is accompanied by the multisystem systemic disorders of cyanotic congenital heart disease (see Chapter 17).[78,79] Isotonic exercise with an Eisenmenger's ductus causes *leg fatigue without dyspnea* because an exercise-induced increase in right-to-left shunt is channeled into the descending aorta (Figures 20-2 and 20-11) distal to the respiratory center and the carotid body, precluding hypoxia-induced stimulation.[78–81] Hypertrophic osteoarthropathy is confined to the lower extremities.[82–84] In an Eisenmenger's ductus, left ventricular failure is absent because volume overload of the left heart is curtailed. A dilated hypertensive pulmonary trunk may cause hoarseness by compressing the recurrent laryngeal nerve. Angina and syncope are not features of nonrestrictive patent ductus with reserved shunt because right ventricular pressure cannot exceed systemic.[79] Cyanosis is missed if the feet are not examined (see section Physical Appearance). A young girl came to attention because she noticed that when she sat in a warm bath, her toes were blue but her fingers were pink.

Constriction or closure of the *fetal ductus* deprives the right ventricle of its only outlet, so neonates present with massive tricuspid regurgitation and right-to-left interatrial shunts.[24] Salicylates cause constriction of the fetal ductus, so the history should include enquiries about maternal use of aspirin. Salicylate levels can be determined on umbilical cord blood.[85]

PHYSICAL APPEARANCE

Maternal rubella is characterized by low birth weight and failure to thrive, irrespective of ductal patency, ductal size, or shunt volume.[86,87] An underdeveloped

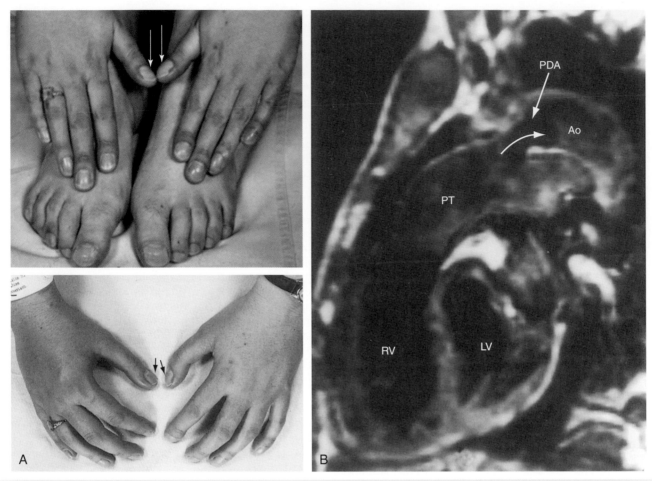

FIGURE 20-11 A, Photographs of a 28-year-old woman with patent ductus arteriosus, suprasystemic pulmonary vascular resistance, and reversed shunt. The upper photograph shows the patient sitting with her hands placed on the dorsum of her feet. The right hand is acyanotic, and the digits are not clubbed. The left hand is mildly cyanotic, and the thumb is clubbed. The toes are cyanotic and clubbed. In the close-up (lower photograph), the right hand is acyanotic, and the thumb is not clubbed (arrow). The left hand is mildly cyanotic, and the thumb is clubbed (arrow). **B,** Magnetic resonance image from a 29-year-old woman with a nonrestrictive patent ductus and reversed shunt (curved arrow) from the pulmonary trunk (PT) through a nonrestrictive patent ductus arteriosus (PDA) into the aorta (Ao). (RV/LV = right ventricle/ left ventricle.)

child with a patent ductus should therefore be examined for cataracts, deafness, and mental retardation (see Figure 20-9).[86,87] Another distinctive phenotype is the clinodactly (overlapping fingers), rocker bottom feet, and lax skin of *Trisomy 18* (Figure 20-12).[88,89] *Char syndrome* is an inherited disorder that maps to chromosome 6p12-p21 and is characterized by ptosis, a flat profile, a very short philtrum, patulous duck-bill lips, facial dysmorphism, and abnormalities of the hands.[90–93] The recurrence rate in offspring of an affected parent is 50%.[92]

Differential cyanosis and clubbing are important physical signs of patent ductus with reversed shunt (see Figures 20-2 and 20-11; see previous).[79,94] The toes are cyanosed and clubbed because unsaturated blood is selectively delivered to the lower extremities. A small amount of unsaturated blood often enters the left subclavian artery, so the digits of the left hand, especially the thumb, are mildly cyanosed and clubbed (see Figure 20-11A) The fingers of the right hand are normal because unsaturated blood does not reach the right subclavian artery. In the rare presence of *bilateral* patent ductuses with reversed shunt, the *right* arm is cyanosed because the right subclavian artery receives desaturated blood from the pulmonary artery via the right ductus arteriosus.[12]

Patients who are old enough to follow instructions should be examined sitting or squatting with their hands placed alongside their feet or on the dorsum of their feet to facilitate comparison of fingers and toes (see Figure 20-11A). The right and left thumbs should be compared (see Figure 20-11A). Differential cyanosis is exaggerated by isotonic exercise or by warming the hands and feet, which are maneuvers that increase skin blood flow and exaggerate the color differences. In neonates with persistent fetal circulation, the right-to-left ductal shunt may cause distinctive differential cyanosis confined to the head, right shoulder, and right arm with a demarcation line that runs obliquely from above the left shoulder to below the right axilla.[18]

Healthy individuals, especially young women, may have *peripheral* cyanosis of the feet because of

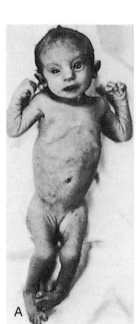

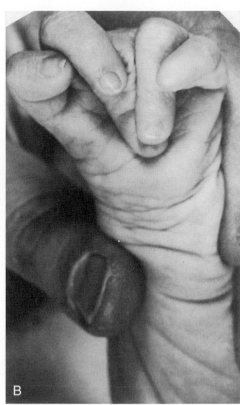

FIGURE 20-12 A, Photographs of a female infant with patent ductus arteriosus, ventricular septal defect, and the physical appearance of trisomy 18 with lax skin and overlapping fingers (clinodactly). **B,** Rocker-bottom feet in **A** are shown.

vasoconstriction, a mechanism that is suspected when the feet are cold. Diagnostic error is prevented by warming the extremities, which abolishes peripheral cyanosis but exaggerates central cyanosis.

ARTERIAL PULSE

Wide systemic pulse pressure is an important physical sign of patent ductus arteriosus with a large left-to-right shunt.[40,94] This sign is especially useful in symptomatic neonates without a ductus murmur. However, the arterial pulse may be weak in preterm infants in whom systemic flow is reduced by the *steal* effect associated with aortopulmonary shunting (see previous).[37,38] The typical pulse is characterized by a brisk rise, a single or bisferiens peak, and a rapid collapse (Figure 20-13). Diastolic flow from aortic root into pulmonary trunk lowers the aortic *diastolic* pressure, and a large left ventricular stroke volume with forceful left ventricular contraction maintains or elevates aortic *systolic* pressure. The carotid, brachial, femoral, and even dorsalis pedis pulses can be bounding.[94] The superficial palmar arch as it crosses the heads of the metacarpals is sometimes evident as a visible pulsation. In a child with a large patent ductus, an erythematous wheal caused by a mosquito bite blushed and blanched synchronously with the pulse.[95]

When pulmonary vascular disease reverses the shunt, the arterial pulse is usually normal. However, in the presence of pulmonary hypertensive *pulmonary* regurgitation, the aortic diastolic pressure is lowered and the pulse pressure widens because diastolic flow is from the aorta through the ductus into the pulmonary artery, across the incompetent pulmonary valve, and into the right ventricle.

JUGULAR VENOUS PULSE

Congestive heart failure is accompanied by a rise in mean jugular venous pressure with an increase in the A and V waves. When suprasystemic pulmonary vascular resistance reverses the shunt, the A wave is relatively unimpressive because the right ventricle adapts to systemic vascular resistance without augmented right atrial contraction.

PRECORDIAL MOVEMENT AND PALPATION

George A. Gibson[96] wrote, "When the ductus arteriosus is permanently patent, a very distinct thrill is to be felt—a thrill which distinctly follows the systole of the heart and persists until the diastolic phase has existed for some time."[2]

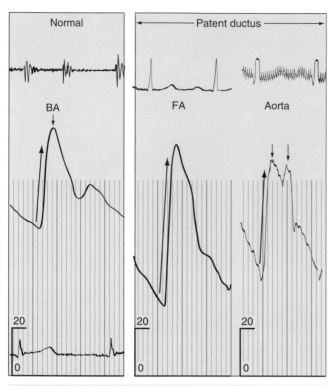

FIGURE 20-13 Femoral arterial (FA) and central aortic pulses in two patients aged 18 months and 22 months, both with a nonrestrictive patent ductus arteriosus and large left-to-right shunts. Pulse pressures are wide with a brisk rate of rise, a single or bisferiens (twin) peak, and a rapid collapse. A normal brachial arterial pulse in the left panel is shown for comparison.

A *moderately* restrictive patent ductus is accompanied by volume overload of the left ventricle and a dynamic left ventricular impulse. A right ventricular impulse is relatively unimpressive because pressure overload of the right ventricle is only moderate.

A *nonrestrictive ductus* with low pulmonary vascular resistance results in appreciable volume overload of the left ventricle and systemic systolic pressure in the right ventricle. The left ventricular impulse is hyperdynamic, and the right ventricular impulse is sustained. A dilated pulmonary trunk and a loud pulmonary closure sound are palpable together. If a thrill is present, it is likely to be confined to systole (see section Auscultation). When flow through the ductus is reversed, pulmonary hypertension exists without volume overload of the left ventricle, so palpation detects only a right ventricular impulse. Symptomatic infants with a nonrestrictive patent ductus and low pulmonary vascular resistance have a hyperdynamic volume-overloaded left ventricular impulse accompanied by the conspicuous impulse of a hypertensive failing right ventricle.

AUSCULTATION

In 1900, Gibson[96] characterized the murmur of patent ductus arteriosus:"It persists through the second sound and dies away gradually during the long pause. The murmur is rough and thrilling. It begins softly and increases in intensity so as to reach its acme just about, or immediately after the incidence of the second sound, and from that point gradually wanes until its termination."

Gibson's description cannot be improved on. Although he was not the first to describe the continuous murmur of patent ductus, he precisely characterized the murmur and confidently established the clinical diagnosis based on that characterization.[2] The classic murmur of uncomplicated patent ductus arteriosus rises to a peak in latter systole; continues without interruption through the second sound, which it envelops; and then declines in intensity during the course of diastole (Figures 20-14, 20-15, and 20-16). The murmur can occupy the entire cardiac cycle (see Figure 20-14), or the end of diastole or early systole can be murmur-free (see Figure 20-15). The term continuous is best applied to the uninterrupted progression of the murmur through the second heart sound and not to the presence of murmur throughout the cardiac cycle.[94] The ductus murmur is therefore considered continuous even when late diastole and early systole are murmur-free.

High-velocity flow through a restrictive ductus generates a relatively soft high-frequency continuous murmur. A moderately restrictive ductus generates a loud coarse

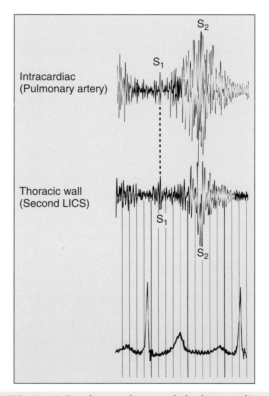

FIGURE 20-14 Simultaneously recorded phonocardiograms from within the pulmonary artery and on the thoracic wall at the second left intercostal space of a 7-year-old girl with a moderately restrictive patent ductus arteriosus and a 2 to 1 left-to-right shunt. In Gibson's words, the murmur "begins softly and increases in intensity so as to reach its acme just about, or immediately after the incidence of the second heart sound, and from that point gradually wanes until its termination."[96]

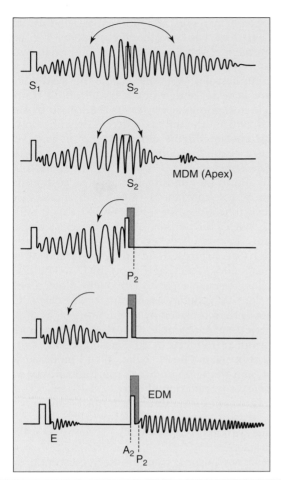

FIGURE 20-15 Schematic sequential modifications of the murmur of patent ductus from a nonpulmonary hypertensive left-to-right shunt (top) to a pulmonary hypertensive right-to-left shunt (bottom). (MDM = mid-diastolic murmur; EDM = early diastolic murmur; A₂/P₂= aortic and pulmonary components of the second heart sound.)

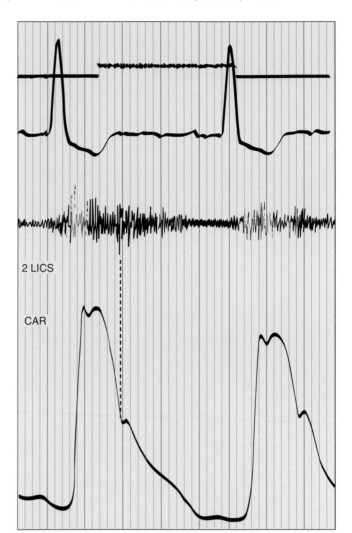

FIGURE 20-16 Tracings from an 84-year-old woman with a moderately restrictive patent ductus arteriosus (see x-ray in Figure 20-38). The murmur in the second left intercostal space (2 LICS) continues through the second heart sound that was timed by the dicrotic notch of the carotid pulse (CAR). The continuous murmur then faded, rendering late diastole murmur-free.

machinery murmur punctuated with *eddy sounds* that are randomly distributed in the second half of systole and in the first half of diastole (Figure 20-17A).[44,94] Intracardiac phonocardiography records the maximal intensity of the ductus murmur in the pulmonary artery at the pulmonary ostium of the ductus (see Figure 20-14). Intraoperative phonocardiograms from the surface of the pulmonary trunk are in accord with this localization,[97] and these observations coincide with the chest wall position of the ductus murmur, which is loudest in the first or second intercostal space or beneath the left clavicle as Gibson originally stated.[2]

Occasionally, a short large ductus is devoid of murmur despite a substantial left-to-right shunt (Figure 20-18). Ductal murmurs are often absent in infants with a nonrestrictive patent ductus and congestive heart failure (see Figure 20-10) and in a significant number of preterm infants with respiratory distress.[98] Failure to detect a murmur, a silent but patent ductus, does not necessarily mean that the ductus has closed (see section The History).[17,43,99] A relatively rare auscultatory variation is *intermittent disappearance and*

reappearance of an otherwise typical continuous ductal murmur.[52,100,101] Interruption of flow has been ascribed to acute angulations of an elongated ductus[100,101] or to a valve or veil-like structure within the ductus (see previous).[52] A similar mechanism has been proposed for the transient diastolic ductal murmur of the neonate.[102] Reappearance of a continuous murmur long after ductal closure has been ascribed to reopening caused by a tear in the valve of the ductus[50] or to spontaneous intramural dissection.

The shape, length, and timing of the murmur of patent ductus arteriosus depend on instantaneous differences in pressure and flow between the aorta and pulmonary trunk (see Figure 20-15).[103,104] At the beginning of systole, flow into the pulmonary artery is derived from the right ventricle rather than the ductus. During the course of systole, the flow contribution from the ductus

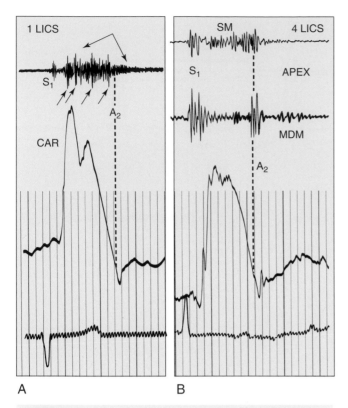

A   B

FIGURE 20-17 Tracings from an 18-year-old woman with a nonrestrictive patent ductus arteriosus and increased pulmonary vascular resistance, but a 2.3 to 1 left-to-right shunt. **A,** The ductus murmur in the first left intercostal space (1 LICS) continued (paired arrows) for a short time after the aortic component of the second heart sound (A_2). Eddy sounds (lower arrows) punctuate the murmur. (CAR = carotid pulse.) **B,** In the fourth left intercostal space (4 LICS), the ductus murmur is holosystolic (SM) and devoid of eddy sounds. The short, low-frequency, mid-diastolic murmur (MDM) at the apex was caused by augmented flow across the mitral valve.

progressively increases, and during diastole, flow into the pulmonary artery is from the ductus alone.[94,105] *Systolic reinforcement* of the ductus murmur described by Skoda occurs because flow from aorta into pulmonary trunk is greater in systole, especially when the systemic pulse pressure is wide, and because systolic flow from right ventricle into pulmonary artery is reinforced by simultaneous flow from the ductus, whereas diastolic flow is derived from the ductus alone. As pulmonary vascular resistance rises, the pulmonary arterial and aortic diastolic pressures equalize (Figure 20-19) and diastolic ductal flow diminishes and finally vanishes, so the diastolic portion of the continuous murmur disappears, leaving a holosystolic murmur (Figures 20-15, 20-20, and 20-21). With a further increase in pulmonary vascular resistance, the systolic portion of the ductus murmur shortens (see Figures 20-15 and 20-21) and ultimately disappears altogether (see Figure 20-15). The ductus is then silent because right-to-left ductal flow, a reversed shunt, does not generate a murmur.[105] The classic Gibson murmur is then replaced by auscultatory signs of pulmonary hypertension: namely, a short pulmonary midsystolic murmur introduced by an ejection sound, a single or closely split second heart sound, a loud pulmonary component, and the Graham Steell murmur of hypertensive pulmonary regurgitation (Figures 20-15 and 20-22).[105] The diagnosis of patent ductus arteriosus cannot be based on auscultatory signs but can confidently be based on *differential cyanosis* (see Figure 20-11; see section Physical Appearance).

In the newborn, a transient soft crescendo systolic murmur from left-to-right flow through the ductus is sometimes detected before normal physiologic closure.[106-108] The murmur ends with the second sound or continues just beyond it.[106] These harmless transient neonatal murmurs are physiologically analogous to the not so harmless murmurs that appear when patent ductus

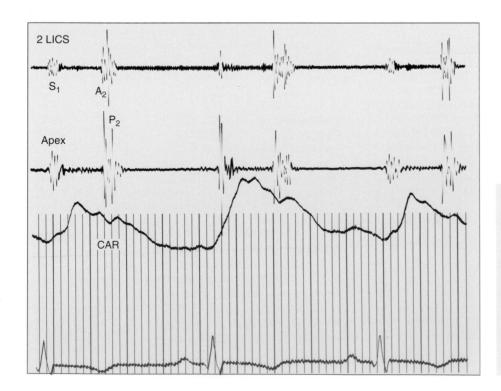

FIGURE 20-18 Tracings from a 30-year-old man with an unusually large, short patent ductus. Despite a 2 to 1 left-to-right shunt, a ductus murmur was neither heard nor recorded. (2 LICS = second left intercostal space.) Relatively wide expiratory splitting of the second heart sound was caused by delay in the loud pulmonary component (P_2) that was transmitted to the apex. (S_1 = first heart sound; A_2 = aortic component of the second sound; CAR = carotid pulse.)

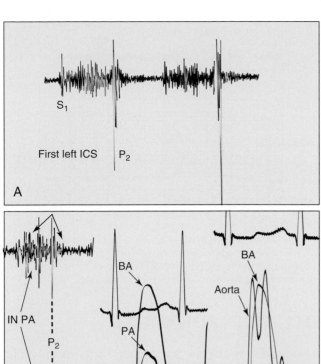

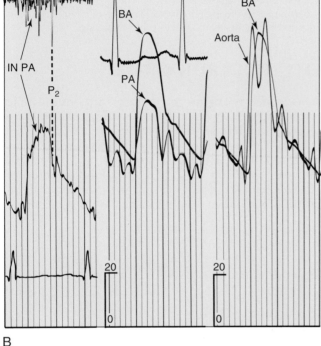

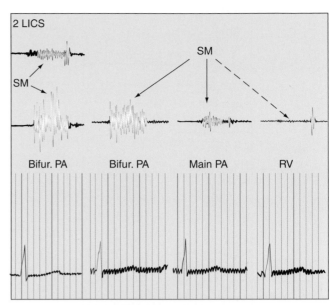

FIGURE 20-20 Phonocardiograms from an 11-year-old girl with a nonrestrictive patent ductus arteriosus and increased pulmonary vascular resistance, but a 2 to 1 left-to-right shunt. The upper left panel shows a holosystolic ductal murmur (SM) in the second left intercostal space (2 LICS). A louder holosystolic ductal murmur was recorded from within the pulmonary artery at its bifurcation (Bifur. PA). The remaining panels show the intracardiac the murmur fading then vanishing as the catheter tip microphone was withdrawn from the bifurcation of the pulmonary artery to the main pulmonary artery and into right ventricle (RV).

FIGURE 20-19 Tracings from a 15-year-old boy with a nonrestrictive patent ductus arteriosus and increased pulmonary vascular resistance, but a 2 to 1 left-to-right shunt. **A,** The ductus murmur in the first left intercostal space (ICS) continued through the timing of the second heart sound (paired arrows) but faded well before the subsequent first heart sound (S₁). **B,** An identical murmur was recorded within the pulmonary artery (IN PA) at its bifurcation. The brachial arterial (BA) and pulmonary arterial (PA) pulses diverge in systole but converge in diastole (center panel), so the ductus murmur is maximal in systole and minimal in diastole (left panel). The right panel shows relatively low diastolic pressures in the brachial artery and in the aorta with a bisferiens (twin-peaked) pulse in the central aorta.

When the left-to-right shunt is large, apical mid-diastolic murmurs are generated by increased flow across the mitral valve.[105] These murmurs cannot not heard unless the diastolic portion of the continuous murmur is attenuated by an increase in pulmonary vascular resistance (Figures 20-15, 20-17, and 20-23).[105] In patent ductus arteriosus with *reversed* shunt, a mid-diastolic murmur has been attributed to a *right-sided Austin Flint* mechanism associated with *pulmonary* regurgitation.[109] *To-and-fro murmurs* over the cranium of infants with a nonrestrictive patent ductus arteriosus have been ascribed to accelerated forward flow followed by rapid diastolic runoff.

The second heart sound is occasionally paradoxically split when the left-to-right shunt is large.[110] Prolonged left ventricular ejection and short right ventricular ejection are held responsible.[40,110] A loud continuous murmur punctuated by eddy sounds obscures the second heart sound. An increase in pulmonary vascular resistance renders the second sound audible because the diastolic portion of the continuous murmur softens or disappears (see Figures 20-15, 20-17, and 20-19). When the shunt is reversed, the second sound is single or closely split, and the pulmonary component is loud (see Figure 20-15). The second sound is widely split when depressed right ventricular contractility and prolonged right ventricular ejection delay the pulmonary component (see Figures 20-22 and 20-23).

arteriosus is subsequently accompanied by a rise in pulmonary vascular resistance. Even when a ductus is destined to remain patent, the neonatal ductal murmur is initially systolic and becomes continuous only after pulmonary vascular resistance has fallen sufficiently to permit both systolic *and* diastolic ductal flow.

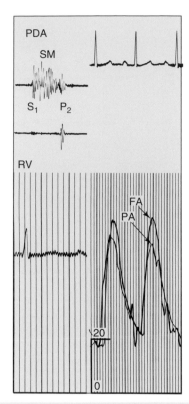

FIGURE 20-21 Tracings from a 3-year-old girl with a nonrestrictive patent ductus and increased pulmonary vascular resistance but a 2.7 to 1 left-to-right shunt. The intracardiac microphone recorded a decrescendo holosystolic murmur *within the lumen* of the patent ductus arteriosus (PDA). The right ventricle (RV) was silent except for the pulmonary component of the second heart sound (P₂). The femoral arterial (FA) and pulmonary arterial (PA) pulses diverge in systole but are identical in diastole, so the ductus murmur was confined to systole.

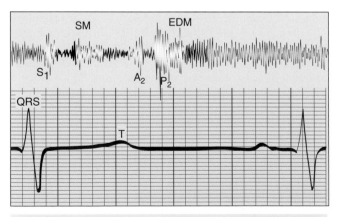

FIGURE 20-22 Phonocardiogram from the second left intercostal space of a 26-year-old woman with a nonrestrictive patent ductus, suprasystemic pulmonary vascular resistance, and reversed shunt. A midsystolic murmur (SM) originated in the dilated hypertensive pulmonary trunk. A Graham Steell murmur (EDM) issued from a loud delayed pulmonary component of the second heart sound (P₂). (S₁ = first heart sound; A₂ = aortic component of the second sound.)

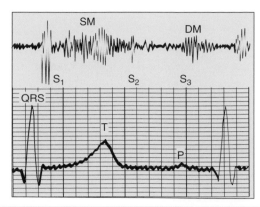

FIGURE 20-23 Phonocardiogram at the apex of a 5-year-old girl with a nonrestrictive patent ductus and a 3 to 1 left-to-right shunt. The systolic portion of the ductus murmur (SM) was transmitted to the apex where a prominent middiastolic murmur (DM) was caused by augmented flow across the mitral valve.

ELECTROCARDIOGRAM

A *moderately restrictive* patent ductus arteriosus with increased pulmonary blood flow is accompanied by a prolonged bifid left atrial P wave in one or more limb leads and in right precordial leads (Figures 20-24 and 20-25). The PR interval is prolonged in 10% to 20% of cases (see Figure 20-24).[111] Atrial fibrillation occurs in older patients. The QRS axis is usually normal, but an occasional infant has right axis deviation, especially

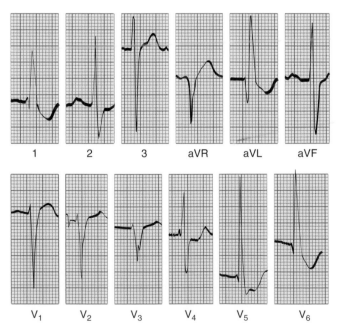

FIGURE 20-24 Electrocardiogram from a 37-year-old woman with a moderately restrictive patent ductus arteriosus, a 2.8 to 1 left-to-right shunt, and a pulmonary arterial pressure of 48/18 mm Hg (see x-ray in Figure 20-32). There is a broad bifid left atrial P wave in lead 2. The PR interval is 200 msec. The QRS is prolonged, and the axis is horizontal. Left ventricular volume overload is manifested by prominent q waves in leads aVL and V₆ and by tall R waves and ST-T wave changes in lead aVL and in leads V₄₋₆.

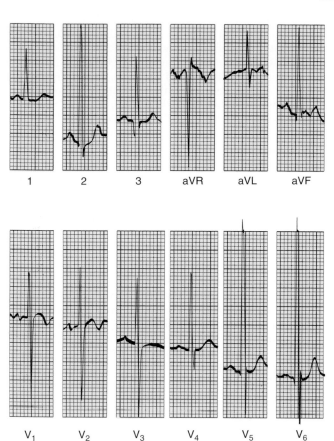

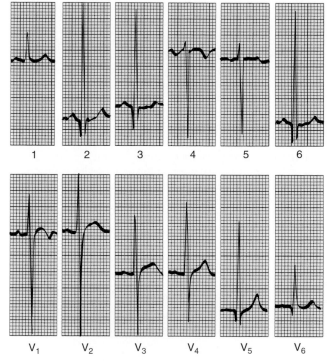

FIGURE 20-25 Electrocardiogram from a 19-month-old male with a moderately restrictive patent ductus, a 3 to 1 left-to-right shunt, and a pulmonary arterial pressure of 45/22 mm Hg (see x-ray in Figure 20-31). There are biphasic left atrial P waves in leads V_{1-2}. Because the QRS axis is normal, the tall R waves of left ventricular volume overload appear in leads 2 and aVF. Volume overload of the left ventricle is also manifested by tall R waves and upright T waves in leads V_{5-6}. Right ventricular hypertrophy is manifested by prominent S waves in leads V_{5-6} and a prominent R wave in lead V_1. Leads V_{2-3} are half standardized and exhibit large RS complexes of biventricular hypertrophy.

FIGURE 20-26 Electrocardiogram from a 16-year-old boy with a moderately restrictive patent ductus, pulmonary arterial pressure of 80/50 mm Hg, and a 2 to 1 left-to-right shunt. The QRS axis is normal and depolarization is clockwise, so prominent q waves and tall R waves of left ventricular volume overload appear in leads 2, 3, and aVF. Volume overload of the left ventricle is also manifested by the deep S wave in lead V_1 and by prominent q waves, tall R waves, and peaked upright T waves in leads V_{5-6}. Biventricular hypertrophy is reflected in the large RS complexes in leads V_{2-4}, which are half standardized.

neonates with respiratory distress. Rare examples of left axis deviation have been reported.[112] The rubella syndrome may be associated with an unusually superior QRS axis directed upward and either to the left or right.[113]

A *nonrestrictive* patent ductus with low pulmonary vascular resistance is associated with biatrial P waves and combined ventricular hypertrophy. Large equidiphasic RS complexes appear in most if not all precordial leads, with tall R waves and prominent S waves in leads V_{5-6} (Figures 20-25 and 20-26). Volume overload of the left ventricle is responsible for tall R waves, prominent q waves, and tall peaked T waves in leads V_{5-6} (see Figures 20-25 and 20-26).

Patent ductus with *pulmonary vascular disease and reversed shunt* is accompanied by peaked right atrial P waves in leads 2, 3, and V_1 (Figure 20-27). Right ventricular hypertrophy is manifested by right axis deviation, tall R waves in lead V_1, and inverted right precordial T waves and is prominent in left precordial leads S waves (see Figure 20-27). R waves in leads V_{5-6} imply that a left-to-right shunt previously existed (see Figure 20-27).

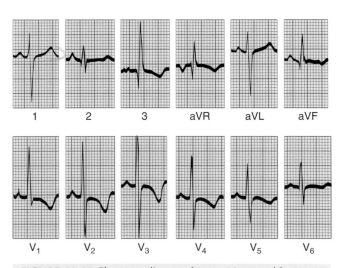

FIGURE 20-27 Electrocardiogram from a 28-year-old woman with a non-restrictive patent ductus, suprasystemic pulmonary vascular resistance, and reversed shunt. Peaked right atrial P waves are present in lead 2 and leads V_{1-2}. Isolated right ventricular hypertrophy is manifested by right axis deviation, tall monophasic R waves, and inverted T waves in leads V_{1-4} and prominent S waves in left precordial leads.

X-RAY

The ductus itself is occasionally seen in the frontal projection as an inconspicuous soft convexity between the aortic knob and the pulmonary artery segment (Figures 20-5A and 20-28).[114] A striking exaggeration of this inconspicuous shadow is an aneurysm of a nonpatent ductus (see Figure 20-6). Calcium appears in the ductus of older patients (Figure 20-29; see Figure 20-38A).[115]

A *moderately restrictive* patent ductus with low pulmonary vascular resistance results in increased pulmonary arterial vascularity, enlargement of the pulmonary trunk and its proximal branches, and enlargement of the left atrium and left ventricle (Figures 20-30, 20-31 and 20-32).[114] Asymmetric pulmonary vascularity is occasionally represented by a hyperlucent left lung.[116] In infants, the ascending aorta is inconspicuous because intrauterine ductal flow does not traverse the aorta (see

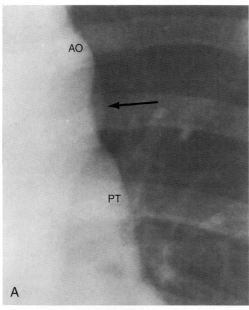

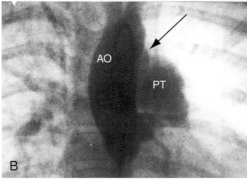

FIGURE 20-28 **A,** Close-up of a portion of the chest x-ray in the 14-year-old girl whose aortogram is shown in Figure 20-3. The soft convex shadow of the patent ductus (arrow) is located between the aortic knuckle (AO) and pulmonary trunk (PT). The convex shadow represents the dilated aortic end of the conical ductus shown in the aortogram of Figure 20-3. **B,** Aortogram in a 5-year-old girl. The convex shadow of a conical ductus (arrow) located between the aortic knuckle (AO) and the pulmonary trunk (PT). Compare with Figure 20-5.

Figures 20-5 and 20-30). After birth, left-to-right ductal flow recirculates through the aortic root, so the ascending aorta becomes prominent (see Figure 20-3).[117] In infants and children with a *nonrestrictive* patent ductus and low pulmonary vascular resistance, pulmonary arterial vascularity is markedly increased and all four cardiac chambers are enlarged (Figure 20-33).

The x-ray of a *nonrestrictive patent ductus with reversed shunt* exhibits reduced pulmonary vascularity, dilation of the pulmonary trunk and its proximal branches, a normal or near normal left ventricle and left atrium, and an hypertrophied but not significantly dilated right ventricle (Figure 20-34).

ECHOCARDIOGRAM

Echocardiography with color flow imaging and Doppler interrogation establishes the size of the patent ductus (Figure 20-35), the flow dynamics through the ductus, and the physiologic consequences of persistent ductal patency.[103,104,118] Transesophageal echocardiography improves diagnostic accuracy.[119] When the shunt is entirely left-to-right, the flow disturbance within the ductus is continuous, with the peak velocity reinforced in latter systole as forward flow from the right ventricle coincides with shunt flow through the ductus (Figure 20-36).[103,104] Systolic forward flow in the aorta distal to the orifice of the ductus is followed by reversed diastolic flow (Figure 20-37). In the presence of large ductal flow, the velocities across the aortic isthmus and in the descending aorta are substantially increased.[120] The color flow pattern in the pulmonary trunk consists of a ductal jet that adheres the lateral wall, travels toward the pulmonary valve, and then reverses itself to travel up the medial wall (Figure 20-38 and Video 20-1). Alternatively, a jet directed toward the pulmonary valve adheres to the medial wall of the pulmonary trunk (Figure 20-39).

Color flow imaging with Doppler interrogation identifies a clinically silent nonrestrictive patent ductus in premature infants[33,42] and detects the tiny clinically silent ductus in adults (Figure 20-40 and Video 20-2).[67] *In utero* ductal closure can be recognized with fetal echocardiography.[121,122] The reversed shunt in a nonrestrictive patent ductus with suprasystemic pulmonary vascular resistance can be identified with Doppler interrogation[103] and contrast echocardiography.[123] Right ventricular systolic pressure and pulmonary arterial diastolic pressure are estimated with continuous-wave Doppler interrogation of the jets of tricuspid and pulmonary regurgitation and with Doppler velocities across the ductus.

SUMMARY

Clinical suspicion of patent ductus arteriosus is heightened by premature birth, maternal rubella, or birth at high altitude. In most patients with a *moderately restrictive* patent ductus, the clinical signs are unmistakable. The arterial pulse is brisk, the pulse pressure is wide, the left

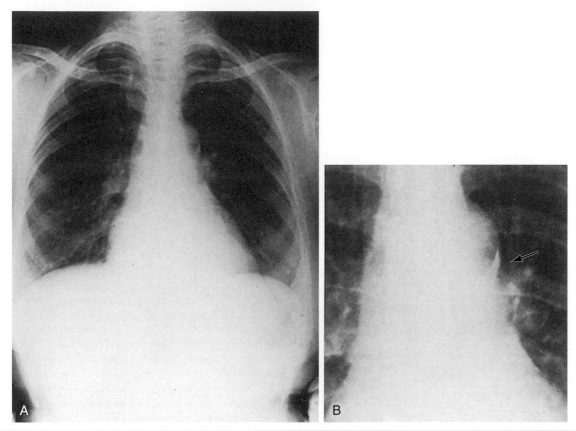

FIGURE 20-29 X-ray from a 63-year-old woman with a restrictive patent ductus and a left-to-right shunt of 1.3 to 1. **A,** Ductal calcification is the comma-like density between the aortic knuckle and the main pulmonary artery segment. **B,** Close-up of the ductal calcification (arrow). The x-ray was otherwise normal.

ventricular impulse is dynamic, and auscultation detects the distinctive continuous Gibson murmur that peaks around the second heart sound and is punctuated by eddy sounds. The electrocardiogram reflects volume overload of the left ventricle, and the x-ray shows increased pulmonary arterial vascularity with enlargement of the left

ventricle, left atrium, ascending aorta, and pulmonary trunk. Echocardiography with color flow imaging and Doppler interrogation establishes the size of the ductus and the flow dynamics within the ductus and within the contiguous aorta and pulmonary trunk and establishes the hemodynamic consequences of ductal patency.

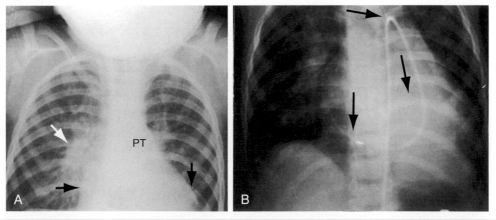

FIGURE 20-30 X-rays from a 13-month-old female with a moderately restrictive patent ductus arteriosus, pulmonary arterial pressure of 39/15 mm Hg, and a 2.3 to 1 left-to-right shunt. **A,** Pulmonary vascularity is increased and the pulmonary trunk (PT) and its right branch (white arrow) are prominent, but the ascending aorta is inconspicuous. The left cardiac border formed by a dilated left ventricle (vertical black arrow) and the right cardiac border is formed by a dilated right atrium (horizontal black arrow). **B,** The femoral artery catheter passed through the ductus (first acute bend, horizontal arrow), into the pulmonary trunk, across the pulmonary valve into the right ventricle (right vertical arrow), and finally across the tricuspid valve into the right atrium where the tip lies (left vertical arrow).

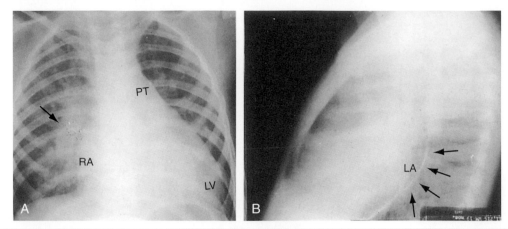

FIGURE 20-31 X-rays from a 19-month-old male with a nonrestrictive patent ductus and a 3 to 1 left-to-right shunt. The electrocardiogram is shown in Figure 20-25. **A,** The increased pulmonary vascularity is both arterial and venous. The pulmonary trunk (PT) and its right branch (arrow) are dilated. The apex is formed by an enlarged left ventricle (LV), and the right cardiac border is formed by a dilated right atrium (RA). **B,** The lateral barium esophagram outlines a moderately enlarged left atrium (LA).

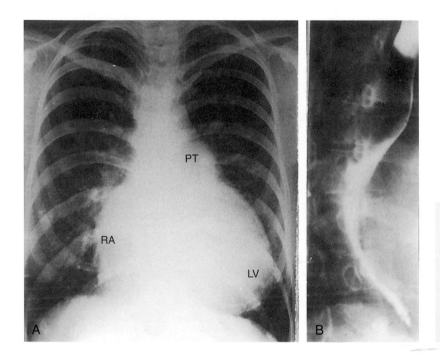

FIGURE 20-32 **A,** X-rays from a 37-year-old woman with a moderately restrictive patent ductus and a 2.8 to 1 left-to-right shunt. The electrocardiogram is shown in Figure 20-24. Pulmonary vascularity is increased, the pulmonary trunk (PT) is prominent, the apex is occupied by a dilated convex left ventricle (LV), and the right cardiac border is formed by a dilated right atrium (RA). **B,** Lateral barium esophagram outlines an enlarged left atrium.

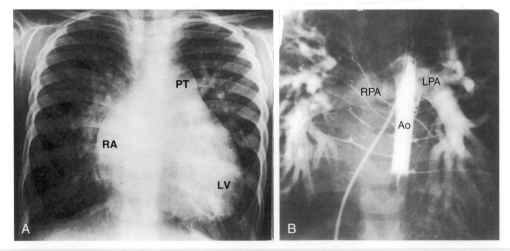

FIGURE 20-33 **A,** X-ray from a 3-year-old boy with a nonrestrictive patent ductus, low pulmonary vascular resistance, and a 3 to 1 left-to-right shunt (see Figure 20-5 for angiocardiograms). Pulmonary blood flow is increased, the pulmonary trunk (PT) is dilated, an enlarged left ventricle (LV) occupies the apex, and an enlarged right atrium (RA) forms the right cardiac border. **B,** The right pulmonary artery (RPA) and left pulmonary artery (LPA) are visualized through the patent ductus after contrast material was injected into the balloon-occluded descending aorta (Ao). The intrapulmonary arteries are strikingly enlarged. Compare with the increased pulmonary vascularity in **A.**

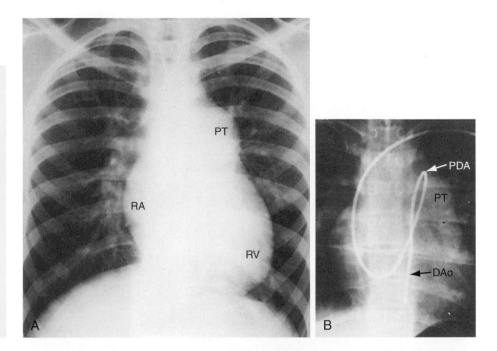

FIGURE 20-34 X-rays from a 14-year-old boy with a nonrestrictive patent ductus, suprasystemic pulmonary vascular resistance, and reversed shunt. **A,** Pulmonary vascularity is decreased, the pulmonary trunk (PT) and its proximal branches are enlarged, the right atrium (RA) is prominent, and the hypertrophied right ventricle (RV) forms an acute angle with the left hemidiaphragm. **B,** A catheter from the left median basilic vein entered the pulmonary trunk (PT), crossed the ductus, and came to rest in the descending aorta (DAo). The course of the catheter represents the pathway taken by unoxygenated blood through a reversed ductal shunt (see Figure 20-2, *lower,* and Figure 20-11A).

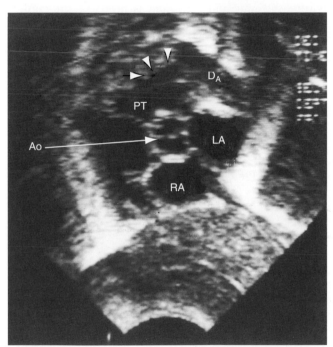

FIGURE 20-35 Echocardiogram of a moderately restrictive patent ductus (three arrowheads) in a 2-month-old infant. (Ao = aortic valve; PT = pulmonary trunk; DA = descending aorta; RA/LA = right atrium and left atrium.)

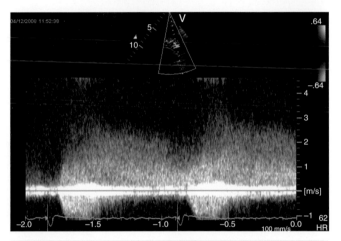

FIGURE 20-36 Continuous-wave Doppler scan from a 7-month-old female with a moderately restrictive patent ductus.

In infants, a *nonrestrictive* patent ductus with low pulmonary vascular resistance presents with congestive heart failure. An incriminating ductus murmur is often absent, but the arterial pulses are bounding and the left and right ventricular impulses are hyperdynamic. Echocardiography establishes the diagnosis.

In a *nonrestrictive* patent ductus with suprasystemic pulmonary vascular resistance and *reversed* shunt, the ductus murmur is absent, but the diagnosis is confidently made based on distinctive differential cyanosis. The toes are cyanosed and clubbed, but the fingers are spared. The clinical signs are those of pure pulmonary hypertension. The electrocardiogram shows right ventricular hypertrophy with little or no volume overload of the left ventricle. The x-ray exhibits normal or reduced pulmonary vascularity, dilation of the pulmonary trunk, and an unimpressive cardiac silhouette. Echocardiography with color flow and contrast imaging confirms the diagnosis.

AORTOPULMONARY WINDOW

In a lecture delivered in 1830 at the St Thomas Hospital, London, Professor John Elliotson[124] described the first known case of aortopulmonary window, often called aortopulmonary or aorticopulmonary septal defect. This uncommon malformation consists of a communication,

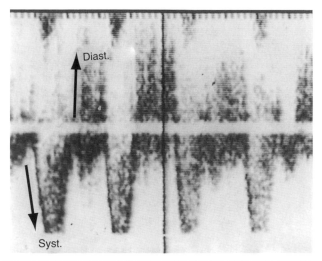

FIGURE 20-37 Pulsed Doppler scan from a 6-month-old female with a moderately restrictive patent ductus and a 2.8 to 1 left-to-right shunt. Sample volume in the descending aorta distal to the ductus recorded systolic flow (Syst.) *down* the aorta and diastolic flow (Diast.) in the opposite direction.

usually nonrestrictive, between adjacent walls of the ascending aorta and pulmonary trunk. During early embryogenesis, two opposing proximal truncal cushions rapidly enlarge and fuse to form the *truncal septum* that partitions the truncus arteriosus into aortic and pulmonary channels.[125–127] The distal truncoaortic sac is then divided by the *aortopulmonary septum*. Maldevelopment of the truncal and aortopulmonary septum results in three morphologic types of aortopulmonary window, namely[125]: (1) nonfusion of the embryonic aortopulmonary septum and the truncal septum that results in a moderate-sized circular defect located about midway between the great arterial valves and the bifurcation of the pulmonary trunk; (2) malalignment of the embryonic aortopulmonary septum and truncal septum that results in a defect similarly located but helical-shaped; and (3) complete absence of the embryonic aortopulmonary septum that results in a nonrestrictive defect. The morphogenesis of an aortopulmonary window is unrelated to the morphogenesis of a patent ductus arteriosus, but the physiologic consequences and clinical manifestations of the two malformations are similar if not identical,[128,129] so inclusion in this chapter is appropriate.

Because an aortopulmonary window tends to be nonrestrictive, it is often mistaken for a nonrestrictive patent ductus, which is the most frequent coexisting anomaly, estimated to have an incidence rate of 12% (Figure 20-41).[129] When pulmonary vascular resistance is suprasystemic and the shunt is reversed, the clinical picture is indistinguishable from a nonrestrictive ventricular septal defect with Eisenmenger's syndrome (see Chapter 17).[79] An aortopulmonary window and a ventricular septal defect can coexist, albeit rarely.[130]

Aortopulmonary window is somewhat more frequent in males in contrast to patent ductus.[128] Also in contrast

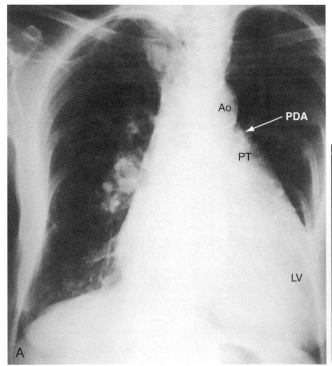

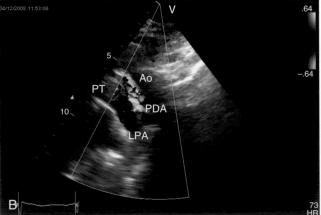

FIGURE 20-38 A, X-ray from the 84-year-old woman with a moderately restrictive patent ductus arteriosus (PDA) whose phonocardiogram is shown in Figure 20-16. The pulmonary trunk (PT) and its right branch are dilated. A thin rim of calcium appears in the transverse aorta (Ao). An enlarged left ventricle (LV) occupies the apex, and an enlarged right atrium occupies the lower right cardiac border. **B,** Notch view of ductal flow going from aorta (Ao) to pulmonary trunk (PT) (Video 20-1). (LPA = left pulmonary artery.)

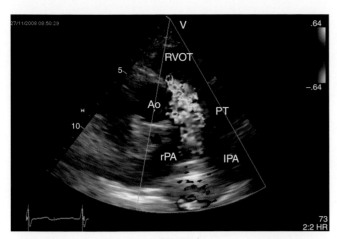

FIGURE 20-39 Color Doppler flow in a 64-year-old man with a restrictive patent ductus. Ductal flow tracts along the medial wall of the pulmonary trunk (PT) and downward toward the pulmonary valve. (rPA = right pulmonary artery; lPA = left pulmonary artery; RVOT = right ventricular outflow tract; Ao = aorta.)

to patent ductus is the rarity of infective endocarditis.[128] An appreciable percentage of infants with a nonrestrictive aortopulmonary window die of congestive heart failure in infancy or early childhood.[128] Only a minority reach teenage or young adulthood, but occasional survivals have been reported in the fourth or fifth decade.[128,131] Survival improves when the shunt is limited by a restrictive defect or curtailed by a rise in pulmonary vascular resistance. The patient referred to in Figure 20-41 lived to age 58 years with a nonrestrictive aortopulmonary window and Eisenmenger's syndrome.

A bounding arterial pulse and a wide pulse pressure are analogous to nonrestrictive patent ductus with low pulmonary vascular resistance (Figure 20-42). When an aortopulmonary window is accompanied by suprasystemic pulmonary vascular resistance and a reversed shunt, unoxygenated blood enters the ascending aorta so differential cyanosis does not occur. The clinical picture is then indistinguishable from nonrestrictive ventricular septal defect with Eisenmenger's syndrome (see Chapter 17).

A *moderately restrictive* aortopulmonary window generates a continuous murmur indistinguishable from a moderately restrictive patent ductus arteriosus.[128,132] The physiologic mechanisms responsible for variations in the murmur of a nonrestrictive aortopulmonary window are analogous to those that apply to a nonrestrictive patent ductus arteriosus (see Figure 20-15). In 80% of patients, the murmur is systolic rather than continuous (see Figure 20-42)[128] and is punctuated by eddy sounds (see Figure 20-42). When the murmur is continuous, its diastolic portion is likely to be shortened (Figure 20-43). A nonrestrictive aortopulmonary window with *suprasystemic pulmonary vascular resistance and reversed shunt* is accompanied by auscultatory signs of pulmonary hypertension. No murmur is generated across the defect. A Graham Steell murmur may appear before the shunt is reversed because of dilation of the hypertensive pulmonary trunk.

Systolic or continuous murmurs generated by an aortopulmonary window are typically maximal in the third left intercostal space.[131] A prominent *systolic* murmur at the mid to lower left sternal border invites the mistaken diagnosis of ventricular septal defect, but eddy sounds and a bounding arterial pulse should prevent error (see Figure 20-42). Apical mid-diastolic murmurs represent increased flow across the mitral valve (see Figure 20-43).

The *electrocardiogram* of a nonrestrictive aortopulmonary window with low pulmonary vascular resistance

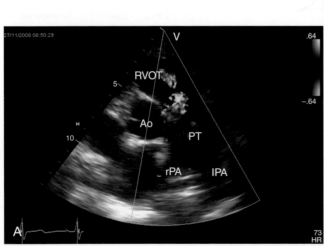
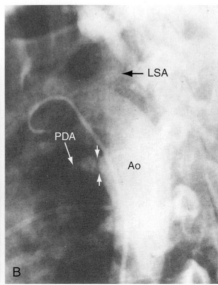

FIGURE 20-40 A, Color Doppler image from a 35-year-old man with patent ductus arteriosus. In the short-axis view, ductal flow is seen entering the pulmonary trunk (PT) toward the right ventricular outflow tract (RVOT). (Ao = aorta; rPA = right pulmonary artery; lPA = left pulmonary artery.) **B,** Lateral aortogram showing a conical ductus arteriosus (PDA) that was patent at its aortic end (Ao, paired white arrows) but was a virtual thread at its pulmonary arterial end (Video 20-2). (LSA = left subclavian artery.)

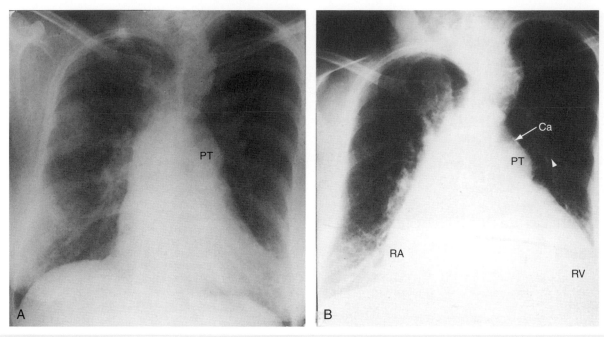

FIGURE 20-41 A, X-ray from a 51-year-old cyanotic woman with an aortopulmonary window, suprasystemic pulmonary vascular resistance, and a reversed shunt. Pulmonary vascularity is normal. The pulmonary trunk (PT) and its proximal branches are moderately enlarged, but the cardiac size and configuration are virtually normal. **B,** X-ray 5 years later after the advent of atrial fibrillation. The right ventricle (RV) and right atrium (RA) are markedly enlarged. The rim of calcium (Ca) above the dilated pulmonary trunk (PT) proved to be in a restrictive patent ductus. The unmarked arrowhead adjacent to the pulmonary trunk identifies the cross section of a dilated intrapulmonary artery. The patient died in her 58th year.

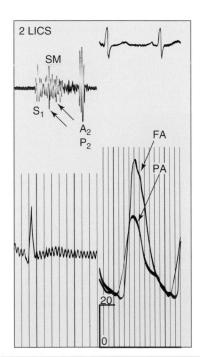

FIGURE 20-42 Tracings from a 2-year-old boy with an aortopulmonary window and a 3.4 to 1 left-to-right shunt. The phonocardiogram in the second left intercostal space (2 LICS) shows a decrescendo holosystolic murmur (SM) punctuated by eddy sounds (paired arrows). The single second heart sound is loud because the pulmonary component (P_2) was increased. The femoral arterial (FA) and pulmonary arterial (PA) pressure pulses diverge in systole but are identical in diastole, so the murmur is confined to systole. (S_1 = first heart sound; A_2 = aortic component of the second sound.)

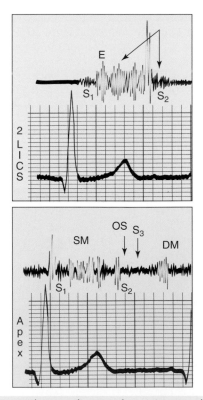

FIGURE 20-43 Phonocardiograms from a 14-year-old boy with an aortopulmonary window and a 3 to 1 left-to-right shunt. The systolic murmur (SM) in the second left intercostal space (2 LICS) continues just beyond the second heart sound (S_2, see paired arrows). (E = pulmonary ejection sound.) At the apex, a soft third heart sound (S_3) and a mid-diastolic murmur (DM) were the result of increased flow across the mitral valve. There was a faint mitral opening sound (OS).

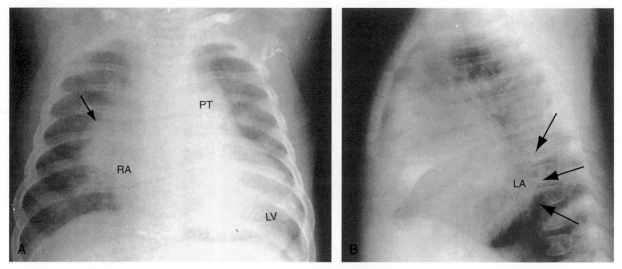

FIGURE 20-44 X-rays from a 5-month-old female with an aortopulmonary window and a 3.5 to 1 left-to-right shunt. **A,** Pulmonary vascularity is increased, pulmonary venous congestion is evident at the right hilus (arrow), the pulmonary trunk (PT) is prominent, and a dilated left ventricle (LV) occupies the apex. **B,** Lateral view shows an enlarged left atrium (LA).

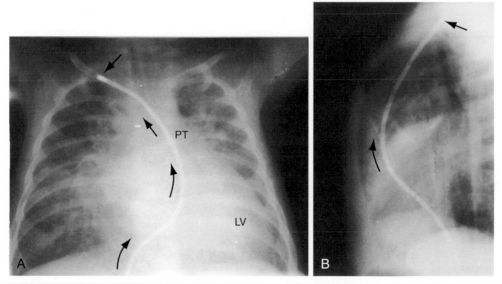

FIGURE 20-45 X-rays from a 6-month-old male with an aortopulmonary window and a 3.5 to 1 left-to-right shunt. **A,** Pulmonary arterial and pulmonary venous vascularity are markedly increased. A dilated left ventricle (LV) occupies the apex. The course of the femoral venous catheter is into the right atrium (lower left arrow), across the right ventricular outflow tract into the pulmonary trunk (PT), through the aortopulmonary window into the ascending aorta (smaller oblique arrow), and into the right subclavian artery. **B,** The lateral projection shows the catheter passing from the pulmonary trunk (curved arrow) across the aortopulmonary window into the aorta and into the right subclavian artery (upper arrow).

reflects combined ventricular hypertrophy in response to volume overload of the left ventricle and pressure overload of the right ventricle, analogous to a nonrestrictive patent ductus with low pulmonary vascular resistance (see Figure 20-25). When pulmonary vascular resistance is suprasystemic and the shunt is reversed, the electrocardiogram is analogous to nonrestrictive patent ductus with Eisenmenger's syndrome (see Figure 20-27).

The x-ray cannot distinguish a nonrestrictive aortopulmonary window with low pulmonary vascular resistance from a nonrestrictive patent ductus with large left-to-right shunt (Figures 20-44 and 20-45). When the shunt is reversed (see Figure 20-41), the x-ray resembles a nonrestrictive patent ductus with Eisenmenger's syndrome (seeFigure 20-34).

Echocardiography localizes the aortopulmonary window between the ascending aorta and pulmonary trunk just proximal to the bifurcation (Figure 20-46 and Video 20-3)[129,133,134] and determines whether a patent ductus coexists. Color flow imaging identifies the shunt as left-to-right, right-to-left (Figure 20-47 and Video 20-3), or bidirectional.

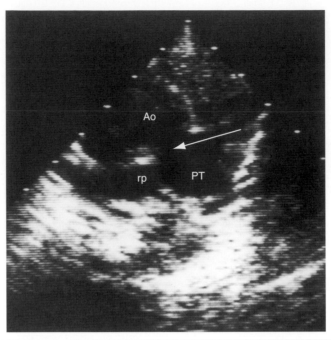

FIGURE 20-46 Echocardiogram (parasternal short-axis) from a 5-month-old female with an aortopulmonary window (arrow) between the ascending aorta (Ao) and the pulmonary trunk (PT) (Video 20-3). (rp = right pulmonary artery.)

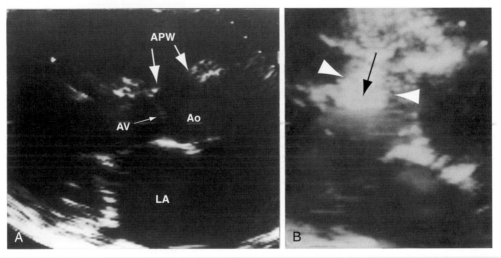

FIGURE 20-47 **A,** Echocardiogram (parasternal long-axis) from the 51-year-old patient whose x-rays are shown in Figure 20-41. Paired arrows identify the aortopulmonary window (APW). (Ao = aorta; AV = aortic valve; LA = left atrium.) **B,** Black-and-white print of a parasternal long-axis color flow image. Large white arrowheads bracket a right-to-left shunt (black arrow) through the aortopulmonary window (Video 20-3).

SUMMARY

Aortopulmonary window is an uncommon malformation that should be considered in acyanotic patients with clinical evidence of a nonrestrictive patent ductus and a large left-to-right shunt. The murmur is usually systolic rather than continuous and is maximal in the third left intercostal space. The relatively low location of the murmur arouses suspicion of ventricular septal defect, but eddy sounds and a bounding arterial pulse should prevent this error. A moderately restrictive aortopulmonary window is accompanied by a continuous murmur and clinical signs indistinguishable from a moderately restrictive patent ductus except for the relatively low precordial location of the murmur. An aortopulmonary window with suprasystemic pulmonary vascular resistance and reversed shunt is clinically indistinguishable from a nonrestrictive ventricular septal defect with Eisenmenger's syndrome. Echocardiography with color flow imaging and Doppler interrogation make the distinction.

REFERENCES

1. Castiglioni A. *A history of medicine.* New York: Alfred A. Knopf; 1947.
2. Marquis RM. The continuous murmur of persistence of the ductus arteriosus—an historical review. *Eur Heart J.* 1980;1:465–478.
3. Carlgren LE. The incidence of congenital heart disease in children born in Gothenburg 1941–1950. *Br Heart J.* 1959;21:40–50.
4. Gittenberger-De Groot AC, Strengers JL, Mentink M, Poelmann RE, Patterson DF. Histologic studies on normal and persistent ductus arteriosus in the dog. *J Am Coll Cardiol.* 1985;6:394–404.
5. Jager BV, Wollenman OJ. An anatomical study of the closure of the ductus arteriosus. *Am J Pathol.* 1942;18:595–613.
6. Dyamenahalli U, Smallhorn JF, Geva T, et al. Isolated ductus arteriosus aneurysm in the fetus and infant: a multi-institutional experience. *J Am Coll Cardiol.* 2000;36:262–269.
7. Acherman RJ, Siassi B, Wells W, et al. Aneurysm of the ductus arteriosus: a congenital lesion. *Am J Perinatol.* 1998;15:653–659
8. Sachdeva R, Smith C, Greenberg BS, Jaquiss RDB. Giant ductal aneurysm in an asymptomatic 4-year-old girl. *Ann Thorac Surg.* 2009;87:946–948.
9. Siu BL, Kovalchin JP, Kearney DL, Fraser CD, Fenrich AL. Aneurysmal dilatation of the ductus arteriosus in a neonate. *Pediatr Cardiol.* 2001;22:403–405.
10. Quiroga C. Partial persistence of the ductus arteriosus. *Acta Radiol.* 1961;55:103–108.
11. Freedom RM, Moes CA, Pelech A, et al. Bilateral ductus arteriosus (or remnant): an analysis of 27 patients. *Am J Cardiol.* 1984;53:884–891.
12. Keagy KS, Schall SA, Herrington RT. Selective cyanosis of the right arm. Isolation of right subclavian artery from aorta with bilateral ductus arteriosus and pulmonary hypertension. *Pediatr Cardiol.* 1982;3:301–303.
13. Spencer H, Dworken HJ. Congenital aortic septal defect with communication between aorta and pulmonary artery. *Circulation.* 1950;2:880–885.
14. Fu M, Hung JS, Liao PK, Chang CH. Isolated right-sided patent ductus arteriosus in right-sided aortic arch. Report of two cases. *Chest.* 1987;91:623–625.
15. Garti IJ, Aygen MM, Vidne B, Levy MJ. Right aortic arch with mirror-image branching causing vascular ring. A new classification of the right aortic arch patterns. *Br J Radiol.* 1973;46:115–119.
16. Festic E, Steiner RM, Spatz E. Aortic dissection with extension to a patent ductus arteriosus. *Int J Cardiovasc Imaging.* 2005;21:459–462.
17. Mahoney LT, Coryell KG, Lauer RM. The newborn transitional circulation: a two-dimensional Doppler echocardiographic study. *J Am Coll Cardiol.* 1985;6:623–629.
18. Gersony WM. Persistence of the fetal circulation: a commentary. *J Pediatr.* 1973;82:1103–1106.
19. Slomp J, Van Munsteren JC, Poelmann RE, De Reeder EG, Bogers AJ, Gittenberger-De Groot AC. Formation of intimal cushions in the ductus arteriosus as a model for vascular intimal thickening. An immunohistochemical study of changes in extracellular matrix components. *Atherosclerosis.* 1992;93:25–39.
20. Wilson RR. Post-mortem observations on contraction of the human ductus arteriosus. *Br Med J.* 1958;1:810–812.
21. Gittenberger-De Groot AC. Persistent ductus arteriosus: most probably a primary congenital malformation. *Br Heart J.* 1977;39:610–618.
22. Gittenberger-De Groot AC, Moulaert AJ, Hitchcock JF. Histology of the persistent ductus arteriosus in cases of congenital rubella. *Circulation.* 1980;62:183–186.
23. Heymann MA, Berman Jr W, Rudolph AM, Whitman V. Dilatation of the ductus arteriosus by prostaglandin E1 in aortic arch abnormalities. *Circulation.* 1979;59:169–173.
24. Levin DL, Mills LJ, Weinberg AG. Hemodynamic, pulmonary vascular, and myocardial abnormalities secondary to pharmacologic constriction of the fetal ductus arteriosus. A possible mechanism for persistent pulmonary hypertension and transient tricuspid insufficiency in the newborn infant. *Circulation.* 1979;60:360–364.
25. Moss AJ, Emmanouilides G, Duffie Jr ER. Closure of the ductus arteriosus in the newborn infant. *Pediatrics.* 1963;32:25–30.
26. Michelakis E, Rebeyka I, Bateson J, Olley P, Puttagunta L, Archer S. Voltage-gated potassium channels in human ductus arteriosus. *Lancet.* 2000;356:134–137.
27. Hirsimaki H, Kero P, Saraste M, Ekblad H, Korvenranta H, Wanne O. Grading of left-to-right shunting ductus arteriosus in neonates with bedside pulsed Doppler ultrasound. *Am J Perinatol.* 1991;8:247–250.
28. Gittenberger-De Groot AC, Van Ertbruggen I, Moulaert AJ, Harinck E. The ductus arteriosus in the preterm infant: histologic and clinical observations. *J Pediatr.* 1980;96:88–93.
29. Tananari Y, Maeno Y, Takagishi T, Sasaguri Y, Morimatsu M, Kato H. Role of apoptosis in the closure of neonatal ductus arteriosus. *Jpn Circ J.* 2000;64:684–688.
30. Danilowicz D, Rudolph AM, Hoffman JI. Delayed closure of the ductus arteriosus in premature infants. *Pediatrics.* 1966;37:74–78.
31. Reller MD, Colasurdo MA, Rice MJ, Mcdonald RW. The timing of spontaneous closure of the ductus arteriosus in infants with respiratory distress syndrome. *Am J Cardiol.* 1990;66:75–78.
32. Reller MD, Ziegler ML, Rice MJ, Solin RC, Mcdonald RW. Duration of ductal shunting in healthy preterm infants: an echocardiographic color flow Doppler study. *J Pediatr.* 1988;112:441–446.
33. Van De Bor M, Verloove-Vanhorick SP, Brand R, Ruys JH. Patent ductus arteriosus in a cohort of 1338 preterm infants: a collaborative study. *Paediatr Perinat Epidemiol.* 1988;2:328–336.
34. Bishop RC. Delayed closure of the ductus arteriosus. *Am Heart J.* 1952;44:639–644.
35. Campbell M. Natural history of persistent ductus arteriosus. *Br Heart J.* 1968;30:4–13.
36. Carboni MP, Ringel RE. Ductus arteriosus in premature infants beyond the second week of life. *Pediatr Cardiol.* 1997;18:372–375.
37. Alverson DC, Eldridge MW, Johnson JD, et al. Effect of patent ductus arteriosus on left ventricular output in premature infants. *J Pediatr.* 1983;102:754–757.
38. Martin CG, Snider AR, Katz SM, Peabody JL, Brady JP. Abnormal cerebral blood flow patterns in preterm infants with a large patent ductus arteriosus. *J Pediatr.* 1982;101:587–593.
39. Miller E, Cradock-Watson JE, Pollock TM. Consequences of confirmed maternal rubella at successive stages of pregnancy. *Lancet.* 1982;2:781–784.
40. Rudolph AM, Scarpelli EM, Golinko RJ, Gootman NL. Hemodynamic basis for clinical manifestations of patent ductus arteriosus. *Am Heart J.* 1964;68:447–458.
41. Whitaker W, Heath D, Brown JW. Patent ductus arteriosus with pulmonary hypertension. *Br Heart J.* 1955;17:121–137.
42. Hammerman C, Strates E, Valaitis S. The silent ductus: its precursors and its aftermath. *Pediatr Cardiol.* 1986;7:121–127.
43. Bennhagen RG, Benson LN. Silent and audible persistent ductus arteriosus: an angiographic study. *Pediatr Cardiol.* 2003;24:27–30.
44. Hubbard TF, Neis DD. The sounds at the base of the heart in cases of patent ductus arteriosus. *Am Heart J.* 1960;59:807–815.
45. Chiles NH, Smith HL, Christensen NA, Geraci JE. Spontaneous healing of subacute bacterial endarteritis with closure of patent ductus arteriosus. *Proc Staff Meet Mayo Clin.* 1953;28:520–525.
46. Gibb WT. Acute bacterial endarteritis of a patent ductus arteriosus. *N Y State J Med.* 1941;41:1861–1863.
47. Foulis J. On a case of patent ductus arteriosus with aneurysm of the pulmonary artery. *Edinburgh Med J.* 1884;29:1117.
48. Jager BV. Noninfectious thrombosis of a patent ductus arteriosus: report of a case, with autopsy. *Am Heart J.* 1940;20:236–243.
49. Fay JE, Travill A. The "valve" of the ductus arteriosus—an enigma. *Can Med Assoc J.* 1967;97:78–80.
50. Wagner O. Beitrag zur pathologie des ductus arteriosus (Botalli). *Dtsch Arch Klin Med.* 1903;79:90.
51. Taussig HB. *Congenital Malformations of the Heart.* New York: The Commonwealth Fund; 1947.
52. Keith TR, Sagarminaga J. Spontaneously disappearing murmur of patent ductus arteriosus. A case report. *Circulation.* 1961;24:1235–1238.
53. Umebayashi Y, Taira A, Morishita Y, Arikawa K. Abrupt onset of patient ductus arteriosus in a 55-year-old man. *Am Heart J.* 1989;118:1067–1069.

54. Ng AS, Vlietstra RE, Danielson GK, Smith HC, Puga FJ. Patent ductus arteriosus in patients more than 50 years old. *Int J Cardiol.* 1986;11:277–285.

55. Wilkins JL. Risks of offspring of patients with patent ductus arteriosus. *J Med Genet.* 1969;6:1–4.

56. Lamy M, De Grouchy J, Schweisguth O. Genetic and non-genetic factors in the etiology of congenital heart disease: a study of 1188 cases. *Am J Hum Genet.* 1957;9:17–41.

57. Lynch HT, Grissom RL, Magnuson CR, Krush A. Patent ductus arteriosus. Study of two families. *JAMA.* 1965;194:135–138.

58. Martin RP, Banner NR, Radley-Smith R. Familial persistent ductus arteriosus. *Arch Dis Child.* 1986;61:906–907.

59. Patterson DF, Detweiler DK. Hereditary transmission of patent ductus arteriosus in the dog. *Am Heart J.* 1967;74:289–290.

60. Emmanouilides GC, Linde LM, Crittenden IH. Pulmonary artery stenosis associated with ductus arteriosus following maternal rubella. *Circulation.* 1964;29(suppl):514–522.

61. Gregg NM. Congenital cataract following German measles in the mother. *Trans Ophthalmol Soc Aust.* 1941;3:35–46.

62. Rutstein DD, Nickerson RJ, Heald FP. Seasonal incidence of patent ductus arteriosus and maternal rubella. *AMA J Dis Child.* 1952;84:199–213.

63. Alzamora-Castro V, Battilana G, Abugattas R, Sialer S. Patent ductus arteriosus and high altitude. *Am J Cardiol.* 1960;5: 761–763.

64. Hays JT. Spontaneous aneurysm of a patent ductus arteriosus in an elderly patient. *Chest.* 1985;88:918–920.

65. Jayakrishnan AG, Loftus B, Kelly P, Luke DA. Spontaneous postpartum rupture of a patent ductus arteriosus. *Histopathology.* 1992;21:383–384.

66. Sardesai SH, Marshall RJ, Farrow R, Mourant AJ. Dissecting aneurysm of the pulmonary artery in a case of unoperated patent ductus arteriosus. *Eur Heart J.* 1990;11:670–673.

67. Houston AB, Gnanapragasam JP, Lim MK, Doig WB, Coleman EN. Doppler ultrasound and the silent ductus arteriosus. *Br Heart J.* 1991;65:97–99.

68. Bejar R, Merritt TA, Coen RW, Mannino F, Gluck L. Pulsatility index, patent ductus arteriosus, and brain damage. *Pediatrics.* 1982;69:818–822.

69. Lipman B, Serwer GA, Brazy JE. Abnormal cerebral hemodynamics in preterm infants with patent ductus arteriosus. *Pediatrics.* 1982;69:778–781.

70. Hay JD. Population and clinic studies of congenital heart disease in Liverpool. *Br Med J.* 1966;2:661.

71. Aiken JE, Bifulco E, Sullivan Jr JJ. Patent ductus arteriosus in the aged. Report of this disease in a 74-year-old female. *JAMA.* 1961; 177:330–331.

72. Boe J, Humerfelt S. Patent ductus arteriosus Botalli in an octogenarian followed for fifty years. *Acta Med Scand.* 1960; 167:73–75.

73. Hornsten TR, Hellerstein HK, Ankeney JL. Patent ductus arteriosus in a 72-year-old woman. Successful corrective surgery. *JAMA.* 1967;199:580–582.

74. Woodruff 3rd WW, Gabliani G, Grant AO. Patent ductus arteriosus in the elderly. *South Med J.* 1983;76:1436–1437.

75. Zarich S, Leonardi H, Pippin J, Tuthill J, Lewis S. Patent ductus arteriosus in the elderly. *Chest.* 1988;94:1103–1105.

76. Kong MH, Corey GR, Bashore T, Harrison JK. Clinical problem-solving. A key miscommunication—an 81-year-old woman presented to the emergency department with increasing abdominal distention, nausea, and vomiting. *N Engl J Med.* 2008;358: 1054–1059.

77. White PD, Mazurkie SJ, Boschetti AE. Patency of the ductus arteriosus at 90. *N Engl J Med.* 1969;280:146–147.

78. Perloff JK. Cyanotic congenital heart disease: a multisystem systemic disorder. In: Perloff JK, Child JS, Aboulhosn J, eds. *Congenital heart disease in adults.* 3rd ed. Philadelphia: Saunders/Elsevier; 2008.

79. Wood P. The Eisenmenger syndrome or pulmonary hypertension with reversed central shunt. I. *Br Med J.* 1958;2:701–709.

80. Adams Jr P, Anderson RC, Varco RL. Patent ductus arteriosus with reversal of flow; clinical study of ten children. *Pediatrics.* 1956;18:410–423.

81. Sietsema KE, Perloff JK. Cyanotic congenital heart disease: dynamics of oxygen uptake and control of ventilation during

exercise. In: Perloff JK, Child JS, eds. *Congenital heart disease in adults.* 2nd ed. Philadelphia: W.B. Saunders Company; 1998.

82. Dailey FH, Genovese PD, Behnke RH. Patent ductus arteriosus with reversal of flow in adults. *Ann Intern Med.* 1962;56:865.

83. Martinez-Lavin M, Bobadilla M, Casanova J, Attie F, Martinez M. Hypertrophic osteoarthropathy in cyanotic congenital heart disease: its prevalence and relationship to bypass of the lung. *Arthritis Rheum.* 1982;25:1186–1193.

84. Williams B, Ling JT, Leight L, Mc GC. Patent ductus arteriosus and osteoarthropathy. *Arch Intern Med.* 1963;111:346–350.

85. Arcilla RA, Thilenius OG, Ranniger K. Congestive heart failure from suspected ductal closure in utero. *J Pediatr.* 1969;75:74–78.

86. Korones SB, Ainger LE, Monif GR, Roane J, Sever JL, Fuste F. Congenital rubella syndrome: study of 22 infants. Myocardial damage and other new clinical aspects. *Am J Dis Child.* 1965; 110:434–440.

87. Robertson SE, Featherstone DA, Gacic-Dobo M, Hersh BS. Rubella and congenital rubella syndrome: global update. *Rev Panam Salud Publica.* 2003;14:306–315.

88. Lin AE, Perloff JK. Upper limb malformations associated with congenital heart disease. *Am J Cardiol.* 1985;55:1576–1583.

89. Rohde RA, Hodgman JE, Cleland RS. Multiple congenital anomalies in the E1-trisomy (group 16–18) syndrome. *Pediatrics.* 1964;33:258–270.

90. Satoda M, Pierpont ME, Diaz GA, Bornemeier RA, Gelb BD. Char syndrome, an inherited disorder with patent ductus arteriosus, maps to chromosome 6p12-p21. *Circulation.* 1999;99: 3036–3042.

91. Satoda M, Zhao F, Diaz GA, et al. Mutations in TFAP2B cause Char syndrome, a familial form of patent ductus arteriosus. *Nat Genet.* 2000;25:42–46.

92. Bertola DR, Kim CA, Sugayama SM, Utagawa CY, Albano LM, Gonzalez CH. Further delineation of Char syndrome. *Pediatr Int.* 2000;42:85–88.

93. Trip J, Van Stuijvenberg M, Dikkers FG, Pijnenburg MWH. Unilateral charge association. *Eur J Pediatr.* 2002;161:78–80.

94. Perloff JK. *Physical examination of the heart and circulation.* 4th ed. Shelton, Connecticut: People's Medical Publishing House; 2009.

95. Holden JD, Jones RC, Akers WA. Patent ductus arteriosus diagnosed by a mosquito bite or the cutis Quincke. *Arch Derm.* 1966;94:742.

96. Gibson GA. Persistence of the arterial duct and its diagnosis. *Edinburgh Med J.* 1900;8:1.

97. Magri G, Jona E, Messina D, Actisdato A. Direct recording of heart sounds and murmurs from the epicardial surface of the exposed human heart. *Am Heart J.* 1959;57:449–459.

98. Baylen B, Meyer RA, Korfhagen J, Benzing 3rd G, Bubb ME, Kaplan S. Left ventricular performance in the critically ill premature infant with patent ductus arteriosus and pulmonary disease. *Circulation.* 1977;55:182–188.

99. Urquhart DS, Nicholl RM. How good is clinical examination at detecting a significant patent ductus arteriosus in the preterm neonate? *Arch Dis Child.* 2003;88:85–86.

100. Kohler CM, Mcnamara DG. Elongated patent ductus arteriosus with intermittent shunting. *Pediatrics.* 1967;39:446–448.

101. Shapiro W, Said SI, Nova PL. Intermittent disappearance of the murmur of patent ductus arteriosus. *Circulation.* 1960;22:226–231.

102. Papadopoulos GS, Folger Jr GM. Diastolic murmurs in the newborn of benign nature. *Int J Cardiol.* 1983;3:107–109.

103. Hiraishi S, Horiguchi Y, Misawa H, et al. Noninvasive Doppler echocardiographic evaluation of shunt flow dynamics of the ductus arteriosus. *Circulation.* 1987;75:1146–1153.

104. Liao PK, Su WJ, Hung JS. Doppler echocardiographic flow characteristics of isolated patent ductus arteriosus: better delineation by Doppler color flow mapping. *J Am Coll Cardiol.* 1988;12: 1285–1291.

105. Perloff JK. Auscultatory and phonocardiographic manifestations of pulmonary hypertension. *Prog Cardiovasc Dis.* 1967;9:303–340.

106. Braudo M, Rowe RD. Auscultation of the heart: early neonatal period. *Am J Dis Child.* 1961;101:575–586.

107. Burnard ED. A murmur from the ductus arteriosus in the newborn baby. *Br Med J.* 1958;1:806–810.

108. Hallidie-Smith KA. Murmur of persistent ductus arteriosus in premature infants. *Arch Dis Child.* 1972;47:725–730.

109. Green EW, Agruss NS, Adolph RJ. Right-sided Austin Flint murmur. Documentation by intracardiac phonocardiography, echocardiography and postmortem findings. *Am J Cardiol.* 1973;32:370–374.
110. Gray IR. Paradoxical splitting of the second heart sound. *Br Heart J.* 1956;18:21–28.
111. Mirowski M, Arevalo F, Medrano GA, Cisneros FA. Conduction disturbances in patent ductus arteriosus. A study of 20 cases before and after surgery with determination of the P-R index. *Circulation.* 1962;25:807–813.
112. Cruze K, Elliott LP, Schiebler GL, Wheat Jr MW. Unusual manifestations of patent ductus arteriosus in infancy. *Dis Chest.* 1963;43:563–571.
113. Halloran KH, Sanyal SK, Gardner TH. Superiorly oriented electrocardiographic axis in infants with the rubella syndrome. *Am Heart J.* 1966;72:600–606.
114. Steinberg I. Roentgenography of patent ductus arteriosus. *Am J Cardiol.* 1964;13:698–707.
115. Currarino G, Jackson JH. Calcification of the ductus arteriosus and ligamentum botalli. *Radiology.* 1970;94:139–142.
116. Sang Oh K, Bowen AD, Park SC, Galvis AG, Young LW. Patent ductus arteriosus: its occurrence with unequal pulmonary vascularity and hyperlucent left lung. *Am J Dis Child.* 1981;135:637–639.
117. Castellanos A, Hernandez FA. Size of ascending aorta in congenital cardiac lesions and other heart diseases. *Acta Radiol Diagn (Stockh).* 1967;6:49–64.
118. Vick 3rd GW, Huhta JC, Gutgesell HP. Assessment of the ductus arteriosus in preterm infants utilizing suprasternal two-dimensional/Doppler echocardiography. *J Am Coll Cardiol.* 1985;5:973–977.
119. Shyu KG, Lai LP, Lin SC, Chang H, Chen JJ. Diagnostic accuracy of transesophageal echocardiography for detecting patent ductus arteriosus in adolescents and adults. *Chest.* 1995;108:1201–1205.
120. Guntheroth WG, Forster FK. Large ductal flow may cause high velocity in the descending aorta without coarctation: improved diagnosis using the continuity equation. *Am J Cardiol.* 2001;87:493–495, A498.
121. Mielke G, Steil E, Breuer J, Goelz R. Circulatory changes following intrauterine closure of the ductus arteriosus in the human fetus and newborn. *Prenat Diagn.* 1998;18:139–145.
122. Leal SD, Cavalle-Garrido T, Ryan G, Farine D, Heilbut M, Smallhorn JF. Isolated ductal closure in utero diagnosed by fetal echocardiography. *Am J Perinatol.* 1997;14:205–210.
123. Sohn DW, Kim YJ, Zo JH, et al. The value of contrast echocardiography in the diagnosis of patent ductus arteriosus with Eisenmenger's syndrome. *J Am Soc Echocardiogr.* 2001;14:57–59.
124. Elliotson J. Case of malformation of the pulmonary artery and aorta. *Lancet.* 1830;1:247–251.
125. Kutsche LM, Van Mierop LH. Anatomy and pathogenesis of aorticopulmonary septal defect. *Am J Cardiol.* 1987;59:443–447.
126. Richardson JV, Doty DB, Rossi NP, Ehrenhaft JL. The spectrum of anomalies of aortopulmonary septation. *J Thorac Cardiovasc Surg.* 1979;78:21–27.
127. Van Praagh R, Van Praagh S. The anatomy of common aorticopulmonary trunk (truncus arteriosus communis) and its embryologic implications. A study of 57 necropsy cases. *Am J Cardiol.* 1965;16:406–425.
128. Morrow AG, Greenfield LJ, Braunwald E. Congenital aortopulmonary septal defect. Clinical and hemodynamic findings, surgical technic, and results of operative correction. *Circulation.* 1962;25:463–476.
129. Rice MJ, Seward JB, Hagler DJ, Mair DD, Tajik AJ. Visualization of aortopulmonary window by two-dimensional echocardiography. *Mayo Clinic Proc.* 1982;57:482–487.
130. Tandon R, Da Silva CL, Moller JH, Edwards JE. Aorticopulmonary septal defect coexisting with ventricular septal defect. *Circulation.* 1974;50:188–191.
131. Downing DF. Congenital aortic septal defect. *Am Heart J.* 1950;40:285–292.
132. Shepherd SG, Park FR, Kitchell JR. A case of aorto-pulmonic communication incident to a congenital aortic septal defect: discussion of embryologic changes involved. *Am Heart J.* 1944;27:733–738.
133. Garver KA, Hernandez RJ, Vermilion RP, Martin Goble M. Images in cardiovascular medicine. Correlative imaging of aortopulmonary window: demonstration with echocardiography, angiography, and MRI. *Circulation.* 1997;96:1036–1037.
134. Satomi G, Nakamura K, Imai Y, Takao A. Two-dimensional echocardiographic diagnosis of aorticopulmonary window. *Br Heart J.* 1980;43:351–356.

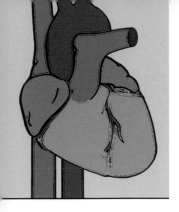

Chapter 21

Anomalous Origin of the Left Coronary Artery from the Pulmonary Trunk

In 1886, St. John Brooks[1] described two cases of "an abnormal coronary artery arising from the pulmonary artery." The diagnosis was subsequently called into question when the abnormal communication was attributed to a coronary arterial fistula. The seminal report of Bland, White, and Garland[2] in 1933 referred to Maude Abbott's case of a 60-year-old woman with anomalous origin of the left coronary artery from the pulmonary trunk (Figure 21-1B). *Bland, White,* and *Garland* remain with us as eponyms.[3] In 1962, Fontana and Edwards[4] reported a series of 58 postmortem specimens.

Anomalous origin of the left coronary artery from the pulmonary trunk is the most common major congenital malformation of the coronary circulation, with an incidence rate estimated at 1 in 300,000 live births.[5–8] More rarely, the right coronary artery (Figure 21-2), the left anterior descending coronary artery,[9] the *circumflex coronary artery,*[10–12] *both coronary arteries,*[13–15] or a *single coronary artery*[16] arises from the pulmonary trunk or its right or left branch.[11,17] Stenosis of the ostium of the anomalous left coronary artery has been reported,[18] and rarely, the anomalous artery courses within the aortic wall (intramural).[19]

No single terminology encompasses all of these many variations. *ALCAPA* (Anomalous Left Coronary Artery from the Pulmonary Artery) has been used as a general designation, but the *ALCA* does not include an anomalous *right* coronary artery and the *PA* does not distinguish the pulmonary trunk from its right or left branch. In this chapter, the designation *anomalous origin of the left coronary artery from the pulmonary trunk* applies to the most prevalent variation, and the less or least prevalent variations are described individually.

The *anomalous left coronary artery* is a thin-walled vessel that resembles a venous channel (Figures 21-1, 21-3, and 21-4).[20,21] The *right coronary artery* originates from its normal aortic sinus, is dilated and tortuous (see Figures 21-1 and 21-4), and, on rare occasions, is aneurysmal.[22] The portion of left ventricle perfused by the anomalous left coronary artery is thin, scarred, and dilated[21] and occasionally forms a ventricular aneurysm. Conversely, the hypoperfused but viable portion of left ventricle *increases* its mass, often appreciably,[20] because immature cardiomyocytes replicate in response to the hypoxemic stimulus.[23] The left ventricular endocardium exhibits fibroelastosis and rarely is focally calcified. Interestingly, in adults with typical ischemic heart disease, newly formed elastic fibers appear within 3 or 4 weeks

after a myocardial infarction and culminate in endocardial fibroelastosis in the vicinity of the infarct.[24]

Three theories have been proposed to explain the origin of a coronary artery from the pulmonary trunk.[15] The first two theories are related to division of the embryologic truncus arteriosus.[25] In the early embryo, two opposing truncal cushions enlarge and fuse to form the truncal septum, which divides the truncus arteriosus into aortic and pulmonary channels.[25] Assuming that the coronary arteries originate as two endothelial buds (see Chapter 32), displacement of the origin of one or both of these buds could assign either or both coronary arteries to the portion of the truncus arteriosus destined to become the pulmonary artery. Alternatively, faulty division of the truncus could incorporate one or both coronary artery buds into the pulmonary artery. The higher incidence of anomalous origin of the *left* rather than the *right* coronary artery from the pulmonary trunk has been attributed to the proximity of the left aortic sinus to the truncal septum, so a relatively small displacement of the left coronary artery anlage suffices to cause the left coronary artery ostium to lie within the pulmonary artery.[15] These theories presuppose that human coronary arteries originate as two endothelial buds that develop before or simultaneously with the division of the truncus arteriosus (see Chapter 32).[15] Nor do these theories explain the presence of a third (accessory) coronary artery or anomalous origin of one branch of the left coronary artery from the pulmonary trunk or explain why the relative sizes of the pulmonary artery, the aorta, and their valves are not altered by the proposed displacement of the truncal septum.[15] The *involution and persistence* theory postulates that there are originally *six* coronary artery anlagen: three from the aorta, and three from the pulmonary artery (see Chapter 32).[15] The coronary arteries that are destined to originate normally are believed to arise from two persistent anlagen in two separate aortic sinuses, whereas the anlage in the third aortic sinus, in addition to all three anlagen in the pulmonary sinuses, undergo involution.[15] According to this theory, anomalous origin of one or both coronary arteries could result from persistence of pulmonary artery coronary anlagen together with involution of the normally persistent aortic coronary anlagen.[15] In the presence of a bicuspid aortic valve, anomalous origin of the left coronary artery from the pulmonary trunk is believed to be the expression of a single morphogenic defect.[26,27] In the Syrian hamster, a relationship has been proposed between anomalous origin of the left coronary artery and the developmental morphology of the semilunar valves.[26,27]

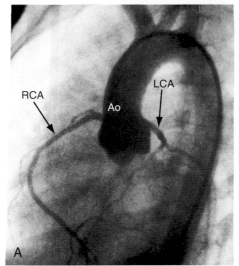

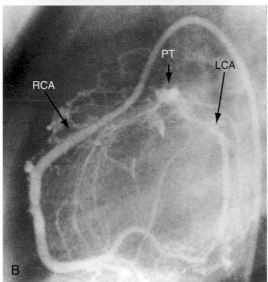

FIGURE 21-1 **A,** Aortogram (left anterior oblique) from a healthy 5-year-old girl with a normal right coronary artery (RCA) and a normal left coronary artery (LCA). **B,** Right coronary arteriogram (lateral projection) from a 4-year-old girl with anomalous origin of the left coronary artery (LCA) from the pulmonary trunk (PT). A dilated right coronary artery originates from the aorta. Intercoronary anastomoses communicate with the left coronary artery that originates from the pulmonary trunk. The direction of flow is from the right coronary artery through intercoronary anastomoses into the left coronary artery then into the pulmonary trunk. (Ao = aorta.)

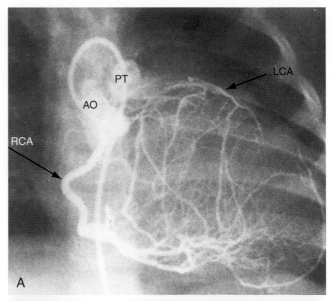

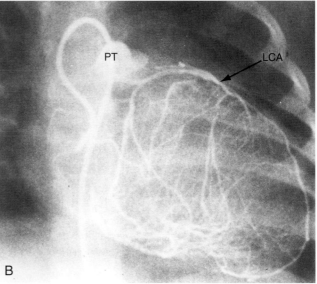

FIGURE 21-2 **A,** Aortogram from a 4-year-old girl with anomalous origin of the left coronary artery (LCA) from the pulmonary trunk (PT). The enlarged right coronary artery (RCA) originated from its appropriate aortic sinus. (Ao = aorta.) **B,** Intercoronary anastomoses from the left coronary artery (LCA) filled the right coronary artery. Flow was *into* the pulmonary trunk (PT).

Myocardial ischemia is a serious sequela of anomalous origin of the left coronary artery from the pulmonary trunk.[28] Ischemia does not stem from the fact that only *one* coronary artery originates from the aorta because the functional consequences of a congenitally single coronary artery are benign,[29-31] with few exceptions (see Chapter 32).[32,33] Nor is perfusion of the anomalous coronary artery by unoxygenated blood from the pulmonary trunk a satisfactory explanation because in *cyanotic* congenital heart disease the oxygen content of coronary arterial blood can be exceedingly low without producing myocardial ischemia. Why then does cardiac muscle become ischemic when the left coronary artery arises from the pulmonary trunk? The answer lies in the *direction* of blood flow through the coronary bed,[34,35] as illustrated in the circulatory patterns of Figure 21-5. In fetal and early neonatal life, relatively high pulmonary arterial pressure results in *antegrade* blood flow *into* the anomalous left coronary artery (see Figure 21-5, *first panel*). The subsequent fall in pulmonary arterial pressure is accompanied by a parallel fall in blood flow into the anomalous left coronary (see Figure 21-5, *middle panel*). During this crucial transition, myocardial perfusion depends almost entirely on perfusion from the right coronary artery (see Figure 21-3).[35,36] Myocardial ischemia is unavoidable unless adequate circulation from right to left coronary artery is established via intercoronary anastomoses, on which survival largely depends (see

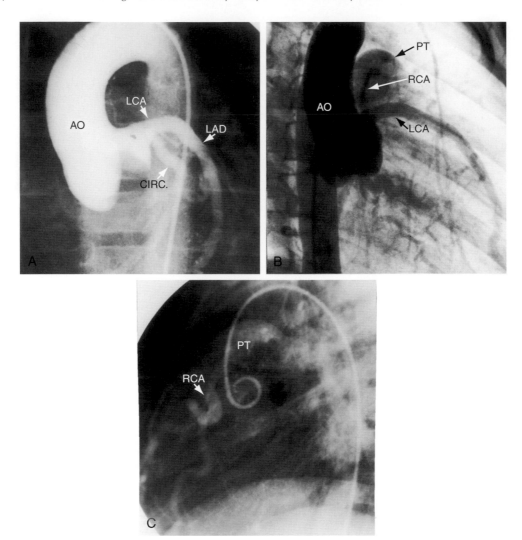

FIGURE 21-3 Aortogram (anteroposterior projection) from a 4-year-old boy with anomalous origin of the *right* coronary artery from the pulmonary trunk. **A,** The left coronary artery (LCA) originates from its aortic (AO) sinus and divides into the left anterior descending (LAD) and circumflex (CIRC) arteries. **B,** Intercoronary anastomoses visualize the left coronary artery (LCA) that originates from the pulmonary trunk as illustrated in Figure 21-5. **C,** Lateral projection shows the right coronary artery (RCA) entering the pulmonary trunk (PT).

Figure 21-3B).[21,35,37] Intercoronary anastomoses represent low-resistance pathways between the aorta and pulmonary trunk, in essence, *arteriovenous fistulae*,[34] that have two opposing effects: (1) a desirable effect of reestablishing left coronary arterial perfusion; and (2) the undesirable effect of a coronary steal that bypasses the capillary bed and deprives the myocardium of oxygen.[34,35,38] The idea of retrograde flow through an anomalous left coronary artery was originally proposed by 1886 by St. John Brooks:

> *"Here are two arteries belonging to the different circulations—the pulmonary and the systemic— anastomosing with each other. In these circulations, as is well known, the arterial pressure is very much greater in the systemic than in the pulmonary; how then did the blood flow in the anomalous coronary artery? There cannot be a doubt that it acted very much after the manner of a vein, and that blood flowed through it towards the pulmonary artery, and from thence into the lungs."[1]*

Physiologic, pathologic, and clinical derangements arise from the ischemic consequences of the transition from decreased antegrade perfusion of the anomalous left coronary artery, to flow from the right coronary artery through the low-resistance intercoronary anastomoses into the left coronary artery, followed by retrograde flow into the pulmonary trunk (see Figure 21-5). Ischemia causes the left ventricle to labor under three handicaps: first, viable myocardium is compromised, so contractility is depressed[39]; second, mitral regurgitation occurs as a consequence of ischemic papillary muscle dysfunction[40] that adds to the hemodynamic burden (Figure 21-6); and third, flow via the intercoronary anastomoses constitutes a left-to-right shunt that is occasionally large enough to impose volume overload on the left ventricle.[41] Although regional abnormalities of wall motion characterize anomalous origin of the left coronary artery from the pulmonary trunk,[42,43] infants tend to exhibit global hypokinesis.[42,43]

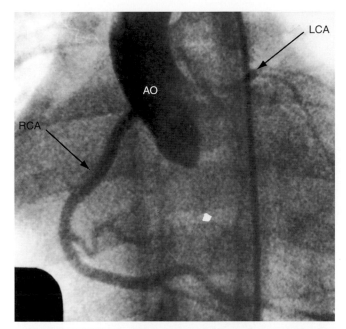

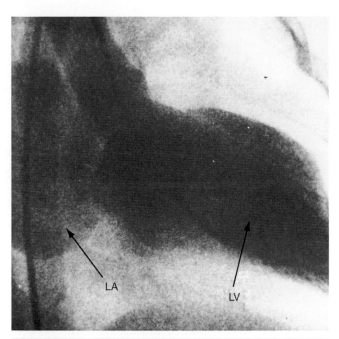

FIGURE 21-4 Anteroposterior aortogram from a 4-month-old female with an enlarged right coronary artery (RCA) that originated from the aorta (AO) and communicated through intercoronary anastomoses with the left coronary artery (LCA) that took origin from the pulmonary trunk. The direction of flow was from the right coronary artery through intercoronary anastomoses into the left coronary artery, then into the pulmonary trunk.

FIGURE 21-6 Left ventriculogram (right oblique projection) from a 5-year-old girl with anomalous origin of the left coronary artery from the pulmonary trunk. Papillary muscle dysfunction caused mitral regurgitation, which was responsible for dilation of the left atrium (LA) and left ventricle (LV).

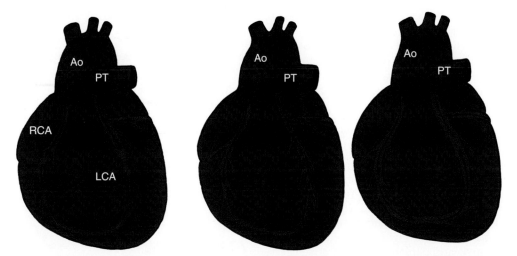

FIGURE 21-5 Flow patterns in anomalous origin of the left coronary artery from the pulmonary trunk. In first illustration (fetus and early neonate), high pressure in the pulmonary trunk (PT) generates flow *into* the anomalous left coronary artery (LCA), and the normally originating right coronary artery (RCA) is perfused from the aorta. Intercoronary anastomoses are not yet functional. In the second illustration, a fall in neonatal pulmonary arterial pressure is accompanied by a parallel fall in flow into the anomalous left coronary artery. Intercoronary anastomoses are still not functional. When the pressures in the pulmonary trunk and anomalous left coronary artery fall *below* the pressure in the right coronary artery, flow proceeds from the right coronary artery into the *left* coronary artery through intercoronary anastomoses. The left coronary artery then drains *into* the pulmonary trunk, and does not receive blood from it. *(Modified from Edwards JE: Editorial: the direction of blood flow in coronary arteries arising from the pulmonary trunk. Circulation 1964;29:163.)*

HISTORY

The outlook is most grave when *both* coronary arteries originate from the pulmonary trunk[13–15] and is most favorable when the right coronary artery alone, or a left anterior descending or circumflex coronary artery alone, originates anomalously.[10–12] The clinical course is a continuum that ranges from death in infancy to asymptomatic adult survival, with all gradations in between.[35,44–47] Nevertheless, there are three general patterns: (1) serious symptoms in early infancy with death before 1 year of age; (2) early symptoms followed by gradual attenuation or disappearance; and (3) absence or virtual absence of early symptoms with asymptomatic survival to adulthood. Adult survival, even to age 90 years,[48] has been reported and is much more likely with anomalous origin of the *right* coronary artery from the pulmonary trunk, which, however, is not necessarily benign.

Eighty percent to 90% of patients with anomalous origin of the left coronary artery from the pulmonary trunk die in their first year.[21,47] Presentation in the neonate is unusual because elevated pulmonary arterial pressure results in *forward flow* into the anomalous left coronary artery.[49] Accordingly, infants appear healthy at birth and often remain so for about 2 months, after which symptoms usually begin.[47] Irritability, dyspnea, wheezing, cough, diaphoresis, and ashen gray pallor are precipitated or aggravated by feeding, crying, or a bowel movement.[47,50] Occasionally, the initial symptom is hoarseness thought to be caused by impingement of a dilated pulmonary artery on the recurrent laryngeal nerve.[51] Chronic congestive heart failure is responsible for poor growth and development and is usually the cause of death. More than a third of patients presents with sudden cardiac death,[52] in which case the diagnosis is necessarily post mortem. Symptomatic infants occasionally have improvement[53] only to die suddenly during a relatively asymptomatic childhood or adolescence. One of the first known patients with the anomaly was the 60-year-old woman described by Maude Abbott[54] in 1908. An elderly asymptomatic man played football in his youth and presented at age 67 years with sustained ventricular fibrillation.[55] Angina may be delayed until the teens, or the anomaly may be discovered in asymptomatic children[56] or adults because of mitral regurgitation (Figures 21-6 and 21-7). A 39-year-old mother of three presented with exertional fatigue.[57] About 15% of individuals with anomalous origin of the left coronary artery survive to adulthood,[58] some reaching the seventh or eighth decade.[22,59] The malformation reveals itself in adults because of detection of the murmur of mitral regurgitation,[22,59,60] because of a continuous murmur mistaken for a patent ductus (see Figure 21-7), or because of angina pectoris, myocardial infarction, congestive heart failure, atrial fibrillation, ventricular tachyarrhythmias, cardiac arrest, or sudden cardiac death.[34,45,46,61–64]

PHYSICAL APPEARANCE

An acutely ill infant presents a dramatic clinical picture with rapid labored breathing, weak cry, cough, and diaphoresis and pallor, which accompany episodes of symptomatic myocardial ischemia (angina). Infants with chronic congestive heart failure are catabolic.

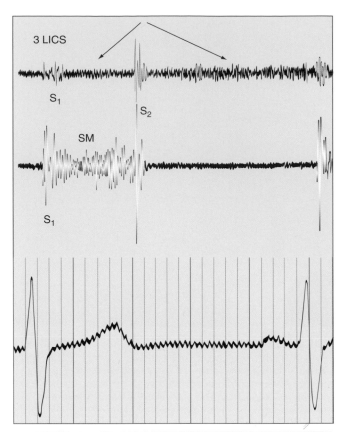

FIGURE 21-7 Phonocardiogram from a 13-year-old boy with anomalous origin of the left coronary artery from the pulmonary trunk. The continuous murmur in the third left intercostal space (3 LICS, arrows) is louder in diastole. A holosystolic murmur of mitral regurgitation (SM) was recorded at the apex. Lead 2 of the electrocardiogram shows left axis deviation.

ARTERIAL PULSE, JUGULAR VENOUS PULSE, PRECORDIAL MOVEMENT, AND PALPATION

Pulsus alternans results from left ventricular failure.[21] Diastolic pressure is occasionally low because of an aortic runoff through the fistulous communication.[41] The jugular venous pulse is elevated in the presence of congestive heart failure but cannot be clinically assessed in symptomatic infants. A left parasternal impulse is the result of an enlarged left atrium that expands in systole in response to mitral regurgitation.

AUSCULTATION

Anomalous origin of the left coronary artery from the pulmonary trunk is accompanied by systolic, diastolic, or continuous murmurs or by no murmur at all. The holosystolic murmur of mitral regurgitation (see Figure 21-7) is the consequence of ischemic papillary muscle dysfunction (see previous).[20,65,66] Short apical mid-diastolic murmurs are analogous to mid-diastolic murmurs in other forms of mitral regurgitation.[66]

Continuous murmurs are generated by flow through intercoronary anastomoses (Figures 21-7 and 21-8).[41]

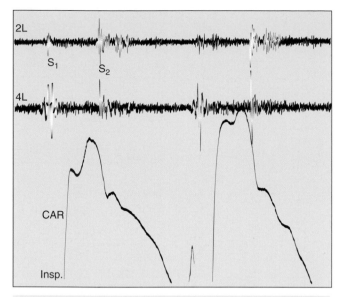

FIGURE 21-8 Phonocardiogram from a 33-year-old woman with anomalous origin of the left coronary artery from the pulmonary trunk misdiagnosed in childhood as patent ductus arteriosus. The continuous murmur in the second (2L) and fourth (4L) left intercostal spaces was maximal *after* second heart sound (S₂). (Car = carotid; S₁ = first heart sound.)

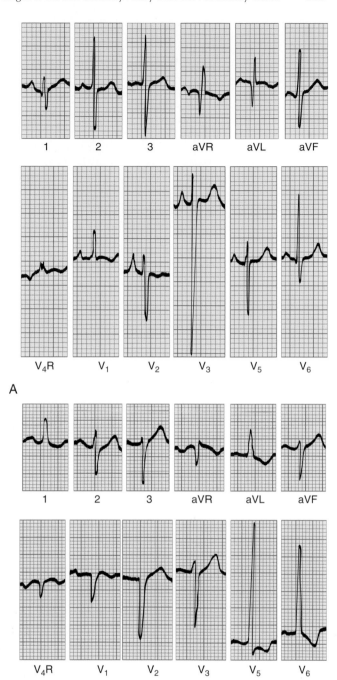

A

B $\longleftarrow \frac{1}{2}$ STD $\longrightarrow$

FIGURE 21-9 A, Electrocardiogram from a symptomatic 4-month-old female with anomalous origin of the left coronary artery from the pulmonary trunk. The QRS axis is indeterminate (equidiphasic complexes in all six limb leads). A small but abnormal q wave is present in lead 1, and a deep narrow q wave appears in lead aVL. Left ventricular hypertrophy is indicated by the deep S wave in lead V_3 and the prominent R wave in lead V_6. **B,** Same patient at age 5 years. There is a left atrial P terminal force in lead V_4R. Left axis deviation is now present, and infarct q waves have developed in leads V_4R through V_2. Left ventricular hypertrophy is represented by voltage and repolarization criteria in leads V_{5-6}. The precordial leads are all half standardized.

Their configuration and location are only occasionally similar to patent ductus arteriosus,[67] which only rarely coexists.[68] The continuous murmur of the intercoronary anastomoses does not peak around the second heart sound but is softer in systole and louder in diastole (see Figures 21-7 and 21-8) because transmural systolic pressure generated by ventricular contraction reduces intercoronary systolic flow. The occasional *isolated diastolic* murmur has been attributed to a reduction in systolic intercoronary flow caused by elevated pulmonary arterial pressure provoked by left ventricular failure or mitral regurgitation.[41]

The continuous murmurs are located at the base of the heart or somewhat lower either to the left or right of the sternum, but usually along the left sternal border (see Figures 21-7 and 21-8). An isolated diastolic murmur along the sternal edge is occasionally mistaken for semilunar valve regurgitation. Third heart sounds coincide with left ventricular failure and mitral regurgitation.

ELECTROCARDIOGRAM

Three features characterize the scalar electrocardiogram of anomalous origin of the left coronary artery from the pulmonary trunk: (1) deep narrow q waves; (2) left ventricular hypertrophy; and (3) left axis deviation. In healthy infants and children, q waves are consistently absent in leads 1 and aVL. In anomalous origin of the left coronary artery from the pulmonary trunk, deep narrow q waves are present in these leads (Figures 21-9A and 21-10)[8] and are in striking contrast to the shallow broad q waves of adult ischemic heart disease. The depth of the q wave

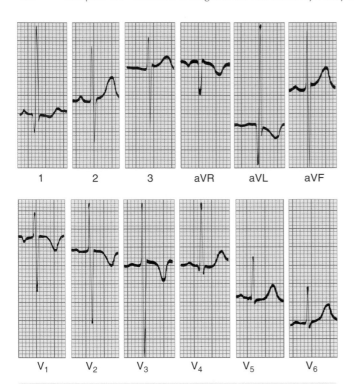

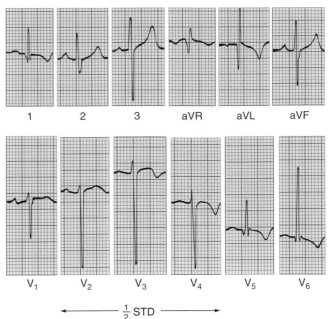

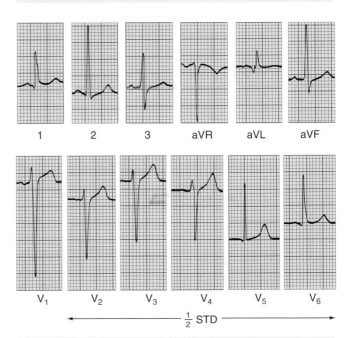

FIGURE 21-10 Electrocardiogram from a 9-year-old boy with anomalous origin of the left coronary artery from the pulmonary trunk. The QRS axis is leftward (–15 degrees). A deep narrow q wave is present in lead 1 and is especially evident in lead aVL. Left ventricular hypertrophy is indicated by the tall R wave and inverted T wave in lead aVL.

FIGURE 21-11 Electrocardiogram from a 15-year-old boy with anomalous origin of the left coronary artery from the pulmonary trunk. A small narrow q wave in lead 1 is especially evident in lead aVL. The QRS axis is leftward (–10 degrees). Voltage and repolarization criteria for left ventricular hypertrophy are present in the precordial leads. Leads V_{2-4} are half standardized.

FIGURE 21-12 Electrocardiogram from a 19-year-old woman with anomalous origin of the left coronary artery from the pulmonary trunk. There is an unusual broad notched q wave in lead aVL. Left ventricular hypertrophy is reflected in the deep S wave in lead V_1 and the tall R waves in leads V_{5-6}. Leads V_{2-6} are half standardized.

in lead aVL can equal or exceed the height of the R wave (Figures 21-9A and 21-11). In infants, these q waves can be small or absent but become progressively more prominent. An abnormal tracing may improve with age[69] or may become more abnormal (see Figure 21-9A, B). Q waves are rarely present in right precordial leads (see Figure 21-9B).

The second electrocardiographic characteristic, *left ventricular hypertrophy*,[7,20,21] was in the title of the original Bland, White, and Garland[2] publication, "Report of an Unusual Case Associated with Cardiac Hypertrophy." Although heart weights are increased, it is the *posterobasal* region of the left ventricle that is selectively increased in mass (see previous).[20,23] From the gross morphologic point of view, this regional increase in mass is *hypertrophy*, but from the cell biologic point of view, the posterobasal increase in mass is *hyperplasia* (i.e., *replication* of cardiomyocytes).[23] The basis for this cellular pattern is the capacity of immature cardiomyocytes to replicate in response to hypoxemia that is a feature of the hypoperfused but viable posterobasal left ventricular wall (see previous).[23]

In the electrocardiogram, left ventricular hypertrophy is represented by typical voltage and repolarization criteria (Figures 21-11 and 21-12).[69] However, in leads aVL and V_6, the deep narrow q waves may reflect the initial force deformity of the congenital coronary artery anomaly rather than left ventricular hypertrophy (Figure 21-13). Electrocardiograms recorded during angina pectoris or exercise stress testing disclose ischemic ST segment depressions and T wave inversions.

Left axis deviation is the third electrocardiographic characteristic of anomalous origin of the left coronary

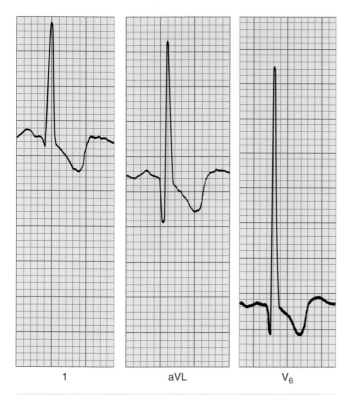

FIGURE 21-13 Leads 1, aVL, and V₆ from a 3-year-old asymptomatic girl with anomalous origin of the left coronary artery from the pulmonary trunk. The small but abnormal q wave in lead 1 and the deep narrow q waves in leads aVL and V₆ reflect initial force deformities of the congenital coronary anomaly rather than left ventricular hypertrophy, which is represented by tall R waves and inverted T waves.

artery from the pulmonary trunk (see Figure 21-9B).[70] The mechanism has been attributed to a disproportionate increase in posterobasal left ventricular muscle mass that results a left superior direction of the major depolarization vector.[20,70]

Left atrial P wave abnormalities occur because of mitral regurgitation (see Figure 21-9B), which is responsible for occasional atrial fibrillation.

X-RAY

The cardiac silhouette varies from massive cardiomegaly in symptomatic infants (Figure 12–14) to normal or nearly so in an occasional older child or adult (Figure 21-15). The most consistent radiologic features are enlargement of the left ventricle (see Figure 21-14)[37,71] and left atrium (see Figures 21-6, 21-14, and 21-15).[37,71] Increased vascularity represents the pulmonary venous congestion of left ventricular failure (see Figure 21-14). Dystrophic calcification of the left ventricle has been described but is not visible in the x-ray.

ECHOCARDIOGRAM

Echocardiography establishes the aortic origins of the left and right coronary arteries (Figure 21-16), identifies the origin of an anomalous left coronary artery from the pulmonary trunk (Figure 21-17 and Video 21-1), and defines the flow patterns. Color flow imaging establishes the presence of diastolic or continuous flow entering the pulmonary trunk just distal to the pulmonary valve[72] and adhering to the medial wall of the pulmonary trunk (Figure 21-18).[73–75] Although a coronary arterial fistula

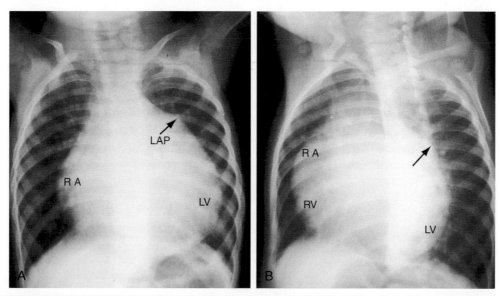

FIGURE 21-14 X-rays from a 10-month-old female with anomalous origin of the left coronary artery from the pulmonary trunk. **A,** The left atrial appendage (LAP) is conspicuous, a dilated left ventricle (LV) occupies the apex, and an enlarged right atrium (RA) occupies the right cardiac border. **B,** Left anterior oblique projection. The anterior border of the heart is formed by the right atrium and right ventricle (RV), the posterior border is formed by the dilated left ventricle, and a large left atrium lies beneath the left bronchus (arrow).

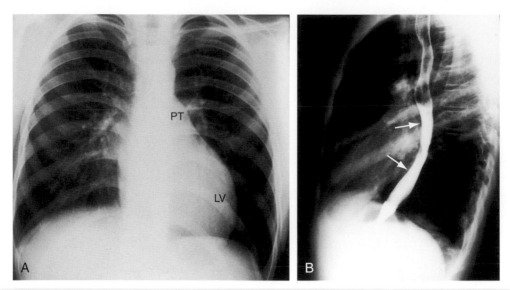

FIGURE 21-15 X-rays from the 13-year-old boy whose phonocardiogram is shown in Figure 21-7. A convex left ventricle (LV) occupies the apex, and there is mild prominence of the pulmonary trunk (PT). The lateral view shows displacement of the barium-filled esophagus (arrows) by a moderately enlarged left atrium.

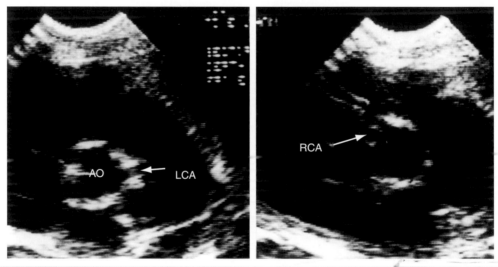

FIGURE 21-16 Echocardiograms in the short axis show normal origin of the left coronary artery (LCA) and normal origin of the right coronary artery (RCA). (Ao = aorta.)

into the pulmonary artery can exhibit similar flow patterns (see Chapter 22), two coronary arteries are identified originating in their normal respective aortic sinuses.[75,76] Patent ductus arteriosus is characterized by color flow that enters near the *left* pulmonary artery, adheres to the *lateral* wall of the pulmonary trunk, and is directed *toward* the pulmonary valve (see Chapter 20). In a 72-year-old woman, the diagnosis was made with both echocardiographic myocardial blush and coronary arteriography.[77] Echocardiography also determines left ventricular size, wall motion, and ejection fraction, and color flow imaging quantifies mitral regurgitation. Echogenic left ventricular papillary muscles indicate ischemic scarring (Figure 21-19)

Echocardiography coupled with scalar electrocardiography is a particularly useful diagnostic combination.[7]

More recent imaging techniques include multislice computed tomography (CT),[78,79] magnetic resonance imaging,[80] and CT coronary angiography.[81]

SUMMARY

Infants with anomalous origin of the left coronary artery from the pulmonary trunk are healthy at birth, and may remain so as neonates, but subsequently develop irritability, pallor, fatigue, cough, weak cry, dyspnea, and diaphoresis from ischemic pain and cardiac failure precipitated or aggravated by feeding, crying, or a bowel movement. Severity ranges from death in infancy (the dominant theme) to relatively asymptomatic adult survival.

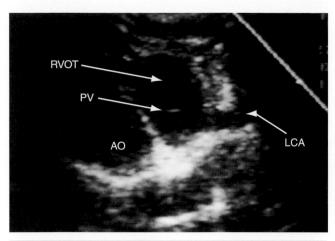

FIGURE 21-17 Echocardiogram in the short axis from a 4-year-old boy. The left coronary artery (LCA) originates anomously from the pulmonary trunk just above the pulmonary valve (PV) (Video 21-1). (AO = aorta; RVOT = right ventricular outflow tract.)

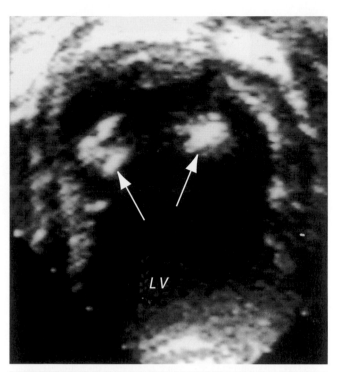

FIGURE 21-19 Echocardiogram from a 9-year-old girl with anomalous origin of the left coronary artery from the pulmonary trunk. Arrows point to left ventricular (LV) papillary muscles that are echogenic because of ischemic scarring.

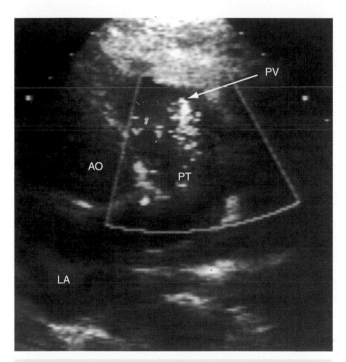

FIGURE 21-18 Black and white rendition of a color flow image in the short axis from a 22-year-old woman with anomalous origin of the left coronary artery from the pulmonary trunk. Flow from the anomalous left coronary artery entered the pulmonary trunk (PT) just above the pulmonary valve (PV). (Ao = aorta; LA = left atrium.)

and left axis deviation. The x-ray varies from massive cardiomegaly from left ventricular and left atrial enlargement in symptomatic infants and children to normal or nearly normal x-rays in an occasional older child or young adult. Color flow imaging and Doppler interrogation identify the origin of the left coronary artery from the pulmonary trunk with retrograde flow. Left ventricular regional wall motion can be determined, ejection fraction can be established, and mitral regurgitation can be quantified.

REFERENCES

1. Brooks HSJ. Two cases of an abnormal coronary artery aising from the pulmonary artery. *J Anat Physiol*. 1886;20:26.
2. Bland EF, White PD, Garland J. Congenital anomalies of the coronary arteries: report of an unusual case associated with cardiac hypertrophy. *Am Heart J*. 1933;8:787–801.
3. Gasul BM, Loeffler F. Anomalous origin of the left coronary artery from the pulmonary artery (Bland-White-Garland syndrome) report of four cases. *Pediatrics*. 1949;4:498–507.
4. Fontana RS, Edwards JE. *Congenital cardiac disease: a review of 357 Case studies pathologically*. Philadelphia: WB Saunders; 1962.
5. Lee AC, Foster E, Yeghiazarians Y. Anomalous origin of the left coronary artery from the pulmonary artery: a case series and brief review. *Congenit Heart Dis*. 2006;1:111–115.
6. Lin C-P, Chen Y-P, Chen T-H, et al. Anomalous origin of the left main coronary artery from the main pulmonary artery in a young adult. *Circulation*. 2001;104:1575–1576.
7. Angelini P, Velasco JA, Flamm S. Coronary anomalies: incidence, pathophysiology, and clinical relevance. *Circulation*. 2002;105:2449–2454.
8. Teixeira AM, Pereira J, Anjos R. Anomalous origin of the left coronary artery from the pulmonary trunk. *Cardiol Young*. 2004;14:439–440.
9. Subban V, Jeyaram B, Sankardas MA. Anomalous origin of the left anterior descending artery from the pulmonary artery. *Heart*. 2010;96:170.

Precordial palpation detects a left ventricular impulse and occasionally anterior movement at the left sternal border as a result of systolic expansion of an enlarged left atrium. Auscultation reveals the systolic murmur of mitral regurgitation and a continuous murmur that tends to be softer in systole and is associated with flow through intercoronary anastomoses. The three characteristic electrocardiographic features include deep but narrow q waves in leads 1 and aVL, left ventricular hypertrophy,

10. Evans JJ, Phillips JF. Origin of the left anterior descending artery from the pulmonary artery. 3 year angiographic follow-up after saphenous vein bypass graft and proximal ligation. *J Am Coll Cardiol.* 1984;3:219–224.

11. Garcia CM, Chandler J, Russell R. Anomalous left circumflex coronary artery from the right pulmonary artery: first adult case report. *Am Heart J.* 1992;123:526–528.

12. Tamer DF, Mallon SM, Garcia OL, Wolff GS. Anomalous origin of the left anterior descending coronary artery from the pulmonary artery. *Am Heart J.* 1984;108:341–345.

13. Bharati S, Szarnicki RJ, Popper R, Fryer A, Lev M. Origin of both coronary arteries from the pulmonary trunk associated with hypoplasia of the aortic tract complex: a new entity. *J Am Coll Cardiol.* 1984;3:437–441.

14. Colmers RA, Siderides CI. Anomalous origin of both coronary arteries from pulmonary trunk. Myocardial infarction in otherwise normal heart. *Am J Cardiol.* 1963;12:263–269.

15. Heifetz SA, Robinowitz M, Mueller KH, Virmani R. Total anomalous origin of the coronary arteries from the pulmonary artery. *Pediatr Cardiol.* 1986;7:11–18.

16. Ogden JA. Origin of a single coronary artery from the pulmonary artery. *Am Heart J.* 1969;78:251–253.

17. Bharati S, Chandra N, Stephenson LW, Wagner HR, Weinberg PM, Lev M. Origin of the left coronary artery from the right pulmonary artery. *J Am Coll Cardiol.* 1984;3:1565–1569.

18. Legendre A, Ou P, Bonnet D. Ostial stenosis of an anomalous left coronary artery from the pulmonary artery in a teenager. *Pediatr Cardiol.* 2009;30:1194–1195.

19. Goldberg SP, Mitchell MB, Campbell DN, Tissot C, Lacour-Gayet F. Anomalous left coronary artery from the pulmonary artery with an intramural course within the aortic wall: report of 3 surgical cases. *J Thorac Cardiovasc Surg.* 2008;135:696–698.

20. Burch GE, Depasquale NP. The anomalous left coronary artery: an experiment of nature. *Am J Med.* 1964;37:159–161.

21. Case RB, Morrow AG, Stainsby W, Nestor JO. Anomalous origin of the left coronary artery; the physiologic defect and suggested surgical treatment. *Circulation.* 1958;17:1062–1068.

22. Arsan S, Naseri E, Keser N. An adult case of Bland White Garland syndrome with huge right coronary aneurysm. *Ann Thorac Surg.* 1999;68:1832–1833.

23. Perloff JK. Normal myocardial growth and the development and regression of increased ventricular mass. In: Perloff JK, Child JS, Aboulhosn J, eds. *Congenital heart disease in adults.* 3rd ed. Philadelphia: Saunders/Elsevier; 2009.

24. Hutchins GM, Bannayan GA. Development of endocardial fibroelastosis following myocardial infarction. *Arch Pathol.* 1971;91:113–118.

25. Kutsche LM, Van Mierop LH. Anatomy and pathogenesis of aorticopulmonary septal defect. *Am J Cardiol.* 1987;59:443–447.

26. Cardo M, Fernandez B, Duran AC, Fernandez MC, Arque JM, Sans-Coma V. Anomalous origin of the left coronary artery from the dorsal aortic sinus and its relationship with aortic valve morphology in Syrian hamsters. *J Comp Pathol.* 1995;112:373–380.

27. Cardo M, Fernandez B, Duran AC, Arque JM, Franco D, Sans-Coma V. Anomalous origin of the left coronary artery from the pulmonary trunk and its relationship with the morphology of the cardiac semilunar valves in Syrian hamsters. *Basic Res Cardiol.* 1994;89:94–99.

28. Browne LP, Kearney D, Taylor MD, et al. ALCAPA: the role of myocardial viability studies in determining prognosis. *Pediatr Radiol.* 2010;40:163–167.

29. Dent Jr ED, Fisher RS. Single coronary artery: report of two cases. *Ann Intern Med.* 1956;44:1024–1030.

30. Murphy ML. Single coronary artery. *Am Heart J.* 1967;74:557–561.

31. Smith JC. Review of single coronary artery with report of 2 cases. *Circulation.* 1950;1:1168–1175.

32. Newton Jr MC, Burwell LR. Single coronary artery with myocardial infarction and mitral regurgitation. *Am Heart J.* 1978;95:126–127.

33. Pachinger O, Vandenhoven P, Judkins M. Single coronary artery-a cause of angina pectoris. *Eur J Cardiol.* 1974;2:161–165.

34. Baue AE, Baum S, Blakemore WS, Zinsser HF. A later stage of anomalous coronary circulation with origin of the left coronary artery from the pulmonary artery. Coronary artery steal. *Circulation.* 1967;36:878–885.

35. Edwards JE. The direction of blood flow in coronary arteries arising from the pulmonary trunk. *Circulation.* 1964;29:163–166.

36. Armer RM, Shumacker HB, Lurie PR, Fisch C. Origin of the left coronary artery from the pulmonary artery without collateral circulation. *Report of a case with a suggested surgical correction Pediatrics.* 1963;32:588–593.

37. Sabiston Jr DC, Neill CA, Taussig HB. The direction of blood flow in anomalous left coronary artery arising from the pulmonary artery. *Circulation.* 1960;22:591–597.

38. Rudolph AM. The effects of postnatal circulatory adjustments in congenital heart disease. *Pediatrics.* 1965;36:763–772.

39. Menke JA, Shaher RM, Wolff GS. Ejection fraction in anomalous origin of the left coronary artery from the pulmonary artery. *Am Heart J.* 1972;84:325–329.

40. Hofmeyr L, Moolman J, Brice E, Weich H. An unusual presentation of an anomalous left coronary artery arising from the pulmonary artery (ALCAPA) in an adult: anterior papillary muscle rupture causing severe mitral regurgitation. *Echocardiography.* 2009;26:474–477.

41. Rudolph AM, Gootman NL, Kaplan N, Rohman M. Anomalous left coronary artery arising from the pulmonary artery with large left-to-right shunt in infancy. *J Pediatr.* 1963;63:543–549.

42. Carvalho JS, Redington AN, Oldershaw PJ, Shinebourne EA, Lincoln CR, Gibson DG. Analysis of left ventricular wall movement before and after reimplantation of anomalous left coronary artery in infancy. *Br Heart J.* 1991;65:218–222.

43. Rein AJ, Colan SD, Parness IA, Sanders SP. Regional and global left ventricular function in infants with anomalous origin of the left coronary artery from the pulmonary trunk: preoperative and postoperative assessment. *Circulation.* 1987;75:115–123.

44. Jameson AG, Ellis K, Levine OR. Anomalous left coronary artery arising from pulmonary artery. *Br Heart J.* 1963;25:251–256.

45. Letcher JR, Mccormick D, Tendler S, Ross Jr J, Chandrasekaran K, Brockman S. Left main coronary artery arising from the pulmonary trunk in a 56-year-old patient presenting with acute myocardial infarction. *Am J Cardiol.* 1991;68:1257–1258.

46. Suzuki Y, Murakami T, Kawai C. Detection of anomalous origin of left coronary artery from pulmonary artery by real-time Doppler color flow mapping in a 53-year-old asymptomatic female. *Int J Cardiol.* 1992;34:339–342.

47. Talner NS, Halloran KH, Mahdavy M, Gardner TH, Hipona F. Anomalous origin of the left coronary artery from the pulmonary artery: a clinical spectrum. *Am J Cardiol.* 1965;15:689–695.

48. Cronk ES, Sinclair JG, Rigdon RH. An anomalous coronary artery arising from the pulmonary artery. *Am Heart J.* 1951;42:906–911.

49. Garty Y, Guri A, Shinwell ES, Matitiau A. An unusual neonatal presentation of anomalous origin of the left coronary artery arising from the pulmonary artery. *Neonatology.* 2008;93:248–250.

50. Castaneda AR, Indeglia RA, Varco RL. Anomalous origin of the left coronary artery from the pulmonary artery. Certain therapeutic considerations. *Circulation.* 1966;33:I52–56.

51. Allen DR, Schieken RM, Donofrio MT. Hoarseness as the initial clinical presentation of anomalous left coronary artery from the pulmonary artery. *Pediatr Cardiol.* 2005;26:668–671.

52. Moustafa SE, Zehr K, Mookadam M, Lorenz EC, Mookadam F. Anomalous interarterial left coronary artery: an evidence based systematic overview. *Int J Cardiol.* 2008;126:13–20.

53. Ihenacho HN, Singh SP, Astley R, Parsons CG. Anomalous left coronary artery. Report of an unusual case with spontaneous remission of symptoms. *Br Heart J.* 1973;35:562–565.

54. Abbott M. Congenital cardiac disease. In: Osler W, McCrae T, eds. *Modern medicine, its theory and practice.* Philadelphia: Lea & Febiger; 1908:323–425.

55. Facciorusso A, Lanna P, Vigna C, et al. Anomalous origin of the left coronary artery from the pulmonary artery in an elderly patient, football player in youth. *J Cardiovasc Med (Hagerstown).* 2008;9:1066–1069.

56. Irving C, Wren C. Asymptomatic anomalous origin of the left coronary artery from the pulmonary artery. *Pediatr Cardiol.* 2009;30:385–386.

57. Maeder M, Vogt PR, Ammann P, Rickli H. Bland-White-Garland syndrome in a 39-year-old mother. *Ann Thorac Surg.* 2004;78:1451–1453.

58. Lampe CF, Verheugt AP. Anomalous left coronary artery. Adult type. *Am Heart J.* 1960;59:769–776.

59. Fierens C, Budts W, Denef B, Van De Werf F. A 72 year old woman with ALCAPA. *Heart.* 2000;83:E2.
60. Kerwin RW, Westaby S, Davies GJ, Blackwood RA. Anomalous left coronary artery from the pulmonary artery presenting with infective endocarditis in an adult. *Eur Heart J.* 1985;6:545–547.
61. Agustsson MH, Gasul BM, Lundquist R. Anomalous origin of the left coronary artery from the pulmonary artery (adult type). A case report. *Pediatrics.* 1962;29:274–282.
62. Alexi-Meskishvili V, Berger F, Weng Y, Lange PE, Hetzer R. Anomalous origin of the left coronary artery from the pulmonary artery in adults. *J Card Surg.* 1995;10:309–315.
63. Frapier JM, Leclercq F, Bodino M, Chaptal PA. Malignant ventricular arrhythmias revealing anomalous origin of the left coronary artery from the pulmonary artery in two adults. *Eur J Cardiothorac Surg.* 1999;15:539–541.
64. Harthorne JW, Scannell JG, Dinsmore RE. Anomalous origin of the left coronary artery. Remediable cause of sudden death in adults. *N Engl J Med.* 1966;275:660–663.
65. Cayler GG, Smeloff EA, Miller Jr GE. A new clinical sign of anomalous coronary artery. *Dis Chest.* 1969;55:163–166.
66. Perloff JK, Roberts WC. The mitral apparatus. Functional anatomy of mitral regurgitation. *Circulation.* 1972;46:227–239.
67. Davis Jr C, Dillon RF, Fell EH, Gasul BM. Anomalous coronary artery simulating patent ductus arteriosus. *J Am Med Assoc.* 1956; 160:1047–1050.
68. Jurishica AJ. Anomalous left coronary artery; adult type. *Am Heart J.* 1957;54:429–436.
69. Puri PS, Rowe RD, Neill CA. Varying vectorcardiographic patterns in anomalous left coronary artery arising from pulmonary artery. *Am Heart J.* 1966;71:616–626.
70. Perloff JK, Roberts NK, Cabeen Jr. WR. Left axis deviation: a reassessment. *Circulation.* 1979;60:12–21.
71. Sabiston Jr DC, Pelargonio S, Taussig HB. Myocardial infarction in infancy. The surgical management of a complication of congenital origin of the left coronary artery from the pulmonary artery. *J Thorac Cardiovasc Surg.* 1960;40:321–336.
72. Kudo Y, Suda K, Koteda Y. Pitfalls of echocardiographic evaluation of anomalous origin of the left coronary artery from the pulmonary trunk. *Cardiol Young.* 2008;18:537–538.
73. Houston AB, Pollock JC, Doig WB, et al. Anomalous origin of the left coronary artery from the pulmonary trunk: elucidation with colour Doppler flow mapping. *Br Heart J.* 1990;63:50–54.
74. Schmidt KG, Cooper MJ, Silverman NH, Stanger P. Pulmonary artery origin of the left coronary artery: diagnosis by two-dimensional echocardiography, pulsed Doppler ultrasound and color flow mapping. *J Am Coll Cardiol.* 1988;11:396–402.
75. Swensson RE, Murillo-Olivas A, Elias W, Bender R, Daily PO, Sahn DJ. Noninvasive Doppler color flow mapping for detection of anomalous origin of the left coronary artery from the pulmonary artery and for evaluation of surgical repair. *J Am Coll Cardiol.* 1988; 11:659–661.
76. Hsu SY, Lin FC, Chang HJ, Yeh SJ, Wu D. Multiplane transesophageal echocardiography in diagnosis of anomalous origin of the left coronary artery from the pulmonary artery: a case report. *J Am Soc Echocardiogr.* 1998;11:668–672.
77. Kandzari DE, Harrison JK, Behar VS. An anomalous left coronary artery originating from the pulmonary artery in a 72-year-old woman: diagnosis by color flow myocardial blush and coronary arteriography. *J Invasive Cardiol.* 2002;14:96–99.
78. Ichikawa M, Lim Y-J, Komatsu S, et al. Detection of Bland-White-Garland Syndrome by multislice computed tomography in an elderly patient. *Int J Cardiol.* 2007;114:288–290.
79. Sato Y, Inoue F, Matsumoto N, et al. Detection of anomalous origins of the coronary artery by means of multislice computed tomography. *Circ J.* 2005;69:320–324.
80. Komocsi A, Simor T, Toth L, et al. Magnetic resonance studies in management of adult cases with Bland-White-Garland syndrome. *Int J Cardiol.* 2007;123:e8–e11.
81. Rha SW, Yong HS, Park CG. Anomalous origin of the left coronary artery from the pulmonary artery in an elderly patient visualised by three dimensional multidetector CT coronary angiography. *Heart.* 2005;91:947.

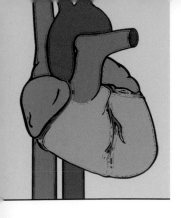

Chapter 22

Congenital Coronary Arterial Fistula

Coronary arterial fistulas are the most frequent functionally significant congenital malformations of the coronary circulation; they comprise 14% of all congenital coronary artery anomalies and 0.2% to 0.4% of all congenital cardiac defects (see Chapter 32). The right and left coronary arteries arise from their appropriate aortic sinuses, but a fistulous branch of one or more than one drains into a cardiac chamber or into the pulmonary trunk, coronary sinus, vena cava, or a pulmonary vein.[1] When the fistula drains into a right cardiac chamber or into the pulmonary *trunk*, it is *arteriovenous*, an appropriate term because the communication allows arterialized systemic blood—*arterio*—to mix with unoxygenated blood in the right side of the heart—*venous*. When the fistula drains into the *left atrium* or *left ventricle*, the appropriate term is coronary *arterial* rather than arteriovenous.

Congenital coronary arterial fistula was described by Krause[2] in 1865 and confirmed by Abbott in 1908[3] and by Trevor in 1912.[4] Approximately half of these fistulas arise from the *right* coronary artery, somewhat less from the *left* coronary artery, and only 5% from *both* coronary arteries.[5] Even more rarely, all three coronary arteries are involved,[6] or multiple fistulas arise from one coronary artery[7] or from a single coronary artery.[8] Isolated reports have appeared of fistulas from the conus artery to the right atrium,[9] from the coronary sinus to the left ventricle,[10] from the left circumflex to the coronary sinus[11,12] or to the pulmonary artery,[13] or from the microfistulae to the left ventricle.[14] A significant minority of these fistulas are *acquired* (i.e., traumatic) because of intravascular, interventional, or surgical procedures.[15–17] The contralateral coronary artery is absent in about 3% of congenital cases.

The *drainage site* of a coronary arterial fistula is more important than its site of origin and consists of a single vascular channel, multiple channels, or a maze of fine channels that form a diffuse network or plexus (spongy myocardium), a pattern especially likely when the left ventricle receives the fistula (see Figure 22-6B).[14] More than 90% of congenital coronary arterial fistulas drain into the *right* side of the heart and are therefore *arteriovenous*. A substantial majority, in approximate order of frequency, enter the right ventricle (40%) or right atrium (25%) (Figure 22-1A); less commonly, the pulmonary trunk (15%; Figures 22-2 and 22-3) or coronary sinus (7%; Figure 22-1B)[18]; and rarely, the hepatic vein[19] or superior vena cava.[20–22] A dual right coronary artery has been accompanied by a fistulous communication.[23] The coronary sinus that receives a fistula can be aneurysmal,

especially if it receives fistulas from *two* coronary arteries (see Figure 22-7).[5] A giant right coronary artery–to–superior vena caval fistula has been reported,[24] as has an aneurysmal coronary artery fistula in which the left main coronary connected to the right atrium.[25] *Bilateral* coronary arterial fistulas usually drain into the pulmonary trunk. The relatively few that do not communicate with the right side of the heart drain into the left atrium (5%; Figure 22-4), left ventricle (3%; Figures 22-5 and 22-6),[26,27] pulmonary veins, or *both* ventricles. A *coronary artery–to–left ventricular fistula* is not the same as an *aortic–to–left ventricular tunnel* (see Chapter 6).[27,28] Small coronary arterial fistulas without clinical evidence of their presence have been unexpectedly discovered during routine echocardiography (see Figure 22-18) and are incidental findings in 0.1% to 0.26% of patients undergoing routine coronary angiography (see Figure 22-3B).[29] In a series of 14,708 coronary arteriograms, 19 congenital coronary arterial fistulas were found; and in a series of 11,000 coronary angiograms, 13 fistulas were identified.[30] These incidentally found fistulas are characterized by one or more small channels that originate from the left anterior descending coronary artery and form networks that communicate at sites in the pulmonary trunk (see Figure 22-3B).

The coronary artery that gives rise to the fistula is characteristically dilated, elongated, and tortuous (see Figure 22-2),[31] and the coronaries distal to the fistula are of normal caliber (see Figure 22-3A). A fistulous coronary artery may contain saccular aneurysms that reach an astonishing size and may rupture (see previous).[32,33]

An estimated 1% to 2% of coronary arterial fistulas close *spontaneously* in infants, children, and adults.[34,35] Occlusion of an atherosclerotic coronary artery proximal to the fistula was responsible for closure in a 44-year-old woman. Occasionally, calcification of the wall of the fistula and thrombi with embolization are seen.

The *embryogenesis* of coronary arterial fistulas is uncertain. Fistulas that enter the *right ventricle* have been related to persistence of primitive intramyocardial sinusoids[36] or to the development of a rectiform vascular network in the distal branches of the involved coronary artery.[18] Fistulas that enter the left ventricle are thought to result from direct flow through thebesian venous channels.[37] Interestingly, the veins of Thebesius were cited as evidence of direct passage of blood from one side of the heart to the other before William Harvey discovered the circulation (see Chapter 32).

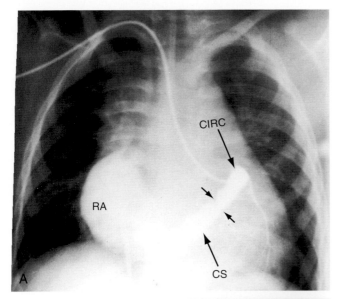

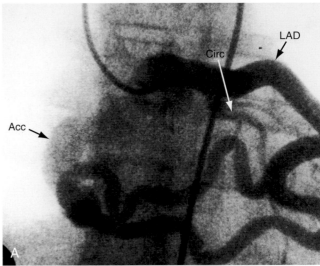

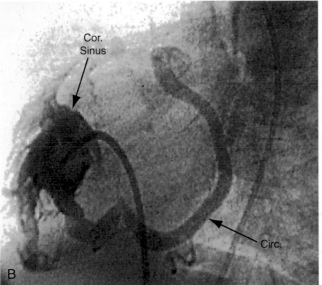

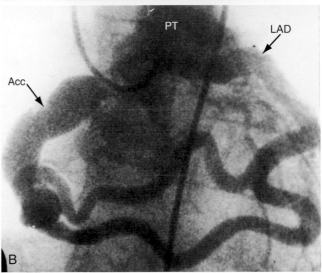

FIGURE 22-1 A, Left coronary arteriogram in an 8-year-old boy. The dilated circumflex coronary artery (CIRC) is narrow (unlabeled paired arrows) as it joins the coronary sinus (CS), which drains into a dilated right atrium (RA). **B,** Left coronary arteriogram in an 18-year-old woman with a coronary arterial fistula from a dilated circumflex artery (Circ.) to a dilated coronary sinus (Cor. Sinus).

FIGURE 22-2 A, Selective left coronary arteriogram from a 10-year-old girl with a coronary arterial fistula from the left anterior descending coronary artery (LAD) to an accessory coronary artery (Acc). The vascular channels that form the fistula are large, dilated, and tortuous. Uninvolved branches of the circumflex system (Circ) are small. **B,** A later frame showing a large accessory coronary artery (Acc) draining into the pulmonary trunk (PT).

Of the six coronary anlagen in the embryo, three are in the developing aorta and three are in the developing pulmonary artery (see Chapter 21).[38] These anlagen are normally involute, except for the two from the right and left aortic sinuses. The relatively high incidence of *bilateral* coronary arterial–to–pulmonary arterial fistulas is in accord with this observation. A *coronary arterial–to–pulmonary artery fistula* may result from persistence of one or more of the pulmonary arterial anlagen, hence the term *accessory* coronary artery, which is either a single large channel (see Figure 22-2), one or more smaller channels, multiple tortuous channels, or a plexiform arrangement.

The *physiologic consequences* of coronary arterial fistulas depend on the volume of blood flowing through them, the chamber or vascular bed into which they drain, and the myocardial ischemia that results from a *coronary steal* caused by low-resistance vascular channels. About 10% of blood from the aortic root normally enters the coronary circulation, but in the presence of a coronary arterial fistula, the volume is considerably larger. A fistula that drains into the right atrium, right ventricle, or coronary sinus constitutes a *left-to-right* shunt. If drainage is into the right ventricular outflow tract, pulmonary trunk (see Figures 22-2 and 22-3), left atrium (see Figure 22-6), or left ventricle (see Figures 22-4 and 22-5), the hemodynamic burden is borne by the left ventricle alone.[26] A fistulous coronary artery receives blood during systole when its stoma is large.[26,39] If the fistula drains into

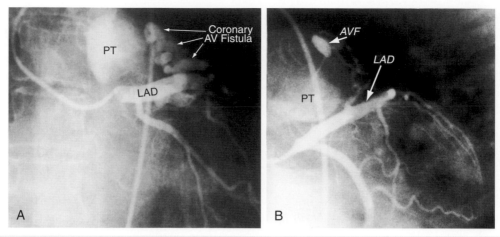

FIGURE 22-3 **A,** Left coronary arteriogram from a 62-year-old woman. A dilated left anterior descending artery (LAD) gave rise to a coronary arteriovenous fistula (Coronary AV Fistula) that drained into the pulmonary trunk (PT). Coronary arterial branches distal to the fistula are of normal caliber. **B,** Left coronary arteriogram from a 58-year-old man in whom a small coronary arterial fistula (AVF) from the left anterior descending artery (LAD) to the pulmonary trunk (PT) was found during routine coronary angiography.

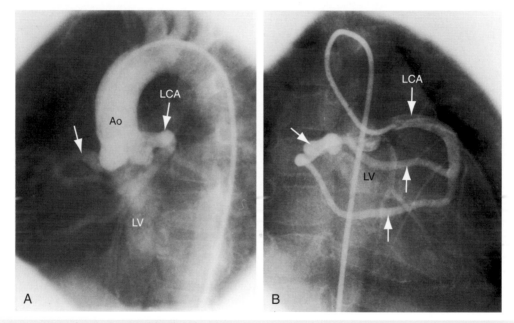

FIGURE 22-4 **A,** Aortogram from a 5-year-old girl with a coronary arterial fistula that originated from the proximal left coronary artery (LCA) and drained into the left ventricle (LV). The proximal left coronary is dilated because it fed the fistula (unmarked left arrow) (Ao=aorta). **B,** A left coronary arteriogram (LCA) visualized the dilated tortuous fistula (unmarked white arrows) that drained into the left ventricle (LV).

the *inflow tract* of the right ventricle, volume overload of the right ventricle coexists. If drainage is *directly* into the right atrium or *indirectly* through the coronary sinus (see Figure 22-1), volume overload of right ventricle exists in addition to overload of the left side of the heart.

Pulmonary-to-systemic flow ratios are typically small, even negligible, regardless of patient age. Shunts in excess of 2:1 are unusual, but an occasional neonate experiences congestive heart failure (see Figure 22-17) when an exceptionally large fistula drains into the left or right side of the heart.[36,39]

Myocardial ischemia is incurred when a coronary arterial fistula functions as a low-resistance pathway that constitutes a *coronary steal*.[26] The coronary artery gives rise to the fistula and then assumes an important role because

steal from a major branch of the *left* coronary artery is more significant than steal from a smaller right coronary artery. Acquired coronary artery stenosis *distal* to a congenital coronary arterial fistula aggravates the perfusion deficit because the fistula acts as a low-resistance alternative to the acquired obstruction.

HISTORY

The initial suspicion of a congenital coronary arterial fistula in an asymptomatic child or young adult is likely to be a continuous murmur. A small acoustically silent coronary arterial fistula is usually discovered during routine

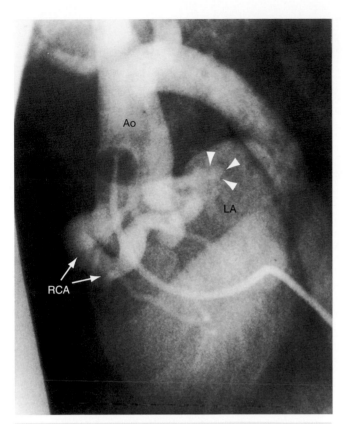

FIGURE 22-5 Aortogram from an 11-month-old male with a coronary arterial fistula that arose from the right coronary artery (RCA) and drained into the left atrium (LA) (Ao = aorta).

be heard but misinterpreted. Coronary arterial fistulas are mistaken for patent ductus arteriosus (Figure 22-8), which occasionally coexists.[40,41] A coronary arteriovenous fistula may present with angina,[26,42] and occasionally with a pericardial effusion[13] or infective endocarditis.[22]

The male:female ratio is about equal. Survival into adulthood is expected, but lifespan is not normal.[18] Longevity has been reported in the sixth to ninth decade (see Figure 22-16),[13,43] and the diagnosis has been made as late as the seventh to ninth decade.[44] A 68-year-old professional athlete was undiagnosed until acquired coronary artery disease prompted coronary angiography, which disclosed bilateral coronary arterial fistulas.

Most patients, especially those less than 20 years of age, are asymptomatic when the coronary arterial fistula is first diagnosed.[18] An uncommon, if not rare, exception is the infant with an exceptionally large fistula (see Figure 22-17).[36,39] Symptoms and complications, in approximate order of frequency, include dyspnea, fatigue, myocardial ischemia,[26] congestive heart failure, sudden death,[45] infective endocarditis,[22,46] and rupture.[47] Obstruction of the superior vena cava has been caused by a large fistulous saccular aneurysm, one of which ruptured at age 82 years.[48] Atrial fibrillation that accompanies drainage into the right or left atrium or coronary sinus heralds congestive heart failure (see Figure 22-16).

A coronary steal may be the cause of myocardial ischemia and angina pectoris (see previous), and ischemia has an undesirable effect on left ventricular function.[26,49] Spontaneous closure of a coronary arterial fistula is uncommon but not rare (see previous).[34,35]

PHYSICAL APPEARANCE

Catabolic effects of congestive heart failure are reserved for the rare occurrence of large fistulas in infants.

ARTERIAL PULSE

The arterial pulse is normal because flow through the fistula is usually small. However, when the right ventricle, right atrium, or left atrium receives a large fistula, the

echocardiography or coronary angiography (see previous). When a coronary arterial fistula drains into the low-pressure right or left atrium, the continuous murmur dates from birth because the pressure gradient responsible for the murmur is present *in utero*. Conversely, coronary arterial fistulas that drain into the right ventricle or pulmonary trunk do not generate continuous murmurs until after the neonatal fall in pulmonary vascular resistance. The continuous murmur is overlooked when it is soft and localized to an atypical site. An isolated *diastolic* murmur may

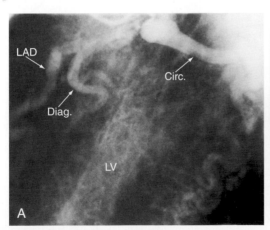
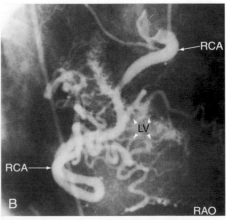

FIGURE 22-6 Coronary arteriograms from a 70-year-old asymptomatic woman who came to medical attention because of a diastolic murmur at the left sternal border. Left ventricular ejection fraction was 58%. **A,** The left anterior descending (LAD), diagonal (Diag.), circumflex (Circ.), and right coronary artery (RCA; see Figure 22B) were all dilated. **B,** The three dilated coronary arteries gave rise to a maze of tortuous fistulae that drained into the left ventricle (LV) through a fine intramural plexus. (RAO = right anterior oblique.)

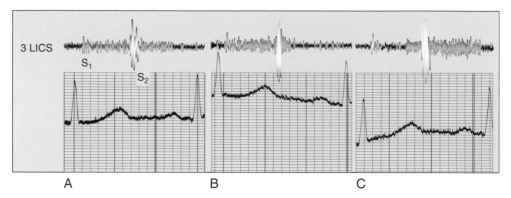

A   B   C

FIGURE 22-7 Phonocardiograms from a 37-year-old woman with a coronary arterial fistula between the right coronary artery and outflow tract of the right ventricle. A continuous murmur that peaked before and after the second heart sound (S$_2$) was mistaken for a patent ductus murmur even though the maximum location was the third left intercostal space (3 LICS) and even though the murmur changed configuration from beat to beat (**A, B, C**).

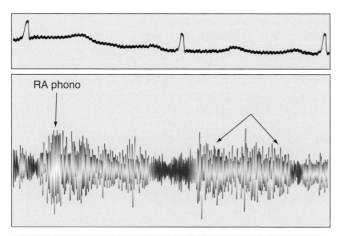

FIGURE 22-8 Phonocardiogram from within the right atrium (RA phono) of a 27-year-old man with a coronary arterial fistula between the right coronary artery and right atrium. In the first cycle, the continuous murmur is louder in systole (vertical arrow). In the second cycle, the murmur is equal in systole and diastole (paired arrows).

arterial pulse is brisk and the pulse pressure is wide because a fall in aortic *diastolic* pressure caused by flow into low-pressure drainage sites is accompanied by a rise in *systolic* pressure caused by an increase in left ventricular stroke volume and ejection velocity (Figure 22-9). When a large fistula drains into the left ventricle, the hemodynamic response is analogous to aortic regurgitation.

JUGULAR VENOUS PULSE

The jugular pulse is normal even when a small or moderate-sized fistula drains directly into the right atrium. With the advent of congestive heart failure induced by a large fistula (see Figure 22-16B), the mean right atrial pressure rises. Obstruction of the superior vena by the saccular aneurysm of a fistula that drained into the right atrium elevated the mean jugular venous pressure and damped the A and V waves. A giant left atrium caused by a large coronary arterial–to–left atrial fistula in a 64-year-old man contributed to *inferior* vena caval obstruction.

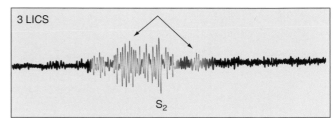

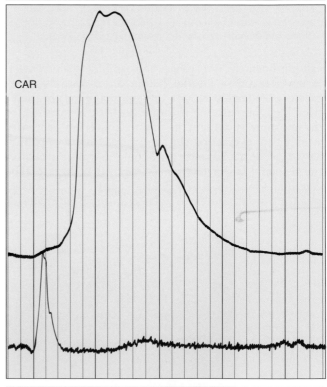

FIGURE 22-9 Phonocardiogram and carotid pulse (CAR) from a 47-year-old man with a coronary arterial fistula between the right coronary artery and outflow tract of the right ventricle. The continuous murmur was much louder in systole (paired arrows) and was maximal in the third left intercostal space (3 LICS). (S$_2$=second heart sound.) The pulse pressure was wide (170/68 mm Hg). Pulmonary-to-systemic flow ratio was 1.7 to 1.

PRECORDIAL MOVEMENT AND PALPATION

A large fistula results in a hyperdynamic left ventricular impulse because left ventricular volume overload accompanies *all* drainage sites. If the fistula drains into the left atrium or left ventricle, or into the pulmonary artery, an *isolated* left ventricular impulse is palpated. If the fistula drains into the right atrium or into the right ventricular inflow tract, volume overload is imposed on *both* ventricles, so right *and* left ventricular impulses are both palpated.

AUSCULTATION

A continuous murmur that is an auscultatory hallmark of coronary arterial fistulas (Figures 22-10, 22-11, and 22-12)[50–53] may be mistaken for the continuous murmur of patent ductus arteriosus.[40,41] The distinction is based on the configuration of the murmur (see Figure 22-8) and on its precordial location that is determined by the drainage site of the fistula, not by its coronary artery of origin (Figure 22-13). Whether the fistula drains *directly* into the right atrium or drains into the right atrium *indirectly* through the coronary sinus (see Figure 22-1), intracardiac phonocardiography records the murmur within the right atrial cavity (see Figure 22-10) and the thoracic wall site is topographically appropriate at the *right* upper or lower

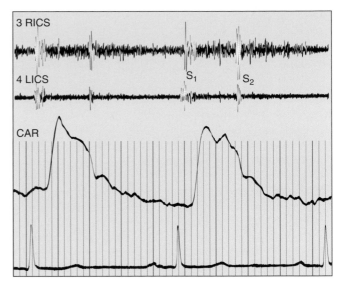

FIGURE 22-11 Phonocardiograms from a 23-year-old woman with a right coronary arterial fistula to the right atrium. A continuous murmur was loudest in the third *right* intercostal space (3 RICS). (S_1 and S_2 = first and second heart sounds; 4 LICS = fourth left intercostal space; CAR = carotid pulse.)

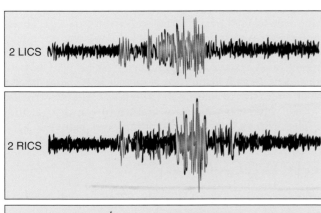
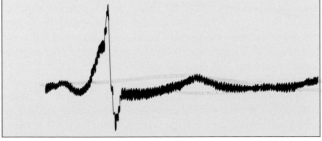

FIGURE 22-10 Phonocardiograms from an 8-year-old boy with a coronary arterial fistula from the circumflex coronary artery to the coronary sinus (see angiogram, Figure 22-3A). The continuous murmur was louder in systole and maximal in the second and third *right* intercostal spaces (2 RICS), which was topographically appropriate for the drainage site. (2 LICS = second left intercostal space). The electrocardiogram shows an incidental delta wave.

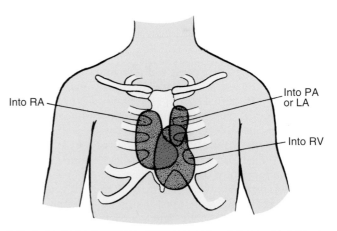

FIGURE 22-12 Schematic illustration of precordial murmur locations as determined by the site of coronary arterial fistula drainage. (*Adapted from Sakakibara S, et al. Coronary arteriovenous fistula. American Heart Journal 1966;72:307.*)

sternal border or over the sternum (see Figure 22-12).[35,40] When a left circumflex coronary arterial fistula drains into the coronary sinus (see Figure 22-1A), the continuous murmur is heard in the back between the spine and left scapula. When the fistula drains into the inflow tract of the right ventricle, the murmur sites are along the mid to lower *left* sternal border, over the *lower sternum*, or *subxyphoid* (see Figure 22-13). When the fistula drains into the outflow tract of the right ventricle, the murmur is maximal along the upper to mid left sternal border (see Figures 22-8 and 22-13).[51] With drainage into the pulmonary trunk, the continuous murmur is prominent at the upper left sternal border (see Figure 22-13).[50] A small or plexiform pulmonary arterial fistula discovered incidentally at coronary angiography (see Figure 22-3B) is

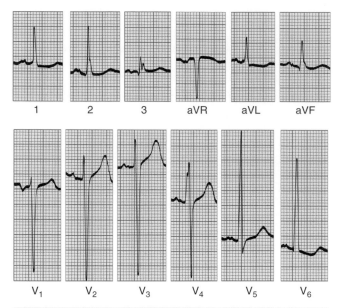

FIGURE 22-13 Electrocardiogram from a 47-year-old man with a right coronary arterial fistula that entered the outflow tract of the right ventricle. The phonocardiogram and carotid pulse are shown in Figure 22-8. P waves are slightly bifid in leads 1, 2, and aVR, and the P terminal force is abnormal in lead V_1. There are voltage and repolarization criteria for left ventricular hypertrophy in leads V_{5-6}.

not accompanied by a chest wall murmur. When a fistula drains into the left atrium, the murmur is maximal along the upper left sternal border (see Figure 22-13) and may radiate toward the left anterior auxiliary line. A fistula that drains into a left superior vena cava is accompanied by a continuous murmur at the upper to mid left sternal edge.[21,22] The coronary arterial fistulas that are especially mistaken for patent ductus arteriosus are those that drain into the pulmonary trunk, left atrium, or right ventricular outflow tract. Because most coronary arterial fistulas drain into the body of the right ventricle or into the right atrium, the accompanying continuous murmur is heard at sites *remote* from the ductus location. Spontaneous closure of a coronary arterial fistula (see previous) is accompanied by diminution or disappearance of the murmur.[34]

Coronary arterial fistulas that drain into the right atrium, left atrium, or right ventricle generate continuous murmurs because pressure differences between the aortic root and the low-pressure receiving chambers are continuous (i.e., without interruption from systole into diastole). The *configurations* of continuous murmurs from these different fistulous sources differ from each other and differ from the continuous murmur of patent ductus arteriosus. When the fistula drains into the right atrium, coronary sinus, or left atrium, pressure gradients between aortic root and receiving chamber are much larger during systole than during diastole, so the murmur is louder in systole (see Figure 22-11). When the fistula communicates with the pulmonary trunk, the continuous murmur may envelope the second heart sound as in patent ductus, but there no *eddy sounds*.[52,53] Flow patterns are more complex when the fistula drains into the right ventricle because right ventricular contraction compresses the fistula during its

transmural course (see Figure 22-8). Compression that is sufficient to reduce systolic flow softens the systolic portion of the murmur (see Figure 22-8C). Less compression increases the intramural systolic gradient, so the systolic portion of the continuous murmur is louder (see Figures 22-8B, and 22-9).[54] A wide aortic pulse pressure (high systolic, low diastolic) reinforces the systolic portion of the continuous murmur (see Figure 22-9). When congestive heart failure elevates right ventricular diastolic pressure, a continuous murmur becomes only systolic because elevated diastolic pressure decreases diastolic flow.

An early diastolic murmur is generated when a fistula drains into the left ventricle. Blood flow *into* the fistula during systole may generate a systolic murmur when a large fistulous stoma remains widely patent during left ventricular contraction. When drainage is through thebesian venous channels, a coronary arterial–to–left ventricular fistula is silent.[37]

Because coronary arterial fistulas usually deliver relatively small blood volumes through narrow pathways, the accompanying continuous murmur is relatively localized, medium to moderately high-frequency, and grade 3 or less. Large fistulas generate coarse harsh rough murmurs that radiate and are accompanied by thrills. The Valsalva's maneuver causes a coronary arterial–to–right ventricular fistulous murmur to soften as systolic pressure in the right ventricle rises. Occasionally, a coronary arterial–to–right atrial fistulous continuous murmur diminishes appreciably during held inspiration and becomes tumultuous during exhalation.

The second heart sound splits normally during respiration even when the right atrium receives the fistula. This is so for two reasons: *first*, the shunt volume is shared equally by the right and left sides of the heart because shunted blood must traverse *both* ventricles on its way back to the aorta; *second*, inspiration results in an *increase* in right ventricular stroke volume and a *decrease* in left ventricular stroke volume because the shunt into the right atrium occurs with an intact atrial septum (see Chapter 15).

ELECTROCARDIOGRAM

Electrocardiographic abnormalities are related chiefly to the chamber receiving the shunt and to the volume of blood flowing through the fistula. Fistulas that drain into the right atrium or coronary sinus result in biatrial P wave abnormalities; drainage into the right ventricle, pulmonary trunk, or left atrium results in left atrial P wave abnormalities (Figure 22-14); and drainage into the right atrium or coronary sinus results in right atrial P wave abnormalities. Atrial fibrillation occasionally occurs in older patients when fistulas drain into the right atrium, left atrium, or coronary sinus (see Figure 22-16B).[5] Fistulas into the right ventricular outflow tract, pulmonary trunk, left atrium, or left ventricle cause left ventricular hypertrophy (see Figure 22-14). Biventricular hypertrophy occurs with drainage into the right atrium or into the body of the right ventricle because shunted blood circulates through *both* ventricles. A *coronary steal* (see previous) induces ischemic ST segment and T wave changes at rest or during exercise stress testing. An ischemic pattern is more likely to occur if the coronary steal involves a major branch of the *left* coronary artery. Myocardial infarction is rarely a feature of the electrocardiogram, although a fistula may aggravate the perfusion deficit of coexisting acquired coronary artery disease (see previous).

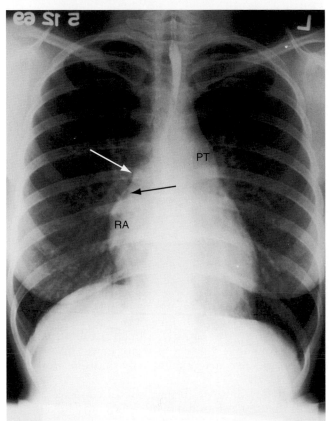

FIGURE 22-14 X-ray from a 23-year-old woman with a right coronary arterial fistula that drained into the right atrium (RA). The fistula reveals itself as a shadow to the right of the vertebral column (white and black arrows). The pulmonary trunk (PT) is moderately dilated. The phonocardiogram is shown in Figure 22-11.

X-RAY

The radiologic features of coronary arterial fistulas reflect the volume and duration of flow and the site of drainage. Young patients with small fistulas have normal x-rays. Infants with large fistulas and congestive heart failure have appreciable cardiomegaly.[36,39] A large fistula that drains into the right atrium or coronary sinus is accompanied by increased pulmonary vascularity and a convex pulmonary trunk with biventricular and biatrial enlargement (Figures 22-15 and 22-16 and Video 22-1).[18] Drainage into the right ventricle results in a similar picture but without dilation of the right atrium. When a coronary arterial fistula drains into the pulmonary trunk or left atrium, chamber enlargement is confined to the left ventricle and left atrium. A giant left atrium was reported in a 64-year-old man with a right coronary arterial–to–left atrial fistula.

Multiple saccular aneurysms of an enlarged tortuous coronary arterial fistula are occasionally recognized in the x-ray as an irregular silhouette along the right or left cardiac border. A giant aneurysm associated with a left coronary artery–to–pulmonary artery fistula presented as a calcified mediastinal mass.[55] Calcification in the wall of a fistula is only occasionally visible.

ECHOCARDIOGRAM

Transthoracic and transesophageal echocardiography with color flow imaging and Doppler interrogation are used to identify the origin and drainage site of coronary arterial fistulas and assess their functional consequences.[56–58] The stoma of a fistulous coronary artery considerably exceeds in size the origin of a normal coronary artery (Figure 22-17 and Videos 22-2A and 22-2B).[57] The *drainage site* can be identified with color flow imaging (Figures 22-18 [Video 22-3] and 22-19),[56] and Doppler interrogation is used to establish systolic and diastolic

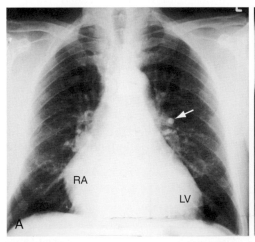
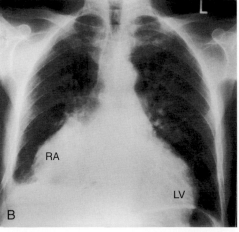

FIGURE 22-15 A, X-ray from a 64-year-old man with a large right coronary arterial–to–right atrial fistula. Pulmonary vascularity is increased. The unmarked white arrow identifies the prominent cross section of an intrapulmonary artery that reflects increased flow. A dilated right atrium (RA) occupies the lower right cardiac border, and a moderately dilated left ventricle (LV) occupies the apex. **B,** X-ray from the same patient after the onset of atrial fibrillation at age 75 years. The size of the right atrium (RA) has increased dramatically. The left ventricle (LV) is much larger and extends below the left hemidiaphragm. There is a small right pleural effusion.

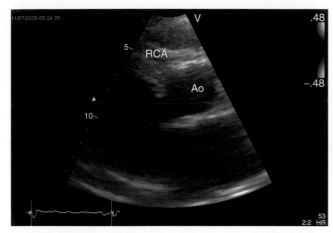

FIGURE 22-16 Echocardiogram (short axis) from a female neonate with congestive heart failure caused by a large right coronary arterial fistula that drained into outflow tract of the right ventricle. The proximal right coronary artery (RCA) is markedly dilated (Video 22-1). (Ao = aorta; PT = pulmonary trunk; PV = pulmonary valve.)

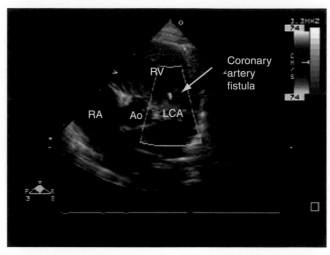

FIGURE 22-18 Color flow images of a silent coronary arterial–to–pulmonary arterial fistula (Video 22-3). (RV = right ventricle; RA = right atrium; Ao = aorta; LCA = left coronary artery.)

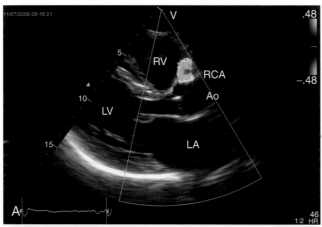

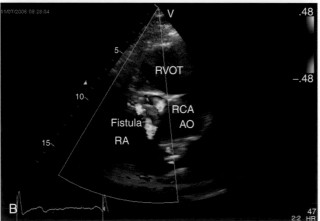

FIGURE 22-17 A, Echocardiogram showing a large coronary arterial fistula that drained into the right ventricle (RV). The proximal right coronary artery (RCA) is dilated. (Ao = aorta; LA = left atrium; LV = left ventricle) **B,** color flow image showing flow from the aorta into the large right coronary artery, from which the fistula originated (Videos 22-2A and 22-2B).

flow patterns[57] that shed light on the configuration of accompanying murmurs.

Coronary arterial fistulas drain into the pulmonary trunk immediately distal to the pulmonary valve, and flow proceeds upward along the medial wall (see Figure 22-18). Alternatively, a small fistula that drains into the pulmonary artery at a site more distal to the pulmonary valve may exhibit only diastolic flow (see Figure 22-18).

Color flow imaging distinguishes a coronary arterial fistula that drains into the right atrium or right ventricle from a ruptured sinus of Valsalva aneurysm (see Chapter 23). A coronary arterial fistula that drains into the pulmonary trunk can be distinguished from a patent ductus arteriosus (see Chapter 20) and from anomalous origin of the left coronary artery from the pulmonary trunk (see Chapter 21), and a fistula that drains into the left ventricle can be distinguished from an aortic–to–left ventricular tunnel (see Chapter 6).

Echocardiography characterizes the hemodynamic response to flow through a coronary arterial fistula and characterizes the response of the left ventricle to potential ischemic effects of a coronary steal. The coronary sinus is dilated when it receives one or more fistulas (see Figures 22-1B, and 22-7). Left ventricular ejection fraction reflects the volume overload delivered through the fistula, and global and regional wall motion reflect potentially adverse ischemic effects of a coronary steal.

SUMMARY

The physical appearance, arterial pulse, and jugular venous pulse are usually normal. Precordial palpation detects the impulse of either or both ventricles, depending on the drainage site of the fistula. A precordial continuous murmur located inappropriately for a patent ductus arteriosus is often the first index of suspicion of a

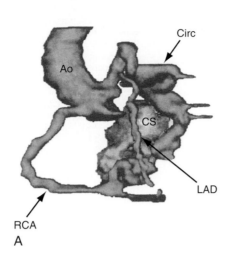

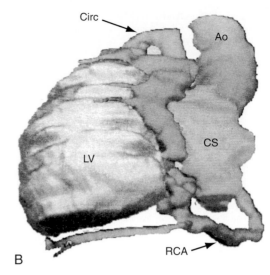

FIGURE 22-19 **A,** Anterior view of a three-dimensional magnetic resonance image obtained with sequential acquisitions in transaxial planes in a 44-year-old man with coronary arterial fistulas from the right coronary artery (RCA) and the circumflex coronary artery (Circ), both of which entered an aneurysmal coronary sinus (CS). (Ao=aorta; LAD=left anterior descending artery.) **B,** Posterior view shows the aneurysmal coronary sinus to better advantage. (LV=left ventricle.)

A

B

congenital coronary arterial fistula in an asymptomatic child or young adult. Suspicion is heightened if the murmur peaks in either systole or diastole, but not immediately before and after the second heart sound. The electrocardiogram reflects the volume of blood delivered through the fistula to individual recipient chambers. Angina from a coronary steal stands out in young patients. The x-ray reflects the response of individual chambers to the volume of the left-to-right shunt. Distinctive, but rarely seen, in the x-ray are the shadows of saccular aneurysms of a coronary arterial fistula as it courses along the right or left cardiac border. Echocardiography identifies the origin and drainage site of the fistula and establishes the physiologic consequences of the left-to-right shunt and the potential ischemic effects of a coronary steal.

REFERENCES

1. Liberthson RR, Sagar K, Berkoben JP, Weintraub RM, Levine FH. Congenital coronary arteriovenous fistula. Report of 13 patients, review of the literature and delineation of management. *Circulation.* 1979;59:849–854.
2. Krause W. Ueber den ursprung einer accessorischen A. Coronaria Cordis ausder. *A Pulmonis Z Rationelle Med.* 1865;24:225.
3. Abbott M. Anomalies of the coronary arteries. In: Osier W, ed. *Modern medicine.* Philadelphia: Lea & Febiger; 1908.
4. Trevor RS. Aneurysm of the descending branch of the right coronary artery, situated in the wall of the right ventricle, and opening into the cavity of the ventricle, associated with great dilatation of the right coronary artery and non-valvular infective endocarditis. *Proc R Soc Med.* 1912;5:20–26.
5. Duerinckx AJ, Perloff JK, Currier JW. Arteriovenous fistulas of the circumflex and right coronary arteries with drainage into an aneurysmal coronary sinus. *Circulation.* 1999;99:2827–2828.
6. Reddy K, Gupta M, Hamby RI. Multiple coronary arteriosystemic fistulas. *Am J Cardiol.* 1974;33:304–306.
7. Schamroth CL, Sareli P, Curcio A, Barlow JB. Multiple coronary artery-right ventricle fistulas. *Am Heart J.* 1985;109:1388–1390.
8. Gupta PD, Rahimtoola SH, Miller RA. Single coronary artery–right ventricle fistula. *Br Heart J.* 1972;34:755–757.
9. Lipoff JI. Anomalous origin of the left main coronary artery from the right sinus of Valsalva with coronary AV fistula of the conus artery. *Chest.* 1988;93:203–204.
10. Gnanapragasam JP, Houston AB, Lilley S. Congenital fistula between the left ventricle and coronary sinus: elucidation by colour Doppler flow mapping. *Br Heart J.* 1989;62:406–408.
11. Aoyagi S, Fukunaga S, Ishihara K, Egawa N, Hosokawa Y, Nakamura E. Coronary artery fistula from the left circumflex to the coronary sinus. *Int Heart J.* 2006;47:147–152.
12. Hayabuchi Y. Coronary arteriovenous fistula: direct connection of the proximal circumflex artery to the coronary sinus. *Pediatr Cardiol.* 2010;31:168–169.
13. Bellisarii FI, Marchetti M, Caputo M, De Caterina R. Coronary arteriovenous fistula presenting as chronic pericardial effusion. *J Cardiovasc Med.* 2006;7:449–453.
14. Cartoni D, Salvini P, De Rosa R, Cortese A, Nazzaro MS, Tanzi P. Images in cardiovascular medicine. Multiple coronary artery-left ventricle microfistulae and spongy myocardium: the eagerly awaited link? *Circulation.* 2007;116:e81–e84.
15. Tabrah F, Aintablian A, Hamby RI. Coronary arteriovenous fistula complicating aortocoronary bypass surgery. *Am Heart J.* 1973;85:534–537.
16. Wexberg P, Gottsauner-Wolf M, Kiss K, Steurer G, Glogar D. An iatrogenic coronary arteriovenous fistula causing a steal phenomenon: an intracoronary Doppler study. *Clin Cardiol.* 2001;24:630–632.
17. Renard VP, Vandenbogaerde J. Fistula between the left internal thoracic artery and the coronary sinus. *N Engl J Med.* 2000;343:149–150.
18. Ogden JA. Congenital anomalies of the coronary arteries. *Am J Cardiol.* 1970;25:474–479.
19. Gorgulu S, Nurkalem Z, Eren M. Right coronary artery hepatic vein fistula: a case report. *Echocardiography.* 2006;23:869–871.
20. Galbraith AJ, Werner D, Cutforth RH. Fistula between left coronary artery and superior vena cava. *Br Heart J.* 1981;46:99–100.
21. Marcus B, Sivazlian K, Gordon LS. Echocardiographic detection of left circumflex coronary artery to left superior vena cava fistula by use of Doppler color flow mapping. *J Am Soc Echocardiogr.* 1991;4:405–407.
22. Stansel Jr HC, Fenn JE. Coronary arteriovenous fistula between the left coronary artery and persistent left superior vena cava complicated by bacterial endocarditis. *Ann Surg.* 1964;160:292–296.
23. Huang Z-Q, Chen S-J, Chen J. Dual right coronary artery associated coronary artery fistula. *Eur Heart J.* 2008;29:968.
24. Lapenna E, Torracca L, De Bonis M, Alfieri O. A giant right coronary artery-to-superior vena cava fistula. *Eur J Cardiothorac Surg.* 2007;31:546.
25. Shiga Y, Tsuchiya Y, Yahiro E, et al. Left main coronary trunk connecting into right atrium with an aneurysmal coronary artery fistula. *Int J Cardiol.* 2008;123:e28–e30.
26. Cheng TO. Left coronary artery-to-left ventricular fistula: demonstration of coronary steal phenomenon. *Am Heart J.* 1982;104:870–872.

27. Takeda K, Okuda Y, Matsumura K, Sakuma H, Tagami T, Nakagawa T. Giant fistula between the right coronary artery and the left ventricle: diagnostic significance of right posterior oblique chest radiograph. *AJR Am J Roentgenol.* 1992;159:1087–1090.

28. Sung CS, Leachman RD, Zerpa F, Angelini P, Lufschanowski R. Aortico-left ventricular tunnel. *Am Heart J.* 1979;98:87–93.

29. Phillips PA, Libanoff AJ. Arteriovenous communication associated with obstructive arteriosclerotic coronary artery disease and myocardial infarction. *Chest.* 1974;65:106–108.

30. Said SA, Landman GH. Coronary-pulmonary fistula: long-term follow-up in operated and non-operated patients. *Int J Cardiol.* 1990;27:203–210.

31. Muir CS. Coronary arterio-cameral fistula. *Br Heart J.* 1960;22:374–384.

32. Braudo JL, Javett SN, Zion MM, Adler DI. Congenital coronary arteriovenous fistula. *Br Med J.* 1962;1:601–604.

33. Lim CH, Tan NC, Tan L, Seah CS, Tan D. Giant congenital aneurysm of the right coronary artery. *Am J Cardiol.* 1977;39:751–753.

34. Mahoney LT, Schieken RM, Lauer RM. Spontaneous closure of a coronary artery fistula in childhood. *Pediatr Cardiol.* 1982;2:311–312.

35. Farooki ZQ, Nowlen T, Hakimi M, Pinsky WW. Congenital coronary artery fistulae: a review of 18 cases with special emphasis on spontaneous closure. *Pediatr Cardiol.* 1993;14:208–213.

36. Verani MS, Lauer RM. Echocardiographic findings in right coronary arterial-right ventricular fistula. Report of a neonate with fatal congestive heart failure. *Am J Cardiol.* 1975;35:444–447.

37. Cha SD, Singer E, Maranhao V, Goldberg H. Silent coronary artery-left ventricular fistula: a disorder of the thebesian system? *Angiology.* 1978;29:169–173.

38. Heifetz SA, Robinowitz M, Mueller KH, Virmani R. Total anomalous origin of the coronary arteries from the pulmonary artery. *Pediatr Cardiol.* 1986;7:11–18.

39. Starc TJ, Bowman FO, Hordof AJ. Congestive heart failure in a newborn secondary to coronary artery-left ventricular fistula. *Am J Cardiol.* 1986;58:366–367.

40. Bosher Jr LH, Vasli S, Mc CC, Belter LF. Congenital coronary arteriovenous fistula associated with large patent ductus. *Circulation.* 1959;20:254–261.

41. Shaffer AB, St Ville J, Mackler SA. Coronary arteriovenous fistula with patent ductus arteriosus. *Am Heart J.* 1963;65:758–765.

42. Said SaM, Van Der Werf T. Dutch survey of coronary artery fistulas in adults: congenital solitary fistulas. *Int J Cardiol.* 2006;106:323–332.

43. Brack MJ, Hubner PJ, Firmin RK. Successful operation on a coronary arteriovenous fistula in a 74 year old woman. *Br Heart J.* 1991;65:107–108.

44. Ben-Gal T, Herz I, Solodky A, Snir E, Birnbaum Y. Coronary artery-main pulmonary artery fistula. *Clin Cardiol.* 1999;22:310.

45. Lau G. Sudden death arising from a congenital coronary artery fistula. *Forensic Sci Int.* 1995;73:125–130.

46. Tsagaris TJ, Hecht HH. Coronary artery aneurysm and subacute bacterial endarteritis. *Ann Intern Med.* 1962;57:116–121.

47. Habermann JH, Howard ML, Johnson ES. Rupture of the coronary sinus with hemopericardium. A rare complication of coronary arteriovenous fistula. *Circulation.* 1963;28:1143–1144.

48. Bauer HH, Allmendinger PD, Flaherty J, Owlia D, Rossi MA, Chen C. Congenital coronary arteriovenous fistula: spontaneous rupture and cardiac tamponade. *Ann Thorac Surg.* 1996;62:1521–1523.

49. Said SaM, Van Der Werf T. Dutch survey of congenital coronary artery fistulas in adults: coronary artery-left ventricular multiple micro-fistulas multi-center observational survey in the Netherlands. *Int J Cardiol.* 2006;110:33–39.

50. Biorck G, Crafoord C. Arteriovenous aneurysm on the pulmonary artery simulating patent ductus arteriosus botalli. *Thorax.* 1947;2:65–74.

51. Davis Jr C, Dillon RF, Fell EH, Gasul BM. Anomalous coronary artery simulating patent ductus arteriosus. *J Am Med Assoc.* 1956;160:1047–1050.

52. Ernst CB, Klassen KP, Ryan JM. Vascular malformation overlying the pulmonary artery simulating a patent ductus arteriosus. *Circulation.* 1961;23:759–761.

53. Nunn DB, Thrower WB, Boone JA, Lipton M. Coronary arteriovenous fistula simulating patent ductus arteriosus. *Am Surg.* 1962;28:476–482.

54. Puyau FA, Collins HA. Congenital coronary arteriovenous fistula. *Am J Dis Child.* 1963;106:65–72.

55. Okita Y, Miki S, Kusuhara K, et al. Aneurysm of coronary arteriovenous fistula presenting as a calcified mediastinal mass. *Ann Thorac Surg.* 1992;54:771–773.

56. Trask JL, Bell A, Usher BW. Doppler color flow imaging in detection and mapping of left coronary artery fistula to right ventricle and atrium. *J Am Soc Echocardiogr.* 1990;3:131–134.

57. Velvis H, Schmidt KG, Silverman NH, Turley K. Diagnosis of coronary artery fistula by two-dimensional echocardiography, pulsed Doppler ultrasound and color flow imaging. *J Am Coll Cardiol.* 1989;14:968–976.

58. Zahn EM, Smallhorn JF, Egger G, Burrows PE, Rebecca IM, Freedom RM. Echocardiographic diagnosis of fistula between the left circumflex coronary artery and the left atrium. *Pediatr Cardiol.* 1992;13:178–180.

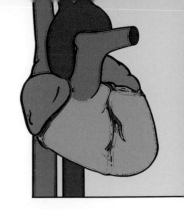

Chapter 23

Congenital Aneurysms of the Sinuses of Valsalva

Antonio Maria Valsalva, anatomist and pathologist, was born in 1666 in the historic Emilia-Romagna region of northern Italy. The sinuses that bear Valsalva's name consist of three small outpouchings in the wall of the aorta immediately above the attachments of each aortic cusp (Figure 23-1). In 1839, James Hope[1] published an account of a *ruptured* congenital aneurysm of a sinus of Valsalva, "a case of aneurysmal pouch of the aorta bursting into the right ventricle." A year later, John Thurnam[2] expanded Hope's report by adding examples of *unruptured* aortic sinus aneurysms and by naming the sinuses according to their relationship to the coronary arteries as the *right* coronary sinus, the *left* coronary sinus, and the *noncoronary* sinus (see Figure 23-1). These designations appeared in Quain's *Elements of Anatomy*[3] and remain in use today.[4]

Aneurysms of the sinuses of Valsalva account for 1% of congenital anomalies of the heart and circulation.[5] The aneurysms tend to be single, although exceptionally, more than one sinus is involved.[6,7] An aneurysm may arise from each sinus of a *bicuspid* aortic valve,[6,8] from each sinus of a *trileaflet* aortic valve,[7] and rarely, from a *quadricuspid* aortic valve.[9]

The anatomic relationship of the sinuses of Valsalva to adjacent structures determines the site into which a given congenital aneurysm ruptures.[4] Ninety percent to 95% originate in the *right* or *noncoronary* sinus and project into the *right ventricle* or *right atrium*, and less than 5% originate in the left coronary sinus (Figure 23-2).[4,10,11] Those that arise in the *noncoronary* sinus almost always rupture into the *right atrium* (see Figure 23-2), and those that arise in the *right coronary* sinus rupture into the *right ventricle* or occasionally into the *right atrium* (see Figure 23-2).[4] Rarely, rupture is into the pulmonary artery,[10,12] left ventricle,[4] left atrium,[4] or pericardial space.[4,13] Also rarely, a sinus aneurysm dissects into the interventricular septum, where it remains unruptured or perforates and ruptures into the left or right ventricle.[5,14–16] A congenital etiology is questionable when an aneurysm originates in the *left* coronary sinus and ruptures into the *left* side of heart.[4]

A sinus of Valsalva aneurysm can cause *aortic regurgitation* by interfering with aortic leaflet coaptation, can enter the right atrium and cause *tricuspid regurgitation*,[17] or can enter the right ventricular outflow tract and cause subpulmonary obstruction. A congenital aortic sinus aneurysm that is the site of infective endocarditis can be difficult to distinguish from *aortic valve* infective endocarditis that caused the aortic sinus to perforate.[4,18–20] A large unruptured aneurysm can compress the superior vena cava, the right atrium, the right ventricle,[21] or a coronary artery.

A congenital sinus of Valsalva aneurysm begins as a blind pouch or diverticulum at a localized site in an aortic sinus and then protrudes as a finger-like or nipple-like projection that ruptures at its tip (Figure 23-3).[4,22,23] The fundamental histologic fault responsible for a coronary sinus aneurysm is discontinuity of the elastic layer in the aortic media at the juncture between the ascending aorta and aortic valve annulus, which sets the stage for avulsion and aneurysm formation.[23,24] The histologic fault is present at birth, but with rare exception, the aneurysm is not.[18,25,26] Marfan syndrome is associated with dilation of the ascending aorta and the sinuses of Valsalva, but dissection or rupture is in the ascending aorta, not in the sinuses.[27] An aorticocameral communication is a tortuous channel that originates the ascending aorta above the left sinus of Valsalva and terminates in the right atrium without involving the aortic sinuses.[28]

The *physiologic consequences* of rupture depend on three factors: 1, the amount of blood flowing through the rupture; 2, the rapidity with which the rupture develops; and 3, the chamber that receives the rupture. Irrespective of the right-sided receiving site, shunted blood must flow through the pulmonary circulation, the left atrium, and the left ventricle before returning to the aorta. When the right atrium receives the rupture, all four cardiac chambers are volume overloaded. A sudden large rupture provokes congestive failure because the heart cannot adapt rapidly to the acute hemodynamic burden. Conversely, small insidious perforations initially go unnoticed (Figure 23-4). Deformity of aortic cusps caused by a ruptured or unruptured aneurysm causes regurgitation *through the valve* (Figure 23-5), and rupture of a sinus aneurysm into the left ventricle causes regurgitation *through the rupture*.[29] Aneurysms that originate in the right sinus of Valsalva are typically associated with a supracristal ventricular septal defect (see Figure 23-5).[4,23,30–32]

Unruptured congenital sinus of Valsalva aneurysms were recognized by Thurnam (see previous).[2] Before the advent of echocardiography, approximately 20% of unruptured aneurysms were chance findings at necropsy or at cardiac surgery.[33] However, occult unruptured congenital aortic sinus aneurysms are now readily imaged, even in older adults (see Figure 23-17).[28,34] An unruptured aneurysm can compress a proximal coronary artery

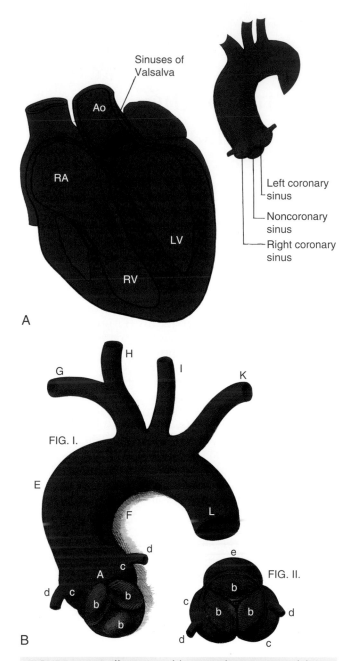

FIGURE 23-1 A, Illustration of the normal aortic root with locations of the sinuses of Valsalva. (RA = right atrium; Ao = aorta; LV = left ventricle; RV = right ventricle.) **B,** Illustration of the aortic sinuses from Antonio Valsalva's *Opera,* published in 1740.

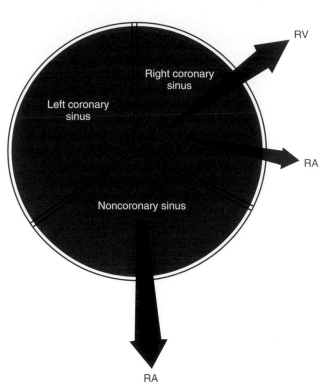

FIGURE 23-2 Illustration of the three sinuses of Valsalva and the chambers that receive a rupture. Ninety percent to 95% of congenital sinus of Valsalva aneurysms originate in the right or noncoronary sinus and rupture into the right ventricle (RV) or right atrium (RA).

or can dissect into the ventricular septum and cause complete heart block.[34] Protrusion of an aneurysm into the left ventricle is occasionally responsible for aortic regurgitation (see previous),[29] less commonly for obstruction to left ventricular outflow.

HISTORY

Ruptured aortic sinus aneurysms typically announce themselves in young males after puberty but before age 30 years. The male:female ratio is as high as 4:1.[22] Rupture rarely occurs in infancy or early childhood[25,26,35]

or as late as the seventh decade[36,37] and rarely occurs during pregnancy.[38] The average age of rupture was 34 years in one large series, with an age range of 11 years to 67 years.[36] An *unruptured* congenital aneurysm of the right coronary sinus was an incidental necropsy finding in a 82-year-old man,[33] and an 85-year-old man came to attention because an occult unruptured aortic sinus aneurysm in the right ventricular outflow tract caused a to-and-fro murmur (see Figure 23-17). Death from congestive heart failure typically occurs within a year after rupture.[36] *Sudden* death follows perforation into the pericardium, and syncope and sudden death are occasional sequelae of complete heart block caused by a ruptured[15] or unruptured[34] aneurysm that dissects into the base of the ventricular septum.[15,39] Conversely, long survival sometimes follows a small slowly progressive perforation (see Figure 23-4). One such individual lived for 30 years, and another lived for 17 years;[40] a 65-year-old man died of gastric carcinoma 10 years after rupture,[37] and rupture in infancy was followed by surgical repair 15 years later. Small perforations come to attention because of a continuous murmur (see Figure 23-4),[41] because of a diastolic murmur caused by aortic regurgitation, because of infective endocarditis,[4,19] or during a diagnostic study for ventricular septal defect.[42] A large unruptured saccular aneurysm filled with laminated thrombus came to light because of a prominent paracardiac density on a routine chest x-ray, and another unruptured aneurysm announced itself with

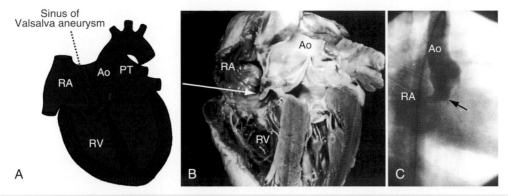

FIGURE 23-3 A, Schematic illustration of a sinus of Valsalva aneurysm projecting into the right atrium (RA). The sinus itself is not dilated. The aneurysm appears as a finger-like or nipple-like projection with a perforation at its tip. (Ao = aorta; PT = pulmonary trunk; RV = right ventricle.) **B,** Specimen from a 27-year-old woman whose heart was sectioned to correspond with the anatomic features in the schematic illustration. The ruptured sinus of Valsalva aneurysm (arrow) projects into the right atrium (RA). **C,** Aortogram from a 20-year-old woman with a congenital aneurysm (arrow) of the right sinus of Valsalva that ruptured into the right atrium (RA).

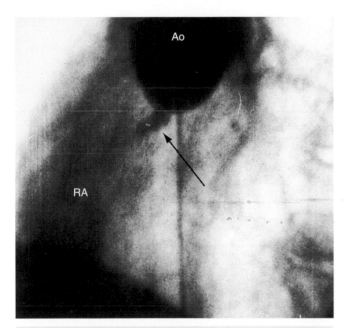

FIGURE 23-4 Left anterior oblique aortogram from an asymptomatic 35-year-old man with a continuous murmur. A small rupture of an aneurysm of the noncoronary sinus of Valsalva (arrow) entered the right atrium (RA). (Ao = aorta.)

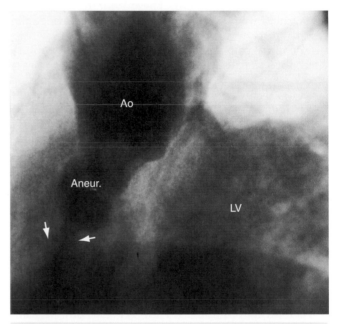

FIGURE 23-5 Aortogram from a 31-year-old woman with an asymptomatic restrictive ventricular septal defect and mild to moderate aortic regurgitation. Sudden dyspnea, orthopnea, and a coarse continuous murmur were caused by rupture of an aneurysm (Aneur., arrows) of the right sinus of Valsalva into the right ventricle. The left ventricle (LV) visualized because of aortic regurgitation. The echocardiogram is shown in Figure 23-14. (Ao = aorta.)

cerebral and retinal emboli.[43] Compression of a coronary artery by an unruptured aneurysm is a rare cause of angina pectoris or myocardial infarction (see previous). In 1957, a 27-year-old soldier with a large acute rupture underwent the first successful surgical repair with a polyvinyl prosthesis shaped as a golf tee. Three decades later, the patient had dramatic reperforation (see second case history subsequent).[44]

Congenital sinus of Valsalva aneurysms come to attention because of the *acute* development of a *large* perforation, *gradual* progression of a *small* perforation, or an asymptomatic or symptomatic *unruptured* aneurysm. An *large acute rupture* is announced by the dramatic onset of severe retrosternal or upper abdominal pain and intractable dyspnea.[31,36] The rupture often but not necessarily follows physical stress. The acute symptoms last for hours or days, sometimes subsiding gradually, leaving the patient's condition temporarily improved, but congestive heart failure appears and progresses relentlessly. The following case histories are illustrative.

The first history describes a 45-year-old truck driver whose work included strenuous lifting of 50-lb to 100-lb sacks of plaster.[31] He was in good health until 3 weeks before an alarming experience. While carrying a 100-lb sack, he suddenly became "out of breath" and fell to the floor. A raw sensation radiated from the epigastrium to the base of the neck. Despite severe weakness and shortness of breath, he carried 20 more sacks before consulting a doctor. When seen by the authors, he was relatively asymptomatic.

The second history is the 27-year-old soldier (see previous) who had been in excellent health and whose physical examinations in the military had been normal. While sitting at his desk, he suddenly experienced shortness of breath, chest pain, and epigastric discomfort. Because the symptoms persisted, he was admitted to an army hospital. The acute symptoms subsided after administration of digitalis and sodium restriction, but congestive heart failure persisted.

The third history is a 21-year-old woman who had previously been well. About 24 hours after her usual weekend hike in woods and hills, and shortly after eating pizza, she had an episode of nausea and retching. Later in the day, she experienced progressive dyspnea with severe retrosternal pressure radiating to the back followed by orthopnea and palpitations. These symptoms remained severe for a week, then gradually subsided, leaving mild residual retrosternal pain and dyspnea.

The initial pain is believed to be related to the rupture itself. Occasionally, the aneurysm compresses a coronary artery, so symptoms of myocardial ischemia or infarction coexist.[45] Rupture may be announced by acute dyspnea rather than pain, or mild chest pain may occur for weeks before the onset of dyspnea and tightness in the upper abdomen. If a patient with a *ventricular septal defect* suddenly develops chest pain, dyspnea, and a continuous murmur, the reason is likely to be rupture of a coexisting aortic sinus aneurysm (see Figure 23-5; see previous).

Small insidious perforations that initially progress gradually go unnoticed (see Figures 23-4 and 23-16). Mild dyspnea without pain sometimes precedes congestive heart failure by months or years.[17] Patients sometimes present during a relatively asymptomatic interval with a continuous murmur mistaken for patent ductus arteriosus.

Congenital aortic sinus aneurysms usually go unrecognized until they rupture.[33] However, unruptured aneurysms can manifest themselves with a to-and-fro murmur from flow in and out of the intact aneurysmal pouch (see Figure 23-17), with the murmur of tricuspid regurgitation, with a midsystolic murmur of right ventricular outflow obstruction, with the pain of myocardial ischemia from coronary artery compression, with aortic regurgitation–caused malapposition of aortic cusps,[29] with superior vena caval obstruction,[21] with a paracardiac mass in the chest x-ray, with systemic emboli,[43] with complete heart block, with syncope, or with sudden death.[15]

PHYSICAL APPEARANCE

Because rupture rarely occurs before puberty (see previous), growth and development are seldom affected by the catabolic effects of congestive heart failure. Aneurysm of the noncoronary sinus of Valsalva has been reported with the Klippel-Feil syndrome, which is characterized by short neck, low posterior hairline, and restricted mobility of the upper spine caused by congenital fusion of any two cervical vertebrae.[46] Giant aneurysms of the left and noncoronary sinuses have been reported with Noonan's syndrome, characterized by hypertelorism, down-slanting eyes, webbed neck, short stature, and chest deformity.[47]

ARTERIAL PULSE

All gradations of an aortic runoff are reflected in the arterial pulse, irrespective of which chamber or side of the heart receives a ruptured sinus of Valsalva aneurysm (Figure 23-6). The pulse pressure may not be wide immediately after perforation because the left ventricle has not had time to adapt to the increase in volume and because left ventricular end diastolic pressure is elevated.[48] If survival permits, the arterial pulse becomes bounding with a rapid rise, a rapid fall, a wide pulse pressure, and a bisferiens configuration. Carotid pulses are visible, Quincke pulses appear in the fingertips, and pistol shot sounds and Duroziez's murmur are heard over the femoral arteries. When an aneurysm penetrates the base of the ventricular septum and causes complete heart block, the arterial pulse is slow.

JUGULAR VENOUS PULSE

The height and waveform of the jugular venous pulse depend on the size and rapidity of the rupture and on the presence and degree of right ventricular failure. A small

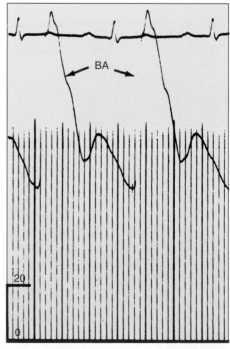

FIGURE 23-6 Brachial arterial (BA) pulse from a 17-year-old boy with a noncoronary sinus of Valsalva aneurysm that ruptured into the right atrium. Pulmonary blood flow was twice systemic. The upstroke of the brachial pulse is brisk. The diastolic pressure is reduced.

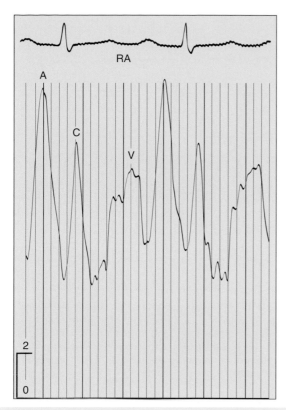

insidious rupture leaves the jugular venous pulse normal, irrespective of which chamber receives the rupture. A large sudden rupture into the right atrium or right ventricle is accompanied by congestive heart failure, an elevated mean jugular venous pressure, and tall A and V waves (Figure 23-7). When an aortic sinus aneurysm projects into the right atrium and causes tricuspid regurgitation (see previous), the V wave is selectively elevated. When an aneurysm causes obstruction of the superior vena cava, the mean jugular venous pressure is elevated, but the wave forms disappear. When an aneurysm results in obstruction to right ventricular outflow, the A wave selectively increases. Complete heart block is accompanied by the distinctive jugular pulse described in Chapter 4.

PRECORDIAL MOVEMENT AND PALPATION

Precordial impulses depend on the size, rapidity, and duration of the rupture rather than on the recipient chamber, except when rupture is directly into the left ventricle. When rupture is into the right atrium or right ventricle, the right and left ventricles are both hyperdynamic because blood from the rupture circulates through all four chambers before reaching the aorta. An aortic sinus aneurysm that ruptures directly into the left ventricle or that causes aortic regurgitation by compromising

aortic cusp coaptation results in an isolated hyperdynamic left ventricular impulse. An unruptured aneurysm that obstructs right ventricular outflow is accompanied by an isolated *right* ventricular impulse and a systolic thrill generated across the obstruction. A continuous thrill that is more prominent in either systole or diastole coincides with a loud coarse murmur and a large acute rupture. The maximal location of thrills varies with murmur sites, as described in the next section.

AUSCULTATION

A hallmark of acute rupture of an aortic sinus aneurysm into the right side of the heart is the sudden appearance of a continuous murmur in a previously healthy individual, usually a young male.[36] In a patient known to have a ventricular septal defect, the sudden appearance of a continuous murmur is a feature of rupture of a coexisting aortic sinus aneurysm (see Figure 23-5).[30,36]

When the right atrium receives the rupture, the continuous murmur is maximal along the right or left sternal border, or over the lower sternum (Figure 23-8). When the rupture enters the body of the right ventricle, the continuous murmur is maximal at the mid to lower left sternal border (Figure 23-9), and rupture into the

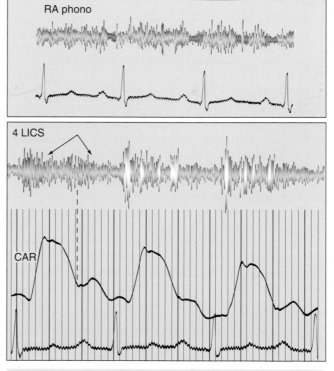

FIGURE 23-8 Right atrial intracardiac phonocardiogram (RA phono) with simultaneous thoracic wall phonocardiogram at the fourth left intercostal space (4 LICS) in the 17-year-old boy with rupture of an aneurysm of the noncoronary sinus of Valsalva into the right atrium (see Figures 23-6 and 23-7). The continuous murmur within the right atrium and on the thoracic wall (4LICS) exhibits systolic or diastolic accentuation from beat to beat but does not peak around the second heart sound. (CAR = carotid pulse).

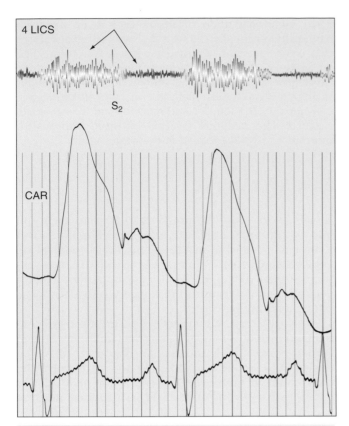

FIGURE 23-9 Phonocardiogram from the fourth left intercostal space (4 LICS) of a 28-year-old man with an aneurysm of the right sinus of Valsalva that ruptured into the right ventricle. The continuous murmur is much louder in systole (paired arrows). (S_2 = second heart sound; CAR = carotid pulse.)

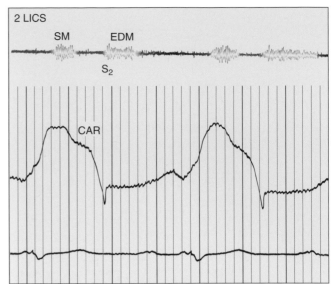

FIGURE 23-10 Phonocardiogram from the second left intercostal space (2 LICS) of a 24-year-old man with a right sinus of Valsalva aneurysm that ruptured into the left ventricle. A short systolic flow murmur (SM) is found in early systole, and an early diastolic murmur of aortic regurgitation (EDM) is seen. (CAR = carotid pulse.)

outflow tract of the right ventricle results in a continuous murmur at the upper left sternal edge. The *systolic* component of continuous murmurs tends to be louder at *higher* thoracic sites, and the *diastolic* component tends to be louder at *lower* thoracic sites.

The quality, loudness, and configuration of the continuous murmur accompanying a sudden large rupture were well stated in early reports. Hope described "a very loud, superficial sawing murmur prolonged continuously over the first and second heart sounds (probably weaker during the period of repose)."[1] Thurnam called attention to "a superficial, harsh murmur and a peculiarly intense sawing or blowing sound accompanied by an equally marked or purring tremor heard over the varicose orifice and in the circulation beyond it; this sound is continuous but is loudest during systole, less loud during diastole."[2] These descriptions carry an important message: namely, that the continuous murmur of a ruptured aortic sinus aneurysm *does not peak around the second heart sound*, in contrast to the continuous murmur of patent ductus arteriosus (Figures 23-9 and 23-10). Either the systolic or the diastolic portion of the murmur tends to be louder. Intensity may diminish around the second heart sound only to increase in diastole, creating a to-and-fro cadence. From time to time, the continuous murmur exhibits either systolic or diastolic accentuation (see Figure 23-9). An aneurysm may be compressed by

right ventricular contraction, by impeding systolic flow, and by accounting for diastolic accentuation of the continuous murmur. Rupture directly into the left ventricle results in an early diastolic murmur of aortic regurgitation and in a short midsystolic murmur from augmented flow into the aorta (see Figure 23-10). An unruptured aneurysm may cause an isolated diastolic murmur of aortic regurgitation by compromising aortic cusp coaptation (see previous).[29]

Variations in murmur patterns are better understood with examination of intracardiac phonocardiograms recorded at sites in and around the rupture (see Figure 23-8). Continuous murmurs are recovered from within the aneurysm itself. The systolic component might be more prominent in the proximal aortic portion of the aneurysm, and the diastolic component may be more prominent in the distal right atrial or right ventricular portion.

Tricuspid regurgitation,[17] mitral regurgitation, and ventricular septal defect[30] result in holosystolic murmurs. Short midsystolic murmurs are generated by rapid ejection across the aortic and pulmonary valves. An aneurysm may protrude into the right ventricular outflow tract and cause a longer midsystolic murmur or may compromise aortic cusp coaptation and cause the murmur of aortic regurgitation. However, these systolic and diastolic murmurs tend to be obscured by the louder continuous murmur through the rupture.

Unperforated aortic sinus aneurysms can be accompanied by prominent murmurs in both phases of the cardiac cycle as blood flows into and out of the unruptured aneurysmal pouch. These to-and-fro murmurs are auscultatory counterparts of the phasic expansion and relaxation of unruptured aneurysms imaged with two-dimensional echocardiography (see Figure 23-17) and with signals recorded with pulsed Doppler echocardiography.[34] An unperforated aneurysm that obstructs the right ventricular outflow tract results in a midsystolic murmur across the obstruction, and an unperforated aneurysm that projects into the right atrium can result in the murmur of tricuspid regurgitation. An unruptured aneurysm that protrudes into the left ventricular outflow tract or into the base of the ventricular septum can cause murmurs of aortic regurgitation[29] and aortic stenosis.[14]

Third heart sounds originate in the right or left ventricle because of biventricular failure and increased atrioventricular flow. The second heart sound splits normally. The pulmonary component is loud because pulmonary artery pressure is elevated.

ELECTROCARDIOGRAM

Small, slowly progressive aortic sinus ruptures are accompanied by normal electrocardiograms. The rhythm is normal sinus even when a large rupture is into the right atrium. The PR interval tends to be prolonged (Figure 23-11). The QRS axis is normal or rightward, and occasionally leftward. Atrioventricular conduction defects, including complete heart block,[49] right or left bundle branch block, and bifascicular block, occur when a ruptured or unruptured aneurysm penetrates the base of the ventricular septum and injures the atrioventricular node or His bundle.[49] A right atrial P wave abnormality is generated when the right atrium receives the rupture, or when an aortic sinus aneurysm

causes tricuspid regurgitation. Increased flow through the left atrium accounts for a left atrial P wave abnormality.

Rupture into the right atrium or right ventricle results in volume overload of both ventricles, but the electrocardiogram usually shows *left* ventricular hypertrophy by voltage criteria and ST segment/T wave abnormalities (see Figure 23-11).[36] Right ventricular hypertrophy may coexist, but does not occur alone,[36] except with aneurysms that cause right ventricular outflow obstruction. An aneurysm that compresses a proximal coronary artery results in electrocardiographic changes of myocardial ischemia or infarction.[45]

X-RAY

Because most patients with ruptured congenital aortic sinus aneurysms are otherwise healthy, previous x-rays are often available for comparison. Small insidious perforations leave the x-ray unchanged. Large acute ruptures are followed by pulmonary venous congestion because of the steep rise in end diastolic pressure in an unprepared left ventricle (Figure 23-12). Increased pulmonary arterial blood flow results in enlargement of the pulmonary trunk (Figure 23-13).[42,50] Moderate left atrial enlargement is seen in the lateral projection; and in the anteroposterior view, a right atrial convexity appears at the right lower cardiac border and a moderately dilated

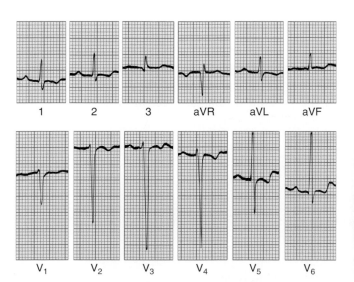

FIGURE 23-11 Electrocardiogram from the 17-year-old boy with an aneurysm of the noncoronary sinus of Valsalva that ruptured into the right atrium (see Figures 23-6, 23-7, and 23-8). The PR interval is prolonged. The QRS axis is normal. Left ventricular hypertrophy is characterized by deep S waves in leads V_{2-4} and prominent R waves and ST segment/T wave abnormalities in leads V_{5-6}.

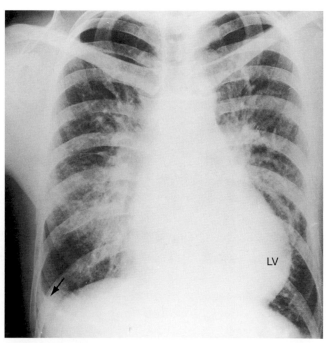

FIGURE 23-12 X-ray from a 21-year-old man with a right sinus of Valsalva aneurysm that ruptured into the right ventricle. Pulmonary venous congestion is evident. There is a small right pleural effusion (arrow). A moderately dilated left ventricle (LV) occupies the apex.

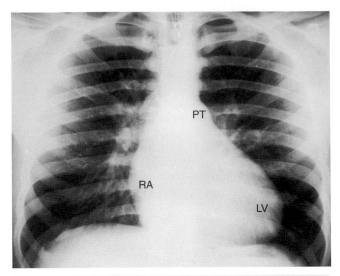

FIGURE 23-13 X-ray from the 17-year-old boy with a noncoronary sinus of Valsalva aneurysm that ruptured into the right atrium (see Figures 23-6, 23-7, and 23-8). Increased venous vascularity is evident in the inner third of the lung fields. The pulmonary trunk (PT) is moderately dilated. An enlarged right atrium (RA) occupies the right lower cardiac border, and a dilated left ventricle (LV) occupies the apex.

increased pulmonary arterial blood flow, and with a selective increase in left ventricular size. Rarely, calcium is seen in the aneurysm. Also rarely, an aneurysm of the *left* aortic sinus presents as a localized convex radiologic prominence immediately below the pulmonary trunk, or a large saccular aneurysm of the *right* aortic sinus presents as a prominent right paracardiac density.

ECHOCARDIOGRAM

Echocardiography with color flow imaging and Doppler interrogation establish the diagnosis of a ruptured or unruptured sinus of Valsalva aneurysm (Figures 23-14 through 23-18) and establish the presence of associated abnormalities that are either intrinsic features of the aneurysm or that are in addition to the aneurysm.[51,52] Echocardiography identifies insidious asymptomatic ruptures manifested only by a continuous murmur (see Figures 23-4 and 23-16). Two-dimensional imaging identifies the aneurysmal sac (see Figures 23-14, 23-15, and 23-18A, B), the aortic sinus of origin (see Figures 23-14, 23-15, and 23-18B), the two normal sinuses, and a normal aorta above the aneurysm. Color flow imaging identifies flow into the recipient chamber (see Figures 23-16B, and 23-18A). Pulsed Doppler (see Figure 23-15) and continuous wave Doppler (see Figure 32-18C) define the flow patterns in the ruptured aneurysm. A large unruptured aortic sinus aneurysm (see Figure 23-17) is characterized by phasic expansion and relaxation and by to-and-fro pulsed Doppler signals at the site of origin from the aorta but has no evidence of rupture.[11] Doppler interrogation establishes the presence and degree of subpulmonary

left ventricle occupies the apex (see Figure 23-13).[42,50] When an aortic sinus aneurysm ruptures into the right side of the heart, volume overload of both ventricles and congestive heart failure account for the radiologic picture (see Figure 23-12).[42] Rupture is into the left ventricle causes pulmonary venous congestion without

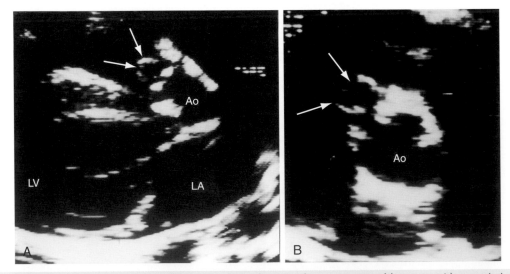

FIGURE 23-14 A, Parasternal long-axis and, **B,** short-axis echocardiograms from a 31-year-old woman with a restrictive perimembranous ventricular septal defect and mild aortic regurgitation. An aneurysm (paired arrows) of the right sinus of Valsalva ruptured into the right ventricle near the attachment of the septal tricuspid leaflet. The aortogram is shown in Figure 23-5. (Ao = aorta; LA = left atrium; LV = left ventricle.)

obstruction when an aneurysm protrudes into the right ventricular outflow tract (see Figure 23-16). The presence and degree of aortic regurgitation are established, a coexisting ventricular septal defect is identified and characterized, and the physiologic consequences of rupture into the right atrium, right ventricle, or left ventricle are determined. Real-time imaging identifies ischemic regional left ventricular wall motion abnormalities that result from compression of a coronary artery by an aortic sinus aneurysm.

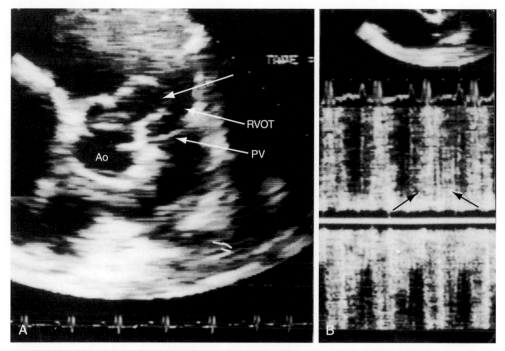

FIGURE 23-15 A, Parasternal short-axis view of a right sinus of Valsalva aneurysm (large unmarked arrow) that ruptured into the right ventricular outflow tract (RVOT) of a 22-year-old man. (PV = pulmonary valve.) **B,** Pulsed Doppler sample volume within the aneurysm shows continuous systolic and diastolic flow (paired arrows).

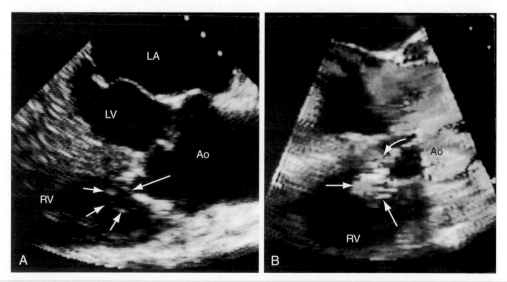

FIGURE 23-16 Transesophageal echocardiogram from an asymptomatic 32-year-old man with a continuous murmur. **A,** The three unmarked oblique arrows (lower left) identify a sinus of Valsalva aneurysm that originated in the right sinus and projected into the right ventricular (RV) outflow tract. (Ao = aorta; LV = left ventricle; LA = left atrium.) **B,** Black-and-white print of a color flow image showing high-velocity flow (oblique arrows) from the right aortic sinus (curved arrow) into the right ventricular outflow tract (RV).

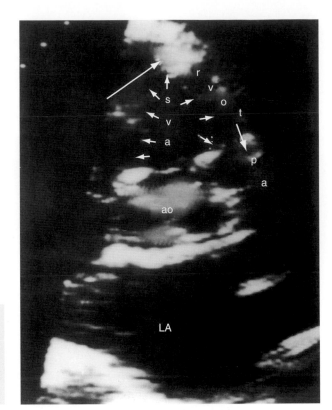

FIGURE 23-17 Black and white print of a color flow image from an asymptomatic 85-year-old man with an unruptured sinus of Valsalva aneurysm (sva) that presented as a to-and-fro murmur. Color flow imaging showed no rupture. Multiple small arrows identify the aneurysm that projected into the right ventricular outflow tract (long arrow, rvot). Color flow imaging showed no rupture. (pa = pulmonary artery; ao = aorta; LA = left atrium.)

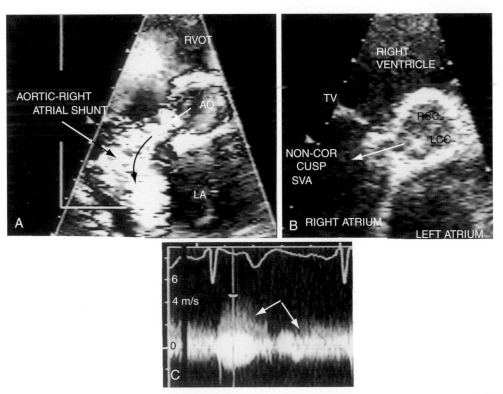

FIGURE 23-18 Echocardiograms with-black-and white images and Doppler interrogation from a 28-year-old man with an initially small asymptomatic rupture of an aneurysm of the noncoronary sinus of Valsalva (SVA) into the right atrium. The rupture gradually increased in size. **A,** Black-and-white print of a color flow image showing the aortic-to-right atrial rupture (large curved arrow). (RVOT = right ventricular outflow tract; Ao = aorta; LA = left atrium.) **B,** Short axis showing origin of the aneurysm from the noncoronary cusp (arrow). The right coronary cusp (RCC) and left coronary cusp (LCC) were normal. (TV = tricuspid valve.) **C,** Continuous wave Doppler within the rupture shows continuous flow that was distinctly greater during systole (larger arrow).

SUMMARY

Acute rupture of a large sinus of Valsalva aneurysm is a clinically dramatic event. A previously healthy, young adult, usually male, has sudden chest pain, dyspnea, and a loud continuous murmur develop. A period of temporary improvement is followed by relentless cardiac failure. The arterial pulse resembles aortic regurgitation, the jugular venous pulse is elevated, and dynamic biventricular impulses are palpable. A continuous murmur is maximal below the third intercostal space along the right or left sternal border, or over the lower sternum. The murmur is louder in either systole or diastole but does not peak around the second heart sound. The electrocardiogram shows biatrial P wave abnormalities and left ventricular or combined ventricular hypertrophy. The x-ray exhibits pulmonary venous congestion followed by increased pulmonary arterial blood flow with dilation of both ventricles and enlargement of the right and left atrium. Echocardiography with color flow imaging and Doppler interrogation establishes the diagnosis of a ruptured or unruptured congenital aortic sinus aneurysm, identifies the chamber that receives the rupture, establishes coexisting abnormalities that are intrinsic to or in addition to the aneurysm, and assesses the physiologic consequences.

Small ruptures that progress slowly are initially unrecognized but ultimately come to light because of a continuous murmur. An *unperforated* aneurysm may generate a to-and-fro murmur because of flow into and out of the aneurysm and can cause obstruction to right ventricular outflow and aortic regurgitation. Ruptured or unruptured aneurysms that penetrate the base of the ventricular septum cause atrioventricular conduction disturbances, syncope, and sudden death.

REFERENCES

1. Hope J. *A treatise on the diseases of the heart and great vessels: comprising a new view of the physiology of the heart's action, according to which the physical signs are explained.* London: J. Churchill & Sons; 1839.
2. Thurnam J. On aneurysms, and especially spontaneous varicose aneurysms of the ascending aorta. *Trans R Med Chir Soc (Glasgow).* 1840;23:323.
3. Walmsley T. The heart. In: *Quain's elements of anatomy.* Vol. 4, Part 3. New York: Longmans, Green & Company; 1929.
4. Sakakibara S, Konno S. Congenital aneurysm of the sinus of Valsalva. Anatomy and classification. *Am Heart J.* 1962;63:405–424.
5. Wells T, Byrd B, Neirste D, Fleurelus C. Images in cardiovascular medicine. Sinus of valsalva aneurysm with rupture into the interventricular septum and left ventricular cavity. *Circulation.* 1999; 100:1843–1844.
6. Chamsi-Pasha H, Musgrove C, Morton R. Echocardiographic diagnosis of multiple congenital aneurysms of the sinus of Valsalva. *Br Heart J.* 1988;59:724–726.
7. Pomerance A, Davies MJ. Congenital aneurysms of all three sinuses of valsalva. *J Pathol Bacteriol.* 1965;89:607–610.
8. Peszek-Przybyla E, Radwan K, Gruszka A, Krejca M, Buszman P, Sosnowski M. Sinus of Valsalva aneurysm. *Cardiology Journal.* 2009;16:455–457.
9. Pitta SR, Kondur A, Afonso L. Quadricuspid aortic valve associated with unruptured sinus of Valsalva aneurysm. *Eur J Echocardiogr.* 2008;9:575–576.
10. Heilman 3rd KJ, Groves BM, Campbell D, Blount Jr. SG. Rupture of left sinus of Valsalva aneurysm into the pulmonary artery. *J Am Coll Cardiol.* 1985;5:1005–1007.
11. Zannis K, Tzvetkov B, Deux J-F, Kirsch EWM. Unruptured congenital aneurisms of the right and left sinuses of Valsalva. *Eur Heart J.* 2007;28:1565.
12. Scagliotti D, Fisher EA, Deal BJ, Gordon D, Chomka EV, Brundage BH. Congenital aneurysm of the left sinus of Valsalva with an aortopulmonary tunnel. *J Am Coll Cardiol.* 1986;7: 443–445.
13. Watanabe M, Aoki M, Fujiwara T. Rare type of congenital aneurysm of the right sinus of Valsalva protruding superiorly into the pericardial space. *General Thoracic & Cardiovascular Surgery.* 2009;57: 151–152.
14. Hands ME, Lloyd BL, Hung J. Cross-sectional echocardiographic diagnosis of unruptured right sinus of Valsalva aneurysm dissecting into the interventricular septum. *Int J Cardiol.* 1985;9:380–383.
15. Onat A, Ersanli O, Kanuni A, Aykan TB. Congenital aortic sinus aneurysms with particular reference to dissection of the interventricular septum. *Am Heart J.* 1966;72:158–164.
16. Raffa H, Mosieri J, Sorefan AA, Kayali MT. Sinus of Valsalva aneurysm eroding into the interventricular septum. *Ann Thorac Surg.* 1991;51:996–998.
17. Taylor FH, Sanger PW, Robicsek F, Ibrahim K. Herniation of ruptured sinus valsalva aneurysm through the tricuspid orifice: case report. *Am Surg.* 1965;31:171–174.
18. Bardy GH, Valenstein P, Stack RS, Baker JT, Kisslo JA. Two-dimensional echocardiographic identification of sinus of Valsalva-right heart fistula due to infective endocarditis. *Am Heart J.* 1982;103:1068–1071.
19. Datta BN, Berry JN, Khattri HN. Infected aneurysm of sinus of Valsalva. Report of a case with involvement of all three sinuses. *Br Heart J.* 1971;33:323–325.
20. Jick H, Kasarjian PJ, Barsky M. Rupture of aneurysm of aortic sinus of Valsalva associated with acute bacterial endocarditis. *Circulation.* 1959;19:745–749.
21. Okita Y, Miki S, Kusuhara K, et al. A giant aneurysm of the non-coronary sinus of Valsalva. *Thorac Cardiovasc Surg.* 1987;35: 316–317.
22. Perloff JK. Sinus of Valsalva-right heart communications due to congenital aortic sinus defects. *Am Heart J.* 1960;59:318–321.
23. Angelini P. Aortic sinus aneurysm and associated defects: can we extrapolate a morphogenetic theory from pathologic findings? *Tex Heart Inst J.* 2005;32:560–562.
24. Edwards JE, Burchell HB. Specimen exhibiting the essential lesion in aneurysm of the aortic sinus. *Proc Staff Meet Mayo Clin.* 1956; 31:407–412.
25. Ainger LE, Pate JW. Rupture of a sinus of Valsalva aneurysm in an infant. Surgical correction. *Am J Cardiol.* 1963;11:547–551.
26. Perry LW, Martin GR, Galioto Jr. FM, Midgley FM. Rupture of congenital sinus of Valsalva aneurysm in a newborn. *Am J Cardiol.* 1991;68:1255–1256.
27. Milewicz DM, Dietz HC, Miller DC. Treatment of aortic disease in patients with Marfan syndrome. *Circulation.* 2005;111:e150–e157.
28. Tsai YC, Wang JN, Yang YJ, Wu JM. Aortico-cameral communication from left sinus Valsalva aneurysm to right atrium via a tortuous tunnel with aneurysmal dilatation. *Pediatr Cardiol.* 2002;23:108–109.
29. London SB, London RE. Production of aortic regurgitation by unperforated aneurysm of the sinus of Valsalva. *Circulation.* 1961;24:1403–1406.
30. Sakakibara S, Konno S. Congenital aneurysm of the sinus of Valsalva associated with ventricular septal defect. Anatomical aspects. *Am Heart J.* 1968;75:595–603.
31. Szweda JA, Drake EH. Ruptured congenital aneurysms of the sinuses of Valsalva: a report of two cases treated surgically. *Circulation.* 1962;25:559.
32. Ishii M, Masuoka H, Emi Y, Mori T, Ito M, Nakano T. Ruptured aneurysm of the sinus of valsalva coexisting with a ventricular septal defect and single coronary artery. *Circ J.* 2003;67:470–472.
33. Fishbein MC, Obma R, Roberts WC. Unruptured sinus of Valsalva aneurysm. *Am J Cardiol.* 1975;35:918–922.
34. Dev V, Shrivastava S. Echocardiographic diagnosis of unruptured aneurysm of the sinus of Valsalva dissecting into the ventricular septum. *Am J Cardiol.* 1990;66:502–503.
35. Gleason MM, Hardy C, Chin AJ, Pigott JD. Ruptured sinus of Valsalva aneurysm in childhood. *Am Heart J.* 1987;114:1235–1238.
36. Sakakibara S, Konno S. Congenital aneurysms of sinus of Valsalva. A clinical study. *Am Heart J.* 1962;63:708–719.

37. Sorensen EW, Kolsaker L. Ruptured aneurysm of sinus of Valsalva. Report of two cases. *Acta Med Scand.* 1962;172:369–374.

38. Cripps T, Pumphrey CW, Parker DJ. Rupture of the sinus of Valsalva during pregnancy. *Br Heart J.* 1987;57:490–491.

39. Krieger OJ, Lee EB, Lee NK. Congenital aneurysm of the noncoronary sinus of Valsalva leading to complete heart block: case report. *Ann Intern Med.* 1956;45:525–534.

40. Jones AM, Langley FA. Aortic sinus aneurysms. *Br Heart J.* 1949;11:325–341.

41. Peters P, Juziuk E, Gunther S. Doppler color flow mapping detection of ruptured sinus of Valsalva aneurysm. *J Am Soc Echocardiogr.* 1989;2:195–197.

42. Guo DW, Cheng TO, Lin ML, Gu ZQ. Aneurysm of the sinus of Valsalva: a roentgenologic study of 105 Chinese patients. *Am Heart J.* 1987;114:1169–1177.

43. Wortham DC, Gorman PD, Hull RW, Vernalis MN, Gaither NS. Unruptured sinus of Valsalva aneurysm presenting with embolization. *Am Heart J.* 1993;125:896–898.

44. Hemp JR, Young JN, Harrell Jr. JE, Woodworth GR. Late recurrent rupture of a sinus of Valsalva aneurysm. *Am J Cardiol.* 1989;63:761–762.

45. Chipps HD. Aneurysm of the sinus of Valsalva causing coronary occlusion. *Arch Pathol.* 1941;31:627–630.

46. Kawano Y, Tamura A, Kadota J. Klippel-Feil syndrome accompanied by an aneurysm of the non-coronary sinus of Valsalva. *Intern Med.* 2006;45:1191–1192.

47. Purnell R, Williams I, Von Oppell U, Wood A. Giant aneurysms of the sinuses of Valsalva and aortic regurgitation in a patient with Noonan's syndrome. *Eur J Cardiothorac Surg.* 2005;28:346–348.

48. Morganroth J, Perloff JK, Zeldis SM, Dunkman WB. Acute severe aortic regurgitation. Pathophysiology, clinical recognition, and management. *Ann Intern Med.* 1977;87:223–232.

49. Ahmad RA, Sturman S, Watson RD. Unruptured aneurysm of the sinus of Valsalva presenting with isolated heart block: echocardiographic diagnosis and successful surgical repair. *Br Heart J.* 1989;61:375–377.

50. Davidsen HG, Petersen O, Thomsen G. Roentgenologic findings in five cases of congenital aneurysm of the aortic sinuses (sinuses of Valsalva). *Acta Radiol.* 1958;49:205–217.

51. Chiang CW, Lin FC, Fang BR, Kuo CT, Lee YS, Chang CH. Doppler and two-dimensional echocardiographic features of sinus of Valsalva aneurysm. *Am Heart J.* 1988;116:1283–1288.

52. Sahasakul Y, Panchavinnin P, Chaithiraphan S, Sakiyalak P. Echocardiographic diagnosis of a ruptured aneurysm of the sinus of Valsalva: operation without catheterisation in seven patients. *Br Heart J.* 1990;64:195–198.

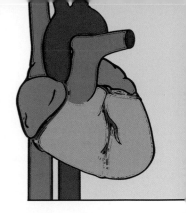

Chapter 24

Pulmonary Atresia with Intact Ventricular Septum

Thomas Peacock,[1] in his first edition of *Malformations of the Human Heart*, wrote:

"... the orifice or trunk of the pulmonary artery is entirely impervious. A case of this description was described by John Hunter in 1783.[2] The child was born at the eighth month, was very livid ... and died in convulsions on the thirteenth day. The pulmonary artery was found entirely impervious. The septum of the ventricles was entire, and the right ventricle had scarcely any cavity left, while the left ventricle was large and powerful. The foramen ovale continued open, and the pulmonary branches received their supply of blood from the aorta, through the medium of the arterial duct."

Peacock referred to what is now called *pulmonary atresia with intact ventricular septum*, a malformation in which an imperforate pulmonary valve completely obstructs forward flow into the pulmonary trunk (Figure 24-1). The ventricular septum is, by definition, intact, and a restrictive interatrial communication is the only exit from the right atrium. The imperforate pulmonary valve consists of three fused but well-formed cusps with triradiate commissural ridges that converge at the center of a sealed orifice that is structurally similar, if not identical, to pinpoint pulmonary valve stenosis (see Chapter 11).[3] Less commonly, commissural ridges are confined to the periphery of the valve, which has an imperforate dimple at the center.[3] The atresia is *valvular* (i.e., membranous) in 75% of cases and *muscular* (i.e., infundibular) in the remainder.[4,5] Muscular obliteration within the right ventricle results in a "unipartite, bipartite, or tripartite" ventricular chamber with an obliterated apex.[4,5]

The reported incidence rate of pulmonary atresia with intact ventricular septum is 1 per 22,000 live births[6] to 4.2 per 100,000 live births.[5,7] A well-developed pulmonary trunk (see Figure 24-1) implies that forward flow once occurred across a pulmonary valve that was stenotic but patent during much, if not most, of fetal life. A normally formed ductus arteriosus implies that intrauterine blood flow was from the right ventricle into the pulmonary trunk through the ductus and into the aorta (see Figure 24-5), in contrast to Fallot's tetralogy with pulmonary atresia in which a long tortuous ductus functions *in utero* as a systemic artery that carries blood from the aorta into the pulmonary artery (see Chapter 18).

The *normal right ventricle* consists of an *inlet portion* that is part of the diastolic filling mechanism and a trabecular and an infundibular portion that are parts of the systolic pump mechanism. More than three quarters of cases of pulmonary atresia with intact ventricular septum are characterized by a small thick-walled right ventricle (Figures 24-1A and 24-2A, B) that is equipped with all three of these morphologic portions (see Figures 24-1A and 24-2A, B),[8,9] together with fiber disarray, capillary disorganization, and endocardial fibroelastosis.[10,11] Pinpoint pulmonary valve stenosis in the neonate occasionally exists with a diminutive right ventricular cavity analogous to pulmonary atresia with intact ventricular septum.

When the right ventricle is small and thick-walled, the tricuspid annulus is also small and houses a small, thickened valve with poorly delineated chordal attachments and hypoplastic papillary muscles. When the right ventricle is dilated and thin-walled, the tricuspid valve is incompetent and either resembles Ebstein's malformation or is dysplastic with normally attached tricuspid leaflets. *Functional* pulmonary atresia has been applied when a dilated mechanically inadequate right ventricle with tricuspid regurgitation cannot generate sufficient systolic pressure to open a stenotic but nonatretic pulmonary valve.[12] Functional pulmonary atresia also occurs during transient neonatal tricuspid regurgitation.[13] In a small subset of patients with florid tricuspid regurgitation, the right ventricle and right atrium are enormous—"wall-to-wall hearts" (see section X-Ray).[14] Rarely, a suprasystemic right ventricle causes leftward displacement of the ventricular septum and obstruction to left ventricular outflow.[15,16]

The coronary circulation in pulmonary atresia with intact ventricular septum and small right ventricle has long been the focus of lively interest.[11,17–24] *Intramyocardial sinusoids* were described in 1926[25] and play important roles in the pathogenesis of right ventricular-to-coronary artery communications (see Figure 24-2).[17,18] Morphogenetic studies have shed new light on coronary vascular bed abnormalities in this malformation (see Chapter 32).[19,26] The normal coronary circulation develops in an orderly sequence of blood islands, coronary venous connections, and coronary artery-to-aortic connections. The blood islands proliferate and coalesce to form networks of vascular channels that have no connection with other blood islands or with the ventricular cavity. Suprasystemic systolic pressure from the small isovolumetrically contracting right ventricle drives blood through primitive vascular channels that are composed of

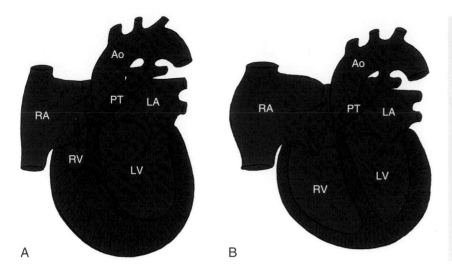

FIGURE 24-1 Illustrations of two varieties of pulmonary atresia with intact ventricular septum. In both varieties, the pulmonary valve is, by definition, imperforate. The pulmonary trunk (PT) is well-formed. A restrictive foramen ovale is the only exit from the right atrium (RA). Pulmonary blood flow depends on tenuous patency of a ductus arteriosus. **A,** In this more common variety, the right ventricle (RV) is small and thick-walled, the tricuspid valve is small but competent, and the right atrium is moderately enlarged. (Ao = aorta; LA = left atrium; LV = left ventricle.) **B,** In this less common variety, the right ventricle is thin-walled and normal in size or enlarged. The tricuspid valve is incompetent because of an Ebstein's-like malformation, so the right atrium is dilated.

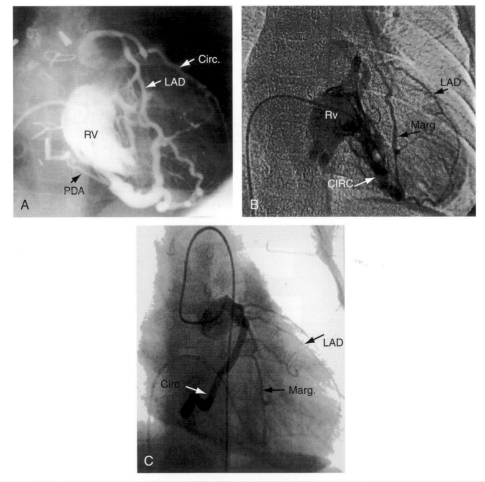

FIGURE 24-2 A, Right ventriculogram from a 3-year-old girl with pulmonary atresia and intact ventricular septum. The metal sutures are from a bidirectional Glenn operation. The small right ventricle (RV) ends blindly. The left anterior descending (LAD), circumflex (Circ.), and posterior descending (PDA) coronary arteries are visualized through ventriculocoronary arterial communications. The luminal irregularities were nonobstructive. The circumflex coronary artery outlines an enlarged left ventricle. **B** and **C,** Angiograms from a 4-year-old boy with pulmonary atresia, intact ventricular septum, and a small right ventricle (RV). **B,** The large circumflex coronary artery (CIRC), left anterior descending (LAD), and marginal (Marg) coronary arteries were visualized through right ventricular sinusoids. **C,** Contrast material injected into the left aortic sinus visualized the large circumflex coronary artery (Circ) and the left anterior descending (LAD) and marginal coronary arteries (Marg.)

thickened intima and fibroelastic walls[19] and that connect the right ventricular cavity to epicardial coronary arteries (see Figure 24-2A, B).[18,19] Abnormalities of the coronary vascular bed occur in 50% of patients with pulmonary atresia, intact ventricular septum, and a small right ventricle and are either secondary to the hemodynamic derangements of the malformation or are co-existing morphologic abnormalities,[18,23] such as ostial atresia[24,27] or fibromuscular dysplasia with focal luminal narrowing.[17] Myocardial sinusoids are rarely primary developmental faults.[28] Epicardial veins may be prominent and thick-walled.[19] Ventriculocoronary arterial connections are located chiefly in the region of the apex of right ventricle and communicate chiefly with the distal left anterior descending coronary arterial system (see Figure 24-2A, B).[19] Intramyocardial channels that end blindly punctuate the endocardium of the thick-walled right ventricle, creating the appearance of a highly trabeculated muscular wall (Figures 24-3 and 24-4).[19]

Ventriculocoronary arterial communications have been found in the *inverted left ventricle* of congenitally corrected transposition of the great arteries with pulmonary atresia and intact ventricular septum.[29,30] Left ventricular–to–coronary arterial connections in *aortic* atresia with intact ventricular septum differ from right ventricular–to–coronary arterial connections in pulmonary atresia with intact ventricular septum (see Chapters 31 and 32).[19,31,32]

Myocardial ischemia is an important sequel of ventriculocoronary arterial connections.[18,19] Large unobstructed connections (see Figure 24-2A, C) function as a fistulous steal because blood from the aortic root flows freely into the right ventricular cavity during diastole. More commonly and more importantly, ischemia and occasionally myocardial infarction result from obstructing luminal abnormalities that range from mild medial and intimal thickening to luminal obliteration and that extend from the origins of the intramyocardial connections to the coronary artery ostia in the aortic sinuses.[17–19] Luminal obstructive lesions that originate in the fetus and neonate can evolve into severe stenoses or obliteration.[18,19] *Proximal*

discontinuity of a coronary artery is the most egregious form of this prejudicial coronary circulation and is the result of acquired ostial obliteration or congenital atresia of an aortic sinus ostium. Left ventricular aneurysm[9] and right ventricular rupture[33,34] are consequences of myocardial ischemia and infarction that are largely responsible for the high mortality rate.[18] Proximal discontinuity and luminal obstruction set the stage for a *right ventricular–dependent coronary circulation* in which suprasystemic systolic pressure is required to generate retrograde coronary blood flow on which myocardial perfusion depends.[33] The right atrium enlarges only moderately when the right ventricle is diminutive, but when the right ventricle is dilated and tricuspid regurgitation is severe, the right atrium can be aneurysmal (see Figure 24-4). The *left atrium* enlarges because

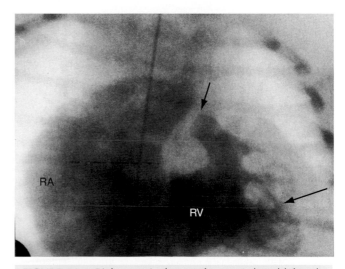

FIGURE 24-4 Right ventriculogram from a 1-day-old female with pulmonary atresia, intact ventricular septum, and a normal-sized right ventricle (RV) that contained an inlet portion, a trabecular portion (lower right arrow), and a blind infundibular portion (upper arrow). Severe tricuspid regurgitation filled a huge right atrium (RA).

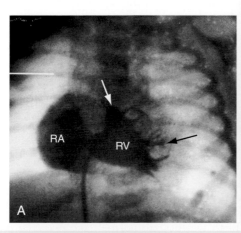

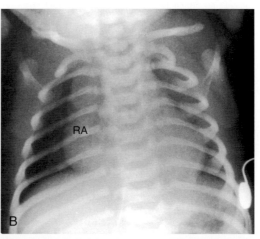

FIGURE 24-3 **A,** Right ventriculogram from a 1-day-old male with pulmonary atresia (upper arrow), intact ventricular septum, and a moderate-sized right ventricle (RV) that contained an inlet portion, a trabecular portion, and a well-formed infundibulum. Intramyocardial sinusoids end blindly (lower right arrow). Tricuspid regurgitation filled a large right atrium (RA). **B,** X-ray from the same patient shows oligemic lung fields, a large right atrium (RA), and a well-formed left ventricle at the apex.

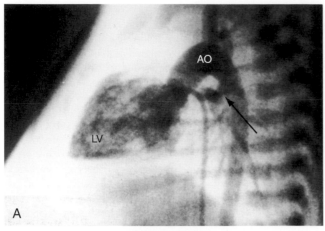

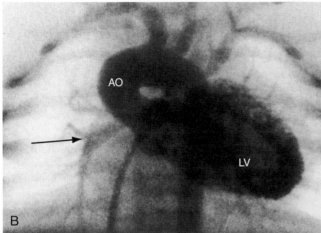

FIGURE 24-5 **A,** Lateral left ventriculogram from a 3-day-old female with pulmonary atresia, intact ventricular septum, a diminutive right ventricle, and a large left ventricle (LV). The arrow on the right identifies a normally formed ductus arteriosus that narrowed at its pulmonary insertion. (Ao = aorta.) **B,** Left ventriculogram showing the large left ventricle (LV) and prominent ascending aorta (Ao). Pulmonary arteries (arrow) filled through the patent ductus.

it receives venous return from both the systemic and the pulmonary circulations. The left ventricle is initially large and powerful as Peacock[1] described (Figure 24-5), but its compliance and ejection fraction diminish because it pumps the entire output for both circulations.[35] The course of the atrioventricular conduction system is normal.[36]

The *physiologic derangements* in pulmonary atresia with intact ventricular septum are implicit consequences of the anatomic features of the malformation. Physiologic classification is based on the tripartite morphology of the right ventricle and on whether the right ventricular hypoplasia is mild, moderate, or severe. Venous blood reaches the systemic circulation via an interatrial communication that is usually a restrictive patent foramen ovale, which is the only exit from the right atrium (see Figure 24-1; see previous). Unoxygenated right atrial blood mixes with oxygenated left atrial blood and flows into the left ventricle and into the aorta, so systemic arterial oxygen saturation is reduced. Blood from the aorta reaches the pulmonary circulation through a tenuously patent ductus arteriosus on which survival depends (see Figures 24-1

and 24-5).[37] When the ductus closes, effective pulmonary blood flow ceases.[37] Systemic-to-pulmonary collaterals are inadequate for survival.[37]

These physiologic pathways from the right atrium to the left side of the heart are relatively constant from patient to patient, but the patterns in the *right* side of the heart vary considerably. When the right ventricle is small, little blood enters or leaves its cavity because the diminutive chamber and the diminutive tricuspid valve obstruct right atrial flow, which is further compromised by a thick ventricular wall and endocardial fibroelastosis. Whatever blood enters the right ventricle during diastole is trapped during systole, except for the small portion that exits through ventriculocoronary arterial connections. When the right ventricle is dilated and thin-walled, and the tricuspid valve is incompetent, right atrial blood copiously enters the ventricular cavity during diastole, only to be returned to the right atrium during the next systole. Systolic pressure is comparatively low when the right ventricle and right atrium communicate freely across an incompetent tricuspid valve. Although right atrial blood readily flows *into* the right ventricle, no useful purpose is served because forward flow into the pulmonary trunk is impossible. Back-and-forth movement of blood across the tricuspid orifice results in progressive enlargement of the right side of the heart, which becomes massive (see previous).[14]

HISTORY

Pulmonary atresia with intact ventricular septum is equally prevalent in males and females.[38] Reports exist of the malformation in siblings,[39,40] in first cousins,[41] and in monozygotic twins,[42] but familial recurrence is rare. More than half of newborns die in the first month of life, a considerable majority die within the first 3 months, and very few live beyond the first year. Survival hinges on tenuous patency of the ductus arteriosus and on the adequacy of the interatrial communication, which is usually restrictive.[37] Cyanosis begins immediately after birth, and the degree depends on patency of the ductus arteriosus.[37] Pulmonary blood flow diminishes as the ductus involutes, and when the ductus closes, pulmonary blood flow ceases. Despite this ominous outlook, isolated examples of survival have been reported to age 3.5 years[43] and 14 years,[44] and four patients lived for 20 to 21 years.[45–48] The 21-year-old patient had a closed ductus arteriosus at necropsy and had instead a sizable connection between the aortic root and pulmonary trunk and a large atrial septal defect.[48] Another 21-year-old woman survived without a patent ductus because the anterior descending branch of the left coronary artery originated from the pulmonary trunk and provided pulmonary blood flow via intercoronary anastomoses.[49]

PHYSICAL APPEARANCE

Birth weights are normal, and neonatal physical appearance is normal except for cyanosis. Survival beyond the newborn period is accompanied by increasing cyanosis, progressive dyspnea, right-sided heart failure, and physical underdevelopment.

ARTERIAL PULSE AND JUGULAR VENOUS PULSE

The arterial pulse is normal or diminished. Large A waves are generated by powerful right atrial contraction when the right ventricle and tricuspid valve are small. Large systolic venous waves are not necessarily generated when an Epstein's tricuspid valve is incompetent because a very large right atrium damps the venous pressure pulse.

PRECORDIAL MOVEMENT AND PALPATION

A right ventricular impulse is necessarily absent when pulmonary atresia with intact ventricular septum occurs with a small right ventricle. The impulse of an enlarged left ventricle occupies the apex (see Figure 24-5). When the right ventricle is dilated and the tricuspid valve is incompetent, a right ventricular impulse is readily palpable. The thrill of tricuspid regurgitation may be present at the lower left sternal edge. A very large right atrium with severe tricuspid regurgitation generates a visible and palpable systolic impulse at the right sternal border and over the liver.

AUSCULTATION

When the right ventricle is small, the hypoplastic tricuspid valve mechanism generates no closure sound, so the first heart sound consists of the single mitral component. When the right ventricle is dilated, audibility of the tricuspid component of the first heart sound depends on mobility of the anterior leaflet, as in Ebstein's anomaly (Figure 24-6).

A soft transient systolic murmur has been ascribed to flow through the patent ductus before its involution, and a soft midsystolic aorta flow murmur occasionally results

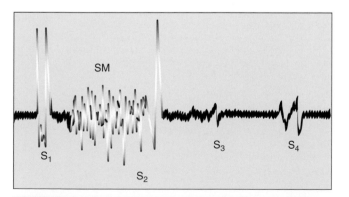

FIGURE 24-6 Phonocardiogram recorded at the lower left sternal border of a 2-day-old male with pulmonary atresia, intact ventricular septum, a normal-sized right ventricle, and tricuspid regurgitation. A long crescendo systolic murmur (SM) goes up to a prominent single second heart sound (S_2), which was aortic valve closure. (S_1 = first heart sound; S_3 = third heart sound; S_4 = fourth heart sound.)

from increased left ventricular stroke volume.[37] The murmur of tricuspid regurgitation is present at birth when the right ventricle is dilated and the malformed tricuspid valve is incompetent (see Figure 24-6). The murmur is medium frequency and decrescendo because right ventricular systolic pressure is relatively low. Maximal intensity is along the lower left sternal edge toward the apex, topographically coinciding with the displaced tricuspid valve, but the murmur may radiate to the right side of the chest and even to the right axilla when a very large right atrium receives tricuspid regurgitant flow (see Figure 24-4).

Continuous murmurs that originate in the ductus arteriosus are rare because ductal patency is transient. In the 21-year-ld woman referred to previously, a continuous murmur was generated, not by a ductus but by flow through intercoronary anastomoses between the right coronary artery and the anterior descending branch of the left coronary artery.[49] In the other 21-year-old woman, a systolic/diastolic murmur originated in a communication between the aortic root and the pulmonary trunk.[48] A 2-month-old girl with bidirectional ventriculocoronary arterial flow had a to-and-fro murmur.[50]

The second heart sound is necessarily single because there is only one functional semilunar valve. Third and fourth heart sounds occur with tricuspid regurgitation because of rapid mid-diastolic filling and an increased force of right atrial contraction transmitted into an unobstructed right ventricle (see Figure 24-6).

ELECTROCARDIOGRAM

The electrocardiogram is a key to the clinical recognition of pulmonary atresia with intact ventricular septum and a small right ventricle because it calls attention to the combination of *cyanosis* with a dominant *left ventricle*. The electrocardiogram also distinguishes this malformation from tricuspid atresia, which it physiologically resembles (see Chapter 25).

When the right ventricle is small, peaked right atrial P waves appear in limb leads and in right precordial leads (Figures 24-7 and 24-8).[51] Biatrial P waves occasionally emerge because the left atrium receives systemic *and* pulmonary venous return.[51] The QRS *mean axis* is normal or rightward with *clockwise deplorization* (see Figures 24-7 and 24-8),[51] which is a useful means of distinguishing pulmonary atresia with intact ventricular septum and small right ventricle from tricuspid atresia, which is characterized by *left* axis deviation and *counterclockwise depolarization* of the QRS.[51] Precordial leads display an adult QRS pattern (see Figures 24-7 and 24-8).[8,51] Right ventricular hypertrophy is conspicuously absent. The small right ventricle does not generate large precordial QRS amplitudes despite its thick wall because the cavity contains so little blood.[51] Similar electrocardiographic patterns can occur in neonates with pinpoint pulmonary stenosis and diminutive right ventricle (see Chapter 11). Left ventricular hypertrophy is manifested by the voltage,[51] but ST segment abnormalities reflect left ventricular ischemia rather than hypertrophy.

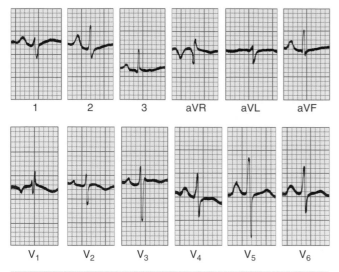

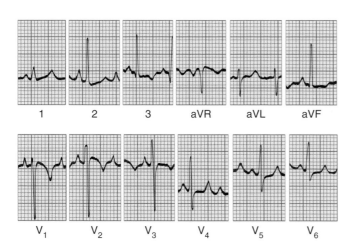

FIGURE 24-7 Electrocardiogram from a 15-hour-old male with pulmonary atresia, intact ventricular septum, and a diminutive right ventricle. There is a tall peaked right artial P wave in lead 2. The QRS axis is rightward, depolarization is clockwise, and there is adult progression of the QRS in the precordial leads.

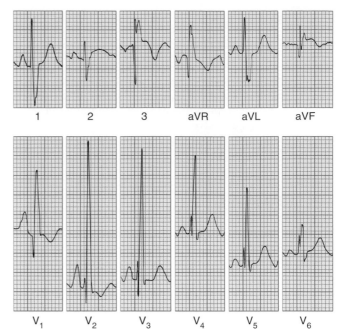

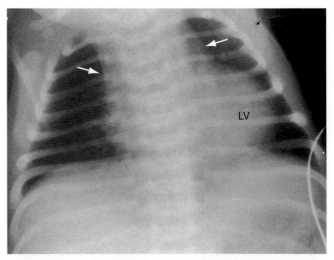

FIGURE 24-9 Electrocardiogram from a 1-day-old female with pulmonary atresia, intact ventricular septum, a dilated right ventricle, severe tricuspid regurgitation, and a large right atrium. Exceptionally tall right atrial P waves appear in lead 1 and in right precordial leads. Right atrial enlargement is indicated by the qR pattern in lead V_1. Tall R waves in V_{1-3} reflect the enlarged right ventricle.

X-RAY

When the right ventricle is small, the cardiac silhouette at birth may be normal or nearly so (Figure 24-10).[52] The pulmonary artery segment is normal because the pulmonary trunk develops normally despite pulmonary valve atresia (Figure 24-11). The ascending aorta is enlarged

FIGURE 24-8 Electrocardiogram from a 2-week-old female with pulmonary atresia, intact ventricular septum, and a small right ventricle. There are tall peaked right atrial P waves in lead 2 and in leads V_{1-3}. The QRS axis is vertical, depolarization is clockwise, and there is adult QRS progression in the precordial leads.

In the first week of life, the electrocardiogram does not reliably distinguish pulmonary atresia with intact ventricular septum and *small* right ventricle from pulmonary atresia with intact ventricular septum and a *large* right ventricle. Soon, however, the electrocardiogram associated with a dilated right ventricle and tricuspid regurgitation reveals itself because of a rightward QRS axis and right ventricular hypertrophy in precordial leads (Figure 24-9).[8,51,52] Right atrial enlargement is reflected in exceptionally tall P waves and a qR complex in lead V_1 (see Figure 24-9).

FIGURE 24-10 X-ray from a 2-day-old female with pulmonary atresia, intact ventricular septum, and a diminutive right ventricle. The lung fields are oligemic. An enlarged convex left ventricle (LV) occupies the apex. Thymus (arrows) obscures the base of the heart.

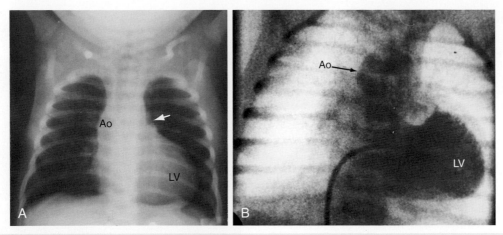

FIGURE 24-11 A, X-ray from a 3-week-old female with pulmonary atresia, intact ventricular septum, and a small right ventricle. The lung fields are oligemic. The ascending aorta (Ao) is enlarged, the main pulmonary artery segment (arrow) is normal, and an enlarged convex left ventricle (LV) occupies the apex. **B,** Angiogram visualizes the enlarged left ventricle (LV) and dilated ascending aorta (Ao).

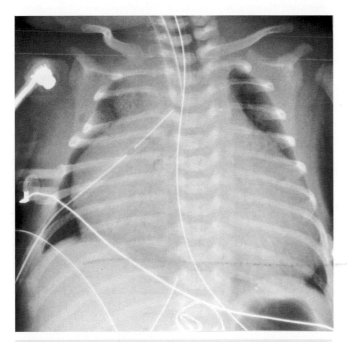

FIGURE 24-12 X-ray from a 5-month-old male with pulmonary atresia, intact ventricular septum, a dilated right ventricle, and severe tricuspid regurgitation. The immense cardiac silhouette—literally, wall-to-wall—is the result of remarkable enlargement of the right atrium and right ventricle. The largely obscured lung fields are oligemic.

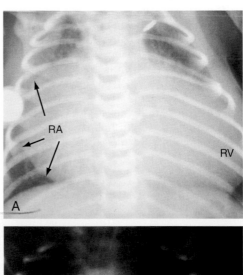

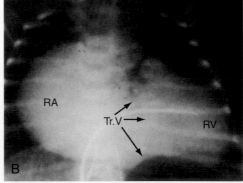

FIGURE 24-13 A, X-ray from a 7-day-old female with pulmonary atresia, intact ventricular septum, a dilated right ventricle, and severe tricuspid regurgitation. The cardiac silhouette is immense because of striking enlargement of the right atrium (RA) and right ventricle (RV). **B,** Contrast injection into the right ventricle (RV) identified the displaced tricuspid valve leaflets (Tr.V) and the huge right atrium (RA).

(see Figures 24-5B, and 24-11).[43] The right atrial shadow is moderately prominent (see Figure 24-11). A well-formed convex left ventricle occupies the apex (see Figures 24-5, 24-10, and 24-11).[43]

The x-ray differs appreciably when the right ventricle is dilated and the tricuspid valve is incompetent.[43] The cardiac silhouette virtually fills the chest—"wall-to-wall"[14]—because of remarkable enlargement of the right atrium and right ventricle (Figures 24-12 and 24-13).

ECHOCARDIOGRAM

Echocardiography with color flow imaging and Doppler interrogation establishes the diagnosis of pulmonary atresia with intact ventricular septum, identifies the atretic pulmonary valve and the well-formed pulmonary trunk, and distinguishes a small right ventricle with a small tricuspid valve from a dilated right ventricle with tricuspid regurgitation.[12,13,38] The malformation can be recognized *in utero*.[53]

Hypoplasia of the right ventricle is judged as mild, moderate, or severe (Figure 24-14 and Video 24-1), and the inlet, trabecular, and outlet portions can be imaged.[38] Deep endocardial recesses represent blind penetrations of the proximal segments of ventriculocoronary arterial communications (see Figure 24-14). Retrograde flow into the aorta is detected with pulsed Doppler or can be suspected because of dilation of a proximal coronary artery. Color flow imaging with Doppler interrogation confirms the absence of flow across the atretic pulmonary valve, which appears as an immobile dense line that moves but fails to open. Initial patency of the ductus is identified with color flow imaging, which also detects a right-to-left shunt across a restrictive interatrial communication.

When the right ventricle is dilated, echocardiography identifies the Ebstein's-like malformation of the tricuspid valve with displacement and immobility of the septal and posterior leaflets (Figures 24-15A and 24-16A). Color flow imaging establishes the degree of tricuspid regurgitation (Figures 24-15B, and 24-16B). The right atrium can be immense (see Figures 24-15A, and 24-16A). Ebstein's anomaly with *functional* pulmonary atresia in which a patent but stenotic pulmonary valve fails to open can be distinguished from *anatomic* pulmonary atresia and a malformed Ebstein's-like tricuspid valve.[12]

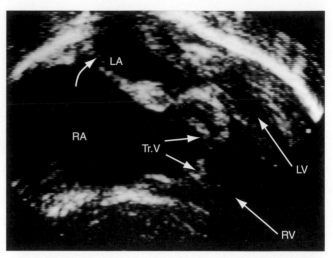

FIGURE 24-15 Echocardiogram from a 6-day-old male with pulmonary atresia, intact ventricular septum, a dilated right ventricle, and severe tricuspid regurgitation. The Ebstein's-like tricuspid valve (TrV) is apically displaced into the enlarged right ventricle (RV). The right atrium (RA) is huge. The left atrium (LA) and left ventricle (LV) are normal. An unmarked curved arrow between the right and left atrium identifies a restrictive patent foramen ovale.

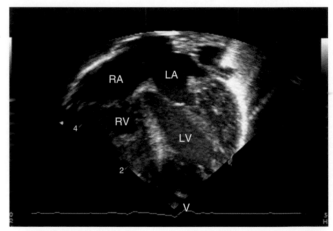

FIGURE 24-16 A, Echocardiogram (four-chamber view) from a 2-day-old female with pulmonary atresia, intact ventricular septum, a moderate sized right ventricle, and severe tricuspid regurgitation. The tricuspid valve (TV) is thickened and recessed into the right ventricle (RV), whose apex is filled with hypertrophied muscle.

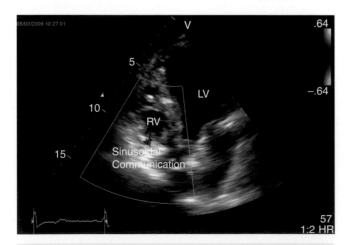

FIGURE 24-14 Echocardiogram (apical four-chamber view) from an infant with pulmonary atresia, intact ventricular septum, and a diminutive right ventricle (RV). Blind ventriculocoronary arterial sinusoids penetrated the right ventricular wall. The left ventricle (LV) was normal (Video 24-1).

SUMMARY

Pulmonary atresia with intact ventricular septum is a diagnostic consideration in neonates and infants with *cyanosis*, a *dominant left ventricle*, and *reduced pulmonary blood flow*. When the right ventricle is small, the physical examination reveals an isolated left ventricular impulse and either no murmur at all or a soft aortic midsystolic flow murmur. The electrocardiogram shows right atrial

P waves, a vertical QRS axis with clockwise depolarization, and adult QRS progression in the precordial leads. An initially normal radiologic cardiac silhouette increases because of moderate enlargement of the right atrium and left ventricle. The lung fields are oligemic, and the main pulmonary artery segment is normal. Echocardiography with color flow imaging and Doppler interrogation identifies an imperforate pulmonary valve, a well-formed pulmonary trunk, a small thick-walled right ventricle, a small tricuspid valve, and moderate enlargement of the right atrium and left ventricle.

A *dilated right ventricle with tricuspid regurgitation* is characterized on physical examination by a right ventricular impulse and a tricuspid regurgitant murmur that radiates to the right of the sternum. The electrocardiogram shows strikingly tall peaked right atrial P waves. The QRS axis is rightward with clockwise depolarization. Right ventricular hypertrophy is reflected in tall right precordial R waves. The x-ray reveals a cardiac silhouette that virtually fills the chest because of massive dilation of the right atrium and right ventricle. The echocardiogram with color flow imaging and Doppler interrogation identifies a dilated right ventricle, an Ebstein's-like malformation of the tricuspid valve, severe tricuspid regurgitation, and striking enlargement of the right atrium.

REFERENCES

1. Peacock TB. *On malformations of the human heart: with original cases.* London: John Churchill & Sons; 1858.
2. Hunter J. *Medical observations and inquiries: Society of Physicians in London.* 1784.
3. Braunlin EA, Formanek AG, Moller JH, Edwards JE. Angiopathological appearances of pulmonary valve in pulmonary atresia with intact ventricular septum. Interpretation of nature of right ventricle from pulmonary angiography. *Br Heart J.* 1982;47:281–289.
4. Daubeney PEF, Delany DJ, Anderson RH, et al., United K, Ireland Collaborative Study of Pulmonary Atresia with Intact Ventricular S. Pulmonary atresia with intact ventricular septum: range of morphology in a population-based study. *J Am Coll Cardiol.* 2002;39:1670–1679.
5. Shinebourne EA, Rigby ML, Carvalho JS. Pulmonary atresia with intact ventricular septum: from fetus to adult: congenital heart disease. *Heart.* 2008;94:1350–1357.
6. Daubeney PE, Sharland GK, Cook AC, Keeton BR, Anderson RH, Webber SA. Pulmonary atresia with intact ventricular septum: impact of fetal echocardiography on incidence at birth and postnatal outcome. UK and Eire Collaborative Study of Pulmonary Atresia with Intact Ventricular Septum. *Circulation.* 1998;98:562–566.
7. Ekman J, Sunnegardh J, Hanseus K. Outcome of children born with pulmonary atresia and intact septum in Sweden from 1980 to 1990. *Scand Cardiovasc J.* 2001;35:192.
8. Shams A, Fowler RS, Trusler GA, Keith JD, Mustard WT. Pulmonary atresia with intact ventricular septum: report of 50 cases. *Pediatrics.* 1971;47:370–377.
9. Zuberbuhler JR, Anderson RH. Morphological variations in pulmonary atresia with intact ventricular septum. *Br Heart J.* 1979;41:281–288.
10. Bulkley BH, D'Amico B, Taylor AL. Extensive myocardial fiber disarray in aortic and pulmonary atresia. Relevance to hypertrophic cardiomyopathy. *Circulation.* 1983;67:191–198.
11. Oosthoek PW, Moorman AF, Sauer U, Gittenberger-De Groot AC. Capillary distribution in the ventricles of hearts with pulmonary atresia and intact ventricular septum. *Circulation.* 1995;91:1790–1798.
12. Smallhorn JF, Izukawa T, Benson L, Freedom RM. Noninvasive recognition of functional pulmonary atresia by echocardiography. *Am J Cardiol.* 1984;54:925–926.
13. Gewillig M, Dumoulin M, Van Der Hauwaert LG. Transient neonatal tricuspid regurgitation: a Doppler echocardiographic study of three cases. *Br Heart J.* 1988;60:446–451.
14. Freedom RM, Jaeggi E, Perrin D, Yoo S-J, Anderson RH. The "wall-to-wall" heart in the patient with pulmonary atresia and intact ventricular septum. *Cardiol Young.* 2006;16:18–29.
15. Amin P, Levi DS, Likes M, Laks H. Pulmonary atresia with intact ventricular septum causing severe left ventricular outflow tract obstruction. *Pediatr Cardiol.* 2009;30:851–854.
16. Peraira Moral JR, Burguens Valero M, Garcia-Guereta Silva L. Pulmonary valve atresia with intact ventricular septum and severe aortic stenosis. *Pediatr Cardiol.* 2005;26:117–118.
17. L'Ecuyer TJ, Poulik JM, Vincent JA. Myocardial infarction due to coronary abnormalities in pulmonary atresia with intact ventricular septum. *Pediatr Cardiol.* 2001;22:68–70.
18. Kasznica J, Ursell PC, Blanc WA, Gersony WM. Abnormalities of the coronary circulation in pulmonary atresia and intact ventricular septum. *Am Heart J.* 1987;114:1415–1420.
19. O'Connor WN, Stahr BJ, Cottrill CM, Todd EP, Noonan JA. Ventriculocoronary connections in hypoplastic right heart syndrome: autopsy serial section study of six cases. *J Am Coll Cardiol.* 1988;11:1061–1072.
20. Craver RD, Caspi J. Pulmonary atresia, intact ventricular septum, right ventricle-dependent coronary artery circulation, and systemic collateral arteries supplying the left coronary artery. *Pediatr Dev Pathol.* 2006;9:152–156.
21. Dyamenahalli U, Mccrindle BW, Mcdonald C, et al. Pulmonary atresia with intact ventricular septum: management of, and outcomes for, a cohort of 210 consecutive patients. *Cardiol Young.* 2004;14:299–308.
22. L'Ecuyer TJ, Poulik JM, Vincent JA. Myocardial infarction due to coronary abnormalities in pulmonary atresia with intact ventricular septum. *Pediatr Cardiol.* 2001;22:68–70.
23. Sandor GGS, Cook AC, Sharland GK, Ho SY, Potts JE, Anderson RH. Coronary arterial abnormalities in pulmonary atresia with intact ventricular septum diagnosed during fetal life. *Cardiol Young.* 2002;12:436–444.
24. Sarkola T, Boldt T, Happonen J-M, Karikoski R, Eronen M. Atresia of proximal coronary arteries in pulmonary atresia with intact ventricular septum: fetal and neonatal findings. *Fetal Diagn Ther.* 2008;24:413–415.
25. Grant R. An unusual anomaly of the coronary vessels in the malformed heart of a child. *Heart.* 1926;13:273–283.
26. Hutchins GM, Kessler-Hanna A, Moore GW. Development of the coronary arteries in the embryonic human heart. *Circulation.* 1988;77:1250–1257.
27. Wald RM, Juraszek AL, Pigula FA, Geva T. Echocardiographic diagnosis and management of bilateral coronary ostial atresia in a patient with pulmonary atresia and intact ventricular septum. *J Am Soc Echocardiogr.* 2006;19:939.e931–939.e933.
28. Engberding R, Bender F. Identification of a rare congenital anomaly of the myocardium by two-dimensional echocardiography: persistence of isolated myocardial sinusoids. *Am J Cardiol.* 1984;53:1733–1734.
29. Shimizu T, Ando M, Takao A. Pulmonary atresia and intact ventricular septum and corrected transposition of the great arteries. *Br Heart J.* 1981;45:471–474.
30. Steeg CN, Ellis K, Bransilver B, Gersony WM. Pulmonary atresia and intact ventricular septum complicating corrected transposition of the great vessels. *Am Heart J.* 1971;82:382–386.
31. Baffa JM, Chen SL, Guttenberg ME, Norwood WI, Weinberg PM. Coronary artery abnormalities and right ventricular histology in hypoplastic left heart syndrome. *J Am Coll Cardiol.* 1992;20:350–358.
32. Sauer U, Gittenberger-De Groot AC, Geishauser M, Babic R, Buhlmeyer K. Coronary arteries in the hypoplastic left heart syndrome. Histopathologic and histometrical studies and implications for surgery. *Circulation.* 1989;80:I168–I176.
33. Powell AJ, Mayer JE, Lang P, Lock JE. Outcome in infants with pulmonary atresia, intact ventricular septum, and right ventricle-dependent coronary circulation. *Am J Cardiol.* 2000;86:1272–1274, A1279.
34. Hubbard JF, Girod DA, Caldwell RL, Hurwitz RA, Mahony LA, Waller BF. Right ventricular infarction with cardiac rupture in an infant with pulmonary valve atresia with intact ventricular septum. *J Am Coll Cardiol.* 1983;2:363–368.
35. Scognamiglio R, Daliento L, Razzolini R, et al. Pulmonary atresia with intact ventricular septum: a quantitative cineventriculographic

study of the right and left ventricular function. *Pediatr Cardiol.* 1986;7:183–187.

36. Ansari A, Goltz D, Mccarthy KP, Cook A, Ho SY. The conduction system in hearts with pulmonary atresia and intact ventricular septum. *Ann Thorac Surg.* 2003;75:1502–1505.

37. Venables AW. The patterns of pulmonary circulation in pulmonary atresia. *Br Heart J.* 1964;26:760–769.

38. Leung MP, Mok CK, Hui PW. Echocardiographic assessment of neonates with pulmonary atresia and intact ventricular septum. *J Am Coll Cardiol.* 1988;12:719–725.

39. Chitayat D, Mcintosh N, Fouron JC. Pulmonary atresia with intact ventricular septum and hypoplastic right heart in sibs: a single gene disorder? *Am J Med Genet.* 1992;42:304–306.

40. Eriksen NL, Buttino Jr. L, Juberg RC. Congenital pulmonary atresia with intact ventricular septum, tricuspid insufficiency, and patent ductus arteriosus in two sibs. *Am J Med Genet.* 1989;32:187–188.

41. Grossfeld PD, Lucas VW, Sklansky MS, Kashani IA, Rothman A. Familial occurrence of pulmonary atresia with intact ventricular septum. *Am J Med Genet.* 1997;72:294–296.

42. De Stefano D, Li P, Xiang B, Hui P, Zambrano E. Pulmonary atresia with intact ventricular septum (PA-IVS) in monozygotic twins. *Am J Med Genet.* 2008; Part A 146A:525–528.

43. Kieffer SA, Carey LS. Radiological aspects of pulmonary atresia with intact ventricular septum. *Br Heart J.* 1963;25:655–662.

44. Allanby KD, Brinton WD, Campbell M, Garnder F. Pulmonary atresia and the collateral circulation to the lungs. *Guys Hosp Rep.* 1950;99:110–152.

45. Abbott M. *Atlas of Congenital Cardiac Diseases.* New York: American Heart Association; 1936.

46. Bostoen H, Robicsek F, Sanger PW. Atresia of the pulmonary valve with normal pulmonary artery and intact ventricular septum in a 21 year old woman. *Coll Works Cardiopulm Dis.* 1966;11: 753–758.

47. Costa A. Atresia congenita dell'ostio della polmonare, con setto interventricolare chiuso e dotto di Botallo persistente in uomodi 20 anni. *Clin Med Ital.* 1930;61:567.

48. Robicsek F, Bostoen H, Sanger PW. Atresia of the pulmonary valve with normal pulmonary artery and intact ventricular septum in a 21-year-old woman. *Angiology.* 1966;17:896–901.

49. Mcarthur JD, Munsi SC, Sukumar IP, Cherian G. Pulmonary valve atresia with intact ventricular septum. Report of a case with long survival and pulmonary blood supply from an anomalous coronary artery. *Circulation.* 1971;44:740–745.

50. Ogden JA. Secondary coronary arterial fistulas. *J Pediatr.* 1971;78: 78–85.

51. Gamboa R, Gersony WM, Nadas AS. The electrocardiogram in tricuspid atresia and pulmonary atresia with intact ventricular septum. *Circulation.* 1966;34:24–37.

52. Celermajer JM, Bowdler JD, Gengos DC, Cohen DH, Stuckey DS. Pulmonary valve fusion with intact ventricular septum. *Am Heart J.* 1968;76:452–465.

53. Patel CR, Shah DM, Dahms BB. Prenatal diagnosis of a coronary fistula in a fetus with pulmonary atresia with intact ventricular septum and trisomy 18. *J Ultrasound Med.* 1999;18:429–431.

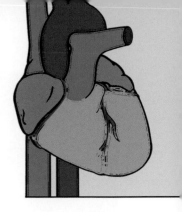

Chapter 25

Tricuspid Atresia

Tricuspid atresia was described in 1817,[1] but almost a century elapsed before the great arterial relationships were defined.[2] Because of the morphologic heterogeneity of the malformation, "manifold anatomic combinations can result in this haemodynamic arrangement."[3,4] The incidence rate has been estimated at 0.06 per 1000 live births, with a prevalence rate of 1% to 3% of congenital heart disease.[5,6] An unguarded tricuspid orifice is different again.[7] This chapter is concerned with hearts in *situs solitus* without ventricular inversion in which a physiologic or anatomic connection does not exist between the morphologic right atrium and the morphologic right ventricle. In 95% of patients, *absence of the right atrioventricular connection* is the result of fibro-fatty tissue that is interposed between the muscular floor of the right atrium and the parietal wall of the ventricular mass.[8] In the remaining 5%, atresia is produced by an *imperforate tricuspid valvular membrane*.[4,8] Systemic venous return cannot directly reach the ventricular portion of the heart but instead crosses the atrial septum from a morphologic right atrium into a morphologic left atrium, where it mixes with pulmonary venous return before traversing a solitary atrioventricular valve into a morphologic left ventricle, which is the only pumping chamber for the pulmonary and systemic circulations (Figure 25-1).[3] This arrangement has been referred to as a "functionally" univentricular heart.[4] Atresia of the tricuspid valve with Ebstein's anomaly and atresia of the right atrioventricular valve with single ventricle are dealt with in Chapters 13 and 26.

Tricuspid atresia, as just defined, has certain anatomic features that consistently recur and certain features that are variable.[6,9,10] Consistent features include: (1), physiologic and anatomic absence of a connection between the morphologic right atrium and the morphologic right ventricle; (2), hypoplasia of the morphologic right ventricle; (3), an interatrial communication; and (4), a morphologic left ventricle equipped with a morphologic mitral valve. The variable features provide the rationale for a clinical classification based on three gross morphologic features[4,6,9–11]: (1), transposed or nontransposed great arteries; (2), the presence or absence of pulmonary stenosis (Figures 25-2 and 25-3); and (3), the size of the coexisting ventricular septal defect. An embryologic classification is based on two microscopic features: (1), rudiments of an atretic tricuspid apparatus that create a dimple on the floor of the right atrium that can be localized with transillumination by a light source placed within the hypoplastic right ventricle[10,12,13]; and (2), a fibrous

atrioventricular remnant that forms a microscopic tract from the right atrium to a tiny inlet component of the subjacent right ventricle.[14] Failure of expansion of this exceedingly small inlet component during early embryogenesis is believed to be the pathogenetic mechanism responsible for most cases of tricuspid atresia.[14] *Congenital tricuspid stenosis* is a less severe form of the malformation in which a well-formed tricuspid valve joins the small inlet portion of the right ventricle (Figure 25-4).[12]

In approximately three fourths of cases, an interatrial communication exists in the form of a restrictive patent foramen ovale.[15] The valve of the foramen ovale occasionally protrudes aneurysmally as the obstructed right atrium vainly seeks an exit.[16,17] The aneurysmal protrusion can obstruct left atrial flow.[17] A much less common form of interatrial communication is an atrial septal defect that is almost always ostium secundum.[9,15]

The great arteries are nontransposed in approximately 90% of cases.[11,15] Pulmonary blood flow then depends on the condition of the ventricular septum (see Figure 25-2). The arrangement at birth is usually a restrictive ventricular septal defect (see Figure 25-2B) that constitutes a zone of *subpulmonary stenosis*, which is physiologically advantageous when blood flow to the lungs is adequate but not excessive. The advantage is lost in about 40% of cases because the defect decreases in size or closes altogether—acquired pulmonary atresia (see Figures 25-2A, and 25-6).[15,18–20] The time course of spontaneous closure is similar to that of isolated perimembranous ventricular septal defects (see Chapter 17), with most that are destined to close doing so in the first year of life.[15,18–20] Rarely, the ventricular septum is *congenitally intact* and the *pulmonary valve is atretic*, an arrangement that completely denies the left ventricle access to the pulmonary circulation (see Figure 25-2A). Also rarely, obstruction is exclusively at valve level because a bicuspid pulmonary valve is stenotic.[21] A *nonrestrictive ventricular septal defect* (Figures 25-2C, and 25-5) permits unobstructed flow from left ventricle to main pulmonary artery. The right ventricle is well-developed, and the pulmonary valve is normally formed. Pulmonary blood flow is regulated by pulmonary vascular resistance.[6]

Tricuspid atresia with complete transposition of the great arteries typically occurs with a nonrestrictive ventricular septal defect without pulmonary stenosis (see Figure 25-3).[11,15] Left ventricular blood has unobstructed access to the transposed aorta through a well-developed right ventricle. Pulmonary blood flow is regulated by

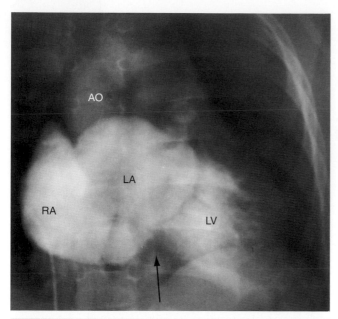

FIGURE 25-1 Angiocardiogram from an 8-year-old boy with tricuspid atresia, normally related great arteries, and an initially restrictive ventricular septal defect that closed spontaneously. Contrast material injected into the right atrium (RA) sequentially filled the left atrium (LA), left ventricle (LV), and aorta (AO). The right ventricle (unmarked arrow) remains unopacified as a wedge-shaped area of negative contrast.

pulmonary vascular resistance because the transposed pulmonary trunk originates from the left ventricle (see Figure 25-3). Pulmonary vascular disease usually develops in the first year of life (Figures 25-7 and 25-8).[15] A decrease in size or spontaneous closure of the

ventricular septal defect constitutes a zone of subaortic stenosis because the transposed aorta arises from the right ventricle.[22] Pulmonary stenosis is infrequent, and pulmonary atresia is rare (see Figure 25-3).[23]

Distribution of the coronary arteries in tricuspid atresia is analogous to, if not identical with, that of univentricular hearts with a single morphologic left ventricle and an outlet chamber (see Chapters 26 and 32).[24] The rudimentary right ventricle of tricuspid atresia and the right ventricular remnant of single ventricle are both delimited by coronary arteries.[24]

Additional anatomic variables associated with tricuspid atresia involve the mitral valve,[25] the ductus arteriosus, the ascending aorta, the aortic isthmus, the atrial appendages, and the pulmonary valve.[26] Abnormalities of the mitral valve are represented by myxomatous, redundant, or prolapsing leaflets; a cleft anterior leaflet; and direct attachment of leaflets to papillary muscles.[25] When the great arteries are nontransposed and the ventricular septum is congenitally intact, which is *physiologic* pulmonary atresia, the fetal ductus arteriosus functions as a small malformed aortic tributary.[27] The ascending aorta and isthmus are large because the aorta receives the entire cardiac output. When the great arteries are transposed and the ventricular septal defect is restrictive, left ventricular blood is diverted into the pulmonary trunk, so the ductus arteriosus enlarges while the ascending aorta and isthmus are underfilled and hypoplastic.[15,28] Very rarely, the pulmonary valve is absent.[26] Juxtaposition of the atrial appendages, a condition in which both appendages lie on one side of the great arteries,[15,29–31] almost always means that the great arteries are transposed (see Chapter 27). Juxtaposition is present in about 50% of patients with tricuspid atresia and complete transposition.

TRICUSPID ATRESIA WITHOUT TRANSPOSITION

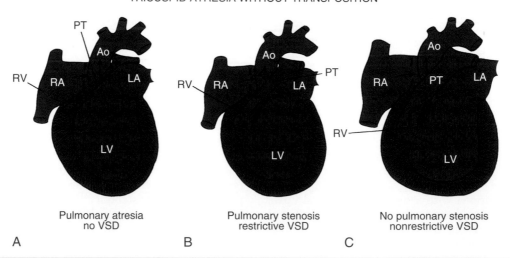

A — Pulmonary atresia no VSD

B — Pulmonary stenosis restrictive VSD

C — No pulmonary stenosis nonrestrictive VSD

FIGURE 25-2 Illustrations of three principal varieties of tricuspid atresia without transposition of the great arteries. Anatomic arrangements proximal to the mitral valve are similar. An interatrial communication provides the right atrium (RA) with its only exit. Anatomic arrangements distal to the mitral valve vary. **A,** Pulmonary atresia is represented by an intact ventricular septum. All left ventricular blood enters the aorta (Ao). The pulmonary trunk (PT) is hypoplastic. Pulmonary blood flow depends on patency of the ductus arteriosus or on systemic arterial collaterals. The left atrium (LA) and left ventricle (LV) are normal-sized. **B,** Subpulmonary stenosis is represented by a restrictive ventricular septal defect between the normal-sized left ventricle and the small right ventricle (RV). The pulmonary trunk is normal or small. **C,** A nonrestrictive ventricular septal defect permits unobstructed blood flow into the pulmonary trunk. When pulmonary vascular resistance is low, pulmonary blood flow is increased, so the left atrium and left ventricle dilate.

TRICUSPID ATRESIA WITH TRANSPOSITION

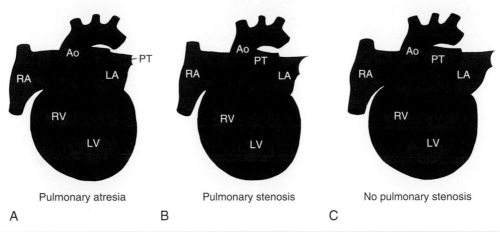

Pulmonary atresia   Pulmonary stenosis   No pulmonary stenosis

A   B   C

FIGURE 25-3 Illustration of three principal varieties of tricuspid atresia with complete transposition of the great arteries. The anatomic arrangements proximal to the mitral valve are similar. An interatrial communication provides the right atrium (RA) with its only exit. A nonrestrictive ventricular septal defect permits unobstructed blood flow from the left ventricle (LV) into the transposed aorta (Ao). Anatomic arrangements distal to the mitral valve vary. **A,** With atresia of the pulmonary valve, all left ventricular blood enters the aorta through the nonrestrictive ventricular septal defect. The right ventricle (RV) is well-formed, but the pulmonary trunk (PT) is hypoplastic. Pulmonary blood flow depends on patency of the ductus arteriosus or on systemic arterial collaterals. The left atrium (LA) and left ventricle (LV) are normal-sized. **B,** Valvular or subvalvular pulmonary stenosis regulates pulmonary blood flow. The pulmonary trunk is well-developed. The left atrium and left ventricle remain normal-sized. **C,** With no pulmonary stenosis and low pulmonary vascular resistance, pulmonary blood flow is increased, so the left atrium and left ventricle enlarge.

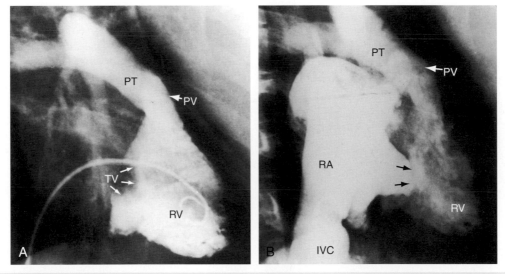

FIGURE 25-4 A, Right ventriculogram (RV) from a 50-year-old woman with congenital tricuspid stenosis, well-formed right ventricles, and no obstruction to right ventricular outflow. The stenotic tricuspid valve (TV) domes in diastole. (PV = pulmonary valve; PT = pulmonary trunk). **B,** Contrast material injected into the right atrium (RA) identifies diastolic doming of the stenotic tricuspid valve (unmarked paired arrows). Negative contrast faintly visualizes a normal pulmonary valve (PV). The inferior vena cava (IVC) is visualized because right atrial (RA) pressure was elevated.

The physiologic consequences of tricuspid atresia begin with the obligatory right-to-left shunt at the atrial level. The left atrium receives the normal *pulmonary* venous return together with the *systemic* venous return across the interatrial communication.[32] The left atrial mixture flows across a morphologic mitral valve into a morphologic left ventricle, which is the sole pumping chamber for the systemic and pulmonary circulations.

When the *great arteries are not transposed*, pulmonary blood flow is reduced because a restrictive ventricular septal defect constitutes a zone of subpulmonary stenosis (see Figures 25-2 and 25-6). This arrangement accounts for about 90% of cases. Left ventricular volume overload is curtailed at the price of increased cyanosis. When the ventricular septal defect is nonrestrictive and pulmonary vascular resistance is low, pulmonary blood flow and left

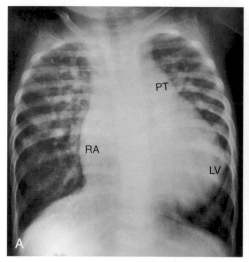
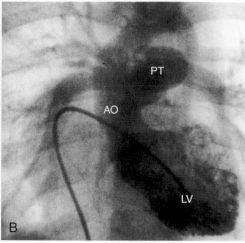

FIGURE 25-5 **A,** X-ray from a 6-year-old girl with tricuspid atresia, normally related great arteries, a nonrestrictive ventricular septal defect, low pulmonary vascular resistance, and a large ostium secundum atrial septal defect (see Figure 25-2C). Pulmonary blood flow is markedly increased, the pulmonary trunk (PT) is prominent, the right atrium (RA) is enlarged, and a dilated left ventricle (LV) occupies the apex. **B,** Left ventriculogram from a 4-year-old girl with tricuspid atresia, normally related great arteries, a nonrestrictive ventricular septal defect, and low pulmonary vascular resistance. The pulmonary trunk (PT) and its branches are dilated, and the left ventricle is enlarged. Compare with Figure 25-2C.

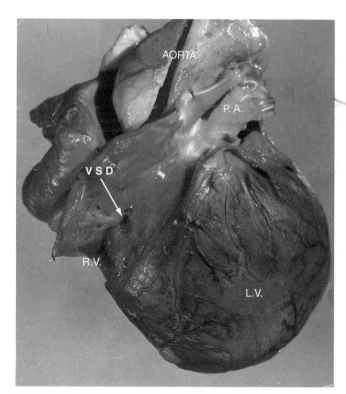

FIGURE 25-6 Necropsy specimen from a 2-year-old boy with tricuspid atresia, normally related great arteries, and a slit-like ventricular septal defect (VSD) as seen from the cavity of the small right ventricle (R.V.). The pulmonary valve and main pulmonary artery (P.A.) were normally formed, which implies that a previously advantageous ventricular septal defect had decreased in size. The left ventricle (L.V.) is moderately enlarged.

ventricular volume overload are excessive, and cyanosis is mild (see Figure 25-5). When the *great arteries are transposed,* the ventricular septal defect is usually nonrestrictive and pulmonary stenosis is usually absent (see Figure 25-3). Low pulmonary vascular resistance results in increased pulmonary blood flow, mild cyanosis, and left ventricular volume overload.[33,34] The degree of pulmonary vascular resistance that achieves adequate but not excessive pulmonary blood flow is a delicate balance that is seldom realized (see Figures 25-7 and 25-8).[15]

HISTORY

When tricuspid atresia occurs with *normally related great arteries,* males and females are equally represented,[15] but when the great arteries are transposed, males predominate[15] unless there is juxtaposition of the atrial appendages.[31] Tricuspid atresia has been reported in siblings,[35–37] in families,[38] and in experimental animals.[39]

In about 6% of infants with tricuspid atresia, birth is premature.[5] Survival depends on an adequate interatrial communication and adequate regulation of pulmonary blood flow.[15,23] Increased longevity incurs the risk of infective endocarditis, paradoxical emboli, and brain abcess.[15,22,40] Life span is less than 6 months when tricuspid atresia occurs with normally related great arteries and pulmonary atresia (see Figure 25-2A), but exceptional survivals have been recorded at age 21 years[41] and 22 years.[42] Acquired pulmonary atresia takes the form of spontaneous closure of the ventricular septal defect (see previous), an eventuality that usually occurs in the first year of life.[15,19] Survival then depends on patency

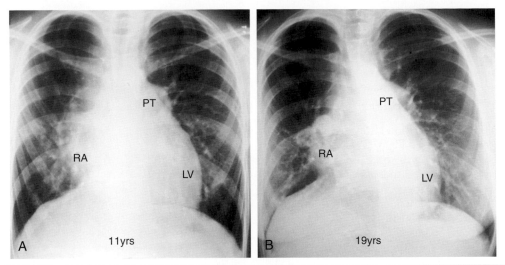

FIGURE 25-7 X-rays from a female with tricuspid atresia, normally related great arteries, a nonrestrictive ventricular septal defect, and a large ostium secundum atrial septal defect. **A,** At age 11 years, pulmonary vascular resistance was below systemic, pulmonary vascularity was increased, the left ventricle (LV) was enlarged, and the pulmonary trunk (PT) and right atrium (RA) were dilated. **B,** At age 19 years, the pulmonary vascular resistance was suprasystemic, pulmonary vascularity was normal, and the pulmonary trunk and right atrium remained dilated, but the left ventricle was no longer enlarged. Overlying breast tissue accounts for prominent lower lung field radiodensities.

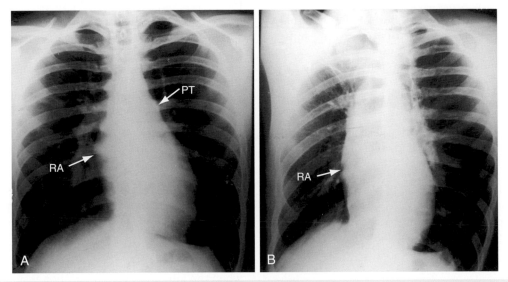

FIGURE 25-8 X-rays from an 18-year-old man with tricuspid atresia, complete transposition of the great arteries, a nonrestrictive ventricular septal defect, and suprasystemic pulmonary vascular resistance. **A,** Pulmonary vascularity is diminished, and the dilated hypertensive posterior pulmonary trunk is border-forming (PT). The right cardiac silhouette is hump-shaped because a prominent superior border is caused by an enlarged right atrium (RA) and a receding inferior border, which is caused by a hypoplastic right ventricle. **B,** Left anterior oblique projection highlights the hump-shaped right superior border.

of the ductus arteriosus, an advantage that is seldom realized. Exceptional survivals have nevertheless been reported at age 8 years (see Figure 25-1), 18 years,[15] and 27 years,[20] in addition to a 21-year-old woman who survived because adequate pulmonary blood flow was achieved by an anomalous artery connecting the ascending aorta to the pulmonary trunk.[3] The most exceptional survival was a 65-year-old man with tricuspid atresia, pulmonary atresia, an ostium secundum atrial septal defect, and large aortic-to-pulmonary arterial collaterals.[43]

Most patients with *tricuspid atresia and normally related great arteries* die in the first year because an already restrictive ventricular septal defect decreases in size or closes altogether.[15] When the ventricular septal defect adequately regulates pulmonary blood flow, survivals have been realized from the second into the fifth decade.[44,45] Two patients lived to 57 years of age,[23] and a 30-year-old woman had a relatively uneventful pregnancy and a dysmature but otherwise healthy offspring.[46] If the ventricular septal defect is nonrestrictive (see Figure 25-2C), increased pulmonary blood flow results in excessive volume overload of the left ventricle and congestive heart failure. However, one such patient was alive at age 6 years (see Figure 25-5), and survivals have been reported to age 32 years and 45 years,[40,47] with an exceptional survival to age 57 years.[48]

The same longevity patterns occur with tricuspid atresia, complete transposition of the great arteries, and a nonrestrictive ventricular septal defect (see Figure 25-3C) in which regulation of pulmonary blood flow depends on pulmonary vascular resistance (see Figure 25-8). Exceptional survivals have been reported to the mid and late teens.[15,49] Satisfactory regulation of pulmonary blood flow is more likely to be achieved by pulmonary stenosis (see Figure 25-3B)[15] with which isolated patients have lived into the second, third, and fourth decades,[21,23,40] with one patient dying at age 56 years.[50]

Survival in congenital *tricuspid stenosis* depends on the degree of obstruction and on an adequate interatrial communication.[51,52] A 20-year-old woman was acyanotic (see Figure 25-11),[52] a cyanotic patient underwent surgical repair at age 50 years (see Figure 25-4), and a cyanotic man survived to age 57 years.[51]

Hypoxic spells precipitated by a reduction in size or spontaneous closure of a restrictive ventricular septal defect are characterized by sudden deepening of cyanosis followed by paroxysmal dyspnea, lethargy, and syncope.[6,15,52] Older children squat for relief of breathlessness.[23,44] Syncope has been attributed to intermittent occlusion of the interatrial communication by a large spinnaker-like valve of the sinus venosus.[53]

PHYSICAL APPEARANCE

Physical appearance in tricuspid atresia reflects the cyanosis of venoarterial mixing and decreased pulmonary blood flow and the catabolic effects of congestive heart failure and excessive pulmonary blood flow. A left precordial bulge does not occur because the right ventricle is underdeveloped. The *cat-eye syndrome* is a distinctive although uncommon appearance characterized by fissures of the iris (congenital coloboma) and an oblong pupillary shape.[54]

ARTERIAL PULSE

The arterial pulse is normal (Figure 25-9B) unless pulmonary blood flow is excessive and the left ventricle has failed. The pulses are feeble if not undetectable when tricuspid atresia occurs with transposition of the great arteries, a restrictive ventricular septal defect, and systemic hypoperfusion.[55]

JUGULAR VENOUS PULSE

The A wave is increased when a restrictive interatrial communication obstructs egress from the right atrium (Figure 25-10). Large A waves are also features of congenital tricuspid stenosis (Figure 25-11). The Y descent is slow when a restrictive interatrial communication impedes right atrial flow during the passive filling phase.

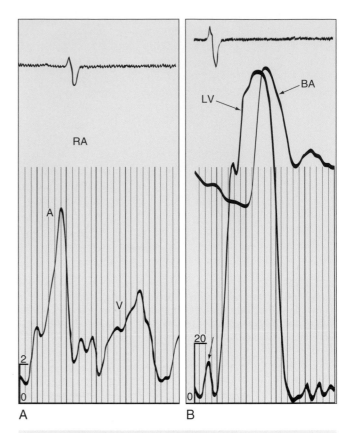

FIGURE 25-9 Tracings from an 18-year-old man with tricuspid atresia, complete transposition of the great arteries, and pulmonary vascular disease. X-rays are shown in Figure 25-8. **A,** Right atrial (RA) pressure pulse showing a prominent A wave. **B,** Presystolic distention of the left ventricle (unmarked lower left arrow) reflected the prominent right atrial A wave that was transmitted into the left ventricle (LV) through a nonrestrictive atrial septal defect. (BA = brachial artery pulse.)

The A wave increases when a thick-walled left ventricle resists right atrial contraction (see Figure 25-9A). A and V waves are both increased when left ventricular failure provokes a rise in mean pressure in a left atrium that is in continuity with the right atrium. Large V waves of mitral regurgitation are transmitted into the right atrium when the interatrial communication is nonrestrictive.[44]

PRECORDIAL MOVEMENT AND PALPATION

A key to the clinical recognition of tricuspid atresia is the combination of a *left ventricular impulse* in a *cyanotic patient* in whom a *right ventricular impulse* is conspicuously *absent*. The left ventricle remains palpable even when pulmonary blood flow is reduced because the chamber handles the entire output of the systemic and pulmonary circulations. When pulmonary blood flow is increased, the impulse of the volume overload left ventricle is also increased.[33] A gentle right ventricular impulse is reserved for the occasional patient with a nonrestrictive ventricular septal defect and a relatively well-developed right ventricle.

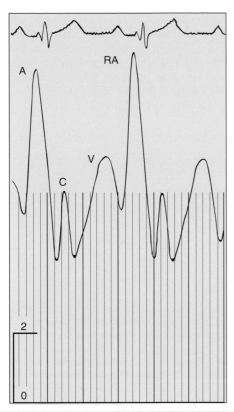

FIGURE 25-10 Right atrial pressure pulse (RA) from a 9-month-old female with tricuspid atresia, normally related great arteries, a restrictive ventricular septal defect, and a patent foramen ovale. The A wave is prominent. The C and V waves are normal.

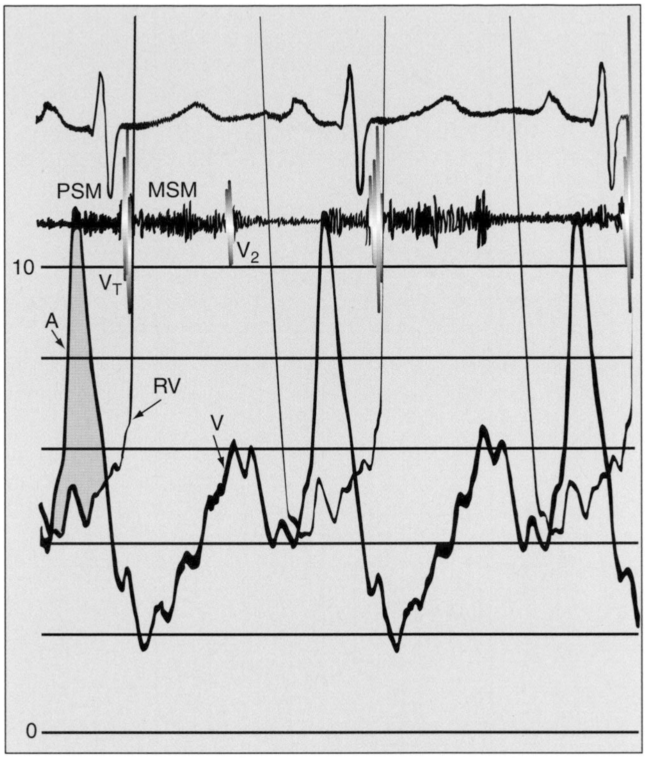

FIGURE 25-11 Right ventricular (RV) and right atrial pressure pulses with phonocardiogram at the lower left sternal border of a 20-year-old woman with congenital tricuspid stenosis and pulmonary valve stenosis. The large right atrial A wave exceeded right ventricular end-diastolic pressure (shaded area) and resulted in a presystolic murmur (PSM). A midsystolic murmur (MSM) was generated across the stenotic pulmonary valve. The height of the V wave was normal. (A2 = aortic component of second heart sound.)

AUSCULTATION

Auscultatory signs are determined by the anatomic variations beyond the mitral valve. The single first heart sound is necessarily the mitral component because the tricuspid valve is atretic.[56] When the great arteries are not transposed, a holosystolic systolic murmur is generated across the restrictive ventricular septal defect (Figures 25-12, 25-13, and 25-14). The murmur is maximal at the mid to lower left sternal edge but radiates to the second left intercostal space when the left ventricle ejects through the ventricular septal defect into the pulmonary trunk (see Figure 25-13). When the ventricular septal defect decreases in size or closes spontaneously, the holosystolic murmur becomes early systolic before vanishing altogether.[18] The second heart sound is represented by the aortic component, although a soft delayed pulmonary component is occasionally detected because the restrictive ventricular septal defect is functionally subpulmonary stenosis (see Figure 25-13). When the ventricular septum is intact from birth (functional congenital pulmonary atresia; see Figure 25-2A), there is either no murmur at all or a short midsystolic murmur into a dilated aortic root. Continuous murmurs through aortopulmonary collaterals are exceptional (Figure 25-15).[20]

Tricuspid atresia with transposition of the great arteries (see Figure 25-3C) is accompanied by a holosystolic murmur that is generated across the ventricular septal defect, which is usually nonrestrictive (Figure 25-16). A single loud second heart sound is aortic because the transposed aorta is anterior (see Figure 25-16). A third heart sound introduces a mid-diastolic murmur generated by increased flow across the mitral valve (see Figure 25-16). When elevated pulmonary vascular resistance reduces pulmonary blood flow, left ventricular stroke volume falls, the ventricular septal defect murmur decreases or disappears (Figure 25-17), and a soft midsystolic murmur is generated into the anterior aortic root. The second heart sound is audibly split because the hypertensive dilated posterior pulmonary trunk generates a loud pulmonary component (see Figure 25-17). Pulmonary or subpulmonary stenosis generates a midsystolic murmur, the loudness and length of which *vary inversely* with the degree of obstruction because the more severe the stenosis, the more left ventricular blood is diverted into the aorta via the ventricular septal defect (see Figure 25-3B). Flow across the stenotic sites falls reciprocally, so the pulmonary stenotic murmur softens and shortens (Figure 25-18). The posterior position of the pulmonary trunk decreases the murmur still further.

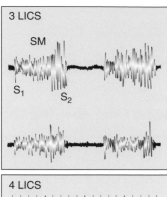

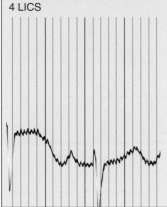

FIGURE 25-12 Phonocardiogram from a 20-month-old boy with tricuspid atresia and normally related great arteries. A holosystolic murmur (SM) in the third and fourth left intercostal spaces (3 LICS/4 LICS) originated at a slitlike ventricular septal defect that constituted a zone of subpulmonary stenosis. (S₁ = single first heart sound; S₂ = second heart sound.)

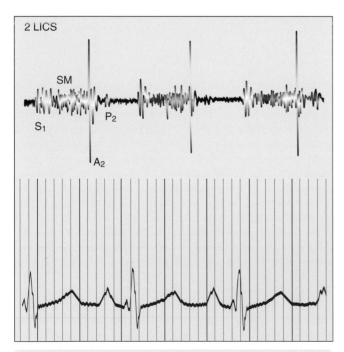

FIGURE 25-13 Phonocardiogram from a 9-month-old female with tricuspid atresia, normally related great arteries, and a restrictive ventricular septal defect. A holosystolic murmur (SM) radiated to the second left interspace (2 LICS) because the left ventricle ejected across the ventricular septal defect into the pulmonary trunk. The pulmonary closure sound (P₂) is soft and delayed. The first heart sound (S₁) is single. (A₂ = aortic component of the second heart sound.)

Left ventricular fourth heart sounds occur when the interatrial communication is nonrestrictive and the increased force of right atrial contraction is transmitted into the left ventricle. Presystolic murmurs are expected in congenital tricuspid stenosis (Figure 25-19)[52] and are possible in tricuspid atresia when powerful right atrial contraction is exerted against a restrictive interatrial communication.

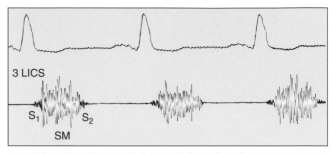

FIGURE 25-14 Phonocardiogram from the third left intercostal space (3 LICS) of a 28-year-old man with tricuspid atresia, normally related great arteries, a restrictive ventricular septal defect, and stenosis of the pulmonary valve and infundibulum. The variation in configuration of the murmur (SM) was caused by the combined effects of a holosystolic murmur of ventricular septal defect and a midsystolic murmur of pulmonaty stenosis. (S₁ = first heart sound; S₂ = second heart sound.)

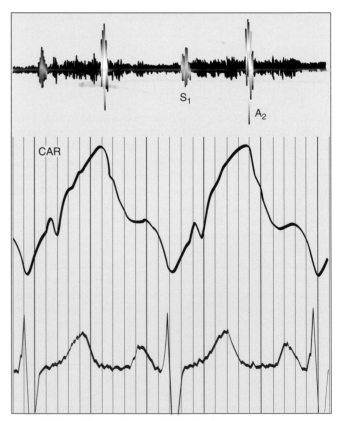

FIGURE 25-15 Phonocardiogram from the right anterior chest of a 7-year-old boy with tricuspid atresia, pulmonary atresia, normally related great arteries, and a continuous murmur from systemic to pulmonary arterial collaterals. (S₁ = first heart sound; A₂ = aortic component of the second heart sound; CAR = carotid pulse.)

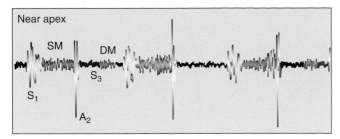

FIGURE 25-16 Phonocardiogram from a 13-month-old boy with tricuspid atresia, transposition of the great arteries, a nonrestrictive ventricular septal defect, and low pulmonary vascular resistance. A holosystolic murmur (SM) originated at the ventricular septal defect. The mid-diastolic murmur (DM) and the third heart sound (S_3) were caused by increased flow across the mitral valve. The aortic component of the second heart sound (A_2) was prominent because the transposed aorta was anterior. (S_1=single first heart sound.)

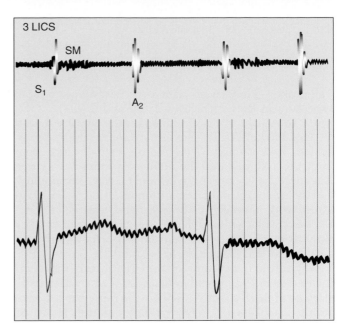

FIGURE 25-18 Phonocardiogram from the third left intercostal space (3 LICS) of an 18-month-old boy with tricuspid atresia, transposition of the great arteries, and severe pulmonary stenosis. The pulmonary stenotic murmur (SM) was trivial because left ventricular blood was diverted away from the pulmonary trunk across a nonrestrictive ventricular septal defect into the transposed aorta (see Figure 25-3B). The aortic component of the second heart sound was prominent (A_2) because the transposed aorta was anterior.

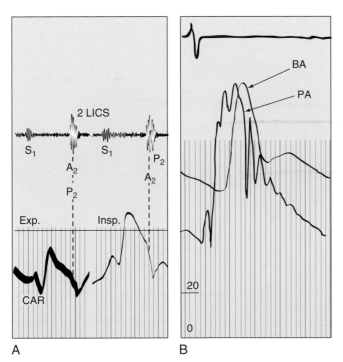

A   B

FIGURE 25-17 Tracings from an 18-year-old man with tricuspid atresia, complete transposition of the great arteries, and pulmonary vascular disease. His x-rays are shown in Figure 25-8. **A,** Phonocardiogram from the second left intercostal space (2 LICS) recorded a single first heart sound (S_1) and no murmur. There was close inspiratory splitting of the second heart sound (A_2/P_2) because pulmonary vascular resistance was lower than systemic resistance (see diastolic pressures in panel B). The pulmonary component of the second sound was prominent because the posterior pulmonary trunk was dilated and hypertensive. (CAR=carotid.) **B,** Brachial arterial (BA) and pulmonary arterial (PA) pressures were equal during systole but diverged during diastole.

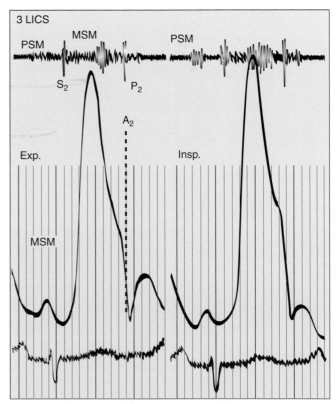

FIGURE 25-19 Phonocardiogram from the third left intercostal space (3 LICS) of the 20-year-old woman with tricuspid stenosis and pulmonary stenosis. Her right atrial and right ventricular pressure pulses are shown in Figure 25-11. The presystolic murmur of tricuspid stenosis (PSM) increased during inspiration (Insp.). The midsystolic murmur (MSM) was across the stenotic pulmonary valve. (CAR=carotid pulse; Exp.=expiration.)

ELECTROCARDIOGRAM

Tall peaked "Himalayan" right atrial P waves are typical, especially in lead 2 (Figures 25-20 and 25-21).[15,57–60] The P terminal force can be dramatically negative in lead V_1 (see Figure 25-21). The left atrium is seldom represented, even though it receives the entire return from both the systemic and the pulmonary veins.[57,58] There is no necessary relationship between P wave morphology and the size of the interatrial communication.[57] Tricuspid atresia with normally related great arteries and a restrictive ventricular septal defect is suspected when *left axis deviation* and *left ventricular hypertrophy* occur in a *cyanotic* patient (see Figures 25-20 and 25-21).[15,57–59,61]

The left axis deviation of tricuspid atresia was commented on in 1929,[62] and its diagnostic value was emphasized by Helen Taussig[63] in 1936. The cause has not been firmly established,[57,64–66] but left anterior fascicular block is not the mechanism.[64,66] The central fibrous body is abnormally formed whether or not the great arteries are transposed.[64] A fibrous strand has been traced to the cavity of the rudimentary right ventricle,[14] and the atrioventricular node pierces the central fibrous body to form the His bundle.[64] The left bundle branches originate close to the atrioventricular (AV) node/His bundle junction and undergo early arborization, whereas the right bundle branch is elongated.[58] It is doubtful that early arborization of the left bundle accounts for left axis deviation, which appears to depend largely on the relative masses

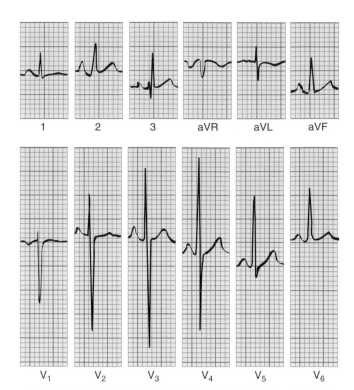

FIGURE 25-21 Electrocardiogram from a 7-year-old boy with tricuspid atresia, normally related great arteries, and "pulmonary atresia" as the result of spontaneous closure of a restrictive ventricular septal defect. Biatrial abnormalities are manifested by tall right atrial P waves in leads 1 and 2 and bifid left atrial P waves in mid and left precordial leads. There is left axis deviation with adult progression of the precordial QRS. Left ventricular hypertrophy is manifested by the tall R wave and inverted T wave in lead aVL and deep S waves in right precordial leads.

of the right and left ventricles. Aborization patterns of the bundle branches are the same in all varieties of tricuspid atresia.[57,58] Left axis deviation and adult progression of the precordial QRS pattern coexist (see Figures 25-20 and 25-21).[58,59] Left ventricular hypertrophy is represented by deep S waves in right precordial leads and tall R waves with repolarization abnormalities in leads aVL and V_{5-6} (see Figures 25-20 and 25-21).

Tricuspid atresia with *complete transposition of the great arteries* typically occurs with a nonrestrictive ventricular septal defect and a well-developed right ventricle. Increased pulmonary blood flow adds materially to left atrial volume. Left and right atrial enlargement coexist, so the P waves are broad, bifid, and peaked (Figure 25-22).[15,57,58,61] The relatively well-developed right ventricle contributes to the normal QRS axis and probably influences the QRS pattern in the precordial leads.[15,58,59]

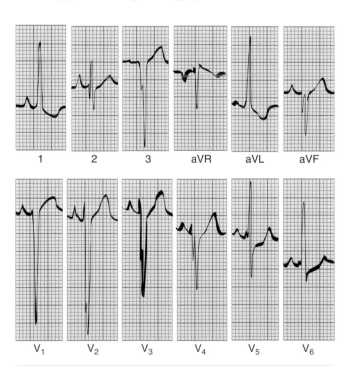

FIGURE 25-20 Electrocardiogram from a 9-month-old female with tricuspid atresia, normally related great arteries, and a slitlike ventricular septal defect. Tall peaked right atrial P waves appear in lead 2 and in right precordial leads. There is left axis deviation with adult progression of the precordial QRS. Left ventricular hypertrophy is manifested by the tall R wave and inverted T wave in lead aVL and the deep S waves in right precordial leads.

X-RAY

The cardiac silhouette can be distinctive in *tricuspid atresia* with a *restrictive ventricular septal defect* and *normally related great arteries* (Figures 25-23 and 25-24).[21] The right cardiac contour exhibits a distinctive, prominent

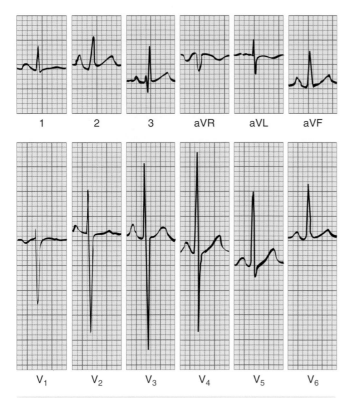

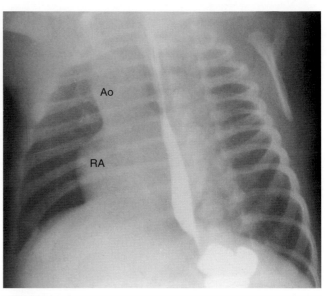

FIGURE 25-24 Left anterior oblique x-ray from a 4-month-old boy with tricuspid atresia, normally related great arteries, and a restrictive ventricular septal defect. The right atrium (RA) is distinctively hump-shaped. The appearance is highlighted by the prominent ascending aorta (Ao). (Also see Figure 25-23.)

FIGURE 25-22 Electrocardiogram from a 32-month-old boy with tricuspid atresia, transposition of the great arteries, a nonrestrictive ventricular septal defect, and low pulmonary vascular resistance. Biatrial P wave abnormalities are manifested by tall peaked right atrial P waves in leads 2, aVF, and V_3 and a bifid left atrial P wave in lead aVL. The QRS axis is normal. Precordial leads show adult progression with large biphasic RS complexes of biventricular hypertrophy in leads V_{3-4}.

superior border caused by enlargement of the right atrium and its appendage and accentuated by a flat receding inferior border that reflects absence of the right ventricle (Figures 25-23B, 25-24, and 25-25B). A convex left ventricle occupies the apex (see Figures 25-23A, and 25-25A). Pulmonary vascularity is reduced and the main pulmonary artery segment is inconspicuous, but the ascending aorta is relatively prominent (see Figures 25-23

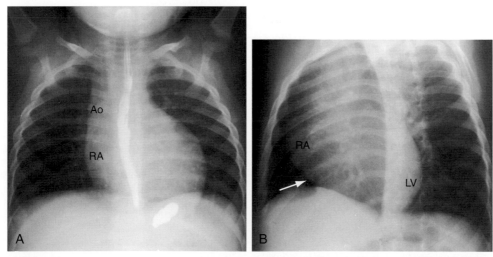

FIGURE 25-23 **A,** X-ray from a 10-month-old boy with tricuspid atresia, normally related great arteries, and a restrictive ventricular septal defect (see Figure 25-2B). Pulmonary vascularity is reduced, the ascending aorta (Ao) is prominent, the main pulmonary artery segment is inconspicuous, the dilated right atrium (RA) recedes acutely because of absence of the right ventricle, and a large left ventricle occupies the apex. **B,** Shallow left anterior oblique projection highlights the hump-shaped appearance caused by right atrial enlargement (RA) in the absence of a right ventricle (arrow). (LV = left ventricle.)

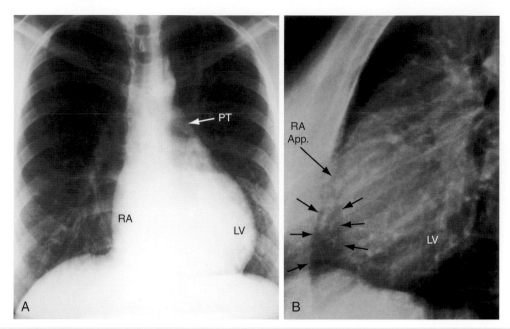

FIGURE 25-25 A, X-ray from a 25-year-old woman with tricuspid atresia, normally related great arteries, and a moderately restrictive ventricular septal defect. Congestive heart failure in infancy improved as the ventricular septal defect decreased in size. Pulmonary vascularity and the pulmonary trunk (PT) are normal, the right atrium (RA) is moderately dilated, and a large convex left ventricle (LV) occupies the apex. **B,** Lateral projection shows the right atrial appendage (RA App.) against the sternum and a receding inferior border because the right ventricle is absent (unmarked arrows). Left ventricular enlargement is confirmed.

and 25-25). When a congenitally intact ventricular septum causes functional pulmonary atresia (see Figure 25-2A), the ascending aorta is more conspicuous, and the lung fields exhibit the lacy vascular pattern of systemic arterial collaterals (Figure 25-26).[21] When the ventricular septal defect is nonrestrictive and pulmonary vascular resistance is low (see Figure 25-2C), pulmonary vascularity is increased, the pulmonary trunk and the left and right atria are enlarged, and a prominent left ventricle is apex-forming (see Figures 25-5A, and 25-7).

The x-ray in tricuspid atresia with *complete transposition of the great arteries*, a *nonrestrictive ventricular septal defect*, and *low pulmonary vascular resistance* (see Figure 25-3C) is characterized by increased pulmonary vascularity, enlargement of the left and right atria, and a prominent apex-forming left ventricle. The vascular pedicle is narrow because the great arteries are transposed. The x-ray resembles uncomplicated complete transposition of the great arteries with analogous pulmonary vascular resistance (see Chapter 27). The left cardiac border is straight if there is left-sided juxtaposition of the atrial appendages. When pulmonary vascular resistance is increased, the lungs are oligemic and the heart size is normal or nearly so, but the right cardiac border may retain its hump-shaped contour even though the right ventricle is not rudimentary (see Figure 25-8).[15]

The x-ray in tricuspid atresia with *transposition of the great arteries* and *pulmonary stenosis* (Figures 25-3B, and 25-27) shows normal or reduced pulmonary vascularity, a prominent right atrium, a convex left ventricle, and a narrow vascular pedicle because of the transposed great arteries.

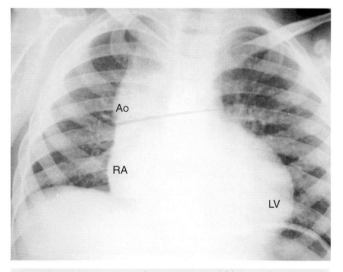

FIGURE 25-26 A, X-ray from a 7-year-old boy with tricuspid atresia, normally related great arteries, and "pulmonary atresia" as a result of a congenitally intact ventricular septum. The lung fields exhibit the lacy appearance of collateral arterial circulation. The main pulmonary artery segment is concave, the ascending aorta is conspicuously dilated (Ao), an enlarged convex left ventricle (LV) extends below the left hemidiaphragm, and a dilated right atrium (RA) occupies the lower right cardiac border.

ECHOCARDIOGRAM

Echocardiography with color flow imaging and Doppler interrogation establishes the diagnosis of tricuspid atresia, the positions of the great arteries, the condition of

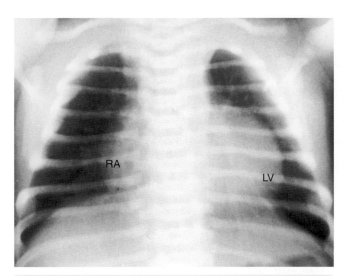

FIGURE 25-27 X-ray from a 10-month-old girl with tricuspid atresia, transposition of the great arteries, and severe pulmonary stenosis. Pulmonary vascularity is decreased, a main pulmonary artery segment is not seen, a prominent right atrium (RA) occupies the lower right cardiac border, and an enlarged convex left ventricle (LV) occupies the apex.

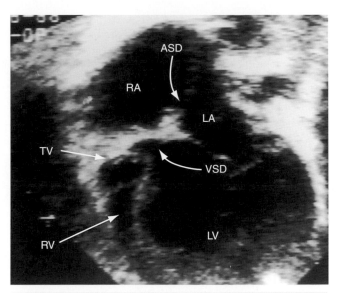

FIGURE 25-28 Echocardiogram (four-chamber view) from a 4-year-old boy with tricuspid atresia, normally related great arteries, and a restrictive ventricular septal defect. The atretic tricuspid valve (TV) is represented by a dense band of bright echoes. The right ventricle (RV) is small, and the left ventricle (LV) is dilated. There was a left-to-right shunt (lower curved arrow) across the ventricular septal defect (VSD) and a right-to-left shunt (upper arrow) across an ostium secundum atrial septal defect (ASD). (RA = right atrium; LA = left atrium.)

the ventricular septum, and the nature of the interatrial communication (Figures 25-28 and 25-29 and Video 25-1).[8,67] Computed tomography provides similar information.[68] An echodense band produced by fibrofatty tissue in the right atrioventricular groove represents absence of the right AV connection that characterizes tricuspid atresia (see Figures 25-28 and 25-29). When the great arteries are not transposed, the right ventricular cavity is small, the ventricular septal defect is restrictive, and the left ventricle is moderately enlarged (see Figure 25-28). When the interatrial communication is restrictive, the right atrium is enlarged and the atrial septum is shifted to the left. When the great arteries are transposed and pulmonary resistance is low, echocardiography identifies a nonrestrictive ventricular septal defect, a well-formed right ventricle, enlarged right and left atria, and a dilated volume-overloaded left ventricle (see Figure 25-29). Structural abnormalities of the mitral valve can be characterized.[25] Color flow mapping with Doppler interrogation establishes the size of the interatrial communication and the condition of the ventricular septum. When the great arteries are transposed, continuous wave Doppler scan interrogates the left ventricular outflow tract for the presence and degree of pulmonary stenosis.

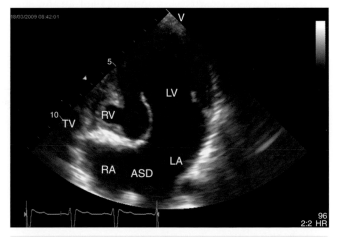

FIGURE 25-29 Echocardiogram from an 18-month-old boy with tricuspid atresia, transposition of the great arteries, a nonrestrictive ventricular septal defect. The atretic tricuspid valve is represented by a dense band of echoes between the right ventricular cavity (RV) and the right atrium (RA). A normal mitral valve lies between the left ventricle (LV) and the left atrium (LA). An atrial septal defect (ASD) is shown between both atria (Video 25-1).

SUMMARY

Tricuspid atresia *without transposition of the great arteries* and with a *restrictive ventricular septal defect* presents with neonatal cyanosis and a clinical picture dominated by hypoxemia. A right ventricular impulse is absent. A left parasternal holosystolic systolic murmur is generated through the restrictive ventricular septal defect that is functionally

subpulmonary stenosis. The electrocardiogram exhibits tall peaked right atrial P waves, left axis deviation, counterclockwise depolarization, and adult progression of the precordial QRS pattern. The x-ray discloses a distinctive hump-shaped appearance of the right cardiac border. Echocardiography with color flow imaging and Doppler interrogation identifies an echodense band at the site of the atretic tricuspid valve, a restrictive ventricular septal defect, a small right ventricle, normally related great arteries, and an interatrial communication that is usually restrictive. Tricuspid atresia *with complete transposition of the great arteries*, a nonrestrictive ventricular septal defect, and low pulmonary vascular resistance presents with mild cyanosis and a clinical picture dominated by congestive heart failure. A left ventricular impulse is prominent, and a right ventricular impulse is present but less conspicuous. A systolic murmur is generated through the ventricular septal defect, and an apical mid-diastolic murmur is generated by increased flow across the mitral valve. The electrocardiogram shows biatrial P wave abnormalities and a normal or vertical axis with adult progression of the precordial QRS. The x-ray is characterized by increased pulmonary blood flow, a narrow vascular pedicle, enlargement of the right and left atria, and enlargement of the left ventricle. Echocardiography with color flow imaging and Doppler interrogation identifies the atretic tricuspid valve, a nonrestrictive ventricular septal defect, a well-formed right ventricle, and enlargement of the left atrium, right atrium, and left ventricle. When pulmonary stenosis coexists, cyanosis ranges from mild to severe, the left ventricle is palpable but not dynamic, and the length and loudness of the pulmonary stenotic murmur vary inversely with severity. The electrocardiogram shows right atrial P waves, a normal or vertical QRS axis, and adult progression of the precordial QRS pattern. The x-ray shows a narrow vascular pedicle, normal or decreased pulmonary vascularity, a prominent right atrium, and a convex left ventricle. The echocardiogram identifies the atretic tricuspid valve, transposed great arteries, and a nonrestrictive ventricular septal defect. Continuous wave Doppler scan establishes the presence and degree of pulmonary stenosis.

REFERENCES

1. Rashkind WJ. Tricuspid atresia: a historical review. *Pediatr Cardiol.* 1982;2:85–88.
2. Kuhne M. Uber zwei falle kongenitaler atresia des ostium venosum dextrum. *Jahrb Kinderheild Physi Erziehung.* 1906;63:225.
3. Anderson RH, Rigby ML. The morphologic heterogeneity of tricuspid atresia. *Int J Cardiol.* 1987;16:67–73.
4. Anderson RH, Ho SY, Rigby ML. The morphologic variability in atrioventricular valvar atresia. *Cardiol Young.* 2000;10:32–41.
5. Report of the New England Regional Infant Cardiac Program. *Pediatrics.* 1980;65:375–461.
6. Sade RM, Fyfe DA. Tricuspid atresia: current concepts in diagnosis and treatment. *Pediatr Clin North Am.* 1990;37:151–169.
7. Mohan JC, Passey R, Arora R. Echocardiographic spectrum of congenitally unguarded tricuspid valve orifice and patent right ventricular outflow tract. *Int J Cardiol.* 2000;74:153–157.
8. Martinez RM, Anderson RH. Echo-morphological correlates in atrioventricular valvar atresia. *Cardiol Young.* 2006;16(suppl 1):27–34.
9. Edwards JE, Burchell HB. Congenital tricuspid atresia; a classification. *Med Clin North Am.* 1949;33:1177–1196.
10. Rao PS. A unified classification for tricuspid atresia. *Am Heart J.* 1980;99:799–804.
11. Tandon R, Edwards JE. Tricuspid atresia. A re-evaluation and classification. *J Thorac Cardiovasc Surg.* 1974;67:530–542.
12. Riker WL, Potts WJ, Grana L, Miller RA, Lev M. Tricuspid stenosis or atresia complexes. A surgical and pathologic analysis. *J Thorac Cardiovasc Surg.* 1963;45:423–433.
13. Rosenquist GC, Levy RJ, Rowe RD. Right atrial-left ventricular relationships in tricuspid atresia: position of the presumed site of

14. the atretic valve as determined by transillumination. *Am Heart J.* 1970;80:493–497.
14. Wenink AC, Ottenkamp J. Tricuspid atresia. Microscopic findings in relation to "absence" of the atrioventricular connexion. *Int J Cardiol.* 1987;16:57–73.
15. Dick M, Fyler DC, Nadas AS. Tricuspid atresia: clinical course in 101 patients. *Am J Cardiol.* 1975;36:327–337.
16. Freedom RM, Rowe RD. Aneurysm of the atrial septum in tricuspid atresia: diagnosis during life and therapy. *Am J Cardiol.* 1976;38:265–267.
17. Reder RF, Yeh HC, Steinfeld L. Aneurysm of the interatrial septum causing pulmonary venous obstruction in an infant with tricuspid atresia. *Am Heart J.* 1981;102:786–789.
18. Rao PS. Natural history of the ventricular septal defect in tricuspid atresia and its surgical implications. *Br Heart J.* 1977;39:276–288.
19. Rao PS, Sissman NJ. Spontaneous closure of physiologically advantageous ventricular septal defects. *Circulation.* 1971;43:83–90.
20. Roberts WC, Morrow AG, Mason DT, Braunwald E. Spontaneous closure of ventricular septal defect, anatomic proof in an adult with tricuspid atresia. *Circulation.* 1963;27:90–94.
21. Kieffer SA, Carey LS. Tricuspid atresia with normal aortic root: roentgen-anatomic correlation. *Radiology.* 1963;80:605–615.
22. Patel R, Fox K, Taylor JF, Graham GR. Tricuspid atresia. Clinical course in 62 cases (1967–1974). *Br Heart J.* 1978;40:1408–1414.
23. Jordan JC, Sanders CA. Tricuspid atresia with prolonged survival. A report of two cases with a review of the world literature. *Am J Cardiol.* 1966;18:112–119.
24. Deanfield JE, Tommasini G, Anderson RH, Macartney FJ. Tricuspid atresia: analysis of coronary artery distribution and ventricular morphology. *Br Heart J.* 1982;48:485–492.
25. Ottenkamp J, Wenink AC. Anomalies of the mitral valve and of the left ventricular architecture in tricuspid valve atresia. *Am J Cardiol.* 1989;63:880–881.
26. Litovsky S, Choy M, Park J, et al. Absent pulmonary valve with tricuspid atresia or severe tricuspid stenosis: report of three cases and review of the literature. *Pediatr Dev Pathol.* 2000;3:353–366.
27. Rudolph AM, Heymann MA, Spitznas U. Hemodynamic considerations in the development of narrowing of the aorta. *Am J Cardiol.* 1972;30:514–525.
28. Gyepes MT, Marcano BA, Desilets DT. Tricuspid atresia, transposition, and coatation of the aorta. *Radiology.* 1970;97:633–636.
29. Becker AE, Becker MJ. Juxtaposition of atrial appendages associated with normally oriented ventricles and great arteries. *Circulation.* 1970;41:685–688.
30. Charuzi Y, Spanos PK, Amplatz K, Edwards JE. Juxtaposition of the atrial appendages. *Circulation.* 1973;47:620–627.
31. Deutsch V, Shem-Tov A, Yahini JH, Neufeld HN. Juxtaposition of atrial appendages: angiocardiographic observations. *Am J Cardiol.* 1974;34:240–244.
32. Rao PS. Left to right atrial shunting in tricuspid atresia. *Br Heart J.* 1983;49:345–349.
33. La Corte MA, Dick M, Scheer G, La Farge CG, Fyler DC. Left ventricular function in tricuspid atresia. Angiographic analysis in 28 patients. *Circulation.* 1975;52:996–1000.
34. Nishioka K, Kamiya T, Ueda T, et al. Left ventricle volume characteristics in children with tricuspid atresia before and after surgery. *Am J Cardiol.* 1981;47:1105–1110.
35. Lin AE, Rosti L. Tricuspid atresia in sibs. *J Med Genet.* 1998;35:1055–1056.
36. Kumar A, Victorica BE, Gessner IH, Alexander JA. Tricuspid atresia and annular hypoplasia: report of a familial occurrence. *Pediatr Cardiol.* 1994;15:201–203.
37. Weigel TJ, Driscoll DJ, Michels VV. Occurrence of congenital heart defects in siblings of patients with univentricular heart and tricuspid atresia. *Am J Cardiol.* 1989;64:768–771.
38. Bonnet D, Fermont L, Kachaner J, et al. Tricuspid atresia and conotruncal malformations in five families. *J Med Genet.* 1999;36:349–350.
39. Svensson EC, Huggins GS, Lin H, et al. A syndrome of tricuspid atresia in mice with a targeted mutation of the gene encoding Fog-2. *Nat Genet.* 2000;25:353–356.
40. Patterson W, Baxley WA, Karp RB, Soto B, Bargeron LL. Tricuspid atresia in adults. *Am J Cardiol.* 1982;49:141–152.

41. Breisch EA, Wilson DB, Laurenson RD, Mazur JH, Bloor CM. Tricuspid atresia (type Ia): survival to 21 years of age. *Am Heart J.* 1983;106:149–151.
42. Voci G, Diego JN, Shafia H, Alavi M, Ghusson M, Banka VS. Type Ia tricuspid atresia with extensive coronary artery abnormalities in a living 22 year old woman. *J Am Coll Cardiol.* 1987;10: 1100–1104.
43. Beaver TR, Shroyer KR, Muro-Cacho CA, Miller GJ, Blount SG. Survival to age 65 years with tricuspid and pulmonic valve atresia. *Am J Cardiol.* 1988;62:165–166.
44. Brown JW, Heath D, Morris TL, Whitaker W. Tricuspid atresia. *Br Heart J.* 1956;18:499–518.
45. Cooley RN, Sloan RD, Hanlon CR, Bahnson HT. Angiocardiography in congenital heart disease of cyanotic type. II. Observations on tricuspid stenosis or atresia with hypoplasia of the right ventricle. *Radiology.* 1950;54:848–868.
46. Hatjis CG, Gibson M, Capeless EL, Auletta FJ, Anderson GG. Pregnancy in a patient with tricuspid atresia. *Am J Obstet Gynecol.* 1983;145:114–115.
47. Hart AS, Vacek JL. Prolonged survival in tricuspid atresia with Eisenmenger's physiology. *Clin Cardiol.* 1984;7:555–556.
48. Patel MM, Overy DC, Kozonis MC, Hadley-Fowlkes LL. Long-term survival in tricuspid atresia. *J Am Coll Cardiol.* 1987;9: 338–340.
49. Shariatzadeh AN, King H, Girod D, Shumacker HB. Tricuspid atresia. A review of 68 cases. *Chest.* 1977;71:538–540.
50. Fontana R, Edwards J. *Congenital cardiac disease: a review of 357 cases studied pathologically.* Philadelphia: W.B. Saunders; 1962.
51. Karalis DG, Chandrasekaran K, Victor MF, Mintz GS. Prolonged survival despite severe cyanosis in an adult with right ventricular hypoplasia and atrial septal defect. *Am Heart J.* 1990; 120:701–703.
52. Steelman RB, Perloff JK, Cochran PT, Ronan JA. Congenital stenosis of the pulmonic and tricuspid valves. Clinical, hemodynamic and angiographic observations in a 20 year old woman. *Am J Med.* 1973; 54:788–792.
53. Jones RN, Niles NR. Spinnaker formation of sinus venosus valve. Case report of a fatal anomaly in a ten-year-old boy. *Circulation.* 1968;38:468–473.
54. Freedom RM, Gerald PS. Congenital cardiac disease and the "cat eye" syndrome. *Am J Dis Child.* 1973;126:16–18.
55. Folger Jr. GM. Systemic hypoperfusion in a neonate with tricuspid atresia and transposition of the great arteries. Similarity to the hypoplastic left heart syndrome. *Angiology.* 1980;31:721–724.
56. Perloff JK. *Physical examination of the heart and circulation.* 4th ed. Shelton, Connecticut: People's Medical Publishing House; 2009.
57. Davachi F, Lucas Jr. RV, Moller JH. The electrocardiogram and vectorcardiogram in tricuspid atresia. Correlation with pathologic anatomy. *Am J Cardiol.* 1970;25:18–27.
58. Guller B, Titus JL, Dushane JW. Electrocardiographic diagnosis of malformations associated with tricuspid atresia: correlation with morphologic features. *Am Heart J.* 1969;78:180–188.
59. Somlyo AP, Halloran KH. Tricuspid atresia. An electrocardiographic study. *Am Heart J.* 1962;63:171–179.
60. Reddy SC, Zuberbuhler JR. Images in cardiovascular medicine. Himalayan P-waves in a patient with tricuspid atresia. *Circulation.* 2003;107:498.
61. Gamboa R, Gersony WM, Nadas AS. The electrocardiogram in tricuspid atresia and pulmonary atresia with intact ventricular septum. *Circulation.* 1966;34:24–37.
62. Rihl J, Terplan K, Weiss F. Uber einen fall von agenesie der tricuspidalklappe. *Medizinische Klinik.* 1923;25:1543.
63. Taussig HB. The clinical and pathological findings in congenital malformations of the heart due to defective development of the right ventricle associated with tricuspid atresia or hypoplasia. *Bulletin of the Johns Hopkins Hospital.* 1936;435.
64. Bharati S, Lev M. The conduction system in tricuspid atresia with and without regular (d-) transposition. *Circulation.* 1977;56: 423–429.
65. Perloff JK, Roberts NK, Cabeen Jr. WR. Left axis deviation: a reassessment. *Circulation.* 1979;60:12–21.
66. Schatz J, Krongrad E, Malm JR. Left anterior and left posterior hemiblock in tricuspid atresia and transposition of the great vessels: observations and electrocardiographic nomenclature and electrophysiologic mechanisms. *Circulation.* 1976;54:1010–1013.
67. Orie JD, Anderson C, Ettedgui JA, Zuberbuhler JR, Anderson RH. Echocardiographic-morphologic correlations in tricuspid atresia. *J Am Coll Cardiol.* 1995;26:750–758.
68. Mochizuki T, Ohtani T, Higashino H, et al. Tricuspid atresia with atrial septal defect, ventricular septal defect, and right ventricular hypoplasia demonstrated by multidetector computed tomography. *Circulation.* 2000;102:E164–E165.

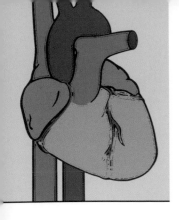

Chapter 26

Univentricular Heart

In 1858, Thomas Peacock described hearts in which "The auricular sinuses are separated by a more or less complete septum, and there are generally two auriculo-ventricular apertures, while the ventricle is either wholly undivided or presents only a very rudimentary septum. The arteries which are given off are usually two in number—an aorta and a pulmonary artery."[1]

These cases correspond to hearts that consist of two auricles and only one ventricle. A case described by Chemineau in 1699 appears to have been of this description.[2]

The univentricular heart is unique in its complexity and scope and has sparked intense debate about terminology and embryology.[2] Nearly a century and a half after Peacock's[1] description, there is still no consensus about the terminology for hearts with *one ventricle*.[3–6] *Single ventricle* and *univentricular* are synonymous (*single = uni = one*), so these terms are interchangeable and are appropriate when two atria are related entirely or almost entirely to one ventricular compartment that qualifies on purely morphologic grounds as a left, right, or indeterminate ventricle.

Univentricular atrioventricular connection or double inlet ventricle is characterized according to *gross morphologic features* of the ventricular mass and according to the *atrioventricular connections* to that mass.[4,5,7] Clinically undetectable and clinically irrelevant developmental considerations are important to the morphologist[4] but should not determine clinical terminology. It is best to avoid inherently contradictory terms such as *ventricular septal defect*[8] and *interventricular communication* that imply the presence of two anatomically definitive ventricles divided by a septum. To say that a ventricular septal defect exists in a heart with a single ventricle and "not a trace of an inter-ventricular septum"[1] strikes most readers as contradictory irrespective of theoretic arguments to the contrary. The term "functionally" univentricular as applied to the hypoplastic left heart should be regarded as a separate category.[9] In this chapter, *univentricular* and *single ventricle* refer to hearts in which one ventricular chamber receives the entire flow from the right atrium and the left atrium, both of which together with the entire atrioventricular junction are related to the single ventricle.

In 80% to 90% of cases, the ventricular chamber that receives the atrioventricular connections is a morphologic *left ventricle* that incorporates at its base an *outlet chamber* that is devoid of a sinus or inlet component, that is devoid or virtually devoid of trabeculae, and that is remote from the crux of the heart (Figures 26-1 through 26-4).[7] In 10% to 25% of cases, the ventricular chamber that receives the atrioventricular connections has *right ventricular* morphologic features and incorporates within its mass a rudimentary compartment—a left ventricular remnant or *trabecular pouch*—that varies in size from well-formed to microscopic (see Figures 26-31 and 26-32).[3,7] The trabecular pouch occupies a posterior, inferior, or lateral position within the ventricular mass and may or may not communicate with the cavity. In less than 10% of cases, the univentricular heart has *indeterminate* morphologic features and incorporates neither an outlet chamber nor a trabecular pouch. Because an indeterminate ventricle does not contain remnants of either a rudimentary morphologic right ventricle or a rudimentary morphologic left ventricle, the term *univentricular heart* or *single ventricle* is unassailable on morphologic grounds.

The *atrioventricular connections* that guard the inlet of a univentricular heart consist of either two separate valves, one patent valve with atresia of the other valve, or a common atrioventricular valve.[10,11] It is customary to refer to *right* atrioventricular or *left* atrioventricular valves, rather than *tricuspid* and *mitral* valves, because tricuspid and mitral morphologic features are not necessarily evident.[8] An atrioventricular (AV) valve is likely to be abnormal when it is *concordant* with the ventricular loop (*right* AV valve with *noninverted* outlet chamber, *left* AV valve with *inverted* outlet chamber).[8,10,12] When the outlet chamber is *inverted*, the *left* AV valve tends to be stenotic, and when the outlet chamber is *noninverted*, the *right* atrioventricular valve tends to be incompetent.[8] A *common atrioventricular valve* is usually equipped with four leaflets,[11] and right atrial isomerism is the usual pattern.[11] Straddling of a right or a left AV valve or a common AV valve refers to attachments of tensor apparatus to both sides of an outlet foramen or to both sides of a trabecular pouch.[7,8,10,12,13]

In univentricular hearts that are morphologically *left ventricular*, the outlet chamber is anterosuperior and either to the right or left of midline. *Noninverted* applies to a *right* anterosuperior position of the outlet chamber, and *inverted* applies to a *left* anterosuperior position (see Figures 26-1 through 26-4). The outlet chamber is either smooth-walled and devoid of trabeculations (see Figure 26-4) or contains scanty ill-defined trabeculations (see previous). The aorta arises discordantly from the outlet chamber, and the pulmonary trunk arises discordantly from the single morphologic left ventricle

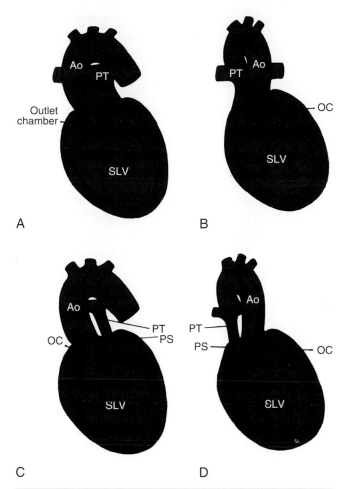

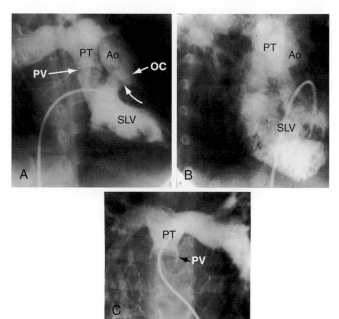

FIGURE 26-1 Illustrations of the most frequent types of univentricular heart represented by a single morphologic left ventricle (SLV). The anterosuperior outlet chamber (OC) is located at the base of the single ventricle and is either right-sided (noninverted; **A** and **C**) or left-sided (inverted; **B** and **D**). Pulmonary stenosis (PS) is absent (**A** and **B**) or present (**C** and **D**). (PT = pulmonary trunk; Ao = aorta.)

FIGURE 26-2 Angiocardiograms from a 7-year-old boy with univentricular heart of left ventricular morphology. **A,** The aorta (Ao) originates from an inverted outlet chamber (OC) that joins the single left ventricle (SLV) through a nonrestrictive outlet foramen (unmarked curved arrow). The pulmonary trunk (PT) originates from the single ventricle. Pulmonary stenosis was caused by a mobile stenotic pulmonary valve (PV) shown in **C. B,** Lateral ventriculogram showing the fine trabecular pattern of a morphologic left ventricle. The great arteries are side-by-side with the aorta (Ao) anterior to the pulmonary trunk (PT). **C,** Pulmonary arteriogram showing the mobile dome stenotic pulmonary valve (PV).

(see Figures 26-1 through 26-4),[7] so *the great arteries are transposed* (see Chapter 27).

In 1824, Andrew Fernando Holmes, who would later become the first Dean of the Medical Faculty at McGill University, published autopsy observations on a 21-year-old man who died with chronic cyanosis and congestive failure. In the uncommon Holmes heart, the aorta arises concordantly from the morphologic left ventricle and the pulmonary trunk arises concordantly from the outlet chamber (see Figure 26-20). William Osler urged Maude Abbott to republish the case, which was included in her seminal atlas of 1936.[14,15] Andrew Fernando Holmes was Canadian, but his 1824 publication on single ventricle was published in a Scottish journal[16] because he trained at the University of Edinburgh. Rarely, the outlet chamber gives rise to both great arteries, to neither great artery, or to a common arterial trunk. In univentricular hearts characterized by a *single morphologic right ventricle*, both great arteries originate from the right ventricle, an arrangement that is a form of *double outlet right ventricle* (see Chapter 19). Occasionally, the pulmonary trunk originates concordantly from a single

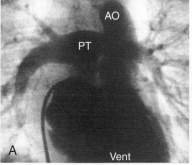

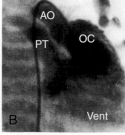

FIGURE 26-3 A, Ventriculogram from a 3-year-old girl with single morphologic left ventricle (Vent) and pulmonary stenosis (gradient, 60 mm Hg). An inverted outlet chamber gives rise to the aorta (AO), which is convex to the left. The posteromedial pulmonary trunk (PT) is not border-forming. **B,** Ventriculogram from a 5-week-old female with single morphologic left ventricle and mild pulmonary stenosis (gradient, 25 mm Hg). The inverted outlet chamber (OC) forms a striking leftward convexity that gives rise to the aorta (AO). The morphologic left ventricle (Vent) is finely trabeculated.

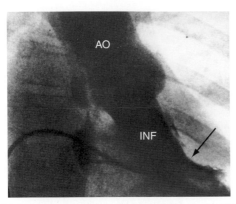

FIGURE 26-4 Ventriculogram from a 9-year-old boy with a univentricular heart of the left ventricular type and an inverted outlet chamber (INF) that is devoid of trabeculations and that gives rise to the aorta (AO). The outlet foramen (unmarked arrow) is nonrestrictive.

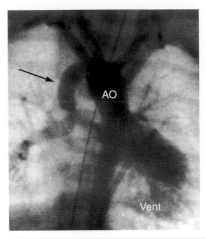

FIGURE 26-5 Ventriculogram from a 1-day-old female with single ventricle (Vent) of the left ventricular type and pulmonary atresia. An enlarged aorta (AO) originates from an inverted outlet chamber. An large anomalous systemic arterial collateral (unmarked arrow) communicated with the right pulmonary artery.

right ventricle, and the aorta originates concordantly from the trabecular pouch, which is a left ventricular remnant. A *morphologically indeterminate* single ventricle incorporates neither an outlet chamber nor a trabecular pouch (see previous), so both great arteries necessarily arise from the indeterminate single ventricle.

The orifice that joins a single left ventricle to an outlet chamber has been variously referred to as a bulboventricular foramen, a ventricular septal defect,[8] and an interventricular communication. *Bulboventricular foramen* assumes that the embryologic foramen is the communication that exists in the univentricular heart, which is not necessarily the case. The terms *ventricular septal defect* and *interventricular communication* are discouraged as inherently contradictory (see previous). *Outlet foramen* is a simple descriptive term that is used herein to refer to the orifice between a single left ventricle and the outlet chamber. A restrictive outlet foramen is a form of subaortic stenosis that can be acquired[8] or present at birth[7] and tends to coexist with coarctation of the aorta.[7]

When the pulmonary trunk originates from a single morphologic left ventricle, the accompanying *pulmonary stenosis* is either subpulmonary or in a bicuspid pulmonary valve (see Figures 26-1, 26-2C, and 26-3).[7] Pulmonary stenosis is a feature of the Holmes heart (see Figure 26-20)[16] and usually results from obstruction of the outlet foramen of the concordant subpulmonary outlet chamber.[14,15,17,18] The degree of stenosis ranges from mild to severe (see Figures 26-2 and 26-3) to atresia (Figure 26-5), a spectrum recognized by Peacock:

> *"The case of Fleischmann differed in some degree ... as though the heart consisted of three cavities, the ventricle only gave rise to one vessel, the orifice of the pulmonary artery being impervious. The child had lived twenty one weeks."*[1]

Coronary artery origins in univentricular hearts of left ventricular morphology depend on the location of the outlet chamber (see Chapters 6 and 32). A major branch of each coronary artery usually outlines or *delimits* the surface boundaries of the outlet chamber.

The *morphogenesis* of univentricular hearts is believed to reside in an abnormality of the ventricular trabecular components of the developing heart.[7,19] The *left ventricular* trabecular component is normally derived from the inlet portion of the embryonic heart tube, and the *right ventricular* trabecular component is derived from the outlet portion. As the ventricular mass develops, the atrioventricular junction is shared between the left ventricular trabecular component and the right ventricular trabecular component. When the atrioventricular junction retains its connection to the *left* ventricular trabecular component, the result is double inlet to a morphologic *left* ventricle. When the atrioventricular junction retains its connection to the *right* ventricular trabecular component, the result is double inlet to a morphologic *right* ventricle. When right and left ventricular trabecular components fail to develop, the result is double inlet to an *indeterminate* ventricle.

The *physiologic derangements* associated with univentricular hearts are related to six variables: (1) the inherent mechanics of a single ventricle[20–23]; (2) the mechanics of a morphologic right ventricle versus a morphologic left ventricle[24]; (3) the morphology and functional state of the atrioventricular valves that guard the inlet to a single ventricle; (4) the degree of mixing within the single ventricle; (5) the pulmonary vascular resistance; and (6) the presence and degree of pulmonary stenosis or subaortic stenosis.[18,25]

In hearts with two ventricles, each ventricle augments the function of the other ventricle.[20,21] *Ventricular-ventricular interaction* is an integral part of cardiac mechanics and results from coupling of the two ventricles through the interventricular septum and through an anatomic continuum that joins the mural myocardium of the two ventricles.[20,21] Ventricular interdependence does not occur unless a right ventricle contributes to left ventricular function and a left ventricle contributes to right ventricular function. Accordingly, ventricular interdependence does not exist in univentricular hearts. The result is abnormal systolic and diastolic function, irrespective of the morphology of the single ventricle.[26,27] Because a single ventricle is the pump that serves both the systemic and the pulmonary circulations, the volume handled by a univentricular heart is increased and provokes an adaptive increase in ventricular mass.[26-28] In univentricular hearts of *right ventricular morphology*, the indices that reflect an adaptive increase in ventricular mass are significantly reduced, including mass *per se*, wall thickness, ratio of wall thickness to transverse ventricular diameter, and ratio of ventricular mass to end-diastolic volume.[28] Inadequate mass relative to chamber volume reflects poor adaptation of univentricular hearts of right ventricular morphology.[24,28]

The *physiology of the circulation* in univentricular hearts is materially influenced by atrioventricular valve structure and function. Incompetence, stenosis, or atresia of an atrioventricular valve affects flow into the single ventricle and modifies its loading conditions. Atrioventricular valve regurgitation adds to the volume overload of the single ventricle. Atresia of the right or left atrioventricular valve results in a single inlet that does not disturb the circulation, provided there is free access to the single ventricle via a nonrestrictive interatrial communication and across the contralateral atrioventricular valve. However, when the right atrioventricular valve is atretic and the interatrial communication is restrictive, the right atrium is obstructed.[29] Similarly, the *left* atrium is obstructed when the left atrioventricular valve is atretic and the interatrial communication is restrictive.

Right atrial venous blood and left atrial arterialized blood remain remarkably separate within the single ventricular chamber.[25] Separation of the streams is greater when pulmonary resistance is low and when the outlet chamber is inverted.[25] Unoxygenated blood from the systemic venous atrium selectively finds its way into the pulmonary trunk, and oxygenated blood from the pulmonary venous atrium selectively finds its way into the aorta. Subaortic stenosis diverts even more blood into the pulmonary circulation, so cyanosis is mild and occasionally absent. However, the benefits of increased pulmonary blood flow are achieved at the price of volume overload of the single ventricle.

Pulmonary vascular disease and *pulmonary stenosis* curtail pulmonary blood flow and adversely affect streaming within the single ventricle. When pulmonary stenosis or pulmonary vascular disease are severe, cyanosis is conspicuous because a smaller volume of oxygenated blood reaches the left atrium and because there is greater mixing of unoxygenated and oxygenated blood within the single ventricle.[18]

Because 80% to 90% of univentricular hearts are characterized by a single morphologic left ventricle with an outlet chamber, the following sections deal principally with this anatomic arrangement.

HISTORY

The male:female ratio in univentricular hearts is between 2:1 and 4:1.[30] Recurrence in siblings is rare.[31] Neonates or infants come to attention because of congestive heart failure, cyanosis, or a murmur. The type of presentation and the survival patterns depend on the pulmonary vascular resistance, the presence and degree of pulmonary stenosis, the morphology of the single ventricle, and the presence and degree of subaortic stenosis. Fifty percent of patients with univentricular hearts of left ventricular morphology die within 14 years, with an annual attrition rate of 4.8%.[32] Fifty percent of patients with univentricular hearts of right ventricular morphology are dead within 4 years.[32]

Infants with increased pulmonary blood flow present with congestive heart failure, mild cyanosis, and poor growth and development.[18] When subaortic stenosis augments already excessive pulmonary blood flow, congestive failure is refractory. Pulmonary vascular resistance seldom achieves satisfactory regulation of pulmonary flow. The oldest reported survivor with a single morphologic left ventricle and pulmonary vascular disease was a 59-year-old man.[33] An exceptional case similar, if not identical, to the 24-year-old man (referred to in Figure 26-18), was described by Peacock[1] in a 24-year-old man.

The heart was very greatly enlarged, and the walls of the ventricle were fully three times their usual thickness. There was not a trace of interventricular septum, but the positions of the vessels of the heart were natural and the orifices were somewhat dilated.

Pulmonary stenosis is more effective than pulmonary vascular resistance in regulating pulmonary blood flow (see Figures 26-2 and 26-3). Peacock described a patient with single ventricle and pulmonary stenosis who suffered from *morbus caeruleus* but lived to age 11 years: "The heart was found to have two auricles and one ventricle, and from the latter cavity the aorta and pulmonary artery arose."[1] Survival into adolescence and early adulthood is not rare. Longevity occasionally extends into the fourth or fifth decade (see Figures 26-15 and 26-24).[14,16,17,34-38] One patient reached 56 years of age, and another reached age 73 years of age and endured three pregnancies despite mild hypoxia.[39] Moderate pulmonary stenosis is physiologically desirable, but severe pulmonary stenosis or atresia results in deep even profound cyanosis (see Figure 26-5). Squatting may attenuate dyspnea. Hypoxic spells are rare.

Subaortic stenosis caused by a restrictive outlet foramen has an adverse effect on longevity by augmenting pulmonary blood flow and augmenting volume overload of the single ventricle. Restriction of the outlet foramen can be progressive.[8]

The multisystem systemic disorders associated with cyanotic congenital heart disease and Eisenmenger's syndrome are important features in the history of patients with univentricular hearts (see Chapter 17).[34]

PHYSICAL APPEARANCE

An underdeveloped, diaphoretic, mildly cyanotic tachypneic infant is the expected appearance associated with increased pulmonary blood flow and congestive heart failure. Profound cyanosis is the expected appearance with severe pulmonary stenosis or atresia.

ARTERIAL PULSE

In neonates and infants with congestive heart failure, the arterial pulses are small and the rate is rapid. In single left ventricle with subaortic stenosis, the brachial and femoral pulses should be compared because of the incidence of coarctation of the aorta.

JUGULAR VENOUS PULSE

The height and waveform of the jugular pulse are normal when moderate pulmonary stenosis curtails excessive pulmonary blood flow (Figure 26-6). Incompetence of the right atrioventricular valve increases the V wave. Atresia of the *right* atrioventricular valve increases the A wave, provided the interatrial communication is restrictive. Atresia of the *left* atrioventricular valve results in a large jugular venous A wave, provided the atrial septal defect is nonrestrictive.

PRECORDIAL MOVEMENT AND PALPATION

Single ventricle of left ventricular morphology generates a precordial impulse analogous to a morphologic left ventricle in a biventricular heart. When pulmonary blood flow is increased, the impulse of the volume-overloaded single

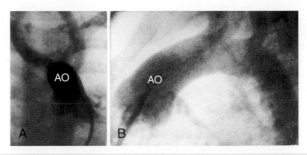

FIGURE 26-7 Aortograms from a 2-year-old boy with single morphologic left ventricle and pulmonary stenosis (gradient, 55 mm Hg). An inverted outlet chamber gave rise to the aorta (Ao), which is convex to the left **(A)** and anterior **(B)**.

left ventricle is hyperdynamic. A visible and palpable systolic impulse in the third left intercostal space is a result of the leftward and anterior position of an inverted outlet chamber (see Figure 26-2A,B). The second heart sound is loud and palpable because the aorta is anterior whether the outlet chamber is inverted or noninverted (Figure 26-7B). A systolic thrill at the mid left sternal border is evidence of subaortic stenosis caused by a restrictive outlet foramen. Potential pulmonary stenotic thrills are attenuated by the posterior position of the pulmonary trunk. A *single morphologic right ventricle* imparts an impulse at the mid to lower left sternal border and subzyphoid area analogous to a morphologic right ventricular impulse in a biventricular heart. There is no impulse in the third left intercostal space because there is no underlying outlet chamber.

AUSCULTATION

A pulmonary ejection sound that might originate in a mobile stenotic pulmonary valve (see Figure 26-2C) is attenuated because of the posterior position of the pulmonary trunk, and pulmonary ejection sounds do not occur with subpulmonary stenosis (see Figure 26-3). An *aortic ejection sound* is generated in the dilated anterior ascending aorta in patients with pulmonary atresia (see Figures 26-5 and 26-25).

A prominent systolic murmur at the mid left sternal border originates in the outlet foramen when pulmonary blood flow is increased. The murmur begins early because flow into the outlet chamber commences before the aortic valve opens. The murmur is decrescendo, ending before the aortic component of the second heart sound because forward flow decelerates and stops before the aortic valve closes.

Pulmonary stenotic murmurs are prominent at the mid or lower left sternal border when the stenosis is subpulmonary, and vary inversely in length and loudness according to the degree of stenosis (Figures 26-8, 26-9, and 26-10). As stenosis increases, more blood is diverted into the aorta and less blood enters the pulmonary trunk, so the stenotic murmur softens and shortens. The murmur is damped still further because of the posterior position of the pulmonary trunk (see previous).

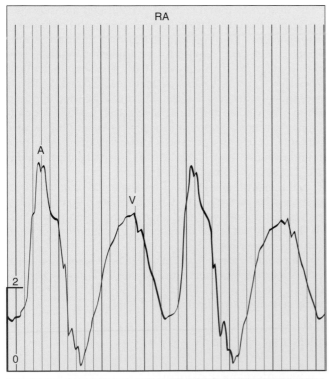

FIGURE 26-6 Right atrial pressure pulse (RA) from an 18-year-old man with single morphologic left ventricle and pulmonary stenosis (gradient, 50 mm Hg). The pressure pulse is normal in height and wave form.

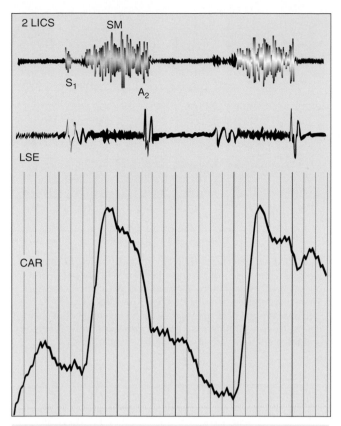

FIGURE 26-8 Phonocardiogram and carotid pulse (CAR) from a 6-year-old girl with single morphologic left ventricle, pulmonary stenosis (gradient, 85 mm Hg), and an inverted outlet chamber. A prominent pulmonary stenotic murmur (SM) was maximal in the second left intercostals space (2 LICS). The single second heart sound (A_2) was aortic because the aorta was anterior to the pulmonary trunk. (LSE = left sternal edge.)

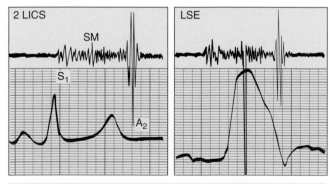

FIGURE 26-9 Tracings from an 8-year-old boy with single morphologic left ventricle and severe pulmonary stenosis (gradient, 100 mm Hg). The pulmonary stenotic murmur (SM) in the second left intercostal space (2 LICS) and at the lower left sternal edge (LSE) is soft and short. The second heart sound (A_2 = aortic component) was loud because an anterior aorta arose from an inverted outlet chamber. The pulmonary component was inaudible because the pulmonary valve was posterior to the aorta. Lower right tracing, carotid pulse.

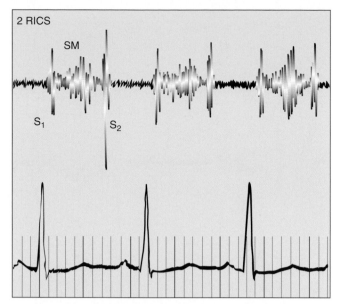

FIGURE 26-10 Phonocardiogram from a 2-month-old male with single morphologic left ventricle and a restrictive outlet foramen (subaortic gradient, 30 mm Hg). The midsystolic stenotic murmur (SM) radiated to the second *right* intercostal space (2 RICS) because the outlet chamber was noninverted and gave rise to an aorta with a rightward convexity. (S_1 = first heart sound; S_2 = second heart sound.)

The murmur of subaortic stenosis caused by a restrctive outlet foramen is midsystolic and radiates from the mid left sternal border to the left or right base depending on whether the outlet chamber is inverted or noninverted (Figure 26-11). Ventricular failure decreases the gradient across the outlet foramen and decreases the subaortic murmur. Because coarctation of the aorta tends to coexist with subaortic stenosis, posterior auscultation should include the interscapular area over the spine in search of the systolic murmur of coarctation (see Chapter 8).

The *second heart sound* splits normally. A rise in pulmonary vascular resistance abolishes the split. The aortic component is loud because the aorta is anterior. Audibility of the pulmonary component improves when the posterior pulmonary trunk is hypertensive and dilated. In the presence of pulmonary stenosis, the loud single second heart sound is aortic. In the presence of subaortic stenosis, the second heart sound tends to be single because the aortic component is attenuated and a prominent pulmonary component originates in the hypertensive posterior pulmonary trunk (see Figure 26-11). In a single morphologic right ventricle, the aortic component of the second sound is loud because the aorta is anterior to the pulmonary trunk or side-by-side.

Two types of diastolic murmurs occur with univentricular hearts. When pulmonary blood flow is increased, a large volume of blood enters the left atrium and flows across the left atrioventricular valve, generating a middiastolic murmur. A rise in pulmonary vascular resistance attenuates the mid-diastolic flow murmur and results in a high-frequency early diastolic Graham Steell murmur of pulmonary hypertensive pulmonary regurgitation.

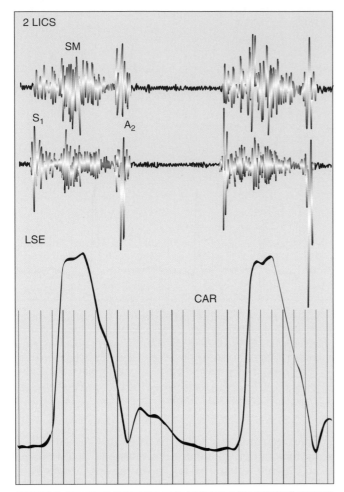

ELECTROCARDIOGRAM

With a *single morphologic left ventricle*, a ventricular septal structure is lacking at the inlet portion of the ventricular mass. The QRS axis is directed *inferior and to the right*, away from the inverted outlet chamber and toward the main ventricular mass (Figures 26-12 and 26-13).[40]

The posterior AV node is hypoplastic and does not form a His bundle or establish a ventricular connection.[41–43] Instead, a well-developed *anterior accessory* AV node gives rise to the His bundle and establishes atrioventricular connections.

When the outlet chamber is *noninverted*, a long nonbranching penetrating bundle runs down the right parietal wall of the single ventricle toward the outlet foramen before bifurcating into right and left bundle branches.[41] When the outlet chamber is *inverted*, the penetrating bundle encircles the outflow tract of the single ventricle before branching at the outlet foramen. The left bundle

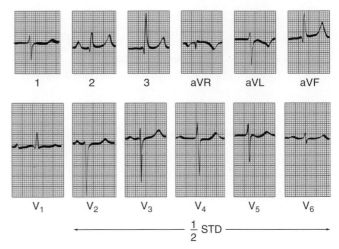

$$\frac{1}{2} \text{STD}$$

FIGURE 26-12 Electrocardiogram from a 30-year-old cyanotic woman with single morphologic left ventricle, inversion of the outlet chamber, and pulmonary stenosis (gradient, 85 mm Hg). There is complete heart block with narrow QRS complexes. The QRS axis is rightward, appropriate for an inverted outlet chamber. In leads V_2 through V_5, the rS complexes are stereotyped and the amplitudes are increased (half standardized).

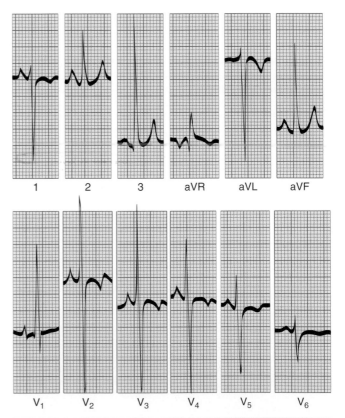

FIGURE 26-13 Electrocardiogram from an 18-year-old man with single morphologic left ventricle, inversion of the outlet chamber, and pulmonary stenosis (gradient, 50 mm Hg). There are tall peaked right atrial P waves in leads 2, aVF, and V_{1-5}. The QRS axis is rightward, which is appropriate for an inverted outlet chamber. The RS complexes are stereotyped in leads V_2 through V_5, with increased amplitude in leads V_{2-4}. There is a tall monophasic R wave in lead V_1 despite a morphologic left ventricle.

branch is concordant with left ventricular morphology of the single left ventricle, and the right bundle branch is concordant with the outlet chamber.[41] The *QRS axis is directed inferior and to the right*, away from the inverted outlet chamber and toward the main ventricular mass (see Figures 26-12 and 26-13).[40]

An inlet septum is also lacking in univentricular hearts with a *morphologic right ventricle* and a rudimentary posterior trabecular pouch. However, the ventricular segment between the morphologic right ventricle and the trabecular pouch extends to the crux where a regular posterior AV node and His bundle are formed.[44] Distribution of the bundle branches apparently depends on the right/left orientation of the trabecular pouch.

When a univentricular heart is morphologically *indeterminate* (no outlet chamber, no trabecular pouch), neither the inlet septum nor trabecular septal tissue reaches the crux. Accordingly, the AV node is anterior or anterolateral, and the penetrating bundles descend as single fascicles among free-running trabeculae.

Diversity in the electrocardiogram reflects the diversity of the anatomic variations of univentricular hearts.[45–47] Electrocardiographic interpretations become clearer when related to specific morphologic types of single ventricles and their physiologic derangements.

When pulmonary blood flow is *increased* (Figure 26-14), P waves show left atrial or biatrial abnormalities. When pulmonary blood flow is *reduced* (Figure 26-15), P waves show right atrial abnormalities. The PR interval tends to be normal with normal atrioventricular conduction despite an elongated nonbranching penetrating bundle (Figure 26-16).

When the outlet chamber is *noninverted* and the single ventricle is a *morphologic left ventricle*, the QRS axis tends to be directed leftward and superior—*left axis deviation axis deviation* (see Figures 26-14 and 26-15).[40] Initial depolarization is anterior and leftward, so small Q waves occasionally appear in left precordial leads (see Figure 26-14).[40] Left ventricular hypertrophy is noteworthy and is especially striking when pulmonary blood flow is increased and the single ventricle is volume overloaded (see Figure 26-14). Precordial QRS complexes then exhibit voltages of remarkably great amplitude (see Figures 26-14 and 26-16) and patterns that are stereotyped (see Figures 26-14 and 26-16).[40,45]

When the outlet chamber is *inverted*, the QRS axis is inferior and to the right, directed away from the inverted outlet chamber toward the main ventricular mass (see Figures 26-12 and 26-13).[40]

Conduction is *triventricular* and often abnormal. PR interval prolongation occasionally culminates in complete heart block.[41] The P wave axis shifts to the left, so tall peaked right atrial P waves appear in mid and left precordial leads (see Figure 26-13). This pattern also occurs with noninversion of the outlet chamber (see Figure 26-15).

Ventricular depolarization is clockwise, so Q waves appear in leads 2, 3, and aVF. Because initial forces of ventricular depolarization are posterior and *leftward*, Q waves may be present in right precordial leads but not in left precordial leads (see Figures 26-12 and 26-13).[40,45] Even though the univentricular heart is morphologically a left

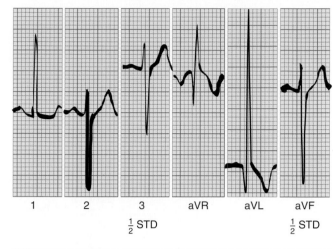

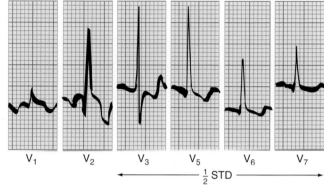

FIGURE 26-14 Electrocardiogram from a 6-year-old boy with single morphologic left ventricle, a noninverted outlet chamber, low pulmonary vascular resistance, and increased pulmonary blood flow. The left atrial P wave abnormality is represented by broad negative terminal forces in leads V_{1-2}. There is left axis deviation with counterclockwise depolarization. The QRS pattern is stereotyped in leads V_{2-7}. The QRS amplitude is strikingly increased in limb leads and in the mid precordium. Leads 3, aVF, and V_{3-7} are half standardized. Small Q waves appear in right and left precordial leads. In lead aVL, the tall R wave and inverted T wave patterns indicate left ventricular hypertrophy.

ventricle, precordial leads may show a dominant R wave in lead V_1 and large equidisphasic RS complexes in midprecordial leads (see Figure 26-13).

In univentricular hearts with a *morphologic right ventricle* and a trabecular pouch, atrioventricular conduction is normal because a regular posterior AV node and His bundle are formed at the crux.[44] Right axis deviation and tall stereotyped precordial R waves are also features of single morphologic right ventricle (Figure 26-17). The QRS axis is usually rightward (see Figure 26-17) but occasionally is leftward and superior.

X-RAY

The location of the outlet chamber is a key diagnostic feature of the x-ray. An *inverted* outlet chamber forms a localized convexity at the upper left cardiac border and gives rise to an aorta that is convex to the left or rises

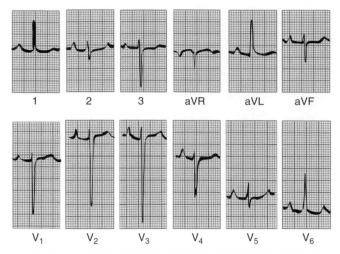

FIGURE 26-15 Electrocardiogram from a 45-year-old woman with single morphologic left ventricle, a noninverted outlet chamber, and pulmonary stenosis (gradient, 80 mm Hg). The PR interval is prolonged. Tall peaked right atrial P waves appear in leads 2, aVF, and V$_{2-6}$. There is left axis deviation with counterclockwise depolarization. The rS patterns in leads V$_{1-4}$ are stereotyped.

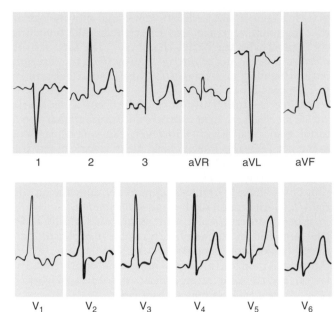

FIGURE 26-17 Electrocardiogram from a 19-year-old man with single morphologic right ventricle and pulmonary stenosis (gradient, 50 mm Hg). There is coarse atrial fibrillation. The QRS axis is rightward, which is appropriate for an inverted outlet chamber. The amplitude of QRS complexes is increased in the limb leads. The Rs pattern is stereotyped in leads V$_1$ through V$_6$.

vertically (Figures 26-2A, 26-3, 26-18, and 26-19),[48,49] as in congenitally corrected transposition of the great arteries (see Chapter 6).[49] In the Holmes heart, the inverted outlet chamber is distinctively convex and, by definition, gives rise to a concordant pulmonary trunk (Figure 26-20 and Video 26-1).[18] A *noninverted* outlet chamber gives rise to an aorta that is convex to the right but is not border-forming (Figure 26-1A), as is the case in complete transposition of the great arteries (see Chapter 27).[49] With the exception of the Holmes heart

(see Figure 26-20),[16,18,40,49] the great arteries are transposed, with the aorta originating discordantly from the outlet chamber and the pulmonary trunk originating discordantly from the morphologic left ventricle (see Figure 26-1). A transposed posteromedial pulmonary trunk may lift its dilated right branch and create a

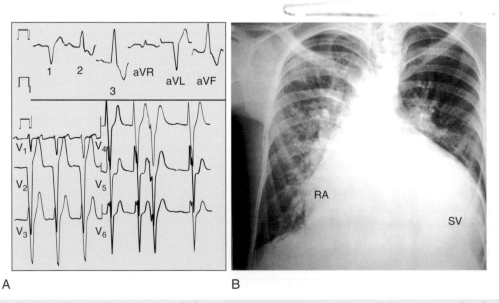

FIGURE 26-16 A, Electrocardiogram from a 7-year-old boy with single morphologic left ventricle, noninverted outlet chamber, and pulmonary vascular disease. The PR interval is 267 msec. The QRS axis is rightward despite noninversion of the outlet chamber. There is an intraventricular conduction defect with a QRS duration of 164 msec. The amplitude of the QRS complexes is striking in limb and precordial leads, all of which are half standardized. Leads V$_1$ through V$_6$ are stereotyped. **B,** X-ray from the same patient showing pulmonary venous congestion and a narrow vascular pedicle caused by noninversion of the outlet chamber and a posterior non border forming pulmonary trunk. The single ventricle (SV) is strikingly dilated, and the right atrium (RA) is appreciably enlarged.

waterfall appearance (see Figure 26-18).[48,49] *Absence of a thymic* shadow is an important radiologic feature of complete transposition of the great arteries in biventricular hearts (see Chapter 27) but is not a feature of complete transposition with univentricular hearts (Figure 26-21B).

The size of the cardiac silhouette increases in response to excessive pulmonary blood flow and volume overload of the single ventricle (see Figures 26-16B, and 26-31A).[10,30,48] Left atrial enlargement is best seen in lateral films or with a barium esophagram[48] because what appears to be left a atrial appendage in the posteroanterior projection is likely to represent an inverted outlet chamber (Figures 26-18 and 26-19). Right atrial dilation accompanies congestive heart failure, which is reinforced by subaortic stenosis (Figures 26-16B, and 26-21A).

The size of the heart is norma,l or nearly so, in *single morphologic left ventricle* with *severe pulmonary stenosis,* but an inverted outlet chamber reveals itself as a bulge at the left upper cardiac border (Figures 26-22, 26-23, and 26-24). Also distinctive is a dilated aorta that arises from an inverted outlet chamber and presents as a convexity to the left (see Figure 26-20) or that ascends vertically and is not border-forming on either side (see Figure 26-24). Pulmonary *atresia* with an inverted outlet chamber has a box-like cardiac silhouette, with the dilated ascending aorta forming the left upper border that merges with a small underfilled ventricle below and the vertebral column forming the straight right border (Figure 26-25).

In univentricular hearts of *right ventricular* morphology, both great arteries necessarily arise from the single right ventricle, so the malformation is a form of double outlet right ventricle (see Chapter 19). The vascular pedicle is narrow because the aorta is anterior and the pulmonary trunk is posterior or side-by-side. Pulmonary stenosis is common, so pulmonary vascularity is normal or reduced and the heart size is not significantly increased.

ECHOCARDIOGRAM

Echocardiography with color flow imaging and Doppler interrogation identifies a single morphologic left ventricle with an outlet chamber at its base.[8,10,50] The internal architecture of the single ventricle can be characterized (Figures 26-26 and 26-27) with two separate patent atrioventricular valves that are usually present (Figure 26-28 and Videos 26-2A and 26-2B). Right and left AV valve morphology is concordant with inversion or noninversion of the outlet chamber.[8] An atrioventricular valve can be incompetent, stenotic, or imperforate, and part of the tensor apparatus can straddle the outlet foramen.[8,13] Color flow imaging establishes the presence and degree of incompetence of the right or left AV valve. A common atrioventricular valve is a feature of atrial isomerism with a univentricular heart (see Chapter 3).

Echocardiography identifies an inverted or noninverted outlet chamber (Figures 26-26 through 26-30) from which the aorta arises discordantly and identifies

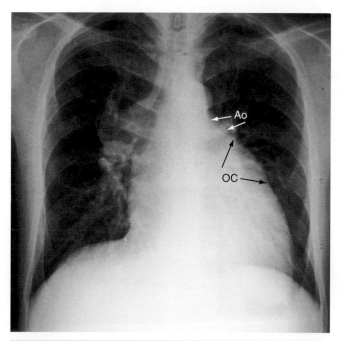

FIGURE 26-18 X-ray from a 24-year-old man with single morphologic left ventricle and pulmonary vascular disease. Pulmonary vascularity was not increased because pulmonary resistance was elevated. An inverted outlet chamber (OC) forms a convex bulge at the left upper cardiac border and gives rise to the aorta (Ao). The large right pulmonary artery is tilted upward, creating a *waterfall* appearance. The single ventricle and right atrium are moderately dilated.

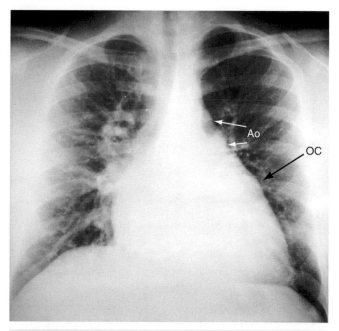

FIGURE 26-19 X-ray from a 19-year-old man with single morphologic left ventricle, pulmonary stenosis (gradient, 50 mm Hg), and increased pulmonary blood flow. The inverted outlet chamber (OC) forms a convex bulge at the upper left cardiac border and gives rise to the aorta (Ao). The single ventricle and right atrium are significantly dilated.

a single left ventricle from which the pulmonary trunk arises discordantly (see Figures 26-27, 26-29 [and Videos 26-3A and 26-3B], and 26-30). In the Holmes heart, the outlet chamber is concordant with the pulmonary trunk and the aorta is concordant with the single morphologic left ventricle (Figure 26-20B). Color flow imaging with continuous wave Doppler scan establishes the presence and degree of pulmonary stenosis or subaortic stenosis caused by a restrictive outlet foramen. When subaortic stenosis exists from infancy, the aortic arch should be interrogated with two-dimensional imaging and color flow and continuous wave Doppler scan because of the increased incidence of coarctation of the aorta and arch hypoplasia.

A univentricular heart of *right ventricular* morphology is recognized by the morphologic characteristics of the ventricular endocardium and the posterior trabecular pouch (Figures 26-31 and 26-32A), which may be straddled by the tensor apparatus of the atrioventricular valve. Two-dimensional echocardiography with color flow imaging shows two side-by-side great arteries arising from the single right ventricle (Figures 26-32B,C). Continuous-wave Doppler scan identifies the presence and degree of pulmonary stenosis.

A univentricular heart of *indeterminate* morphology can be suspected by its endocardial morphology and by the absence of both an outlet chamber and a trabecular pouch.

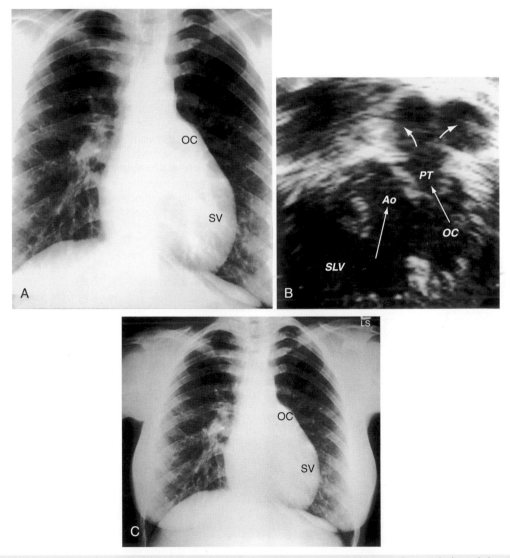

FIGURE 26-20 A, X-ray from a 20-month-old male with the Holmes heart characterized by a single morphologic left ventricle (SV) that gave rise to a concordant aorta and an inverted outlet chamber (OC) that gave rise to a concordant pulmonary trunk. Subpulmonary stenosis was caused by the restrictive ostium of the outlet chamber. **B,** Echocardiogram from the same patient showing the aorta (Ao) arising concordantly from the single left ventricle (SLV) and the pulmonary trunk (PT) arising concordantly from the inverted outlet chamber (OC). **C,** X-ray from a 20-year-old woman with the Holmes heart. The cardiac silhouette is virtually identical to that of the 20-month-old male shown in **A.**

Continued

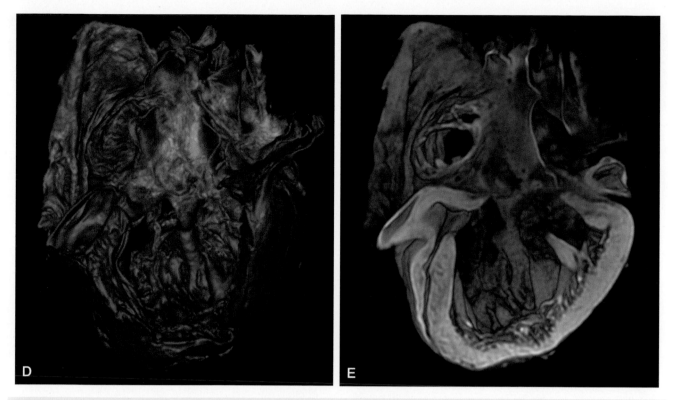

FIGURE 26-20—cont'd   D and **E,** Three-dimensional renderings of the Holmes heart as imaged in its original glass container using a 1.5-Tesla magnet with a standard 3D-SPGR sequence. **D,** A three-dimensional rendering with color mapping of the Holmes heart. **E,** A thick-slab volumetric rendering revealing the depth of vestigial chamber beyond the bulboventricular foramen (Video 26-1). *(Panels D and E courtesy Dr. Luc Jutras, Division of Cardiology, Department of Pediatrics, Montreal Children's Hospital of the McGill University Health Centre.)*

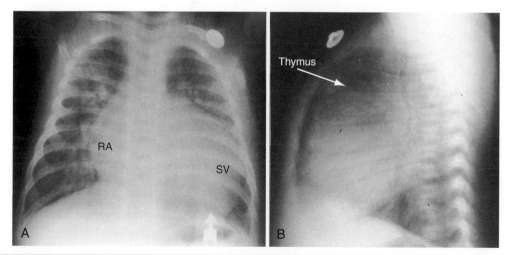

FIGURE 26-21 X-rays from a 3-week-old neonate with a single morphologic left ventricle and a noninverted outlet chamber. **A,** The posteroanterior projection shows a narrow vascular pedicle appropriate for complete transposition of the great arteries. Pulmonary venous congestion is marked, and the single ventricle (SV) and right atrium (RA) are strikingly dilated. **B,** The lateral projection shows a thymic shadow, which implies that complete transposition is occurring with a single ventricle and not as an isolated malformation.

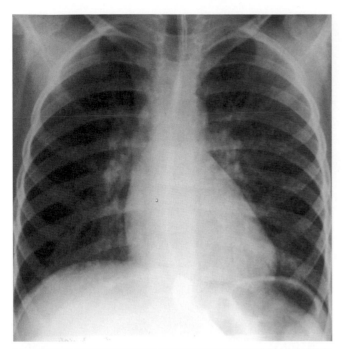

FIGURE 26-22 X-ray from a 7-year-old girl with single morphologic left ventricle and severe pulmonary stenosis (gradient, 105 mm Hg). Pulmonary arterial vascularity is reduced. The vascular pedicle is narrow because a noninverted outlet chamber gave rise to an anterior aorta that ascended vertically and the posterior pulmonary trunk was not border-forming. The size and shape of the heart are virtually normal.

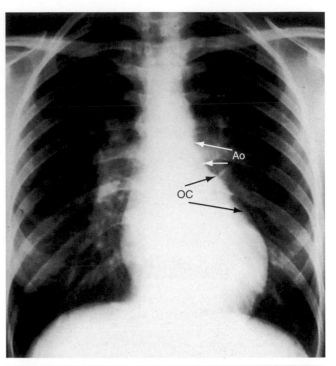

FIGURE 26-24 X-ray from a 30-year-old woman with single morphologic left ventricle, pulmonary stenosis (gradient, 85 mm Hg), inversion of the outlet chamber, and a normal heart size. Pulmonary vascularity is reduced. The vascular pedicle is narrow because the pulmonary trunk was posterior and the inverted outlet chamber (OC) gave rise to an aorta (Ao) that was anterior and ascended vertically.

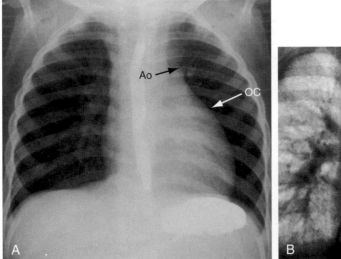
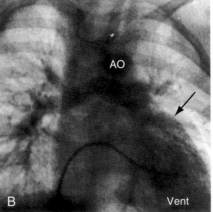

FIGURE 26-23 A, X-ray from a 1-year-old boy with single morphologic left ventricle, an inverted outlet chamber, and pulmonary stenosis (gradient, 65 mm Hg). The straight left upper cardiac border is caused by the inverted outlet chamber (OC) and contiguous ascending aorta (Ao). The size and shape of the heart are otherwise virtually normal. **B,** Ventriculogram from the same patient showing the fine trabecular pattern of a morphologic left ventricle (Vent). The aorta (Ao) arises from an inverted outlet chamber (unmarked arrow).

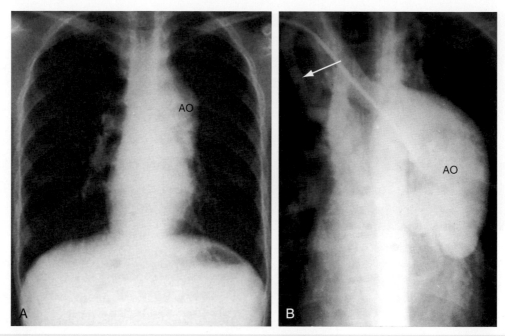

FIGURE 26-25 X-rays from a 22-year-old man with single morphologic left ventricle and pulmonary atresia. **A,** Pulmonary vascularity markedly is reduced. The cardiac silhouette has a box-like configuration, with the left upper border of the box formed by a dilated aorta that ascends vertically from the inverted outlet chamber and the straight right border of the box formed by the vertebral column above and a barely visible right atrium below. **B,** The aortogram shows the dilated convex ascending aorta (AO) and a nonfunctional right Blalock-Taussig shunt (arrow).

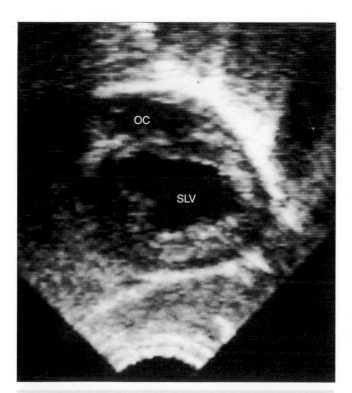

FIGURE 26-26 Echocardiogram (short-axis view) from a 16-month-old boy with a finely trabeculated single morphologic left ventricle (SLV). (OC = outlet chamber.)

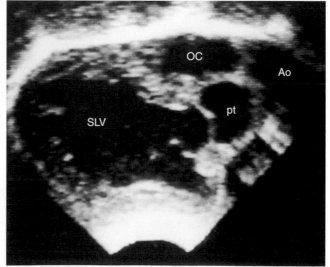

FIGURE 26-27 Echocardiogram (subcostal) from a 10-month-old male with a finely trabeculated single morphologic left ventricle (SLV) from which the pulmonary trunk (pt) originates. The aorta (Ao) originates from an outlet chamber (OC).

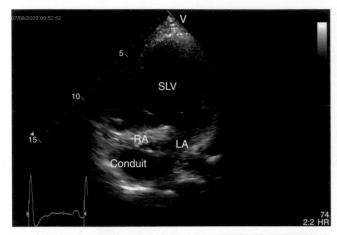

FIGURE 26-28 Echocardiogram (apical view) from a 1-month-old male with single morphologic left ventricle (SLV) and separate right and left atrioventricular valves. The atrial septum is intact (Videos 26-2A and 26-2B). (RA = right atrium; LA=left atrium.)

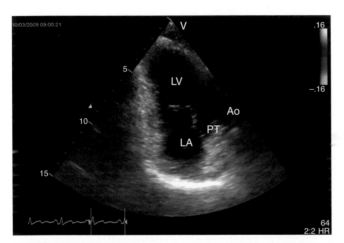

FIGURE 26-29 Echocardiogram (parasternal long-axis view) from a 13-year-old boy with a single morphologic left ventricle (SLV) from which the pulmonary trunk (pt) originates. The aorta originates from a noninverted outlet chamber (OC) (Videos 26-3A and 26-3B). (AV = aortic valve.)

SUMMARY

Single ventricular or *univentricular* refers to hearts with atrioventricular connections that are exclusively or primarily assigned one main ventricular chamber that is morphologically a left, right, or indeterminate ventricle. This chapter is concerned with the three major types of univentricular or single ventricular hearts in which atrioventricular connections are exclusively or primarily assigned one main ventricular chamber: (1) a single morphologic *left* ventricle with an anterobasal outlet chamber

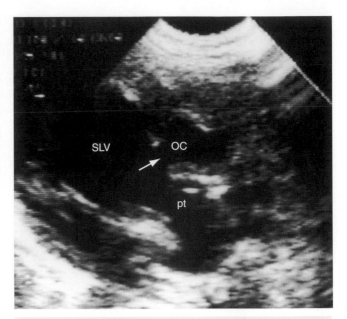

FIGURE 26-30 Echocardiogram (parasternal long-axis view) from a 1-month-old male with single morphologic left ventricle (SLV) from which the pulmonary trunk (pt) originates and an inverted outlet chamber (OC) from which the aorta originates. The outlet foramen (arrow) was restrictive with continuous wave Doppler scan.

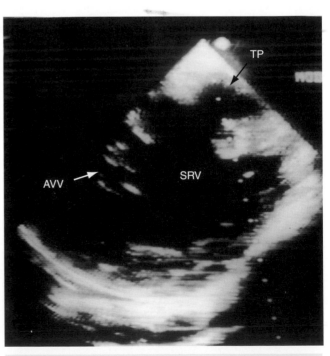

FIGURE 26-31 Transesophageal echocardiogram from a 36-year-old man with a coarsely trabeculated single morphologic right ventricle (SRV). A trabecular pouch (TP) arises from the posteroinferior wall of the single ventricle. The atrioventricular valve (AVV) tensor apparatus did not straddle the trabecular pouch.

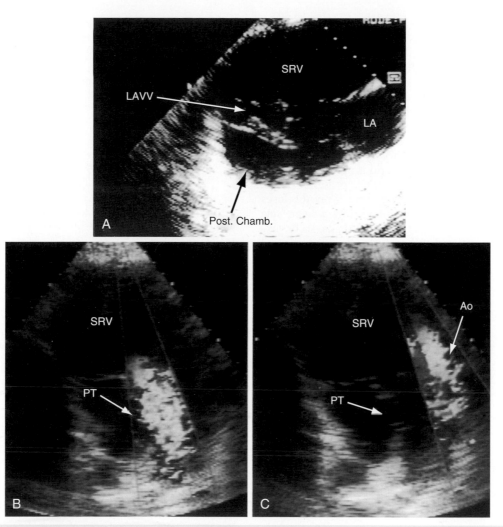

FIGURE 26-32 Echocardiogram (parasternal long-axis view) from a 29-year-old woman with a single morphologic right ventricle (SRV) and pulmonary stenosis (gradient, 65 mm Hg). **A,** The trabecular pouch arose from the posterior wall (Post. Chamb.) of the single ventricle. Tensor apparatus from the left atrioventricular valve (LAVV) did not straddle the trabecular pouch. **B,** Black-and-white print of a color flow image showing flow from the single right ventricle (SRV) into the pulmonary trunk (PT). **C,** Black-and-white print of a color flow image showing flow from the single right ventricle into the aorta (Ao). The aorta and pulmonary trunk (PT) are side by side.

that is either inverted or noninverted; (2) a single morphologic *right* ventricle with a rudimentary trabecular pouch (left ventricular remnanent) that is directly posterior or posteroinferior and left-sided or right-sided; and (3) a single ventricle that is morphologically *indeterminate* and devoid of either an outlet chamber or a trabecular pouch.

The physiologic derangements and clinical manifestations depend on the absence, presence, and degree of pulmonary vascular disease, pulmonary stenosis, or subaortic stenosis and on the morphology and functional state of the artioventricular connections. Because univentricular atrioventricular connections to a single morphologic *left* ventricle with an outlet chamber represent 80% to 90% of cases, this chapter and this summary deal chiefly with that arrangement.

Single morphologic left ventricle with increased pulmonary blood flow presents in infancy with mild cyanosis and congestive heart failure. Physical appearance reflects the poor growth and development caused by the catabolic effects of congestive heart failure. Arterial pulses are

sometimes useful because subaortic stenosis (restrictive outlet foramen) is associated with coarctation of the aorta. Precordial palpation identifies a ventricular impulse with left ventricular characteristics together with a visible and palpable left basal impulse of an inverted outlet chamber. Auscultation detects a prominent long decrescendo systolic murmur at the mid left sternal border as a result of flow through the outlet foramen. Electrocardiographic features associated with a *noninverted* outlet chamber include left axis deviation, left ventricular hypertrophy, QRS complexes of great amplitude, and stereotyped precordial patterns. Electrocardiographic features associated with an *inverted* outlet chamber include PR interval prolongation, an inferior or rightward QRS axis, absent left precordial Q waves, QRS complexes of great amplitude, and stereotyped precordial patterns. The chest x-ray exhibits increased pulmonary vascularity and an inverted convex outlet chamber with an aorta that is convex to the left. Echocardiography with color flow imaging and Doppler interrogation identifies two atrioventricular valves that enter a single ventricle with left ventricular morphology and that incorporate at its base an inverted or noninverted outlet chamber from which the aorta arises discordantly.

A *single morphologic left ventricle* with *pulmonary stenosis* presents with cyanosis rather than congestive heart failure. The ventricular impulse is modest compared with the dynamic impulse of a volume-overloaded single ventricle. Auscultation detects a pulmonary stenotic murmur with loudness and length that vary inversely with severity. A loud single second heart sound is aortic. The electrocardiogram does not reveal either the presence or the degree of pulmonary stenosis. The chest x-ray discloses normal or decreased pulmonary blood flow, a heart size that is normal or nearly normal, and the left basal convexity of an inverted outlet chamber. Color flow imaging and continuous wave Doppler interrogation establish the degree of pulmonary stenosis. In the presence of pulmonary atresia, a dilated ascending aorta is dramatically border-forming, and the cardiac silhouette is box-like.

Univentricular hearts of *right ventricular morphology* are more likely to present with cyanosis than with congestive heart failure because of coexisting pulmonary stenosis. The length and intensity of the pulmonary stenotic murmur vary inversely with the degree of stenosis. Precordial QRS complexes are stereotyped with right ventricular hypertrophy patterns of increased amplitude. The chest x-ray discloses a narrow vascular pedicle because the aorta is side-by-side or anterior to the pulmonary trunk. An outlet chamber is conspicuously absent. Pulmonary vascularity and heart size vary inversely with the severity of pulmonary stenosis and the degree of pulmonary vascular disease.

REFERENCES

1. Peacock TB. On *malformations of the human heart*. London: John Churchill; 1858.
2. Khairy P, Poirier N, Mercier L-A. Univentricular heart. *Circulation*. 2007;115:800–812.
3. Thies WR, Soto B, Diethelm E, Bargeron Jr LM, Pacifico AD. Angiographic anatomy of hearts with one ventricular chamber: the true single ventricle. *Am J Cardiol*. 1985;55:1363–1366.
4. Cook AC, Anderson RH. The anatomy of hearts with double inlet ventricle. *Cardiol Young*. 2006;16(suppl 1):22–26.
5. Jacobs ML, Anderson RH. Nomenclature of the functionally univentricular heart. *Cardiol Young*. 2006;16(suppl 1):3–8.
6. Cook AC, Anderson RH. The functionally univentricular circulation: anatomic substrates as related to function. *Cardiol Young*. 2005;15(suppl 3):7–16.
7. VanPraagh R, Ongley PA, Swan HJ. Anatomic types of single or common ventricle in man. Morphologic and geometric aspects of 60 necropsied cases. *Am J Cardiol*. 1964;13:367–386.
8. Bevilacqua M, Sanders SP, Van PS, Colan SD, Parness I. Double-inlet single left ventricle: echocardiographic anatomy with emphasis on the morphology of the atrioventricular valves and ventricular septal defect. *J Am Coll Cardiol*. 1991;18:559–568.
9. Jacobs JP, Anderson RH, Weinberg PM, et al. The nomenclature, definition and classification of cardiac structures in the setting of heterotaxy. *Cardiol Young*. 2007;17(suppl 2):1–28.
10. Freedom RM, Picchio F, Duncan WJ, Harder JR, Moes CA, Rowe RD. The atrioventricular junction in the univentricular heart: a two-dimensional echocardiographic analysis. *Pediatr Cardiol*. 1982;3:105–117.
11. Stein JI, Smallhorn JF, Coles JG, Williams WG, Trusler GA, Freedom RM. Common atrioventricular valve guarding double inlet atrioventricular connexion: natural history and surgical results in 76 cases. *Int J Cardiol*. 1990;28:7–17.
12. Tandon R, Becker AE, Moller JH, Edwards JE. Double inlet left ventricle. Straddling tricuspid valve. *Br Heart J*. 1974;36:747–759.
13. Rice MJ, Seward JB, Edwards WD, et al. Straddling atrioventricular valve: two-dimensional echocardiographic diagnosis, classification and surgical implications. *Am J Cardiol*. 1985;55:505–513.
14. Abbott ME. *Atlas of congenital cardiac disease*. New York: The American Heart Association; 1936.
15. Jutras LC. Magnetic resonance of hearts in a jar: breathing new life into old pathological specimens. *Cardiol Young*. 2010;20:275–283.
16. Holmes AE. Case of malformation of the heart. *Transaction of the Medico-Chirurgical Society of Edinburgh*. 1824;1:252.
17. Klaus AP, Smith RM, Schneider AB, Parker BM. Single ventricle with normal relationship of the great vessels and pulmonic stenosis. A case report of an adult with the "Holmes heart" *Am Heart J*. 1969;78:530–536.
18. Marin-Garcia J, Tandon R, Moller JH, Edwards JE. Common (single) ventricle with normally related great vessels. *Circulation*. 1974;49:565–573.
19. De La Cruz MV, Markwald RR, Krug EL, et al. Living morphogenesis of the ventricles and congenital pathology of their component parts. *Cardiol Young*. 2001;11:588–600.
20. Fogel MA, Weinberg PM, Fellows KE, Hoffman EA. A study in ventricular-ventricular interaction. Single right ventricles compared with systemic right ventricles in a dual-chamber circulation. *Circulation*. 1995;92:219–230.
21. Fogel MA, Weinberg PM, Gupta KB, et al. Mechanics of the single left ventricle: a study in ventricular-ventricular interaction II. *Circulation*. 1998;98:330–338.
22. Damiano Jr RJ, La Jr FP, Cox JL, Lowe JE, Santamore WP. Significant left ventricular contribution to right ventricular systolic function. *Am J Physiol*. 1991;261:H1514–H1524.
23. Williams RV, Ritter S, Tani LY, Pagoto LT, Minich LL. Quantitative assessment of ventricular function in children with single ventricles using the Doppler myocardial performance index. *Am J Cardiol*. 2000;86:1106–1110.
24. Piran S, Veldtman G, Siu S, Webb GD, Liu PP. Heart failure and ventricular dysfunction in patients with single or systemic right ventricles. *Circulation*. 2002;105:1189–1194.
25. Macartney FJ, Partridge JB, Scott O, Deverall PB. Common or single ventricle. An angiocardiographic and hemodynamic study of 42 patients. *Circulation*. 1976;53:543–554.
26. Akagi T, Benson LN, Green M, et al. Ventricular performance before and after Fontan repair for univentricular atrioventricular connection: angiographic and radionuclide assessment. *J Am Coll Cardiol*. 1992;20:920–926.
27. Parikh SR, Hurwitz RA, Caldwell RL, Girod DA. Ventricular function in the single ventricle before and after Fontan surgery. *Am J Cardiol*. 1991;67:1390–1395.
28. Sano T, Ogawa M, Yabuuchi H, et al. Quantitative cineangiographic analysis of ventricular volume and mass in patients with single ventricle: relation to ventricular morphologies. *Circulation*. 1988;77:62–69.
29. Cabrera A, Azcuna JI, Bilbao F. Single primitive ventricle with D-transposition of the great vessels and atresia of the left A-V valve. *Am Heart J*. 1974;88:225–228.
30. Hallermann FJ, Davis GD, Ritter DG, Kincaid OW. Roentgenographic features of common ventricle. *Radiology*. 1966;87:409–423.
31. Shapiro SR, Ruckman RN, Kapur S, et al. Single ventricle with truncus arteriosus in siblings. *Am Heart J*. 1981;102:456–459.
32. Moodie DS, Ritter DG, Tajik AJ, O'Fallon WM. Long-term follow-up in the unoperated univentricular heart. *Am J Cardiol*. 1984;53:1124–1128.
33. Habeck JO, Reinhardt G, Findeisen V. A case of double inlet left ventricle in a 59-year-old man. *Int J Cardiol*. 1991;30:119–120.
34. Niwa K, Perloff JK, Kaplan S, Child JS, Miner PD. Eisenmenger syndrome in adults: ventricular septal defect, truncus arteriosus, univentricular heart. *J Am Coll Cardiol*. 1999;34:223–232.
35. Chambers WN, Criscitiello MG, Goodale F. Cor triloculare biatriatum. Survival to adult life. *Circulation*. 1961;23:91–101.
36. Ammash NM, Warnes CA. Survival into adulthood of patients with unoperated single ventricle. *Am J Cardiol*. 1996;77:542–544.
37. Mehta JB, Hewlett RF. Cor triloculare biauriculare: an unusual adult heart. *Br Heart J*. 1945;7:41–44.

38. Sagar KB, Mauck HP. Univentricular heart in adults: report of nine cases with review of the literature. *Am Heart J*. 1985;110: 1059–1062.
39. Chen MS, Younoszai A, Gurm HS, Asher CR. Images in cardiovascular medicine. Univentricular heart. *Circulation*. 2004;109:2030.
40. Davachi F, Moller JH. The electrocardiogram and vectorcardiogram in single ventricle. Anatomic correlations. *Am J Cardiol*. 1969;23: 19–31.
41. Anderson RH, Arnold R, Thapar MK, Jones RS, Hamilton DI. Cardiac specialized tissue in hearts with an apparently single ventricular chamber (double inlet left ventricle). *Am J Cardiol*. 1974;33:95–106.
42. Bharati S, Lev M. The course of the conduction system in single ventricle with inverted (L-) loop and inverted (L-) transposition. *Circulation*. 1975;51:723–730.
43. Wenink AC. Development of the human cardiac conducting system. *J Anat*. 1976;121:617–631.
44. Essed CE, Ho SY, Hunter S, Anderson RH. Atrioventricular conduction system in univentricular heart of right ventricular type with right-sided rudimentary chamber. *Thorax*. 1980;35:123–127.
45. Elliott LP, Ruttenberg HD, Eliot RS, Anderson RC. Vectorial analysis of the electrocardiogram in common ventricle. *Br Heart J*. 1964;26:302–311.
46. Freireich AW, Nicolson GB. A rare electrocardiographic finding occasionally seen in single ventricle hearts; report of two cases of cor triloculare biatriatum. *Am Heart J*. 1952;43:526–532.
47. Neill CA, Brink AJ. Left axis deviation in tricuspid atresia and single ventricle; the electrocardiogram in 36 autopsied cases. *Circulation*. 1955;12:612–619.
48. Carey LS, Ruttenberg HD. Roentgenographic features of common ventricle with inversion of the infundibulum: corrected transposition with rudimentary left ventricle. *Am J Roentgenol Radium Ther Nucl Med*. 1964;92:652–668.
49. Elliott LP, Gedgaudas E. The roentgenologic findings in common ventricle with transposition of the great vessels. *Radiology*. 1964; 82:850–865.
50. Child JS. Transthoracic and transesophageal echocardiographic imaging: anatomic and hemodynamic assessment. In: Perloff JK, Child JS, Aboulhosn J, eds. *Congenital heart disease in adults*. 3rd ed. Philadelphia: Saunders/Elsevier; 2009.

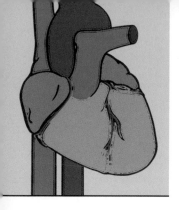

Chapter 27

Complete Transposition of the Great Arteries

In 1797, Matthew Baillie called attention to "a singular malformation in which the pulmonary artery arises from the left ventricle and the aorta from the right ventricle."[1] Seventeen years later, John Farre[2] used the term transposition to characterize Baillie's singular malformation. Each great artery is *placed across* the ventricular septum: *positio* means *placed*, *trans* means *across*. The term *transposition of the great arteries* is used herein in its original sense to signify that the aorta arises from the morphologic right ventricle and the pulmonary trunk arises from the morphologic left ventricle—ventriculoarterial discordance (Figures 27-1 through 27-4).[3–6] The designation "*complete*" means that *ventriculoarterial discordance* is associated with *atrioventricular concordance*. The single discordance between ventricles and great arteries makes the transposition *physiologically complete*. These alignments result in a unique extrauterine circulation in which two independent circulations function in parallel (Figure 27-5). Congenitally corrected transposition (see Chapter 6) refers to atrioventricular and ventriculoarterial discordance. The double discordance physiologically corrects the transposition, which is therefore not complete. Accordingly, there is one circulation in series, as in the normal heart. The term *malposition of the great arteries* refers to abnormal spatial relations but concordant ventricular alignments.[7,8]

d-Transposition and *complete transposition* are synonymous. Because d- refers to a dextro (rightward) bend in the bulboventricular loop, the designation is appropriate because virtually all examples of complete transposition of the great arteries are accompanied by a d-ventricular loop (see Figures 27-2A, and 27-4A). Segmental analysis identifies situs solitus (S), a dextro-ventricular loop (d), and a rightward (d) and anterior aorta (see Figures 27-2A, 27-3, and 27-4). In about one third of cases, the aorta is anterior and to the left, directly anterior, or rarely, posterior to the pulmonary trunk.[3,5] The great arteries rise in parallel and do not cross, as in the normal heart (see Figures 27-1, 27-34, and 27-35).[9] Anomalous origin of the left subclavian artery from the pulmonary artery has been reported in association with a right aortic arch.[10]

The origin and course of the coronary arteries are physiologically unimportant but anatomically pivotal because of the arterial switch operation (see Chapter 32).[11–14] In complete transposition with *situs solitus*, the morphologic right coronary artery is concordant with the morphologic right ventricle and the morphologic left coronary artery is concordant with the morphologic left ventricle.[15] Two aortic sinuses face the right ventricular outflow tract

(Figure 27-6), irrespective of the spatial relations between the ascending aorta and the pulmonary artery.[13,14] The two facing sinuses are the left sinus and the posterior sinus.[13,14] The right aortic sinus does not face the right ventricular outflow tract (see Figure 27-6). Rarely, both coronary arteries are intramural.[16] In complete transposition with *situs inversus*, the anatomy of the coronary arteries has not been well established.[17]

Dual sinus origin indicates that a coronary artery arises from each of the two facing sinuses (see Figure 27-6) and accounts for about 90% of cases; in most of these cases, the left main coronary artery arises from the left aortic sinus and gives rise to the anterior descending and circumflex coronary arteries, and the right coronary artery arises by a single ostium from the posterior aortic sinus (see Figure 27-6A). In the less common type of dual sinus origin, the left anterior descending coronary artery originates from the left aortic sinus, and the circumflex and right coronary arteries originate by a single ostium in the posterior aortic sinus (see Figure 27-6B.) Single sinus origin indicates that both coronary arteries arise from one of the two, but not both, facing sinuses by a single ostium or by multiple ostia. In a small minority of cases of single sinus origin, the left anterior descending, circumflex, and right coronary arteries arise by ostia in the posterior aortic sinus. The sinus node artery originates from the proximal right coronary artery and courses upward and to the right, partially embedded in the limbus of the atrial septum. An aberrant anterior descending coronary artery may pass intramurally between the aortic root and pulmonary trunk.[18]

The incidence rate of complete transposition of the great arteries is estimated at 1 in 2300 to 1 in 5100 live births.[19] The malformation represents approximately 5% to 8% of congenital cardiac malformations but accounts for 25% of deaths from congenital heart disease in the first year of life. The morphogenesis of the ventriculoarterial discordance that characterizes complete transposition focuses on the conus as the crucial connection between the ventricles and the great arteries.[20] The segmental components of the heart, the atria, the ventricles, and the great arteries, appear at different developmental stages.[3] The straight heart tube is formed from primordia of the trabeculated portions of both ventricles. During looping, the atria are at the caudal end of the embryonic tube, and the conus is at the cephalic end of the tube. When the truncus appears, the developing heart has three segments: atrial, ventricular, and arterial.[3] The

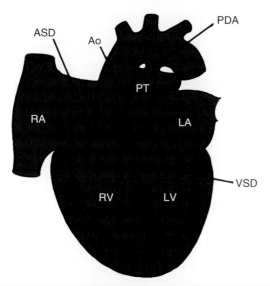

FIGURE 27-1 Illustration of complete transposition of the great arteries. The aorta (Ao) arises from the morphologic right ventricle (RV), is convex to the right, and is positioned to the right of and anterior to the pulmonary trunk (PT), which arises from the morphologic left ventricle (LV). The great arteries are parallel to each other and do not cross. The systemic and pulmonary circulations are joined by three types of communications: atrial septal defect (ASD), ventricular septal defect (VSD), and patent ductus arteriosus (PDA). (LA = left atrium; RA = right atrium.)

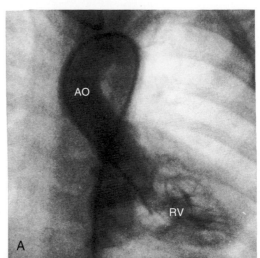

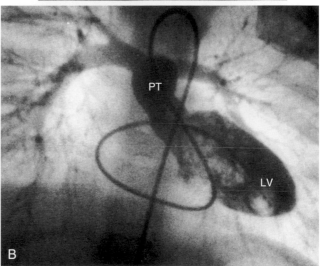

FIGURE 27-2 Ventriculograms from an 8-month-old male with complete transposition of the great arteries, patent foramen ovale, an intact ventricular septum, and a closed ductus arteriosus. A balloon atrial septostomy was performed at 6 days of age. **A,** The right ventricle (RV) gives rise to the ascending aorta (AO), which is convex to the right. **B,** The left ventricle (LV) gives rise to a centrally placed pulmonary trunk (PT) with a rightward inclination. The great arteries are parallel to each other and do not cross. Blood flow in the left pulmonary artery is less than blood flow in the right pulmonary artery.

ventral end of the arterial segment is continuous with the conus, and the dorsal end is continuous with the aortic arches. The spiral division that develops within the truncus progresses from the aortic arches toward the truncal ridges. Conal development then becomes pivotal.[20] Rarely, the aortic arch is double.[21] The subaortic portion of the conus persists in complete transposition of the great arteries, and the subpulmonary conus is absorbed (conal inversion). The aortic valve moves anteriorly, and the pulmonary valve moves inferoposteriorly into fibrous continuity with the mitral valve. The maldeveloped conus is inappropriate for the ventricular loop, so the great arteries are discordant relative to their ventricles of origin. Pulmonary/mitral continuity exists because a left-sided subpulmonary conus is absent, and aortic/tricuspid discontinuity exists because a right-sided subaortic conus is present. Aortic/tricuspid discontinuity causes the aortic valve to lie superior to the pulmonary valve and causes the ascending aorta to lie parallel to the pulmonary trunk.

The ductus arteriosus is usually closed or insignificantly patent in complete transposition (Figures 27-3, 27-4, and 27-7)[22] but is occasionally widely open (Figure 27-8).[23] Interatrial communications take the form of a patent foramen ovale or an ostium secundum atrial septal defect.[5,6,24] Rarely, the foramen ovale closes prematurely.[25] Ventricular septal defects are inlet, muscular, perimembranous, or infundibular.[26] Inlet defects caused by malalignment with the atrial septum result in straddling of the tricuspid valve. Perimembranous ventricular septal defects extend into the inlet septum and into the muscular septum. Infundibular septal defects result from malalignment of the infundibular

septum, which is shifted leftward and posterior or rightward and anterior, and the malaligned defect can be subaortic, subpulmonary, or doubly committed.[26]

Pulmonary stenosis is represented by obstruction to *left ventricular outflow* and occurs in approximately 15% of cases of complete transposition.[5,27] Fixed subpulmonary stenosis is characterized by a circumferential fibrous membrane or diaphragm (Figure 27-9A), a fibromuscular ridge, herniation of tricuspid leaflet tissue, anomalous septal attachments of the mitral valve, accessory mitral leaflet tissue, tissue tags from the membranous septum, or hypertrophy of the anterolateral muscle bundle.[5,27] Leftward and posterior deviation of the infundibular septum causes tunnel or tubular subpulmonary stenosis.[26] Pulmonary valve stenosis is uncommon.[27]

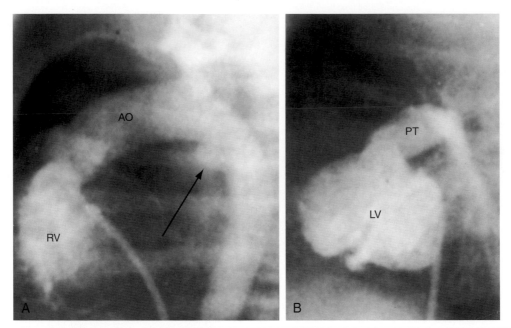

FIGURE 27-3 Lateral ventriculograms from a 4-day-old male with complete transposition of the great arteries, patent foramen ovale, and an intact ventricular septum. A balloon atrial septostomy was performed at 4 days of age. **A,** The aortic root (AO) curves anteriorly as it arises from the morphologic right ventricle (RV), so the plane of the aortic valve is tilted upward. Arrow points to a dimple at the aortic site of the closed ductus. **B,** The posterior pulmonary trunk (PT) arises from a morphologic left ventricle (LV).

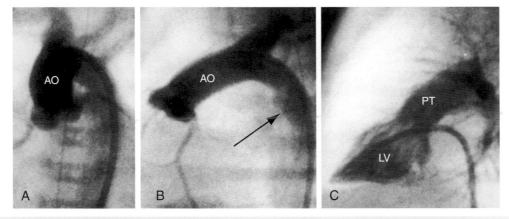

FIGURE 27-4 Angiocardiograms from a 3-day-old male with complete transposition of the great arteries, patent foramen ovale, an intact ventricular septum, and a closed ductus arteriosus. **A,** Aortogram (anteroposterior) shows a midline ascending aorta (AO) with slight rightward convexity. **B,** Lateral aortogram shows the anterior position of the aortic root with the plane of the aortic valve tilted upward. Arrow points to a dimple at the aortic site of the closed ductus. **C,** Lateral left ventriculogram showing the posterior pulmonary trunk (PT) arising from the morphologic left ventricle (LV).

Dynamic subpulmonary stenosis develops during the first few weeks of life and is associated with systolic anterior motion of the anterior mitral leaflet (see Figures 27-9B, and 27-36).[28] The obstruction is dynamic because the degree varies spontaneously and is augmented by isoproterenol and reduced by beta blockade.[28] The development of dynamic subpulmonary stenosis coincides with a fall in pulmonary vascular resistance and a fall in left ventricular systolic pressure in the face of persistent systemic systolic pressure in the adjacent right ventricle. Systemic right ventricular pressure results in systolic movement of the base of the ventricular septum into the outflow tract of the adjacent low-pressure left ventricle. Systolic anterior motion of the anterior mitral leaflet is then caused by the Venturi effect that is generated by

hyperkinetic ejection of a volume-overloaded left ventricle into a low-resistance pulmonary vascular bed (see Figure 27-9B).

Subaortic stenosis is the result of rightward and anterior deviation of a malaligned infundibular septum.[26,29,30] Aortic arch anomalies are represented by hypoplasia, coarctation, and interruption and have been attributed to reduced flow during morphogenesis.[31]

Juxtaposition of the atrial appendages refers to an anomaly in which both atrial appendages or the left appendage and part of the right appendage are adjacent to each other (juxtaposed) on the same side of the heart. Juxtaposition is a rare anomaly that is strongly associated with complete transposition of the great arteries[32–35] and occurs in 2% to 6% of cases of anatomically corrected

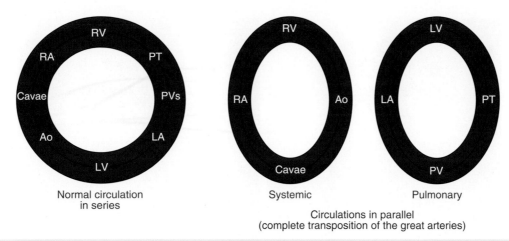

FIGURE 27-5 Illustrations of the normal circulation and the distinctive circulation in transposition of the great arteries. In the normal heart, there is a single circulation in series with flow from the right ventricle (RV) into the pulmonary trunk (PT), pulmonary veins (PV), left atrium (LA), left ventricle (LV), aorta (Ao), systemic venous bed, vena cavae, and right atrium (RA) and back to the right ventricle. In complete transposition of the great arteries, two circulations are in parallel. The systemic circulation is characterized by flow from the right ventricle into the aorta, systemic venous bed, vena cavae, and right atrium and back to the right ventricle. The pulmonary circulation is characterized by flow from left ventricle into pulmonary trunk, pulmonary veins, left atrium, and back to the left ventricle.

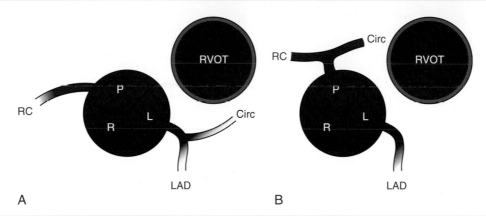

FIGURE 27-6 Illustrations of the coronary artery origins in complete transposition of the great arteries. The left sinus (L) and the posterior sinus (P) face the right ventricular outflow tract (RVOT). The right (R) sinus does not face the right ventricular outflow tract. **A,** The left main coronary artery arises from left sinus and branches into the circumflex (Circ) and left anterior descending (LAD) arteries. The right coronary artery (RC) arises from the posterior sinus (P). **B,** The left main coronary artery arises from the posterior sinus (P) and branches into the right coronary artery (RC) and the circumflex coronary artery (Circ). The left anterior descending coronary artery (LAD) arises from the left sinus (L).

malpositions.[32] Juxtaposition reduces the size and volume of the right atrium. Left-sided juxtaposition is six times as frequent as right-sided juxtaposition. There is female preponderance with juxtaposition of the atrial appendages, in contrast to marked male preponderance in complete transposition of the great arteries without juxtaposition (see section History).[34]

Tricuspid valve abnormalities occur in about 30% of patients with complete transposition and inlet ventricular septal defects.[36] These abnormalities include straddling or overriding of chordae, overriding of the tricuspid annulus, abnormal chordal attachments, and less commonly, tricuspid valve dysplasia, accessory tricuspid tissue, and double orifice tricuspid valve.[36] Mitral valve abnormalities occur in 20% to 30% of necropsy specimens of complete transposition and include a cleft anterior leaflet, straddling of the mitral valve, abnormal size or position, anomalous mitral tissue strands, redundant mitral valve tissue, and abnormal papillary muscles.[37,38]

Matthew Baillie[1] described the *anatomic* features of a singular malformation. The malformation is even more singular in *physiologic* terms. The *normal heart* is associated with a *single circulation in series* (see previous and Figure 27-5), with sequential flow from the right ventricle into the pulmonary artery, pulmonary veins, left atrium, left ventricle, aorta, systemic venous bed, venae cavae, and right atrium and back to the right ventricle. Blood at any given location must traverse both sides of the circulation before returning to that location (see Figure 27-5). In complete transposition of the great arteries, *two circulations are in parallel* (see Figure 27-5). The *systemic circulation* is characterized by flow from the right ventricle into the aorta, systemic venous bed, venae cavae, and right atrium and back to the right ventricle. The *pulmonary circulation* is characterized by flow from the left ventricle into the pulmonary artery, pulmonary capillary bed, pulmonary veins, and left atrium and back to the left ventricle. Blood within the systemic circulation

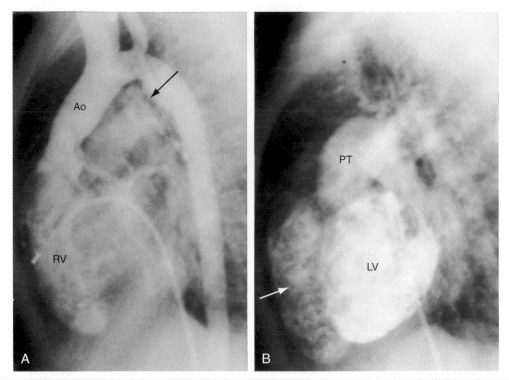

FIGURE 27-7 Lateral angiocardiograms from an 18-month-old girl with complete transposition of the great arteries, an atrial septal defect, a nonrestrictive ventricular septal defect, and a restrictive ductus arteriosus. **A,** The right ventricle (RV) gives rise to an anterior aorta (Ao) with a valve that lies in a horizontal plane. Arrow points to a small patent ductus. **B,** The left ventricle (LV) gives rise to a posterior pulmonary trunk (PT). The right ventricle (arrow) is opacified through the ventricular septal defect. This patient, who remains unoperated, is alive and functional at the age of 43 years despite pulmonary vascular disease.

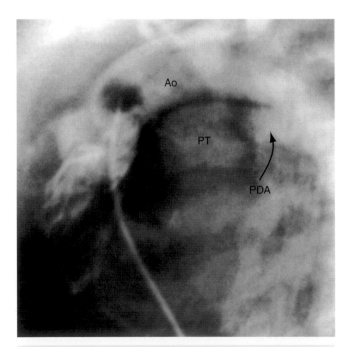

FIGURE 27-8 Lateral aortogram from a 3-day-old female with complete transposition of the great arteries and a large patent ductus arteriosus (PDA, arrow) that was the only communication between the two circulations. Shunting was essentially unidirectional from the anterior aorta (Ao) through the ductus into the posterior pulmonary trunk (PT).

recirculates within the systemic circulation, and blood within the pulmonary circulation recirculates within the pulmonary circulation. The two circulations do not cross unless they are joined by communications at the atrial, ventricular, or great arterial level, on which survival depends. These communications permit blood from the systemic circulation to enter the pulmonary circulation for oxygenation and permit oxygenated blood from the pulmonary circulation to enter the systemic circulation.

The net volume of blood exchanged between the systemic and pulmonary circulations must be isovolumetric over short periods of time or the donor circulation is rapidly depleted and the recipient circulation is rapidly overloaded. The amount of blood exchanged between the two parallel circulations is small relative to the volume that recirculates within each circulation. The volume of effective bidirectional mixing depends on the location and size of the communication that joins the two circulations and on the magnitude of pulmonary blood flow.[39] Survival is tightly coupled to the delicate interplay between the intercirculatory communications and the pulmonary blood flow. In a neonate with complete transposition, a restrictive foramen ovale, and a nonpatent ductus arteriosus, the circulations are in parallel, as illustrated in Figure 27-5. The tendency for neonatal pulmonary vascular resistance to fall prompts an increase in pulmonary blood flow, but that advantage is lost because the oxygenated blood cannot enter the systemic vascular bed. The value of an adequate interatrial communication

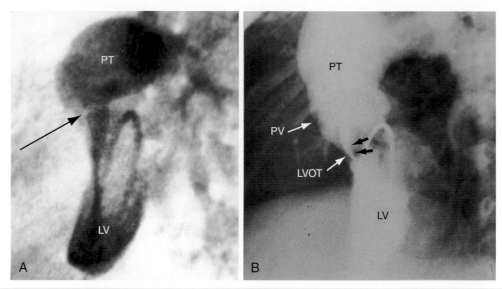

FIGURE 27-9 A, Lateral left ventriculogram (LV) from a 9-month-old female with complete transposition of the great arteries and intact ventricular septum. Arrow points to a subpulmonary membrane or diaphragm. Left ventricular systolic pressure was 60 mm Hg, and pulmonary artery systolic pressure was 18 mm Hg. The pulmonary trunk (PT) is dilated. **B,** Left ventriculogram from a 3-week-old male neonate with complete transposition of the great arteries, intact ventricular septum, and dynamic subpulmonary stenosis. Systolic anterior motion of the anterior mitral leaflet (paired black arrows) caused obstruction of the left ventricular outflow tract (LVOT). (PT = pulmonary trunk; PV = pulmonary valve.)

is dramatized by the immediate response to balloon atrial septostomy.[40,41] An adequate interatrial communication permits quantitatively equal bidirectional shunting that is right-to-left during ventricular diastole and left-to-right during ventricular systole.[39,42,43]

An adequately sized ventricular septal defect permits bidirectional shunting that is determined by instantaneous pressure differences between the two ventricles. When pulmonary vascular resistance is low, there is preferential right-to-left systolic shunting into the low resistance pulmonary circulation and preferential left-to-right diastolic shunting away from the volume-loaded left ventricle. A large patent ductus arteriosus (see Figure 27-8) is initially accompanied by bidirectional flow that is replaced by virtually exclusive systemic-to-pulmonary flow as pulmonary vascular resistance falls.[23] The temporary value of ductal patency is witnessed by the response to prostaglandin-induced ductal dilation as a pharmacologic bridge to balloon septostomy.[44] Because ductal flow is essentially unidirectional, the pulmonary circulation becomes volume overloaded with no egress except a through restrictive foramen ovale.

Low pulmonary vascular resistance with an increase in pulmonary blood flow provides a large volume of oxygenated blood for intercirculatory mixing.[39] Elevated pulmonary vascular resistance and pulmonary stenosis decrease pulmonary blood flow and result in a smaller volume of oxygenated blood for intercirculatory mixing. The increase in left ventricular afterload incurred by pulmonary vascular disease or pulmonary stenosis results in a reduction in left ventricular compliance that adversely affects intracardiac mixing.[39,42] Hypoxemia provokes a fall in systemic vascular resistance and an increase in the volume of unsaturated blood recirculating in the systemic vascular bed.[39,42]

The geometry of the left ventricle in complete transposition is governed by the volume overload imposed by increased pulmonary blood flow and the pressure overload imposed by increased pulmonary vascular resistance or pulmonary stenosis. Right ventricular free wall thickness exceeds normal in the neonate and outstrips left ventricular wall thickness. Septal thickness and right ventricular free wall thickness then increase in parallel, so the septum becomes disproportionately thick relative to the left ventricular wall.[45–49] When the ventricular septum bows into a low-pressure left ventricle, the right ventricle becomes spherical and the left ventricle resembles a prolate ellipsoid.[50]

When left ventricular pressure is elevated, the septum flattens or bows into the right ventricle, resulting in a more normal septal position and better left ventricular function.[45] During the first few weeks of life, left ventricular function is normal, but mass does not increase in proportion to volume,[51] a discrepancy that is responsible for decreased left ventricular function. The right ventricle performs normally at birth, but its contractility and ejection fraction then decline.[51,52] A morphologic subaortic right ventricle is ill-equipped to support the systemic circulation because of the adverse effects of its mass, geometry, and the coronary circulation (see Chapter 6).

Pulmonary vascular disease is prevalent in patients with complete transposition of the great arteries, especially in the presence of a nonrestrictive ventricular septal defect[53–55] or a large patent ductus arteriosus.[23] Grade 3 or 4 Heath-Edwards changes of pulmonary vascular disease are found in 20% of infants before 2 months of age, and in about 80% after 1 year.[56] A reduction in number of intra-acinar pulmonary arteries has been identified with quantitative morphomeric studies.[57,58] Vasoconstriction of pulmonary arterioles induced by hypoxemic blood carried in the systemic arterial collaterals accelerates the pulmonary vascular disease.[59] Early pulmonary vascular disease is more prevalent with a nonrestrictive ventricular septal defect and complete transposition than with an equivalent isolated ventricular septal defect.[56,59,60] Even with an isolated atrial septal defect, the incidence rate of pulmonary vascular disease is about 6%, although progression is slower.[53,61]

HISTORY

Males outnumber females with a ratio as high as 4:1,[5,62] unless there is juxtaposition of the atrial appendages.[34] Complete transposition of the great arteries seldom occurs in firstborns; but in offspring of mothers who have had three or more pregnancies, a twofold increase in incidence rate has been reported. Familial recurrence of concordant cardiac defects within affected family members supports monogenic or oligogenic inheritance in selected pedigrees.[63] Complete transposition and congenitally corrected transposition sometimes segregate in the same family, probably because of monogenic transmission, which supports a pathogenetic link between complete transposition and disorders of looping.[63]

Cyanosis begins as early as the first day of life in more than 90% of infants with an intact ventricular septum.[19] Severe pulmonary stenosis or atresia results in intense neonatal cyanosis. Mild cyanosis with delayed onset is a feature of complete transposition with a nonrestrictive ventricular septal defect[64] or a patent ductus arteriosus.[23] A large isolated ductus (see Figure 27-8) is associated with severe congestive heart failure in the first few days of life, and spontaneous closure results in a sudden fall in systemic arterial oxygen saturation, rapid clinical deterioration, and death.[23] Dynamic subpulmonary stenosis or a rise in pulmonary vascular resistance curtails pulmonary blood flow and alleviates congestive heart failure, but at the expense of increasing hypoxemia. Pulmonary stenosis is occasionally responsible for hypercyanotic spells characterized by intense cyanosis, tachypnea, extreme irritability, and hypothermia but seldom by loss of consciousness.[28] Squatting is rare. Neonatal survival is tightly coupled to the delicate interplay between the intercirculatory communications and pulmonary blood flow.[65] An older infant depends for survival on adequate pulmonary blood flow. Outcome is bleak, with an overall death rate of 30% in the first week, 50% in the first month, and 90% in the first year.[24,66,67]

Survival is poorest when the foramen ovale is restrictive, the ventricular septum is intact, and the ductus is closed. The salutary effect of an adequately sized interatrial communication is underscored by the immediate response to balloon septostomy (see previous),[41] after which 75% of patients survive for 6 months, 65% survive for 1 year, and many survive into their teens.[40] A nonrestrictive ventricular septal defect with pulmonary vascular disease carries a 6-month survival rate of about 30% and a 1-year survival rate of about 20%. Moderate pulmonary stenosis improves longevity by regulating pulmonary blood flow, with three quarters of patients surviving for a year or more. Most of those who reach their teens have a nonrestrictive ventricular septal defect with pulmonary vascular disease or pulmonary stenosis. Sporadic examples of unusual longevity have been recorded in the third, fourth, and fifth decades (see Figure 27-7),[31,68,69] and

complete transposition was confirmed at necropsy in a 56-year-old patient.[70] Brain abscess is rare in patients younger than 2 years of age but is believed to have a predilection for complete transposition of the great arteries and Fallot's tetralogy.[71]

PHYSICAL APPEARANCE

Birth weights in infants with complete transposition average greater than normal, with a substantial proportion above 8 pounds,[72] in contrast to newborns with other forms of congenital heart disease whose birth weights average less than normal for gestational age. The illusion of robust health is soon dispelled by the catabolic effects of congestive heart failure (Figure 27-10). Increased anteroposterior chest dimensions are associated with hyperinflation of the lungs (see section X-Ray). Intense early cyanosis reflects poor intercirculatory mixing and low pulmonary blood flow. Cyanosis that is mild and delayed indicates good intercirculatory mixing and increased pulmonary blood flow. Complete transposition with a large patent ductus, pulmonary vascular disease, and an intact ventricular septum is associated with *reversed differential cyanosis*—the feet are less cyanotic than the hands—because oxygenated blood from the pulmonary artery enters the aorta distal to the left subclavian artery and flows selectively to the lower extremities (see Chapter 20).[23] Deeply cyanotic patients with pulmonary vascular disease or severe pulmonary stenosis have varicosities of the scalp and arms because of the large volume of highly unsaturated blood in the systemic circulation.

ARTERIAL PULSE

In 1957, Cleland and associates[73] described peripheral arterial pulses of remarkably full volume (Figure 27-11) with visible pulsations of the dorsalis pedis and posterior tibial arteries. Shaher[69] attributed the bounding pulses, the scalp varices, and the warm extremities to the large volume of highly unsaturated blood recirculating in the hyperkinetic low-resistance systemic vascular bed (see previous). Bounding pulses are not associated with patent ductus arteriosus because ductal flow is essentially systolic from aorta into pulmonary trunk and does not enter the right ventricle from which the aorta and systemic arteries arise.[23] Diminished femoral pulses call attention to coexisting coarctation of the aorta with anterior and rightward deviation of the infundibular septum (subaortic stenosis).

JUGULAR VENOUS PULSE

The jugular venous pulse is elevated under two widely divergent physiologic circumstances. The first and most common is congestive heart failure that accompanies a nonrestrictive ventricular septal defect with low pulmonary vascular resistance. The second circumstance is right ventricular failure in deeply cyanotic patients with a large volume of unsaturated blood recirculating through the right ventricle and right atrium (Figure 27-12).

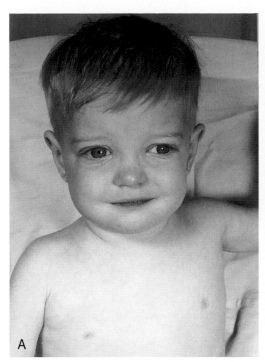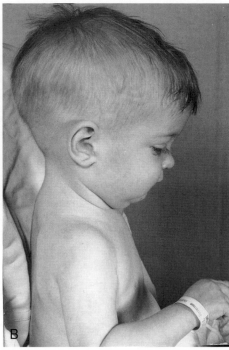

FIGURE 27-10 Physical appearance of a 15-month-old boy with complete transposition of the great arteries. Birth weight was 9 pounds 2 ounces. The child's head is large, although his body and arms have lost the robust appearance with which he was born.

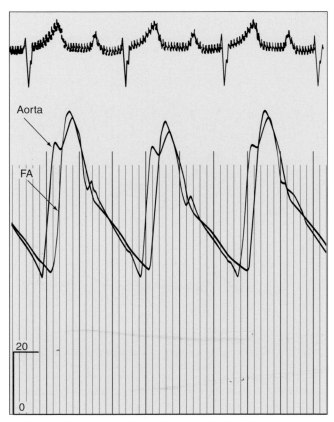

FIGURE 27-11 Aortic and femoral artery pulses (FA) from a deeply cyanosed 15-month-old boy with complete transposition of the great arteries, a ventricular septal defect, and severe pulmonary stenosis. The pulse pressure is wide because the diastolic pressure is low. The rate of the rise is brisk, and the aortic pulse (upper arrow) is bisferiens (twin peaked).

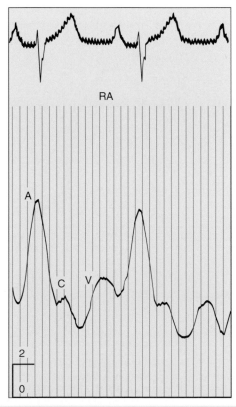

FIGURE 27-12 Right atrial pressure pulse (RA) from the deeply cyanotic 15-month-old boy referred to in Figure 27-11. The A wave is dominant, and the mean right atrial pressure is elevated.

PRECORDIAL MOVEMENT AND PALPATION

The right ventricular impulse is transiently normal or nearly so in neonates with complete transposition. The impulse becomes prominent in response to congestive heart failure that accompanies a nonrestrictive ventricular septal defect and is especially prominent when the right ventricle is overloaded by the large volume of unoxygenated blood that recirculates in a hypervolemic hyperdynamic systemic vascular bed.

A loud palpable second heart sound at the left base originates in the aortic valve (Figure 27-13) because the transposed aorta is anterior. A dilated hypertensive posterior pulmonary trunk does not transmit its impulse or closure sound. A right aortic arch occurs in about 8% of patients with complete transposition and occasionally reveals itself as a right sternoclavicular impulse, especially when the aortic root is pulsatile and hyperkinetic in deeply cyanotic patients.[74]

A left ventricular impulse is not identified in neonates and is overshadowed by the right ventricular impulse in older patients. The left ventricle is palpable when a nonrestrictive ventricular septal defect exists with low pulmonary vascular resistance because the left ventricle is both volume-overloaded and pressure-overloaded. The left ventricle is seldom palpable despite volume overload when there is a nonrestrictive atrial septal defect and an intact ventricular septum (see Figure 27-28) because ejection is at a low systolic pressure.

AUSCULTATION

Pulmonary ejection sounds (Figure 27-14) originate in the dilated hypertensive posterior pulmonary trunk (Figure 27-15).[75] The ejection sound does not selectively decrease during inspiration because the transposed pulmonary trunk arises from the left ventricle. Aortic ejection sounds occasionally occur when complete transposition is accompanied by a dilated aortic root with leftward and posterior malalignment of the infundibular septum (subaortic stenosis).

Midsystolic flow murmurs originate in the transposed anterior aorta, especially when the systemic circulation is hypervolemic and hyperkinetic. Midsystolic flow murmurs potentially originate in a dilated posterior pulmonary trunk (see Figure 27-15) but are inherently soft and are likely to be rendered inaudible by interposition of the anterior aorta (Figures 27-13 and 27-16).

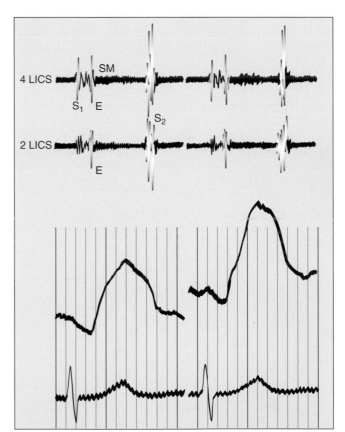

FIGURE 27-14 Tracings from a 5-year-old girl with complete transposition of the great arteries, a nonrestrictive ventricular septal defect, and pulmonary vascular disease. The soft decrescendo systolic murmur (SM) at the fourth left intercostal space (4 LICS) was caused by systolic shunting across the ventricular septal defect. The pulmonary ejection sound (E) originated in a dilated hypertensive posterior pulmonary trunk. (2 LICS = second left intercostal space.) The second heart sound (S2) was single because of synchronous closure of the aortic and pulmonary valves and was loud because of amplification caused by the anterior position of the aortic root in conjunction with amplification caused by the dilated hypertensive posterior pulmonary trunk. Carotid pulse is shown below.

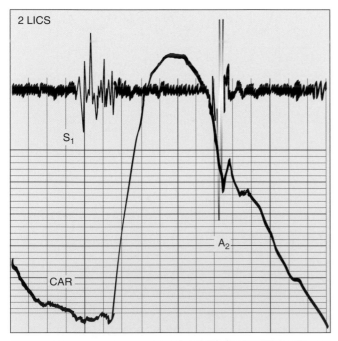

FIGURE 27-13 Phonocardiogram and carotid pulse (CAR) from a 2-year-old boy with complete transposition of the great arteries, a nonrestrictive atrial defect, low pulmonary vascular resistance, and increased pulmonary blood flow. The aortic component of the second heart sound (A2) was loud because the aortic root was anterior. There were no murmurs. (2 LICS = second left intercostal space; S1 = first heart sound.)

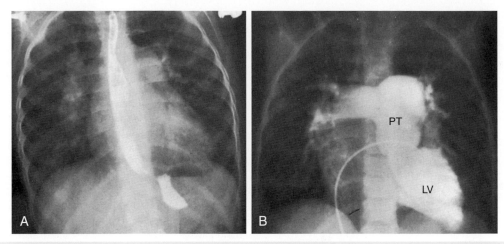

FIGURE 27-15 X-ray and angiocardiogram from a 7-year-old boy with complete transposition of the great arteries, a nonrestrictive atrial septal defect, an intact ventricular septum, and pulmonary vascular disease. **A,** The hypertensive posterior pulmonary trunk is sufficiently dilated to be border-forming on the left. **B,** Angiocardiogram shows the dilated hypertensive pulmonary trunk (PT) arising from a morphologic left ventricle (LV).

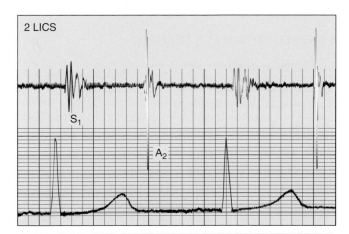

FIGURE 27-16 Phonocardiogram from the second left intercostal space (2 LICS) of an 18-month-old girl with complete transposition of the great arteries, a nonrestrictive atrial septal defect, low pulmonary vascular resistance, and increased pulmonary blood flow. There were no murmurs. The second heart sound was loud because the aortic component (A_2) originated in an anterior aortic root.

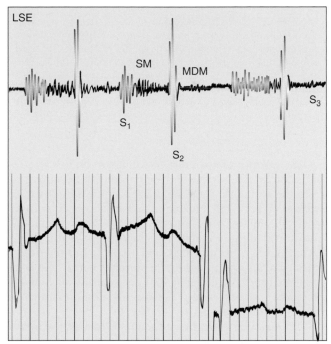

FIGURE 27-17 Phonocardiogram at the lower left sternal edge (LSE) of a 10-month-old male with complete transposition of the great arteries, a nonrestrictive ventricular septal defect, low pulmonary vascular resistance, and increased pulmonary blood flow. The decrescendo holosystolic murmur (SM) originated across the ventricular septal defect. The second heart sound (S2) was the aortic component that was loud because the aortic root was anterior. A mid-diastolic murmur (MDM) and a third heart sound (S3) resulted from augmented flow across the mitral valve.

A holosystolic murmur of ventricular septal defect awaits the neonatal fall in pulmonary vascular resistance (Figure 27-17; see Chapter 17).[75] A subsequent rise in pulmonary resistance shortens and ultimately abolishes the murmur,[76] as in patients with Eisenmenger's syndrome (see Figure 27-14). A restrictive ventricular septal defect generates a holosystolic murmur or a soft early systolic murmur that disappears when the defect spontaneously closes.

The midsystolic murmur of fixed pulmonary stenosis is present at birth. The midsystolic murmur of dynamic obstruction to left ventricular outflow appears after the first few weeks of life and progressively increases in length and loudness. Pulmonary stenotic murmurs are heard best in the third left intercostal space at the sternal border because the stenosis is usually subvalvular. The murmur radiates upward and to the right because of the rightward course of the transposed pulmonary trunk (see Figure 27-2B). The midsystolic murmur of pulmonary stenosis with a nonrestrictive ventricular septal defect varies inversely in length and loudness with the degree of stenosis, as in Fallot's tetralogy (see Chapter 18). A soft pulmonary stenotic murmur is rendered inaudible by the anterior aortic root (Figure 27-18).

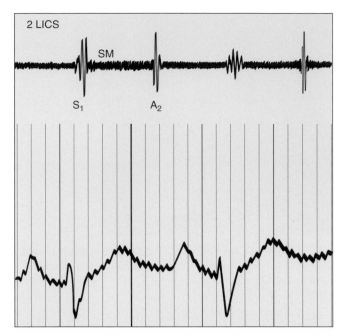

FIGURE 27-18 Phonocardiogram from a deeply cyanotic 13-month-old boy with complete transposition of the great arteries, a nonrestrictive ventricular septal defect, and severe fixed subpulmonary stenosis. A pulmonary stenotic murmur (SM) was virtually absent because flow was reduced and the pulmonary trunk was posterior. (2 LICS = second left intercostal space; S_1 = first heart sound; A_2 = aortic component of the second heart sound.)

The murmur of a nonrestrictive patent ductus arteriosus is confined to systole and not continuous because flow from the aorta into the pulmonary trunk is almost exclusively systolic.[23] High neonatal pulmonary vascular resistance eliminates the diastolic portion of a continuous murmur by curtailing diastolic flow (see Chapter 20).[76] A continuous murmur that could originate in a restrictive patent ductus is damped by the anterior aorta. The large systemic arterial collaterals that occasionally accompany complete transposition seldom cause continuous murmurs (see previous).

Mid-diastolic murmurs are generated across the mitral valve when pulmonary blood flow is increased (see Figure 27-17).[75] Mid-diastolic murmurs across the tricuspid valve are generated in deeply cyanotic patients because the systemic circulation is hypervolemic and hyperkinetic.[75] A high-frequency early diastolic Graham Steell murmur of pulmonary hypertensive pulmonary regurgitation is difficult to hear because of the posterior position of the pulmonary trunk.

A loud and single second heart sound is the aortic component because the aorta is anterior (see Figures 27-13, 27-14, 27-16, and 27-17). The sequence of semilunar valve closure is normal because the aortic component precedes the pulmonary component despite ventriculoarterial discordance. Low pulmonary vascular resistance and increased pulmonary capacitance result in normal timing or in only a slight delay of the pulmonary arterial dicrotic notch.[77] Right bundle branch block causes paradoxical splitting of the second sound because

the aortic component is delayed until after the pulmonary component.[78] Pulmonary hypertension increases audibility of the pulmonary component, provided the pulmonary vascular resistance remains sufficiently low to permit inspiratory splitting. When pulmonary and systemic resistances equalize, the semilunar valves close simultaneously, the second sound is single, and its intensity is reinforced, as in Eisenmenger's syndrome with a ventricular septal defect (see Figure 27-14; see Chapter 17). With pulmonary stenosis, splitting is not audible because the inherently soft pulmonary component is further attenuated by the posterior position of the pulmonary trunk.

A left ventricular third heart sound is generated in mildly cyanotic patients when increased pulmonary blood flow causes volume overload of the left ventricle, especially when the left ventricle fails (see Figure 27-17). A right ventricular third heart sound is generated in deeply cyanotic patients when increased systemic blood flow causes volume overload of the right ventricle, especially when the right ventricle fails.

ELECTROCARDIOGRAM

The electrocardiogram can be normal in the first few days of life (Figure 27-19).[79,80] Tall peaked right atrial P waves soon emerge because mean right atrial pressure is increased (congestive heart failure) or because right atrial volume is increased (hypervolemic systemic circulation;

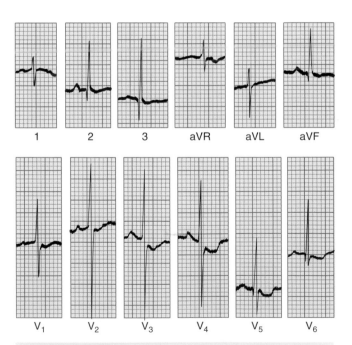

FIGURE 27-19 Electrocardiogram from a 7-day-old female with complete transposition of the great arteries and a nonrestrictive ventricular septal defect. For the first few days of life, the electrocardiogram was normal; and as shown, the electrocardiogram is virtually normal here except for nonspecific ST segment and T waves changes in leads V_{5-6}. The QRS axis is +90 degrees. Compare with Figure 27-20, which is the electrocardiogram from the same patient at 4 years of age.

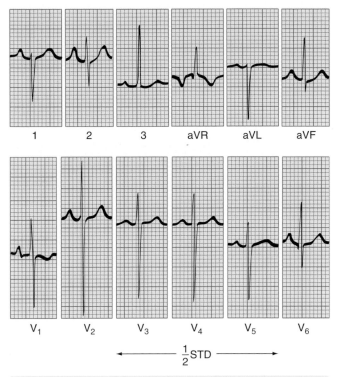

$\longleftarrow \frac{1}{2}STD \longrightarrow$

FIGURE 27-20 Electrocardiogram at 4 years of age from the patient whose normal neonatal electrocardiogram is shown in Figure 27-19. Tall peaked right atrial P waves are present in lead 2 and in leads V_{1-2}. Precordial leads exhibit combined ventricular hypertrophy reflected in the large R/S complexes in leads V_{2-5}, which are half standardized. Left ventricular volume overload is manifested by the Q wave and the well-developed R wave in lead V_6. Right ventricular pressure overload is manifested by right axis deviation, a monophasic R wave in lead aVR, and a prominent S wave in lead V_6.

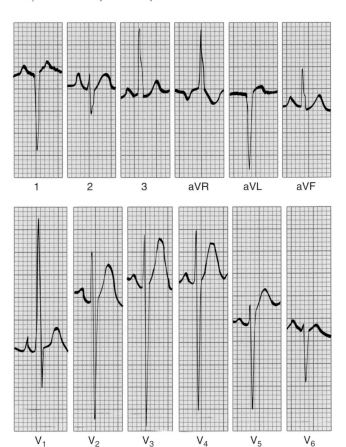

FIGURE 27-21 Electrocardiogram from a deeply cyanotic 15-month-old boy with complete transposition of the great arteries, a nonrestrictive ventricular septal defect, and severe fixed subpulmonary stenosis. Peaked right atrial P waves appear in leads 2 and aVF and in lead V_1. Pure right ventricular hypertrophy is reflected in marked right axis deviation, tall monophasic R waves in leads aVR and V_1, and deep S waves in left precordial leads. T waves are taller in right precordial leads than in left precordial leads.

Figures 27-20 and 27-21.)[81,82] Left atrial P wave abnormalities are reserved for patients with a large atrial septal defect and increased pulmonary blood flow (Figure 27-22).

Right axis deviation is moderate or absent when the left ventricle is volume-overloaded in the presence of a nonrestrictive ventricular septal defect and increased pulmonary blood flow. Right axis deviation occurs when left ventricular volume overload is curtailed by pulmonary vascular disease or pulmonary stenosis (Figures 27-21 and 27-23). Right axis deviation is most striking when an atrial septal defect occurs with increased pulmonary blood flow, normal pulmonary artery pressure, and pure right ventricular hypertrophy (see Figure 27-22). Left precordial R waves are small, and Q waves are absent, despite left ventricular volume overload (see Figure 27-22). Pure right ventricular hypertrophy also occurs when pulmonary stenosis or a nonrestrictive ventricular septal defect with pulmonary vascular disease reduces left ventricular volume and when a hypervolemic systemic circulation increases right ventricular volume (see Figures 27-21 and 27-23). Biventricular hypertrophy is evidence of a nonrestrictive ventricular septal defect with low pulmonary vascular resistance and both volume and pressure overload of the left ventricle (see

Figure 27-20).[80] Right precordial T waves are seldom deeply inverted, even when the systemic right ventricle is volume-overloaded. Right precordial T waves often are not only positive but also tend to be distinctly taller than left precordial T waves (see Figures 27-21 and 27-22).

X-RAY

An initially normal neonatal x-ray assumes typical features of complete transposition as pulmonary vascular resistance falls and pulmonary blood flow increases.[19] Increased pulmonary vascularity is sometimes evident within the first few days of life (see Figures 27-24 and 27-25). The distribution of pulmonary blood flow favors the right lung because of the rightward direction of the pulmonary trunk (see Figures 27-2B, and 27-25B).[9,83] A progressive increase in flow into the right lung may culminate in a substantial decrease in flow to the left lung.[9] The crural portions of the hemidiaphragms are low when the lungs are hyperinflated.

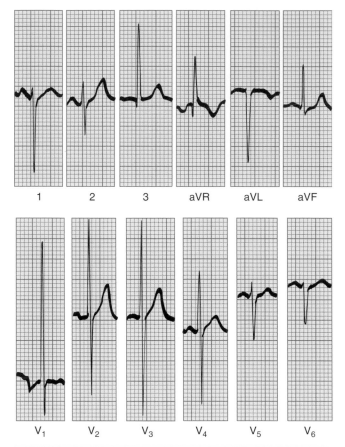

FIGURE 27-22 Electrocardiogram from a 2-year-old girl with complete transposition of the great arteries, a nonrestrictive atrial septal defect, low pulmonary vascular resistance, and increased pulmonary blood flow. The broad deep P terminal force in lead V_1 indicates a left atrial abnormality. Except for large equidiphasic RS complexes in leads V_{2-3}, there is pure right ventricular hypertrophy manifested by marked right axis deviation, a tall monophasic R wave in lead V_1, and rS complexes in leads V_{5-6}. The T wave amplitude is much greater in lead V_2 than in lead V_6.

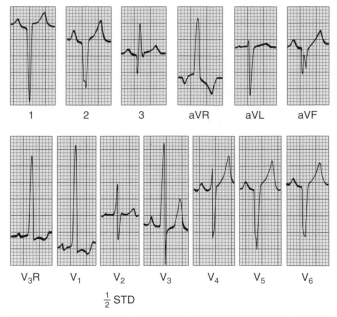

FIGURE 27-23 Electrocardiogram from a 16-month-old boy with complete transposition of the great arteries, a nonrestrictive ventricular septal defect, and suprasystemic pulmonary vascular resistance. There are tall peaked right atrial P waves in leads 1, 2, and aVF. Pure right ventricular hypertrophy is manifested by marked right axis deviation, tall monophasic R waves in leads V_3R and V_1, and the deep S waves in leads V_{4-6}.

Thymic shadow is almost always absent after the first 12 hours of life (see Figure 27-24A), so the distinctive radiologic appearance of the narrow vascular pedicle is seldom obscured (Figures 27-24 through 27-27). The pulmonary trunk is posterior and medial (see Figures 27-2B, 27-3B, and 27-25B).[84] The pedicle is narrowest when the ascending aorta courses vertically upward directly anterior to the pulmonary trunk (Figure 27-28). The aortic root is seldom sufficiently rightward to be border-forming (see Figures 27-2A, and 27-4), except when the ascending aorta enlarges in the presence of leftward and posterior malalignment of the infundibular septum

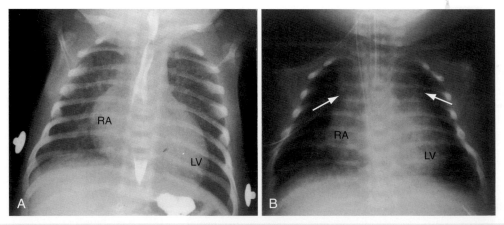

FIGURE 27-24 A, X-ray from a 4-day-old male with complete transposition of the great arteries and a nonrestrictive ventricular septal defect. The thymus is characteristically absent, disclosing a narrow vascular pedicle. The right atrium (RA) is prominent, and a convex left ventricle (LV) occupies the apex. Pulmonary vascularity is increased even in this overpenetrated film. B, X-ray from another 4-day-old male with complete transposition of the great arteries and an uncharacteristically present thymus (arrows) that obscures the vascular pedicle.

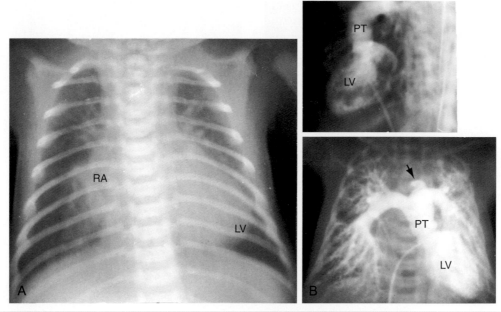

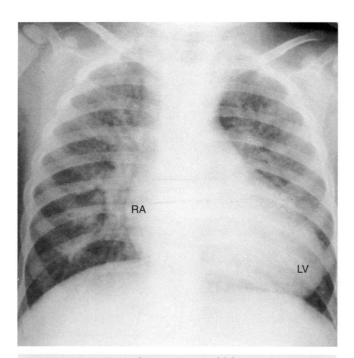

FIGURE 27-25 X-ray and angiocardiograms from a 5-day-old male with complete transposition of the great arteries, a patent foramen ovale, an intact ventricular septum, and a large patent ductus arteriosus. **A,** Increased pulmonary blood flow is evident even at this young age. Absence of a thymic shadow discloses a narrow vascular pedicle. The right atrium (RA) is prominent, and a dilated left ventricle (LV) occupies the apex. **B,** Contrast material injected into the left ventricle (LV). The lateral projection (top) shows the pulmonary trunk (PT) arising from the left ventricle. The frontal projection (bottom) shows the pulmonary trunk arising from the left ventricle and proceeding rightward with disproportionate flow into the right pulmonary artery. Relatively little contrast material enters the ductus (arrow).

FIGURE 27-26 X-ray from a 1-year-old boy with complete transposition of the great arteries, a nonrestrictive ventricular septal defect, and increased pulmonary vascularity. The vascular pedicle is narrow, and a distinctive egg-shaped cardiac silhouette results from an enlarged right atrium (RA) at the right cardiac border and an enlarged left ventricle (LV) at the apex.

(Figure 27-29). The vascular pedicle also widens when a dilated hypertensive posterior pulmonary trunk is convex to the left (Figure 27-30). When pulmonary stenosis and ventricular septal defect coexist, a right aortic arch is present in 11% to 16% cases.[5,74,84–86]

The size and shape of the heart are determined chiefly by the magnitude of pulmonary blood flow. When pulmonary vascular resistance is low and pulmonary blood flow is increased, the cardiac silhouette often has the distinctive appearance of a tilted egg lying on its side pointing downward and to the left (see Figures 27-26 and 27-27).[84] The blunter right border of the egg consists of the right atrium, and the convex left border is the left ventricle. In the lateral projection, the heart assumes a circular appearance because an enlarged right ventricle merges with the anterior aorta, and an enlarged left ventricle merges with the dilated posterior left atrium (see Figure 27-3). Juxtaposition of the atrial appendages is recognized by a localized bulge along the mid left cardiac border that represents the contiguous mass of the two appendages.[87]

As pulmonary vascular resistance increases, lung vascularity decreases, the size of the left ventricle and left atrium decrease, and a dilated hypertensive posterior pulmonary trunk emerges at the left base (Figures 27-15, 27-30, and 27-31). Severe fixed pulmonary stenosis is associated with decreased pulmonary vascularity, a small left ventricle, a small left atrium, and enlargement of the right ventricle and right atrium because of the hypervolemic systemic circulation (see Figure 27-29).[6]

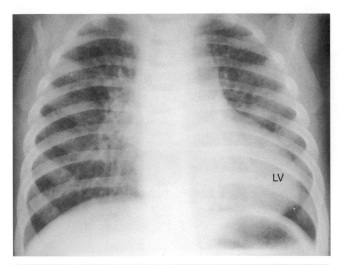

FIGURE 27-27 X-ray from a 9-month-old male with complete transposition of the great arteries, patent foramen ovale, and an intact ventricular septum. An atrial septostomy was performed at 2 days of age. Pulmonary vascularity is increased, the vascular pedicle is narrow, and an enlarged convex left ventricle (LV) occupies the apex.

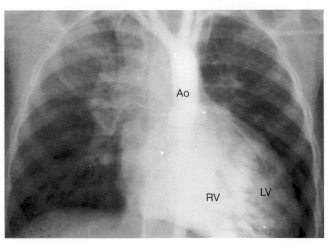

FIGURE 27-28 Angiocardiogram from a 29-month-old boy with complete transposition of the great arteries and a nonrestrictive atrial septal defect. The aorta (Ao) originates from the right ventricle (RV) and arises vertically. An enlarged unopacified left ventricle (LV) occupies the apex.

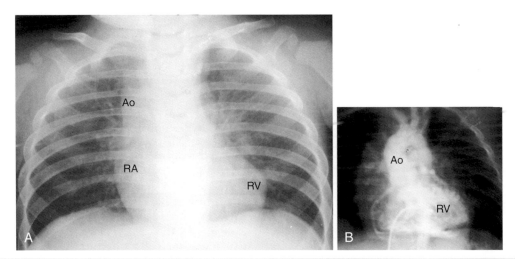

FIGURE 27-29 **A,** X-ray from a 15-month-old boy with complete transposition of the great arteries, a nonrestrictive ventricular septal defect, and severe fixed subpulmonary stenosis caused by posterior and leftward deviation of the infundibular septum. Pulmonary vascularity is reduced. The vascular pedicle is uncharacteristically wide because the ascending aorta (Ao) is dilated. The right atrium (RA) is moderately enlarged, but the apex-forming right ventricle (RV) is not dilated. **B,** The right ventriculogram discloses a dilated ascending aorta (Ao) with a rightward convexity, accounting for an uncharacteristically wide vascular pedicle.

ECHOCARDIOGRAM

Echocardiography with color flow imaging and Doppler interrogation establishes the ventricular origins of the great arteries (ventriculoarterial discordance), their spatial relationships, the presence of a ventricular septal defect or an atrial septal defect, and the presence and degree of obstruction to ventricular outflow.[88–90] The spiral relationship of the aorta and main pulmonary artery segment is normally represented in the short axis by an anterior "sausage," which is the right ventricular outflow tract and main pulmonary artery segment transected tangentially, and a posterior circle, which is the aorta. In complete transposition, the great arteries appear as double circles, with the aorta anterior and to the right or side-by-side and to the right of the main pulmonary artery (Figure 27-32A and Video 27-1). Identification of each great artery rests more securely on imaging the right and left branches of the main pulmonary artery (Figures 27-32B, and 27-33) and on imaging the brachiocephalic branches of the aortic arch with continuation as the descending thoracic aorta (Figure 27-34 and Video 27-2). The anterior aortic root and posterior pulmonary trunk run parallel to each other (see Figure 27-34 and Video 27-2) and do not cross

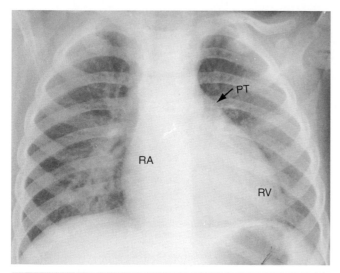

FIGURE 27-30 X-ray from a 16-month-old boy with complete transposition of the great arteries, a nonrestrictive ventricular septal defect, and pulmonary vascular disease. A dilated hypertensive posterior pulmonary trunk (PT) extends to the left (arrow). The right ventricle (RV) occupies the apex, and the right atrium (RA) occupies the right lower cardiac border.

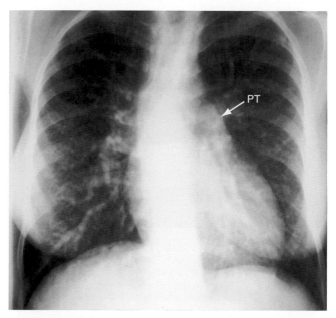

FIGURE 27-31 X-ray from a 30-year-old woman with complete transposition of the great arteries, a nonrestrictive ventricular septal defect, and pulmonary vascular disease. The lung fields have the lacy pattern of neovascularity. A dilated hypertensive posterior pulmonary trunk (PT) reveals itself at the left base. The left branch is obscured, but the dilated right branch is evident. The right atrium is slightly convex, and a moderately enlarged right ventricle occupies the apex.

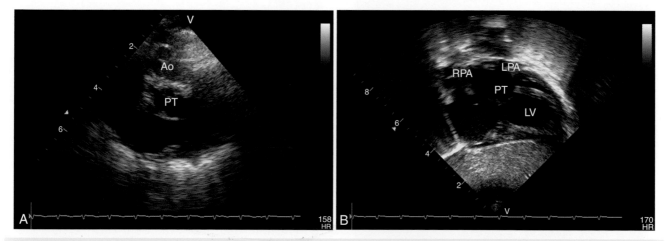

FIGURE 27-32 Echocardiograms from a 3-month-old male with complete transposition of the great arteries, patent foramen ovale, and an intact ventricular septum. An atrial septostomy was performed at 4 days of age. **A,** The great arteries are characteristically represented in the short axis by two circles, with the aorta (Ao) anterior and rightward and the pulmonary trunk (PT) posterior and leftward. **B,** The subxiphoid image shows alignment of the morphologic left ventricle (LV) with the pulmonary trunk (PT), which is identified by its bifurcation into right and left branches (Video 27-1). (RPA = right pulmonary artery; LPA = left pulmonary artery.)

as in the normal heart. The ventricle of origin of each discordant great artery can be properly assigned (see Figures 27-32, 27-33, and 27-34). An important role of echocardiography is in determining the origin and course of the coronary arteries.[11] Commissural malalignment of the facing sinus can be established.[91]

Echocardiography with color flow imaging and Doppler interrogation establishes the presence of a ventricular septal defect or an atrial septal defect. Visualization of

the left ventricular outflow tract determines the absence (see Figures 27-32 and 27-33), presence, and degree of obstruction as well as its morphologic type (Figures 27-35 and 27-36),[89,90,92] and continuous wave Doppler interrogation establishes the magnitude of the gradient. Fixed obstruction to left ventricular outflow is represented by pulmonary valve stenosis (see Figure 27-35) or posterior and leftward malalignment of the infundibular septum.[90,92] Dynamic obstruction to left ventricular

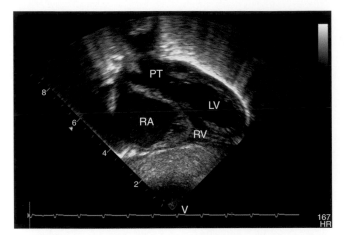

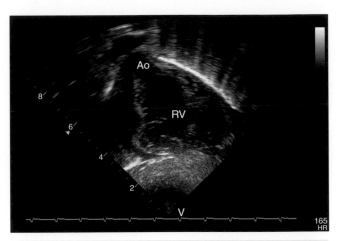

FIGURE 27-33 Echocardiogram (subcostal) from a male neonate with complete transposition of the great arteries, a patent foramen ovale, and an intact ventricular septum. The left ventricle (LV) gives rise to the pulmonary trunk (PT). A normal left ventricular outflow tract is delineated beneath delicate pulmonary valve echoes. Compare with the angiocardiogram in Figure 27-2B. (RA = right atrium; RV = right ventricle.)

FIGURE 27-35 Echocardiogram (subcostal) from a 2-month-old male with complete transposition of the great arteries showing the aorta (Ao) originating from the right ventricle (RV).

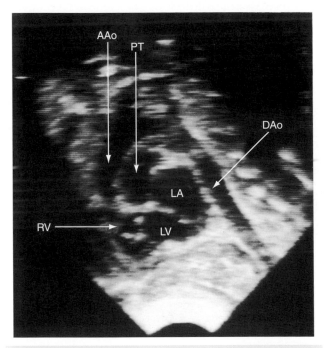

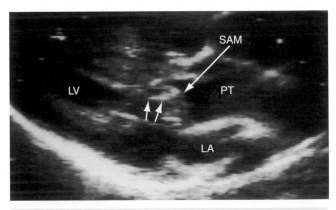

FIGURE 27-36 Echocardiogram (parasternal long-axis view) from an 8-week-old male with dynamic subpulmonary stenosis caused by systolic anterior motion (SAM) of the anterior mitral leaflet (paired arrows). (LA = left atrium; LV = left ventricle; PT = pulmonary trunk.)

FIGURE 27-34 Echocardiogram (subcostal) from a male neonate with complete transposition of the great arteries, a patent foramen ovale, and an intact ventricular septum. The ascending aorta (AAo) is anterior, rising vertically from the right ventricle (RV) and giving off the brachiocephalic arteries before continuing as the descending aorta (DAo). Compare with the angiocardiogram in Figure 27-2A. The left ventricle (LV) gives rise to the pulmonary trunk (PT), which is posterior and parallel to the ascending aorta (Video 27-2). (LA = left atrium.)

movement of the base of the ventricular septum, and a hyperkinetic left ventricular free wall conspire to produce the left ventricular outflow gradient of dynamic subpulmonary stenosis.[89,90]

Juxtaposition of the atrial appendages is recognized in the two-dimensional echocardiogram by malposition of the right atrial appendage with an abnormal plane of the atrial septum.[93] Tricuspid valve anomalies can be identified, especially straddling or overriding.

outflow is characterized by systolic anterior movement of the anterior mitral leaflet that can be recognized with two-dimensional real time imaging (see Figure 27-36A).[09] The combination of systolic anterior movement of the anterior mitral leaflet, abnormal systolic

SUMMARY

The clinical recognition of complete transposition of the great arteries is based on the following features: (1), male gender; (2), large birth weight; (3), neonatal cyanosis, (4), radiologic evidence of increased pulmonary blood flow in the presence of cyanosis and an egg-shaped cardiac silhouette with a narrow vascular pedicle; (5), absent thymic shadow; and (6), echocardiographic identification of aortic alignment with the morphologic right ventricle, pulmonary trunk alignment with the morphologic left ventricle, right atrial alignment with right ventricle, and left atrial alignment with left ventricle.

Complete transposition with a restrictive foramen ovale presents with rapidly progressive cyanosis that begins on the first day of life. The electrocardiogram and x-ray can be transiently normal, and apart from conspicuous cyanosis, the physical signs are disarmingly unimpressive, with a normal arterial pulse, a moderate right ventricular impulse, and no cardiac murmur.

Complete transposition with nonrestrictive ventricular septal defect presents with relatively mild cyanosis and congestive heart failure that coincides with the neonatal fall in pulmonary vascular resistance. A right ventricular impulse is accompanied by a palpable left ventricle. There is a loud holosystolic left parasternal murmur, the electrocardiogram shows moderate right axis deviation and biventricular hypertrophy, and the x-ray shows increased pulmonary blood flow and an egg-shaped cardiac silhouette with a narrow vascular pedicle. Pulmonary vascular disease causes a decrease in pulmonary blood flow, progressive cyanosis, a decrease in size of the left ventricle and left atrium, loss of the left ventricular impulse, a pulmonary ejection sound, an inconspicuous or absent midsystolic murmur, a loud single second sound, and a Graham Steell murmur. The electrocardiogram shows pure right ventricular hypertrophy. The vascular pedicle is narrow, but a dilated posterior pulmonary trunk may emerge at the left base.

Dynamic subpulmonary stenosis reveals itself several weeks after birth. The midsystolic murmur increases in length and loudness as the dynamic obstruction to left ventricular outflow progresses. Neonates with *fixed subpulmonary stenosis* and a nonrestrictive ventricular septal defect present with conspicuous cyanosis and a pulmonary stenotic murmur that varies inversely in loudness length with the degree of obstruction. The pulmonary stenotic murmur radiates upward and to the right because of the rightward direction taken by the pulmonary trunk. The second heart sound is loud because the aorta is anterior and is single because the pulmonary component is inaudible as a result of the posterior position of the pulmonary trunk. The right ventricle is palpable, but not the left ventricle. Arterial pulses are bounding because the systemic circulation is hypervolemic and hyperkinetic. The vascular pedicle widens because of rightward convexity of a dilated aortic root. The electrocardiogram shows pure right ventricular hypertrophy and marked right axis deviation.

Complete transposition with a nonrestrictive atrial septal defect is associated with mild cyanosis and a conspicuous right ventricular impulse but no left ventricle impulse. The pulmonary midsystolic flow murmur is damped by the anterior aorta and is followed by the loud second sound of aortic valve closure. The electrocardiogram shows marked right axis deviation with pure right ventricular hypertrophy. The x-ray is similar to that of complete transposition with a nonrestrictive ventricular septal defect and increased pulmonary blood flow, but the left ventricle is less dilated.

Complete transposition with a nonrestrictive patent ductus arteriosus presents in neonates with mild to moderate cyanosis and tachypnea, but without bounding pulses and without a continuous murmur.

REFERENCES

1. Baillie M. *Morbid anatomy of some of the most important parts of the human body.* 2nd ed. London: Johnson and Nicol; 1797.
2. Farre JR. *On malformations of the human heart.* London: Longman, Hurst, Rees, Orme, and Brown; 1814.
3. De La Cruz MV, Arteaga M, Espino-Vela J, Quero-Jimenez M, Anderson RH, Diaz GF. Complete transposition of the great arteries: types and morphogenesis of ventriculoarterial discordance. *Am Heart J.* 1981;102:271–281.
4. De La Cruz MV, Berrazueta JR, Arteaga M, Attie F, Soni J. Rules for diagnosis of arterioventricular discordances and spatial identification of ventricles. Crossed great arteries and transposition of the great arteries. *Br Heart J.* 1976;38:341–354.
5. Elliott LP, Neufeld HN, Anderson RC, Adams P, Edwards JE. Complete transposition of the great vessels: I. An anatomic study of sixty cases. *Circulation.* 1963;27:1105.
6. Lev M, Rimoldi HJ, Paiva R, Arcilla RA. The quantitative anatomy of simple complete transposition. *Am J Cardiol.* 1969;23:409–416.
7. Anderson RH, Becker AE, Losekoot TG, Gerlis LM. Anatomically corrected malposition of great arteries. *Br Heart J.* 1975;37:993 1013.
8. Van Praagh R, Durnin RE, Jockin H, et al. Anatomically corrected malposition of the great arteries (S, D, L). *Circulation.* 1975;51:20–31.
9. Muster AJ, Paul MH, Van Grondelle A, Conway JJ. Asymmetric distribution of the pulmonary blood flow between the right and left lungs in d-transposition of the great arteries. *Am J Cardiol.* 1976;38:352–361.
10. Mosieri J, Chintala K, Delius RE, Walters 3rd HL, Hakimi M. Abnormal origin of the right subclavian artery from the right pulmonary artery in a patient with D-transposition of the great vessels and left juxtaposition of the right atrial appendage: an unusual anatomical variant. *J Card Surg.* 2004;19:41–44.
11. Sim EK, Van Son JA, Edwards WD, Julsrud PR, Puga FJ. Coronary artery anatomy in complete transposition of the great arteries. *Ann Thorac Surg.* 1994;57:890–894.
12. Elliott LP, Amplatz K, Edwards JE. Coronary arterial patterns in transposition complexes. Anatomic and angiocardiographic studies. *Am J Cardiol.* 1966;17:362–378.
13. Gittenberger-De Groot AC, Saucer U, Oppenheimer-Dekker A, Quaegebeur J. Coronary arterial anatomy in transposition of the great arteries: a morphological study. *Pediatr Cardiol.* 1983;4:15.
14. Rossi MB, Ho SY, Anderson RH, Rossi Filho RI, Lincoln C. Coronary arteries in complete transposition: the significance of the sinus node artery. *Ann Thorac Surg.* 1986;42:573.
15. Li J, Tulloh RM, Cook A, Schneider M, Ho SY, Anderson RH. Coronary arterial origins in transposition of the great arteries: factors that affect outcome. A morphological and clinical study. *Heart.* 2000;83:320–325.
16. Padalino MA, Ohye RG, Devaney EJ, Bove EL. Double intramural coronary arteries in D-transposition of the great arteries. *Ann Thorac Surg.* 2004;78:2181–2183.
17. Chiu I-S, Wang J-K, Wu M-H. Coronary artery anatomy in complete transposition of the great arteries with situs inversus. *Am J Cardiol.* 2002;89:94–95.
18. Gittenberger-De Groot AC, Sauer U, Quaegebeur J. Aortic intramural coronary artery in three hearts with transposition of the great arteries. *J Thorac Cardiovasc Surg.* 1986;91:566–571.
19. Levin DL, Paul MH, Muster AJ, Newfeld EA, Waldman JD. d-Transposition of the great vessels in the neonate. A clinical diagnosis. *Arch Intern Med.* 1977;137:1421–1425.
20. Chuaqui B. Doerr's theory of morphogenesis of arterial transposition in light of recent research. *Br Heart J.* 1979;41:481–485.

21. Kondrachuk O, Yalynska T, Tammo R, Yemets I. D-transposition of the great arteries and double aortic arch. *Eur J Cardiothorac Surg.* 2009;35:729.

22. Al-Naami GH, Al-Mesned AA. Transposition of great arteries with constrictive ductus arteriosus revisited. *Pediatr Cardiol.* 2008;29:827–829.

23. Waldman JD, Paul MH, Newfeld EA, Muster AJ, Idriss FS. Transposition of the great arteries with intact ventricular septum and patent ductus arteriosus. *Am J Cardiol.* 1977;39:232–238.

24. Boesen I. Complete transposition of the great vessels: importance of septal defects and patent ductus arteriosus. Analysis of 132 patients dying before age 4. *Circulation.* 1963;28:885–887.

25. Chiou H-L, Moon-Grady A, Rodriguez R, Konia T, Parrish M, Milstein J. A rare lethal combination of premature closure of the foramen ovale and d-transposition of the great arteries with intact ventricular septum. *Int J Cardiol.* 2008;130:e57–e59.

26. Milanesi O, Ho SY, Thiene G, Frescura C, Anderson RH. The ventricular septal defect in complete transposition of the great arteries: pathologic anatomy in 57 cases with emphasis on subaortic, subpulmonary, and aortic arch obstruction. *Hum Pathol.* 1987;18:392–396.

27. Shrivastava S, Tadavarthy SM, Fukuda T, Edwards JE. Anatomic causes of pulmonary stenosis in complete transposition. *Circulation.* 1976;54:154–159.

28. Aziz KU, Paul MH, Idriss FS, Wilson AD, Muster AJ. Clinical manifestations of dynamic left ventricular outflow tract stenosis in infants with d-transposition of the great arteries with intact ventricular septum. *Am J Cardiol.* 1979;44:290–297.

29. Schneeweiss A, Motro M, Shem-Tov A, Neufeld HN. Subaortic stenosis: an unrecognized problem in transposition of the great arteries. *Am J Cardiol.* 1981;48:336–339.

30. Waldman JD, Schneeweiss A, Edwards WD, Lamberti JJ, Shem-Tov A, Neufeld HN. The obstructive subaortic conus. *Circulation.* 1984;70:339–344.

31. Messeloff CR, Weaver JC. A case of transposition of the large vessels in an adult who lived to the age of 38 years. *Am Heart J.* 1951;42:467–471.

32. Becker AE, Becker MJ. Juxtaposition of atrial appendages associated with normally oriented ventricles and great arteries. *Circulation.* 1970;41:685–688.

33. Charuzi Y, Spanos PK, Amplatz K, Edwards JE. Juxtaposition of the atrial appendages. *Circulation.* 1973;47:620–627.

34. Deutsch V, Shem-Tov A, Yahini JH, Neufeld HN. Juxtaposition of atrial appendages: angiocardiographic observations. *Am J Cardiol.* 1974;34:240–244.

35. Hunter AS, Henderson CB, Urquhart W, Farmer MB. Left-sided juxtaposition of the atrial appendages. Report of 4 cases diagnosed by cardiac catheterization and angiocardiography. *Br Heart J.* 1973;35:1184–1189.

36. Huhta JC, Edwards WD, Danielson GK, Feldt RH. Abnormalities of the tricuspid valve in complete transposition of the great arteries with ventricular septal defect. *J Thorac Cardiovasc Surg.* 1982;83:569–576.

37. Moene RJ, Oppenheimer-Dekker A. Congenital mitral valve anomalies in transposition of the great arteries. *Am J Cardiol.* 1982;49:1972–1978.

38. Rosenquist GC, Stark J, Taylor JF. Congenital mitral valve disease in transposition of the great arteries. *Circulation.* 1975;51:731–737.

39. Mair DD, Ritter DG. Factors influencing intercirculatory mixing in patients with complete transposition of the great arteries. *Am J Cardiol.* 1972;30:653–658.

40. Powell TG, Dewey M, West CR, Arnold R. Fate of infants with transposition of the great arteries in relation to balloon atrial septostomy. *Br Heart J.* 1984;51:371–376.

41. Rashkind WJ, Miller WW. Creation of an atrial septal defect without thoracotomy. A palliative approach to complete transposition of the great arteries. *JAMA.* 1966;196:991–992.

42. Mair DD, Ritter DG. Factors influencing systemic arterial oxygen saturation in complete transposition of the great arteries. *Am J Cardiol.* 1973;31:742–748.

43. Satomi G, Nakazawa M, Takao A, et al. Blood flow pattern of the interatrial communication in patients with complete transposition of the great arteries: a pulsed Doppler echocardiographic study. *Circulation.* 1986;73:95–99.

44. Lang P, Freed MD, Bierman FZ, Norwood Jr WI, Nadas AS. Use of prostaglandin E1 in infants with d-transposition of the great arteries and intact ventricular septum. *Am J Cardiol.* 1979;44:76–81.

45. Graham Jr TP, Atwood GF, Boucek Jr RJ, Boerth RC, Nelson JH. Right heart volume characteristics in transposition of the great arteries. *Circulation.* 1975;51:881–889.

46. Huhta JC, Edwards WD, Feldt RH, Puga FJ. Left ventricular wall thickness in complete transposition of the great arteries. *J Thorac Cardiovasc Surg.* 1982;84:97–101.

47. Keane JF, Ellison RC, Rudd M, Nadas AS. Pulmonary blood flow and left ventricular volumes in transposition of the great arteries and intact ventricular septum. *Br Heart J.* 1973;35:521–526.

48. Maroto E, Fouron JC, Douste-Blazy MY, et al. Influence of age on wall thickness, cavity dimensions and myocardial contractility of the left ventricle in simple transposition of the great arteries. *Circulation.* 1983;67:1311–1317.

49. Smith A, Wilkinson JL, Arnold R, Dickinson DF, Anderson RH. Growth and development of ventricular walls in complete transposition of the great arteries with intact septum (simple transposition). *Am J Cardiol.* 1982;49:362–368.

50. Van Doesburg NH, Bierman FZ, Williams RG. Left ventricular geometry in infants with d-transposition of the great arteries and intact interventricular septum. *Circulation.* 1983;68:733–739.

51. Daliento L, Cuman G, Isabella G, et al. Ventricular development and function in complete transposition: angiocardiographic evaluation. *Int J Cardiol.* 1986;12:341–352.

52. Hurwitz RA, Caldwell RL, Girod DA, Mahony L, Brown J, King H. Ventricular function in transposition of the great arteries: evaluation by radionuclide angiocardiography. *Am Heart J.* 1985;110:600–605.

53. Newfeld EA, Paul MM, Muster AJ, Idriss FS. Pulmonary vascular disease in complete transposition of the great arteries: a study of 200 patients. *Am J Cardiol.* 1974;34:75–82.

54. Wagenvoort CA, Nauta J, Van Der Schaar PJ, Weeda HW, Wagenvoort N. The pulmonary vasculature in complete transposition of the great vessels, judged from lung biopsies. *Circulation.* 1968;38:746–754.

55. Yamaki S, Tezuka F. Quantitative analysis of pulmonary vascular disease in complete transposition of the great arteries. *Circulation.* 1976;54:805–809.

56. Haworth SG, Radley-Smith R, Yacoub M. Lung biopsy findings in transposition of the great arteries with ventricular septal defect: potentially reversible pulmonary vascular disease is not always synonymous with operability. *J Am Coll Cardiol.* 1987;9:327–333.

57. Dick 2nd M, Heidelberger K, Crowley D, Rosenthal A, Hees P. Quantitative morphometric analysis of the pulmonary arteries in two patients with D-transposition of the great arteries and persistence of the fetal circulation. *Pediatr Res.* 1981;15:1397–1401.

58. Rabinovitch M, Haworth SG, Castaneda AR, Nadas AS, Reid LM. Lung biopsy in congenital heart disease: a morphometric approach to pulmonary vascular disease. *Circulation.* 1978;58:1107–1122.

59. Aziz KU, Paul MH, Rowe RD. Bronchopulmonary circulation in d-transposition of the great arteries: possible role in genesis of accelerated pulmonary vascular disease. *Am J Cardiol.* 1977;39:432–438.

60. Viles PH, Ongley PA, Titus JL. The spectrum of pulmonary vascular disease in transposition of the great arteries. *Circulation.* 1969;40:31–41.

61. Newfeld EA, Paul MH, Muster AJ, Idriss FS. Pulmonary vascular disease in transposition of the great vessels and intact ventricular septum. *Circulation.* 1979;59:525–530.

62. Flyer DC. Report of the New England Regional Infant Cardiac Program. *Pediatrics.* 1980;65:375–461.

63. Digilio MC, Casey B, Toscano A, et al. Complete transposition of the great arteries: patterns of congenital heart disease in familial precurrence. *Circulation.* 2001;104:2809–2814.

64. Shaher RM, Kidd L. Acid-base balance in complete transposition of the great vessels. *Br Heart J.* 1967;29:207–211.

65. Maeno YV, Kamenir SA, Sinclair B, Van Der Velde ME, Smallhorn JF, Hornberger LK. Prenatal features of ductus arteriosus constriction and restrictive foramen ovale in d-transposition of the great arteries. *Circulation.* 1999;99:1209.

66. Schmaltz AA, Knab I, Seybold-Epting W, Apitz J. Prognosis of children with transposition of the great arteries, treated in a regional heart centre between 1967 and 1979. *Eur Heart J.* 1982;3:570–576.

67. Sterns LP, Baker RM, Edwards JE. Complete transposition of the great vessels. Unusual longevity in a case with subpulmonary stenosis. *Circulation.* 1964;29(suppl):610–613.

68. Nichol AD, Segal AJ. Complete transposition of the main arterial stems; report of a case. *J Am Med Assoc.* 1951;147:645–648.
69. Shaher RM. Prognosis of transposition of the great vessels with and without atrial septal defect. *Br Heart J.* 1963;25:211–218.
70. Kato K. Congenital transposition of cardiac vessels: a clinical and pathologic study. *Arch Pediatr Adolesc Med.* 1930;39:363.
71. Fischbein CA, Rosenthal A, Fischer EG, Nadas AS, Welch K. Risk factors of brain abscess in patients with congenital heart disease. *Am J Cardiol.* 1974;34:97–102.
72. Rosenthal GL, Wilson PD, Permutt T, Boughman JA, Ferencz C. Birth weight and cardiovascular malformations: a population-based study. The Baltimore-Washington Infant Study. *Am J Epidemiol.* 1991;133:1273–1281.
73. Cleland WP, Goodwin JF, Steiner RE, Zoob M. Transposition of the aorta and pulmonary artery with pulmonary stenosis. *Am Heart J.* 1957;54:10–22.
74. Mathew R, Rosenthal A, Fellows K. The significance of right aortic arch in D-transposition of the great arteries. *Am Heart J.* 1974;87:314–317.
75. Wells B. The sounds and murmurs in transposition of the great vessels. *Br Heart J.* 1963;25:748–754.
76. Perloff JK. Auscultatory and phonocardiographic manifestations of pulmonary hypertension. *Prog Cardiovasc Dis.* 1967;9:303–340.
77. Fouron JC, Douste-Blazy MY, Ducharme G, Van Doesburg N, Davignon A. Hang-out time of pulmonary valve in d-transposition of great arteries. *Br Heart J.* 1982;47:277–280.
78. Zuberbuhler JR, Bauersfeld SR, Pontius RG. Paradoxic splitting of the second sound with transposition of the great vessels. *Am Heart J.* 1967;74:816–819.
79. Calleja HB, Hosier DM, Grajo MZ. The electrocardiogram in complete transposition of the great vessels. *Am Heart J.* 1965;69:31–40.
80. Shaher RM, Deuchar DC. The electrocardiogram in complete transposition of the great vessels. *Br Heart J.* 1966;28:265–275.
81. Elliott LP, Anderson RC, Tuna N, Adams Jr P, Neufeld HN. Complete transposition of the great vessels: II. An electrocardiographic analysis. *Circulation.* 1963;27:1118.
82. Khoury GH, Shaher RM, Fowler RS, Keith JD. Preoperative and postoperative electrocardiogram in complete transposition of the great vessels. *Am Heart J.* 1966;72:199–205.
83. Vidne BA, Duszynski D, Subramanian S. Pulmonary blood flow distribution in transposition of the great arteries. *Am J Cardiol.* 1976;38:62–66.
84. Carey LS, Elliott LP. Complete transposition of the great vessels. Roentgenographic findings. *Am J Roentgenol Radium Ther Nucl Med.* 1964;91:529–543.
85. Jue KL, Adams Jr P, Pryor R, Blount Jr SG, Edwards JE. Complete transposition of the great vessels in total situs inversus. Anatomic, electrocardiographic and radiologic observations. *Am J Cardiol.* 1966;17:389–394.
86. Schneeweiss A, Blieden LC, Shem-Tov A, Fiegal A, Neufeld HN. Wide vascular pedicle on thoracic roentgenogram in complete transposition of the great arteries. *Clin Cardiol.* 1982;5:75–77.
87. Bream PR, Elliott LP, Bargeron Jr LM. Plain film findings of anatomically corrected malposition: its association with juxtaposition of the atrial appendages and right aortic arch. *Radiology.* 1978;126:589–595.
88. Pasquini L, Sanders SP, Parness IA, et al. Conal anatomy in 119 patients with d-loop transposition of the great arteries and ventricular septal defect: an echocardiographic and pathologic study. *J Am Coll Cardiol.* 1993;21:1712–1721.
89. Moro E, Ten Cate FJ, Tirtaman C, Leonard JJ, Roelandt J. Doppler and two-dimensional echocardiographic observations of systolic anterior motion of the mitral valve in d-transposition of the great arteries: an explanation of the left ventricular outflow tract gradient. *J Am Coll Cardiol.* 1986;7:889–893.
90. Vitarelli A, D'Addio AP, Gentile R, Burattini M. Echocardiographic evaluation of left ventricular outflow tract obstruction in complete transposition of the great arteries. *Am Heart J.* 1984;108:531–538.
91. Kim SJ, Kim WH, Lim C, Oh SS, Kim YM. Commissural malalignment of aortic-pulmonary sinus in complete transposition of great arteries. *Ann Thorac Surg.* 2003;76:1906–1910.
92. Riggs TW, Muster AJ, Aziz KU, Paul MH, Ilbawi M, Idriss FS. Two-dimensional echocardiographic and angiocardiographic diagnosis of subpulmonary stenosis due to tricuspid valve pouch in complete transposition of the great arteries. *J Am Coll Cardiol.* 1983;1:484–491.
93. Rice MJ, Seward JB, Hagler DJ, Edwards WD, Julsrud PR, Tajik AJ. Left juxtaposed atrial appendages: diagnostic two-dimensional echocardiographic features. *J Am Coll Cardiol.* 1983;1:1330–1336.

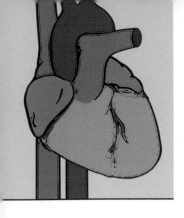

Chapter 28

Truncus Arteriosus

Truncus arteriosus was recognized in 1798,[1] and the clinical and necropsy findings were described in 1864.[2] Humphreys summarized the reports up to 1932, and Lev and Saphir[3] critically reviewed published accounts during the following decade. The malformation accounts for approximately 1% to 2% of cases of congenital heart disease at necropsy and approximately 0.7% to 1.2% of all congenital cardiac malformations.[4]

Truncus arteriosus is characterized by a single great artery with a single semilunar valve that leaves the base of the heart and gives rise to the coronary, pulmonary, and systemic circulations.[4-7] A second semilunar valve is neither present nor implied. The single arterial trunk receives the output from both ventricles, so a ventricular septal defect is obligatory.[4,5,8] Type IV, or pseudotruncus with a biventricular aorta and an atretic pulmonary valve, is now uniformly considered to be a form of pulmonary atresia with ventricular septal defect rather than truncus arteriosus (see Chapter 18).[9] Edwards, with disarming candor, stated, "Twenty-eight years after the introduction of the term, we doubt that the condition which Collett and Edwards had called truncus Type IV exists."[5] Similarly, a solitary pulmonary trunk referred to in 1814 by Farrell[10] is considered to be a variety of aortic atresia.[11,12] *Hemitruncus*, a term no longer used, referred to a rare anomaly in which one pulmonary artery branch arose from the ascending aorta just above the aortic sinuses and in which the main pulmonary artery with the other branch arose in its normal position.[13,14] Rarely, the main pulmonary artery arises anteriorly and proximally at the level of the sinus of the common arterial trunk.[15]

The truncus is large because it accepts the entire output of both systemic and pulmonary circulations (Figures 28-1 and 28-2A), although inherent medial abnormalities contribute to the dilation.[16] Agenesis of the ductus arteriosus occurs in 50% to 75% of cases,[4,7,17] which is not surprising because a fetal ductus is not needed to channel pulmonary arterial blood into the aorta.[18]

The greatest anatomic variability is in the branching patterns of the common trunk.[19,20] In 1949, Collett and Edwards[5] classified truncus arteriosus into four types based on the origins of the pulmonary arteries. The first three types were reconsidered by van Praagh and van Praagh[7] in 1965 and form the basis of current terminology (Figure 28-3). Type 4 is now regarded as pulmonary atresia with ventricular septal defect (see previous and see Chapter 18). The most common variety is type 1, which is characterized by a short main pulmonary artery that originates from the truncus and gives rise to the right and left pulmonary arteries (Figures 28-2A, 28-4, and 28-5).[7] Type 2 and type 3 of Collett and Edwards were originally defined by right and left pulmonary arteries that arose from separate ostia at either the side or the back of the truncus (see Figure 28-3).[4,5] These two types are now grouped within a single category referred to as type 2 (see Figures 28-1B, and 28-3).[7] In about 15% of cases, the right or left pulmonary artery is absent or hypoplastic (Figure 28-4B). An absent[21] or hypoplastic pulmonary artery is usually concordant with the side of the aortic arch,[22] which is right-sided in as many as 30% of patients with truncus arteriosus (see Figures 28-1 and 28-5).[4,7,19,23] Rarely, there is a double aortic arch[24,25] or an interrupted aortic arch.[26]

In approximately two thirds of patients, the truncal valve has three leaflets, and its has either two leaflets (bicuspid) or four leaflets (quadricuspid) in most of the others. Very rarely, the valve is pentacuspid or hexacuspid (see Figures 28-10 and 28-22).[19] A normal trileaflet aortic valve differs from a trileaflet truncal valve because of the presence of truncal raphes and cuspal inequality and because trileaflet truncal valves tend to be thickened and focally or diffusely dysplastic.[17,27,28] A trileaflet truncal valve with raphes and cusps in excess of three represents a morphogenetic combination of aortic and pulmonary valves.[7] Truncal valves are poorly supported therefore and are frequently incompetent.[4,29] Stenotic truncal valves are less common,[4,27,30,31] may be dysplastic,[32] and may calcify in older adults.[33]

The *coronary arteries in truncus arteriosus* are defined by their relationship to the truncal sinuses and by their epicardial courses (see Figure 32-12).[7,8,34–36] Coronary arterial ostia appear after division of the embryonic truncus is complete during normal morphogenesis.[37] There are initially six coronary artery anlagen (primordia), three from the aorta and three from the pulmonary artery.[38] Anlagen in the three pulmonary sinuses and in one of the aortic sinus normally undergo involution, leaving two coronary arteries that arise from two persistent anlagen in the right and left aortic sinuses. In truncus arteriosus, the sinus substrates to which coronary arteries are assigned are influenced by failure of septation of the embryonic truncus and by developmental abnormalities of the truncal valve.[34,36] The left coronary artery tends to arise from the left posterior aspect of the truncus, and the right coronary artery tends to arise from the right anterior aspect of the truncus,

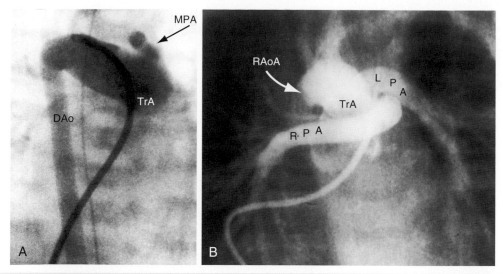

FIGURE 28-1 A, Angiogram from a week-old female with truncus arteriosus type 1 (TrA). A main pulmonary artery (MPA) arose from the truncus that continued as a right aortic arch and a right descending aorta (DAo). **B,** Angiogram from a 4-month-old female with truncus arteriosus type 2. Separate right and left pulmonary arteries (RPA, LPA) arose by separate ostia from the truncus, which continued as a right aortic arch (RAoA).

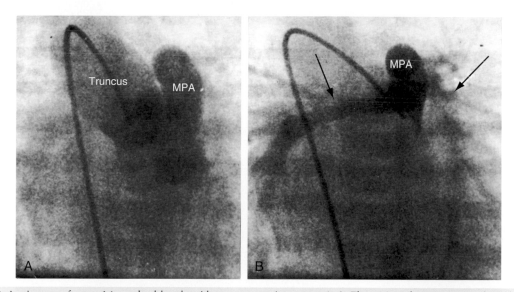

FIGURE 28-2 Angiograms from a 14-week-old male with truncus arteriosus type 1. **A,** The main pulmonary artery (MPA) arose directly from the truncus. **B,** The right and left branches (two unmarked arrows) arose from the main pulmonary artery.

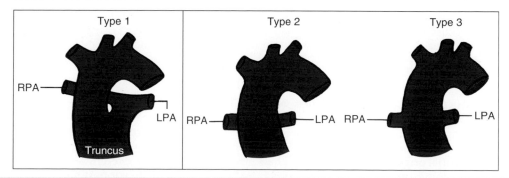

FIGURE 28-3 Illustrations of three anatomic types of truncus arteriosus. Type 1: A short main pulmonary artery originates from the truncus and gives rise to right and left pulmonary arteries (RPA, LPA). Type 2 and type 3: Right and left pulmonary arteries arise by separate ostia directly from the posterior or lateral wall of the truncus. Type 2 and type 3 are now considered as one category.

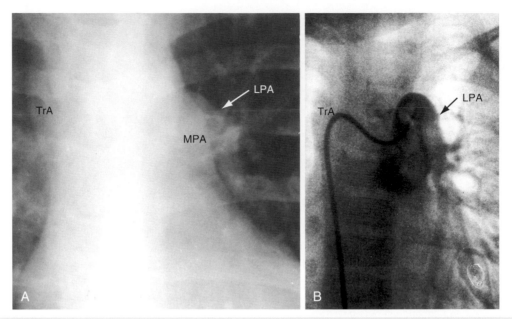

FIGURE 28-4 X-rays from a 7-year-old boy with truncus arteriosus type 1. **A,** The truncus (TrA) formed a right aortic arch. A main pulmonary artery (MPA) arose directly from the truncus and bifurcated into a left pulmonary artery (LPA) and a right pulmonary artery (not shown). The left pulmonary artery formed a hilar comma, which was delineated in the accompanying angiogram. **B,** Angiogram from a 16-month-old boy with truncus arteriosus type 1 and a right aortic arch. The left pulmonary artery (LPA) formed a distinctive hilar comma. The right pulmonary artery was absent.

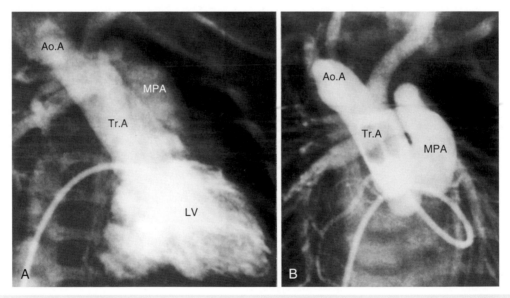

FIGURE 28-5 Angiocardiograms from a male neonate with truncus arteriosus type 1 and DiGeorge syndrome (see Figure 28-6). **A,** The left ventriculogram (LV) visualized the truncus (Tr.A) that continued as a right aortic arch (AoA). The main pulmonary artery (MPA) originated directly from the truncus. **B,** Contrast material into the truncus delineated a main pulmonary artery originating directly from the truncus and continuing as a right aortic arch (AoA).

whether the truncal valve is bicuspid, tricuspid, or quadricuspid (see Figure 32-12).[8] When the truncal valve is quadricuspid, which is usually the case, coronary artery orifices originate in opposite sinuses rather than in adjacent sinuses, and high ostial origins are frequent.[8,36] The right coronary artery is dominant in about 85% of cases; the conus branch of the right coronary artery is large, and the left anterior descending artery is small.[8] There is an increased incidence of single coronary artery (see

Chapter 32).[34,36] An ostial membrane of the left coronary artery has been reported.[39]

A ventricular septal defect results from absence or deficiency of the infundibular septum and is almost always nonrestrictive and roofed by the truncal valve, setting the stage for inadequate support and truncal valve regurgitation.[40] The biventricular truncal valve is assigned equally to the two ventricles, or predominantly to the right ventricle but only infrequently to the left ventricle.[4,6,17]

Cardiovascular anomalies commonly associated with truncus arteriosus include a right aortic arch (see previous and see Figures 28-1 and 28-5), truncal valve abnormalities (see previous and see Figures 28-10 and 28-22), anomalies of origin and distribution of the coronary arteries (see previous and see Figure 32-12), absence of the right or left pulmonary artery (see Figure 28-4B), and atresia of the ductus arteriosus. *Abnormalities that occur sporadically* include single ventricle, aberrant subclavian artery, left superior vena cava, and total anomalous pulmonary venous connection.[41,42] When truncus arteriosus occurs with complete interruption of the aortic arch, the interruption is distal to the origin of the left carotid artery.[17] The left subclavian artery arises from the descending aorta, and a patent ductus provides continuity from truncus to descending aorta.[17]

A common arterial trunk is a feature of normal early embryogenesis, an understanding of which sheds light on the morphogenesis of persistent truncus arteriosus.[43,44] Septation of the arterial pole of the normal heart begins with the appearance of two opposing truncal cushions that rapidly enlarge and fuse to form the truncal septum. The proximal truncal septum normally fuses with the distal infundibular septum, a process that completes the spiral division of the truncus arteriosus and establishes left ventricular origin of the aorta and right ventricular origin of the pulmonary trunk. The aortic and pulmonary valves and their sinuses develop from truncal tissue at the line of fusion of the truncal and infundibular septa. In persistent truncus arteriosus, the truncal septum fails to develop. The infundibular septum is deficient or absent, which is responsible for a nonrestrictive ventricular septal defect roofed by the truncal valve. Vestigial development of the distal truncal septum is responsible for a short main pulmonary artery that arises from the truncus. When the truncal septum is absent altogether with no vestigial remnant, the main pulmonary artery is also absent, so the right and left pulmonary arteries arise directly from the truncus by separate ostia.

Physiologic consequences of truncus arteriosus depend on the size of the pulmonary arteries and on the pulmonary vascular resistance. Right ventricular pressure is identical with systemic because both ventricles communicate directly with the biventricular truncus via the nonrestrictive ventricular septal defect. When a main pulmonary artery arises directly from the truncus, blood flow from the left and right ventricles tends to cross, so oxygen content is higher in the aorta than in the pulmonary artery. Systemic arterial oxygen saturation is high when pulmonary resistance is low and pulmonary blood flow is increased, an advantage purchased at the price of volume overload of the left ventricle and congestive heart failure. Truncal valve regurgitation or truncal valve stenosis adds to the hemodynamic burden of the volume-overloaded left ventricle[4,30] and to the hemodynamic derangements that are imposed on the right ventricle because of the biventricular truncus. As pulmonary vascular resistance rises, pulmonary blood flow falls. Volume overload of the left ventricle is curtailed at the price of increased cyanosis. Occasionally, pulmonary blood flow is adequately regulated by mild to moderate hypoplasia of both pulmonary arteries. In patients with truncus arteriosus and an absent right or left pulmonary artery, early vascular disease develops in the contralateral pulmonary artery (see Figure 28-16A).[22]

HISTORY

Truncus arteriosus occurs with equal frequency in males and females.[17] Isolated examples have been reported in siblings[17,45–47] and in twins,[48–50] and a relatively high incidence rate of congenital cardiac malformations is found in siblings of children with truncus arteriosus. Familial recurrence of nonsyndromic truncus with interrupted aortic arch has been described.[51] Truncus arteriosis has been reported with chromosome 22q11 deletion,[15,52] trisomy 18,[53] and trisomy 21.

Truncus arteriosus comes to attention in the first few weeks of life because of tachypnea, diaphoresis, poor feeding, and failure to thrive. As pulmonary resistance falls, pulmonary blood flow increases and neonatal cyanosis diminishes or may virtually vanish. Truncal valve regurgitation is responsible for biventricular failure because regurgitant flow is received by both ventricles. A systolic murmur awaits the fall in neonatal pulmonary vascular resistance analogous to the time course with ventricular septal defect (see Chapter 17).

Infants with truncus arteriosus seldom reach their first birthday.[5,17,54] Most die of congestive heart failure in the first few months of life. In van Praagh and van Praagh's[7] necropsy series, mean age at death was 5 weeks. A rise in pulmonary vascular resistance occasionally regulates pulmonary blood flow and relieves the volume-overloaded left ventricle, so symptoms of congestive heart failure improve while cyanosis deepens. A small but not insignificant number of patients reach their third, fourth, or fifth decade (see Figures 28-15 through 28-18),[5,54–57] with an occasional survival into the sixth[58,59] or seventh decade.[60] A patient with truncus arteriosus "type 4" survived to age 54 years.[61] Patients with truncus arteriosus and Eisenmenger's syndrome are subject to the multisystem systemic disorders described in Chapter 17. Rarely, death is from sudden intramural dissection and rupture of the common trunk.[62] Morbidity and mortality are also influenced by a host of noncardiac abnormalities that coexist with truncus arteriosus, as described subsequently.

PHYSICAL APPEARANCE

Infants with increased pulmonary blood flow and congestive heart failure are frail and have poor development. Cyanosis is inconspicuous or absent. When truncus arteriosus occurs with hypoplasia of a pulmonary artery, the ipsilateral hemithorax tends to be small (see Figure 28-16A).[4] A distinctive appearance in truncus arteriosus is DiGeorge syndrome, which includes hypertelorism, low-set ears, micrognathia, a small fishlike mouth, a short philtrum, short down-slanting palpebral fissures, deformed or absent pinnae, cleft lip, a high-arched or cleft palate, a malformed nose, and bilateral cataracts (Figure 28-6).[63–66] Extracardiac congenital abnormalities involve the limbs, kidneys, and intestines.[64] Infants experience hypocalcemic

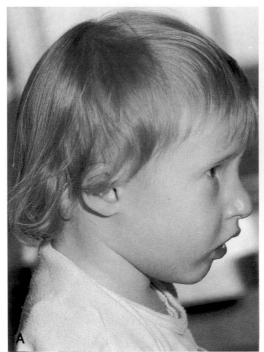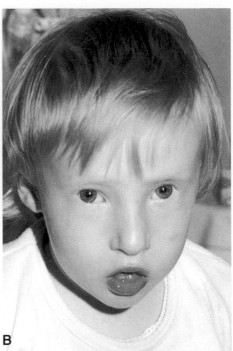

FIGURE 28-6 A 2-year-old girl with truncus arteriosus, DiGeorge syndrome, and facial dysmorphism represented by hypertelorism, low-set ears, micrognathia, a small fish-like mouth, a short philtrum, a malformed nose, and down-slanting palpebral fissures. (From Radford DJ, Perkins L, Lachman R, Thong YH. Spectrum of Di George syndrome in patients with truncus arteriosus: expanded Di George syndrome, *Pediatric Cardiology* 1988;9:95.)

seizures and severe infections as a result of deficient cell-mediated immunity and absence of the thymus and parathyroid glands.[64] The CHARGE association includes coloboma, heart disease, choanal atresia, retardation of growth and of mental development, genital hypoplasia, and ear anomalies.[67] Conotruncal anomalies, especially truncus arteriosus, have been reported in 42% of patients with CHARGE association.[67]

ARTERIAL PULSE

The pulse pressure is wide because low pulmonary vascular resistance permits a diastolic runoff from the truncus into the pulmonary bed (Figure 28-7). The rate of rise of the arterial pulse is brisk because of rapid ejection of a large left ventricular stroke volume. A brisk arterial pulse is especially noteworthy in the context of left ventricular failure and pulsus alternans (see Figure 28-7). Truncal valve regurgitation independently causes a bounding arterial pulse analogous to the water-hammer pulse of aortic regurgitation.[4,29]

JUGULAR VENOUS PULSE

In infants with congestive heart failure, the jugular veins are distended, the liver is enlarged, and waveform or a liver pulse cannot be identified. In adults with truncus arteriosus and Eisenmenger's syndrome, the jugular venous pulse is normal or nearly so, analogous to the jugular pulse in Eisenmenger's syndrome with nonrestrictive ventricular septal defect (see Chapter 17).

PRECORDIAL MOVEMENT AND PALPATION

The impulse of a volume-overloaded hyperdynamic left ventricle is accompanied by a parasternal and subxiphoid impulse of a systemic right ventricle. Both impulses are augmented by regurgitant flow across an incompetent biventricular truncal valve. The main pulmonary artery of type 1 truncus arteriosus can be palpated in the second left intercostal space. The second heart sound is palpable because the truncal valve closes at systemic pressure and because truncal dilation brings the valve closer to the chest wall. A systolic thrill appears at the left midsternal edge as neonatal pulmonary vascular resistance falls and the left ventricle ejects a large stroke volume through the ventricular septal defect. A right sternoclavicular impulse indicates a right aortic arch.

In adults with truncus arteriosus and pulmonary vascular disease, the left ventricle is not volume-overloaded and right ventricular pressure remains systemic, so the precordial impulse is from the right ventricle alone. Biventricular regurgitation across the truncal valve makes both ventricles palpable irrespective of pulmonary vascular resistance.

AUSCULTATION

A normal first heart sound is followed by a high-pitched ejection sound generated within the dilated truncus (Figures 28-8 and 28-9).[68] The systolic murmur through

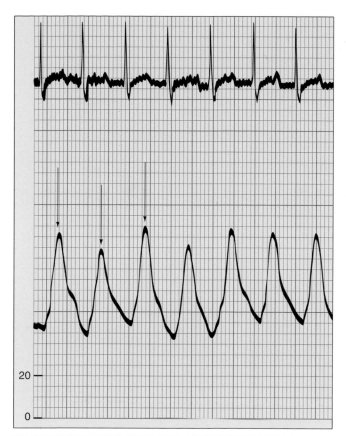

FIGURE 28-7 Aortic pressure pulse from an 18-day-old female with truncus arteriosus type 1. A short main pulmonary artery arose directly from the truncus and bifurcated into large right and left branches. The pulse pressure is wide. The rate of rise is brisk despite depressed left ventricular function indicated by pulsus alternans (arrows).

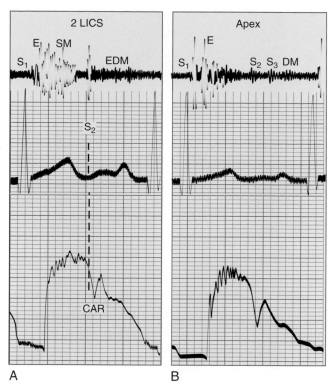

FIGURE 28-9 Phonocardiograms from an 11-year-old boy with truncus arteriosus type 2. The right and left pulmonary arteries arose directly from the truncus. **A,** In the second left intercostal space (2 LICS), an ejection sound (E) was recorded followed by a prominent decrescendo systolic murmur (SM) that ends before a loud single second sound (S_2). A decrescendo early diastolic murmur (EDM) of truncal valve regurgitation issued from the single second heart sound. (CAR = carotid; S_1 = first heart sound.) **B,** The third heart sound (S_3) and short mid-diastolic murmur (DM) were recorded at the apex, together with the transmitted ejection sound and systolic murmur.

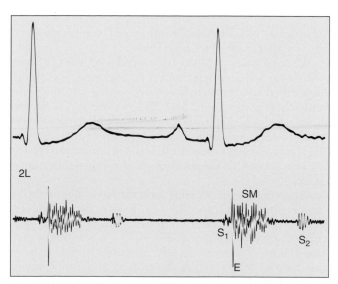

FIGURE 28-8 Phonocardiogram in the second left intercostal space (2L) of a 3-week-old male with truncus arteriosus type 2. The first heart sound (S_1) is followed by an ejection sound (E) and an early systolic decrescendo murmur (SM) that ended well before the second heart sound (S_2).

the ventricular septal defect and into the truncus is decrescendo, beginning with the ejection sound and ending before the second heart sound (see Figures 28-8 and 28-9).[68] The murmur is harsh, blowing, and usually grade 3/6 to 4/6, with maximal intensity in the third or fourth left intercostal space. Radiation is upward and to the right because a truncus takes the course of an ascending aorta (see Figure 28-5). The murmur is more prominent when the biventricular truncus arises chiefly above the right ventricle and is less prominent and often midsystolic when the truncus arises chiefly above the left ventricle, or when pulmonary vascular disease minimizes the shunt. Flow is then across the truncal valve rather than across the ventricular septal defect. When the truncal valve is thickened, dysplastic, or stenotic, the murmur is midsystolic, as in aortic stenosis (see Chapter 7).

Murmurs that are confined to systole, or continuous murmurs that are louder in systole, are generated at the origins of hypoplastic pulmonary arteries as they emerge from the truncus. Continuous murmurs are seldom generated by the systemic arterial collaterals that supply the ipsilateral lung when a pulmonary artery is absent.

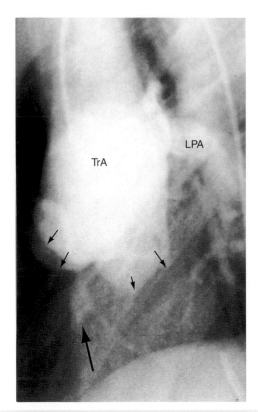

FIGURE 28-10 Lateral angiocardiogram from a 6-year-old boy with type 2 truncus arteriosus (TrA) and an incompetent quadricuspid truncal valve (four small arrows). (LPA [large arrow] = left pulmonary artery.)

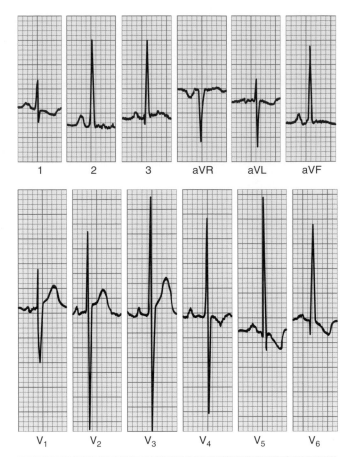

FIGURE 28-11 Electrocardiogram from a 3-week-old male with truncus arteriosus type 1. Peaked right atrial P waves appear in leads 2 and aVF and in mid precordial leads. The QRS axis is normal. Left ventricular hypertrophy is indicated by tall R waves and inverted T waves in leads V_{5-6}. Biventricular hypertrophy is reflected in the large equidiphasic RS complexes in leads V_{2-4}.

The truncal valve closure sound is prominent because the enlarged truncus is closer to the chest wall and because the truncal valve closes at systemic pressure (see Figure 28-9). Splitting is not be possible because the truncus is equipped with only one valve. However, the second heart sound arising from a truncal valve that is equipped with three or more well-formed cusps may be impure or reduplicated, but phonocardiograms show that the vibrations merge and do not separate into two distinct sounds separated by an interval. On the other hand, the phonocardiogram occasionally records two components that have been attributed to cuspal inequality with asynchronous closure of tricuspid or quadricuspid truncal valves.[68]

A high-frequency blowing early diastolic murmur is caused by truncal valve regurgitation (Figures 28-9A and 28-10).[4,29] An apical mid-diastolic murmur introduced by a third heart sound (Figure 28-9B) results from increased mitral valve flow in response to increased pulmonary blood flow. Mid-diastolic or presystolic Austin Flint murmurs are thought to be associated with severe truncal valve regurgitation.

ELECTROCARDIOGRAM

Tall peaked right atrial P waves appear in limb leads and in precordial leads (Figures 28-11 and 28-12) and are often accompanied by notched bifid left atrial P waves.[69]

Infants may exhibit isolated left atrial P waves generated by increased pulmonary blood flow.

When pulmonary blood flow is reduced, the QRS axis is rightward and depolarization is clockwise because an underfilled left ventricle is coupled with a systemic right ventricle (Figures 28-12 and 28-13). The axis is normal or leftward when increased pulmonary blood flow overloads the left ventricle (see Figure 28-11).[4] However, the conduction system and QRS axis in truncus arteriosus are also related to the location of the ventricular septal defect.[70]

Precordial leads exhibit biventricular hypertrophy (see Figures 28-11 and 28-12). Pure right ventricular hypertrophy is reserved for adults with pulmonary vascular disease (see Figure 28-13).[4,59] When pulmonary blood flow is increased, left precordial leads exhibit the deep Q waves, tall R waves, and inverted T waves of left ventricular hypertrophy, and right precordial leads continue to display the tall R waves of right ventricular hypertrophy (see Figures 28-11 and 28-12). Large equidiphasic QRS complexes in central chest leads indicate combined ventricular hypertrophy (see Figure 28-11).

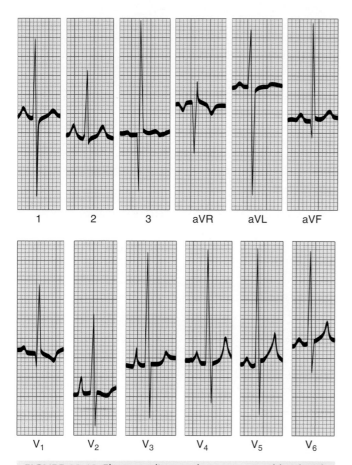

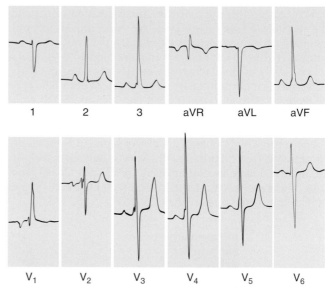

FIGURE 28-13 Electrocardiogram from a 42-year-old man with truncus arteriosus type 1 and pulmonary vascular disease. His x-rays are shown in Figure 28-18. The P wave in lead 2 is slightly peaked. The negative P terminal force in lead V_1 is a right atrial abnormality. There is right axis deviation. Right ventricular hypertrophy is manifested by a tall monophasic R wave in lead V_1, by deep S waves in left precordial leads, and by increased amplitude of the R waves in leads 3 and aVF. The R waves in leads V_{4-5} indicate that the left ventricle is well-developed.

FIGURE 28-12 Electrocardiogram from a 2-year-old girl with truncus arteriosus type 1 and absent left pulmonary artery. Tall peaked right atrial P waves appear in lead 2 and in leads V_{2-4}. The Q wave in lead V_1 reflects right atrial enlargement. The QRS axis is +90 degrees. Right ventricular hypertrophy is manifested by the tall monophasic R wave in lead V_1 and by the prominent S waves in leads V_{4-6}. Left ventricular hypertrophy is manifested by the tall R waves and peaked T waves in leads V_{4-6} and by tall R waves in leads 3 and aVF.

X-RAY

Increased pulmonary vascularity is a combination of both pulmonary arterial blood flow and pulmonary venous congestion (Figure 28-14). The main pulmonary artery segment is absent when right and left pulmonary arteries arise directly from the truncus (see Figure 28-14B). The concave profile stands out in the right anterior oblique projection (see Figure 28-17B). A dilated left pulmonary

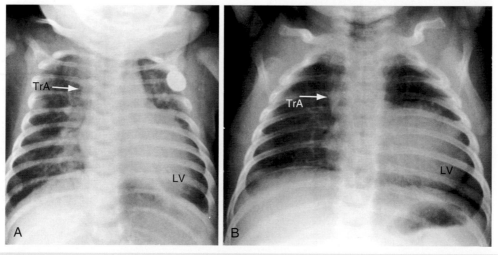

FIGURE 28-14 A, X-ray from a 3-week-old male with truncus arteriosus type 1 that revealed itself at the right base (TrA, arrow). Pulmonary vascularity is increased, and the left ventricle (LV) is markedly dilated. **B,** X-ray from a 2-month-old male with truncus arteriosus type 2. The truncus is evident at the right base (TrA, arrow). A main pulmonary artery is conspicuously absent. Pulmonary vascularity is increased. The left ventricle (LV) is strikingly dilated.

artery may occupy the concavity, but its shadow can usually be recognized (see Figure 28-17A). A prominent left pulmonary artery may reveal itself as a high shadow that curves upward to form a left hilar comma (see Figure 28-4), which is especially evident when the aortic arch is right-sided.[4] The convex main pulmonary artery segment of truncus type 1 tends to arise at a higher level (see Figure 28-18) compared with other forms of pulmonary artery dilation. In older adults with pulmonary vascular disease, the dilated hypertensive main pulmonary artery segment is especially prominent (see Figure 28-18). A large truncus arteriosus resembles a large ascending aorta (see Figure 28-14) that may continue as a right aortic arch (see Figure 28-5) and a high transverse aorta (Figure 28-15).

The left ventricle dilates in response to volume overload–associated increased pulmonary blood flow (see Figures 28-14 and 28-15A). Enlargement of the right ventricle and right atrium accompany congestive heart failure and occur when the right ventricle receives regurgitant flow across an incompetent biventricular truncal valve. Hypoplasia or absence of a pulmonary artery results in reduced pulmonary vascularity and a smaller ipsilateral hemithorax (Figure 28-16A). Absence of a pulmonary artery is usually on the same side as the aortic arch (see Figure 28-4B),[71] in contrast to Fallot's tetralogy (see Chapter 18).

In adults with high pulmonary vascular resistance, the x-ray shows decreased pulmonary vascularity, increased

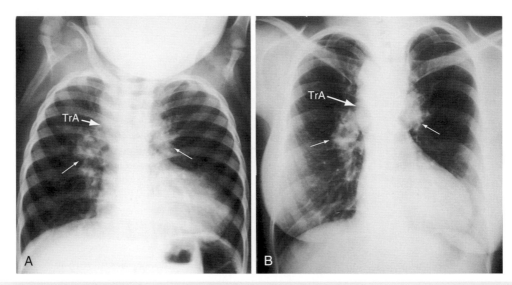

FIGURE 28-15 X-rays at 18 months and at 21 years of age from the same female patient with truncus arteriosus type 2. **A,** The truncus (TrA) continued as a right aortic arch and a high transverse aorta. Two separate pulmonary arteries (unmarked arrows) originated directly from the truncus by separate ostia. Pulmonary vascularity is increased, and the volume-overloaded left ventricle is dilated. **B,** Twenty years later, pulmonary vascular resistance was suprasystemic. Large right and left pulmonary arteries (unmarked arrows) stand out in bold relief against clear lung fields of reduced pulmonary blood flow. The left ventricle remained enlarged because of truncal valve regurgitation.

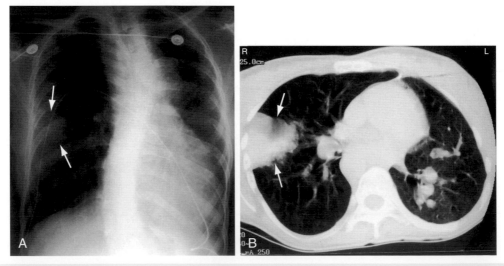

FIGURE 28-16 A, X-ray and, **B,** magnetic resonance image from a 32-year-old woman with truncus arteriosus type 2. Scoliosis rotated the heart into a partial right anterior oblique position. The left pulmonary artery was hypoplastic, the left lung was hypoperfused, and the left hemithorax was small. The right pulmonary artery was normally formed. There was pulmonary vascular disease in the right lung. Arrows bracket a density that the magnetic resonance image identified as intrapulmonary hemorrhage.

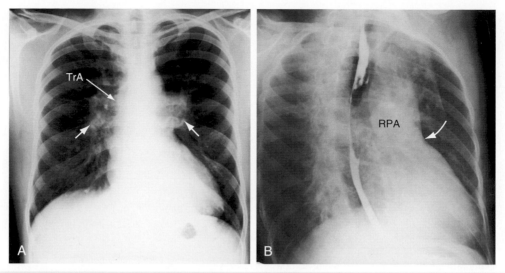

FIGURE 28-17 A, X-rays from a 30-year-old man with truncus arteriosus type 2 (TrA). Pulmonary vascularity was reduced by pulmonary vascular disease. The hypertensive right and left pulmonary arteries are huge (unmarked arrows). **B,** The right anterior oblique projection highlights the absence of a main pulmonary artery segment (unmarked curved arrow) in contrast to enlargement of the pulmonary artery branches. The dilated right pulmonary artery (RPA) is shown end-on.

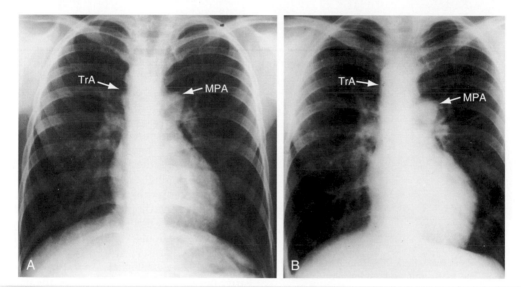

FIGURE 28-18 X-rays at age 10 years **(A)** and at age 42 years **(B)** from the same man with truncus arteriosus type 1 and pulmonary vascular disease. His electrocardiogram is shown in Figure 28-13. The two films are virtually identical except for body size. A dilated main pulmonary artery (MPA) originated from the truncus (TrA) and gave rise to enlarged hypertensive right and left branches. The truncus continued as a right aortic arch, a high transverse aorta, and a right descending aorta. Pulmonary vascularity was reduced because of pulmonary vascular disease. The left ventricle is convex but of normal size.

prominence of the main pulmonary artery and its right and left branches, and a relatively normal left ventricle (Figures 28-17 and 28-18).

ECHOCARDIOGRAM

Echocardiography with color flow imaging and Doppler interrogation establish the type of truncus arteriosus, the relationship of the truncus to the left and right ventricles, the morphologic and functional derangements of the truncal valve, and the physiologic consequences of

the malformation.[19,72,73] A single great arterial trunk overrides a nonrestrictive ventricular septal defect in the infundibular septum (Figures 28-19 and 20-20, and Video 28-1). The truncal valve forms the roof of the defect (see Figure 28-20). Right and left pulmonary arteries either arise from a short main pulmonary artery (see Figures 28-19 and 28-20) or arise directly from the truncus by separate ostia. Biventricular unbalanced right or left ventricular origin of the truncus can be determined (see Figure 28-20), and the morphology of the truncal valve can be established (Figure 28-21). Color flow imaging determines the presence and degree

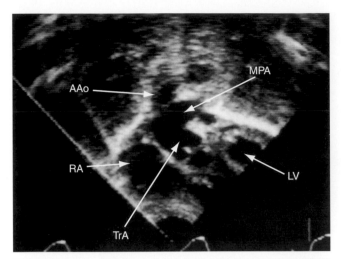

FIGURE 28-19 Echocardiogram (subcostal) showing truncus arteriosus type 1 (TrA) communicating with a main pulmonary artery (MPA) that gave rise to right and left branches. (AAo = ascending aorta; RA = right atrium; LV = left ventricle.)

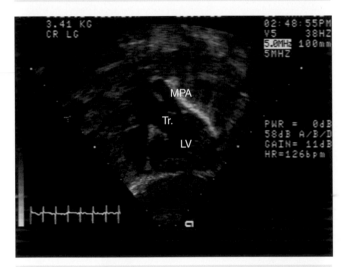

FIGURE 28-20 Echocardiogram (subcostal) from a 3-year-old boy with truncus arteriosus type 1. The biventricular truncus (Tr.) arises above a nonrestrictive ventricular septal that is roofed by the truncal valve. The main pulmonary artery (MPA) arises directly from the truncus (Video 28-1). (LV = left ventricle.)

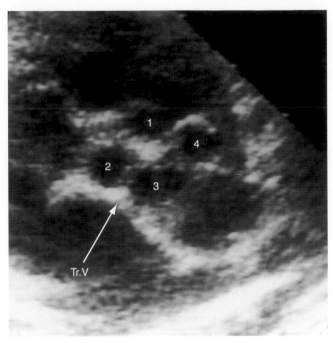

FIGURE 28-21 A quadricuspid truncal valve (Tr.V) in the short axis.

of truncal valve regurgitation, and continuous wave Doppler scan determines the presence and degree of truncal valve stenosis.

SUMMARY

Truncus arteriosus typically comes to attention in early infancy because of the consequences of congestive heart failure caused by increased pulmonary blood flow. Cyanosis is mild or absent. A systolic murmur across the ventricular septal defect becomes evident as neonatal pulmonary vascular resistance falls. The arterial pulse is bounding despite congestive heart failure. Left and right ventricular impulses are conspicuous, and in type 1 truncus, a main pulmonary artery impulse is palpable. Auscultation reveals an ejection sound and a relatively long decrescendo systolic murmur maximal in the third left intercostal space with radiation upward and to the right. A mid-diastolic murmur reflects augmented mitral valve flow. When the shunt across the ventricular septal defect is reduced by increased pulmonary vascular resistance, a soft midsystolic murmur emerges across the truncal valve. The midsystolic truncal murmur is louder and longer when the valve is dysplastic or stenotic. The second heart sound is loud, single, and reduplicated. An early diastolic murmur is caused by truncal valve regurgitation.

The electrocardiogram records right atrial or biatrial P waves, and the QRS pattern exhibits varying degrees of combined ventricular hypertrophy. Pure right ventricular hypertrophy is reserved for adults with elevated pulmonary vascular resistance. The x-ray shows increased vascularity because of increased pulmonary arterial blood flow and pulmonary venous congestion. The truncus often continues as a right aortic arch with a high transverse segment. The main pulmonary artery is prominent in type 1 truncus but is concave when the right and left pulmonary arteries arise directly from the truncus by separate ostia. The left pulmonary artery may form a distinctive hilar comma. The left and right ventricles dilate because of congestive heart failure and in response to biventricular truncal valve regurgitation. In adults with pulmonary vascular disease, the lungs are oligemic and the main pulmonary artery segment and the left and right branches are prominent, but the heart size is normal or nearly so unless the truncal valve is regurgitant or stenotic. Echocardiography with color flow imaging and Doppler interrogation establish the type of truncus arteriosus, the relationship of the truncus to the right and left ventricles, the morphology and functional derangements of the truncal valve, and the physiologic consequences of the malformation.

REFERENCES

1. Wilson J. A description of a very unusual malformation of the human heart. *Philosophical Transactions of the Royal Society of London*. 1798;88:346–356.
2. Buchanan A. Malformation of heart. Undivided truncus arteriosus. Heart otherwise double. *Transactions of the Pathologic Society of London*. 1864;15:89.
3. Lev M, Saphir O. Truncus arteriosus communis persistens. *J Pediatr*. 1942;20:74–88.
4. Calder L, Van Praagh R, Van Praagh S, et al. Truncus arteriosus communis. Clinical, angiocardiographic, and pathologic findings in 100 patients. *Am Heart J*. 1976;92:23–38.
5. Collett RW, Edwards JE. Persistent truncus arteriosus; a classification according to anatomic types. *Surg Clin North Am*. 1949;29: 1245–1270.
6. Van Praagh R. Editorial: classification of truncus arteriosus communis (TAC). *Am Heart J*. 1976;92:129–132.
7. Van Praagh R, van Praagh S. The anatomy of common aorticopulmonary trunk (truncus arteriosus communis) and its embryologic implications. A study of 57 necropsy cases. *Am J Cardiol*. 1965; 16:406–425.
8. Anderson KR, McGoon DC, Lie JT. Surgical significance of the coronary arterial anatomy in truncus arteriosus communis. *Am J Cardiol*. 1978;41:76–81.
9. Kapoor A, Gupta N. Adult survival of persistent truncus arteriosus type IV. *Int J Cardiol*. 2003;88:323; author reply 325.
10. Farrell JR. *Pathological researches. Essay 1. On malformation of the human heart*. London: Longman; 1814.
11. Allwork SP, Bentall RH. Truncus solitarius pulmonalis. *Br Heart J*. 1973;35:977–980.
12. Sennari E, Nishiguchi T, Okishima T, et al. Truncus solitarius pulmonalis. *Pediatr Cardiol*. 1990;11:50–53.
13. Fong LV, Anderson RH, Siewers RD, Trento A, Park SC. Anomalous origin of one pulmonary artery from the ascending aorta: a review of echocardiographic, catheter, and morphological features. *Br Heart J*. 1989;62:389–395.
14. Fontana GP, Spach MS, Effmann EL, Sabiston Jr DC. Origin of the right pulmonary artery from the ascending aorta. *Ann Surg*. 1987; 206:102–113.
15. Phelps CM, Da Cruz E, Fagan T, Younoszai AK, Tissot C. Images in cardiovascular medicine. Anterior origin of the main pulmonary artery from the arterial valvar sinus: unusual truncus arteriosus. *Circulation*. 2009;119:624–627.
16. Niwa K, Perloff JK, Bhuta SM, et al. Structural abnormalities of great arterial walls in congenital heart disease: light and electron microscopic analyses. *Circulation*. 2001;103:393–400.
17. Butto F, Lucas Jr RV, Edwards JE. Persistent truncus arteriosus: pathologic anatomy in 54 cases. *Pediatr Cardiol*. 1986;7:95–101.
18. Mello DM, Mcelhinney DB, Parry AJ, Silverman NH, Hanley FL. Truncus arteriosus with patent ductus arteriosus and normal aortic arch. *Ann Thorac Surg*. 1997;64:1808–1810.
19. Colon M, Anderson RH, Weinberg P, et al. Anatomy, morphogenesis, diagnosis, management, and outcomes for neonates with common arterial trunk. *Cardiol Young*. 2008;18(suppl 3):52–62.
20. Jacobs ML. Congenital Heart Surgery Nomenclature and Database Project: truncus arteriosus. *Ann Thorac Surg*. 2000;69:S50–S55.
21. Wong MNL, Kirk R, Quek SC. Persistent truncus arteriosus with absence of right pulmonary artery. *Heart*. 2003;89:549.
22. Fyfe DA, Driscoll DJ, Di Donato RM, et al. Truncus arteriosus with single pulmonary artery: influence of pulmonary vascular obstructive disease on early and late operative results. *J Am Coll Cardiol*. 1985;5:1168–1172.
23. Hastreiter AR, D'cruz IA, Cantez T, Namin EP, Licata R. Right-sided aorta. I. Occurrence of right aortic arch in various types of congenital heart disease. II. Right aortic arch, right descending aorta, and associated anomalies. *Br Heart J*. 1966; 28:722–739.
24. Bhan A, Gupta M, Kumar MJS, Kothari SS, Gulati GS. Persistent truncus arteriosus with double aortic arch. *Pediatr Cardiol*. 2006; 27:378–380.
25. Huang S-C, Wang C-J, Su W-J, Chu J-J, Hwang M-S. The rare association of truncus arteriosus with a cervical double aortic arch presenting with left main bronchial compression. *Cardiology*. 2008;111:16–20.
26. Verhaert D, Arruda J, Thavendiranathan P, Cook SC, Raman SV. Truncus arteriosus with aortic arch interruption: cardiovascular magnetic resonance findings in the unrepaired adult. *J Cardiovasc Magn Reson*. 2010;12:16.
27. Ledbetter MK, Tandon R, Titus JL, Edwards JE. Stenotic semilunar valve in persistent truncus arteriosus. *Chest*. 1976;69:182–187.
28. Marino B, Digilio MC, Dallapiccola B. Severe truncal valve dysplasia: association with DiGeorge syndrome? *Ann Thorac Surg*. 1998; 66:980.
29. Deely WJ, Hagstrom JW, Engle MA. Truncus insufficiency: common truncus arteriousus with regurgitant truncus valve. Report of four cases. *Am Heart J*. 1963;65:542–548.
30. Burnell RH, Mcenery G, Miller GA. Truncal valve stenosis. *Br Heart J*. 1971;33:423–424.
31. Lee MH, Bellon EM, Liebman J, Perrin EV. Truncal valve stenosis. *Am Heart J*. 1973;85:397–400.
32. Elzein C, Ilbawi M, Kumar S, Ruiz C. Severe truncal valve stenosis: diagnosis and management. *J Card Surg*. 2005;20:589–593.
33. MacGilpin Jr HH. Truncus arteriosus communis persistence. *Am Heart J*. 1950;39:615–625.
34. De La Cruz MV, Cayre R, Angelini P, Noriega-Ramos N, Sadowinski S. Coronary arteries in truncus arteriosus. *Am J Cardiol*. 1990;66: 1482–1486.
35. Shrivastava S, Edwards JE. Coronary arterial origin in persistent truncus arteriosus. *Circulation*. 1977;55:551–554.
36. Suzuki A, Ho SY, Anderson RH, Deanfield JE. Coronary arterial and sinusal anatomy in hearts with a common arterial trunk. *Ann Thorac Surg*. 1989;48:792–797.
37. Heifetz SA, Robinowitz M, Mueller KH, Virmani R. Total anomalous origin of the coronary arteries from the pulmonary artery. *Pediatr Cardiol*. 1986;7:11–18.
38. Hackensellner HA. Ueber akessorische, von der Arteria Pulmonalis abgehende Herzgefaesse und ihre bei den Tung fuer das Verstaendis der formalen Genese des Ursprunges einer oder belder Coronarterien von der Lungenschlagader. *Frankf Z Pathol*. 1955;66:263.
39. Van Son JA, Autschbach R, Hambsch J. Congenital ostial membrane of left coronary artery in truncus arteriosus. *J Thorac Cardiovasc Surg*. 1999;118:1132–1134.
40. Rosenquist GC, Bharati S, McAllister HA, Lev M. Truncus arteriosus communis: truncal valve anomalies associated with small conal or truncal septal defects. *Am J Cardiol*. 1976;37:410–412.
41. Litovsky SH, Ostfeld I, Bjornstad PG, Van Praagh R, Geva T. Truncus arteriosus with anomalous pulmonary venous connection. *Am J Cardiol*. 1999;83:801–804 A810.
42. Paris YM, Bhan I, Marx GR, Rhodes J. Truncus arteriosus with a single left ventricle: case report of a previously unrecognized entity. *Am Heart J*. 1997;133:377–380.
43. Orts-Llorca F, Puerta Fonolla J, Sobrado J. The formation, septation and fate of the truncus arteriosus in man. *J Anat*. 1982;134:41–56.
44. Yu IT, Hutchins GM. Truncus arteriosus malformation: a developmental arrest at Carnegie stage 14. *Teratology*. 1996;53:31–37.
45. Brunson SC, Nudel DB, Gootman N, Aftalion B. Truncus arteriosus in a family. *Am Heart J*. 1978;96:419–420.
46. Goodyear JE. Persistent truncus arteriosus in two siblings. *Br Heart J*. 1961;23:194–196.
47. Shapiro SR, Ruckman RN, Kapur S, et al. Single ventricle with truncus arteriosus in siblings. *Am Heart J*. 1981;102:456–459.
48. Benesova D, Sikl H. A rare concordant malformation in monochoriate twins; persistent common arterial trunk. *J Pathol Bacteriol*. 1954;67:367–370.
49. Lang MJ, Aughton DJ, Riggs TW, Milad MP, Biesecker LG. Dizygotic twins concordant for truncus arteriosus. *Clin Genet*. 1991;39:75–79.
50. Mas C, Delatycki MB, Weintraub RG. Persistent truncus arteriosus in monozygotic twins: case report and literature review. *Am J Med Genet*. 1999;82:146–148.
51. Digilio MC, Marino B, Musolino AM, Giannotti A, Dallapiccola B. Familial recurrence of nonsyndromic interrupted aortic arch and truncus arteriosus with atrioventricular canal. *Teratology*. 2000; 61:329–331.
52. Momma K, Ando M, Matsuoka R. Truncus arteriosus communis associated with chromosome 22q11 deletion. *J Am Coll Cardiol*. 1997;30:1067–1071.
53. Moore JW, Wight NE, Jones MC, Krous HF. Truncus arteriosus associated with trisomy 18. *Pediatr Cardiol*. 1994;15:154–156.

54. Guenther F, Frydrychowicz A, Bode C, Geibel A. Cardiovascular flashlight. Persistent truncus arteriosus: a rare finding in adults. *Eur Heart J*. 2009;30:1154.

55. Carr FB, Goodale RH, Rockwell AEP. Persistent truncus arteriosus in a man aged thirty-six years. *Arch Pathol*. 1935;19:833.

56. Hicken P, Evans D, Heath D. Persistent truncus arteriosus with survival to the age of 38 years. *Br Heart J*. 1966;28:284–286.

57. Silverman JJ, Scheinesson GP. Persistent truncus arteriosus in a 43 year old man. *Am J Cardiol*. 1966;17:94–96.

58. Carter JB, Blieden LC, Edwards JE. Persistent truncus arteriosus. Report of survival to age of 52 years. *Minn Med*. 1973;56:280–282.

59. Niwa K, Perloff JK, Kaplan S, Child JS, Miner PD. Eisenmenger syndrome in adults: ventricular septal defect, truncus arteriosus, univentricular heart. *J Am Coll Cardiol*. 1999;34:223–232.

60. Menon SC, Julsrud PR, Cetta F. Late diagnosis of common arterial trunk. *Cardiol Young*. 2007;17:333–335.

61. Bodi V, Insa L, Sanchis J, et al. Persistent truncus arteriosus type 4 with survival to the age of 54 years. *Int J Cardiol*. 2002;82:75–77.

62. Gutierrez PS, Binotto MA, Aiello VD, Mansur AJ. Chest pain in an adult with truncus arteriosus communis. *Am J Cardiol*. 2004;93:272–273.

63. Freedom RM, Rosen FS, Nadas AS. Congenital cardiovascular disease and anomalies of the third and fourth pharyngeal pouch. *Circulation*. 1972;46:165–172.

64. Radford DJ, Perkins L, Lachman R, Thong YH. Spectrum of Di George syndrome in patients with truncus arteriosus: expanded Di George syndrome. *Pediatr Cardiol*. 1988;9:95–101.

65. Van Mierop LH, Kutsche LM. Cardiovascular anomalies in DiGeorge syndrome and importance of neural crest as a possible pathogenetic factor. *Am J Cardiol*. 1986;58:133–137.

66. Farrell MJ, Stadt H, Wallis KT, et al. HIRA, a DiGeorge syndrome candidate gene, is required for cardiac outflow tract septation. *Circ Res*. 1999;84:127–135.

67. Lin AE, Chin AJ, Devine W, Park SC, Zackai E. The pattern of cardiovascular malformation in the CHARGE association. *Am J Dis Child*. 1987;141:1010–1013.

68. Victorica BE, Gessner IH, Schiebler GL. Phonocardiographic findings in persistent truncus arteriosus. *Br Heart J*. 1968;30:812–816.

69. Portillo B, Perez Martin R. Truncus arteriosus communis. Electrocardiographic study in 17 cases. *Arch Inst Cardiol Mex*. 1960;30:609–620.

70. Bharati S, Karp R, Lev M. The conduction system in truncus arteriosus and its surgical significance. A study of five cases. *J Thorac Cardiovasc Surg*. 1992;104:954–960.

71. Mair DD, Ritter DG, Danielson GK, Wallace RB, McGoon DC. Truncus arteriosus with unilateral absence of a pulmonary artery. Criteria for operability and surgical results. *Circulation*. 1977;55:641–647.

72. Duke C, Sharland GK, Jones AM, Simpson JM. Echocardiographic features and outcome of truncus arteriosus diagnosed during fetal life. *Am J Cardiol*. 2001;88:1379–1384.

73. Child JS. Transthoracic and transesophageal echocardiographic imaging: Anatomic and hemodynamic assessment. In: Perloff JK, Child JS, eds. *Congenital heart disease in adults*. 2nd ed. Philadelphia: W.B. Saunders Company; 1998:91.

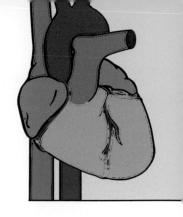

Chapter 29

Congenital Anomalies of Vena Caval Connection

Anomalous vena caval connections comprise a wide range of malformations that vary from minor to major and that occur in isolation or with coexisting congenital heart disease. Persistent left superior vena cava occurs in 0.3% of the general population and in 4.3% of congenital heart disease.[1] A left-sided inferior vena cava occurs in 0.2% to 0.5% of the general population.[1] This chapter focuses on *isolated* anomalous vena caval connections in *situs solitus* hearts (Table 29-1). Anomalies of vena caval connection with cardiac malpositions or with atrial isomerism are dealt with in Chapter 3.

In early embryonic development, the common cardinal veins are bilaterally symmetric and are potentially responsible for bilateral superior vena cavae.[2] The *left common cardinal vein* initially drains into the left portion of the sinus venosus, which becomes the coronary sinus.[2] Failure of obliteration of the left common cardinal vein results in persistent connection of a left superior vena cava to the coronary sinus (Figure 29-1),[2] a relatively common anomaly estimated at 0.3% to 0.5% of the general population and 1.5% to 10% of patients with congenital heart disease.[3] An isolated left superior vena cava in itself produces no physiologic derangements when it drains harmlessly into the right atrium via the coronary sinus (see Figure 29-1). However, the coronary sinus dilates sometimes appreciably,[4] especially if there is atresia of its right atrial orifice[5] or absence of the right superior vena vava.[6,7] When the right superior cava is absent, the sinus node pacemaker is absent because the pacemaker is normally located at the junction of the right superior vena cava and the morphologic right atrium.[8-11] A persistent left superior vena cava is a significant anomaly when it connects to the left atrium (Figures 29-2 and 29-3).[12-14] The coronary sinus is usually absent[15] with partial or complete unroofing of its anterosuperior wall. Unroofing results in a connection between the left atrium and the right atrium—a coronary sinus type of atrial septal defect (see Chapter 15).[16] A right-to-left shunt coexists through the left superior vena caval to left atrial connection.[14,17] An absent coronary sinus with bilateral superior vena cavae (right superior cava connected to the right atrium, left superior cava connected to the left atrium) is thought to represent a developmental complex.[18] If the right superior vena cava is absent or atretic (see Figure 29-3), the innominate vein crosses the midline and terminates in the left superior vena cava.[19] The left atrium occasionally receives the azygos vein, the hepatic vein, or the coronary sinus,[14] variations that are not considered in this chapter.

Direct connections between vena cavae and left atrium are uncommon.[7,20,21] Rarely, a right superior vena cava connects to the left atrium.[22-24] Still more rarely, a right superior vena cava connects to the left atrium, and a left superior vena cava connects to the right atrium.[25] *Connection* of a right superior vena cava to the left atrium must be distinguished from *drainage* of a right superior vena cava into both atria caused by a contiguous superior vena caval sinus venosus atrial septal defect (see Chapter 15).[20] When a right superior vena cava is congenitally absent (see Figure 29-3), brachiocephalic veins join a left superior vena cava that connects to the coronary sinus.[6,26]

Bilateral superior vena cavae[3] are illustrated in Figure 29-2. The innominate bridge that connects the two superior cavae may be widely patent, narrow, or atretic (see Figure 29-2), and the size of the left superior vena cava ranges from large to rudimentary.[3] Bilateral superior vena cavae with atrial isomerism are dealt with in Chapter 3.

Anomalous connection of the inferior vena cava to the left atrium consists of a morphogenetic spectrum represented by combinations of persistence of the valve of the right sinus venosus, fusion of the valve with the septum secundum, and incomplete development of the atrial septum.[27] The inferior vena cava penetrates the diaphragm at its expected site. An enlarged azygos vein may arise from the anomalous inferior cava and convey inferior caval blood into the right atrium (Figure 29-4).[21,28,29] An isolated left-sided abdominal inferior vena cava usually crosses to the right after receiving the renal veins, then penetrates the diaphragm and enters the right atrium at the normal site. A distinction must be made between *connection* of the inferior vena cava to the left atrium and anomalous inferior vena caval *drainage* into the left atrium from persistence of a large Eustachian valve (right valve of the sinus venosus) that directs flow toward a patent foramen ovale or across an ostium secundum atrial septal defect (see Chapter 15).[27]

Inferior vena caval interruption with azygous continuation is rare as an isolated malformation and is of no physiologic significance but can be mistaken for the descending thoracic aorta (Figure 29-5).[30] Interruption is immediately proximal to the renal veins and continues into a dilated azygos vein that enters the thorax to the right of the aorta, runs in the posterior mediastinum, and connects to a right superior vena cava (see Figure 29-5). There is an association with congenital

Table 29-1 **Congenital Anomalies of Vena Caval Connection**

Left superior vena cava:
- Connected to coronary sinus
- Connected to left atrium

Right superior vena cava:
- Absent
- Connected to left atrium

Bilateral superior vena cavae

Inferior vena cava:
- Connected to left atrium
- Interruption with azygous continuation

Superior and inferior vena cavae both connected to left atrium (total anomalous systemic venous connection)

absence of the portal vein.[31] Inferior vena caval interruption with azygos continuation and left isomerism are dealt with in Chapter 3.

Anomalous connection of either vena cava to the left atrium is rare enough, but connection of the right superior vena cava *and* the inferior vena cava to the left atrium—total anomalous systemic venous connection—is even rarer (Figures 29-6 and 29-7). [7,20,32] Survival depends on adequate mixing through an interatrial communication.

The *physiologic consequences* of anomalous vena caval connections to the left atrium take into account two variables: (1), the direction and volume of blood flow through the connection; and (2), the effect of the connection on the amount of blood flow entering the right and left sides of the heart. Flow patterns are complex when a persistent left superior vena cava communicates with the left atrium

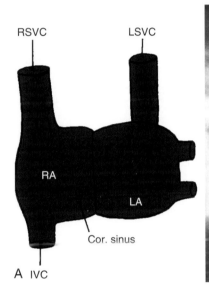

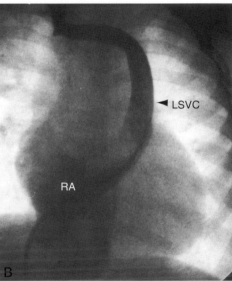

FIGURE 29-1 **A,** Persistent left superior vena cava (LSVC) draining into the right atrium (RA) via the coronary sinus. The right superior vena cava (RSVC) and the inferior vena cava (IVC) drain normally into the right atrium. **B,** Left superior vena cava draining into the coronary sinus in a 3-year-old child.

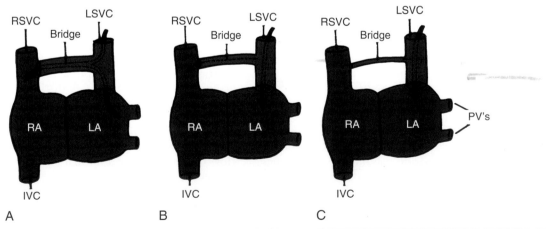

FIGURE 29-2 **A,** Persistent left superior vena cava (LSVC) communicating directly with the left atrium (LA). The right superior vena cava (RSVC) and the inferior vena cava (IVC) drain normally into the right atrium (RA). The bilateral superior vena cavae communicate through a large innominate bridge. The direction of blood flow is *from* the left atrium *into* the anomalous left superior vena cava and then across the innominate bridge into the right superior vena cava. These pathways constitutes a left to right shunt. **B,** Restrictive innominate bridge offers resistance so that left superior vena caval blood is diverted into the left atrium with only a small portion flowing across the bridge. **C,** An atretic innominate bridge diverts left superior vena caval blood entirely into the left atrium. (PV's = pulmonary veins.)

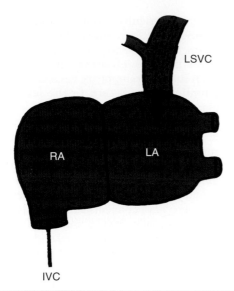

FIGURE 29-3 Persistent left superior vena cava (LSVC) connecting directly to the left atrium (LA). The right superior vena cava is absent. The inferior vena cava (IVC) drains normally into the right atrium (RA).

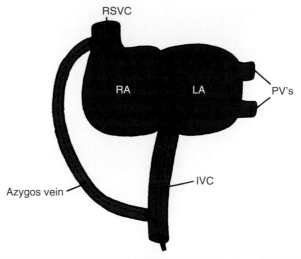

FIGURE 29-4 Inferior vena cava (IVC) connecting directly to the left atrium (LA). An anomalous inferior vena cava gives rise to an enlarged azygos vein that joins a normal right superior vena cava (RSVC). A small portion of inferior vena caval blood is diverted through the azygos vein into the right superior vena cava and into the right atrium (RA; see curved arrow). (PV's = pulmonary veins.)

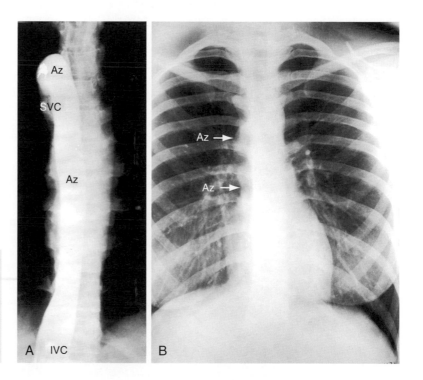

FIGURE 29-5 **A,** Inferior vena cavagram from a 28-year-old woman with isolated inferior vena caval interruption (IVC) and azygos (Az) continuation to a right superior vena cava (SVC). **B,** X-ray from same patient showing the azygos vein ascending along the right side of the vertebral column (lower Az) and forming a knuckle as it joins the right superior cava (upper Az).

(see Figure 29-2).[14,17] The left superior vena cava may be the *only* superior cava (see Figure 29-3), or bilateral superior cavae may fail to communicate with each other because of stenosis or atresia of the innominate bridge (see Figures 29-2B and C). All or nearly all of left superior vena caval blood is then channeled *into* the left atrium (Figure 29-2B and C), so cyanosis is obligatory. Alternatively, when bilateral superior vena cavae communicate freely through a nonrestrictive innominate bridge, the

direction of blood flow is *from* the left atrium *into* the anomalous left superior vena cava, across the innominate bridge and *into* the right superior vena cava (Figure 29-2A).[17,33] The pathway constitutes a left-to-right shunt, so cyanosis is absent.[14] With this exception, communications between vena cavae and left atrium result in right-to-left shunts and in a decrease in systemic arterial oxygen saturation. When a right superior vena cava connects to the left atrium, caval blood flow is *into* the left atrium, so cyanosis is

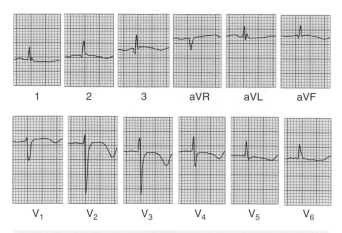

FIGURE 29-6 Electrocardiogram from a 28-year-old woman in whom the superior and inferior vena cavae both joined the left atrium—*total anomalous systemic venous connection*. A large ostium secundum atrial septal defect permitted interatrial mixing on which survival depended. The sinus node was absent because a junction between the superior vena cava and right atrium was absent. The P wave axis is directed upward and to the left, indicating an ectopic atrial focus. Broad notched P waves in leads 1, 3, and aVL reflect total caval drainage into the left atrium. The T wave abnormalities are nonspecific.

inevitable. When the inferior vena cava connects to the left atrium, unoxygenated blood is directed into the left atrium despite a large azygos vein, so cyanosis is obligatory (see Figure 29-4).

Now consider the relative volume of blood flowing through the two sides of the heart in the presence of vena caval–to–left atrial connections. Normally, the entire systemic venous return from the superior and inferior vena cavae enters the *right* side of the heart, and the entire pulmonary venous return from the pulmonary veins enters the left side of the heart. If one vena cava connects to the left atrium, the right side of the heart is effectively

bypassed, so right ventricular output and pulmonary blood flow fall reciprocally.[34] Left ventricular output theoretically remains unchanged because the increment in anomalous caval flow into the left atrium is matched by the reciprocal decrement in pulmonary venous flow. Accordingly, as systemic venous return to the left atrium increases, pulmonary venous return to the left atrium decreases by the same amount, so total blood flow to the left side of the heart remains unchanged. In the absence of compensatory mechanisms, anomalous caval connections to the left atrium should be associated with reduced *pulmonary* flow and normal *systemic* flow,[34] patterns that should pertain irrespective of whether the superior or inferior vena cava connects anomalously. Do these circulatory patterns really exist? Clinical and experimental observations indicate that right atrial and right ventricular pressures are normal or low[34] and pulmonary blood flow is usually,[34] but not always, reduced. Necropsy descriptions of a small right atrium and a small right ventricle are relevant.[35] However, *left* ventricular output tends to be moderately *increased*.[34] The mechanisms responsible for these deviations from theoretical blood flow patterns are not known.

When the superior vena cava and inferior vena cava *both* connect to the left atrium *(total anomalous systemic venous connection)*, flow patterns are modified by obligatory mixing at atrial level. The left atrium receives blood from both cavae *and* from the pulmonary veins. Part of this mixture reaches the left ventricle directly across the mitral valve, and the remainder enters the right side of the heart across an atrial septal defect. Pulmonary blood flow is not increased even in the presence of a nonrestrictive atrial septal defect and normal pulmonary vascular resistance (see Figure 29-7).

The inferior vena cava normally carries about twice the volume of systemic venous return as the superior vena cava. Accordingly, an anomalously connecting *inferior* cava delivers a larger proportion of blood to the left

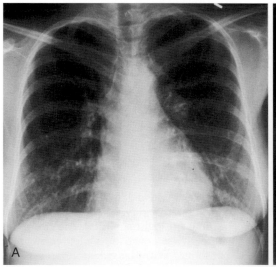
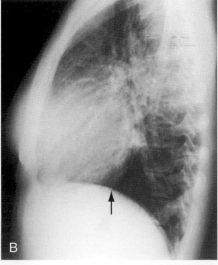

FIGURE 29-7 X-rays from the 28-year-old woman with total anomalous systemic venous connection whose electrocardiogram is shown in Figure 29-6. **A,** The size and configuration of the heart are normal. Pulmonary vascularity is not reduced. Increased markings in the left lower lung fields are superimposed breast tissue. **B,** In the lateral projection, the inferior vena caval shadow is absent (arrow).

atrium than an anomalously connecting *superior* vena cava. However, the magnitude of systemic blood flow (cardiac output) does not depend on which vena cava delivers its return to the left atrium, provided that pulmonary venous return falls by an equivalent amount.

HISTORY

Isolated anomalous vena caval connection to the left atrium has an equal gender distribution. Cyanosis dates from birth or infancy[20,27] unless bilateral superior cavae are connected by a nonrestrictive innominate bridge (see Figure 29-2A). Despite conspicuous cyanosis, there is a paucity of symptoms.[21,27] the syndrome of cyanosis and clubbing with normal heart. Adult survival is expected, with longevities recorded in the sixth, seventh, and eighth decades.[12,20] Effort intolerance, dyspnea, and light-headedness develop late if at all and are generally mild.[20,21] One man tolerated training in the armed forces.[27] Brain abscess and paradoxical embolus have been reported.[20,23]

The cause of death is usually unrelated to the isolated congenital anomalies of vena caval connection. However, unexplained sudden death has been reported with isolated left superior vena caval connection to the coronary sinus, especially if the right superior vena cava is absent.[9]

PHYSICAL APPEARANCE

Cyanosis and clubbing are the only abnormalities of physical appearance.[20] Cyanosis increases with effort because caval venous return increases. Cyanosis is greater when the *inferior* vena cava connects to the left atrium because approximately twice as much blood is delivered to the heart via the inferior vena cava (see previous).[34,36] A large azygos venous system allows substantial inferior vena caval flow into the right atrium and proportionately less flow into the left atrium (see Figure 29-4), so cyanosis is relatively mild.[21] A superior vena cava that connects to the left atrium (see Figure 29-3) is accompanied by conspicuous cyanosis. When a nonrestrictive innominate bridge joins bilateral superior vena cavae, cyanosis is absent because the direction of flow is *from* the left atrium *into* the anomalous left superior vena cava (see Figure 29-2A).[17]

ARTERIAL PULSE AND JUGULAR VENOUS PULSE

The *arterial pulse* is normal because left ventricular stroke volume increases little if at all.

Attention has been called to a *new physical sign:* namely, relative prominence of the *left* internal jugular venous pulse because of persistence of the *left* superior vena cava. When there is congenital absence of the *right* superior vena cava, the jugular venous pulse is *confined* to the left side of the neck.

PRECORDIAL MOVEMENT AND PALPATION

The left ventricular impulse is normal or only moderately increased, which reflects the normal or only moderate increase in systemic output. A right ventricular impulse is absent. These physical signs indicate that *cyanosis* is occurring with a dominant *left* ventricle, an important observation in the clinical recognition of cyanotic congenital heart disease (see Box 1-1).

AUSCULTATION

Left ventricular stroke volume is seldom sufficient to generate a flow murmur into the aorta.[20,21] The second heart sound is single because decreased right ventricular stroke volume and decreased pulmonary capacitance result in early pulmonary valve closure and synchrony or near synchrony of the two components.[20] The intensity of the pulmonary component is normal or reduced because pulmonary arterial pressure is normal or low.[34]

ELECTROCARDIOGRAM

When a left superior vena cava connects to the coronary sinus (see Figure 29-1), the atrial rhythm may be ectopic and abnormalities of atrioventricular conduction may coexist.[2,8,9] When a right superior vena cava is absent or connects to the left atrium, the sinus node is absent, so the atrial focus is ectopic and the P wave axis is abnormal (see Figure 29-6).[11] Atresia or absence of the segment of superior vena cava adjacent to the right atrium is accompanied by developmental abnormalities of the sinus node and an ectopic atrial focus.[9]

The QRS pattern is normal with vena caval–to–left atrial connections (Figure 29-8). Adult survival anticipates age-related electrocardiographic abnormalities.[12,20,21] Right ventricular hypertrophy is absent because flow into the right side of the heart is normal or reduced. Left ventricular electrical forces retain their normal adult dominance (Figures 29-6 and 29-9), but the modest increment in left ventricular volume is seldom sufficient to cause hypertrophy.

X-RAY

The size and configuration of the heart are normal (see Figure 29-8),[20,21,35] even when both superior *and* inferior vena cavae connect to the left atrium (see Figure 29-7). A left superior vena cava may form a concave or crescentic shadow as it emerges from beneath the middle third of the left clavicle.[14,17,37] When the *inferior* vena cava communicates with the *left* atrium, the inferior vena caval shadow is absent from its expected location at the angle formed by the posterior cardiac silhouette and the diaphragm (see Figure 29-7B). An inferior vena caval shadow is also absent when there is inferior caval interruption

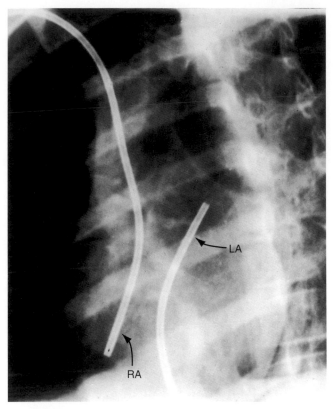

FIGURE 29-8 Left anterior oblique projection from a 9-year-old girl with isolated inferior vena caval connection to the left atrium. One catheter entered the right atrium (RA) from the superior vena cava, and a second catheter entered the left atrium (LA) from the inferior vena cava (see Figure 29-6 for electrocardiogram). *(With permission, from Venables AW. Isolated drainage of the inferior vena cava to the left atrium. British Heart Journal 1963;25:545.)*

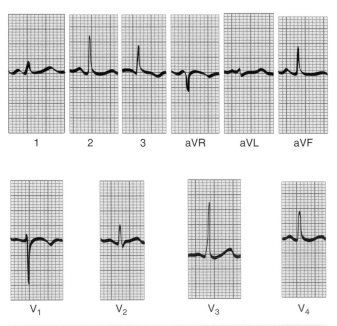

FIGURE 29-9 Normal electrocardiogram from a 9-year-old girl with isolated connection of the inferior vena cava to the left atrium. *(With permission, from Venables AW. Isolated drainage of the inferior vena cava to the left atrium. British Heart Journal 1963;25:545.)*

with azygos continuation (see Figure 29-5). The azygos vein ascends along the right edge of the vertebral column, forming a knuckle as it courses anteriorly to join the right superior vena cava (see Figure 29-5).

ECHOCARDIOGRAM

Echocardiography with color flow and contrast imaging establishes the diagnoses of most if not all anomalies of vena caval connection described in this chapter,[1,16,38–43] including intrauterine.[44] A dilated coronary sinus in the parasternal long-axis view arouses suspicion of a hitherto unsuspected connection of a left superior vena cava to the coronary sinus (Figure 29-10 and Video 29-1).[45] The coronary sinus is absent when a left superior vena cava connects directly to the left atrium (see Figure 29-2). Color flow imaging confirms the course of a persistent left superior vena cava (Figure 29-11 and Video 29-2), which can sometimes be visualized together with the innominate bridge associated with bilateral cavae (see Figure 29-2). When the right superior vena cava is absent, a persistent left superior vena cava is imaged along the left side of the aorta.[46,47]

Contrast echocardiography identifies specific vena caval to left atrial connections.[38,40,48] When a left superior vena cava connects directly to the left atrium, injection of echo contrast into the left antecubital vein is followed by immediate opacification of the left atrium.[38] Conversely, when a right superior vena cava connects directly to the left atrium, injection of contrast into the right antecubital vein promptly opacifies the left atrium.[38] Contrast echocardiography is more complex when the inferior vena caval connects to the left atrium[49] because contrast material injected into the femoral vein may appear in the right as well as the left atrium depending on the size of the azygos vein that leaves the inferior vena cava and joins the right atrium via a right superior

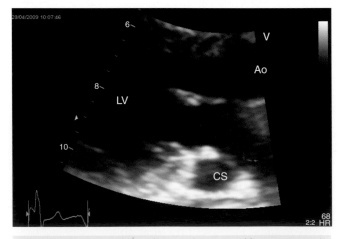

FIGURE 29-10 A, Echocardiogram (parasternal long-axis view) from a healthy 9-month-old male with a coronary sinus (CS) that was dilated by connection to a persistent left superior vena cava. The large size of the coronary sinus is evident when compared with the cross-section of the descending aorta (Ao) (Video 29-1). (LV = left ventricle, LA = left atrium.)

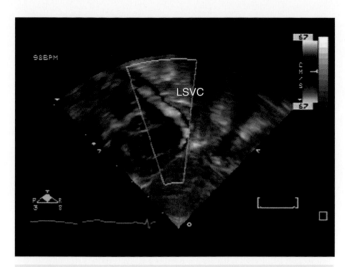

FIGURE 29-11 Color flow image showing the course of a persistent left superior vena cava (LSVC) that communicated with a dilated coronary sinus in a 3-day-old male with an ostium secundum atrial septal defect (Video 29-2).

vena cava (see Figure 29-4). When a right superior vena cava and an inferior connect both connect to the left atrium (see Figure 29-7), injection of contrast into the right antecubital vein and into the femoral vein result in a combination of the patterns just described.

SUMMARY

A left superior vena cava can connect anomalously to the coronary sinus or left atrium. A right superior vena cava can connect anomalously to the left atrium or can be absent altogether. Bilateral superior vena cavae can be connected by an innominate bridge that is either widely patent, narrow, or atretic. An inferior vena cava can connect to the left atrium or can be interrupted with azygous continuation. Superior and inferior vena cavae can both connect to the left atrium—total anomalous systemic venous connection.

Persistent left superior vena cava is suspected in the x-ray by a shadow that emerges from beneath the middle third of the left clavicle and passes downward toward the left upper border of the aortic arch. Echocardiography with color flow imaging and echo contrast confirm the diagnosis and determine whether the caval connection is to the coronary sinus or left atrium. A left superior vena cava to coronary sinus connection is often first suspected on routine echocardiography because of dilation of the coronary sinus. Isolated superior vena caval connection to the left atrium is a form of cyanotic congenital heart disease with a dominant left ventricle that is palpable at the apex without a palpable right ventricle. Cyanosis dates from birth or early life, but cardiac symptoms are absent or mild even when cyanosis is conspicuous. The electrocardiogram shows normal adult left ventricular dominance. Echocardiography with color flow and echo contrast imaging identify the left superior vena cava entering the left atrium. A dilated coronary sinus effectively excludes direct connection of a left superior vena cava to the left

atrium. *Bilateral superior vena cavae* and an innominate bridge can be imaged.

Inferior vena caval connection to the left atrium is accompanied by conspicuous cyanosis unless a large azygos vein channels inferior caval return into the right atrium. The inferior vena caval shadow is absent from its expected location in the lateral chest x-ray. Contrast echocardiography with injection into the femoral vein opacifies the left atrium.

REFERENCES

1. Guray Y, Yelgec NS, Guray U, et al. Left-sided or transposed inferior vena cava ascending as hemiazygos vein and draining into the coronary sinus via persistent left superior vena cava: case report. *Int J Cardiol.* 2004;93:293–295.
2. Nsah EN, Moore GW, Hutchins GM. Pathogenesis of persistent left superior vena cava with a coronary sinus connection. *Pediatric Pathol.* 1991;11:261–269.
3. Buirski G, Jordan SC, Joffe HS, Wilde P. Superior vena caval abnormalities: their occurrence rate, associated cardiac abnormalities and angiographic classification in a paediatric population with congenital heart disease. *Clin Radiol.* 1986;37:131–138.
4. Ascuitto RJ, Ross-Ascuitto NT, Kopf GS, et al. Persistent left superior vena cava causing subdivided left atrium: diagnosis, embryological implications, and surgical management. *Ann Thorac Surg.* 1987; 44:546–549.
5. Imai S, Matsubara T, Yamazoe M, et al. Atresia of the right atrial orifice of the coronary sinus with persistent left superior vena cava: a case report. *J Cardiol.* 1999;34:341–344
6. Chan KL, Abdulla A. Images in cardiology. Giant coronary sinus and absent right superior vena cava. *Heart.* 2000;83:704.
7. Winter S. Persistent left superior vena cava. Survey of world literature and report of 30 additional cases. *Angiology.* 1954;5:90.
8. James TN, Marshall TK, Edwards JE. De subitaneis mortibus. XX. Cardiac electrical instability in the presence of a left superior vena cava. *Circulation.* 1976;54:689–697.
9. Lenox CC, Hashida Y, Anderson RH, Hubbard JD. Conduction tissue anomalies in absence of the right superior caval vein. *Int J Cardiol.* 1985;8:251–260.
10. Momma K, Linde LM. Abnormal rhythms associated with persistent left superior vena cava. *Pediatr Res.* 1969;3:210–216.
11. Langford EJ, Sulke AN, Curry PV. Atrial permanent pacing for sinus node dysfunction with absent right superior vena cava. *Int J Cardiol.* 1993;40:177–178.
12. Arsenian MA, Anderson RA. Anomalous venous connection of the superior vena cava to the left atrium. *Am J Cardiol.* 1988;62: 989–990.
13. Kabbani SS, Feldman M, Angelini P, Leachman RD, Cooley DA. Single (left) superior vena cava draining into the left atrium. Surgical repair. *Ann Thorac Surg.* 1973;16:518–525.
14. Taybi H, Kurlander GJ, Lurie PR, Campbell JA. Anomalous ssssystemic venous connection to the left atrium or to a pulmonary vein. *Am J Roentgenol Radium Ther Nucl Med.* 1965;94:62–77.
15. Wiles HB. Two cases of left superior vena cava draining directly to a left atrium with a normal coronary sinus. *Br Heart J.* 1991;65: 158–160.
16. Chen MC, Hung JS, Chang KC, et al. Partially unroofed coronary sinus and persistent left superior vena cava: intracardiac echocardiographic observation. *J Ultrasound Med.* 1996;15:875–879.
17. Odman P. A persistent left superior vena cava communicating with the left atrium and pulmonary vein. *Acta Radiologica.* 1953;40: 554–560.
18. Foster ED, Baeza OR, Farina MF, Shaher RM. Atrial septal defect associated with drainage of left superior vena cava to left atrium and absence of the coronary sinus. *J Thorac Cardiovasc Surg.* 1978;76: 718–720.
19. De Leval MR, Ritter DG, Mcgoon DC, Danielson GK. Anomalous systemic venous connection. Surgical considerations. *Mayo Clin Proc.* 1975;50:599–610.
20. Shapiro EP, Al-Sadir J, Campbell NP, et al. Drainage of right superior vena cava into both atria. Review of the literature and

description of a case presenting with polycythemia and paradoxical embolization. *Circulation*. 1981;63:712–717.

21. Venables AW. Isolated drainage of the inferior vena cava to the left atrium. *Br Heart J*. 1963;25:545–548.

22. Bharati S, Lev M. Direct entry of the right superior vena cava into the left atrium with aneurysmal dilatation and stenosis at its entry into the right atrium with stenosis of the pulmonary veins: a rare case. *Pediatr Cardiol*. 1984;5:123–126.

23. King RE, Plotnick GD. Isolated right superior vena cava into the left atrium detected by contrast echocardiography. *Am Heart J*. 1991; 122:583–586.

24. Tandon R. Anomalous drainage of right superior vena cava into the left atrium. *Indian Heart J*. 1999;51:345.

25. Leys D, Manouvrier J, Dupard T, et al. Right superior vena cava draining into the left atrium with left superior vena cava draining into the right atrium. *Br Med J (Clin Res Ed)*. 1986;293:855.

26. Bartram U, Van Praagh S, Levine JC, et al. Absent right superior vena cava in visceroatrial situs solitus. *Am J Cardiol*. 1997;80: 175–183.

27. Meyers DG, Latson LA, Mcmanus BM, Fleming WH. Anomalous drainage of the inferior vena cava into a left atrial connection: a case report involving a 41-year-old man. *Cathet Cardiovasc Diagn*. 1989;16:239–244.

28. Cabrera A, Arriola J, Llorente A. Anomalous connection of inferior vena cava to the left atrium. *Int J Cardiol*. 1994;46:79–81.

29. Genoni M, Jenni R, Vogt PR, Germann R, Turina MI. Drainage of the inferior vena cava to the left atrium. *Ann Thorac Surg*. 1999;67: 543–545.

30. Blanchard DG, Sobel JL, Hope J, et al. Infrahepatic interruption of the inferior vena cava with azygos continuation: a potential mimicker of aortic pathology. *J Am Soc Echocardiogr*. 1998;11: 1078–1083.

31. Le Borgne J, Paineau J, Hamy A, et al. Interruption of the inferior vena cava with azygos termination associated with congenital absence of portal vein. *Surg Radiol Anat*. 2000;22:197–202.

32. Pugliese P, Murzi B, Redaelli S, Eufrate S. Total anomalous systemic venous drainage into the left atrium. Report of a case of successful surgical correction. *G Ital Cardiol*. 1983;13:62–67.

33. Lam W, Danoviz J, Witham D, Wyndham C, Rosen KM. Left-to-right shunt via left superior vena cava communication with left atrium. *Chest*. 1981;79:700–702.

34. Hultgren HN, Gerbode F. A physiological study of experimental left atrium inferior vena caval anastomoses. *Am J Physiol*. 1954; 177:164–169.

35. Vaquez-Perez J, Frontera-Izquierdo P. Anomalous drainage of the right superior vena cava into the left atrium as an isolated anomaly. Rare case report. *Am Heart J*. 1979;97:89–91.

36. Levy SE, Blalock A. Fractionation of the output of the heart and of the oxygen consumption of normal unanesthetized dogs. *Am J Physiol*. 1937;118:368.

37. Gensini GG, Caldini P, Casaccio F, Blount Jr SG. Persistent left superior vena cava. *Am J Cardiol*. 1959;4:677–685.

38. Foale R, Bourdillon PD, Somerville J, Rickards A. Anomalous systemic venous return: recognition by two-dimensional echocardiography. *Eur Heart J*. 1983;4:186–195.

39. Hibi N, Fukui Y, Nishimura K, et al. Cross-sectional echocardiographic study on persistent left superior vena cava. *Am Heart J*. 1980;100:69–76.

40. Pan C, Chen C, Wang S, Al E. Echocardiographic evidence for drainage of a persistent left supeior vena cava into the left atium. *J Cardiovasc Ultrasonog*. 1984;3:329.

41. Chin AJ. Subcostal two-dimensional echocardiographic identification of right superior vena cava connecting to left atrium. *Am Heart J*. 1994; 127:939–941.

42. Kogon BE, Fyfe D, Butler H, Kanter KR. Anomalous drainage of the inferior vena cava into the left atrium. *Pediatr Cardiol*. 2006;27: 183–185.

43. Miraldi F, Carbone I, Ascarelli A, Barretta A, D'Angeli I. Double superior vena cava: right connected to left atrium and left to coronary sinus. *Int J Cardiol*. 2009;131:e78–e80.

44. Galindo A, Gutierrez-Larraya F, Escribano D, Arbues J, Velasco JM. Clinical significance of persistent left superior vena cava diagnosed in fetal life. *Ultrasound Obstet Gynecol*. 2007;30: 152–161.

45. Gonzalez-Juanatey C, Testa A, Vidan J, et al. Persistent left superior vena cava draining into the coronary sinus: report of 10 cases and literature review. *Clin Cardiol*. 2004;27:515–518.

46. Srivastava V, Mishra P, Kumar S, et al. Persistent left SVC with absent right SVC: a rare anomaly. *J Card Surg*. 2007;22:535–536.

47. Waikar HD, Lahie YKM, De Zoysa L, Chand P, Kamalanesan RPP. Systemic venous anomalies: absent right superior vena cava with persistent left superior vena cava. *J Cardiothorac Vasc Anesth*. 2004;18:332–335.

48. Gorenflo M, Sebening C, Ulmer HE. Anomalous connection of the right superior caval vein to the morphologically left atrium. *Cardiol Young*. 2006;16:184–186.

49. Burri H, Vuille C, Sierra J, et al. Drainage of the inferior vena cava to the left atrium. *Echocardiography*. 2003;20:185–189.

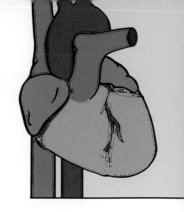

Chapter 30

Congenital Pulmonary Arteriovenous Fistula

In 1897, the British Medical Journal published a necropsy description of *congenital pulmonary arteriovenous fistulae*,[1] and four decades later, the anomaly was recognized in a living subject.[2] Pulmonary arteriovenous fistulae are the result of an embryonic fault in the vascular complex that is responsible for the development of pulmonary arteries and veins.[3] The fistulae can be solitary or multiple, unilateral or bilateral, or minute and diffuse throughout both lungs.[4–6] Approximately 75% of congenital pulmonary arteriovenous fistulae involve the lower lobes or right middle lobe (Figures 30-1 through 30-5)[4,7]; they usually occur without coexisting congenital heart disease. Isolated exceptions have been reported with left isomerism (see Chapter 3)[8,9] and with atrial septal defect (see Chapter 15).[10] Estimated minimal prevalence rate is 1/10,000 births.[11]

In 1865, Babington[12] called attention to familial epistaxis; and in 1876, Legg[13] described recurrent epistaxes and cutaneous telangiectasia in three generations. Twenty years later, Rendu[14] published his classic description of familial epistaxes and telangiectasia (cutaneous angiomatas) of the nose, cheeks, and upper lip. In 1901, Osler[15] reported on a *"family form of recurring epistaxis associated with multiple telangiectases of the skin and mucous membranes"*; and in 1907, Weber[16] reported "multiple hereditary developmental angiomata (telangiectases) of the skin and mucous membranes associated with recurring haemorrhages." In 1909, Hanes[17] referred to the disorder as *hereditary hemorrhagic telangiectasia*,[18] but the eponym *Rendu, Osler, Weber* remains in use without the inclusion of Legg[13] and with no consensus about the most appropriate sequence of names.[19,20] The diagnosis of hereditary hemorrhagic telangiectasia (HHT) is made clinically with the *Curaçao criteria*, which was established in 1999 by the Scientific Advisory Board of the HHT Foundation International. The criteria include recurrent epistaxis; telangiectases of the lips, oral cavity, fingers, and nose; gastrointestinal telangiectasia; and pulmonary, hepatic, cerebral or spinal arteriovenous malformations.[19,21,22]

A fistula consists of either one or more relatively large vascular trunks, a thin aneurysmal sac, or a tangle of distended tortuous vascular channels (Figures 30-1 through 30-7).[18] The arterial supply is through enlarged tortuous branches of a pulmonary artery, and drainage is through dilated pulmonary veins (see Figures 30-1 through 30-4 and 30-6).[3,23] Fistulous rupture results in hemorrhage into the pulmonary parenchyma or into the pleural space.[24] Exceptionally, the arterial supply is from a bronchial, intercostal,

anomalous systemic artery or a coronary artery (see Chapter 22). The fistula is then *systemic* arteriovenous rather than *pulmonary* arteriovenous.[18] A rare anatomic variation consists of a congenital connection between a pulmonary artery and the left atrium, an anomaly in which an initial connection exists between a pulmonary artery and a pulmonary vein; but during vascular development, the pulmonary vein becomes incorporated into the left atrium.[25–29] Extralobar arteriovenous fistulae are represented by pulmonary sequestrations in which the arterial supply and venous drainage are systemic rather than pulmonary. Isolated congenital varicose pulmonary veins are rare and not the result of arteriovenous malformations.[30]

The *physiologic consequences* of pulmonary arteriovenous fistulae depend on the amount of unoxygenated blood delivered through the malformation and on the size of the malformation, which tends to increase with age.[31,32] Although the volume of blood delivered through the fistula is sufficient to cause cyanosis, it is rarely sufficient to impose a physiologic burden (see Figure 30-7). Pulmonary artery pressure is normal, with rare exception.[33] In experimental pulmonary arteriovenous fistulae, cardiac output and left ventricular stroke volume are increased,[34] but in congenital pulmonary arteriovenous fistulae, blood flow through the malformation is increased while flow through uninvolved lung decreases by a comparable amount. Accordingly, the net volume of blood that reaches the left side of the heart is little if at all affected, so left ventricular stroke volume and cardiac output remain normal or nearly so. Rarely, a large pulmonary arteriovenous malformation imposes an excess volume load on the left side of the heart and induces congestive heart failure (see Figure 30-7).

Blood flow through pulmonary arteriovenous fistulae is affected by mechanical factors.[35] Flow through lower lobe fistulae is augmented in the upright position because of increased perfusion of dependent portions of the lungs. A decubitus position compresses the dependent lung and reduces blood flow through an ipsilateral fistula. A case in point was a large pulmonary arteriovenous fistula in an infant in whom ipsilateral chest wall compression was therapeutic, immediately decreasing the cyanosis and relieving the dyspnea (see Figure 30-7). Elevation of the diaphragm during pregnancy can compress a lower lobe fistula and abolish the accompanying murmur, which reappears after delivery.[35]

Acquired pulmonary arteriovenous fistulae are occasional sequelae of cavo-pulmonary shunts, especially

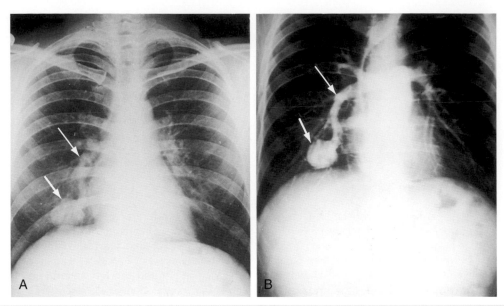

FIGURE 30-1 A, X-ray of a 21-year-old man with a congenital right lower lobe pulmonary arteriovenous fistula (thick arrow). The lobulated density is connected to the hilus (thin arrow) by dilated vessels that enter and leave the fistula. The x-ray is otherwise normal. **B,** Angiocardiogram showing the fistula (thick arrow) with its pulmonary arterial connection (thin arrow).

Glenn shunts.[36,37] Acquired fistulae occur in children with hepatic cirrhosis and portal hypertension, especially with biliary atresia and right isomerism (see Chapter 3),[38,39] and regress after liver transplantation.[38] Large *hepatic* arteriovenous fistulae sometimes occur *without* pulmonary arteriovenous fistulae in Rendu-Osler-Weber disease.[40–42] Hepatic, cerebral, and pulmonary arteriovenous fistulae may coexist.[43]

In 1917, telangiectasia and epistaxes were reported in a patient who died of massive hemothorax and at necropsy had three pulmonary arteriovenous fistulae.[44] The association of hemorrhagic telangiectasias with

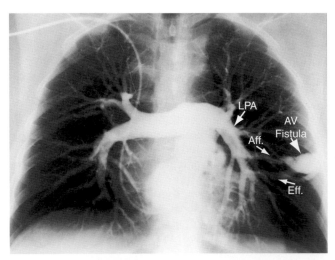

FIGURE 30-2 Pulmonary arteriogram from a 35-year-old woman with a solitary left lower lobe congenital pulmonary arteriovenous fistula (AV Fistula). An afferent channel (Aff.) enters the fistula, and an efferent channel (Eff.) leaves the fistula. (LPA = left pulmonary artery.)

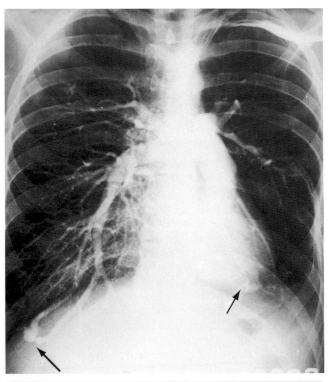

FIGURE 30-3 Angiocardiogram from a 32-year-old man with congenital bilateral pulmonary arteriovenous fistulae of the right and left lower lobes (arrows). Afferent and efferent vascular channels join and leave the fistula and are readily seen on the right. The left lower lobe fistula (lower left arrow) was behind the cardiac apex, inviting a mistaken diagnosis of intracardiac origin. The heart size is normal.

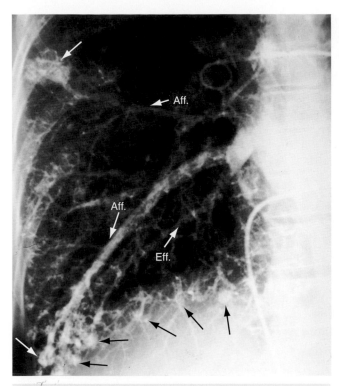

FIGURE 30-4 Right pulmonary arteriogram from a 50-year-old woman with hereditary hemorrhagic telangiectasia and pulmonary arteriovenous fistulae. Afferent (Aff.) and efferent (Eff.) vascular channels enter and leave the fistulae. Unmarked arrows identify multiple fistulae in the right lower and right middle lobes.

pulmonary arteriovenous fistulae has been amply confirmed.[4,5,18,19] Hereditary hemorrhagic telangiectasis is an autosomal dominant vasculopathy.[11] Clinical diagnostic criteria have changed remarkably little in the last century.[19]

Pulmonary arteriovenous fistulae occur in 5% to 30% of patients with telangiectasia, and telangiectasia occur in 30% to 60% of patients with pulmonary arteriovenous fistulae.[45] The incidence rate of pulmonary arteriovenous fistulae with telangiectasia is 1:50,000 with autosomal dominant transmission and a 20% mutation rate. The mucocutaneous lesions are tiny localized arteriovenous fistulae composed of thin dilated vascular membranes with a layer of endothelium and no muscular or elastic coat.[18,46] The lesions are fragile and rupture easily.[18] Telangiectasia are found on the skin, the lips (Figure 30-8), and the nasal, oral and vaginal mucous membranes; beneath the nails; and in the gastrointestinal tract, liver, central nervous system, kidney, and retina.[18,47–49]

HISTORY

Pulmonary arteriovenous fistulae and hereditary hemorrhagic telangiectasia afflict males and females with equal frequency.[18,50,51] The fistulae tend to increase in size and number with the passage of time[31,32] and are seldom recognized until adulthood.[50,52] Symptoms are the same whether the malformations are multiple or single (see Figures 30-1, 30-2, and 30-3), except for minute diffuse fistulous channels (see Figures 30-4 and 30-5). Mean patient age in a large series was 39 years (range, 3 years to 73 years), with a distinct majority over age 20 years. However, the first description of a pulmonary

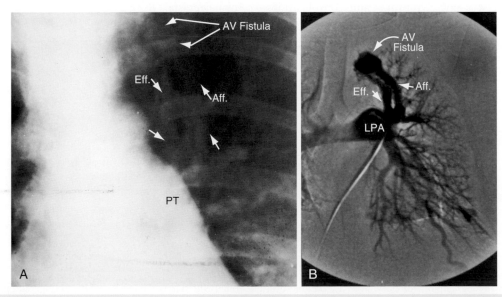

FIGURE 30-5 **A,** Close-up of the chest x-ray of a 26-year-old woman with a single large left upper lobe pulmonary arteriovenous fistula (AV Fistula). She had endured two brain abscesses. The solitary fistula and its afferent (Aff.) and efferent (Eff.) vascular channels are faintly seen. (PT = pulmonary trunk.) **B,** Contrast material selectively injected into the left pulmonary artery (LPA) visualized the afferent channel that entered the fistula and the efferent channel that left the fistula.

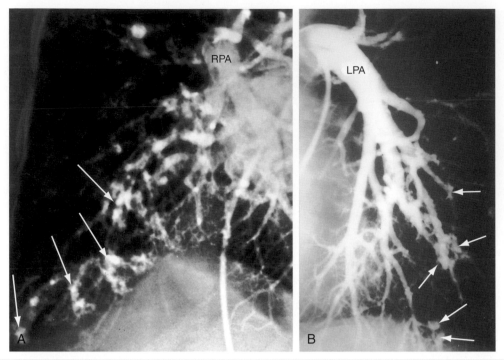

FIGURE 30-6 A, Selective injection of contrast material into the right pulmonary artery (RPA) of a 73-year-old woman with multiple small bilateral congenital pulmonary arteriovenous fistulae but no telangiectasia. Arrows point to at least four fistulae in the right lower lobe. **B,** Contrast material injected into the left pulmonary artery (LPA) of the patient's 71-year-old brother who also had multiple small bilateral pulmonary arteriovenous fistulae and no telangiectasia. Arrows identify at least five left lower lobe fistulae. These siblings represent the rare occurrence of familial congenital pulmonary arteriovenous fistulae without telangiectasia.

arteriovenous fistula was at necropsy in a 12-year-old boy (see previous).[1] Despite adult prevalence, cyanosis is occasionally present shortly after birth,[53] and the malformation is occasionally overtly manifest in childhood (Figure 30-9).[53]

Asymptomatic acyanotic pulmonary arteriovenous fistulae usually come to light because of abnormal shadows on a routine chest x-ray. Symptoms and complications are related to the pulmonary malformation *per se* or to coexisting hereditary hemorrhagic telangiectasia.[34,54] Congestive heart failure is reserved for infants with a rare large fistula (see Figure 30-7). The right-to-left shunt inherent in the fistulous communication results in cyanosis but seldom causes significant symptoms.[53] Dyspnea and fatigue are the result of anemia provoked by bleeding telangiectasia. Rupture of fistulae into a contiguous

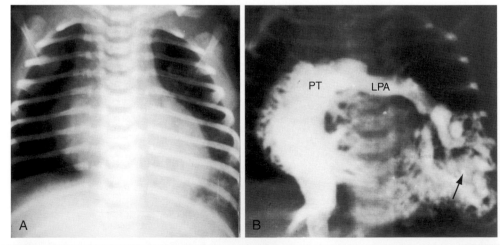

FIGURE 30-7 X-ray and angiocardiogram from a 4-day-old cyanotic infant with a massive left lower lobe congenital pulmonary arteriovenous fistula. **A,** The fistulous mass is seen in the x-ray as a hazy density above the left hemidiaphragm. The cardiac silhouette is enlarged because of congestive heart failure. **B,** Contrast material injected into the inferior vena cava visualized the pulmonary trunk (PT) and an elongated left pulmonary artery (LPA) that entered a large left lower lobe vascular malformation (arrow) that displaced the heart to the right. *(From Hall RJ, et al. Massive pulmonary arteriovenous fistula in the newborn. Circulation 1965;31:762.)*

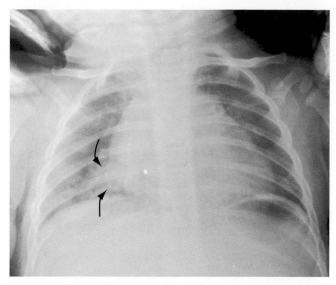

FIGURE 30-8 X-ray of a 6-month-old cyanotic female with a congenital right lower lobe pulmonary arteriovenous fistula that faintly revealed itself (paired arrows). Mucocutaneous telangiectasia were not identified. Cyanosis disappeared after coil embolization.

bronchus causes hemoptysis that varies from mild and occasional to recurrent and massive.[55,56] Fistulae are rarely substrates for infective endocarditis.[23] Chest pain accompanies pleural involvement. Hemothorax results from rupture of a subpleural fistula.[18,23,24,55,57] Intrapulmonary hemorrhage can be massive and fatal.[58] Pregnancy is accompanied by adverse effects that resolve after delivery, including hemothorax,[59] hemoptysis,[60,61] enlargement of existing fistulae, increasing cyanosis,[59,61] and expansion of occult fistulae.[62] However, pregnancy exerts favorable effects, such as compression of lower lobe fistulae, because of elevation of the diaphragm.[35]

Epistaxes are the most frequent and usually the first overt hemorrhagic event.[18] Cutaneous lesions bleed easily, especially when exposed to sunlight.[18] Tracheobronchial telangiectases set the stage for hemoptysis,[18] and appropriately placed lesions elsewhere cause melena, hematuria, intraocular hemorrhage, vaginal bleeding, and cerebrovascular accidents.[18,48,46]

Gastrointestinal endoscopy detects mucosal telangiectases.[22] Cerebral events special deserve comment with reference to a peculiar constellation of symptoms, including dizziness, vertigo, paresthesiae, tinnitus, faintness, visual disturbances, speech defects, headache, weakness of the limbs, hemiplegia, mental confusion, and convulsions.[35,18] Cerebral episodes may be brief or prolonged, isolated or recurrent, and tend to manifest similar patterns with subsequent attacks.[18] Pathogenesis has not been established, but occurrence in acyanotic patients without pulmonary arteriovenous fistulae incriminates telangiectasias,[18] which have been described with a cerebral arteriovenous malformation characterized by a plexiform nidus with an afferent arterial pedicle and a draining vein.[63]

Pulmonary arteriovenous fistulae set the stage for paradoxical emboli, stroke, and brain abscess (see Figure 30-6).[18,32,63–68] Intracranial malformations induce

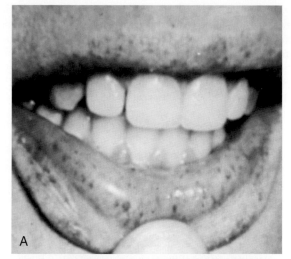

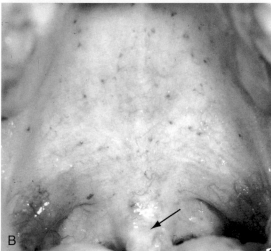

FIGURE 30-9 A, Typical hemorrhagic telangiectasia on the lips of a 25-year-old woman. **B,** Telangiectasia on the palate and uvula (arrow) of a 30-year-old man. Both patients had pulmonary arteriovenous fistulae.

grand mal seizures, which can be fatal.[69] Sudden death results from massive intrapulmonary hemorrhage and massive hemothorax.[18,24,58] A 41-year-old woman whose case was reported in 1906 died of intractable epistaxes.[70] Platypnea-orthodeoxia has been described with pulmonary arteriovenous fistula and a patent foramen ovale.[71]

PHYSICAL APPEARANCE

Cyanosis and clubbing are intense when the fistulous shunt is large.[18,72] Anemia caused by bleeding telangiectasia can virtually abolish the cyanosis, but clubbing persists.[18,72] Cyanosis is absent when *systemic* arteries rather than *pulmonary* arteries feed the fistulae.[18]

However, the most distinctive physical appearance in patients with pulmonary arteriovenous fistulae is the coexisting *mucocutaneous telangiectases*—clusters of tiny ruby lesions on the nasal and oral mucous membranes (see Figure 30-8) and on the face, tongue, skin, retina, and nail beds.[18,20] The lesions blanch with the slightest pressure and bleed with the slightest provocation. Unlike spider angioma, blanching with pressure is usually incomplete. Telangiectases are rarely evident in infants and young children but may be the first evidence of a pulmonary arteriovenous fistula.

An annotation in the *Lancet* vividly described the classic pattern of mucocutaneous telangiectases:

> *"Every large general hospital is certain to have on its list of frequent attenders a small group of unfortunate adults who come to the casualty department complaining of recurrent bleeding from the nose, lips or mouth. The blood is seen to stem from an insignificant leak in the center of a small ruby patch, many of which are usually to be found scattered here and there on the mucous membrane (Figure 30-8). Although the flow of blood is seldom vigorous it may eventually, by its persistence, cause some concern. Its arrest can be infuriatingly difficult. Each ruby patch marks the position of a tiny arteriovenous communication at the capillary level. Presumably these vessels are very close to the surface or else they are abnormally fragile. Whatever the cause, they can be induced to bleed by the most trivial of injuries."*

ARTERIAL PULSE AND JUGULAR VENOUS PULSE

The arterial pulse and the jugular venous pulse are normal because left ventricular stroke volume is normal or only modestly increased, and congestive heart failure is rare. Isolated examples of an increased arterial pulse occur with a massive pulmonary arteriovenous fistula (see Figure 30-7) and when coexisting intrahepatic arteriovenous fistulae cause a hyperdynamic circulatory state.[40,42]

PRECORDIAL MOVEMENT AND PALPATION

The extra amount of blood pumped by the right or left ventricle is relatively small (see Physiologic Consequences), so the impulses of both ventricles are normal.

Precordial impulses are hyperdynamic in the rare event of a massive pulmonary arteriovenous fistula (see Figure 30-7), and hepatic arteriovenous fistulae are accompanied by hyperdynamic ventricular impulses, hepatomegaly, and an hepatic thrill.[40,42]

AUSCULTATION

Pulmonary arteriovenous fistulae transmit murmurs to overlying chest wall sites because the fistulae are close to the periphery of the lungs (Figures 30-1, 30-2, and 30-3).[53] Murmurs are absent when fistulae lie deeply within the lungs or when they are small and diffuse (see Figures 30-4 and 30-5).[10,18] Murmurs are missed when they are faint and are assigned to nonprecordial sites.[53] The clinical diagnosis is untenable in *acyanotic* patients *with no murmur* and *no telangiectases.*

The abdominal location of the murmur is responsible for oversight when arteriovenous fistulae are hepatic.[40,41]

Murmurs are typically less than grade 3 and are therefore rarely accompanied by a thrill.[23] Loud harsh murmurs are exceptional. Auscultation should be carried out in a quiet room with the patient comfortable and the thorax relaxed to avoid the interference of muscle tremor. The entire chest should be examined, in addition to the liver and the cranium. Respiration should be quiet and should include gentle held exhalation. Because 75% of pulmonary arteriovenous fistulae are in the lower lobes and right middle lobe, the relevant overlying chest wall sites warrant special auscultatory attention.[7] Murmurs overlying the lingula of the left lung can be mistaken for intracardiac murmurs (see Figure 30-3).

Pulmonary arteriovenous fistulae generate systolic or continuous murmurs (Figures 30-10 and 30-11).[18,23,73] In the first clinically diagnosed case, the murmur was continuous.[2] The major pressure gradient across the fistula is systolic.[23,73] Diastolic gradients are negligible or absent, so the diastolic portion of the murmur is negligible or absent, which accounts for the high incidence rate of murmurs that are confined to systole (see Figure 30-10). Isolated diastolic murmurs are rare.[73] Fistulae are downstream from the right ventricle, so an interval elapses from the onset of right ventricular ejection to blood flow through the fistula.

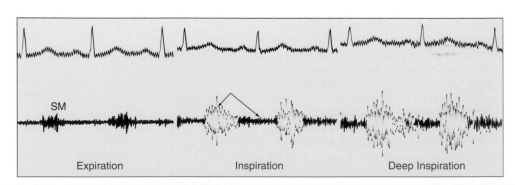

FIGURE 30-10 Phonocardiogram from the left mid axillary line of the 35 year old woman whose solitary left lower lobe pulmonary arteriovenous fistula is shown in Figure 30-2. The systolic murmur (SM) recorded during expiration becomes continuous and increases appreciably during deep inspiration.

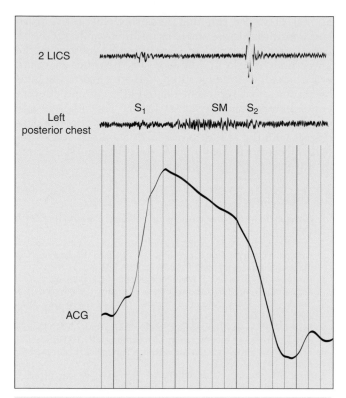

FIGURE 30-11 Phonocardiograms from a 38-year-old woman with a congenital pulmonary arteriovenous fistula of the left lower lobe. Recordings from the second left intercostal space (2 LICS) disclosed no murmur, but recordings from the left posterior chest disclosed a soft delayed systolic murmur (SM). (S_1/S_2 = first and second heart sounds; ACG = apex cardiogram.)

This interval is responsible for the delayed onset and late crescendo exhibited by the murmurs, which begin late and finish after the second heart sound (see Figure 30-11)

The normal inspiratory increase in right ventricular volume is available for forward flow through the fistula, and inspiratory depression of the diaphragm reduces compression of lower lobe fistulae. Accordingly, the murmur decreases during expiration and increases during inspiration, especially during deep held inspiration (see Figure 30-10).[18,23,35,73] The murmur may be heard only at the end of an exaggerated inspiratory effort, so unless this maneuver is performed, the response of the murmur will be missed. Inspiration may also cause a systolic murmur to become continuous (see Figure 30-10). To detect these respiratory effects, auscultation should be carried out at the end of normal expiration and at the height of deep momentarily held inspiration. These maneuvers serve two purposes: namely, to minimize respiratory interference and to provide time for right ventricular blood to reach the fistula. The Valsalva's and Müller's maneuvers exaggerate these effects.[23] Flow through the fistula diminishes during the Valsalva's maneuver, so the murmur softens or vanishes. When straining is released, flow abruptly accelerates and the murmur abruptly intensifies. The Müller's maneuver (forced inspiration against a closed glottis) increases flow through the fistula and increases the intensity of the fistulous murmur. Standing

increases perfusion of the dependent portions of the lungs and increases audibility of lower lobe murmurs.[35] A lateral decubitus position on the side of a fistula compresses the ipsilateral lung and decreases the murmur.[35] Pregnancy elevates the diaphragm, compresses lower lobe fistulae, and decreases or abolishes the murmur (see previous).[35]

ELECTROCARDIOGRAM

The electrocardiogram is typically normal because the hemodynamic burden is modest. Flow through the fistula is associated with a reciprocal decrease in flow through the uninvolved lung, so right ventricular output is normal, and the volume entering the left side of the heart is normal. The increment of blood shunted through the fistula seldom imposes volume load on either ventricle. These circulatory adjustments are less effective when fistulae are large, which may account for the occasional presence of right or left axis deviation.[23,73] When a large pulmonary arteriovenous fistula or a large pulmonary arterial–to–left atrial fistula exists *in utero*, right ventricular blood preferentially flows through the low-resistance fistula and imposes volume overload on the left side of the heart. This mechanism is held responsible for left ventricular hypertrophy and left atrial P wave abnormalities.

X-RAY

The rare large fistula is associated with an increase in heart size (see Figure 30-7),[23] but otherwise, the size and shape of the heart are normal (see Figures 30-1 and 30-2). The most important feature of the x-ray is the abnormal density cast by the fistula itself (see Figures 30-1A, 30-3, 30-6A, 30-7A, and 30-9). Lateral views should be examined to disclose a density hidden by the heart or diaphragm (see Figure 30-3).[4] Multiple small fistulae are hazy radiodensities rather than circumscribed lesions and are difficult to identify in the x-ray.[3,6,18,23] Fistulae in infants are usually poorly defined in the x-ray (see Figure 30-9) but tend to increase in size and radiodensity as the child grows.[31,32] Large fistulae are exceptional (see Figure 30-7).

Pulmonary arteriovenous fistulae can be single or multiple, unilateral or bilateral, and typically involve the lower lobes and right middle lobe (see Figures 30-1 through 30-4; see previous). Upper lobe fistulae are uncommon (see Figure 30-6). The densities vary in size and shape from small focal opacities (see Figures 30-4 and 30-5) to large homogeneous densities that can be mistaken for coin lesions or metastatic carcinoma (see Figures 30-1 and 30-2). The densities are hazy and ill-defined or round or lobulated with well-demarcated edges (see Figures 30-1, 30-2, 30-7,A, and 30-9).[18,20,23] Lateral projections confirm that the opacities are within the lung parenchym.[18] Calcification is exceptional.[74] Hemorrhage may obscure the lesion. Intrapleural rupture is accompanied by painful hemothorax.[18,24]

Vascular shadows that connect the parenchymal density to the hilus establish the lung lesion as pulmonary arteriovenous (see Figures 30-1 through 30-6).[18,23,75] The linear vascular shadows correspond to dilated afferent pulmonary arterial channels that join the fistula and efferent channels that leave the fistula (see Figures 30-1 through 30-4 and 30-6). Rarely, localized notching of ribs is caused by dilated tortuous intercostal arteries that enter the fistula.[23] Subtle variations in size of a fistula can be induced by changes in intrathoracic pressure (see previous).[23] The Valsalva's maneuver diminishes the fistula by decreasing flow. The Müller's maneuver enlarges the fistula by increasing flow.

ECHOCARDIOGRAM

Pulmonary arteriovenous fistulae are seldom imaged with echocardiography because the lesions are within the lung parenchyma. An exception is a solitary large paracardiac fistula.[25] Pulsed Doppler echocardiography can record bidirectional flow into and out of the fistula,[76] and the diagnosis has been made with color Doppler scan and amplitude ultrasound angiography.[77] "Bubble echocardiography" can be a useful diagnostic tool.[78] Contrast echocardiography detects relatively small right-to-left fistulous shunts and establishes the shunts as extracardiac.[25,79,80] Agitated saline solution injected into a peripheral vein, vena cava, or pulmonary artery is promptly detected in pulmonary veins or the left atrium with transthoracic and transesophageal echocardiograpy.[25,32,79,80]

SUMMARY

Pulmonary arteriovenous fistulae are usually discovered in young adults because of abnormal densities on routine chest x-rays or because of cyanosis or mucocutaneous telangiectasia. Dyspnea and fatigue do not correspond to the degree of cyanosis but are related to anemia caused by bleeding hemorrhagic telangiectasia. The history is characterized by recurrent epistaxis, hemoptysis, and bleeding from mouth, lips, and gastrointestinal tract. Cerebral, intrapulmonary, and intrapleural hemorrhage can be lethal. Peculiar cerebral symptoms include dizziness, tinnitus, vertigo, paresthesias, faintness, visual aberrations, speech disturbances, headache, extremity weakness, mental confusion, and seizures. Pulmonary arteriovenous malformations set the stage for paradoxical embolism, stroke, and brain abscess. Physical appearance reflects cyanosis and clubbing but especially clusters of small ruby patches (telangiectases) on the face, nasal and oral mucous membranes, tongue, lips, and skin. The arterial pulse, the jugular venous pulse, and the precordial movements are usually normal. Auscultation detects systolic or continuous murmurs at nonprecordial sites corresponding to the lower lobe or right middle lobe locations of the majority of pulmonary arteriovenous fistulae. Systolic murmurs increase in intensity and become continuous during inspiration, during the Müller's maneuver, or with standing and decrease in intensity during exhalation, during the Valsalva's maneuver, or in an ipsilateral decubitus position. The electrocardiogram is normal, and the size and shape of the heart on x-ray are normal. However, the lung fields show distinctive fistulous densities that are single or multiple, unilateral or bilateral, small or large, and are typically located in the lower lobes or right middle lobe. The densities are round or lobulated, well-demarcated, and attached to the hilus by shadows that represent dilated afferent and efferent vessels entering and leaving the fistula. The radiologic size of a fistula decreases with the Valsalva's maneuver and increases with the Müller's maneuver. Contrast echocardiography confirms small right-to-left fistulous shunts and identifies the shunts as extracardiac.

REFERENCES

1. Churton T. Multiple aneurysms of pulmonary artery. *Br Med J.* 1897;1:1223.
2. Smith HL, Horton BT. Arteriovenous fistula of the lung associated with polycythemia vera: report of a case in which the diagnosis was made clinically. *Am Heart J.* 1939;18:589–592.
3. Anabtawi IN, Ellison RG. Maldevelopment of the pulmonary veins and pulmonary arteriovenous aneurysms. *Am Surg.* 1964;30:770–773.
4. Boczko ML. Pulmonary arteriovenous fistulas. *Mayo Clin Proc.* 1999;74:1305.
5. Brian CA, Payne RM, Link KM, Hundley WG, Warner Jr JG. Pulmonary arteriovenous malformation. *Circulation.* 1999;100:e29–e30.
6. Hales MR. Multiple small arteriovenous fistulae of the lungs. *Am J Pathol.* 1956;32:927–943.
7. Sahn SH, Bluth I, Schub H. Pulmonary arteriovenous fistula: a report of two unusual cases. *Dis Chest.* 1963;44:542–546.
8. Amodeo A, Marino B. Pulmonary arteriovenous fistulas in patients with left isomerism and cardiac malformations. *Cardiol Young.* 1998;8:283–284.
9. Kapur S, Rome J, Chandra RS. Diffuse pulmonary arteriovenous malformation in a child with polysplenia syndrome. *Pediatr Pathol Lab Med.* 1995;15:463–468.
10. Sanders JS, Martt JM. Multiple small pulmonary arteriovenous fistulas. Diagnosis by cardiac catheterization. *Circulation.* 1962;25:383–389.
11. Franzen O, Lund C, Baldus S. Pulmonary arteriovenous fistula in hereditary hemorrhagic telangiectasis. *Clin Res Cardiol.* 2009;98:749–750.
12. Babington BG. Hereditary epistaxis. *Lancet.* 1865;2:362.
13. Legg JW. A case of haemophilia complicated with multiple naevi. *Lancet.* 1876;2:856.
14. Rendu H. Epistaxis répétée chez un sujet porteur de petits angiomes cutanés et muqueaux. *Bull Mem Soc Med Hop Paris.* 1896;13:731.
15. Osler W. On a family form of recurring epistaxis, associated with multiple telangiectases of skin and mucous membranes. *Bull Johns Hopkins Hosp.* 1901;12:333.
16. Weber FP. Multiple hereditary developmental angiomata (telangiectases) of the skin and mucous membranes associated with recurring haemorrhages. *Lancet.* 1907;2:160–162.
17. Hanes FM. Multiple hereditary telangiectases causing hemorrhage (hereditary hemorrhagic) telangiectasia. *Bull Johns Hopkins Hosp.* 1909;20:63–73.
18. Hodgson CH, Burchell HB, Good CA, Clagett OT. Hereditary hemorrhagic telangiectasia and pulmonary arteriovenous fistula: survey of a large family. *N Engl J Med.* 1959;261:625–636.
19. Shovlin CL, Guttmacher AE, Buscarini E, et al. Diagnostic criteria for hereditary hemorrhagic telangiectasia (Rendu-Osler-Weber syndrome). *Am J Med Genet.* 2000;91:66–67.
20. Steinberg I, Mcclenahan J. Pulmonary arteriovenous fistula; angiocardiographic observations in nine cases. *Am J Med.* 1955;19:549–568.
21. Hu S-Y, Tsai C-H, Tsan Y-T. Pulmonary arteriovenous malformation in Osler-Weber-Rendu syndrome. *Eur J Cardiothorac Surg.* 2009;36:395.
22. Yunoki K, Naruko T, Komiyama M, et al. Images in cardiovascular medicine. Hereditary hemorrhagic telangiectasia with pulmonary arteriovenous fistulas. *Circulation.* 2006;114:e48–e49.
23. Le Roux BT. Pulmonary arteriovenous fistulae. *Q J Med.* 1959;28:1.
24. Dalton Jr ML, Goodwin FC, Bronwell AW, Rutledge R. Intrapleural rupture of pulmonary arteriovenous aneurysm. Report of a case. *Dis Chest.* 1967;52:97–100.

25. Jimenez M, Fournier A, Choussat A. Pulmonary artery to the left atrium fistula as an unusual cause of cyanosis in the newborn. *Pediatr Cardiol*. 1989;10:216–220.

26. Kroeker EJ, Adams HD, Leon AS, Pouget JM. Congenital communication between a pulmonary artery and the left atrium. Physiologic observations and review of the literature. *Am J Med*. 1963; 34:721–725.

27. Sheikhzadeh A, Hakim H, Ghabusi P, Ataii M, Tarbiat S. Right pulmonary artery-to-left atrial communication: recognition and surgical correction. *Am Heart J*. 1984;107:396–398.

28. Tirilomis T, Busch T, Aleksic I, et al. Pulmonary arteriovenous fistula drainage into the left atrium. *Thorac Cardiovasc Surg*. 2000;48: 37–39.

29. Tuncali T, Aytac A. Direct communication between right pulmonary artery and left atrium. Report of a case and proposal of a new entity. *J Pediatr*. 1967;71:384–389.

30. Nelson WP, Hall RJ, Garcia E. Varicosities of the pulmonary veins simulating arteriovenous fistulas. *JAMA*. 1966;195:13–17.

31. Swanson KL, Prakash UB, Stanson AW. Pulmonary arteriovenous fistulas: Mayo Clinic experience, 1982-1997. *Mayo Clin Proc*. 1999;74:671–680.

32. Teragaki M, Akioka K, Yasuda M, et al. Hereditary hemorrhagic telangiectasia with growing pulmonary arteriovenous fistulas followed for 24 years. *Am J Med Sci*. 1988;295:545–547.

33. Sapru RP, Hutchison DC, Hall JI. Pulmonary hypertension in patients with pulmonary arteriovenous fistulae. *Br Heart J*. 1969; 31:559–569.

34. Waldhausen JA, Abel FL. The circulatory effects of pulmonary arteriovenous fistulas. *Surgery*. 1966;59:76–80.

35. Hazlett DR, Medina J. Postural effects on the bruit and right-to-left shunt of pulmonary arteriovenous fistula. *Chest*. 1971;60:89–92.

36. Bernstein HS, Brook MM, Silverman NH, Bristow J. Development of pulmonary arteriovenous fistulae in children after cavopulmonary shunt. *Circulation*. 1995;92:II309–II314.

37. Premsekar R, Monro JL, Salmon AP. Diagnosis, management, and pathophysiology of post-Fontan hypoxaemia secondary to Glenn shunt related pulmonary arteriovenous malformation. *Heart*. 1999;82:528–530.

38. Barbe T, Losay J, Grimon G, et al. Pulmonary arteriovenous shunting in children with liver disease. *J Pediatr*. 1995;126:571–579.

39. Hoffbauer FW, Rydell R. Multiple pulmonary arteriovenous fistulas in juvenile cirrhosis. *Am J Med*. 1956;21:450–460.

40. Burckhardt D, Stalder GA, Ludin H, Bianchi L. Hyperdynamic circulatory state due to Osler-Weber-Rendu disease with intrahepatic arteriovenous fistulas. *Am Heart J*. 1973;85:797–800.

41. Danchin N, Thisse JY, Neimann JL, Faivre G. Osler-Weber-Rendu disease with multiple intrahepatic arteriovenous fistulas. *Am Heart J*. 1983;105:856–859.

42. Razi B, Beller RM, Ghidoni J, et al. Hyperdynamic circulatory state due to intrahepatic fistula in Osler-Weber-Rendu disease. *Am J Med*. 1971;50:809–815.

43. Maruyama J, Watanabe M, Onodera S, et al. A case of Rendu-Osler-Weber disease with cerebral hemangioma, multiple pulmonary arteriovenous fistulas and hepatic arteriovenous fistula. *Jpn J Med*. 1989;28:651–656.

44. Wilkens GD. Ein fall von multiplen pulmonalis aneurysmen. *Beitr Klin Tuberk*. 1917;38:1–10.

45. Ehrenhaft JL, Taber RE. Arteriovenous fistulae and arterial aneurysms of the pulmonary arterial tree. *AMA Arch Surg*. 1956;73:567–577.

46. Mestre JR, Andres JM. Hereditary hemorrhagic telangiectasia causing hematemesis in an infant. *J Pediatr*. 1982;101:577–579.

47. Boston LN. Gastric hemorrhage due to familial telangiectasis. *Am J Med Sci*. 1930;180:798.

48. Humphries JE, Frierson Jr HF, Underwood Jr PB. Vaginal telangiectasias: unusual presentation of the Osler-Weber-Rendu syndrome. *Obstet Gynecol*. 1993;81:865–866.

49. Reilly PJ, Nostrant TT. Clinical manifestations of hereditary hemorrhagic telangiectasia. *Am J Gastroenterol*. 1984;79:363–367.

50. Mckusick VA. A genetical view of cardiovascular disease. The Lewis A. Conner memorial lecture. *Circulation*. 1964;30:326–357.

51. Peery WH. Clinical spectrum of hereditary hemorrhagic telangiectasia (Osler-Weber-Rendu disease). *Am J Med*. 1987;82:989–997.

52. Standefer JE, Tabakin BS, Hanson JS. Pulmonary arteriovenous fistulas. Case report with cine-angiographic studies. *Am Rev Respir Dis*. 1964;89:95–99.

53. Husson GS. Pulmonary arteriovenous aneurysm in childhood. *Pediatrics*. 1956;18:871–879.

54. Kraemer N, Krombach GA. Images in clinical medicine. Pulmonary arteriovenous fistula. *N Engl J Med*. 2009;360:1769.

55. Brummelkamp WH. Unusual complication of pulmonary arteriovenous aneurysm: Intrapleural rupture. *Dis Chest*. 1961;39:218.

56. Lyons HA, Mannix Jr EP. Successful resections for bilateral pulmonary arteriovenous fistulas. *N Engl J Med*. 1956;254:969–974.

57. Livingston SO, Carr RE. Hereditary hemorrhagic telangiectasia; report of a case with hemothorax. *J Thorac Surg*. 1956;31:497–503.

58. Ference BA, Shannon TM, White Jr RI, Zawin M, Burdge CM. Life-threatening pulmonary hemorrhage with pulmonary arteriovenous malformations and hereditary hemorrhagic telangiectasia. *Chest*. 1994;106:1387–1390.

59. Freixinet J, Sanchez-Palacios M, Guerrero D, et al. Pulmonary arteriovenous fistula ruptured to pleural cavity in pregnancy. *Scand J Thorac Cardiovasc Surg*. 1995;29:39–41.

60. Bradshaw DA, Murray KM, Mull NHT. Massive hemoptysis in pregnancy due to a solitary pulmonary arteriovenous malformation. *West J Med*. 1994;161:600–602.

61. Esplin MS, Varner MW. Progression of pulmonary arteriovenous malformation during pregnancy: case report and review of the literature. *Obstet Gynecol Surv*. 1997;52:248–253.

62. Wilmshurst P, Jackson P. Arterial hypoxemia during pregnancy caused by pulmonary arteriovenous microfistulas. *Chest*. 1996; 110:1368–1369.

63. Preston DC, Shapiro BE. Pulmonary arteriovenous fistula and brain abscess. *Neurology*. 2001;56:418.

64. Brydon HL, Akinwunmi J, Selway R, Ul-Haq I. Brain abscesses associated with pulmonary arteriovenous malformations. *Br J Neurosurg*. 1999;13:265–269.

65. Chambers WR. Brain abscess associated with pulmonary arteriovenous fistula. *Ann Surg*. 1955;141:276–277.

66. Sajeev CG, Fasaludeen M, Venugopal K. Pulmonary arteriovenous fistula presenting as brain abscess. *Int J Cardiol*. 2005;98:153.

67. Kawano H, Hirano T, Ikeno K, Fuwa I, Uchino M. Brain abscess caused by pulmonary arteriovenous fistulas without Rendu-Osler-Weber disease. *Intern Med*. 2009;48:485–487.

68. Tomelleri G, Bovi P, Carletti M, et al. Paradoxical brain embolism in a young man with isolated pulmonary arteriovenous fistula. *Neurol Sci*. 2008;29:169–171.

69. Byard RW, Schliebs J, Koszyca BA. Osler-Weber-Rendu syndrome–pathological manifestations and autopsy considerations. *J Forensic Sci*. 2001;46:698–701.

70. Kelly AB. Multiple telangiectases of the skin and mucous membranes of the nose and mouth. *Glas Med J*. 1906;65:411–422.

71. Ohara T, Nakatani S, Hashimoto S, et al. A case of platypnea-orthodeoxia syndrome in a patient with a pulmonary arteriovenous fistula and a patent foramen ovale. *J Am Soc Echocardiogr*. 2007;20: 439–440.

72. Dhillon BS, Fawcett AW. Pulmonary arterio-venous fistula; review of world literature and report on two additional cases. *Postgrad Med J*. 1956;32:353–356.

73. Yater WM, Finnegan J, Giffin HM. Pulmonary arteriovenous fistula; review of the literature and report of two cases. *J Am Med Assoc*. 1949;141:581–589.

74. Sloan RD, Cooley RN. Congenital pulmonary arteriovenous aneurysm. *Am J Roentgenol Radium Ther Nucl Med*. 1953;70:183–210.

75. Singleton EB, Leachman RD, Rosenberg HS. Congenital abnormalities of the pulmonary arteries. *Am J Roentgenol Radium Ther Nucl Med*. 1964;91:487–499.

76. Kataoka H, Matsuno O. Rendu-Osler-Weber Disease: transthoracic Doppler ultrasonographic findings. *Circulation*. 2001;103:E36–E38.

77. Wang HC, Kuo PH, Liaw YS, et al. Diagnosis of pulmonary arteriovenous malformations by colour Doppler ultrasound and amplitude ultrasound angiography. *Thorax*. 1998;53:372–376.

78. Sands A, Dalzell E, Craig B, Shields M. Multiple intrapulmonary arteriovenous fistulas in childhood. *Pediatr Cardiol*. 2000;21: 493–496.

79. Ozkutlu S, Saraclar M. Two-dimensional contrast echocardiography in pulmonary arteriovenous fistula. *Jpn Heart J*. 1989;30:425–430.

80. Shub C, Tajik AJ, Seward JB, Dines DE. Detecting intrapulmonary right-to-left shunt with contrast echocardiography. Observations in a patient with diffuse pulmonary arteriovenous fistulas. *Mayo Clin Proc*. 1976;51:81–84.

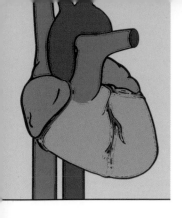

Chapter 31

Hypoplastic Left Heart

In 1952, Lev[1] called attention to congenital hypoplasia of major components of the left side of the heart. In 1958, Noonan and Nadas[2] referred to these malformations as the *hypoplastic left heart syndrome*. At the severe end of the spectrum, the aortic and mitral valves are atretic, and the left ventricle is virtually nonexistent (Figure 31-1).[3,4] At the mild end of the spectrum, the aortic and mitral valves are patent, and there is a lesser degree of left ventricular hypoplasia (Figure 31-2).[4] The hypoplastic left heart syndrome is a genetically heterogeneous disorder that affects 1 in 5000 live births[5] and accounts for 7.5% of infants with congenital heart disease.[6]

Aortic atresia is accompanied by a hypoplastic ascending aorta that serves as a common coronary artery (see Figures 31-1 and 31-2).[7] A hypoplastic but patent mitral valve is accompanied by a hypoplastic but patent left ventricle (see Figure 31-2). Mitral atresia is accompanied by a blind slit-like left ventricular cavity embedded in the ventricular muscle (see Figure 31-1). An experimental model in chick embryos is represented by atresia or hypoplasia of the mitral valve and of the left ventricle, aortic valve, and thoracic aorta.[8] Hypoplasia or atresia of the mitral valve leaves the left atrium without an exit except a restrictive patent foramen ovale (see Figures 31-1 and 31-2), which is further compromised by hypoplasia of the limbus that is rotated and deviated close to the orifice of the superior vena cava.[9] An intact atrial septum is accompanied by either a thick muscular septal wall and a small left atrium or by a thick septum secundum, a thin septum primum, and an enlarged left atrium.[10] Alternative decompression pathways for the obstructed left atrium consist of vascular channels from a levoatrial cardinal vein to the innominate vein, an accessory vein from left atrium to the superior vena cava, a venous connection from left atrium to hepatic veins, a coronary venous connection from left atrium to coronary sinus, and a coronary sinoseptal defect.[10]

Vasoconstriction during early embryogenesis leads to decreased growth and development of pulmonary veins and to alveolar capillary dysplasia, which forces arterial blood to bypass the deficient capillary bed and drain through anomalous bronchial veins.[11] Lymphatics are strikingly enlarged.[10] Dilated pulmonary veins are thick and arterialized with multiple elastic laminae.[10]

The subject of the *first section of this chapter* is aortic atresia with a hypoplastic but perforate mitral valve (see Figure 31-2). The *second section* deals with aortic atresia and mitral atresia (Figure 31-3).

AORTIC ATRESIA WITH HYPOPLASTIC BUT PERFORATE MITRAL VALVE

The pathway to the systemic circulation is a single arterial trunk represented by pulmonary artery/ductus/descending aortic continuity (see Figure 31-2). A hypoplastic ascending aorta serves as a common coronary artery.[3,12] Fifty percent to 75% of cases are accompanied by moderate coarctation of the aorta[13] located either proximal to the ductus (preductal) or distal to the junction of the ductus and aortic arch (paraductal; see Figure 31-3).[13] The right ventricle is hypertrophied because it is the sole pumping chamber for the systemic and pulmonary circulations.[3] It harbors histologic changes of ischemia and infarction.[14] The blind hypoplastic left ventricle is thick-walled and lined with endocardial fibroelastosis.[2,3] Rarely, the left ventricle is characterized by isolated apical hypoplasia with fatty replacement.[15] Isovolumetric contraction causes myofiber disarray but does not cause direct ventriculocoronary artery communications.[16] Pinpoint neonatal aortic stenosis with small left ventricular cavity (see Chapter 7) is associated with intramyocardial sinusoids but not with direct ventriculocoronary arterial communications. The left ventricle is adequately formed in the presence of a ventricular septal defect and a patent aortic valve.[3,17]

The tricuspid valve is abnormal in a distinct minority of patients.[18] The leaflets may be dysplastic with nodular free edges, shortened chordae tendineae, obliterated interchordal spaces, and an accessory orifice, and only two leaflets may be identifiable.[18]

A major concern in hypoplastic left heart syndrome is the brain that is smaller and structurally less mature than normal.[19] The scimitar syndrome has been reported in a child with a hypoplastic left heart.[20]

The *coronary circulation* has been a matter of lively interest.[2,3,7,14,21,22] A hypoplastic ascending aorta functions as a common coronary artery that receives retrograde systolic and diastolic flow from the patent ductus (see Figures 31-2 and 31-3).[2,3,14] The tubular, hypoplastic ascending aorta is not an impediment to retrograde flow into the common coronary artery, but the preductal coarctation (see Figure 31-3) is an impediment.[14] Intramyocardial coronary abnormalities analogous to those of pulmonary atresia with intact ventricular septum can be anticipated (see Chapter 24)

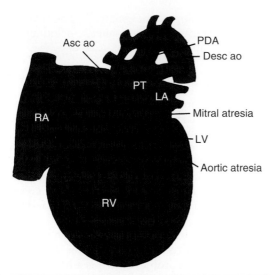

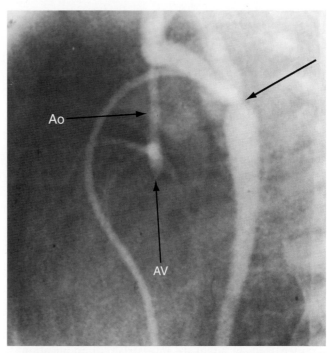

FIGURE 31-1 Illustration of the essential anatomic and physiologic derangements of a hypoplastic left heart with aortic atresia and mitral atresia. The left ventricular cavity (LV) is a rudimentary blind slit. The physiologic derangements are as described in Figure 31-2. (PDA = patent ductus arteriosus; ASC ao = ascending aorta; Desc ao = descending aorta.)

FIGURE 31-3 Lateral aortogram in a male neonate with atresia of the aortic valve (AV) and a hypoplastic but perforate mitral valve. The catheter is across a patent ductus arteriosus. The hypoplastic ascending aorta (Ao) functioned as a common coronary artery. The large unmarked arrow at the upper right identifies coarctation of the aorta.

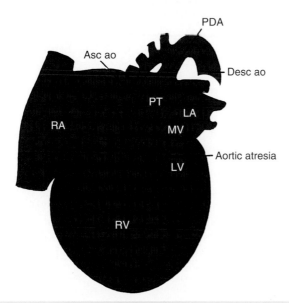

FIGURE 31-2 Illustration of the essential anatomic and physiologic derangements in a hypoplastic left heart with aortic atresia, a hypoplastic but perforate mitral valve (MV), and a hypoplastic left ventricle (LV). There is retrograde filling of the hypoplastic ascending aorta (Asc. ao.) that functions as a common coronary artery. The right ventricle (RV) serves the pulmonary circulation through the pulmonary trunk (PT) and perfuses the systemic circulation through pulmonary trunk/ductus/descending aortic continuity. A patent foramen ovale is the only exit for the left atrium (LA; upper left curved arrow). (RA = right atrium; Desc ao = descending aorta; PDA = patent ductus arteriosus.)

because isovolumetric contraction generates excessive systolic pressure that acts as a driving force for direct ventriculocoronary arterial communications.[7] However, the differences between pulmonary atresia with intact ventricular septum and aortic atresia with a hypoplastic

but patent mitral valve are as great as the similarities.[7] *Myocardial sinusoids* consist of restrictive vascular networks that spare the coronary arteries from the impact of high ventricular systolic pressure delivered through direct ventriculocoronary arterial communications.[7] In aortic atresia with a hypoplastic but patent mitral valve (see Figure 31-2), the intramyocardial communications are sinusoidal.[7] Accordingly, epicardial and subepicardial coronary arteries do not receive the impact of high isovolumetric systolic pressure and are spared the luminal obliterative features of pulmonary atresia with intact ventricular septum (see Chapter 24).[7]

The *physiologic consequences* of hypoplastic left heart with aortic atresia and a hypoplastic but perforate mitral valve are determined by the size of the ductus arteriosus, the pulmonary vascular resistance, and the condition of the atrial septum. Constriction of the ductus compromises flow into the systemic circulation and into the hypoplastic ascending aorta, which functions as a common coronary artery (see previous). Right ventricular function suffers because of the ischemic effects of inadequate coronary blood flow,[14,23] because of pulmonary hypertension caused by the nonrestrictive ductus, because of high pressure in the obstructed left atrium, and because a large left ventricular mass has disadvantageous effects on right ventricular end-diastolic volume and right ventricular wall motion. Competence of the tricuspid valve is important for survival, yet tricuspid dysplasia with a multiple papillary muscles is common (see previous). Low pulmonary vascular resistance permits increased pulmonary arterial blood flow that is received by the obstructed left atrium from which the only effective egress is a restrictive patent foramen ovale (see previous; see Figure 31-2). In the presence of an adequate interatrial communication, increased pulmonary blood flow makes a large volume of oxygenated left atrial blood available for mixing in the right atrium, so systemic arterial oxygen saturation is relatively high. However, preferential blood flow into the lungs through the ductus is accompanied by a reciprocal fall in systemic blood flow and a shock-like state. When pulmonary vascular resistance is high, systemic blood flow is maintained at the price of increasing cyanosis.

History

Hypoplastic left heart comprises 7% to 8% of symptomatic heart disease in the first year of life[24] and is responsible for 25% of cardiac deaths in the first week of life.[6] The malformation has been called the most malignant form of congenital heart disease, a conclusion underscored by an average lifespan of only 5 to 14 days.[3,6,25] Precarious survival depends on three tenuous variables: patency of the ductus arteriosus, pulmonary vascular resistance, and an adequate interatrial communication.[26] Tachypnea, tachycardia, and cyanosis are present during the brief interval of ductal patency.[24] Risk is greatest during the period of normal ductal closure when systemic blood flow and coronary blood flow decrease or cease altogether. A fall in pulmonary vascular resistance diverts blood from the systemic circulation into the pulmonary circulation and augments flow into the obstructed left atrium. A rise in pulmonary vascular resistance improves systemic blood flow, but at the price of hypoxemia. Ninety-five percent of afflicted infants die within the first month of life.[6,27] Two extraordinary survivals include a 22-year-old woman with a large patent ductus arteriosus and an adequate-sized atrial septal defect and a 24-year-old man with a patent ductus arteriosus and a ventricular septal defect.[28]

There is male prevalence of 55% to 70% in *aortic atresia with a hypoplastic but perforate mitral valve*.[2,3,29] Maternal age tends to be above average, with a mean of 31 years. First-degree relatives of probands have an increased prevalence of congenital heart disease.[24] The malformation is occasionally familial[30,31] and has been reported in siblings as an autosomal recessive inheritance.[32] A mosaic chromosomal 22q11 deletion is associated with hypoplastic left heart,[33,34] and genetic disorders include Turner's syndrome (see subsequent), trisomy 13, trisomy 18, and trisomy 21.[35-37] Concordance has been reported in a monochromic twin pregnancy.[38]

Reports of geographic clustering implicate environmental factors.[39] Eastern Wisconsin has increased rates of hypoplastic left heart syndrome,[40,41] a region in Baltimore has twice the expected frequency,[42] and the island of Malta has a *decreased* incidence.[43]

Hypoxemia and hypotension are associated with hypoxic-ischemic cerebral injury and intracranial hemorrhage.[44] Major and minor congenital central nervous system abnormalities include microcephaly, microencephaly, abnormal cortical mantle, agenesis of the corpus callosum, and holoprosencephaly.[45] The overall frequency of extracardiac anomalies, including central nervous system abnormalities, is 12% to 37%.[35]

Physical Appearance

Tachypnea and cyanosis are present even during the brief period of ductal patency (see previous). Cyanosis is mildest when an adequate interatrial communication and a patent ductus are accompanied by low pulmonary vascular resistance and increased pulmonary blood flow. A fall in pulmonary vascular resistance is accompanied by systemic hypoperfusion and a shock-like state. Cyanosis is profound when pulmonary resistance is high and the ductus is restrictive.

The hypoplastic left heart syndrome can be associated with Turner's syndrome (see Chapter 8)[35-37,46]; the Rubenstein-Taybi syndrome, which is a Mendelian dominant disorder characterized by mental retardation, growth retardation, typical facies, cognitive defects, broad thumbs and toes, and short stature[47,48]; the abdominal distension of Hirschsprung's disease[49]; and the Kubuki syndrome, characterized by eversion of the lower lateral eyelids, arched eyebrows with the lateral one third dispersed or sparse, depressed nasal tip, prominent ears, skeletal anomalies, short stature, and mental retardation.[50]

Arterial Pulse, Jugular Venous Pulse, and Precordial Palpation

Brachial and carotid arterial pulses remain palpable because the ascending aortic tubular hypoplasia does not include the arch (see Figures 31-1 and 31-2).[2] Femoral artery pulses are palpable because of pulmonary trunk/ductal/descending aortic continuity (see Figures 31-1 and 31-2) and because coarctation is usually paraductal or mild preductal (see Figure 31-3). When low pulmonary vascular resistance diverts blood from the systemic circulation, all arterial pulses diminish, if not vanish.

Increased right atrial A and V waves are not amenable to clinical assessment. Precordial palpation is dominated by a striking right ventricular impulse and a palpable pulmonary closure sound.

Auscultation

Auscultatory signs are unimpressive in contrast to the dramatic clinical picture. Murmurs are usually absent (Figure 31-4),[2,24] or a soft midsystolic murmur is generated by ejection into the dilated hypertensive pulmonary trunk. A long systolic murmur is likely to be caused by tricuspid regurgitation. The second heart sound is single because the aortic valve is atretic and is loud because of pulmonary hypertension (see Figure 31-4). A triple rhythm is caused by summation of right ventricular third and fourth heart sounds (see Figure 31-4).

Electrocardiogram

Tall peaked right atrial P waves are common (Figures 31-5 and 31-6) but not invariable (Figure 31-7). The PR interval is occasionally prolonged (see Figure 31-5). Left axis

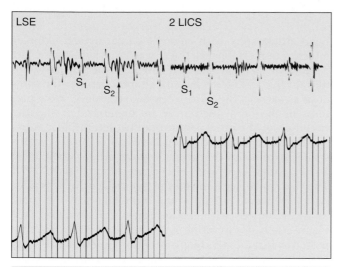

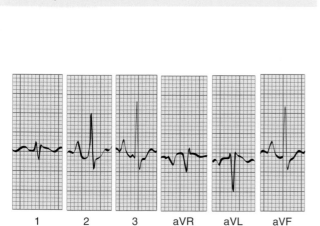

FIGURE 31-4 Phonocardiograms from a 9-day-old male with aortic atresia and a hypoplastic but perforate mitral valve. Necropsy findings were as illustrated in Figure 31-2. A loud filling sound (unmarked arrow) with after-vibrations at the lower left sternal edge (LSE) was caused by summation of right ventricular third and fourth heart sounds. The second heart sound (S$_2$) in the second left intercostal space (2 LICS) was loud because of pulmonary hypertension and single because the aortic valve was atretic. (S$_1$ = first heart sound.)

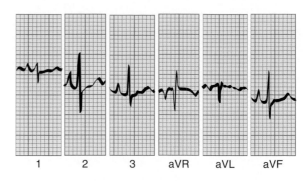

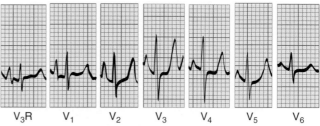

FIGURE 31-6 Electrocardiogram from a 3-week-old male with aortic atresia and a hypoplastic but perforate mitral valve. Necropsy findings were as illustrated in Figure 31-2. Tall peaked right atrial P waves are present in leads 2, 3, aVF, and V$_{1-3}$. Right ventricular dominance is indicated by the prominent R waves in leads V$_{2-4}$, the upright T waves in right precordial leads, and the rightward QRS axis.

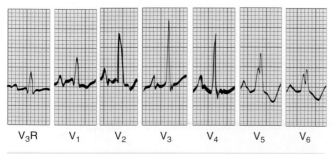

FIGURE 31-5 Electrocardiogram from the 9-day-old male with aortic atresia and a hypoplastic but perforate mitral valve. The phonocardiogram is shown in Figure 31-4. Tall peaked right atrial P waves are present in leads 2, 3, aVF, and V$_{2-4}$. Right atrial enlargement is indicated by qR complexes in leads V$_3$R and V$_1$. The PR interval is prolonged. Right ventricular hypertrophy is reflected in the tall monophasic R waves in right and mid precordial leads and the vertical QRS axis. The splintered QRS in leads V$_{5-6}$ is the result of a right ventricular conduction defect. The left ventricle is not represented.

deviation is uncommon despite abnormalities of the left bundle branch, and left bundle branch block is unknown.[2,51] Alterations in the branching portion of the His bundle and the left bundle branch depend on the size of the left ventricular cavity, with major changes reserved for absence or virtual absence of a cavity.[52] When the left ventricular cavity is small but not slit-like, the left bundle branch has a peripheral Purkinje network and the right bundle branch is normal in size.[52] Wolff-Parkinson-White bypass tracks are rare even though there are persistent connections of the left bundle branch to ventricular septal musculature with abundant Mahaim fibers.[52]

The QRS reflects pure right ventricular hypertrophy (see Figures 31-5 and 31-6). Left ventricular hypertrophy is infrequent despite an increase in mass because of the effect of a low end-diastolic volume on the magnitude of the QRS.[53] Left ventricular forces are absent when the cavity is small but may be present when the cavity is more adequately developed (see Figure 31-7).

X-Ray

Dilation of the right atrium and right ventricle is responsible for cardiac enlargement (Figure 31-8).[54] The shadow of the hypoplastic ascending aorta is necessarily absent, and the shadow of the dilated hypertensive pulmonary trunk is necessarily prominent (see Figure 31-8). Pulmonary venous congestion is the rule,[54] but the amount of lung available for assessment may be limited by remarkable cardiomegaly, even in the first 24 to 48 hours of life.

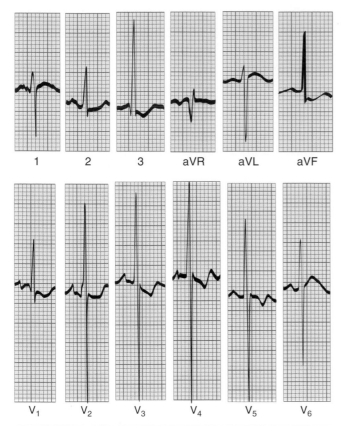

1   2   3   aVR   aVL   aVF

V₁   V₂   V₃   V₄   V₅   V₆

FIGURE 31-7 Electrocardiogram from a 4-week-old male with aortic atresia and a hypoplastic but perforate mitral valve. P waves are normal despite an enlarged right atrium and a high pressure left atrium. Right ventricular hypertrophy is indicated by right axis deviation, a tall R wave in lead V_1, and a deep S wave in lead V_6. Large RS complexes in leads V_{2-5} suggest biventricular hypertrophy. The left ventricle at necropsy was thick-walled with a small cavity lined with endocardial fibroelastosis.

Echocardiogram

Echocardiography with color flow imaging and Doppler interrogation establishes the diagnosis of hypoplastic left heart with aortic atresia and a hypoplastic but perforate mitral valve.[55] Fetal echocardiography permits the diagnosis as early as the 24th week of gestation.[56] Flow patterns in the fetal ductus can be monitored,[57] and the condition of the atrial septum can be determined. A hypoplastic but perforate mitral valve communicates with a small left ventricle that gives rise to an atretic aortic valve and a tubular hypoplastic ascending aorta (Figure 31-9). The ventricular septum and the free wall of the hypoplastic left ventricle are thick and immobile, and the small cavity is lined with endocardial fibroelastosis (see Figure 31-9). Coarctation is identified as a thin discrete posterior ledge extending across the lumen of the aorta at the level of the ductus arteriosus or as kinking and narrowing at the site of ductal insertion. The left atrium is small and thick-walled (see Figure 31-9). Function of the enlarged hypertrophied right ventricle and competence of the tricuspid valve can be established (see Figure 31-9),[58,59] and ductus/pulmonary trunk/descending aortic continuity is confirmed with color flow imaging. Doppler interrogation establishes retrograde flow into the hypoplastic ascending aorta and occasionally identifies biphasic flow in the proximal coronary arteries. Direct ventriculocoronary arterial communications can be identified.[60]

Summary

Hypoplastic left heart represented by aortic atresia and a hypoplastic but perforate mitral valve presents as a listless, tachypneic, often moribund male neonate with mild to profound cyanosis. Brachiocephalic and femoral arterial pulses are palpable. A right ventricular impulse is conspicuous. Auscultation detects a soft pulmonary

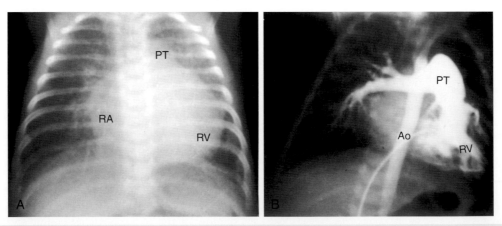

FIGURE 31-8 X-ray and angiocardiogram from a 2-day-old male with aortic atresia and a hypoplastic but perforate mitral valve. Necropsy findings were as illustrated in Figure 31-2. **A,** Pulmonary venous congestion is prominent. The right atrium (RA) and right ventricle (RV) are enlarged, the pulmonary trunk (PT) is dilated, and the ascending aorta is conspicuously absent. **B,** The right ventricular (RV) angiocardiogram visualizes the large pulmonary trunk (PT) with pulmonary artery/ductus /descending aortic continuity. (Ao = descending aorta.)

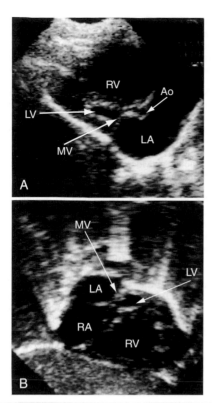

FIGURE 31-9 A, Echocardiogram (parasternal long-axis view) from a male neonate with aortic atresia and a hypoplastic but perforate mitral valve (MV). The hypoplastic left ventricle is lined with endocardial fibroelastosis. The ascending aorta (Ao) is hypoplastic, the left atrium (LA) is thick-walled but not enlarged, and the right ventricle (RV) is dilated. **B,** Subcostal four-chamber view shows a hypoplastic left ventricular cavity with endocardial fibroelastosis, a nondilated left atrium, and a dilated right ventricle (RV) and right atrium (RA). (ASD = atrial septal defect.)

midsystolic murmur, a tricuspid regurgitant murmur, or, more often than not, no murmur at all. The electrocardiogram displays right atrial P waves and right ventricular hypertrophy. The x-ray discloses pulmonary venous congestion, dilation of the right atrium, and right ventricle and pulmonary trunk, but conspicuous absence of the ascending aorta. Echocardiography with color flow imaging and Doppler interrogation identifies a hypoplastic perforate mitral valve, a hypoplastic left ventricle lined with endocardial fibroelastosis, a tubular hypoplastic ascending aorta guarded by an atretic aortic valve, and a single arterial trunk that consists of pulmonary artery/ductus/descending aortic continuity.

HYPOPLASTIC LEFT HEART WITH AORTIC AND MITRAL ATRESIA

The major physiologic derangements are similar to those of aortic atresia with a hypoplastic but perforate mitral valve, but there are anatomic differences and subtle clinical differences. The attachment of the valve of the fossa

ovalis may be malaligned relative to the muscular rim of the fossa. Mitral atresia is represented by an imperforate macroscopic membrane on the floor of the left atrium or a microscopic fibrous remnant between the floor of the left atrium and a putative left ventricular cavity represented by a minute blind slit (see Figure 31-1).[3,61,62] Myofiber disarray does not occur because isovolumetric contraction does not occur.[3,7,62] Because there is no left ventricular cavity to develop excessive systolic pressure, ventriculocoronary arterial connections do not develop, and epicardial and subepicardial coronary arteries are neither thickened nor tortuous.[7] A ventricular septal defect or absence of the right ventricular sinus is associated with a well-formed left ventricle.[3] The physiologic consequences are the same, and longevity patterns are similar,[63] whether aortic atresia is accompanied by mitral atresia or by a hypoplastic but perforate mitral valve (see Figures 31-1 and 31-2). Male gender predominates, although female twins have been reported.[29]

Subtle clinical points favor hypoplastic left heart with mitral atresia. The electrocardiogram shows pure right ventricular hypertrophy devoid of left ventricular potentials because a left ventricular cavity does not exist (Figure 31-10).[53] The left bundle branch does not develop a Purkinje network because there is no left ventricular cavity in which to do so.[52] Mahaim fibers are the only extensions of the left bundle branch that maintain continuity with ventricular septal muscle.[52] The right bundle branch enlarges because it is responsible for conduction

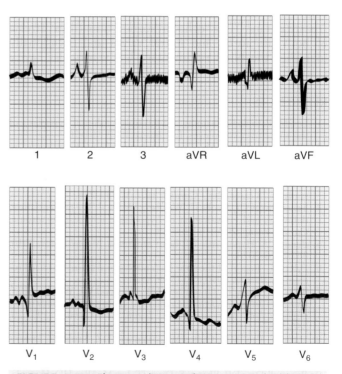

FIGURE 31-10 Electrocardiogram from a 3-week-old male with aortic atresia and mitral atresia. Necropsy findings were as illustrated in Figure 31-1. Peaked right atrial P waves are present in leads 2 and 3. Right atrial enlargement is indicated by the qR pattern in leads V_1. Pure right ventricular hypertrophy is reflected in tall monophasic R waves in leads V_{2-4} and the vertical and superior QRS axis.

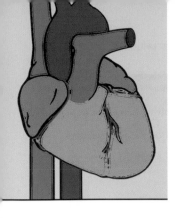

Chapter 32

Congenital Anomalies of the Coronary Circulation

The word coronary is derived from the Latin *coronarius* (pertaining to a crown), translated from the Greek *stephanos* (wreath), which refers to the crown-like or wreath-like arrangement of arteries that encircle the heart.[1] This chapter deals with the coronary circulation—arterial and venous—including morphogenesis, the normal coronary arteries, and the congenital anomalies as classified in Table 32-1.

In 1513, Leonardo da Vinci's anatomic drawings of a bullock's heart identified the coronary arteries (see Figure 32-3A) and the *great cardiac vein* (coronary sinus).[2] Leonardo called attention to *two vessels that arise from two external openings* (aortic sinuses). In 1543, 500 years later, the circulation in the normal heart was characterized,[3] and congenital anomalies of the coronary arteries were recognized.[4] In 1543, Andreas Vesalius, the celebrated 16th century Flemish anatomist, depicted an anomalous right coronary artery originating from the left aortic sinus and passing anterior to the right ventricular outflow tract *(De Humani Corporis Fabrica)*.

Selective coronary angiography was introduced in 1962 by Mason Sones[5] and was a major step forward in imaging coronary artery anatomy in the living beating human heart. Techniques continue to advance and include transesophageal echocardiography, magnetic resonance imaging, computerized axial tomography, electron beam tomography, and three-dimensional reconstruction.[6–8] Concurrently, nomenclature has evolved.[9]

Myocardial morphogenesis begins with the emergence of trabeculations in the luminal ventricular layers that permit an increase mass in the absence of a coronary circulation.[10] Cardiac jelly in the embryonic luminal layer is the primitive site of metabolic exchange between cardiac mesenchyma and blood in the ventricular cavity.[4,11] The human heart begins to beat as early as the 22nd day after conception, and a few days later, an ebb and flow circulation permits metabolic exchange.

The sequence of development of the coronary vascular bed begins with blood islands and coronary venous connections followed by coronary artery–to–aortic connections. Blood islands are epicardial layers of endothelial cells distended by nucleated erythrocytes. The blood islands proliferate, coalesce, and form rudimentary networks of vascular channels with no discernible connections to other islands or to the cavity of the ventricle. The *second stage* of development is a venous connection between the network of vascular channels and the coronary sinus, an arrangement that drains the blood islands

and reduces their size. The distal coronary bed remains a loose intermingling vascular network until myocardial mass develops. In the *third stage* of development, the coronary arteries join the aorta through an arterial connection to the plexus of vascular channels. The third stage is established after aortopulmonary septation and after formation of the semilunar valves. Flow commences from the aorta into the proximal coronary arteries through myocardial capillaries, then into coronary veins and into the coronary sinus. It is unknown why the two coronary arteries originate from the right and left aortic sinuses that face the right ventricular outflow tract (Figure 32-1A). The embryonic great arteries contain six sinuses, three in the aorta and three in the pulmonary trunk. The endothelial outgrowths or anlagen (buds, sprouts) in the third aortic sinus and in all three pulmonary sinuses undergo rapid involution or do not develop. Aortic–to–coronary artery connections become evident before the appearance of precursor connections in the aortic sinuses. It has been speculated that the aortic sinus sites of the two coronary ostia are determined by mural tension that is increased by the catenoid configuration of the right and left sinuses, so that endothelium penetrates the aortic wall preferentially in the right and left sinus sites, establishing connections with the epicardial coronary plexus.

The *capillary bed* interposed between the coronary arterial and coronary venous circulations plays a pivotal role in the transport of oxygen and nutrients to the myocardium. Capillary density, defined as the ratio of the number of capillaries to the number of cardiomyocytes, is basic to the metabolic exchange between blood and tissues. Capillary density depends on angiogenesis—the capacity of capillaries to replicate. Fetal capillaries replicate in response to the hypoxic intrauterine environment. Postnatal angiogenesis is a diminishing continuation of that response.[11]

The coronary circulation includes three separate systems of veins.[12] The largest system terminates in the coronary sinus and drains blood from most of the left ventricle. A second venous system drains most of the blood from the right ventricle. Adam Christian Thebesius, a German anatomist (1686-1732), described a third venous system consisting of tributaries that drain directly into the cardiac chambers.[12] Before the discovery of the pulmonary circulation, Thebesian veins were considered pathways of blood flow from right heart to left heart.

Patterns of *blood flow in the coronary circulation* are different in the right and left ventricles. In the normal

Table 32-1	**Classification of Congenital Anomalies of the Coronary Circulation**

Congenital anomalies of coronary arteries unassociated with
    congenital heart disease
- Anomalous aortic origin
- Anomalous proximal course
- Anomalous distal connection
- Anomalous pulmonary arterial origin
- Anomalies of size: atretic, hypoplastic, ectatic, aneurysmal

Congenital anomalies of coronary arteries associated with
    congenital heart disease

Acquired anomalies of coronary arteries resulting from
    congenital heart disease

Congenital anomalies of the coronary venous circulation

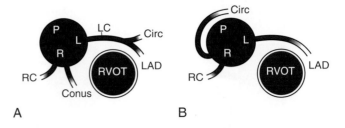

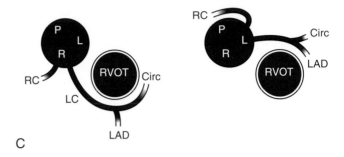

Anterior or posterior to aorta

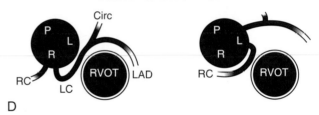

Between aorta and RVOT

FIGURE 32-1   A, Illustration of the normal origin of the left coronary artery (LC) and the right coronary artery (RC). A conus artery arises by a separate ostium from the right aortic sinus. (P = posterior aortic sinus; R = right aortic sinus; L = left aortic sinus.) **B,** The left anterior descending coronary artery (LAD) arises normally from the left aortic sinus, and the circumflex coronary artery (Circ) arises aberrantly from the right aortic sinus. **C,** The first illustration shows an aberrant left coronary artery (LC) passing anterior to the right ventricular outflow tract (RVOT), and the second illustration shows an aberrant right coronary (RC) artery passing posterior to the right ventricular outflow tract. **D,** The first illustration shows an aberrant *left* coronary artery (LC) passing between the aorta and right ventricular outflow tract (RVOT), and the second illustration shows an aberrant *right* coronary artery (RC) passing between the aorta and right ventricular outflow tract.

thin-walled *right ventricle*, coronary flow is continuous because pressure in the aorta continuously exceeds right ventricular intramural pressure. A higher diastolic pressure in the aorta coincides with a diastolic fall in intramyocardial pressure that results in brisk diastolic flow into the epicardial coronary arteries. Isovolumetric left ventricular contraction exerts disproportionate pressure on the subendocardial third of the wall, expressing blood from the subendocardial perforating branches and arresting flow into extramural branches. The pressure in the aorta during ventricular systole generates transient flow into the extramural coronary arteries and into the contiguous subepicardial myocardium because subepicardial pressure is appreciably lower than pressure in the subendocardium.

The round or ovoid ostia of the two coronary arteries are located in the right and left anterior aortic sinuses, which are therefore called the *coronary sinuses*.[1] The posterior aortic sinus is devoid of a coronary ostium and is appropriately called the *noncoronary sinus*.[1] *Normal coronary artery ostia* are located in the middle of an aortic sinus just below the sinotubular junction and just above the upper margin of the aortic cusps. *Abnormally located ostia* originate above the sinotubular junction, in the posterior aortic sinus, or eccentrically near a commissure.

There are typically two coronary ostia, but three or four ostia are considered normal variants. A third ostium usually results from a separate conus branch in the right coronary sinus (see Figure 32-1A). Less commonly, three coronary ostia are the result of origin of the left anterior descending and circumflex coronary arteries from the left aortic sinus and of origin of the right coronary artery from the right aortic sinus, an arrangement that has been designated *absent left main coronary artery* (Figure 32-2A).

Coronary arteries that originate from normally located ostia arise at a right angle from the aortic wall. Coronary arteries that originate from *ectopic ostia* arise from the aortic wall at an acute angle and run tangential to the aortic wall. Normal proximal coronary arteries are epicardial; but in about a quarter of cases, the proximal left anterior descending coronary artery is *intramural* (see previous), which is recognized by angiographic narrowing of the intramyocardial segment.

A relatively large left ventricular mass is served by both the left and the right coronary arteries. Either the right or

the left coronary artery can be dominant, with dominance encompassing a wide range. *Extreme dominance* assumes that the dominant and nondominant coronary arteries arise from separate ostia in separate aortic sinuses, in contrast to dominance that results from a *single coronary artery* that originates from a single coronary ostium in a single aortic sinus (see subsequent).[13]

Congenital anomalies of the coronary arteries are the subject of comprehensive clinical and necropsy reviews.[13–16] The widespread use of selective coronary angiography has gone far in establishing the types and prevalence of these anomalies (see Table 32-1).[13,15,17] The incidence rate was 1.3% in 126,595 coronary

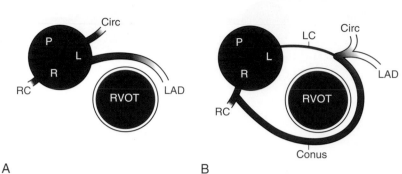

FIGURE 32-2 A, Absent left main coronary artery represented in the left aortic sinus (L) by separate origins of the ostia of the circumflex coronary artery (Circ) and the left anterior descending coronary artery (LAD). **B,** Atresia of the ostium and proximal segment of left main coronary artery (LC). A large conus branch from the right coronary artery (RC) supplies the circumflex coronary artery (Circ) and the left anterior descending coronary artery (LAD).

arteriograms performed at the Cleveland Clinic.[18] Transesophageal echocardiography[19,20] and multislice computed tomographic coronary angiography[21–25]are established procedures for depicting the origin and course of anomalous coronary arteries.

ANOMALOUS AORTIC ORIGINS OF CORONARY ARTERIES UNASSOCIATED WITH CONGENITAL HEART DISEASE

Anomalous origins of coronary arteries that are unassociated with congenital heart disease are shown in Table 32-2.

A normal coronary ostium is located in the middle of the aortic sinus and is considered anomalous when it is located above the sinotubular junction, in the posterior sinus, or in close proximity to an aortic commissure.[4] In 30% to 50% of normal human hearts, a small conus artery arises from the right aortic sinus and is of no functional significance (Figure 32-1A).[17,26] The circumflex coronary artery may arise from a separate ostium in the right aortic sinus and pass behind the aorta (Figure 32-1B) or may arise from the proximal right coronary artery and enter the left atrioventricular groove as if it were a proximal branch of the left coronary artery.[18,27] Anomalous origin of the circumflex coronary artery is regarded as benign, but there is one report of myocardial ischemia in the absence of coronary atherosclerosis. Also regarded as benign is the *absence* of the circumflex coronary artery with a dominant right coronary artery that perfuses the lateral and posterolateral left ventricular walls.[18]

The left anterior descending coronary artery can arise from the right aortic sinus or from the right coronary artery. The anomalous left anterior descending artery usually passes anterior or posterior to the great arteries but occasionally passes *between* the aorta and the right ventricular outflow tract, where it poses a potential risk. Rarely, the left anterior descending coronary artery, the circumflex coronary artery, and right coronary arteries arise by separate ostia from the right aortic sinus.

Origin of the left main coronary artery from the right aortic sinus is uncommon but clinically important.[13,18,26] The right coronary artery and the left main coronary artery can arise from separate ostia in the

Table 32-2 Congenital Anomalies of Coronary Arteries Unassociated with Congenital Heart Disease

Anomalous Aortic Origin
- Eccentric ostium within an aortic sinus
- Ectopic ostium above an aortic sinus
- Conus artery from the right aortic sinus
- Circumflex coronary artery from the right aortic sinus or from the right coronary artery
- Origin of left anterior descending and circumflex coronary arteries from separate ostia in the left aortic sinus (absence of left main coronary artery)
- Atresia of the left main coronary artery
- Origin of the left anterior descending coronary artery from the right aortic sinus or from the right coronary artery
- Origin of the right coronary artery from the left aortic sinus, from posterior aortic sinus, or from left coronary artery
- Origin of a single coronary artery from the right or left aortic sinus
- Anomalous origin from a noncardiac systemic artery

Anomalous Aortic Origin with Anomalous Proximal Course
- Acute proximal angulation
- Ectopic right coronary artery passing between aorta and pulmonary trunk
  - Ectopic left main coronary artery:
  - Between aorta and pulmonary trunk
  - Anterior to the pulmonary trunk
  - Posterior to the aorta
- Within the ventricular septum (intramyocardial)
- Ectopic left anterior descending coronary artery that is anterior, posterior, or between the aorta and pulmonary trunk

Anomalous Origin of a Coronary Artery from the Pulmonary Trunk
- Left main coronary artery
- Left anterior descending coronary artery
- Right coronary artery
- Both right and left coronary arteries
- Circumflex coronary artery
- Accessory coronary artery

right aortic sinus (see Figure 32-1C).[28] The left main coronary artery passes either anterior or posterior to the right ventricular outflow tract (see Figure 32-1C) or between the right ventricular outflow tract and the

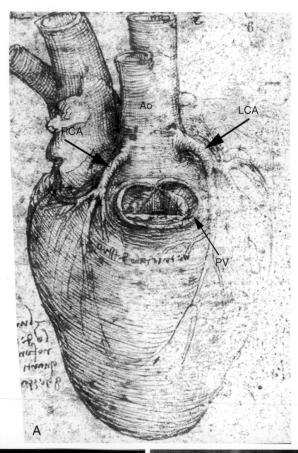

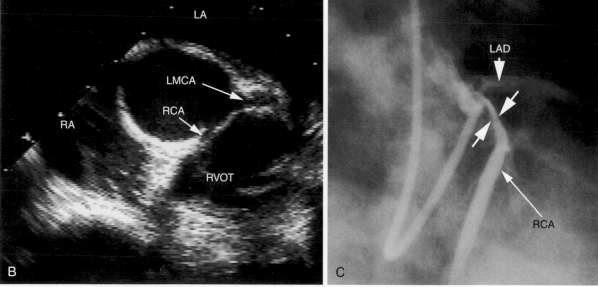

FIGURE 32-3 A, Drawing of a bullock's heart by Leonardo da Vinci, circa 1513, with labels by the author. "*The heart from the right side. The pulmonary artery has been removed to expose the pulmonary orifice and the semilunar valves guarding it. From the aorta spring the right and left coronary arteries.*" **B,** Echocardiogram (short-axis view) from an asymptomatic 23-year-old man in whom the right coronary artery (RCA) originated from the left aortic sinus and passed between the aorta and right ventricular outflow tract. The left main coronary artery (LCA) originated from the left aortic sinus by a separate ostium and divided into the left anterior descending and circumflex coronary arteries (compare with Figure 32-1D, second illustration). (Ao = aorta; LAD = left anterior descending.) **C,** Coronary arteriogram from a 29-year-old woman with angina pectoris. The right coronary artery (RCA) originated from the left aortic sinus and was compressed (paired arrows) as it passed between the aorta and right ventricular outflow tract (compare with Figure 32-1D, second illustration). The left coronary artery originated by a separate ostium from the left aortic sinus and divided into the left anterior descending (LAD) and circumflex coronary arteries.

aorta (see Figure 32-1D) or is within the ventricular septum (intramyocardial).[13,18,26,29] The risk associated with passage of the left main coronary artery between the aorta and the right ventricular outflow tract has been convincingly established (see subsequent).

Absence of a left main coronary artery refers to a rare anomaly in which the left anterior descending and circumflex coronary arteries originate from separate ostia in the left aortic sinus (see Figure 32-2A).[13,18,30] Both arteries are then normally distributed, so the arrangement is functionally benign.[18]

Atresia of the left main coronary artery includes ostial atresia, which is represented by an imperforate dimple, and atresia of the proximal course of the coronary artery, which is represented by a fibrous strand (see Figure 32-2B). A large conus branch originates from the right coronary artery and supplies the left anterior descending and circumflex coronary arteries (see Figure 32-2B).

Origin of the right coronary artery from the left aortic sinus (see Figures 32-1C and D, and 32-3B) represents about one quarter of ectopic coronary artery origins.[13,28] Less common is origin of the right coronary artery from the posterior aortic sinus or from the left coronary artery.[18] The functional significance of these arrangements does not depend on the anomalous origin but on whether the ectopic right coronary artery passes between the aorta and right ventricular outflow tract (see Figures 32-1D, and 32-3B and C).[13,18,28]

Single coronary artery has been known since 1903.[31] The single coronary artery originates from a single ostium in the left or right aortic sinus and gives rise to the entire coronary circulation (Figures 32-4 and 32-5).[13,18] A second coronary ostium is neither present nor implied. A single coronary artery unassociated with congenital heart disease divides into normally formed and normally distributed branches irrespective of the aortic sinus from which it originates (see Figure 32-4C and D).[13,18] A single coronary artery associated with a congenital heart disease is characterized by branching patterns that bear no resemblance to normal.[13] A single coronary artery functions normally unless a major branch is congenitally hypoplastic[32] or passes between the aorta and right ventricular outflow tract (Figure 32-6).

Anomalous origin of a coronary artery from a *systemic artery* is relatively rare (see Table 32-2). The anomalous coronary artery can originate from the innominate, subclavian, internal mammary, or carotid or bronchial artery or from the descending aorta.

The Coronary Artery Surgery Study (1989) asked whether a coronary artery that originated anomalously from an aortic sinus was predisposed to atherosclerosis.[33] The study concluded that atherosclerosis was more prevalent in anomalous circumflex coronary arteries than in matched controls with nonanomalous circumflex arteries.

The courses taken by anomalous coronary arteries and their branches are more important than their ectopic origins.[26,29,34,35] These courses include: (1) passage anterior to the right ventricular outflow tract (see Figure 32-1C); (2) passage posterior to the aorta (see Figure 32-1C); (3) passage between the aorta and

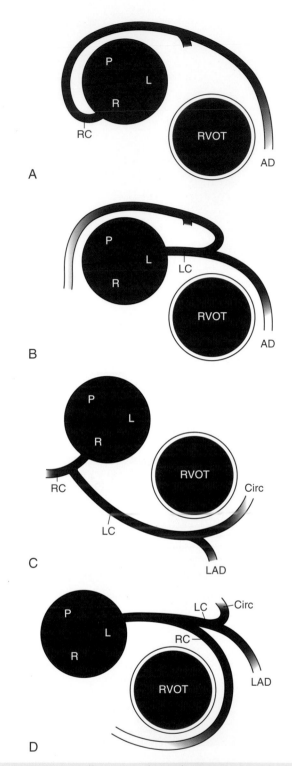

FIGURE 32-4 A, Illustration of a single coronary artery arising from a single ostium in the right aortic sinus (R) then coursing as a right coronary artery (RC). (AD = anterior descending artery.) **B,** A single coronary artery arising from a single ostium in the left aortic sinus (L) then coursing as a left coronary artery. **C,** A single coronary artery arising from a single ostium in the right aortic sinus then branching into the right coronary (RC) and left coronary (LC) artery. **D,** A single coronary artery arising from a single ostium in the left aortic sinus then branching into right coronary (RC) and left coronary (LC) arteries. (Circ = circumflex; LAD = left anterior descending.)

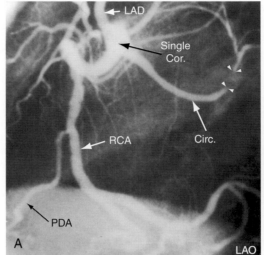

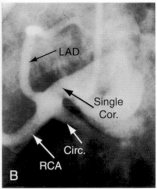

FIGURE 32-5 Coronary arteriograms from a 54-year-old woman. **A,** A single ostium in the right aortic sinus gave rise to a single coronary artery (Single Cor.) from which originated the left anterior descending (LAD), the circumflex (Circ.), and the right coronary artery (RCA). **B,** Injection into the right aortic sinus shows the single coronary artery from which the left anterior descending, circumflex, and right coronary arteries originate.

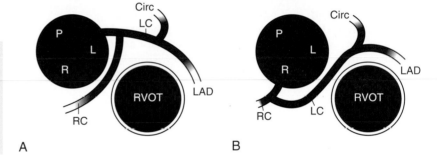

FIGURE 32-6 A, A single coronary artery originates from the left coronary sinus (L). The right coronary artery branch (RC) passes between the aorta and right ventricular outflow tract (RVOT). **B,** A single coronary artery originates from the right coronary sinus (R). The left coronary artery branch (LC) passes between the aorta and the right ventricular ourflow tract.

right ventricular outflow tract (see Figure 32-1D); and (4) intramyocardial passage (bridging).[13,34–38] The clinical significance of bridging is uncertain.[39] Angina pectoris, myocardial infarction, and sudden death are, with few exceptions, reserved for anomalous coronary arteries that pass between the aorta and the right ventricular outflow tract (see previous).[13,26,29,34,40–42]

Ischemic risk is determined by a number of variables in addition to the course of an anomalous coronary artery, namely[13,26,28]: (1) the coronary artery or branch that is involved; (2) the slit-like ostium and acute angulation of the origin of the ectopic coronary artery[34,41,43]; (3) coronary dominance[28]; and (4) the effect of strenuous exercise.[26,34,43,44] Risk is greatest when the *left main coronary artery* arises from the right aortic sinus and courses between the aorta and right ventricular outflow tract (see Figure 32-1D)[26,29,34,42,45] or when the *left branch of a single coronary artery* courses between the aorta and the right ventricular outflow tract (see Figure 32-6B). Risk is less when the right coronary artery originates from the left aortic sinus and passes between the aorta and the right ventricular outflow tract (see Figure 32-1D).[28,41,43] Sudden death typically occurs during or immediately after physical exercise.[26,29,34,42,44] Fatal impairment to coronary blood flow appears to be sporadic in light of the fact that highly trained competitive athletes perform intense physical exercise repeatedly and for many years

before experiencing sudden death.[46] It has been proposed that expansion of the aortic root and pulmonary trunk during exercise is responsible for an increase in acute angulation of the ectopic coronary artery and for flap-like closure of its slit-shaped ostium.[13,26,46] An analogous risk may confront the fetus during the hemodynamic stress of labor and delivery. A stillborn term fetus that died during labor had at necropsy a right coronary artery that originated from the left aortic sinus.[41] Exercise-induced dilation of the aortic root can compress an ectopic coronary artery against the base of the pulmonary trunk to which the infundibular septum is firmly anchored.[13,26] This mechanism may account for sudden death when an ectopic coronary artery is not characterized by acute angulation or a slit-like ostium.[28]

Coronary arteries that originate normally from their respective aortic sinuses can have abnormal distal connections. A small coronary arterial fistula incidentally discovered during routine coronary arteriography is a case in point (see Chapter 22).[18] Another example is a functionally benign distal intercoronary communication in which contiguous peripheral coronary artery branches form an open-ended circulation with bidirectional flow.[18]

Anomalous pulmonary arterial origins of coronary arteries[13,18,47,48] are listed in Table 32-2. Anomalous origin of the left coronary artery from the pulmonary trunk is the most important (see Chapter 21).[24] Anomalous origin of the right coronary artery from the pulmonary trunk is a rare anomaly that was first reported in 1885[49] and may be discovered incidentally at necropsy.[50,51]

CONGENITAL ANOMALIES OF CORONARY ARTERIES UNASSOCIATED WITH CONGENITAL HEART DISEASE

These congenital anomalies are shown in Table 32-2.

Anomalies of coronary arterial size include congenital hypoplasia or atresia, or conversely congenital coronary artery ectasia or aneurysm (Tables 32-1 and 32-3). Atresia of the ostium of the left main coronary artery extends proximally as a fibrous chord from a blind dimple in the left aortic sinus (see Figure 32-2B).[13,52–56] Survival depends on adequate connections between a normally arising right coronary artery and the distal nonhypoplastic portion of the left coronary artery (see Figure 32-2B). Myocardial infarction and death occur from infancy[54] to the teens[56] to 60 years and 71 years of age.[55] The clinical presentation of infants with ostial atresia or left main coronary artery atresia is similar to the presentation of infants with anomalous origin of the left coronary artery from the pulmonary trunk (see Chapter 21).[54]

Hypoplasia of coronary arteries exists when the right coronary artery and left circumflex coronary artery do not go beyond the lateral border of the heart.[57] Hypoplasia of the *left main coronary artery*[57] is analogous to atresia described previously (see Figure 32-2B).

Coronary artery ectasia accompanies cyanotic congenital heart disease (see Figure 32-14). Hereditary hemorrhagic telangiectasia or Rendu-Osler-Weber disease is another association[58] (see Chapter 30). *Congenital aneurysms* in the proximal right or left coronary artery are believed to result from an occult developmental fault.[59]

Table 32-3 **Congenital Anomalies of the Coronary Sinus**
Partial or complete absence:
• Coronary sinus atrial septal defect
• Unroofed coronary sinus
Hypoplasia of the coronary sinus
Stenosis or atresia of the ostium of the coronary sinus
Enlargement of the coronary sinus
• Without left-to-right shunt:
• Persistent left superior vena cava
• Anomalous inferior vena caval drainage
• Partial anomalous hepatic venous connection
• With left-to-right shunt:
• Total anomalous pulmonary venous connection
• Unroofed coronary sinus
• Coronary artery–to–coronary sinus fistula

Modified from Mantini E, Grondin CM, Lillehei CW, Edwards JE: Congenital anomalies involving the coronary sinus. *Circulation* 1966;33:317-327.

CONGENITAL CORONARY ARTERY ANOMALIES ASSOCIATED WITH CONGENITAL HEART DISEASE

Congenital anomalies of the coronary arteries associated with congenital heart disease are shown in Box 32-1.

Congenital and acquired abnormalities of the coronary arteries coexist with congenital malformations of the heart.[60] Routine coronary angiography during catheterization of adults with congenital heart disease has revealed an 11% incidence rate of congenital abnormalities and a 5% incidence rate of acquired lesions.[60]

Fallot's tetralogy is associated with a 10% to 36% incidence rate of anomalies of origin, course, and distribution of coronary arteries (see Chapter 18).[61–63] Most common are origin of a conus artery from the right coronary artery or from the right aortic sinus (Figure 32-7A), origin of a circumflex coronary artery from the right coronary artery, origin of a left anterior descending artery from the right aortic sinus (Figure 32-7B), and origin of a single coronary artery from the right aortic sinus (Figures 32-7C, and 32-8). Less common anomalies include origin of a coronary artery from the posterior aortic sinus, anastomoses between coronary arteries and bronchial arteries,[64,65] fistulas between coronary arteries and pulmonary arteries or right atrium,[64] hypoplastic coronary arteries, and pulmonary arterial origin of the left anterior descending coronary artery.[66] The physiologic consequences of these coronary anomalies are unimportant, but the surgical risk incurred when anomalous coronary arteries cross the right ventricular outflow tract is important indeed (see Figure 32-7B and C).

In *complete transposition of the great arteries* (see Chapter 27), the origins of the coronary arteries are relevant to arterial switch operations.[67–69] Coronary artery morphology and ventricular morphology are concordant (i.e., a morphologic right coronary artery is assigned to the morphologic subaortic right ventricle and a morphologic left coronary is assigned to the morphologic subpulmonary left ventricle). The *left aortic sinus* and the *posterior aortic sinus* face the right ventricular outflow tract (Figure 32-9). The rightward left sinus is designated sinus 1.[69,70] The posterior sinus is leftward and is designated sinus 2 (see Figure 32-9).[69,70] *Dual sinus origin* means

BOX 32-1 **CONGENITAL ANOMALIES OF THE CORONARY ARTERIES ASSOCIATED WITH CONGENITAL HEART DISEASE**
Fallot's tetralogy
Complete transposition of the great arteries
Congenitally corrected transposition of the great arteries
Double outlet ventricle
Univentricular heart
Tricuspid atresia
Truncus arteriosus
Isolated quadricuspid aortic valve
Isolated bicuspid aortic valve

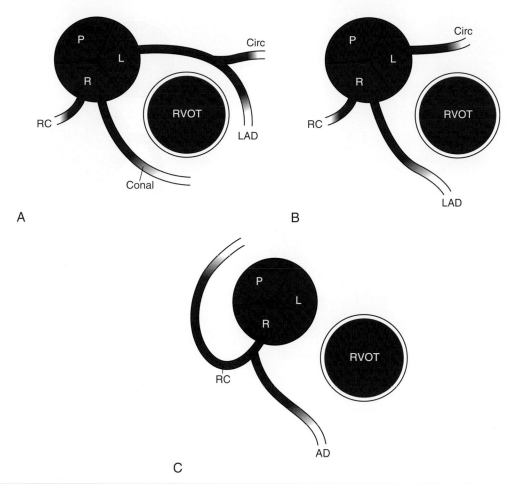

A

B

C

FIGURE 32-7 Illustrations of the coronary artery anomalies in Fallot's tetralogy. **A,** The conal artery arises by a separate ostium from the right aortic sinus (R). **B,** Left anterior descending coronary artery (LAD) arises by a separate ostium from the right aortic sinus and passes anterior to the right ventricular outflow tract (RVOT). **C,** The anterior descending branch (AD) of a single coronary artery passes anterior to the right ventricular outflow tract. (RC = right coronary artery branch.)

that a main coronary artery branch arises from each of the two sinuses that face the right ventricular outflow tract, an arrangement that is present in 90% of cases.[69] Most dual sinus origins are represented by the circumflex coronary artery, the left anterior descending artery arising from left aortic sinus, and the right coronary artery arising from the posterior sinus (Figure 32-9A).[69] Less common is dual sinus origin of circumflex coronary artery and right coronary artery from the posterior sinus and origin of the left anterior descending artery from the left aortic sinus (Figure 32-9B).[69] *Single sinus origin* means that main coronary arterial branches arise from one of the two but not both of the sinuses that face the right ventricular outflow tract.[69] In single sinus origin, the anterior descending, circumflex and right coronary arteries arise from the posterior sinus.[69] Rarely, an anomalous coronary artery is intramyocardial or passes between the aorta and the right ventricular outflow tract.

Congenitally corrected transposition of the great arteries is characterized by morphologic right and morphologic left coronary arteries that are concordant with morphologic right and morphologic left ventricles (see Chapter 6).[67,71] The two aortic sinuses that face the right ventricular outflow tract are designated *right posterior* and *left posterior* (Figure 32-10). The nonfacing anterior sinus is noncoronary (see Figure 32-10). The morphologic right coronary artery originates from the left posterior sinus, and the morphologic left coronary artery originates from the right posterior sinus, arrangements that are *inverted* (see Figure 32-10). The course of the left anterior descending coronary artery establishes the position of the ventricular septum. Coronary anomalies are uncommon, but there are reports of hypoplasia of the circumflex and left anterior descending coronary arteries[72] and of a single coronary ostium arising from the right posterior sinus.[71,72]

In *double outlet right ventricle*, the origin, course, and distribution of the coronary arteries is the same as in the normal heart (see Chapter 19).[56,67] The right coronary artery arises from the right aortic sinus, and the left coronary artery arises from the left aortic sinus (Figure 32-11).[56,67]

Occasionally, both coronary arteries arise from the same aortic sinus, or a single coronary artery arises from a single coronary artery ostium. *Double outlet left ventricle* is associated with a relatively high incidence of congenital anomalies of the origin and course of coronary arteries,

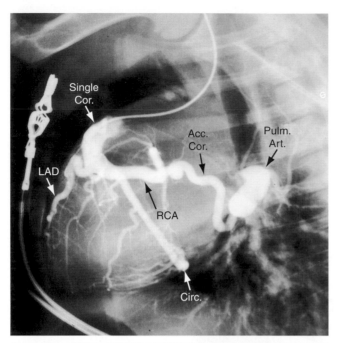

FIGURE 32-8 Coronary arteriogram from a 3-week-old Holstein calf with Fallot's tetralogy confirmed at necropsy. A single coronary artery (Single Cor.) originated from the right aortic sinus and branched into the left anterior descending (LAD), circumflex (Circ.), and right coronary (RCA) arteries. An accessory coronary artery (Acc. Cor.) connected the right coronary artery (RCA) to the pulmonary artery (Pulm. Art.). *(Courtesy Dr Sidney Moise, New York College of Veterinary Medicine, Cornell University, Ithaca, New York.)*

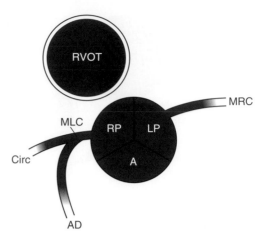

FIGURE 32-10 Illustration of the coronary arteries in congenitally corrected transposition of the great arteries. The left posterior sinus (LP) and the right posterior sinus (RP) face the right ventricular outflow tract (RVOT). The anterior sinus (A) is noncoronary. The morphologic right coronary artery (MRC) arises from the left posterior sinus. The morphologic left coronary artery (MLC) arises from the right posterior sinus and divides into the circumflex coronary artery (Circ) and anterior descending artery (AD).

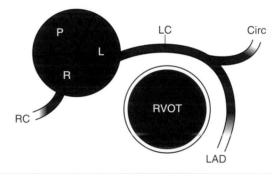

FIGURE 32-11 Illustration of the coronary arteries in double outlet right ventricle. The right coronary artery (RC) arises from the right aortic sinus (R). The left coronary artery (LC) arises from the left aortic sinus (LC) and branches into the left anterior descending coronary artery (LAD) and the circumflex artery (Circ) as in the normal heart.

including single coronary artery, origin of the left anterior descending artery from the right aortic sinus, and origin of both coronary arteries or all three coronary arteries from the right or left aortic sinus.[73] In *univentricular hearts* with left ventricular morphology (see Chapter 26), the aortic sinus from which the right or left coronary artery originates is determined by inversion or noninversion of the outlet chamber. When the outlet chamber is *inverted*, the aortic sinus from which each coronary

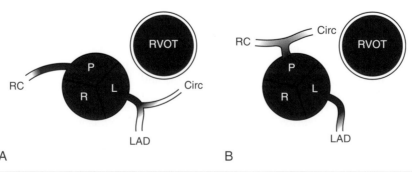

A   B

FIGURE 32-9 Illustrations of the coronary arteries in complete transposition of the great arteries. The two aortic sinuses facing the right ventricular outflow tract (RVOT) are designated the left sinus (L) and the posterior sinus (P). The right sinus (R) does not face the right ventricular outflow tract. **A,** The left coronary artery arises from the left sinus (L) and divides into the circumflex coronary artery (Circ) and the left anterior descending artery (LAD). The right coronary artery (RC) arises from the posterior sinus (P). **B,** The left anterior descending coronary artery arises from the left sinus (L), and a second coronary artery arises in the posterior sinus (P) branches into the right coronary artery (RC) and the circumflex coronary artery (Circ).

artery originates is the same as in congenitally corrected transposition of the great arteries with a biventricular heart (see Figure 32-10), but a major branch of each coronary artery *delimits* or *outlines* the surface boundaries of the outlet chamber.[74] When the outlet chamber is *noninverted,* the aortic sinus from which each coronary artery originates is the same as in complete transposition of the great arteries with a biventricular heart (see Figure 32-9). *Tricuspid atresia* (see Chapter 25) is characterized by *delimiting* coronary arteries that meet at the apex of the rudimentary morphologic right ventricle.[75]

Coronary artery origins in truncus arteriosus (see Chapter 28) correspond to the number and spatial relationships of the quadricuspid, tricuspid, or bicuspid truncal valve (Figure 32-12).[76–78] Truncal cusps that face the atrioventricular orifices lie posterior, and the cusp or cusps that do not face the atrioventricular orifices lie anterior.[76] When the truncal valve is tricuspid, the right coronary artery arises from the right anterior sinus, and the left coronary artery arises from the posterior sinus or the left anterior sinus (see Figure 32-12A). Bicuspid truncal valve cusps are oriented right/left or anterior/posterior (see Figure 32-12B). When the cusps are anterior/posterior, the left coronary artery or a single coronary artery arises from the posterior sinus, and the right coronary artery arises from the anterior sinus (see Figure 32-12B).[76,79] When bicuspid truncal valves are oriented right/left, the right coronary artery arises from the right sinus, and the left coronary artery arises from the left sinus.[76] Quadricuspid truncal valves are associated with two types of coronary artery arrangements. When two of the four truncal cusps are posterior and two are anterior, the left coronary artery arises from the left posterior sinus, and the right coronary artery arises from the right or left anterior sinus (see Figure 32-12C).[76,79] In both of these arrangements, high origins of right and left coronary artery ostia are frequent.[79]

Isolated quadricuspid valves are rare (see Chapter 7).[80,81] In one such patient, a single coronary artery arose from the right anterior sinus.[82] Isolated bicuspid aortic valves are associated with two types of cusp relationships and coronary artery origins (Figure 32-13). The two cusps may be oriented anterior/posterior with both coronary arteries arising from the anterior sinus (see Figure 32-13A), or the cusps may be oriented right/left with the right coronary artery arising from the right sinus and the left coronary artery arising from the left sinus (see Figure 32-13B). Bicuspid aortic valves tend to be associated with left coronary artery dominance and have a relatively high incidence of immediate bifurcation of the left coronary artery into circumflex and left anterior descending arteries.[83–86]

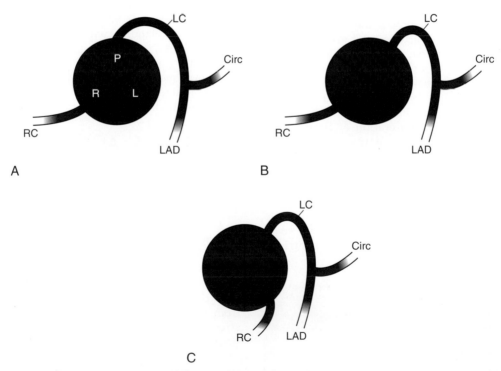

FIGURE 32-12 Illustrations of the coronary arteries in truncus arteriosus. **A,** When the truncal valve is *trileaflet,* the left coronary artery (LC) arises from the posterior sinus and divides into the circumflex coronary artery (Circ), and the left anterior descending artery (LAD). The right coronary artery (RC) arises from the right aortic sinus (R). **B,** When the truncal valve is *bicuspid,* the right coronary artery (RC) arises from the anterior sinus, and the left coronary artery (LC) arises from the posterior sinus and divides into the circumflex coronary artery (Circ) and the left anterior descending artery (LAD). **C,** When the truncal valve is *quadricuspid,* two of the aortic sinuses are posterior and two are anterior. The right coronary artery (RC) arises from the left anterior sinus. The left coronary artery (LC) arises from the left posterior sinus and divides into the circumflex coronary artery (Circ) and the left anterior descending artery (LAD).

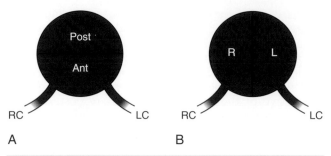

FIGURE 32-13 Illustrations of the coronary arteries when the aortic valve is bicuspid. **A,** When the two cusps are posteroanterior, the right coronary artery (RC) and the left coronary artery (LC) both originate in the sinus of the anterior cusp. **B,** When the two cusps are right/left, the right coronary artery (RC) and the left coronary artery (LC) each arise concordantly from the right coronary sinus (R) and the left coronary sinus (L).

CORONARY ARTERY DISEASE AS A RESULT OF CONGENITAL HEART DISEASE

Anomalies of coronary arteries that result from congenital heart disease are shown in Box 32-2.

Coarctation of the aorta is associated with extramural and intramural abnormalities of the coronary arteries (see Chapter 8), and systemic hypertension causes intimal proliferation and medial thickening, which are risk factors for premature coronary atherosclerosis.[87] Luminal size in coarctation increases in proportion to medial thickness.[88] Intramural coronary arteries and arterioles have thick walls, a rich adventitia, and dense collagen and elastic fibers.[87]

Supravalvular aortic stenosis (see Chapter 7) is associated with extramural coronary artery abnormalities analogous to coarctation of the aorta.[89–92] Ostial obstruction results from aortic medial proliferation or from adherence of an aortic cusp.[90,93] The extramural coronary arteries are exposed to systolic hypertension proximal to the supravalvular stenosis, so they are thick-walled, dilated, tortuous, and prematurely atherosclerotic.

Severe bicuspid aortic regurgitation is accompanied by large smooth-walled extramural coronary arteries appropriate for the increase in left ventricular mass of a magnified geometrically normal left ventricle.

BOX 32-2 ANOMALIES OF CORONARY ARTERIES THAT RESULT FROM CONGENITAL HEART DISEASE

Coarctation of the aorta

Supravalvular aortic stenosis

Aortic regurgitation

Coronary ectasia with cyanotic congenital heart disease

Pulmonary atresia with intact ventricular septum and hypoplastic right ventricle

Aortic atresia with intact ventricular septum and hypoplastic left ventricle

Paradoxical coronary arterial emboli

Coronary artery ectasia refers to elongation, tortuosity, and dilation of extramural coronary arteries in adults with cyanotic congenital heart disease (Figure 32-14).[94–96]

Suprasystemic pressure in the blind hypoplastic right ventricle of pulmonary atresia with intact ventricular septum generates flow through intramural intratrabecular channels with the development of ventriculocoronary artery connections (see Chapter 24).[97–99] Myocardial ischemia is caused by the fistulous steal associated with aortic diastolic runoff into the right ventricle through these large intramural channels. Ischemia is also caused by luminal narrowing of the ventriculocoronary arterial channels that extend from their right ventricular origins to the coronary ostia.[98,99] Narrowing ranges from mild to obliteration to coronary ostial discontinuity.[98,100,101]

In *aortic atresia with mitral atresia*, the coronary circulation is not accompanied by ventriculocoronary arterial channels because the sealed left ventricle cannot generate suprasystemic pressure.[102–105] When the mitral valve is hypoplastic but *perforate*, the small left ventricle receives diastolic flow, contracts isovolumetrically, and generates suprasystemic pressure. Nevertheless, intramyocardial sinusoids with direct ventriculocoronary artery connections do not develop, so suprasystemic left ventricular pressure is not transmitted into epicardial coronary arteries, which are spared the morphologic changes that characterize pulmonary atresia with intact ventricular septum. A sinusoidal/capillary network develops, but coronary arterial abnormalities, if present at all, consist of tortuosity with an increase in wall thickness, but not luminal narrowing.[102] *Paradoxical emboli* to the coronary arteries are rare complications of cyanotic congenital heart disease.[106,107] Right-to-left intracardiac shunts deliver paradoxical emboli from peripheral thromboembolic sources.

CONGENITAL ANOMALIES INVOLVING THE CORONARY SINUS

Congenital anomalies of the coronary sinus are shown in Table 32-3.

The coronary sinus is subject to a variety of congenital abnormalities.[108] *Partial or complete absence* results from loss of the roof, from absence of the entire coronary sinus, or from an atrial septal defect that occupies the site of the ostium of the coronary sinus (see Chapter 15). *Hypoplasia of the coronary sinus* is a response to diversion of blood from the sinus into dilated Thebesian veins. Stenosis or atresia of the sinus ostium is represented by a coronary sinus that is hypoplastic or that ends blindly. A left superior vena cava carries coronary sinus blood retrograde into the left innominate vein.[109] The coronary sinus enlarges when it receives a left superior vena cava or an hepatic vein, when it is joined by a left superior vena cava that receives blood from the inferior vena cava via the hemiazygos vein (see Chapter 29), when it is the drainage site for total anomalous pulmonary venous connection (see Chapter 15), or when there is a coronary artery–to–coronary sinus fistula (see Chapter 22).

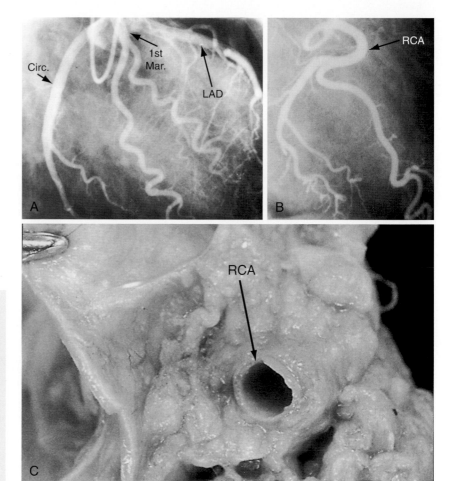

FIGURE 32-14 Coronary arteriograms from a 50-year-old cyanotic man with a nonrestrictive ventricular deptal defect and Eisenmenger's syndrome. **A,** The circumflex coronary artery (Circ.) and the left anterior descending artery (LAD) are dilated, and the first marginal (1st Mar.) is dilated and tortuous. **B,** The right coronary artery (RCA) is dilated and tortuous. **C,** Dilated right coronary artery (RCA) from a 40-year-old cyanotic woman with double outlet right ventricle, a subpulmonary ventricular septal defect (Taussig Bing), and pulmonary vascular disease.

REFERENCES

1. Anderson R, Becker AE. *Cardiac anatomy.* London: Gower Medical Pubishing; 1980.
2. O'Malley C, Saunders JB, Saunders MC, eds. *Translations, text and introduction. Leonardo da Vinci on the Human Body.* New York: Greenwich House; 1982.
3. Baroldi G, Scomazzoni G. *Coronary circulation in the normal heart and in the pathologic heart.* Washington, DC: United States Government Printing Office; 1967.
4. Blake HA, Manion WC, Mattingly TW, Baroldi G. Coronary artery anomalies. *Circulation.* 1964;30:927–940.
5. Sones Jr FM, Shirey EK. Cine coronary arteriography. *Mod Concepts Cardiovasc Dis.* 1962;31:735–738.
6. Ropers D, Moshage W, Daniel WG, Jessl J, Gottwik M, Achenbach S. Visualization of coronary artery anomalies and their anatomic course by contrast-enhanced electron beam tomography and three-dimensional reconstruction. *Am J Cardiol.* 2001;87:193–197.
7. Taylor AM, Thorne SA, Rubens MB, et al. Coronary artery imaging in grown up congenital heart disease: complementary role of magnetic resonance and x-ray coronary angiography. *Circulation.* 2000;101:1670–1678.
8. Fernandes F, Alam M, Smith S, Khaja F. The role of transesophageal echocardiography in identifying anomalous coronary arteries. *Circulation.* 1993;88:2532–2540.
9. Dodge-Khatami A, Mavroudis C, Backer CL. Congenital Heart Surgery Nomenclature and Database Project: anomalies of the coronary arteries. *Ann Thorac Surg.* 2000;69:S270–S297.
10. Sedmera D, Pexieder T, Vuillemin M, Thompson RP, Anderson RH. Developmental patterning of the myocardium. *Anat Rec.* 2000;258:319–337.
11. Tomanek RJ. Age as a modulator of coronary capillary angiogenesis. *Circulation.* 1992;86:320–321.
12. James T. *Anatomy of the coronary arteries.* New York: Paul B. Hoeber; 1961.
13. Roberts WC. Major anomalies of coronary arterial origin seen in adulthood. *Am Heart J.* 1986;111:941–963.
14. Anderson R, Becker A, Lucchesse F, et al. *Morphology of congenital heart disease.* Baltimore: University Park Press; 1983.
15. Greenberg MA, Fish BG, Spindola-Franco H. Congenital anomalies of the coronary arteries. Classification and significance. *Radiol Clin North Am.* 1989;27:1127–1146.
16. Levin DC, Fellows KE, Abrams HL. Hemodynamically significant primary anomalies of the coronary arteries. Angiographic aspects. *Circulation.* 1978;58:25–34.
17. Engel HJ, Torres C, Page Jr HL. Major variations in anatomical origin of the coronary arteries: angiographic observations in 4,250 patients without associated congenital heart disease. *Cathet Cardiovasc Diagn.* 1975;1:157–169.
18. Yamanaka O, Hobbs RE. Coronary artery anomalies in 126,595 patients undergoing coronary arteriography. *Cathet Cardiovasc Diagn.* 1990;21:28–40.
19. Gaither NS, Rogan KM, Stajduhar K, et al. Anomalous origin and course of coronary arteries in adults: identification and improved imaging utilizing transesophageal echocardiography. *Am Heart J.* 1991;122:69–75.
20. Samdarshi TE, Hill DL, Nanda NC. Transesophageal color Doppler diagnosis of anomalous origin of left circumflex coronary artery. *Am Heart J.* 1991;122:571–573.
21. Berbarie RF, Dockery WD, Johnson KB, Rosenthal RL, Stoler RC, Schussler JM. Use of multislice computed tomographic coronary angiography for the diagnosis of anomalous coronary arteries. *Am J Cardiol.* 2006;98:402–406.
22. Datta J, White CS, Gilkeson RC, et al. Anomalous coronary arteries in adults: depiction at multi-detector row CT angiography. *Radiology.* 2005;235:812–818.

23. Duran C, Kantarci M, Durur Subasi I, et al. Remarkable anatomic anomalies of coronary arteries and their clinical importance: a multidetector computed tomography angiographic study. *J Comput Assist Tomogr.* 2006;30:939–948.

24. Friedman AH, Fogel MA, Stephens Jr P, et al. Identification, imaging, functional assessment and management of congenital coronary arterial abnormalities in children. *Cardiol Young.* 2007; 17(suppl 2):56–67.

25. Girzadas M, Varga P, Dajani K. A single-center experience of detecting coronary anomalies on 64-slice computed tomography. *J Cardiovasc Med (Hagerstown).* 2009;10:842–847.

26. Barth 3rd CW, Roberts WC. Left main coronary artery originating from the right sinus of Valsalva and coursing between the aorta and pulmonary trunk. *J Am Coll Cardiol.* 1986;7:366–373.

27. Young-Hyman PJ, Tommaso CL, Singleton RT. A new double coronary artery anomaly: the right coronary artery originating above the coronary sinus giving off the circumflex artery. *J Am Coll Cardiol.* 1984;4:1329–1331.

28. Kragel AH, Roberts WC. Anomalous origin of either the right or left main coronary artery from the aorta with subsequent coursing between aorta and pulmonary trunk: analysis of 32 necropsy cases. *Am J Cardiol.* 1988;62:771–777.

29. Roberts WC, Shirani J. The four subtypes of anomalous origin of the left main coronary artery from the right aortic sinus (or from the right coronary artery). *Am J Cardiol.* 1992;70:119–121.

30. Dicicco BS, McManus BM, Waller BF, Roberts WC. Separate aortic ostium of the left anterior descending and left circumflex coronary arteries from the left aortic sinus of Valsalva (absent left main coronary artery). *Am Heart J.* 1982;104:153–154.

31. Banchi A. Morfologia della arterial coronariae cordiae. *Arch Ital Anat Embriol.* 1903;3.

32. Newton Jr MC, Burwell LR. Single coronary artery with myocardial infarction and mitral regurgitation. *Am Heart J.* 1978;95: 126–127.

33. Click RL, Holmes Jr DR, Vlietstra RE, Kosinski AS, Kronmal RA. Anomalous coronary arteries: location, degree of atherosclerosis and effect on survival—a report from the Coronary Artery Surgery Study. *J Am Coll Cardiol.* 1989;13:531–537.

34. Cheitlin MD, De Castro CM, McAllister HA. Sudden death as a complication of anomalous left coronary origin from the anterior sinus of Valsalva, a not-so-minor congenital anomaly. *Circulation.* 1974;50:780–787.

35. Roberts WC, Dicicco BS, Waller BF, et al. Origin of the left main from the right coronary artery or from the right aortic sinus with intramyocardial tunneling to the left side of the heart via the ventricular septum. The case against clinical significance of myocardial bridge or coronary tunnel. *Am Heart J.* 1982;104:303–305.

36. Arat N, Altay H, Yildirim N, Ilkay E, Sabah I. Noninvasive assessment of myocardial bridging in the left coronary artery by transthoracic Doppler echocardiography. *Eur J Echocardiogr.* 2007;8: 284–288.

37. Herrmann J, Higano ST, Lenon RJ, Rihal CS, Lerman A. Myocardial bridging is associated with alteration in coronary vasoreactivity. *Eur Heart J.* 2004;25:2134–2142.

38. Konen E, Goitein O, Sternik L, Eshet Y, Shemesh J, Di Segni E. The prevalence and anatomical patterns of intramuscular coronary arteries: a coronary computed tomography angiographic study. *J Am Coll Cardiol.* 2007;49:587–593.

39. Kuribayashi S. Multidetector-row computed tomography is a powerful tool in detection of myocardial bridges but clinical significance remains uncertain. *Journal of Cardiovascular Computed Tomography.* 2007;1:84–85.

40. Maron BJ, Roberts WC, McAllister HA, Rosing DR, Epstein SE. Sudden death in young athletes. *Circulation.* 1980;62:218–229.

41. Muus CJ, McManus BM. Common origin of right and left coronary arteries from the region of left sinus of Valsalva: association with unexpected intrauterine fetal death. *Am Heart J.* 1984;107: 1285–1286.

42. Tsung SH, Huang TY, Chang HH. Sudden death in young athletes. *Arch Pathol Lab Med.* 1982;106:168–170.

43. Roberts WC, Siegel RJ, Zipes DP. Origin of the right coronary artery from the left sinus of valsalva and its functional consequences: analysis of 10 necropsy patients. *Am J Cardiol.* 1982; 49:863–868.

44. Liberthson RR. Congenital anomalies of the coronary arteries. *Cardiovascular Medicine.* 1984;9:857.

45. Pelliccia A. Congenital coronary artery anomalies in young patients: new perspectives for timely identification. *J Am Coll Cardiol.* 2001;37:598–600.

46. Basso C, Maron BJ, Corrado D, Thiene G. Clinical profile of congenital coronary artery anomalies with origin from the wrong aortic sinus leading to sudden death in young competitive athletes. *J Am Coll Cardiol.* 2000;35:1493–1501.

47. Heifetz SA, Robinowitz M, Mueller KH, Virmani R. Total anomalous origin of the coronary arteries from the pulmonary artery. *Pediatr Cardiol.* 1986;7:11–18.

48. Sreenivasan VV, Jacobstein MD. Origin of the right coronary artery from the pulmonary trunk. *Am J Cardiol.* 1992;69: 1513–1514.

49. Brooks HS. Two cases of an abnormal coronary artery of the heart arising from the pulmonary artery: with some remarks upon the effect of this anomaly in producing cirsoid dilatation of the vessels. *J Anat Physiol.* 1885;20:26–29.

50. Hekmat V, Rao SM, Chhabra M, Chiavarelli M, Anderson JE, Nudel DB. Anomalous origin of the right coronary artery from the main pulmonary artery: diagnosis and management. *Clin Cardiol.* 1998;21:773–776.

51. Albertal J, Lynch FG, Vaccarino G, Vrancic M, Pichinini F, Albertal M. Anomalous origin of right coronary artery. *Circulation.* 2001;103:E73–E75.

52. Bedogni F, Castellani A, La Vecchia L, et al. Atresia of the left main coronary artery: clinical recognition and surgical treatment. *Cathet Cardiovasc Diagn.* 1992;25:35–41.

53. Beretta L, Lemma M, Santoli C. Isolated atresia of the left main coronary artery in an adult. *Eur J Cardiothorac Surg.* 1990;4: 169–170.

54. Byrum CJ, Blackman MS, Schneider B, Sondheimer HM, Kavey RE. Congenital atresia of the left coronary ostium and hypoplasia of the left main coronary artery. *Am Heart J.* 1980; 99:354–358.

55. Fortuin NJ, Roberts WC. Congenital atresia of the left main coronary artery. *Am J Med.* 1971;50:385–389.

56. Van Der Hauwaert LG, Dumoulin M, Moerman P. Congenital atresia of left coronary ostium. *Br Heart J.* 1982;48: 298–300.

57. Casta A. Hypoplasia of the left coronary artery complicated by reversible myocardial ischemia in a newborn. *Am Heart J.* 1987; 114:1238–1241.

58. Kurnik PB, Heymann WR. Coronary artery ectasia associated with hereditary hemorrhagic telangiectasia. *Arch Intern Med.* 1989; 149:2357–2359.

59. Wong CK, Cheng CH, Lau CP, Leung WH. Asymptomatic congenital coronary artery aneurysm in adulthood. *Eur Heart J.* 1989;10:947–949.

60. Koifman B, Egdell R, Somerville J. Prevalence of asymptomatic coronary arterial abnormalities detected by angiography in grown-up patients with congenital heart disease. *Cardiol Young.* 2001;11:614–618.

61. Fellows KE, Freed MD, Keane JF, Praagh R, Bernhard WF, Castaneda AC. Results of routine preoperative coronary angiography in tetralogy of Fallot. *Circulation.* 1975;51: 561–566.

62. Weber HS, Zangwill SD, Zachary CH, Cyran SE. Transvenous approach to coronary angiography in infants with tetralogy of Fallot. *Am J Cardiol.* 1999;83:630–632 A610–A631.

63. Achenbach S, Dittrich S, Kuettner A. Anomalous left anterior descending coronary artery in a pediatric patient with Fallot tetralogy. *Journal of Cardiovascular Computed Tomography.* 2008;2: 55–56.

64. Dabizzi RP, Caprioli G, Aiazzi L, et al. Distribution and anomalies of coronary arteries in tetralogy of fallot. *Circulation.* 1980;61: 95–102.

65. Zureikat HY. Collateral vessels between the coronary and bronchial arteries in patients with cyanotic congenital heart disease. *Am J Cardiol.* 1980;45:599–603.

66. Yamaguchi M, Tsukube T, Hosokawa Y, Ohashi H, Oshima Y. Pulmonary origin of left anterior descending coronary artery in tetralogy of Fallot. *Ann Thorac Surg.* 1991;52:310–312.

67. Elliott LP, Amplatz K, Edwards JE. Coronary arterial patterns in transposition complexes. Anatomic and angiocardiographic studies. *Am J Cardiol*. 1966;17:362–378.

68. Shaher R, Puddu G. Coronary arterial anatomy in complete transposition of the great vessels. *Am J Cardiol*. 1966;17:355–361.

69. Smith A, Arnold R, Wilkinson JL, Hamilton DI, McKay R, Anderson RH. An anatomical study of the patterns of the coronary arteries and sinus nodal artery in complete transposition. *Int J Cardiol*. 1986;12:295–307.

70. Rossi MB, Ho SY, Anderson RH, Rossi Filho RI, Lincoln C. Coronary arteries in complete transposition: the significance of the sinus node artery. *Ann Thorac Surg*. 1986;42:573–577.

71. Losekoot T, Anderson R, Becker AE, et al., eds. *Congenitally corrected transposition*. Edinburgh: Churchill Livingstone; 1983.

72. Dabizzi RP, Barletta GA, Caprioli G, Baldrighi G, Baldrighi V. Coronary artery anatomy in corrected transposition of the great arteries. *J Am Coll Cardiol*. 1988;12:486–491.

73. Coto E, Jimenez M, Anderson R, et al., eds. *Double outlet left ventricle*. Edinburgh: Churchill Livingstone; 1983.

74. Lev M, Liberthson RR, Kirkpatrick JR, Eckner FA, Arcilla RA. Single (primitive) ventricle. *Circulation*. 1969;39:577–591.

75. Deanfield JE, Tommasini G, Anderson RH, Macartney FJ. Tricuspid atresia: analysis of coronary artery distribution and ventricular morphology. *Br Heart J*. 1982;48:485–492.

76. De La Cruz MV, Cayre R, Angelini P, Noriega-Ramos N, Sadowinski S. Coronary arteries in truncus arteriosus. *Am J Cardiol*. 1990;66:1482–1486.

77. Shrivastava S, Edwards JE. Coronary arterial origin in persistent truncus arteriosus. *Circulation*. 1977;55:551–554.

78. Van Praagh R, Van Praagh S. The anatomy of common aorticopulmonary trunk (truncus arteriosus communis) and its embryologic implications. A study of 57 necropsy cases. *Am J Cardiol*. 1965;16:406–425.

79. Anderson KR, McGoon DC, Lie JT. Surgical significance of the coronary arterial anatomy in truncus arteriosus communis. *Am J Cardiol*. 1978;41:76–81.

80. Kurosawa H, Wagenaar SS, Becker AE. Sudden death in a youth. A case of quadricuspid aortic valve with isolation of origin of left coronary artery. *Br Heart J*. 1981;46:211–215.

81. Lanzillo G, Breccia PA, Intonti F. Congenital quadricuspid aortic valve with displacement of the right coronary orifice. *Scand J Thorac Cardiovasc Surg*. 1981;15:149–151.

82. Kim HS, McBride RA, Titus JL. Quadricuspid aortic valve and single coronary ostium. *Arch Pathol Lab Med*. 1988;112:842–844.

83. Johnson AD, Detwiler JH, Higgins CB. Left coronary artery anatomy in patients with bicuspid aortic valves. *Br Heart J*. 1978;40:489–493.

84. Line DE, Babb JD, Pierce WS. Congenital aortic valve anomaly. Aortic regurgitation with left coronary artery isolation. *J Thorac Cardiovasc Surg*. 1979;77:533–535.

85. Roberts WC. The congenitally bicuspid aortic valve. A study of 85 autopsy cases. *Am J Cardiol*. 1970;26:72–83.

86. Scholz DG, Lynch JA, Willerscheidt AB, Sharma RK, Edwards JE. Coronary arterial dominance associated with congenital bicuspid aortic valve. *Arch Pathol Lab Med*. 1980;104:417–418.

87. Schneeweiss A, Sherf L, Lehrer E, Lieberman Y, Neufeld HN. Segmental study of the terminal coronary vessels in coarctation of the aorta: a natural model for study of the effect of coronary hypertension on human coronary circulation. *Am J Cardiol*. 1982;49:1996–2002.

88. MacAlpin RN, Abbasi AS, Grollman Jr JH, Eber L. Human coronary artery size during life. A cinearteriographic study. *Radiology*. 1973;108:567–576.

89. Neufeld HN, Wagenvoort CA, Ongley PA, Edwards JE. Hypoplasia of ascending aorta. An unusual form of supravalvular aortic stenosis with special reference to localized coronary arterial hypertension. *Am J Cardiol*. 1962;10:746–751.

90. Pansegrau DG, Kioshos JM, Durnin RE, Kroetz FW. Supravalvular aortic stenosis in adults. *Am J Cardiol*. 1973;31:635–641.

91. Roberts WC. Valvular, subvalvular and supravalvular aortic stenosis: morphologic features. *Cardiovasc Clin*. 1973;5:97–126.

92. Underhill WL, Tredway JB, D'Angelo GJ, Baay JE. Familial supravalvular aortic stenosis. Comments on the mechanisms of angina pectoris. *Am J Cardiol*. 1971;27:560–565.

93. Price AC, Lee DA, Kagan KE, Baker WP. Aortic dysplasia in infancy simulating anomalous origin of the left coronary artery. *Circulation*. 1973;48:434–437.

94. Bjork L. Ectasia of the coronary arteries. *Radiology*. 1966;87:33–34.

95. Perloff JK, Urschell CW, Roberts WC, Caulfield Jr WH. Aneurysmal dilatation of the coronary arteries in cyanotic congenital cardiac disease. Report of a forty year old patient with the Taussig-Bing complex. *Am J Med*. 1968;45:802–810.

96. Perloff JK, Rosove MH, Sietsema KE, eds. *Cyanotic congenital heart disease: a multisystem systemic disorder*. 2nd ed. Philadelphia: W.B. Saunders Company; 1998.

97. Bull C, De Leval MR, Mercanti C, Macartney FJ, Anderson RH. Pulmonary atresia and intact ventricular septum: a revised classification. *Circulation*. 1982;66:266–272.

98. Burrows PE, Freedom RM, Benson LN, et al. Coronary angiography of pulmonary atresia, hypoplastic right ventricle, and ventriculocoronary communications. *AJR Am J Roentgenol*. 1990;154:789–795.

99. Calder AL, Co EE, Sage MD. Coronary arterial abnormalities in pulmonary atresia with intact ventricular septum. *Am J Cardiol*. 1987;59:436–442.

100. Lenox CC, Briner J. Absent proximal coronary arteries associated with pulmonic atresia. *Am J Cardiol*. 1972;30:666–669.

101. Ueda K, Saito A, Nakano H, Hamazaki Y. Absence of proximal coronary arteries associated with pulmonary atresia. *Am Heart J*. 1983;106:596–598.

102. Baffa JM, Chen SL, Guttenberg ME, Norwood WI, Weinberg PM. Coronary artery abnormalities and right ventricular histology in hypoplastic left heart syndrome. *J Am Coll Cardiol*. 1992;20:350–358.

103. O'Connor WN, Cash JB, Cottrill CM, Johnson GL, Noonan JA. Ventriculocoronary connections in hypoplastic left hearts: an autopsy microscopic study. *Circulation*. 1982;66:1078–1086.

104. Raghib G, Bloemendaal RD, Kanjuh VI, Edwards JE. Aortic atresia and premature closure of foramen ovale. Myocardial sinusoids and coronary arteriovenous fistula serving as outflow channel. *Am Heart J*. 1965;70:476–480.

105. Roberts WC, Perry LW, Chandra RS, Myers GE, Shapiro SR, Scott LP. Aortic valve atresia: a new classification based on necropsy study of 73 cases. *Am J Cardiol*. 1976;37:753–756.

106. Gerber RS, Sherman CT, Sack JB, Perloff JK. Isolated paradoxical embolus to the right coronary artery. *Am J Cardiol*. 1992;70:1633–1635.

107. Jungbluth A, Erbel R, Darius H, Rumpelt HJ, Meyer J. Paradoxical coronary embolism: case report and review of the literature. *Am Heart J*. 1988;116:879–885.

108. Mantini E, Grondin C, Lillehei C, Edwards J. Congenital anomalies involving the coronary sinus. *Circulation*. 1966;33:317.

109. Gerlis LM, Gibbs JL, Williams GJ, Thomas GD. Coronary sinus orifice atresia and persistent left superior vena cava. A report of two cases, one associated with atypical coronary artery thrombosis. *Br Heart J*. 1984;52:648–653.

Index

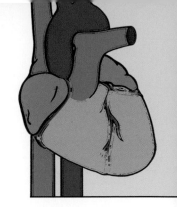

Note: Page numbers followed by *b* indicate boxes, *f* indicate figures and *t* indicate tables.